Lo físico, mental y espiritual
Guía de supervivencia pandémica
Una guía de supervivencia orientada a la familia

Por Mark Wilkins, El profeta de la vida y el Dr. Goose.

Tabla de contenido:

I0085544

A TOPOGRAPHICAL DICTIONARY OF ENGLAND

By Samuel Lewis

VOLUME II

CLEARFIELD

Originally published, London, 1831
Reprinted, four volumes in two, 1996, by
Genealogical Publishing Co., Inc.
Baltimore, Maryland

Reprinted in the original four-volume format, 2018, by
Genealogical Publishing Company for
Clearfield Company
Baltimore, Maryland

ISBN Volume II: 9780806358680
Set ISBN: 9780806315089

A

TOPOGRAPHICAL DICTIONARY

OF

ENGLAND,

COMPRISING THE

SEVERAL COUNTIES, CITIES, BOROUGHS, CORPORATE AND MARKET TOWNS,
PARISHES, CHAPELRIES, AND TOWNSHIPS,
AND THE ISLANDS OF GUERNSEY, JERSEY, AND MAN,

WITH

HISTORICAL AND STATISTICAL DESCRIPTIONS;

ILLUSTRATED BY

MAPS OF THE DIFFERENT COUNTIES AND ISLANDS;

AND EMBELLISHED WITH

ENGRAVINGS OF THE ARMS OF THE CITIES, BISHOPRICKS, UNIVERSITIES, COLLEGES, CORPORATE TOWNS,
AND BOROUGHS; AND OF THE SEALS OF THE SEVERAL MUNICIPAL CORPORATIONS.

BY SAMUEL LEWIS.

IN FOUR VOLUMES.

VOL. II.

LONDON:
PUBLISHED BY S. LEWIS AND CO., 87, ALDERSGATE-STREET.
M.DCCC.XXXI.

A

TOPOGRAPHICAL DICTIONARY

OF

ENGLAND.

DACRE, a parish in LEATH ward, county of CUMBERLAND, 5 miles (S.W. by W.) from Penrith, comprising the townships of Dacre, Great Blencow, Newbiggin, Soulby, and Stainton, and containing 904 inhabitants. The living is a discharged vicarage, in the archdeaconry and diocese of Carlisle, rated in the king's books at £8, endowed with £200 private benefaction, £200 royal bounty, and £1200 parliamentary grant, and in the patronage of the Crown. The church is dedicated to St. Andrew. A school was built in 1749, by subscription, in which four free children are educated, and others at a small charge. A monastery existed here in the time of Bede; and at this place, Constantine, King of Scotland, and Eugenius, King of Cumberland, placed themselves and their kingdom under the authority of King Athelstan. Dacre castle was long the residence of an ancient and noble family of that name: the main body of it, consisting principally of four towers of excellent workmanship, remains in a very perfect state. Lime-stone is obtained here; and at Southwaite, in this parish, is a mineral spring.

DACRE, a township in that part of the parish of RIPON which is in the lower division of the wapentake of CLARO, West riding of the county of YORK, 6½ miles (W.) from Ripley, containing 777 inhabitants. A schoolroom was built in 1695, by William Hardcastle, who endowed it with £100 for the education of children; and in 1778 William Mountain bequeathed £100 in addition to the above, producing together £8. 8. per annum; but from its being generally conceived that the benefit of the school is confined to the descendants of William Hardcastle, the number of free scholars has been very limited. In 1774, Edward Yates bequeathed an estate, now producing £32 per annum, for the endowment of a school; between thirty and forty scholars are educated.

DADLINGTON, a chapelry in the parish of HINCKLEY, hundred of SPARKENHOE, county of LEICESTER, 3 miles (N.W. by N.) from Hinckley, containing 179 inhabitants. The Ashby de la Zouch canal passes through the chapelry.

DAGENHAM, a parish in the hundred of BECONTREE, county of ESSEX, 3½ miles (S. by W.) from Romford, containing 1864 inhabitants. The living is a vicarage, in the archdeaconry of Essex, and diocese of London, rated in the king's books at £19. 10. Mrs. Bonyinge was patroness in 1816. The church is dedicated to St. Peter and St. Paul. The parish is bounded on the south by the Thames. There is a small endowment for the instruction of children. A very destructive irruption of the Thames occurred here in 1707, the waters, rushing in by an opening made by the blowing up of a small sluice for draining the land, overflowed one thousand acres of rich land, and washed nearly one hundred and twenty acres into the river, where a sand-bank was formed almost half-way across its bed; in this state it remained nearly fifteen years, when the breach was stopped, and the land recovered by Captain Perry, at an expense of £40,000.

DAGLINGWORTH, a parish in the hundred of CROWTHORNE and MINETY, county of GLOUCESTER, 2¾ miles (N.W.) from Cirencester, containing 253 inhabitants. The living is a rectory, in the archdeaconry and diocese of Gloucester, rated in the king's books at £8. 6. 3., and in the patronage of the Crown. The church is dedicated to the Holy Rood. The Roman road, called Ermin-street, passes through the parish, and a tesselated pavement has been discovered. There is a school for poor children, supported by an annuity of £4. 10., arising from a bequest of £100 by Jeremiah Hancock, in 1729.

DAGNELL, a chapelry in the parish of EDDLESBOROUGH, hundred of COTTESLOE, county of BUCKINGHAM, 3½ miles (E.) from Ivinghoe, containing 314 inhabitants. The chapel, dedicated to All Saints, has long been in ruins.

DAGWORTH, a hamlet in the parish of OLD NEWTON, hundred of STOW, county of SUFFOLK, 2¼ miles (N.) from Stow-Market. The population is returned with the parish.

DALBURY, a parish in the hundred of APPLETREE, county of DERBY, 6½ miles (W. by S.) from Derby, containing, with the township of Lees, 241 inhabitants. The living is a rectory, in the archdeaconry of Derby, and diocese of Lichfield and Coventry, rated in the king's books at £ 4. 16. 3., and in the patronage of the Crown. The church is dedicated to All Saints.

DALBY, a parish in the Wold division of the wapentake of CANDLESHOE, parts of LINDSEY, county of LINCOLN, 2¼ miles (N.) from Spilsby, containing 99 inhabitants. The living is a perpetual curacy, in the peculiar jurisdiction of the Dean and Chapter of Lincoln, endowed with £200 royal bounty, and £200 parliamentary grant. Lord Monson was patron in 1808.

DALBY, a parish in the wapentake of BULMER, North riding of the county of YORK, 9½ miles (W. by S.) from New Malton, containing, with Skewsby, 169 inhabitants. The living is a discharged rectory, in the archdeaconry of Cleveland, and diocese of York, rated in the king's books at £5. 1. 0½. Mrs. Leybourne was patroness in 1806. The church is dedicated to St. Mary.

DALBY (MAGNA), a parish in the eastern division of the hundred of GOSCOTE, county of LEICESTER, 3¾ miles (S. by W.) from Melton-Mowbray, containing 402 inhabitants. The living is a discharged vicarage, in the archdeaconry of Leicester, and diocese of Lincoln, rated in the king's books at £8. 4. 7., and endowed with £200 royal bounty, and in the patronage of Sir Francis Burdett, Bart. The church is dedicated to St. Swithin.

DALBY (PARVA), a parish in the hundred of FRAMLAND, county of LEICESTER, 4½ miles (S.S.E.) from Melton-Mowbray, containing 185 inhabitants. The living is a vicarage, in the archdeaconry of Leicester, and diocese of Lincoln, rated in the king's books at £9, and in the patronage of E. B. Hartop, Esq. The church is dedicated to St. James.

DALBY on the WOLDS, a parish in the eastern division of the hundred of GOSCOTE, county of LEICESTER, 6½ miles (N.W. by W.) from Melton-Mowbray, containing 357 inhabitants. The living is a perpetual curacy, in the jurisdiction of the peculiar court of Old Dalby, and in the patronage of Lord Feversham. The church is dedicated to St. John the Baptist. A preceptory of Knights Hospitallers was founded, it is supposed, by Robert Bossu, Earl of Leicester, in the reign of Henry II.: at the dissolution its revenue was valued at £91. 2. 8. per annum. Here is a chalybeate spring.

DALDERBY, a parish in the southern division of the wapentake of GARTREE, parts of LINDSEY, county of LINCOLN, 3 miles (S. by W.) from Horncastle, containing 40 inhabitants. The living is a discharged rectory, united in 1731 to the rectory of Scrivelsby, in the archdeaconry and diocese of Lincoln, rated in the king's books at £4. 19. 4½., and in the patronage of H. Dymoke, Esq. The church is dedicated to St. Martin. The river Bane and the Horncastle canal pass through this parish.

DALE-ABBEY, an extra-parochial liberty, in the hundred of MORLESTON and LITCHURCH, county of DERBY, 7 miles (E. by N.) from Derby, containing 418 inhabitants. Here is a chapel within the jurisdiction of the manor and peculiar court of Dale-Abbey. The poor of this liberty are entitled to the benefit of the school at West Hallam, founded by the Rev. John Scargill; and of that at Risley, founded by Mrs. Elizabeth Grey. There are the remains of an abbey of Premonstratensian canons, which was founded about the year 1204, by William Fitz-Rauf, seneschal of Normandy, and his son-in-law Jeffrey de Salicosa Mara, in honour of the Blessed Virgin Mary; at the dissolution its revenue was estimated at £144. 12.

DALE-TOWN, a township in the parish of HAWNBY, wapentake of BIRDFORTH, North riding of the county of YORK, 9½ miles (N.E. by E.) from Thirsk, containing 68 inhabitants.

DALHAM, a parish in the hundred of RISBRIDGE, county of SUFFOLK, 5 miles (E. by S.) from Newmarket, containing 498 inhabitants. The living is a rectory, in the archdeaconry of Sudbury, and diocese of Norwich, rated in the king's books at £15. 10. 5. Sir James Affleck, Bart. was patron in 1823. The church is dedicated to St. Mary.

DALLINGHOO, a parish partly in the hundred of LOES, but chiefly in the hundred of WILFORD, county of SUFFOLK, 2¾ miles (W. by S.) from Wickham-Market, containing 303 inhabitants. The living is a discharged rectory, in the archdeaconry of Suffolk, and diocese of Norwich, rated in the king's books at £13. 6. 8. Edward Moor, Esq. was patron in 1827. The church is dedicated to St. Mary.

DALLINGTON, a parish in the hundred of NOBOTTLE-GROVE, county of NORTHAMPTON, 1¾ mile (N.W.) from Northampton, containing 369 inhabitants. The living is a discharged vicarage, in the archdeaconry of Northampton, and diocese of Peterborough, rated in the king's books at £6. 15. 8. Miss Wrighte was patroness in 1823. The church, dedicated to St. Mary, has portions in the early style of English architecture.

DALLINGTON, a parish in the hundred of NETHERFIELD, rape of HASTINGS, county of SUSSEX, 6 miles (W.N.W.) from Battle, containing 548 inhabitants. The living is a vicarage, in the archdeaconry of Lewes, and diocese of Chichester, rated in the king's books at £8. The Earl of Ashburnham was patron in 1810. The church, dedicated to St. Margaret, is principally in the later style of English architecture.

DALPOOL, a hamlet in the parish of THURSTASTON, hundred of WIRRALL, county palatine of CHESTER, 5 miles (N. W. by N.) from Parkgate. The population is returned with the parish.

DALSCOTE, a hamlet in the parish of PATTISHALL, hundred of TOWCESTER, county of NORTHAMPTON, 4 miles (N. by E.) from Towcester. The population is returned with the parish.

DALSTON, a parish in the ward and county of CUMBERLAND, comprising the chapelry of Ivegill, and the townships of Buckhowbank, Cumdevock, Dalston, Hawkesdale, and Raughton with Gatesgill, and containing 2617 inhabitants, of which number, 955 are in the township of Dalston, 4½ miles (S. S. W.) from Carlisle. The living is a vicarage, in the archdeaconry and diocese of Carlisle, rated in the king's books at £8. 18. 1½., and in the patronage of the Bishop of Carlisle. The church, dedicated to St. Michael, was rebuilt about eighty years ago. There are several cotton and other mills; also an iron and plating forge, where spades and other implements of husbandry are manufactured to a considerable extent. A small customary market is held on Friday. At the eastern end of the village is an ancient cross, raised on a flight of steps, and bearing various coats of arms. There is a commodious school-room, rebuilt by subscription in 1815, and endowed from various sources with about £33 per annum, in which seventy children are instructed: in 1814, Mary

Strong bequeathed £100 for the instruction of girls. From some extensive quarries of free-stone here it is supposed a great part of the stone used for building the Roman wall from Carlisle to Bowness was extracted, and the discovery, about the middle of the last century, of a Roman inscription on the face of a rock, serves to confirm this supposition. Vestiges of three Roman encampments likewise exist in the neighbourhood; and a circle of stones, about thirty yards in circumference, is thought to mark the site of a Druidical place of worship. The old castellated mansion of Dalston has been converted into a farm-house. Rose castle, in this parish, is situated in a beautiful valley, through which winds the river Caldew, and is supposed to have been the principal residence of the bishops of Carlisle from the year 1228. In 1322, it was burned by Robert Bruce, and, about 1366, it was twice attacked and ravaged by the Scots. Before the civil war in the seventeenth century, the building formed a complete quadrangle, had five towers, and was surrounded by a turreted wall; in 1648, being then held for the king, it was attacked by General Lambert, and taken by storm; shortly afterwards, the Duke of Hamilton's army was here reinforced by that under Sir Marmaduke Langdale, and the castle, after having been used as a prison for the royalists, was burnt down by order of Major Cholmley. Since the Restoration it has been rebuilt and improved by successive prelates. The celebrated Dr. Paley was vicar of Dalston from 1774 to 1793.

DALSTON, a hamlet in the parish of HACKNEY, Tower division of the hundred of OSSULSTONE, county of MIDDLESEX, 2½ miles (N. N. E.) from London. The population is returned with the parish.

DALTON, a township in that part of the parish of BURTON in KENDAL which is in the hundred of LONSDALE, south of the sands, county palatine of LANCASTER, 1¼ mile (S. E. by E.) from Burton in Kendal, containing 151 inhabitants. Fairs are held, June 6th for cattle, and October 23rd for cattle, horses, and pedlary.

DALTON, a township in that part of the parish of WIGAN which is in the hundred of WEST DERBY, county palatine of LANCASTER, containing 486 inhabitants.

DALTON, a hamlet in the parish of HEXHAM, southern division of TINDALE ward, county of NORTHUMBERLAND, 4 miles (S. by W.) from Hexham, with which the population is returned.

DALTON, a township in that part of the parish of NEWBURN which is in the eastern division of TINDALE ward, county of NORTHUMBERLAND, 10½ miles (N. W. by W.) from Newcastle upon Tyne, containing 122 inhabitants.

DALTON, a township in that part of the parish of TOPCLIFFE which is in the wapentake of BIRDFORTH, North riding of the county of YORK, 4¼ miles (S.) from Thirsk, containing 235 inhabitants.

DALTON, a township partly in the parish of CROFT, eastern division, but chiefly in the parish of KIRKBY-RAVENSWORTH, western division, of the wapentake of GILLING, North riding of the county of YORK, 3½ miles (S. S. E) from Greta-Bridge, and containing 265 inhabitants. An annuity of £40 is paid by the Master and Wardens of Kirkby-Ravensworth hospital to a schoolmaster in this township, for the education of the poor children, and of those from Newsham; and there is a

small endowment of £3 a year, bequeathed by Thomas Buckton, for which three poor children are instructed. Within the township is a place called Castle-Steeds, where are the remains of a *castra æstiva*, on a slip of land above the conflux of two rivulets, near which passes the Roman Watling-street.

DALTON, a township in the parish of KIRK-HEATON, upper division of the wapentake of AGBRIGG, West riding of the county of YORK, 2 miles (N. E.) from Huddersfield, containing 2289 inhabitants.

DALTON, a township in that part of the parish of ROTHERHAM which is in the southern division of the wapentake of STRAFFORTH and TICKHILL, West riding of the county of YORK, 3 miles (E.) from Rotherham, containing 225 inhabitants.

DALTON le DALE, a parish in the northern division of EASINGTON ward, county palatine of DURHAM, comprising the townships of Dalton le Dale, Dawdon, Cold Hesleton, and East Morton, and containing 211 inhabitants, of which number, 49 are in the township of Dalton le Dale, 6 miles (S.) from Sunderland. The living is a discharged vicarage, in the archdeaconry and diocese of Durham, rated in the king's books at £6. 0. 7., endowed with £200 private benefaction, and £200 royal bounty, and in the patronage of the Dean and Chapter of Durham. The church, dedicated to St. Andrew, is principally in the early style of English architecture: there is a Norman door-way, now closed.

DALTON in FURNESS, a parish in the hundred of LONSDALE, north of the sands, county palatine of LANCASTER, comprising the market town of Dalton, the chapelry of Ireleth, and the townships of Hawcoat-above-town and Yarleside, and containing 2446 inhabitants, of which number, 714 are in the town of Dalton, 25 miles (N.W. by W.) from Lancaster, and 265 (N.W. by N.) from London. This place derives its name from being situated in a dale in the lower part of the district of Furness, of which it was formerly the chief town. According to Tacitus, Agricola, when he had conquered that district, erected a fort here for its protection, and the remains of a Roman road, discovered in 1803 by some workmen, at a considerable depth from the surface, confirm the probability of its having been a Roman station, though there are no other vestiges except some slight traces of the fosse by which it was surrounded. The mount on which the fort was built, upon due examination, was found to be of artificial construction; it was defended on the south and west sides by steep precipices, and on the east by a rampart and ditch; and a brook which flowed at the base supplied the garrison with water. The town derived its principal importance from the erection of the magnificent abbey of Furness, founded in 1127, by Stephen, afterwards king of England, for monks of the Cistercian order, whom he removed from Tulket, in Amounderness, to this valley, where, obtaining valuable grants, they continued to flourish for more than four centuries. The abbots were invested with extensive privileges, and enjoyed large possessions; they held in their own right the woods, pastures, fisheries, and mills of the district, and had considerable shares in the salt-works and mines: the abbey and monastic edifices formed a vast pile of buildings, the character of which was most that of simple magnificence arising from their extent, than of richness and beauty resulting from their style. The chapter-house, which was by far the most elegant of the conventual buildings, was of the early style of English architecture; the church, and most of the other parts, were in the Norman style, partly intermixed with the early English: the revenue of this establishment, at the dissolution, was £966. 7. 10. The remains, an extended mass of ponderous ruins, occupy a considerable part of an area of sixty-five acres, called the Deer park, enclosed with a stone wall, in the sequestered vale of Bekang's Gill, about half a mile west of the town; the approaches are strewed with memorials of its abbots, and mutilated tombs. In the reign of Edward III., a castle, in which during peaceable times the abbots of Furness held their secular courts, was erected here, probably as a place of retreat for the inhabitants, and for the protection of their property from the frequent predatory incursions of the Scots, of whose approach numerous beacons in this part of the country were kept in constant readiness to give notice. In the reign of Henry VIII., Lambert Simnel, the pretended earl of Warwick, landed here, whence he proceeded to assert his claims to the throne; and during the parliamentary war in the reign of Charles I., the town and neighbourhood were the scene of frequent engagements between the hostile parties.

The town is situated on the acclivity of a gradual eminence, and consists principally of one street, at the western extremity of which is the market-place: the houses, in general old, have in some instances given place to others of modern erection: some improvement has been made, but the inhabitants are indifferently supplied with water. The environs are pleasant, and favourable for the sports of the chase; the Dalton Hunt, established in 1703, and noticed in the London Gazette, under the title of the Dalton Rout, and in a contribution to the Tatler, in which the balls and amusements attending its celebration are described, has been discontinued since 1789: a book society, anciently established here, is still continued under judicious regulations. The trade is principally in malt, which is carried on to a great extent; and the iron mines in the vicinity, which have been worked for more than four centuries, produce many thousand tons of excellent ore. A canal, one mile and a half in length, has been constructed, by which vessels may sail up to the town from the sea; and at South End Haws, at the extremity of the Isle of Walney, a light-house, sixty-eight feet in height, was erected in the year 1790. The market is on Saturday: the fairs are, April 28th, June 6th, and October 23d; the first is a statute fair. The parochial affairs are under the direction of twenty-four sidesmen appointed by the parishioners. A court for the recovery of debts under 40s. is held every third week for the barony of Furness; and the lord of the manor holds a court leet twice in the year: the landholders in the parish are customary tenants of the manor; the estates are of the same extent, and pay the same rent, and can neither be partitioned by the tenant, nor devised by will. The castle, erected in the reign of Edward III., and supposed to occupy a portion of the site of the fort built by Agricola, is at present appropriated to the holding of the courts for the liberty, and for the recovery of debts; it is a massive quadrilateral building of three stages, having the principal entrance on the south side, over which is a central window of three lights, surmounted by another of four lights, with flowing tracery in the decorated style.

The living is a discharged vicarage, in the archdeaconry of Richmond, and diocese of Chester, rated in the king's books at £17. 6. 8., endowed with £600 private benefaction, £400 royal bounty, and £1500 parliamentary grant, and in the patronage of the King, as Duke of Lancaster. The church, dedicated to St. Mary, is a neat plain structure of considerable antiquity, built on the declivity of a hill within the precincts of the ancient castellum. There is a place of worship for Wesleyan Methodists. The free grammar school was founded in 1622, by Thomas Boulton, Esq., who bequeathed in trust to the twenty-four sidesmen £220, of which sum, £20 was to be laid out in the erection of the school-room, and the remainder to be invested in the purchase of land for its endowment; with this sum, a farm at Beggar, in the Isle of Walney, has been purchased, producing at present £137 per annum, of which, £100 is paid to the master, who instructs so many of the scholars as require it, in Latin, arithmetic, and the mathematics, and £35 per annum to the assistant, who teaches the rest on Dr. Bell's system. the school is free to all the boys and girls of the parish, and there are, upon the average, eighty scholars attending it. At Ireleth, a chapelry in this parish, there is a similar school. There are various charitable bequests for distribution among the poor. On High Haume, an eminence near the town, is a circular intrenchment which appears to have been a fortified beacon; and on the Pile of Fouldrey, a rocky island separated from the Isle of Walney, are the ruins of a castle, thought by Camden to have been erected in the reign of Edward III., by the abbots of Furness, to defend the approach to the harbour. George Romney, an historical and portrait painter of considerable eminence, was born in this parish, in 1734.

DALTON (NORTH), a parish in the Bainton-Beacon division of the wapentake of HARTHILL, East riding of the county of YORK, comprising the townships of North Dalton and Neswick, and containing 453 inhabitants, of which number, 398 are in the township of North Dalton, 7½ miles (S.W. by W.) from Great Driffield. The living is a perpetual curacy, in the archdeaconry of the East riding, and diocese of York, endowed with £400 private benefaction, £600 royal bounty, and £800 parliamentary grant. James Walker, Esq. was patron in 1827. The church is dedicated to All Saints.

DALTON-PIERCY, a township in the parish of HART, north-eastern division of STOCKTON ward, county palatine of DURHAM, 8½ miles (N. by E.) from Stockton upon Tees, containing 75 inhabitants.

DALTON (SOUTH), a parish in the Hunsley-Beacon division of the wapentake of HARTHILL, East riding of the county of YORK, 6 miles (N.W.) from Beverley, containing 277 inhabitants. The living is a rectory, in the archdeaconry of the East riding and diocese of York, rated in the king's books at £12. Lord Hotham was patron in 1802. The church is dedicated to St. Mary.

DALTON upon TEES, a township in the parish of CROFT, partly within the liberty of ST. PETER of YORK, and partly in the eastern division of the wapentake of GILLING, North riding of the county of YORK, 5 miles (S.) from Darlington, containing 167 inhabitants.

DALWOOD, a chapelry in the parish of STOCKLAND, within the liberty of FORDINGTON, Dorchester division of the county of DORSET, though locally in the hundred of Axminster, county of Devon, 3¾ miles

(W.N.W.) from Axminster, containing 522 inhabitants. The chapel is dedicated to St. Peter. A fair is held on the Wednesday after August 24th.

DAMERHAM (SOUTH), a parish in the southern division of the hundred of DAMERHAM, county of WILTS, 4 miles (N.E. by E.) from Cranbourn, containing 605 inhabitants. The living is a vicarage with the curacy of Martin, in the archdeaconry and diocese of Salisbury, rated in the king's books at £25. 10. 2½., and in the patronage of the Duke of Newcastle. The church is dedicated to St. George.

DANBURY, a parish in the hundred of CHELMSFORD, county of ESSEX, 5½ miles (E. by S.) from Chelmsford, containing, with the hamlet of Russels, which is in the hundred of Dengie, 1005 inhabitants. The living is a rectory, in the archdeaconry of Essex, and diocese of London, rated in the king's books at £20. Sir B. W. Bridges, Bart. was patron in 1793. The church is dedicated to St. John the Baptist. The name is contracted from Danesbury, signifying the town or castle of the Danes. On the summit of Danbury hill is an ancient encampment, about six hundred and eighty yards in circumference; the glacis on the south side is still nearly thirty feet deep, and the lines may be distinctly traced on the other sides. In 1402, the body of the church, and part of the chancel, were destroyed by lightning; and in February, 1750, the upper part of the spire was struck down by a like cause. There is a fair for toys on the 29th of May.

DANBY, a parish in the eastern division of the liberty of LANGBAURGH, North riding of the county of YORK, 9½ miles (S.E.) from Guilsbrough, containing 1373 inhabitants. The living is a perpetual curacy, in the archdeaconry of Cleveland, and diocese of York, endowed with £400 royal bounty, and £1400 parliamentary grant. Lord Viscount Downe was patron in 1781. On a neighbouring hill are the ruins of Danby castle, an edifice of uncertain antiquity.

DANBY-WISK, a parish in the eastern division of the wapentake of GILLING, North riding of the county of YORK, comprising the chapelry of Yafforth, and the township of Danby-Wisk, and containing 477 inhabitants, of which number, 328 are in the township of Danby-Wisk, 3½ miles (N.W.) from North Allerton. The living is a rectory, in the archdeaconry of Richmond, and diocese of Chester, rated in the king's books at £9. 3. 11½. The Rev. William Cust was patron in 1811.

DANTHORPE, a township in the parish of HUMBLETON, middle division of the wapentake of HOLDERNESS, East riding of the county of YORK, 10½ miles (E.N.E.) from Kingston upon Hull, containing 52 inhabitants.

DARENTH, a parish in the hundred of AXTON, DARTFORD, and WILMINGTON, lathe of SUTTON at HONE, county of KENT, 2½ miles (S.E. by S.) from Dartford, containing 574 inhabitants. The living is a discharged vicarage, in the peculiar jurisdiction of the Archbishop of Canterbury, rated in the king's books at £9. 18. 11½., and in the patronage of the Dean and Chapter of Rochester. The church, dedicated to St. Margaret, is principally in the early style of English architecture, and possesses several interesting specimens of the period of its erection, particularly the font, which has attracted much attention. The river Darent passes through the parish, and gives name to it. In 1195, Archbishop Hubert gave this manor to the prior and convent of Rochester, by whom a monastery, dedicated to St. Margaret, was founded here, of which there are still some remains. There are also vestiges of various tumuli, or barrows.

DARESBURY, a chapelry in the parish of RUNCORN, hundred of BUCKLOW, county palatine of CHESTER, 5½ miles (N.E.) from Frodsham, containing 146 inhabitants. The living is a perpetual curacy, in the archdeaconry and diocese of Chester, endowed with £1000 private benefaction, £400 royal bounty, and £900 parliamentary grant, and in the patronage of the Dean and Canons of Christ Church, Oxford. The chapel is dedicated to All Saints. A school, founded by subscription in the reign of Elizabeth, is endowed with the interest of £185, the amount of various benefactions.

DARFIELD, a parish comprising the chapelry of Worsbrough, and the township of Ardsley, in the wapentake of STAINCROSS, and the townships of Billingley, Darfield, Great Houghton, Little Houghton, and Wombwell, in the northern division of the wapentake of STRAFFORTH and TICKHILL, West riding of the county of YORK, and containing 4340 inhabitants, of which number, 512 are in the township of Darfield, 5¼ miles (E. by S.) from Barnesley. The living is a discharged vicarage in the archdeaconry and diocese of York, rated in the king's books at £14. 11. 7., endowed with £600 private benefaction, and £600 royal bounty, and in the patronage of the Master and Fellows of Trinity College, Cambridge: there is also a rectory, one moiety of which is rated at £53. 1. 8., and in the patronage of the Rev. Henry Cooke. The church is dedicated to All Saints. The rivers Drame and Dove run through this parish, and on their banks are some large mills. There are grounds for bleaching linen and yarn, and establishments for weaving cloth, smelting and casting iron, &c. Several trifling endowments have been given for the instruction of children; and an hospital for four widows has been endowed by the Saville family.

DARLASTON, a parish in the southern division of the hundred of OFFLOW, county of STAFFORD, 1½ mile (N.W. by N.) from Wednesbury, containing 5585 inhabitants. The living is a rectory, in the archdeaconry of Stafford, and diocese of Lichfield and Coventry, rated in the king's books at £3. 11. 5½., and in the patronage of the Society for purchasing advowsons. The church is dedicated to St. Lawrence. There are places of worship for Independents and Wesleyan Methodists. A National school is supported by subscription, in which about one hundred and seventy boys and eighty girls are educated. The manufacture of gun-locks is carried on to a considerable extent, and there are some iron-foundries : nails, screws, and hinges are also manufactured. Coal and iron-stone abound, and what is unusual in this mining neighbourhood, there is a good supply of water. The Birmingham canal passes through the parish. On the top of a hill at Berry Bank are ruins of a large castle, fortified with a double vallum and intrenchments, about two hundred and fifty yards in diameter: this, according to tradition, was the seat of Wulpher, King of Mercia, who murdered his two sons for embracing Christianity, and the barrow near it his tomb.

DARLASTON, a liberty in the parish of STONE, southern division of the hundred of PIREHILL, county of STAFFORD, 2 miles (N.W.) from Stone, with which the population is returned.

DARLESTON, a hamlet in the parish of PREES, Whitchurch division of the hundred of BRADFORD (North), county of SALOP, 6 miles (S.S.E.) from Whitchurch. The population is returned with the township of Sandford.

DARLEY, a parish partly in the hundred of WIRKSWORTH, but chiefly in the hundred of HIGH PEAK, county of DERBY, 3 miles (N.W.) from Matlock, containing, with the hamlet of Winsley with Snitterton, which is in Wirksworth hundred, 1830 inhabitants. The living is a rectory, comprising the mediety of North Darley, rated in the king's books at £9. 13. 1½., and the discharged mediety of South Darley, rated at £9. 13. 0½., which were united in 1774 ; it is in the archdeaconry of Derby, and diocese of Lichfield and Coventry, endowed with £2000 parliamentary grant, and in the patronage of the Dean of Lincoln. The church, dedicated to St. Helen, is partly of Norman architecture. There is a school with a small endowment for the education of poor children. Fairs for cattle and sheep are held on the moors in this parish, May 13th and October 27th. Darley is in the honour of Tutbury, duchy of Lancaster, and within the jurisdiction of a court of pleas held at Tutbury every third Tuesday, for the recovery of debts under 40s. A Benedictine abbey was founded here in the reign of Henry I., or in that of Stephen, to the honour of the Blessed Virgin Mary, the annual revenue of which, at the suppression, was valued at £258. 13. 5.

DARLEY, a joint township with Menwith, in the parish of HAMPSTHWAITE, lower division of the wapentake of CLARO, West riding of the county of YORK, 5¼ miles (W. by S.) from Ripley, containing 648 inhabitants.

DARLEY-ABBEY, a chapelry in that part of the parish of ST. ALKMUND, DERBY, which is in the hundred of MORLESTON and LITCHURCH, county of DERBY, 1¼ mile (N.) from Derby, containing 841 inhabitants. The living is a perpetual curacy, in the archdeaconry of Derby, and diocese of Lichfield and Coventry, and in the patronage of Walter Evans, Esq., who, in 1819, built and endowed the church at his sole expense, for the accommodation of his work-people. It is pleasantly situated on the banks of the Derwent, on which are extensive cotton and paper-mills, the proprietors of which have established schools on an extensive scale, for the children of the people in their employment. The abbey was founded in the reign of Henry I., for friars of the order of St. Augustine, and endowed with its privileges confirmed by Henry II. ; at the dissolution its annual revenue was £285. 9. 6½.

DARLINGSCOTT, a hamlet in the parish of TREDINGTON, upper division of the hundred of OSWALDSLOW, county of WORCESTER, though locally in the Kington division of the hundred of Kington, county of Warwick, 2¼ miles (N.W. by W.) from Shipston upon Stour, containing 189 inhabitants.

DARLINGTON, a parochial chapelry in the southeastern division of DARLINGTON ward, county palatine of DURHAM, comprising the market town of Darlington, the townships of Archdeacon-Newton, Blackwell, and Cockerton, and containing 6551 inhabitants, of which number, 5750 are in the town of Darlington, 18½ miles (S.) from Durham, and 236½ (N. N. W.) from London, on the great north road. The name, which is of Saxon etymology, is conjectural only ; by some it is considered to denote the darling, or favourite town ; according to others, who assume Dare as the ancient name of the river Skerne, and ing to signify a meadow, Dare-ing-tun was its appellation, to signify the town in the meadows of the Dare. About the end of the ninth century, Darlington, with its dependencies, was given to St. Cuthbert, under license from Ethelred, by Seir, son of Ulphus ; and in 1082 it became the asylum of the secular clergy, who had been driven from Durham abbey by Bishop Carilepho. About 1164, a mansion-house was erected here by Bishop Pudsey, in which several of his successors resided : the manor-house was subsequently purchased of one of the bishops of Durham, under an act for the redemption of the land tax, and has been converted into a workhouse. From this place, in 1291, Edward I. issued an order to his chief military tenants in the northern counties, to proceed to the war in Scotland. In the reign of Edward III. a skirmish between Archibald, Earl Douglas, and a band of Englishmen, took place here, and proved fatal to many of the latter. In 1504, the Princess Margaret, then betrothed to James of Scotland, slept at the manor-house on her journey northward ; and in 1640 the king's troops rested here, when retreating before the Covenanters, after the battle of Stellahaugh, and were well supplied with provisions under the direction of the Earl of Stafford.

The town is situated in a rich grazing district, on the eastern declivity of an eminence, at the base of which flows the river Skerne, in its course to the Tees, and is crossed by a bridge of three arches ; it is built in the form of a square, with streets leading therefrom in different directions ; the houses in general are modern : several new streets have been formed under an act of parliament obtained in 1823, pursuant to which the town was lighted with oil. From the favourable nature of the surrounding country for the pasturage of sheep, of which there was formerly a considerable number, the Leicestershire breed having been recently introduced, Darlington was formerly noted for the manufacture of tammies, camblets, moreens, harrateens, &c.; to this succeeded the manufacture of linen, which also has much declined. There are mills for spinning wool and flax, and for grinding optical glasses, also an extensive worsted-mill, and two iron-foundries ; the principal employment of the labouring class consists in combing wool, and in other business connected with the mills. The worsted-yarn is used for Brussels and other carpets, which are manufactured here, as well as for the finest imitation Indian shawls. Within half a mile of the town is the main line of a rail-road, which has been constructed from Wilton Park colliery to Stockton, pursuant to an act of parliament obtained in 1821, and is about twenty-five miles in length : coal, lime, and other minerals, are conveyed on it at the rate of three halfpence per ton, and merchandise at three pence per ton, per mile: the line is worked by two fixed locomotive engines, working four inclined planes half a mile in length. On this road coaches pass daily, and are charged at the rate of threepence per mile: it was completed in September, 1825, at the total expense of £125,000, and is the joint property of sixty shareholders. A market for corn is held every Monday, and one for cattle and sheep on every alternate Monday : there are general and cattle fairs on the first Monday in March, Easter-Monday, Whit-Monday, and a fortnight after; on the 9th of November for horses, and 10th for horned cattle and sheep; 13th for hogs, and 23d a hiring and general fair; also on the second Monday after, a fair for cattle, horses, and sheep. The market-house was erected at the expense of Lady Brown. The government of the town is vested in a bailiff appointed by the Bishop of Durham, but he possesses no magisterial authority : the town is divided into four constableries, called the Borough, Bondgate, Prebend-row, Oxenhall, or Oxon le Field: constables for the borough are chosen by house row at the May-day court. The tolls are held for three lives under the see of Durham, by a few respectable inhabitants, who in 1808 rebuilt the town-hall, within which are a house of correction, dispensary, and public library, and near it the shambles, which were erected in 1815. Here the county magistrates hold a petty session every alternate Monday. The old Tolbooth was taken down and rebuilt in 1807.

The living is a perpetual curacy, in the archdeaconry and diocese of Durham, endowed with £1000 private benefaction, £400 royal bounty, and £900 parliamentary grant, and in the patronage of the Marquis of Cleveland. The church was erected about 1160, by Bishop Pudsey, and dedicated to St. Cuthbert; it was formerly collegiate, and had four chantries, besides the free chapel of Badelfielde, or Battlefield, the ecclesiastical body then consisting of a dean, who held a prebend, and four other prebendaries : this society was dissolved in 1550, and the property became vested in the Crown, but at present one part is held by the Marquis of Cleveland, subject to a crown rental, and the remainder distributed amongst other individuals. The church, dedicated to St. Cuthbert, is an elegant cruciform structure in the early English style, having a square embattled tower which stands on four arches, ornamented with the nail-head mouldings, and springing from light fluted columns with richly adorned capitals; it rises from the intersection, and is surmounted by a light spire, the upper part of which, having sustained some injury from lightning on the 17th of July, 1750, was taken down and rebuilt : on each side of the nave is a range of dissimilar columns supporting pointed arches, which separate it from the aisles; a lofty arch leads from the nave to the chancel, and the southern portion of the transept is highly ornamented. There are places of worship for Particular Baptists, the Society of Friends, Independents, and Primitive and Wesleyan Methodists. A new Roman Catholic chapel, dedicated to St. Augustine, was opened in 1827. A free grammar school, endowed by charter of Elizabeth, dated June 15th, 1567, with lands formerly belonging to the chantry established by Robert Marshall, for a master and an usher, is under the superintendence of the four churchwardens of the town, and its annual revenue is upwards of £240. The Blue-coat charity school, founded principally by means of a benefaction by Dame Mary Calverly, of Eryholme, amounting to £1000, made by indenture dated 19th of April, 1715, now possesses funded property to the value of £1392. 9. three per cent. consols., which yields an annual income of £41. 15. 4. A British school, for an unlimited number of boys and one hundred girls, is supported by the Society of Friends, Independents, and Wesleyan Methodists; and a National school affords instruction to about one hundred and fifty boys and one hundred girls. There is also an infant school, supported by Mr. James Backhouse, a member of the Society of Friends, in which the children pay the weekly sum of twopence. In 1631, Francis Forster, of this town, gave, by indenture dated 9th of March, to trustees, two houses in Northgate, as almshouses for six poor men, or women, natives of this place; and in 1641 he gave a field, the rent of which was to be distributed among the poorest persons who had resided three years in the town. In 1636, a bequest in land was made by James Bellasis, Esq., of Owton, for the establishment of a linen and woollen manufactory, for the benefit of the poor of the town and neighbourhood, which was placed under the superintendence of the principal persons in the borough, but this benefaction has been lost, and the rent of the land thus given withheld from the poor ever since 1810. William Middleton, of Blackwall, gave a field of six acres, now let for £18 per annum, to the churchwardens and overseers in trust for apprenticing poor boys. An almshouse was founded by Mrs. Mary Pease, a member of the Society of Friends, in 1820, for four poor widows, each to be at least of the age of fifty, and not belonging to that society; and Richard Lindley, of Darlington, bequeathed £350, to be invested, and the proceeds thereof to be distributed annually amongst the poor, with a similar restriction. There are several minor charities, in small sums and donations of bread, for the relief of the necessitous. A dispensary was established in 1809, and is supported by voluntary contributions; and a savings' bank in 1817; the deposits in which, in 1827, amounted to £36,000. A mechanics' institute and library were commenced in 1825, under the patronage of the Earl of Darlington, J. G. Lambton, Esq., (now Lord Durham,) and the Hon. W. J. F. V. Powlet: the collection of books consists of three hundred volumes. A society for the relief of poor lying-in women was established in 1822.

At Oxen-hall are four celebrated circular pools, called Hell-Kettles; the diameter of the three larger ones is about thirty-eight yards each, and their respective depths nineteen feet and a half, seventeen, and fourteen : the fourth is twenty-eight feet in diameter, and five feet and a half deep; they are always brim full, and although nearly on a level with the Tees, are unaffected by its flood or fall, excepting the smallest, which is now nearly dry : the water is quite cold; it is said to be impregnated with sulphur, and not to mix with milk or soap. Amidst various conjectures as to their formation, the generally received opinion is that they were originally marl pits. A sulphureous spring, discovered in 1805, in the vicinity of the town, is of reputed efficacy in scorbutic disorders, and much resorted to. Mr. John Kendrew, the inventor and patentee of machinery for spinning flax, hemp, &c., also of a machine for grinding and polishing optical glasses, formerly resided here; and the Grange, a neat brick mansion about a mile southward, was the residence of Mr. George Allan, a barrister, who collected very extensive historical and topographical notes, designed to furnish a history of this county, which are now in the possession of John Allan, Esq., of Blackwell: he had also a valuable museum of coins, medals, and paintings, with various other natural curiosities, and a printing-press, whence issued some of Pennant's publications, which are now extremely rare, and various other works.

Darlington confers the title of earl on the Marquis of Cleveland.

DARLTON, a chapelry in the parish of DUNHAM, South-clay division of the wapentake of BASSETLAW, county of NOTTINGHAM, 3¼ miles (N.E. by E.) from Tuxford, containing 153 inhabitants. The chapel is dedicated to St. Giles.

DARNALL, a hamlet in that part of the parish of SHEFFIELD which is in the southern division of the wapentake of STRAFFORTH and TICKHILL, West riding of the county of YORK, 2¼ miles (E.) from Sheffield. The population is returned with the chapelry of Attercliffe.

DARNHALL, a township in the parish of WHITE-GATE, or NEW CHURCH, first division of the hundred EDDISBURY, county palatine of CHESTER, 6 miles (W.S.W.) from Middlewich, containing 207 inhabitants.

DARRAS-HALL, a township in the parish of PON-TELAND, western division of CASTLE ward, county of NORTHUMBERLAND, 7 miles (N.W.) from Newcastle, containing 12 inhabitants.

DARRINGTON, a parish in the upper division of the wapentake of OSGOLDCROSS, West riding of the county of YORK, comprising the townships of Darrington and Stapleton, and containing 619 inhabitants, of which number, 510 are in the township of Darrington, 2¾ miles (S.E. by E.) from Pontefract. The living is a discharged vicarage, in the archdeaconry and diocese of York, rated in the king's books at £16. 11. 3., and in the patronage of the Archbishop of York. The church is dedicated to St. Luke and All Saints.

DARSHAM, a parish in the hundred of BLYTHING, county of SUFFOLK, 5¼ miles (N.E. by N.) from Saxmundham, containing 487 inhabitants. The living is a discharged vicarage, in the archdeaconry of Suffolk, and diocese of Norwich, rated in the king's books at £4. 10. 10., endowed with £200 royal bounty, and in the patronage of the Earl of Stradbroke. The church is dedicated to All Saints. There is a Sunday school, supported by £4 per annum, arising from cottages and land called the Town Estate.

DARTFORD, a market town and parish, in the hundred of AXTON, DARTFORD, and WILMINGTON, lathe of SUTTON at HONE, county of KENT, 15 miles (S. E.) from London, and 22 (N. W.) from Maidstone, on the great road from London to Canterbury and Dover, containing 3593 inhabitants. The name is a contraction of Darent-ford, or the ford on the Darent, on the banks of which river the town is situated. Dartford is mentioned in history as the place where Isabella, sister of Henry III., was married by proxy in 1235, to the German Emperor, Frederick II. Edward III. held a tournament here, on his return from France in 1331; and in 1355 he founded, and afterwards richly endowed, a monastery at Dartford, for nuns of the order of St. Autine, the revenue of which, at the dissolution, was £408. At this town commenced the insurrection under Wat Tyler, in the 5th of Richard II.; and on the neighbouring heath, called Dartford-Brent, the army of Richard, Duke of York, encamped in 1451, while he waited to obtain a conference with King Henry VI., who then lay with his army at Blackheath. Dartford-Brent also was the rendezvous of the parliamentary forces under General Fairfax, in 1648. The town is pleasantly situated in a narrow valley, between two hills, in one of which, towards Crayford, is a number of pits, sunk in the chalky strata of which the hill is composed, from ten to twenty fathoms in depth, and of considerable extent, supposed to have been used by the Saxons as granaries, or store-rooms. The principal street is in the line of the London road, and two smaller streets branch off from it at right angles. There is a bridge over the Darent, built since the commencement of the reign of Edward III., and repaired and improved at the expense of the county about fifty years ago, at which time a new market-house was erected, and the streets were newly paved. The river is navigable up to the town for boats, which sail regularly to London. The numerous mills on the Darent contribute greatly to the trading prosperity of Dartford. Here is an extensive gunpowder manufactory, which occupies the site of the first paper-mill erected in this country, by Sir John Spielman, a German, who died in 1607; and at a short distance is a paper-mill, where formerly stood a mill for rolling and slitting iron, also the first of the kind in England, constructed by Godfrey Box, of Liege, in 1590. Here are also mills for grinding corn, and for extracting oil from seeds; besides a very extensive establishment for the construction of steam-engines, to which is attached a foundry, on a scale of considerable magnitude, where nearly two hundred workmen are constantly employed. The market is on Saturday, which is plentifully supplied with provisions; and a fair is held on the 2nd of August. Here are held the petty sessions for the upper division of the lathe of Sutton at Hone; and a court of requests, for the recovery of debts not exceeding £5, is held, under an act of parliament passed in the 47th of George III., "for the town of Gravesend, and the several hundreds of Toltingtrough, Dartford, Wilmington, and Axtane, in the county of Kent."

The living is a discharged vicarage, in the archdeaconry and diocese of Rochester, rated in the king's books at £18. 11. 3., endowed with £200 private benefaction, and £200 royal bounty, and in the patronage of the Bishop of Rochester. The church, dedicated to the Holy Trinity, is a spacious structure, consisting of a nave, aisles, and chancel, with an embattled tower at the north-west side: it contains many ancient monuments, among which is one in commemoration of the above-mentioned Sir John Spielman. The ancient burying-ground is situated on a high hill, at some distance from the church; and a new one was consecrated a few years since in a more convenient situation. There are places of worship for various denominations of dissenters. A free grammar school was founded here in 1576, for the education of eight boys, and endowed with property producing £48. 15. per annum, which is vested in trustees, by a decree of the commissioners of charitable uses, dated July 5th, 1678. There is also a charity school for boys in connexion with the church, conducted on the National system, and supported chiefly by the income arising from various benefactions, the master of which has a salary of £100 per annum. At Lowfield, in this parish, are four alms-houses, founded in 1572, in pursuance of a bequest by John Byer, who also founded and endowed nine more almshouses in the parish. Traces of the Roman Watling-street appear on the south side of the high road, between Dartford and Dartford-Brent. The Augustine nunnery, after the dissolution, was made a royal residence by Henry VIII. and Elizabeth; and its remains, consisting of an embattled gateway and some other buildings of brick, have been converted into a farm-house. An hospital, dedicated to the Holy Trinity, was founded in the reign of Henry VI.; and an hospital for lepers existed here in the fourteenth century. In the latter part of Elizabeth's reign, the county assizes are said to have been frequently held at Dartford; and a spot at the entrance to Dartford-Brent from the town was the place of execution for malefactors. The Earl of Jersey enjoys the inferior title of Viscount Villiers, of Dartford.

DARTINGTON, a parish in the hundred of Stanborough, county of Devon, 2 miles (N. by W.) from Totness, containing 602 inhabitants. The living is a rectory, in the archdeaconry of Totness, and diocese of Exeter, rated in the king's books at £36. 4. 4½. The trustees of A. Champernowne, Esq., a minor, were patrons in 1799. The church is dedicated to St. Mary.

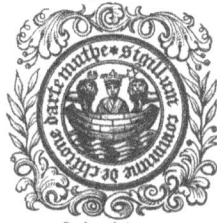
Seal and Arms.

DARTMOUTH, a borough, sea-port, and market town, having separate jurisdiction, locally in the hundred of Coleridge, county of Devon, 30¾ miles (S. by W.) from Exeter, and 204 W. S. W.) from London, containing 4485 inhabitants. This place, which derives its name from being situated at the mouth of the river Dart, appears to have been distinguished at a very early period for the convenience of its harbour, which, in 1190, was the rendezvous of the fleet destined for the Holy Land. In the reign of Richard I. the French effected a landing on this coast, and, after setting fire to the town, retreated with inconsiderable loss. It is stated by Leland to have received a charter of incorporation from King John, but no authentic document exists of a date prior to Edward III.: if not incorporated, it enjoyed many privileges, and, in 1226, the inhabitants obtained the grant of a weekly market and an annual fair. In the reign of Edward I. the town sent members to parliament, and had become a considerable staple for wool, wine, and iron; and in that of Edward III. the port contributed thirty-one ships, and nearly eight hundred men, to the naval armament for the invasion of France. In this reign the town, together with the adjacent villages of Clifton and Hardness, received a regular charter of incorporation, and was exempted from tolls. By act of parliament in the reign of Richard II., the exportation of tin was exclusively restricted to the port of Dartmouth, but the restriction was soon after abolished. In 1404, the French pirates having burnt Plymouth, sailed to this town, but were gallantly repulsed by the male and female inhabitants; De Chastell; their commander, and several of his men were killed, and twenty of the crew taken prisoners. The castle is supposed to have been erected in the reign of Henry VII. During the parliamentary war, Dartmouth was regarded as a very important post, and eagerly contended for by both parties. in 1643, it was taken, after a siege of four weeks, by Prince Maurice, who garrisoned it for the king; and, in 1646, it was taken by storm by General Fairfax, who commanded the assault in person.

The town is beautifully situated on the western shore of the bay formed by the river Dart, near its

influx with the sea. The houses are built on the acclivity of an eminence sloping gently from the margin of the water, and ranged in streets rising above each other at different elevations : they are in general ancient, and some of them are ornamented with grotesque carvings : the governor's house, which occupies a higher site, is a modern adaptation of the ancient style of building which prevails in the town, and forms the front to a naval museum. The streets, though inconveniently narrow, are partially paved by the commissioners, and the inhabitants are supplied with water brought by pipes from springs in the neighbourhood, at the expense of the corporation. A subscription reading-room has been established, and an annual regatta is celebrated, generally in July. The surrounding scenery is strikingly beautiful : the view of the town from the bay is truly picturesque; and the rocks, which are of a purple-coloured slate, are finely contrasted with the verdant foliage of the trees in which the houses are embosomed, extending for nearly a mile along the coast, and interspersed with a rich variety of plants and shrubs. The bay, in several points of view, from which the town and the sea are excluded by projecting rocks, has the appearance of an inland lake, noted for its romantic beauty. The harbour is sufficiently capacious for the reception of five hundred sail of vessels, and is remarkable for its security, and for the depth and tranquillity of its water, the surface of which is undisturbed, while the sea, at the distance only of a quarter of a mile, is in a state of strong agitation. The entrance is on the south, between the ruins of Kingswear castle and the fort and church of St. Petrock, where a battery has been erected for its defence. The port extends from the river Teign to the river Erme, including a range of coast forty miles in length, and is under the superintendence of a governor appointed by the corporation, and paid by the crown. The number of vessels belonging to the port in 1828 was three hundred and forty-eight, averaging seventy-two tons' burden. The trade is principally with Newfoundland, the English coast, and the collieries : in the year ending January 5th, 1827, one hundred and two British and fourteen foreign vessels entered inward from foreign parts; and one hundred and forty-three British and one foreign vessel cleared outward. An artificial quay has been constructed, projecting into the harbour; and there is a custom-house, with requisite offices for the despatch of business. The river Dart is navigable to Totness, ten miles distant; and the passage is highly interesting from the beautiful scenery with which its banks abound throughout. A considerable trade is carried on in ship-building there are commodious dock-yards, in which nineteen vessels were built in the year 1826; but the inhabitants are chiefly engaged in the Newfoundland and other fisheries, in which three thousand persons are employed, of whom a certain number is by law required to be landsmen. The market is on Friday: there are no fairs of any importance. The government, by charter of Edward III., confirmed by succeeding monarchs, and extended by James II., is vested in a mayor, recorder, and twelve aldermen, assisted by a town clerk, coroner, two bailiffs, a receiver, and other officers. The mayor, the late mayor, and recorder, are justices of the peace for the borough, and hold a court of session quarterly, for the trial of all offenders not ac-

C

eused of capital crimes; and a court of record, under a charter of Edward III., for the recovery of debts to any amount, on the Monday in every week, but no writ has issued from it since 1823. The manorial courts for the borough, and also for the parish of Townstall, of which the corporation are lords of the manor, are also held here. The borough prison is a small building, containing two wards, with accommodation for four prisoners. The borough has continued to return two members to parliament since its incorporation in the 24th of Edward III.: the right of election is vested in the freemen generally; the mayor is the returning officer.

Dartmouth comprises the parishes of St. Petrock, St. Saviour, and Townstall, all in the archdeaconry of Totness, and diocese of Exeter. The living of St. Petrock's is a perpetual curacy, endowed with £1000 royal bounty, and £1200 parliamentary grant, and in the patronage of the Rector of Stoke-Fleming: the church is beautifully situated near the entrance to the harbour. The living of St. Saviour's is a perpetual curacy annexed to the vicarage of Townstall, endowed with £200 private benefaction, and £300 parliamentary grant, and in the patronage of the Mayor and Corporation: the church, commonly called the mayor's chapel, is a spacious cruciform structure, possessing little external, but considerable internal, beauty; it is principally in the decorated style of English architecture: the pulpit is of stone, richly sculptured and gilt; the wooden screen is an elaborate and highly enriched specimen of carving, in the decorated style; and the stalls of the corporation are of good modern workmanship: the original ceiling of oak is still preserved. The living of the parish of Townstall is a discharged vicarage, with the perpetual curacy of St. Saviour's, rated in the king's books at £12. 15. 4½., endowed with £15 per annum and £200 private benefaction, £200 royal bounty, and £300 parliamentary grant, and in the patronage of the Mayor and Corporation. The church is dedicated to St. Clement. There are places of worship for Baptists, Independents, and Wesleyan Methodists. Sunday schools in each parish are supported by subscription; and there are some small charitable bequests for the benefit of the poor and the instruction of poor children. Newcomen, the inventor of the steam-engine, was a native of this place. Dartmouth gives the title of earl to the family of Legge.

DARTON, a parish in the wapentake of STAINCROSS, West riding of the county of YORK, comprising the townships of Barugh, Darton, and Kexborough, and containing 2176 inhabitants, of which number, 1340 are in the township of Darton, 3¾ miles (N. W.) from Barnesley. The living is a discharged vicarage, in the archdeaconry and diocese of York, rated in the king's books at £12. 10., endowed with £250 private benefaction, and £200 royal bounty, and in the patronage of G. W. Wentworth, Esq. The church is dedicated to All Saints. In 1668, George Beaumont bequeathed £500 towards supporting a schoolmaster for the free education of the children of the inhabitants; the number is about sixty, and the income £54 a year: the schoolroom was rebuilt in 1800.

DARWEN (LOWER), a township in the parish of BLACKBURN, lower division of the hundred of BLACKBURN, county palatine of LANCASTER, 2¼ miles (S.S.E.) from Blackburn, containing 2238 inhabitants. A chapel is now being erected by the commissioners appointed under the act passed in the 58th of George III., for building additional churches, and of which the Vicar of Blackburn will be patron.

DARWEN (OVER), a chapelry in the parish of BLACKBURN, lower division of the hundred of BLACKBURN, county palatine of LANCASTER, 4¼ miles (S. by E.) from Blackburn, containing 6711 inhabitants. The living is a perpetual curacy, in the archdeaconry and diocese of Chester, endowed with £620 private benefaction, and £600 royal bounty, and in the patronage of the Vicar of Blackburn. The chapel is dedicated to St. James. There are different places of worship for dissenters, and about one thousand five hundred children are instructed in Sunday schools. Print and bleaching-works are extensively carried on, and coal and slate are plentiful. Three annual fairs are held here, on the first Thursday in October, and the first Thursday in May, for cattle and horses, and on Holy Thursday, which is a pleasure fair.

DARWENT, a chapelry in the parish of HATHERSAGE, hundred of HIGH PEAK, county of DERBY, 10 miles (N.N.W.) from Stony-Middleton, containing 123 inhabitants. The living is a perpetual curacy with that of All Saints', Derby, in the archdeaconry of Derby, and diocese of Lichfield and Coventry, endowed with £400 private benefaction, and £600 royal bounty. The chapel is dedicated to St. James. There is an endowment of £5 a year, arising from bequests by Robert Turner, in 1720, and John Eyre, in 1772, for teaching twelve poor children.

DASSETT (AVON), a parish in the Burton-Dassett division of the hundred of KINGTON, county of WARWICK, 5¼ miles (E. by S.) from Kington, containing 242 inhabitants. The living is a rectory, in the peculiar jurisdiction of the Bishop of Lichfield and Coventry, rated in the king's books at £13. 18. 9. Robert Green, Esq. was patron in 1803. The church is dedicated to St. John the Baptist.

DATCHETT, a parish in the hundred of STOKE, county of BUCKINGHAM, 2 miles (E.S.E.) from Eton, containing 839 inhabitants. The living is a discharged vicarage, in the archdeaconry of Buckingham, and diocese of Lincoln, rated in the king's books at £11, endowed with £15 per annum and £200 private benefaction, £200 royal bounty, and £700 parliamentary grant, and in the patronage of the Dean and Canons of Windsor. The church is dedicated to St. Mary. There is a place of worship for Baptists. Datchett is separated from Windsor by the river Thames, over which here was formerly a bridge, built by Queen Anne, but it fell down in 1795, and has not since been rebuilt.

DATCHWORTH, a parish in the hundred of BROADWATER, county of HERTFORD, 3¼ miles (N.E. by E.) from Welwyn, containing 494 inhabitants. The living is a rectory, in the archdeaconry of Huntingdon, and diocese of Lincoln, rated in the king's books at £14. 13. 4., and in the patronage of the Master and Fellows of Clare Hall, Cambridge. The church is dedicated to All Saints.

DAUNTSEY, a parish in the hundred of MALMESBURY, county of WILTS, 4¼ miles (S.E.) from Malmesbury, containing 467 inhabitants. The living is a rectory, in the archdeaconry and diocese of Salisbury, rated in the king's books at £13.6.3. The Earl of Peterborough was patron in 1800. The church, dedicated to St. James, contains a noble monument of white marble to the memory of Henry Danvers, Baron Dauntsey, created Earl of Danby in 1625; he founded here a free school and an almshouse, and the Botanical Garden at Oxford. There is a chapel of ease at Westend, in this parish.

DAVENHAM, a parish in the hundred of NORTHWICH, county palatine of CHESTER, comprising the townships of Bostock, Davenham, Eaton, Leftwich, Moulton, Newhall, Rudheath, Shipbrook, Shurlach, Stanthorne, Wharton, and Whatcroft, and containing 3470 inhabitants, (exclusively of 97 in the township of Great Rudheath, which are returned with the parishes of Great Budworth and Sandbach) of which number, 379 are in the township of Davenham, 2¼ miles (S.) from Northwich. The living is a rectory, in the archdeaconry and diocese of Chester, rated in the king's books at £23. 13. 1½., and in the patronage of R. W. Tomkinson, Esq. The church is dedicated to St. Wilfred. Davenham derives its name from its situation on the river Daven, or Dane. A school, founded more than a century since, is supported by a rent-charge on Shipbrook-hill farm, and other benefactions, amounting together to about £20 per annum. In the lordship of Rudheath, in this parish, an action was fought on the 22d of February, 1643, between the king's troops and the parliamentary forces under Sir William Brereton.

DAVENPORT, a township in that part of the parish of ASTBURY which is in the hundred of NORTHWICH, county palatine of CHESTER, 4½ miles (N.W. by W.) from Congleton, containing 96 inhabitants.

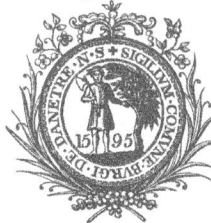
Corporate Seal.

DAVENTRY, a market town and parish having separate jurisdiction, locally in the hundred of Fawsley, county of NORTHAMPTON, 12¼ miles (W. by N.) from Northampton, and 72 (N.W.) from London, on the road to Holyhead, containing, with the hamlet of Drayton, 3326 inhabitants. This place derives its name from the British Dwy-avon-tre, town of the two Avons, denoting its situation between two rivers of that name. About half a mile to the south-east is Borough hill, a lofty eminence, on which is an elliptical intrenchment, including an area of nearly two hundred acres, defended on the south and west by a double trench and rampart, and on the north and east sides by four deep trenches and five ramparts, the entrances to which are on the south and south-east sides. The origin of this camp, which Mr. Pennant considers to have been a post of the Britons when opposed to Ostorius, and after its reduction to have been occupied by that general, as the castra æstiva of his forces, has been by some antiquaries referred to the Danes, by whom it may probably have been occupied during their irruption in 1006, and to whom the building of the town has been ascribed. From this erroneous supposition, strengthened by the contraction of the name to Dantrey, and Daintree, has probably resulted the device of the common seal. At the distance of nearly three hundred yards below this intrenchment is a smaller quadrilateral camp, including an acre of ground, defended by a single intrenchment; below which is another, including six acres, called Burnt Walls, where John of Gaunt is said to have had a palace. This station, which is one of the largest of the kind in the kingdom, was the Bennavenna of the Britons, and the Isanta Varia of Antonine. At the time of the Conquest Daventry was a place of considerable importance. In 1090 a priory was founded here by Hugh de Leycester, for monks of the Cluniac order; it was richly endowed, its revenue amounting to £236. 7. 6., and it was one of those which, by permission of pope Clement VII., were dissolved in the 17th of Henry VIII., and granted to Cardinal Wolsey, for endowing his intended colleges at Ipswich and Oxford: the last remains of the buildings were taken down in 1826. During the parliamentary war, Daventry was the scene of frequent conflicts, in one of which, in the beginning of 1645, Sir William and Sir Charles Compton, brothers of the Earl of Northampton, with three hundred horse, routed four hundred of the parliamentarian cavalry near the town. In the same year, the king having taken Leicester by storm, on his march to relieve Oxford, which was closely besieged, fixed his head-quarters at this town, where he remained for six days, prior to his departure for Market-Harborough where the vanguard of his army was stationed, in the neighbourhood of which place the battle of Naseby was fought on the following day.

The town is pleasantly situated on the acclivity of a gentle eminence, sheltered by other hills to the south and south-east, and consists of two principal streets, intersected by several smaller, lighted and paved by an act passed in the 46th of George III., for that purpose, and also for the rebuilding of the moot-hall. The houses, though irregularly, are neatly and well built, and the inhabitants are supplied with water from a spring on the Borough hill, at the distance of half a mile to the south-east of the town. The only branch of manufacture is that of whips: the support of the trade arises chiefly from its situation as a public thoroughfare, and from its numerous fairs. The Grand Junction canal, at the north angle of the parish, passes through a tunnel two thousand yards in length, to the south of which is the reservoir. The market is on Wednesday: the fairs are on the first Monday in January, the last Monday in February, Tuesday in Easter week, June 6th and 7th, August 3rd, the first Monday in September, October 2nd and 3rd, October 27th, and the last Wednesday in November. The first October fair is on the first day of that month, for cheese; and the second for live stock; the others are generally for horses and cattle. On the two next Wednesdays after Michaelmas are statute fairs for hiring servants. St. Augustine's fair, now held on the 6th and 7th of June, is coeval with the grant of the market, and with it appended to the manor; and the inhabitants, notwithstanding several attempts to emancipate themselves, are still compelled to grind their corn at the lord's mill, and to bake their bread at his oven. The town is supposed to have had a guild-merchant at a very early period: it received a charter of incorporation from King John, which was confirmed by Queen Elizabeth in the eighteenth year of her reign, and subsequently by James I. Under the present charter of the 27th of Charles II. the government is vested in a bailiff, a recorder, (who must be a barrister, and whose appointment is subject to approval by the crown), and a chamberlain, twelve burgesses, twenty common council-men, assisted by a town clerk (who must be a barrister), two wardens, two serjeants at mace, and other officers. The bailiff, who is also clerk of the market, is elected on Michaelmas-day, by the common council-men, from two burgesses nominated by the bailiff and two of the burgesses; the chamberlain and wardens are chosen at the same time by the commonalty, or, on their declining to elect, by the bailiff and burgesses. The bailiff, the late bailiff, who acts as coroner the following year, and the recorder, are justices of the peace for the borough. The corporation hold a general court of session annually; and under the charter of Elizabeth, confirmed and extended by Charles II., a weekly court of record, for the recovery of debts not exceeding £100. 1. is held, in which the bailiff and recorder preside, either in person or by deputy; but from this court no writs have been issued since 1823. The town-hall having become greatly dilapidated, a large house has been purchased and commodiously fitted up for the borough sessions and courts of record; and within the last three years, a new gaol and house of correction for the borough has been erected.

The living is a perpetual curacy, in the archdeaconry of Northampton, and diocese of Peterborough, endowed with £20 per annum private benefaction, and in the patronage of the Dean and Canons of Christ Church, Oxford. The ancient church, dedicated to the Holy Cross, formerly the conventual church of the priory, was taken down in 1752, and the present structure erected on its site, at the expense of £3486. There are places of worship for Independents and Wesleyan Methodists. The free grammar school was founded in 1576, by Mr. William Parker, of London, who endowed it with a rent-charge of £20 per annum, of which £15 per annum was to be paid to the master, and £5 to an usher, for the instruction of fifty poor children of the town; the endowment was farther augmented, in 1729, by Mr. John Farrer, of Daventry, who bequeathed £400 to five trustees, for the purchase of lands, now producing £43 per annum, as a stipend to the master, who must be in holy orders, on condition of his reading evening prayers on Sundays, and morning prayers on Mondays, Tuesdays, Thursdays, and Saturdays, at the parish church. John Sawbridge, Esq., of Daventry, in 1740, bequeathed £150, to which £100 was added by his brother, Edward Sawbridge, Esq., to purchase or build a house for the master; these sums, which are at present invested in the funds, produce £16 per annum. An English charity school was founded in 1736, by Dr. Edward Maynard, who gave £200 to the corporation, in trust for that purpose; it is supported partly by subscription, and is also endowed with £6 per annum, the bequest of Nathaniel, Lord Crewe, Bishop of Durham; £4 per annum, the gift of Edward Sawbridge; £89 per annum, part of the rental of an estate at Cosford, in Northamptonshire, purchased with money arising from several benefactions; and the interest of £700 three per cent. consols., bought with money procured from the sale of timber on the Cosford estate, and occasional savings of income. The master has £67 per annum, besides an allowance of £4. 16. per annum for providing books and stationery: twenty-four boys, who are all supplied with clothing, and some placed apprentices, are educated in this school; the boys' school is now combined with a National school supported by subscription. An academy for dissenters was maintained here by the trustees of William Coward, Esq., of London, till the

year 1789, when it was removed. Mr. John Welch gave the interest of £700, now vested in the South Sea annuities, producing £21 per annum, of which, £9 per annum is paid to the minister of the congregation of Independents, and the remaining £12 towards the support of a charity school for children of both sexes. There are various charitable bequests for distribution among the poor, among which may be noticed £10 per annum by Mr. Parker, the founder of the grammar school, to be distributed quarterly to six beadsmen appointed by the lord of the manor of Ipswich, to which several others have been subsequently added for the same purpose. John Smith, a celebrated engraver in mezzotinto, was born here in 1740. Daventry gives the title of baron to the Earl of Winchelsea.

DAVIDSTOW, a parish in the hundred of Lesnewth, county of Cornwall, 3½ miles (N.E.) from Camelford, containing 363 inhabitants. The living is a vicarage, in the archdeaconry of Cornwall, and diocese of Exeter, rated in the king's books at £8, and in the patronage of the King, as Prince of Wales. The church is dedicated to St. David.

DAVINGTON, a parish in the hundred of Faversham, lathe of Scray, county of Kent, ½ a mile (N.W.) from Faversham, containing 151 inhabitants. The living is a donative, to which T. Bennett, Esq. presented in 1821. The church, dedicated to St. Mary Magdalene, is principally of Norman architecture, and has a beautifully arched door-way. From the numerous remains found here, this is supposed to have been a Roman station. A priory for Benedictine nuns was founded in 1153, probably by Fulk de Newenham, the revenue of which, in the 17th of Edward III., when the society petitioned to be exempted from the payment of taxes on account of poverty, was only £21. 13. 10; having been entirely deserted, it escheated to the crown in the 27th of Henry VIII.: the remains are considerable, and form an interesting ruin, part having been converted into the parish church. Here is a large powder manufactory.

DAWDON, a township in the parish of Dalton le Dale, northern division of Easington ward, county palatine of Durham, 6½ miles (S.S.E.) from Sunderland, containing 35 inhabitants.

DAWLEY (MAGNA), a parish in the Wellington division of the hundred of Bradford (South), county of Salop, 4 miles (W. by S.) from Shiffnal, containing, with the townships of Little Dawley and Malins-Lee, 5147 inhabitants. The living is a perpetual curacy, in the archdeaconry of Salop, and diocese of Lichfield and Coventry, endowed with £400 private benefaction, £400 royal bounty, and £2300 parliamentary grant. J. Oakeley, Esq. and another were patrons in 1792. The church is dedicated to St. Leonard, besides which a chapel is now being erected, toward defraying the expense of which, a grant was made in 1828, by the commissioners appointed under the act of the 58th of George III. for building additional churches. There are extensive coal, iron, lime, and tile, works in the parish, with numerous rail-ways in connexion with them.

DAWLISH, a parish in the hundred of Exminster, county of Devon, 2¾ miles (N.N.E.) from East Teignmouth, containing 2700 inhabitants. This place, at the time of the Norman survey, in which it is noticed under the name Doelis, was an appendage to the see of Exeter: it was an inconsiderable fishing town prior to 1790, about which time the salubrity of its air, the pleasantness of its situation, and the beauty of its environs, made it the resort of invalids, for whose accommodation preparations were progressively made, in proportion to the increase of the visitors, and it is now a fashionable watering-place. The town is beautifully situated in a valley open to the sea on one side, and sheltered on the other by rising grounds in a rich state of cultivation. Ranges of modern houses occupy three sides of a quadrangular area sloping from the shore, tastefully laid out, and intersected by a stream called Dawlish water, which rises in Haldon, an extensive waste adjoining, and after traversing the village, where it is crossed by three bridges for carriages, falls into the sea. The streets are roughly paved, and the inhabitants are amply supplied with water from springs. On the beach are the baths, neatly built of brick, near which are a library, reading-room, and billiard and assembly-rooms; an annual regatta is celebrated generally in August. The environs afford some pleasant walks and rides: the towering cliffs which overhang the sea give an air of grandeur to the scenery, which is finely contrasted with the rich fertility of the vale, and the luxuriant foliage of the wood-crowned heights. A great quantity of mackerel is occasionally taken on the coast; potatoes are extensively cultivated for exportation to Newfoundland, and cider is made in abundance from the orchards which are attached to the farms in the parish. Mines of cobalt have been discovered in the vicinity. It is in contemplation to erect a market-house by subscription, for the supply of the inhabitants: a pleasure fair is held annually on Easter-Monday.

The living is a vicarage, with the curacy of East Teignmouth, rated in the king's books at £25. 5., and in the peculiar jurisdiction and patronage of the Dean and Chapter of Exeter. The church, dedicated to St. Gregory, was rebuilt in 1824, at an expense of £4000: it is a handsome and commodious edifice in the later style of English architecture, with a square embattled tower crowned with pinnacles, the only part remaining of the original structure. At Sedwell and Cofton, hamlets in this parish, are the remains of two ancient chapels; the latter has been disused since 1715, and a grant obtained for rebuilding it, in 1824, has, with the consent of the vicar, been transferred to the parish of Kenton, where a district chapel has been erected. There are places of worship for Independents and Methodists. A National school is supported by subscription; and there are societies for clothing the poor and affording them medical relief. An old house near the churchyard, with walls of extraordinary thickness, is said to have been formerly a monastery.

DAY (ST.), a hamlet in the parish of GWENNAP, hundred of KERRIER, county of CORNWALL, 2¼ miles (E. by N.) from Redruth. The population is returned with the parish. From the mines in the neighbourhood, rail-ways communicate with the English and Bristol channels.

DAYLESFORD, a parish in the upper division of the hundred of OSWALDSLOW, county of WORCESTER, though locally in the upper division of the hundred of Slaughter, county of Gloucester, 3½ miles (E.) from Stow on the Wold, containing 103 inhabitants. The living is a rectory, in the archdeaconry of Gloucester, and diocese of Worcester, rated in the king's books at £7, and in the patronage of Mrs. Hastings. The church is dedicated to St. Peter. The Rev. William Langton bequeathed £14 a year for teaching children, which is paid to a schoolmistress. The culture of cinque-foil was introduced here prior to any other place in England, in 1650. Warren Hastings, Governor General of British India, who was impeached by the parliament on his return to England in 1786, was born here.

DEAL, a sea-port, market town and parish, and a member of the town and port of SANDWICH, in the hundred of BEWSBOROUGH, lathe of ST. AUGUSTINE, county of KENT, on the coast of which it is situated, between the north and south Forelands, 18 miles (S.E.) from Canterbury, and 72 (E. by S.) from London, containing 6811 inhabitants. The origin of the town is buried in obscurity: it has been considered the place where Cæsar landed when he invaded Britain, but this is doubtful. Leland gives the town the Latinized name of *Dela.* Nennius, who probably wrote in the ninth century, says, "Cæsar fought at *Dola,*" which Camden supposes to mean Deal; but there are no records of any town existing here until several centuries after the Romans quitted Britain. Perkin Warbeck, who personated the Duke of York as heir to the crown, made an attempt to land at Deal, July 3d, 1495, but finding that a party which he landed was attacked by his enemies, he returned to Flanders, and afterwards, September 7th, 1497, landed at Whitsun-bay, in Cornwall. In an ordinance of Henry III., dated in 1229, Deal is mentioned as dependent on the port of Sandwich, the jurisdiction of which (as one of the cinque ports) over Deal and Walmer was confirmed by letters patent in the 19th of Henry VI. The town was then governed by a deputy and assistants appointed by the mayor and jurate of Sandwich: in the 11th of William III., notwithstanding the opposition of the corporation of Sandwich, a charter was granted to Deal; but the inhabitants are still obliged to serve on juries at Sandwich as before. Henry VIII. having issued illegal writs for the purpose of raising a subsidy, Deal refused to pay its quota, on which the king annulled its charter, and re-annexed it as a member to Sandwich, There is no harbour; but the sea between the shore and the Goodwin sands forms a fine roadstead, called the Downs, which is of great importance to the country, as it is not only a station for ships of war, but merchant vessels, of which four or five hundred are frequently seen here wind-bound, riding in safety, except during heavy gales from the north and east, when they either proceed on their respective voyages, or put into Ramsgate for shelter. Henry VIII. appreciated the value of this position, and built on the south side of the town, a strong castle, surrounded by a ditch, with a draw-bridge: the castle consists of a round tower, in which are apartments for the captain and other officers. The batteries and martello towers, constructed during the late war, completely command the coast, and defend the town, which consists principally of three long streets running parallel with each other along the shore, and connected by cross streets, in general narrow and inconvenient. The houses are irregularly built, chiefly of brick; but in those which have been recently erected greater attention has been paid to uniformity; particularly since the year 1790, when an act was passed for paving and lighting the streets. Here are a custom-house, a naval store-house, and a naval and military hospital, the latter of which is in the parish of Walmer. The East India Company has a resident agent here, to protect the interests of their shipping when detained in the Downs. The pilots of the cinque-ports are under the direction of the Lord Warden; the Downs pilots are those from Gravesend and London, who are under the direction of the Trinity House. The greater part of the male inhabitants are employed in maritime occupations, and in furnishing supplies for ships lying in the Downs. The pilots of Deal are intrepid and excellent seamen, and particularly active in affording assistance to vessels in distress, which they have often rescued from almost inevitable destruction, and been publicly rewarded for their heroic conduct. The markets, which are well supplied with provisions, are on Tuesday and Saturday : the fairs are, April 5th and October 10th. By charter of the 11th of William III., this was constituted a free town and borough, with a body corporate, consisting of a mayor, recorder, town clerk, twelve jurats, and twenty-four common council-men. The mayor and recorder, or their deputies, and one or two other jurats, are authorised to hold a court of record for the recovery of debts to the amount of £ 100 ; but no writs have been issued since 1823, the charter requiring the recorder or his deputy to be a barrister of three years' standing, and no person thus qualified being resident within eighteen miles of Deal, and no fees allowed for attendance. A court of requests for debts under 40s. is held under an act of parliament passed in the 26th of George III. : its jurisdiction extends over the town and borough of Deal, and the parishes of Ripple, Sutton, Northbourne, Great Mongeham, Little Mongeham, Tilmanstone, Betshanger, Ham, and Sholden, in this county.

The living is a rectory, exempt from the jurisdiction of the archdeacon, rated in the king's books at £ 19. 10., and in the patronage of the Archbishop of Canterbury. The church, dedicated to St. Leonard, is situated about a mile from the sea, in that part of the town called Upper Deal. There is also a chapel of ease in Lower Deal, dedicated to St. George the Martyr, built at the expense of £2554. 12. 4¾., raised partly by subscription, and partly by a duty on coal and culm, levied under an act of parliament obtained in 1712: this chapel was consecrated in 1716. The Baptists, Independents, and Calvinistic and Wesleyan Methodists, have also their places of worship. There is a National school for ninety boys and ninety girls, supported by voluntary contributions. Mrs. Elizabeth Carter, well known in the literary world for her classical attainments, was born here in 1717 ; her ather, the Rev. Nicholas Carter, having been more than fifty-six years curate of the chapel at Lower Deal. Here also was born, in 1735, William Boys, a distinguished naturalist and antiquary.

DEAN, a parish in ALLERDALE ward above Darwent, county of CUMBERLAND, comprising the townships of Branthwaite, Dean, and Ullock with Pardsey and Dean-Scales, and containing 832 inhabitants, of which number, 168 are in the township of Dean, 5 miles (S.W.) from Cockermouth. The living is a rectory, in the archdeaconry of Richmond, and diocese of Chester, rated in the king's books at £ 19. 3. 1½., and in the patronage of the Rev. Henry Sill. The church is dedicated to St. Oswald. A free grammar school was founded in 1596, by John Fox, with an endowment of about £ 10. 17. 6. per annum ;

the school-room was rebuilt in 1615, at the expense of his son. Quarries of red and white free-stone, lime-stone, and black-stone, termed cat-scalp, and coal pits, are interspersed throughout the parish.

DEAN, a parish in the hundred of SALFORD, county palatine of LANCASTER, 1¾ mile (S.W. by W.) from Great Bolton, comprising the chapelries of Farnworth, Little Hilton, Horwick, and West Houghton, and the townships of Heaton, Middle Hilton, Over Hilton, Halliwell, Kearsley, and Rumworth, and containing 18,916 inhabitants. The living is a discharged vicarage, in the archdeaconry and diocese of Chester, rated in the king's books at £4, endowed with £527 private benefaction, £200 royal bounty, and £600 parliamentary grant, and in the patronage of the Crown. The church is dedicated to St. Mary. There are some dissenting places of worship and endowed schools at the different townships in this parish.

DEAN, a hamlet in the parish of SPELSBURY, hundred of CHADLINGTON, county of OXFORD, 3¾ miles (S.E. by S.) from Chipping-Norton. The population is returned with the parish.

DEAN, a parish in the hundred of OVERTON, Kings-clere division of the county of SOUTHAMPTON, 5½ miles (W. by S.) from Basingstoke, containing 157 inhabitants. The living is a rectory, in the archdeaconry and diocese of Winchester, rated in the king's books at £ 10. 8. 11½., and in the patronage of Wither Bramston, Esq. The church is dedicated to All Saints. This parish is within the jurisdiction of the Cheyney Court held at Winchester every Thursday, for the recovery of debts to any amount. It formerly contained within its limits the adjoining parish of Ashe, which was separated and erected into a distinct parish by act of parliament, about two hundred years ago.

DEAN (EAST), a chapelry in the parish of MOTTISFONT, hundred of THORNGATE, Andover division of the county of SOUTHAMPTON, 7¼ miles (N.W. by W.) from Romsey, containing 160 inhabitants. The living is a perpetual curacy annexed to the rectory of Mottisfont, in the archdeaconry and diocese of Winchester. The Salisbury and Southampton canal passes through the parish.

DEAN (EAST), a parish in the hundred of WESTBOURN and SINGLETON, rape of CHICHESTER, county of SUSSEX, 7 miles (S. by E.) from Midhurst, containing 397 inhabitants. The living is a discharged vicarage with the rectory of Singleton, in the archdeaconry of Lewes, and diocese of Chichester, rated in the king's books at £ 5. 4. 4½.

DEAN (EAST), a parish in the hundred of WILLINGDON, rape of PEVENSEY, county of SUSSEX, 2¾ miles (W.S.W.) from East Bourne, containing 296 inhabitants. The living is a vicarage united to the vicarage of Friston, in the archdeaconry of Lewes, and diocese of Chichester, rated in the king's books at £8, and in the patronage of the Dean and Chapter of Chichester.

DEAN (FOREST of), an extra-parochial liberty, in the hundred of ST. BRIAVELL's, county of GLOUCESTER, comprising the divisions of Denby walk, Herbert's walk, Little Dean walk, Speech-House walk, Worcester walk, and York walk, and containing 5535 inhabitants : the centre of the forest is 5 miles (S.W. by W.) from Newnham. There are three chapelries in the Forest of Dean, viz., Christ Church, endowed with £200 private benefaction, and £2300 parliamentary grant; the chapel of the Holy Trinity, endowed with £200 private benefaction, and £2500 parliamentary grant; and St. Paul's, endowed with £2200 parliamentary grant; all of which are perpetual curacies, in the archdeaconry and diocese of Gloucester. This district, extending from north to south twenty miles, from east to west ten miles, and lying between the rivers Severn and Wye, was anciently occupied by the *Silures*, and probably obtained its name either from the contraction of the Gaelic word *Arden*, a wood, or from the British *Danys Coed*, the wood of fallow deer, for which it was famous for many centuries. Within its original bounds were situated the very ancient towns of Tudenham and Wollaston; also on the margin of the Severn, the *Abona* of Antoninus, long since reduced to a small village, called Alvington; and on the Wye, Breulais Castle, embosomed in almost an impenetrable thicket, and now fallen to decay. In the reign of Henry II., so dark and intricate were its tracts or cross ways, that the inhabitants committed the most daring outrages and robberies with impunity, until restrained by the discovery of its rich mines of iron and coal, and the consequent establishment of forges, by authority of parliament, together with the erection of towns and villages for the residence of the miners and manufacturers; before which, the six lodges for the keepers of the several walks were the only houses in it. All the inhabitants are exempted from rates and taxes, with free liberty of pasturage and to cut wood, and the privilege of sinking mines, the sixth part of the produce of which, called the king's gawl, is due to the king, and is collected by the gaveller. The forest, as defined in the 12th of Henry III., the definition having been subsequently confirmed, is stated to comprise twenty-three thousand and fifteen acres, belonging to the crown, exclusively of freeholds obtained by grants. Charles I. conveyed all the coppices and waste soil of the forest, except the Lea Bailey, with all mines and quarries, to Sir John Wyntour, for £10,600, and a fee-farm rent of £1950. 12. 8. for ever, at which time there were standing one hundred and five thousand five hundred and fifty-seven trees, estimated to contain sixty-one thousand nine hundred and twenty-eight tons of timber, and one hundred and fifty-three thousand two hundred and nine cords of wood; but the civil war putting an end to the patent, the enclosures were thrown open, and the whole re-forested; however, a renewal of the grant, excepting the timber fit for naval purposes, was made by Charles II. to the same individual; but, on a survey made by the parliament in 1667, it was discovered that he had made great encroachments upon the property of the crown, to repair which one thousand and one hundred acres were then enclosed and planted; from this plantation the royal dock-yards are chiefly supplied. There are orchards producing a peculiar kind of fruit, called the Styre apple, the cyder made from which is of a superior quality, and bears a high price. It is affirmed that the commander of the Spanish Armada had directions, if he failed in subduing the kingdom, to destroy every tree in the Forest of Dean. The government is vested in a lord warden, who is constable of St. Briavell's Castle; six deputy wardens, four verdurers, chosen by the freeholders, a conservator, seven woodwards, a chief forester in fee, and bow bearer, which united offices are held by the Wyndham family, in right of inheritance; eight foresters in fee, a gaveller, and a steward of the

swainmote, who are empowered to hold a court of attachment every forty days; a court of swainmote thrice a year, and a court called the justice seat, once in three years. The steward presides at the miners' court, and is assisted by a jury of miners, who judge upon the particular laws and customs by which they are governed, to prevent encroachments upon each other in the coal and iron works. These courts are held at the Speech-House, in the centre of the forest, the general aspect of which is picturesque in the extreme, being beautifully diversified with hill and valley, interspersed with the rich and varied foliage of the woods. Pursuant to an act passed in the 36th of George III., new roads have been opened in various directions through the forest, which is also intersected by several railways, communicating with the Severn and the Wye.

DEAN (LITTLE), a parish in the hundred of St. Briavell's, county of Gloucester, 1¾ mile (N.W. by N.) from Newnham, containing, with 123 persons resident in an adjoining extra-parochial district, 807 inhabitants. The living is a perpetual curacy, annexed to the perpetual curacy of Newnham, in the archdeaconry and diocese of Gloucester, endowed with £400 parliamentary grant, and in the patronage of the Mayor and Corporation of Gloucester. The church is dedicated to St. Ethelbert. The village is situated on the verge of the Forest of Dean, in the neighbourhood of which there are considerable mines of coal and iron, in which, and in the manufacture of nails, the inhabitants are principally employed. It had formerly the privilege of a market, which is now disused, but the market cross is still standing, having a low octangular roof spreading from a central shaft, and surmounted by a pinnacle with niches and statues. There are fairs for pedlary on Whit-Monday and November 26th. Dorothy Pyrke, in 1760, bequeathed an annuity of £4. 10. for teaching ten poor children.

DEAN (MITCHELL), a market town and parish in the hundred of St. Briavell's, county of Gloucester, 11 miles (W.) from Gloucester, and 113 (W.) from London, containing 556 inhabitants. This place, the origin of which is anterior to the Conquest, derives its name, denoting its situation in a deep dell, from the Saxon *Dene*, a dell, and its adjunct from *Mycel*, great, in contradistinction to the village of Little Dean, in the neighbourhood: it was the principal town in the Forest of Dean, and consists of three streets, diverging obliquely from the common centre; and was formerly a staple town for the wool trade; at present the manufacture of leather is carried on to a small extent. The market is on Monday: the fairs are on Easter-Monday and October 10th, for horses, cattle, and sheep. The living is a discharged vicarage, in the archdeaconry of Hereford, and diocese of Gloucester, rated in the king's books at £10. 16. 0½., and endowed with £200 royal bounty. M. Colchester, Esq. was patron in 1802. The church, dedicated to St. Michael, is a spacious structure, built at different periods, and exhibiting various styles of English architecture, with a tower, surmounted by an octagonal spire: in the east window of the north aisle are some remains of the original stained glass with which the church appears to have been generally ornamented; the roof, of oak, is decorated with flowers and other ornaments, exquisitely carved; the font appears to have been formed from the inverted capital of a column, which, from its embellishments, has the character of the early English style. A subterraneous passage leads from the church to a wood, about half a mile from the town. A charity school was founded by means of a bequest of £1000, by William Lane, Esq., of Gloucester, in 1789, and one of £300 by his widow, in 1806; these sums being vested by the trustees in the funds, together with other benefactions, produce an annual income of £62, of which the master receives £15 per annum : there are about thirty boys, who are supplied with books : the sum of £5. 5. is paid to the minister for catechising them, and the overplus is bestowed, at the discretion of the trustees, in rewards to the scholars and their teacher. Mr. Jonathan Parker, in 1718, bequeathed £200, the interest of which is applied to the clothing and apprenticing of one poor child; there are also other charitable bequests.

DEAN (NETHER), a parish in the hundred of STODDEN, county of BEDFORD, 3½ miles (W. by S.) from Kimbolton, containing, with the hamlet of Upper Dean, 479 inhabitants. The living is a perpetual curacy, in the archdeaconry of Bedford, and diocese of Lincoln, and in the patronage of the Dean and Chapter of Worcester. The church is dedicated to All Saints. Joseph Neale, in 1702, gave land, now producing £55 a year, for teaching twenty poor boys.

DEAN (PRIOR'S), a chapelry in the parish of COLEMORE, hundred of BARTON-STACEY, Andover division, though locally in the hundred of Selborne, Alton (North) division, of the county of SOUTHAMPTON, 4¾ miles (N. by W.) from Petersfield, containing 150 inhabitants.

DEAN (UPPER), a hamlet in the parish of NETHER DEAN, hundred of STODDEN, county of BEDFORD, 3½ miles (W. N. W) from Kimbolton. The population is returned with the parish.

DEAN (WEST), a parish in the hundred of WESTBOURN and SINGLETON, rape of CHICHESTER, county of SUSSEX, 6½ miles (S. S. W.) from Midhurst, containing 622 inhabitants. The living is a discharged vicarage, in the archdeaconry and diocese of Chichester, rated in the king's books at £6. 12., endowed with £200 private benefaction, and £200 royal bounty, and in the patronage of S. Harrison, Esq. The church is dedicated to St. Andrew.

DEAN (WEST), a parish in the hundred of WILLINGDON, rape of PEVENSEY, county of SUSSEX, 3 miles (E.) from Seaford, containing 163 inhabitants. The living is a discharged rectory, in the archdeaconry of Lewes, and diocese of Chichester, rated in the king's books at £14. 15. 5., and in the patronage of the Dean and Chapter of Chichester. The church is dedicated to All Saints.

DEAN (WEST), a parish in the hundred of ALDERBURY, county of WILTS, 7 miles (E. by S.) from Salisbury, containing, with the chapelry of East Grimstead, 365 inhabitants. The living is a rectory, in the archdeaconry and diocese of Salisbury, rated in the king's books at £19. 4. 4½. Francis Glossop, Esq. was patron in 1820. The church is dedicated to St. Mary.

DEAN-HILL, a hamlet in that part of the parish of SANDBACH which is in the hundred of NANTWICH, county palatine of CHESTER, 1½ mile (S.E. by E.) from Sandbach, with which the population is returned.

DEAN-PRIOR, a parish in the hundred of STANBOROUGH, county of DEVON, 4 miles (S. S. W.) from Ashburton, containing 561 inhabitants. The living is a vicarage, in the archdeaconry of Totness, and diocese of Exeter, rated in the king's books at £21, and in the patronage of W. Y. Buller, Esq. The church is dedicated to St. George the Martyr.

DEAN-RAW, a township in the parish of WARDEN, north-western division of TINDALE ward, county of NORTHUMBERLAND, 8 miles (W.) from Hexham, containing 535 inhabitants. Near the confluence of the Allen and Harsingdale bourn, on the south side of the township, are the remains of an ancient building, called Staward le Peel, which Edward, Duke of York, in 1386, granted to the friars eremites of Hexham, to be held by the annual payment of five marks.

DEAN-ROW, a hamlet in the parish of WILMSLOW, hundred of MACCLESFIELD, county palatine of CHESTER, 6½ miles (N. N. W.) from Macclesfield. The population is returned with the parish.

DEAN-SCALES, a joint township with Ullock and Pardsey, in the parish of DEAN, ALLERDALE ward above Darwent, county of CUMBERLAND, 3¼ miles (S. W.) from Cockermouth, containing 309 inhabitants. There is a manufacture of linen thread at this place.

DEANHAM, a township in that part of the parish of HARTBURN which is in the north-eastern division of TINDALE ward, county of NORTHUMBERLAND, 12½ miles (W. by S.) from Morpeth, containing 53 inhabitants.

DEARHAM, a parish in ALLERDALE ward below Darwent, county of CUMBERLAND, comprising the townships of Dearham, and Ellenborough with Unerigg, and containing 1136 inhabitants, of which number, 515 are in the township of Dearham, 6¼ miles (N. W.) from Cockermouth The living is a discharged vicarage, in the archdeaconry and diocese of Carlisle, rated in the king's books at £4. 13. 4., endowed with £200 private benefaction, £400 royal bounty, and £1000 parliamentary grant, and in the patronage of the Bishop of Carlisle. The church, originally of Norman architecture, was much modernised by repairs in 1814; it has an ancient and curiously carved font, and in the churchyard is a sculptured cross. There are extensive collieries, and a manufactory for pottery-ware in the parish; a considerable quantity of the coal is shipped at Maryport adjoining. Ewan Christian, Esq., in 1715, endowed a school with about £10 per annum. Near Unerigg-hall is the site of an old castle.

DEARNBROOK, a hamlet in that part of the parish of ARNCLIFFE which is in the western division of the wapentake of STAINCLIFFE and EWCROSS, West riding of the county of YORK, 8 miles (N.E.) from Settle. The population is returned with the parish.

DEBACH, a parish in the hundred of WILFORD, county of SUFFOLK, 4¼ miles (N.N.W.) from Woodbridge, containing 113 inhabitants. The living is a discharged rectory, annexed to the rectory of Boulge, in the archdeaconry of Suffolk, and diocese of Norwich. The church is dedicated to All Saints. A trifling sum, out of the rents of the town lands, is paid weekly to the parish clerk, for teaching poor children.

DEBDEN, a parish in the hundred of UTTLESFORD, county of ESSEX, 4¼ miles (N.W. by W.) from Thaxted, containing 940 inhabitants. The living is a rectory, in the archdeaconry of Colchester, and diocese of London, rated in the king's books at £34. R. M. F. Chiswell,

Esq. was patron in 1796. The church, dedicated to St. Mary, has at the east end an octangular chapel, containing several handsome monuments of the Chiswells: the font, an elegant piece of workmanship, adorned with statues, was presented by the late Mr. Chiswell.

DEBDON, a township in the parish of ROTHBURY, western division of COQUETDALE ward, county of NORTHUMBERLAND, 2¼ miles (N.) from Rothbury, containing 18 inhabitants. There is a chalybeate spring, efficacious in scorbutic complaints: several excavations have been made, from which ochre is obtained.

DEBENHAM, a small market town and parish, in the hundred of THREDLING, county of SUFFOLK, 13 miles (N.) from Ipswich, and 83 (N.E. by N.) from London, containing 1535 inhabitants. This town derives its name from being situated near the river Deben: from its standing on the declivity of a hill, the streets are dry and clean, but the roads in the vicinity are usually in bad repair from the miry state of the country. A market for corn is held on Friday, which is but little attended; and there is an annual fair on the 24th of June. The living is a vicarage, in the archdeaconry of Suffolk, and diocese of Norwich, rated in the king's books at £15. 2. 6., and in the patronage of Lord Henniker. The church, dedicated to St. Mary, contains some ancient monuments. Here is a free school for twenty boys, founded in 1643, and endowed by Sir Robert Hitcham, with £20 per annum.

DEBTLING, a parish in the hundred of MAIDSTONE, lathe of AYLESFORD, county of KENT, 2¾ miles (N.E.) from Maidstone, containing 321 inhabitants. The living is a discharged vicarage, in the archdeaconry and diocese of Canterbury, endowed with £400 private benefaction, and £400 royal bounty, and in the patronage of the Archbishop of Canterbury. The church is dedicated to St. Martin.

DECUMAN (ST.), a parish in the hundred of WILLITON and FREEMANNERS, county of SOMERSET, 5¼ miles (E. by S.) from Dunster, containing 1865 inhabitants. The living is a discharged vicarage, rated in the king's books at £10. 10. 5½., and in the peculiar jurisdiction and patronage of the Prebendary of St. Decuman's in the Cathedral Church of Wells. The church, dedicated to St. Peter, is a handsome structure, with a lofty tower. There are three places of worship for Wesleyan Methodists, and two belonging to the Baptists. The parish derives its name from St. Decombes, or Decumanus, who, landing from South Wales, and finding a perfect wilderness, fixed upon this spot in order to seclude himself from the rest of the world; and having been murdered, was dignified by the natives with the title of Saint.

DEDDINGTON, a parish (formerly a market town) in the hundred of WOOTTON, county of OXFORD, containing, with the townships of Clifton and Hempton, 1847 inhabitants, of which number, 1404 are in the town of Deddington, 16 miles (N. by W.) from Oxford, and 69 (N.W.) from London. This place, though formerly of some importance, having sent members to two parliaments in the reign of Edward I., is now an inconsiderable town. According to Dr. Plot, a castle was anciently built here, either by the Saxons or the Danes, but no vestiges of it can be traced, nor is there any thing of importance occurring in the history of the place, except its having been the retreat of Piers

Gavestone, the favourite of Edward II., a short time previous to his capture by the Earl of Warwick, and his decapitation on Blacklow Hill, and subsequently the possession of his successor in that monarch's affections, Hugh de Spencer, who suffered a similar fate. The town, which has been noted for its malt liquor, contains several well-built houses, and is well supplied with water: a branch of the Oxford and London canal passes through the parish. The market has been discontinued; but a fair for cattle is still held on the 22nd of November. A bailiff is annually appointed at the court leet of the lord of the manor.

The living is a discharged vicarage, in the archdeaconry and diocese of Oxford, rated in the king's books at £15. 9. 4., endowed with £600 private benefaction, £200 royal bounty, and £1400 parliamentary grant, and in the patronage of the Dean and Canons of Windsor. The church is dedicated to St. Peter and St. Paul. Parochial schools for boys and girls are supported by subscription. Almshouses for four aged men and four aged women, were founded in 1818, and are endowed with property arising from various benefactions vested in feoffees for the benefit of the poor, producing about £140 per annum. In the neighbourhood are two mineral springs, now neglected, one of which is said to have been highly impregnated with sulphur. Lord Chief Justice Scroggs, who flourished in the reign of Charles II., was a native of this parish; and Sir Thomas Pope, an eminent statesman, and founder of Trinity College, Oxford, is said to have been born here, in 1507.

DEDHAM, a parish in the Colchester division of the hundred of LEXDEN, county of ESSEX, 4 miles (W. by N.) from Manningtree, containing 1651 inhabitants. The living is a vicarage, in the archdeaconry of Colchester, and diocese of London, rated in the king's books at £10. 0. 2½., endowed with £200 private benefaction, and £300 parliamentary grant, and in the patronage of the King, as Duke of Lancaster. The church, dedicated to St. Mary, is a spacious structure in the later style of English architecture, having an embattled tower at the west end, and crowned with octagonal turrets richly pinnacled. Annexed to the church is a lectureship which, in the beginning of the eighteenth century, was endowed with the great tithes, by the Rev. William Birkett, then lecturer, the able and learned commentator on the New Testament; the appointment belongs to the governors of the grammar-school. Dedham is situated in a picturesque valley on the river Stour, over which it has a good bridge, and consists chiefly of one street: it had formerly the privilege of a market on Tuesday: there is a fair for toys on Easter-Tuesday. The clothing trade flourished here so early as the reign of Richard II., but has wholly declined, and the place is now only remarkable for the number of genteel residences in the vicinity. A free grammar school was built by Dame Jane Clarke, prior to 1571, when it was endowed by William Littlebury, with a farm of one hundred and eighty acres, for teaching twenty boys, in aid of which, William Cardinal, in 1593, bequeathed land, now let for £60 per annum, for the maintenance and education of two of the boys at St. John's College, Cambridge, born at Dedham or Much Bromley; the governors of the school, twenty-four in number, were incorporated by charter of Queen Elizabeth, in 1574. The same William Littlebury, also founded and endowed an English school, and some almshouses. John Marsh, in 1642, left an annuity of £6 for teaching two boys in the grammar school, and one in the English school, with a house and land to the English master, in farther augmentation of whose salary a bequest of £4 per annum was made by William Burkitt, in 1698, which the vicar holds in trust.

DEDWORTH, a hamlet in the parish of New Windsor, hundred of Ripplesmere, county of Berks, 2 miles (W. by S.) from New Windsor, with which the population is returned.

DEENE, a parish in the hundred of Corby, county of Northampton, 5½ miles (E. by N.) from Rockingham, containing, with the hamlet of Deenthorpe, 458 inhabitants. The living is a rectory, in the archdeaconry of Northampton, and diocese of Peterborough, rated in the king's books at £24. 3. 6½. The Earl of Cardigan was patron in 1820. The church is dedicated to St. Peter. Here was anciently a priory, a cell to the abbey of Westminster, which was suppressed soon after the Conquest, by consent of the abbot and convent, who accepted an annuity in lieu of its revenues.

DEENTHORPE, a hamlet in the parish of Deene, hundred of Corby, county of Northampton, 6 miles (N. W. by W.) from Oundle, containing 224 inhabitants.

DEEP-DALE, a hamlet in that part of the parish of Arncliffe which is in the eastern division of the wapentake of Staincliffe and Ewcross, West riding of the county of York, 15½ miles (N. N. E.) from Settle. The population is returned with the parish.

DEEPING (MARKET), a market town and parish in the wapentake of Ness, parts of Kesteven, county of Lincoln, 43 miles (S. S. E.) from Lincoln, and 86 (N. by W.) from London, containing, with some extra-parochial places in the fens, 1016 inhabitants. This place derives its name from its situation among deep or low meadows, or pastures, formerly the receptacle of many streams in the lowest part of the fens; and its origin from Richard de Rulos, chamberlain to William the Conqueror, who built several houses on the dykes which he had constructed to confine within its channel the river Welland, which frequently inundated the adjoining lands. The neighbourhood has been greatly improved by draining, which has been successfully and extensively practised; and several tracts of land have been recovered, and rendered fit for culture. The houses are in general old and inconveniently built: there is an ample supply of water from the river Welland, which is navigable, and affords facility for the conveyance of coal, grocery, and other articles of merchandise. The market is on Wednesday: the fairs are on the second Wednesday in May, O. S., and October 10th for cattle and toys. The living is a rectory, in the archdeaconry and diocese of Lincoln, rated in the king's books at £16. 1. 3., and in the patronage of the Crown. The church, dedicated to St. Guthlack, is an ancient structure, containing many portions of its original Norman architecture, though principally in the later style of English architecture There is a free school for sixteen boys, who are taught reading, writing, and arithmetic; the master has a salary of £30 per annum, a house, and a garden. John Warrington, Esq. left £5 each per annum, in half yearly payments, to ten poor widows; and there are several other charitable bequests for distribution among the poor.

DEEPING (ST. JAMES), a parish in the wapentake of Ness, parts of Kesteven, county of Lincoln, ¾ of a mile (E.) from Market-Deeping, containing 1385 inhabitants. The living is a discharged vicarage, in the archdeaconry and diocese of Lincoln, rated in the king's books at £6. 19. 9½., endowed with £400 private benefaction, and £400 royal bounty, and in the patronage of Sir T. Whichcote, Bart. The church, dedicated to St. James, is a handsome edifice, with a tower surmounted by a spire at the west end : it was originally a chapel, erected by the monks of Croyland abbey, and was made parochial by Richard de Rulos. The Wesleyan Methodists have a small place of worship. A school on the National system has been built since 1814, wherein thirty children are taught by a master, who receives an annual stipend out of the income of a discretionary trust estate, consisting of houses and land, which produces upwards of £200 a year, left in 1635, by Robert Tygh. The river Welland, which is navigable for small craft, has been recently restrained from inundating the land on its banks, at a great expense. An ancient stone cross, the base of which is twelve feet square, and its sides divided into compartments, ornamented with shields, was in 1819 converted into a round-house, but the original form is preserved. At the eastern end of the village there is a strong chalybeate spring, the water of which is impregnated with iron. A cell to the Dominican abbey at Thorney was founded in 1139, by Baldwin Wac, or Wake; it was dedicated to St. James, and, as parcel of Thorney abbey, was granted, in the 32nd of Henry VIII., to Thomas, Duke of Norfolk.

DEEPING (WEST), a parish in the wapentake of Ness, parts of Kesteven, county of Lincoln, 1½ mile (W. S. W.) from Market-Deeping, containing 302 inhabitants. The living is a rectory, in the archdeaconry and diocese of Lincoln, rated in the king's books at £9. 17. 11., and in the patronage of the Crown. The church, dedicated to St. Michael, has portions in the early English, with insertions in the decorated and later styles of English architecture; the font is a fine specimen of the early English style.

DEEPING-FEN, an extra-parochial liberty, in the wapentake of Elloe, parts of Holland, county of Lincoln, 6 miles (S. W.) from Spalding, containing 398 inhabitants. This extensive district was enclosed from part of the waste land formerly belonging to several parishes, and is partly held by adventurers, for draining, and partly by persons who are free from drainage expenses by the nature of their tenures; all the land is exempt from the land tax, and from ecclesiastical and all other assessments.

DEEPING-GATE, a hamlet in the parish of Maxey, liberty of Peterborough, county of Northampton, 1¼ mile (S. E.) from Market-Deeping, containing 170 inhabitants.

DEERHURST, a parish partly in the lower division of the hundred of Deerhurst, and partly in the lower division of the hundred of Westminster, county of Gloucester, 2 miles (S. W.) from Tewkesbury, containing, with the hamlets of Apperley with Whitefield, and Deerhurst-Walton, 742 inhabitants. The living is a perpetual curacy, within the jurisdiction of the peculiar court of Deerhurst, endowed with £600 royal bounty, and £1400 parliamentary grant, and in the patronage of the Bishop of Gloucester. The church, dedicated to the Holy

Trinity, and exhibiting portions in the Norman, the early English, and the decorated, styles of architecture, formerly belonged to a priory established about 715, by the Mercian duke, Doddo, one of the founders of Tewkesbury abbey : this priory having been destroyed by the Danes, was re-founded in 980, and given by Edward the Confessor to the Benedictine abbey of St. Denis, in France, to which it became a cell; upon the seizure of Alien priories it was granted to Eton College, but Edward IV., revoking that grant, made it a cell to the abbey of Tewkesbury, and so it remained till the dissolution : the remains of the structure, which have been converted into a farm-house, are in the later style of English architecture, much enriched with decorated tracery. The navigable river Severn flows along the western boundary of the parish. Deerhurst gives the title of viscount to the noble family of Coventry.

DEFFORD, a chapelry in the parish of St. ANDREW, PERSHORE, upper division of the hundred of PERSHORE, county of WORCESTER, 3 miles (S. W.) from Pershore, containing 347 inhabitants. The living is a perpetual curacy, in the archdeaconry and diocese of Worcester, rated in the king's books at £2. 13. 4. The chapel is dedicated to St. James.

DEIGHTON, a chapelry in the parish of NORTHALLERTON, wapentake of ALLERTONSHIRE, North riding of the county of YORK, 5½ miles (N. by E.) from North Allerton, containing 134 inhabitants.

DEIGHTON, a township in the parish of ESCRICK, wapentake of OUZE and DERWENT, East riding of the county of YORK, 5¼ miles (S. by E.) from York, containing 168 inhabitants.

DEIGHTON (KIRK), a parish in the upper division of the wapentake of CLARO, West riding of the county of YORK, comprising the townships of Kirk-Deighton and North Deighton, and containing 512 inhabitants, of which number, 371 are in the township of Kirk-Deighton, 1¾ mile (N. by W.) from Wetherby, and 141 in the adjoining township of North Deighton. The living is a rectory, in the archdeaconry and diocese of York, rated in the king's books at £15. 11. 10½., and in the patronage of the Rev. Dr. Goldart. The church is dedicated to All Saints. The river Nidd forms part of the boundary, and the Warf, a beautiful stream, winds along the southern side of the parish. A vast quantity of lime-stone is burnt for agricultural purposes. A Sunday school was endowed by the late Sir Hugh Palliser with £30 a year, for teaching and clothing poor children.

DELAMERE, a parish in the first division of the hundred of EDDISBURY, county palatine of CHESTER, comprising the townships of Delamere, Eddisbury, and Oakmere, and containing 424 inhabitants, of which number, 262 are in the township of Delamere, 5¾ miles (W.) from Northwich. The living is a rectory not in charge, in the archdeaconry and diocese of Chester, and in the patronage of the Crown. The church was consecrated in 1817. This parish, which includes the ancient and royal forest of Delamere, was almost wholly common land, and extra-parochial, before 1812, when it was enclosed and erected into a parish by act of parliament, certain allotments having been reserved to the crown, and others. On this occasion it first gave the title of Baron Delamere, of Vale Royal, to Thomas Cholmondeley, Esq., the proprietor of the ancient possessions of the Cistercian monks of Vale

Royal, whose sumptuous abbey, completed in 1330 by Edward I., cost £32,000 : it was dedicated to our Lord Jesus Christ, the Virgin Mary, St. Nicholas, and St. Nichasius, and in the 26th of Henry VIII. had a revenue of £540. 6. 2. The sessions for [the division are annually held, on the 22nd of March, also monthly meetings of the county magistrates, at a new inn, called the Abbey Arms, in the centre of the forest. At the time of the meeting in March there are races, termed the Tanfield hunt, at which two cups are given to be run for by the county, and one by the trainers. Delamere Forest, which once contained a great number of red and fallow deer, exhibits a pleasing variety of well-wooded hills, rich vallies for pasturage, meres affording plenty of fish and aquatic fowl, and mosses producing an abundance of turf and peat for fuel. Upon the highest hill stood the Saxon fortress of Finborrow, and near it a city, both of which are said to have been founded by Ethelfleda, daughter of Alfred the Great; the latter, called Eadesbury (the happy town), gave name to the hundred, but the ancient residence of the chief forester is all that now remains; this house is termed the Chamber in the Forest, and at convenient distances around it are neat lodges for the keepers of the several walks. About half of the forest has been planted, and still belongs to the crown, the remainder having been either sold, or allotted to different individuals.

DELAPREE, a hamlet in the parish of HARDINGSTONE, hundred of WYMERSLEY, county of NORTHAMPTON, 1¼ mile (S. by E.) from Northampton, containing, with the hamlets of Far-Cotton and Paper-Mills, 356 inhabitants. An abbey for nuns of the Cluniac order was founded in the reign of Stephen, by Simon Seinliz, Earl of Northampton, and dedicated to St. Mary: at the dissolution it contained ten religious, whose revenue was valued at £119. 9. 7¼. per annum.

DEMBLEBY, a parish in the wapentake of AVELAND, parts of KESTEVEN, county of LINCOLN, 6 miles (N.W. by W.) from Folkingham, containing 58 inhabitants. The living is a discharged rectory, in the archdeaconry and diocese of Lincoln, rated in the king's books at £6. 11. 8., and endowed with £200 royal bounty. The Misses Buckworth were patronesses in 1805. The church is dedicated to St. Lucia.

DENBURY, a parish in the hundred of HAYTOR, county of DEVON, 2½ miles (S.W. by S.) from Newton-Abbots, containing 412 inhabitants. The living is a rectory, in the archdeaconry of Totness, and diocese of Exeter, rated in the king's books at £12. 7. 6. The Duke of Bedford was patron in 1798. The church is dedicated to St. Mary. Denbury, said to have been anciently a borough, belonged, with the manor, to the abbey of Tavistock, the superior of which, in 1285, obtained for it a weekly market and a fair; the market is disused, but there is a cattle fair on the 11th of September. A school-room has been built by subscription, on a plot of ground given by Mr. Bartlett, of Newton-Abbots, the National Society having contributed £25 towards defraying the expense : it is endowed, chiefly from the parish lands, with about £30 per annum, and is conducted upon Dr. Bell's system.

DENBY, a parish in the hundred of MORLESTON and LITCHURCH, county of DERBY, 8 miles (N.N.E.) from Derby, containing 1073 inhabitants. The living is a perpetual curacy, in the archdeaconry of Derby, and diocese of Lichfield and Coventry, endowed with £200 private benefaction, £400 royal bounty, and £1200 parliamentary grant, and in the patronage of the Earl of Chesterfield. The church is dedicated to St. Mary. Jane Massie, in 1728, bequeathed an estate towards erecting and endowing a free school; the income is £47. 10., with a house and garden for the master, who teaches twenty-five children. John Flamsteed, a celebrated mathematician, and Astronomer Royal, was born here in 1646; he died at Greenwich in 1719.

DENBY, a chapelry in the parish of PENISTONE, wapentake of STAINCROSS, West riding of the county of YORK, 7¼ miles (W. by N.) from Barnesley, containing 1412 inhabitants. The living is a perpetual curacy, in the archdeaconry and diocese of York, endowed with £200 private benefaction, £200 royal bounty, and £1200 parliamentary grant, and in the patronage of the Vicar of Penistone. Francis Burdett, in 1731, bequeathed £100, the interest of which, amounting to £6. 3. per annum, is applied towards teaching six children.

DENCHWORTH, a parish in the hundred of WANTAGE, county of BERKS, 2½ miles (N.W. by N.) from Wantage, containing 254 inhabitants. The living is a discharged vicarage, in the archdeaconry of Berks, and diocese of Salisbury, rated in the king's books at £7. 10. 10., endowed with £600 private benefaction, £200 royal bounty, and £600 parliamentary grant, and in the patronage of the Provost and Fellows of Worcester College, Oxford. The church is dedicated to St. James. Richard Gilgrasse, in 1729, bequeathed £50 for the instruction of children, which, with a donation of £50 from another benefactor, produces £8. 16. per annum, applied in aid of a National school.

DENDRON, a chapelry in the parish of ALDINGHAM, hundred of LONSDALE, north of the sands, county palatine of LANCASTER, 2½ miles (S.S.E.) from Dalton. The population is returned with the parish. The living is a perpetual curacy, in the archdeaconry of Richmond, and diocese of Chester; endowed with £200 private benefaction, and £600 royal bounty, and in the patronage of the Rector of Aldingham. The chapel, erected by Robert Dickenson, in 1642, was rebuilt about fifty years ago, at the expense of Thomas Green, Esq., of Gray's Inn, London. Robert Dickenson, in 1644, also founded a school, with an endowment of £200, in augmentation of which, John Simpson, in 1770, bequeathed £10, and Thomas Troughton, in 1774, left the interest of £100: Simpson's endowment has been lost, but the dividends arising from the other bequests are paid to the curate, who keeps the school.

DENERDISTAN, otherwise DENSTON, a parish in the hundred of RISBRIDGE, county of SUFFOLK, 5¾ miles (N.) from Clare, containing 327 inhabitants. The living is a perpetual curacy, in the archdeaconry of Sudbury, and diocese of Norwich, endowed with £400 royal bounty, and £200 parliamentary grant, and in the patronage of General Robinson. The church is dedicated to St. Nicholas.

DENFORD, a parish in the hundred of HUXLOE, county of NORTHAMPTON, 1½ mile (S.) from Thrapston, containing 310 inhabitants. The living is a discharged vicarage with Ringstead, in the archdeaconry of Northampton, and diocese of Peterborough, rated in the king's books at £8. 10., endowed with £200 private bene-

faction, and £200 royal bounty. Thomas Burton, Esq. was patron in 1822. The church, dedicated to the Holy Trinity, is principally in the early style of English architecture, with a tower and spire.

DENGE-MARSH, a member of the town and cinque-port of NEW ROMNEY, in the parish of LYDD, liberty of ROMNEY-MARSH, though locally in the hundred of Langport, lathe of SHEPWAY, county of KENT, 1½ mile (S. by E.) from Lydd. It is bounded by the English channel on the south, where stands Dengeness light-house, for the guidance of mariners, which was projected by a Mr. Allen, of Rye, in the reign of James I.

DENGIE, a parish in the hundred of DENGIE, county of ESSEX, 4 miles (S. by W.) from Bradwell, containing 234 inhabitants. The living is a rectory, in the archdeaconry of Essex, and diocese of London, rated in the king's books at £13. The Rev. J. H. Stephenson was patron in 1825. There is also a sinecure, called Bacon's portion, rated at £4. The church is dedicated to St. James.

DENHAM, a parish in the hundred of STOKE, county of BUCKINGHAM, 2½ miles (N.N.W.) from Uxbridge, containing 1189 inhabitants. The living is a rectory, in the archdeaconry of Buckingham, and diocese of Lincoln, rated in the king's books at £19. 9. 4½. Benjamin Way, Esq. was patron in 1797. The church, dedicated to St. Mary, contains some interesting monuments. There is a place of worship for Wesleyan Methodists. The river Colne and the Grand Junction canal pass through the parish. Sir William Bowyer, in 1721, gave £30 per annum, with a house for a master and a mistress, for instructing fifteen boys and fifteen girls. A school-room has been erected in that part of the village called Cheapside, and was opened in 1826; the children are taught on the British system.

DENHAM, a parish in the hundred of HOXNE, county of SUFFOLK, 2 miles (E.) from Eye, containing 259 inhabitants. The living is a discharged vicarage, to which the vicarage of Hoxne is annexed, in the archdeaconry of Suffolk, and diocese of Norwich, rated in the king's books at £5. 0. 10. T. Maynard, Esq. was patron in 1794. The church is dedicated to St. John the Baptist.

DENHAM, a parish in the hundred of RISBRIDGE, county of SUFFOLK, 7½ miles (W. by S.) from Bury-St. Edmund's, containing 166 inhabitants. The living is a perpetual curacy, in the archdeaconry of Sudbury, and diocese of Norwich. James Farmer, Esq. was patron in 1813.

DENMEAD, a tything in the parish and hundred of HAMBLEDON, Portsdown division of the county of SOUTHAMPTON, 7½ miles (S.E. by E.) from Bishop's Waltham. The population is returned with the parish.

DENNABY, a township in the parish of MEXBOROUGH, southern division of the wapentake of STRAFFORTH and TICKHILL, West riding of the county of YORK, 6¼ miles (N.E. by N.) from Rotherham, containing 141 inhabitants.

DENNEY, a hamlet in the parish of WATERBEACH, hundred of NORTHSTOW, county of CAMBRIDGE, 7½ miles (N.N.E.) from Cambridge. The population is returned with the parish. A cell to the Benedictine abbey of Ely, with a church dedicated to St. James and St. Leonard, was founded here in the twelfth century, and in the next was occupied by the Knights Templars: in the 15th of Edward III., Mary, Dowager Countess of Pembroke, converted it into an abbey for nuns minoresses, to the honour of the Blessed Virgin and St. Clare, to which the monastery at Waterbeach was united: at the dissolution, there were in Denney abbey twenty-five nuns, whose revenue was valued at £218. 0. 1.

DENNINGTON, a parish in the hundred of HOXNE, county of SUFFOLK, 2¾ miles (N.) from Framlingham, containing 938 inhabitants. The living is a rectory, in the archdeaconry of Suffolk, and diocese of Norwich, rated in the king's books at £36. 3. 4. S. Long, Esq. was patron in 1808. The church is dedicated to St. Mary. Nathan Wright, Esq., in 1657, bequeathed land, now producing £10 per annum, for apprenticing poor children. The Earl of Stradbroke enjoys the title of Baron Rous, of Dennington, which was conferred in 1796.

DENNIS (ST.), a parish in the eastern division of the hundred of POWDER, county of CORNWALL, 5¼ miles (S.E. by S.) from St. Columb Major, containing 592 inhabitants. The living is a perpetual curacy annexed to the rectory of St. Michael Carhaise, in the archdeaconry of Cornwall, and diocese of Exeter.

DENSHANGER, a hamlet in the parish of PASSENHAM, hundred of CLELEY, county of NORTHAMPTON, 1¾ mile (S.W.) from Stony-Stratford. The population is returned with the parish.

DENSTON, a township in the parish of ALVETON, southern division of the hundred of TOTMONSLOW, county of STAFFORD, 5½ miles (N.) from Uttoxeter, containing 230 inhabitants.

DENT, a chapelry in the parish of SEDBERGH, western division of the wapentake of STAINCLIFFE and EWCROSS, West riding of the county of YORK, 6 miles (S. E. by S.) from Sedbergh, containing 1782 inhabitants. The living is a perpetual curacy, in the archdeaconry of Richmond, and diocese of Chester, endowed with £400 private benefaction, £200 royal bounty, and £300 parliamentary grant, and in the patronage of the Vicar of Sedbergh. The chapel is dedicated to St. Andrew. There is a place of worship for Independents. A free grammar school was founded for the maintenance of a master and an usher, by charter of James I., who ordained that it should be placed under the direction of fifteen governors, who are a body corporate: it is not known by whom it was endowed, but the income is about £28 a year, and there are from twenty to thirty pupils, some of whom are taught the classics.

DENTON, a chapelry in that part of the parish of GAINFORD which is in the south-eastern division of DARLINGTON ward, county palatine of DURHAM, 5¾ miles (N.W.) from Darlington, containing 125 inhabitants. The chapel, dedicated to St. Mary, was rebuilt about 1810. Denton, now a small village, was anciently a considerable town, vestiges of which are still discernible; it is said to have been burnt by Malcolm, King of Scotland, on his advance to Cleveland.

DENTON, a parish in the hundred of NORMAN-CROSS, county of HUNTINGDON, 1¾ mile (S. W.) from Stilton, containing 90 inhabitants. The living is a discharged rectory, in the archdeaconry of Huntingdon, and diocese of Lincoln, rated in the king's books at £5. 13. 6½., and in the patronage of the Executors of the late Captain Wells, R.N. The church, dedicated to All Saints, was partly rebuilt about 1665, by Sir John Cotton. Sir

Robert Bruce Cotton, Bart., a celebrated antiquary, whose manuscripts, called the Cottonian Manuscripts, are now in the British Museum, was born here in 1570.

DENTON, a parish partly in the hundred of KING-HAMFORD, and partly in that of EASTRY, lathe of ST. AUGUSTINE, county of KENT, 9 miles (S.S.E.) from Canterbury, containing 196 inhabitants. The living is a rectory, in the archdeaconry and diocese of Canterbury, rated in the king's books at £5. 19. 4½., and in the patronage of Sir Egerton Brydges, Bart. The church, dedicated to St. Mary Magdalene, is a small edifice mostly in the early style of English architecture, with an east window in the decorated style.

DENTON, a parish in the hundred of SHAMWELL, lathe of AYLESFORD, county of KENT. The population is returned with the parish of Chalk. The church, which was dedicated to St. Mary, has been long desecrated, and the cemetery converted into a farm-yard.

DENTON, a chapelry in the parish of MANCHESTER, hundred of SALFORD, county palatine of LANCASTER, 3¾ miles (N. E. by N.) from Stockport, containing 2012 inhabitants. The living is a perpetual curacy, in the archdeaconry and diocese of Chester, endowed with £400 private benefaction, £800 royal bounty, and £400 parliamentary grant, and in the patronage of the Earl of Wilton. The church, dedicated to St. James, was erected about 1530, and has portions in the early and decorated styles of English architecture, with some fragments of stained glass in the windows. The Wesleyan Methodists have a place of worship here. A free school has been erected and is supported by subscription, affording the means of instruction to about three hundred children of Denton and Haughton. The village probably derived its name from Dane-town, an etymology countenanced by the appellations Dane-headbank and Daneditch-bourne, places in the neighbourhood. The manufacture of hats, both for home trade and exportation, is carried on upon a very large scale; and coal is obtained at several places within the township.

DENTON, a parish in the soke of GRANTHAM, parts of KESTEVEN, county of LINCOLN, 4 miles (S.W. by W.) from Grantham, containing 577 inhabitants. The living is a rectory, in the archdeaconry and diocese of Lincoln, rated in the king's books at £18. 8. 4., and in the patronage of the Prebendary of North Grantham in the Cathedral Church of Salisbury. The church is dedicated to St. Andrew. About 1727, a mosaic pavement, and several large pieces of Roman bricks, composing part of some ancient foundations, were discovered in Denton fields.

DENTON, a parish in the hundred of EARSHAM, county of NORFOLK, 4¼ miles (N.E.) from Harleston, containing 601 inhabitants. The living is a rectory, in the archdeaconry of Norfolk, and diocese of Norwich, rated in the king's books at £24, and in the patronage of the Archbishop of Canterbury, who appoints a fellow, or one who has been a fellow, of Merton College, Oxford. The church, dedicated to St. Mary, stands on a high hill, at the foot of which is the church-yard and village.

DENTON, a parish in the hundred of WYMERSLEY, county of NORTHAMPTON, 6¼ miles (E. S. E.) from Northampton, containing 475 inhabitants. The living, which may be considered a joint rectory, is divided between the rectors of Whiston and Yardley-Hastings, who perform single duty every alternate year; it is in the archdeaconry of Northampton and diocese of Peterborough. There are two farms in the parish, one of which, containing about one hundred and forty acres was given to the rector of Whiston, and the other, comprising about sixty-four acres, was given to the rector of Yardley-Hastings. The church, dedicated to St. Margaret, has received an addition of one hundred and sixty sittings, of which one hundred and fifty-two are free, the Incorporated Society for the enlargement of churches and chapels having granted £100 toward defraying the expense. Children of this parish are admitted into the free school at Yardley-Hastings.

DENTON, a chapelry in the parish of CUDDESDEN, hundred of BULLINGTON, county of OXFORD, 6½ miles (W. by N.) from Tetsworth, containing 134 inhabitants.

DENTON, a parish in the hundred of BISHOPSTONE, rape of PEVENSEY, county of SUSSEX, 1½ mile (N.E.) from Newhaven, containing 133 inhabitants. The living is a discharged rectory, in the archdeaconry of Lewes, and diocese of Chichester, rated in the king's books at £14. 19. 8., endowed with £200 private benefaction, and £200 royal bounty, and in the patronage of the Crown. The church, dedicated to St. Leonard, is partly in the early English style, and partly in the decorated style of architecture. Denton is within the liberty of the duchy of Lancaster.

DENTON, a chapelry in that part of the parish of OTLEY which is in the lower division of the wapentake of CLARO, West riding of the county of YORK, 5½ miles (N.W. by W.) from Otley, containing 192 inhabitants. The living is a donative, in the patronage of Sir C. C. Ibbetson, Bart. Edward Fairfax, the translator of Tasso, and his descendants, Ferdinando and Thomas, successively Lords Fairfax, and commanders in the parliamentary army, were born here ; the last, in addition to his high military fame, was noted for his attachment to antiquarian pursuits, and was once owner of the Dodsworth MSS. now preserved in the Bodleian library at Oxford.

DENTON (EAST), a township in the parish of NEWBURN, western division of CASTLE ward, county of NORTHUMBERLAND, 3 miles (W.N.W.) from Newcastle upon Tyne, containing 548 inhabitants. The remains of a chapel and cemetery were discovered here about fifty years ago. At Denton Burn are vestiges of the old Roman wall, faced with stone, in the vicinity of which many remarkable coins and medals have been found.

DENTON (NETHER), a parish in ESKDALE ward, county of CUMBERLAND, 5½ miles (E.N.E.) from Brampton, containing 278 inhabitants. The living is a discharged rectory, in the archdeaconry and diocese of Carlisle, rated in the king's books at £4. 5. 2., endowed with £400 private benefaction, and £400 royal bounty, and in the patronage of the Bishop of Carlisle. The church is dedicated to St. Cuthbert. The parish is bounded on the north by the river Irthing, and abounds with free stone and lime-stone, besides a considerable quantity of shell-marl. Denton hall was formerly the seat of the Dentons, the old tower of which has been converted into a farm-house.

DENTON (UPPER), a parish in ESKDALE ward, county of CUMBERLAND, 6½ miles (E.N.E.) from Brampton, containing 100 inhabitants. The living is a perpetual curacy, in the archdeaconry and diocese of Carlisle, endowed with £200 private benefaction, and £800 royal

bounty, and in the patronage of the Earl of Carlisle The parish is bounded on the north and west by the river Irthing.

DENTON (WEST), a township in the parish of NEWBURN, western division of CASTLE ward, county of NORTHUMBERLAND, 3 miles (W. by N.) from Newcastle upon Tyne, containing 404 inhabitants.

DENVER, a parish in the hundred of CLACKCLOSE, county of NORFOLK, 1¼ mile (S.) from Market-Downham, containing 770 inhabitants. The living is a rectory in medieties, viz., St. Peter's Easthall, and St. Michael's Westhall, in the archdeaconry of Norfolk, and diocese of Norwich, rated in the king's books at £10. 13. 4., and in the patronage of the Master and Fellows of Caius College, Cambridge. The church, dedicated to St. Mary, is built of rough stone, with a square embattled tower.

DENWICK, a hamlet in that part of the parish of ALNWICK which is in the southern division of BAMBROUGH ward, county of NORTHUMBERLAND, 1½ mile (E. by N.) from Alnwick, with which the population is returned. There is a handsome arch, erected by the Duke of Northumberland, over which a private road passes into a field, called White Cross Howl, from a cross which formerly stood there, and where persons dying of the plague, which once infected this place, were buried.

DEOPHAM, a parish in the hundred of FOREHOE, county of NORFOLK, 3¾ miles (W. by S.) from Wymondham, containing 471 inhabitants. The living is a discharged vicarage, in the archdeaconry of Norfolk, and diocese of Norwich, rated in the king's books at £5. 7. 11., endowed with £200 private benefaction, and £200 royal bounty, and in the patronage of the Dean and Chapter of Canterbury. The church is dedicated to St. Andrew. There was formerly a petrifying spring at the foot of a remarkable linden tree in the parish.

DEPDEN, a parish in the hundred of RISBRIDGE, county of SUFFOLK, 7¼ miles (S.W.) from Bury-St. Edmund's, containing 319 inhabitants. The living is a rectory, in the archdeaconry of Sudbury, and diocese of Norwich, rated in the king's books at £10. 11. 5½., and in the patronage of the Crown. The church is dedicated to St. Mary.

DEPTFORD, a town partly in the eastern division of the hundred of BRIXTON, county of SURREY, but principally in the hundred of BLACKHEATH, lathe of SUTTON at HONE, county of KENT, 4 miles (E.) from London, containing 20,818 inhabitants. This place, according to Henshall, was at the time of the Norman survey, called Moreton, or town in the marsh; it was afterwards, from its contiguity to Greenwich, called West Greenwich, and Depeford Stronde, from a deep ford on the river Ravensbourne, of which the mouth forms the small æstuary now called Deptford creek. Edward III. frequently resided here, in a place called the Stonehouse; but the town was of little importance till the time of Henry VIII., who, for the better preservation of the royal navy, established a dock-yard, and, in the 4th year of his reign, incorporated the society of the Trinity House, by the title of the "Master, Wardens and Assistants of the guild or fraternity of the most Glorious and Undivided Trinity, and of St. Clement, in the county of Kent," confirming to them the ancient rights and privileges of the company of Mariners of England, together with their possessions at Deptford; and farther grants were afterwards made by Queen Elizabeth and Charles II., which were confirmed by James II., in 1685. In 1671, an inundation took place here, by which a prodigious quantity of cattle was destroyed in the marshes; the cables of ships at anchor were broken, and the water of the Thames rose to the height of ten feet. The houses in the upper part of the town are in general neat and well built; the streets are paved, and lighted with gas, and the inhabitants are amply supplied with water by the Kent Water Works Company. The main support and consequence of Deptford arises from its excellent docks. The royal dock-yard includes a space of about thirty-one acres of land: here the ships of the royal navy were formerly built and repaired, and here the royal yachts are still generally laid up. The old Store-house, which consisted only of the building on the north side of the present quadrangle, was erected in the year 1513. A spacious store-house, parallel with this, and of the same length, was completed about the year 1796; and a long range of smaller store-houses was built in 1780, under the direction of Sir Charles Middleton. This yard contains three slips for building second and third-rate ships, a double and a single wet dock, a basin, and two mast-ponds. Here are also a large smithy for making anchors, &c., mast-houses, sheds for timber, a mould-loft, various workshops, and houses for the officers. The establishment consists of a master-shipwright, master-attendant, store-keeper, clerk of the checque, clerk of the survey, surgeon, &c., the whole being under the inspection of the Navy Board. In the reigns of James I. and Charles I., the treasurer of the navy resided here. A short distance north of the king's yard, by the side of the river, and in the parish of St. Paul, stands the victualling-office, built in 1745, on the north side of the ancient range of store-houses, called the Red House, and new store-houses have since been added. Besides which it has an extensive cooperage and brewhouse, slaughtering-houses, houses for curing beef, pork, &c., bake-houses, and other buildings. Near the victualling office is Deadman's dock-yard, belonging to the Evelyn family, in which ships of seventy-four guns have, at different times, been built; and there are two other private docks in the parish of St. Nicholas. The only branch of manufacture carried on to any great extent is that of earthenware, known by the name of Deptford-ware. There are works for the refining of gold and silver, and a laboratory for the making of sulphuric, nitric, and oxalic acids, and other chemical productions, by a process which, though it has been practised for some years in France, was only introduced into England in 1827, by the present proprietors of these extensive works; which occupy an area of more than fifteen thousand square yards, and comprise a range of building two hundred and seventy feet in length, containing, exclusively of other apparatus, from twelve to fifteen furnaces, and affording employment to from thirty to forty persons, mostly natives of France: the peculiarity of the chemical process consists principally in the use of retorts made of platina, instead of glass, in the distillation of the acids, and in the substitution of sulphuric instead of nitric acid in the solution of the metals. The Grand Surrey canal passes through the upper part of the parish of St. Paul, from which there is a branch to Croydon. The bridge over the Ravensbourne, anciently of wood, was rebuilt with stone in 1628, by Charles I., and has lately been widened at the expense of the county. Another bridge has recently been erected over Deptford creek, near its junction with the Thames, by a company called the Deptford Creek Bridge Company, thus forming a direct communication between the lower part of Deptford and Greenwich.

The town is within the jurisdiction of the county magistrates, who sit daily, and hold a petty session for the division weekly on Saturday; and within that of the court of requests for the recovery of debts not exceeding 40s., held at Greenwich, of which twelve commissioners are appointed from each parish: the banks of the Ravensbourne are under the superintendence of commissioners of sewers, whose jurisdiction extends from its source to Lambard's wall, near Greenwich. In 1730, the town was divided into the two parishes of St. Nicholas and St. Paul, the former of which, including the old town, is small, the latter extends into the county of Surrey: they are in the archdeaconry and diocese of Rochester, and the livings are both in the patronage of Mrs. Mary Drake and Mrs. Ann Drake Tyrwhit Drake. The living of St. Nicholas' is a vicarage, rated in the king's books at £12. 17. 3½.: the church, with the exception of the tower, was re built upon a larger scale in 1697. The living of St. Paul's is a rectory, not in charge: by act of parliament in 1730, £3500, arising from the duty on coal, was allotted to be invested in the purchase of land for the maintenance of the rector; it was also enacted that the churchwardens, in whom are vested four acres of glebe taken out of the old parish, should pay the rector £70 per annum, in lieu of fees for vaults and burials, except when the corpse is carried into the church. The church, erected in the reign of Queen Anne, under an act of parliament for building fifty new churches in and near London, is a fine structure in the Grecian style of architecture, with a tower surmounted by a spire; the roof of the nave is supported by a handsome range of pillars, and the east window is ornamented with modern painted glass. There are places of worship for Baptists, the Society of Friends, Independents, and Wesleyan Methodists. Dr. Robert Breton, in 1672, left £500 for the endowment of a grammar school for the education of thirty children, but a considerable part of the benefaction was lost; the remainder, producing £6. 16. per annum, is paid to a master, who teaches six children of each parish, and who also receives £5 per annum, and £2. 17. for teaching five boys of the parish of St. Nicholas, from a bequest by Mr. Thomas Fellows, who in 1753 left £1000 three per cents, in trust to the minister and churchwardens, from which a schoolmistress also receives £5 per annum for teaching five girls; these children are clothed and provided with books. A charity school was founded in 1722, by Dean Stanhope, then vicar of Deptford; a school-house was built on a plot of land given by Mr. Robert Grandsden; it was subsequently endowed with various benefactions for the instruction and clothing of sixty-five boys and thirty girls. Dean Stanhope also bequeathed to this charity £6 per annum, for apprenticing and clothing the children, which was augmented, in 1790, by a bequest of £150, from Dr. Wilson, vicar of St. Nicholas'; the annual income arising from the property belonging to the school is £212, which sum is greatly increased by subscription.

There are two almshouses belonging to the Corporation of the Trinity House, for decayed pilots and masters of ships, or their widows; one, which adjoins the church-yard, was built in the reign of Henry VIII., and consists of twenty-five apartments; the other which is situated in Church-street, was built about the close of the seventeenth century, and contains fifty-six apartments : it forms a spacious quadrangle, in the centre of which is a statue of Captain Maples, who, in 1680, contributed £1300 towards the building. Here the brethren of the Trinity House hold their annual meeting on Trinity-Monday, when they attend divine service at St. Nicholas' church. The parish of St. Paul has the right of presenting one pensioner to certain almshouses at St. Clements near Oxford, founded by Edmund Boulter, Esq. A dispensary, open to poor invalids belonging to the town and the neighbouring parishes, and a savings-bank, have been established : here is also a mechanics' institution. The Gun Tavern, lately pulled down, is said to have been the residence of the Earl of Nottingham, who was Lord High Admiral in the reign of Elizabeth. Sayes court, the ancient mansion-house of the manor of West Greenwich, so called from its having been possessed in the thirteenth and fourteenth centuries by the family of Say, became (in consequence of his marriage with the daughter of Sir Richard Browne, who then held it under the crown,) the residence of John Evelyn, Esq., the celebrated author of the "Sylva," who, after the Restoration, obtained a lease of Sayes court and the demesne lands, for ninety-nine years. The poet Cowley resided here while composing his six Latin books on plants, in which work the fine gardens belonging to Mr. Evelyn are supposed to have afforded him great assistance. Mr. Evelyn also lent the use of this residence to the Czar Peter, while pursuing the study of naval architecture, in 1698, in the neighbouring dock-yard : the mansion was pulled down in 1728, and the work-house erected on its site.

DEPTFORD, a tything in the parish of WILY, hundred of BRANCH and DOLE, county of WILTS, 8 miles (N.W.) from Wilton. The population is returned with the parish.

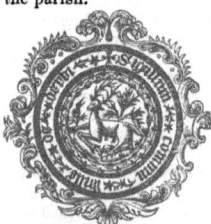

Seal and Arms.

DERBY, a borough and market town, possessing separate jurisdiction, locally in the hundred of MORLESTON and LITCHURCH, county of DERBY, of which it is the capital, 15 miles (W.) from Nottingham, 29 miles (N.W.) from Leicester, and 126 (N.W) from London, on the river Derwent, and on the high road to Manchester, containing 17,423 inhabitants, and, including parts of certain parishes which extend beyond the limits of the borough, 19,648, but the population since the census of 1821 has greatly increased. The origin of this town is not known : by the Saxons it was called Northworthig, and by the Danes Derwentby, but more commonly Deoraby, of which Derby is a corruption, probably referring to its situation on the Derwent. King Egbert constituted the town a royal burgh, and a mint was established in it. It was possessed by the Danes and Saxons alternately during their contests. In 874 it was occupied by Halfolen, a Danish chief, whose head-quarters were at Rippandune, now Repton. Alfred having defeated the Danes, planted a colony here in 880, and constituted this the chief town in the county. The Danes, after a second defeat by the same monarch, regained possession of the place, and retained it till 918, when being taken by surprise, they were completely defeated by the heroic Ethelfleda, Countess of Mercia, and daughter of King Alfred, who, obtaining possession of the town, held it till her death. The Danes, however, retook it soon after her decease, but were again. dispossessed by King Edmund I. in 942. In 1040, during the reign of Edward the Confessor, it contained two hundred and forty-three burgesses, at which time two-thirds of the profits from tolls, &c. belonged to the king, and the remaining third to the Earl of Mercia. In 1066, the king of Norway; at the instigation of Tostig, Harold's brother, invaded the northern parts of England, on which many of the inhabitants of Derby, who were then vassals of Edwin, Earl of Mercia, quitted their homes, and joined the forces of Morcar, Earl of Northumberland, to oppose the invader : but they were defeated with great slaughter, only four days before the latter and his army were destroyed by Harold. On the victor's return to encounter William, Duke of Normandy, he recruited his army at Derby, to which is to be ascribed the diminution of the number of burgesses; for at the time of the Norman survey, they amounted to only one hundred, and of these forty-three were minors. The town was given by the Conqueror to his illegitimate son, William Peverel, and an augmentation of its privileges ensued, which was followed by a revival of industry, and an increase of its population. In the rebellion of 1745, Derby was occupied by Charles James Stuart, son of the Pretender ; but, on the approach of the royal army, commanded by the Duke of Cumberland, he retreated, after levying a contribution of two or three thousand pounds on the inhabitants during his short stay of two days.

Derby is pleasantly situated in a valley which is open to the south, the country in that direction being flat and low : a small brook runs through it under nine stone bridges. The town is large and well built; for, notwithstanding the want of regularity in their appearance, many of the more modern houses are spacious and handsome : it is lighted with gas ; the streets are regularly paved, and considerable improvement has recently taken place. An elegant stone bridge of three elliptical arches, over the river Derwent, forms a handsome entrance to the town from Nottingham. The roads in the neighbourhood have been recently improved under the superintendence of Mr. M Adam, and are in a very good state. Water is abundantly supplied from the Derwent, by means of pipes and machinery.

The Derby Philosophical Society, which has for its object the promotion of scientific knowledge, by occasional meetings and conversation, as well as by the circulation of books, was founded by Dr. Darwin, in 1788 : it has a considerable number of members, who are in possession of an extensive and valuable library. Another flourishing institution was commenced in 1808, under the title of the Derby Literary and Philosophical Society, the objects of which are the pursuit of literary and scientific enquiries, by the production and discussion of papers or essays, which may be written on any subject connected with literature or science, excluding only the practical departments of medicine and surgery, politics and religion; but this institution has been almost wholly discontinued. There are eight or ten other institutions in the town, one of which is devoted exclusively to the cultivation of French literature. An agricultural society was established many years ago, which holds two meetings annually : there are also a mechanics' institution, with a library attached to it ; a permanent subscription library ; a theological book society, &c. The races, which are of considerable repute, are held on a fine course, called the Siddals, and are much frequented. The walks in the vicinity of the town present a variety of scenery, and are very pleasant.

Derby enjoyed, under a license from King John, the exclusive privilege of dyeing cloth, but this has wholly declined : it is nevertheless a place of considerable trade. Until of late years, silk was the principal article of manufacture ; but to that it has added those of cotton and porcelain, which are carried on to a great extent. The first silk-mill erected in England was built here, about 1718, by Mr. John Lombe, who procured in Italy (by means of bribing two workmen, who accompanied him to England,) drawings and models of the silk machinery then in use in that country, for which he took out a patent : its operations are to wind, double, and twist the silk, so as to render it fit for weaving. After the death of Mr. Lombe, about four years afterwards, caused as it is stated by means of poison, administered to him by an Italian female, sent over for that purpose, his cousin Sir Thomas Lombe obtained the patent, in consideration of the sum of £14,000, whereby the manufacture was thrown open, and the trade rapidly increased. The factory stands upon an island in the Derwent, and is built on large piles, over which are turned thirteen arches of stone : the original machinery has been replaced by other less cumbrous, and far more simple in its construction : it is now worked by a water-wheel, twenty-three feet in diameter ; and such has been the progressive increase of this branch of manufacture, that there are now nine silk-mills, worked either by water or steam. The weaving of silk was also introduced here in 1827. The porcelain manufacture was established in 1793, and has been brought to great perfection ; it gives employment to about two hundred persons : the beautiful ornaments, called "white biscuit figures," are the production of this establishment. The machinery for cutting, polishing, and turning the Derbyshire marble spar is worked by steam ; and a variety of sculptured articles, which will bear comparison with those of the best Italian artists, is produced here. In 1756, Mr. Jedediah Strutt invented and introduced " The Derby ribbed stocking-frame," for which he obtained a patent ; and silk, cotton, and fine worsted stockings, are still made. The first fire-proof mill for spinning cotton was erected here in 1793, and there is a considerable trade carried on in cotton-yarn for making bobbin, in net-lace, galloons, ferrets, and tapes, in red and white lead, tin plates, sheet and bar iron, shot, and jewellery. Hot and cold air-stoves, upon what is called "Silvester's principle," by which the most considerable buildings in the country may be warmed and ventilated, are exclusively made here ; it has now become an object of importance in its trade.

The navigation of the Derwent was closed on the completion of the Derby canal ; the latter communicating by branches, each about eight miles in length, with the Trent and Erwash canal, thus rendering the former unnecessary. The company entrusted with the management of the canal were empowered by act of parliament to raise the sum of £90,000, and are required, when the dividend exceeds eight per cent., to reduce the tolls : there is a large and convenient wharf for the purpose of loading and unloading the boats. The market days are Wednesday and Friday ; and on every alternate Tuesday there is one for fat cattle. The fairs are held on the Monday after January 6th, January 25th, March 21st and the two following days, Friday in Easter-week, Friday after May 1st, Friday in Whitsun-week, July 25th, September 27th, and the two following days, and on the Friday before October 4th : those in March and October are great cheese fairs; the others are principally for cattle.

Henry I. granted the town of Derby to Ralph, Earl of Chester, and gave the inhabitants a charter of incorporation ; this charter was materially altered, and their privileges were subsequently enlarged by Henry II., Richard I., and John. James I. gave the corporation authority to hold courts of record, made them independent of any foreign jurisdiction, and empowered them to hold " sessions quarterly, two courts leet, and six fairs yearly." In 1638, mention is first made of a mayor ; the corporation, antecedently to that period, having been styled " the Bailiffs and Burgesses of the town of Derby." In 1680, the charter was surrendered to Charles II., and a new one, now in force, was obtained in 1683, by which the government of the borough is vested in a mayor, nine aldermen, fourteen brethren, and fourteen capital burgesses, who together constitute the common council ; and these appoint a recorder, town-clerk (who is also coroner), chamberlain, four serjeants at mace (one of whom is keeper of the gaol), six constables, and other inferior officers, elected annually on the first Monday after St. Luke's day. The mayor is chosen from among the aldermen, by the aldermen and brethren, and the aldermen from among the brethren, these last being appointed from the capital burgesses. The mayor, the late mayor (who is always deputy mayor, with equal powers), and the four senior aldermen, are justices of the peace : the mayor, aldermen, and burgesses, must reside within the borough, otherwise they can neither locally vote, nor exercise any official function. The freedom of the borough is inherited by all the sons of a freeman born within the borough, or acquired by serving apprenticeship to a resident freeman, or by gift from the corporation. Sessions for the borough are held by the mayor quarterly, on days appointed by himself. A court of record is held every second Tuesday, before the mayor, his deputy, the recorder, and the town-clerk, in which pleas to any amount are cognizable ; and a court of requests, for the recovery of debts under 40s., was established by act of parliament in the 6th of George III., which is held every third Tuesday. Derby has sent two members to parliament ever since 1294 : the right of election is vested in the free burgesses, of whom there are about two thousand ; the mayor is the returning officer. The Duke of Devonshire's influence predominates in parliamentary elections. The old town-hall, erected on the site of the ancient guildhall, about the year 1730, though in itself a

E

good building, was found, from its isolated situation in the market-place, to be a great obstruction to business, and has therefore been taken down : a new one, nearly in a line with the south side of the market-place, has been erected : it presents a handsome appearance, and, being built on arches, is connected with a new market-house built by the corporation. The assizes and general quarter sessions were formerly held in the county-hall, a spacious handsome building of freestone, built in 1660; new courts of a more convenient construction having been subsequently erected. Adjoining the hall, on the right, is a handsome brick building, erected in 1811, for the accommodation of the judges; and on the left an hotel. The town gaol, which until lately was the county prison, is a plain, solid, brick building, erected about 1756; but not admitting of the arrangements required by a late act of parliament, a new county gaol and house of correction, affording ample means of classification, has been erected upon the radiating principle, at an expense of £63,000 : it comprises one hundred and sixty-four cells, and twenty-one courts, a chapel and a house for the governor.

Derby is divided into five parishes, viz., All Saints', St. Werburgh's, St. Alkmund's, St. Peter's, and St. Michael's, of which the last three extend into the hundred of Morleston and Litchurch; they are all in the archdeaconry of Derby, and diocese of Lichfield and Coventry. The living of All Saints' is a perpetual curacy, in the patronage of the Mayor and Corporation. The church, which, prior to the dissolution, was collegiate, is considered the principal architectural ornament of the town : the body, erected in 1725, from a design by Gibbs, at an expense of £4000, is in the Roman Doric style, and the interior particularly light, elegant, and spacious : the tower, one hundred and eighty feet high, erected in the reign of Henry VII., is in the later English style, the upper part being richly ornamented with buttresses, pinnacles, battlements, and tracery. Rich open screen-work of iron, said to have cost £500, separates the east end of the church from the place allotted for divine worship, in the centre of which is an elegant chancel. Over an altar-piece of Derbyshire marble is a fine painting by Rawlinson; and on the southern side of the chancel a monument to the memory of William, Earl of Devonshire, who died in 1628, and his countess, whose figures stand under a dome, nearly twelve feet in height: there is also a splendid mural monument to the memory of the celebrated Countess of Shrewsbury, executed under her own inspection. The living of St. Alkmund's is a vicarage, not in charge, in the patronage of the Mayor and Corporation. The church is supposed to have been originally founded early in the ninth century, in honour of Alkmund, son of Alured, the deposed King of Northumberland, who being slain in battle, while endeavouring to reinstate his father, was first interred at Lilleshall, in Shropshire, but removed thence and deposited in this church. Many pilgrimages were formerly made to his tomb, which, in point of miracles, was exceeded in renown only by that of Thomas à Becket, at Canterbury. The chapelries of Little Eaton and Darley are in this parish, though without the limits of the borough. The living of St. Peter's is a discharged vicarage, rated in the king's books at £8, and in the patronage of the Rev. T. Wright's family, of Market-Bosworth. The church is ancient, but of uncertain date. The living of St. Werburgh's is a discharged vicarage,

rated in the king's books at £5. 12. 8., and in the patronage of the Crown. The original church of St. Werburgh is supposed to have been built prior to the Conquest. From being situated near Markeaton-brook, its foundation was injured by occasional floods; so that in 1601 the tower fell, and within a century afterwards the church having become ruinous, the present edifice was erected. A chapel of ease, dedicated to St. John, capable of accommodating one thousand four hundred persons, has recently been erected in the later English style, at an expense of about £8000, one half of which was defrayed by the parliamentary commissioners, and the other by subscription among the inhabitants. The living of St. Michael's is a discharged vicarage, rated in the king's books at £4. 15., endowed with £400 private benefaction, £400 royal bounty, and £2000 parliamentary grant, and in the patronage of the Crown. The church is very ancient, and of uncertain date. An episcopal chapel, dedicated to St. George, has recently been erected in this parish, capable of seating one thousand persons. There are places of worship for General and Particular Baptists, the Society of Friends, Independents, Wesleyan Methodists (New and Old connexion), Swedenborgians, and Unitarians, and a Roman Catholic chapel.

The free grammar school is said to have been founded in the reign of Henry II., soon after the removal of the canons of the priory of St. Helen's, at Derby, to Darley. Walter Durdant, Bishop of Lichfield, in his charter, makes mention of the school of Derby, as the gift of himself and William de Barba Aprilis. Queen Mary, in the first year of her reign, granted a charter to the corporation, in which provision is made for the support of this school, by the payment of £13. 6. 8. per annum : the queen's grant was also accompanied by the patronage of two of the churches. The sum of £25 is annually paid to the master, by the Master and Fellows of Emanuel College, Cambridge, under the will of Mr. Ash, who also founded ten exhibitions at the same college, for boys educated at this school and at that of Ashby de la Zouch. Mrs. Jane Walton, who died in 1603, also bequeathed the sum of £40 for the benefit of the master and usher, and £100 to the master of St. John's College, Cambridge, towards the maintenance of such of the young men educated here as should be admitted into that college. Flamsteed, the celebrated astronomer, received the elementary part of his education at this institution. In 1812, National schools were established in the parish of St. Werburgh, in which about ninety boys and one hundred girls are instructed; and in 1829, schools upon the same system were opened in the parish of St. Peter, which afford instruction to one hundred boys and seventy girls. There is also a school upon the Lancasterian plan, in which about one hundred and forty boys are taught; also several infant schools.

The Devonshire almshouse was founded by the Countess of Shrewsbury, in the reign of Queen Elizabeth, and endowed with a bequest of £100 a year. In 1777, it was rebuilt in a handsome style, at the expense of the then Duke of Devonshire, who, before his death, added a farther endowment of £50 a year: eight men and four women are now supported in it. About 1716, Edward Large, Esq. endowed an almshouse near the top of Friargate, for five widows of clergymen, each of whom receives about £26 per annum. Robert Willymott, Esq.

of Chaddesden, by will dated September 1st, 1629, founded and endowed ten almshouses, for six men and four women, to be supported by his heirs in perpetuity; these were rebuilt by Sir Robert Wilmot, in 1814. A munificent bequest was also made by Richard Crawshaw, Esq., who died in 1631, of upwards of £4000, for the benefit of the poor of Derby, including the maintenance of lectures, and other laudable purposes : additional bequests have lately been made to this charity, which has now a revenue of £750 per annum. There is an asylum for discharged female prisoners, the object of which is, by the inculcation of moral principles, to restore them to society and to useful employment. Robert Lyversege, dyer, of the parish of St. Peter's, bequeathed various lands and tenements "for good and godly purposes," the present rental of which, about £700, is from the renewal of leases, continually increasing : the poor have also the benefit of numerous small bequests. The general infirmary is situated near the London road, on a healthful, airy, and dry plot of ground : the building is constructed of hard white stone, of a handsome, yet simple elevation of three stories, containing a light central hall, with a double staircase : there are two light and spacious rooms, one for each sex, called day or convalescent rooms : a statue of Æsculapius, indicating its useful design, is placed upon the centre of the dome, which is of iron. The building is calculated to accommodate more than one hundred patients : three physicians, four surgeons, and a house apothecary, are appointed to the institution. It is surrounded by fourteen acres of land, purchased to prevent the near approach of buildings, and cost nearly £18,000. The ordnance depôt, situated near the infirmary, erected according to a design by Mr. Wyatt, in 1805, has been purchased of government, and converted into a silk-mill.

About half a century ago there were vestiges of an ancient castle, but the site is now completely covered with buildings. Remains of St. Mary's chapel, supposed to have been the church of St. Mary given by William the Conqueror to the abbey of Burton, still exist : the chapel, in the time of Charles II., was used by the Presbyterians, but was subsequently converted into small tenements. Of several religious houses which once had existence here there are no traces. Among the eminent natives of Derby may be mentioned Dr. Thomas Linacre, the founder of the College of Physicians in London, of which he was president till his death, in 1524 ; Samuel Richardson, the novelist, in 1689 ; William Hutton, in 1723 ; and Joseph Wright, the celebrated painter, in 1734 : this distinguished artist resided here during the greater part of his life, and died in 1797 ; his view of Ulswater, which is considered to be one of the finest efforts of British genius, in landscape, was purchased by Sir Richard Arkwright, for £315, and is now at Willersley castle, in this county. Thomas Parker, Earl of Macclesfield, and Lord High Chancellor, resided here during the early part of his life ; and while practising in this town as an attorney, laid the foundation of his future fame. John Whitehurst, an ingenious mechanist and philosopher, also resided here about the middle of the last century ; and Dr. Erasmus Darwin here spent the last twenty years of his life, and died in 1802. Derby gives the title of earl to the family of Stanley.

DERBYSHIRE, an inland county, bounded on the east by the counties of Nottingham and Leicester, on the south by that of Leicester, on the west by the counties of Stafford and Chester, and on the north by the county of York ; it extends from 52° 38' to 53° 27' (N. Lat.), and from 1° 13' to 2° 3' 30" (W. Lon.), and contains one thousand and twenty-six square miles, or six hundred and fifty-six thousand six hundred and forty statute acres. The population, in 1821, amounted to 213,333. The tract of country now forming the county of Derby, was, in the time of the Britons, part of the territory occupied by the Coritani, and, under the government of the Romans, was included in Britannia Prima. During the Heptarchy it formed part of the kingdom of Mercia ; and the inhabitants of Derbyshire and Nottinghamshire were called North Mercians, those two counties lying for the most part north of the river Trent. The earliest historical event recorded in connexion with Derbyshire is the invasion by the Danes, in 874, when they expelled Burrhed, King of Mercia, and fixed their head-quarters at his royal residence of Repandune, now Repton, in this county, where they remained until the following year. Derbyshire was recovered from their possession in 918, by Ethelfleda, the celebrated Countess of Mercia. Derby, however, was not long afterwards again in the power of the Danes, and was retaken from them by King Edmund, in 942. In the rebellion of Prince Henry against his father Henry II., the castle of Duffield was held against the king by Robert, Earl Ferrars ; and in the reign of John, William, Earl Ferrars captured Bolsover and Peak castles from the barons. In 1264, Henry III. sent his son, Prince Edward, into Derbyshire, to take vengeance upon Robert, Earl of Derby, then one of the most active of the barons in rebellion against him, with orders to lay waste his manors with fire and sword : the earl made his peace by the promise of a large sum of money, and by taking a fresh oath of allegiance ; notwithstanding which, he again appeared in arms, in 1266, with other barons, and knights, and having assembled a numerous force at Duffield Frith, marched thence to Chesterfield, where being surprised by the king's nephew, Henry, the greater part of them was put to the sword, the earl himself was made prisoner, and such of his adherents as made their escape withdrew into the Forest of the Peak, where they remained leading a predatory life for two years. The earl's life was spared, but his earldom was taken from him, and its extensive possessions being given to Edmund, Earl of Lancaster, eventually furnished a considerable part of the revenue of the duchy of Lancaster. The most remarkable historical circumstance connected with Derbyshire, from this period until the reign of Charles I., is the captivity of Mary, Queen of Scots, who, while in the custody of the Earl of Shrewsbury, resided much in this county, at the seats of that nobleman. Charles I., after having erected his standard at Nottingham, marched to Derby, at which period the inhabitants of the whole county declared for him, so at least Sir John Gell states, in his own Memoirs, in which he also claims the merit of having been the first who appeared in arms in this county for the parliament. Repairing to Hull, in October, 1642, he obtained the command of a regiment of foot, consisting of one hundred and forty men, with which he advanced into Derbyshire ; reaching Chesterfield on the seventeenth, he there raised two hundred men, and marched to Derby, where he collected a

E 2

regiment of horse, and garrisoned the town. At that time, Lord Clarendon observes, there was in Derbyshire no visible party for the king, the whole county being under the power of Sir John Gell, who maintained this ascendancy throughout the war; the transactions of which within the county, though carried on with spirit, consisted chiefly in the attack and defence of small garrisons. It may, however, be particularized, that in the year 1643, Sir Thomas Fairfax came to Derby, and staid there three days, for the purpose of procuring a supply of men from the Derbyshire garrisons, and that, after the battle of Naseby, the king, with three thousand horse, passed from Bewdley into Derbyshire, about the middle of August, 1645, and having defeated Sir John Gell in some skirmishes at Sudbury and Ashbourn, marched through the Peak to Doncaster. In 1745, Charles Edward Stuart, commonly called the young Pretender, having penetrated into the heart of the kingdom, entered Derby with his army on December 4th: his advanced guard secured the passage of the Trent at Swarkston bridge, but on the evening of the fifth he held a council of war, at which, after a warm debate, it was determined, in consequence of the little encouragement he had met with in England, and the near approach of the Duke of Cumberland with a superior force, immediately to commence a retreat northward; which resolution was accordingly carried into effect early the next morning. On the 9th of June, 1817, a number of miserably deluded people of the lowest order broke out into open insurrection at South Winfield, in this county, and proceeded towards Nottingham, within a few miles of which they were met by a party of the military, and speedily dispersed: the well known termination of this affair was the trial at Derby, in October of the same year, by special commission, of a number of the insurgents, when twenty-two of them were convicted of high treason, of whom three were executed at Derby, on the 7th of November following, and the rest were transported for life.

Derbyshire is in the diocese of Lichfield and Coventry, and province of Canterbury; it forms an archdeaconry, comprising the deaneries of Ashbourn, Castillar, Chesterfield, Derby, High Peak, and Repton, and contains one hundred and thirty-seven parishes, of which fifty-two are rectories, fifty-four vicarages, and thirty-one perpetual curacies: there are also fifty dependent chapels. For civil purposes it is divided into the hundreds of Appletree, High Peak, Morleston and Litchurch, Repton and Gresley, Scarsdale, and Wirksworth. It contains the borough and market town of Derby, and the market towns of Alfreton, Ashbourn, Bakewell, Belper, Buxton, Chapel en le Frith, Chesterfield, Cromford, Tideswell, Winster, and Wirksworth. Two knights are returned for the shire, and two representatives for the borough of Derby: the county members are elected at Derby. This county is included in the midland circuit: Derbyshire and Nottinghamshire formed but one shrievalty until the year 1569, and the assizes for both were held at Nottingham until the reign of Henry III. From that period until the division of the shrievalty, they were held at Nottingham and Derby alternately; but since 1569, the assizes for this county have been held uniformly at Derby, except once in the year 1610, when, on account of a commotion at that place, they were removed to Ashbourn. The Epiphany, Eas-

ter, and Michaelmas sessions are held at Derby, and the Midsummer sessions at Chesterfield. A new county gaol and house of correction has recently been erected at Derby, the expense of which, including the purchase of the site, tread-mill, &c. was £63,335. 5. 6.; on its completion, in 1827, prisoners were ordered to be removed to it from the houses of correction at Ashbourn, Chesterfield, Tideswell, and Wirksworth. There are fifty-four acting magistrates. A great part of the county is within the jurisdiction of the duchy of Lancaster court, held at Tutbury, for the recovery of small debts, for determining on trespasses, assaults, &c. Many of the parishes in the hundreds of High Peak, Scarsdale, and Wirksworth, are within the jurisdiction of the Peverel court, of the same nature, held at Lenton in Nottinghamshire. The barmote courts, for regulating the mineral concerns of Derbyshire, and determining all disputes relative to the working of the mines, are held at Monyash, in the Peak, and at Wirksworth. The rates raised in the county for the year ending March 25th, 1827, amounted to £97,532; the expenditure to £99,518. 5., of which sum £76,568. 13. was applied to the relief of the poor.

Derbyshire, as a manufacturing county, ranks next after Lancashire, Staffordshire, and Warwickshire. Cotton spinning is extensively carried on at Belper, Cromford, Calver, Hayfield, New Mills, &c. The woollen manufacture is chiefly in the parish of Glossop, on the Yorkshire border; worsted-spinning at Derby, Melbourne, Tideswell, &c. The silk-mill was introduced at the beginning of the last century, the manufacture being chiefly at Derby. The manufacture of stockings is principally at Derby, Belper, and Chesterfield, and in the villages on the eastern side of the county: this branch of manufacture is carried on for the most part in private dwellings. The manufacture of cotton, excepting that used in making stockings, was first established in this county by Sir Richard Arkwright in 1771, and in 1773 Sir Richard, in conjunction with two other gentlemen, made, at Derby, the first successful attempt to establish the manufacture of calicoes in this kingdom. In 1817, the number of cotton-mills in Derbyshire was one hundred and twelve, of which one half were in the parish of Glossop; several others in the Peak; and others at Matlock, Pleaseley, Wilne, Measham, &c. In the same year, there were forty-three factories for calico-weaving, fifteen bleaching-grounds, four calico-printing works, three factories for weaving cambric, two for fustian, eight for muslin, and two for tape. Machines for the cotton-factories, stocking-frames, &c. are made at Derby, Alfreton, Glossop, Belper, Heanor, Matlock, Butterley, &c. The linen manufacture is not of great extent: flax is spun at Darley dale, and there are linen-yarn mills in the parishes of Ashover and Glossop; linen-weaving is carried on in those of Belper, Turnditch, &c., and lace-weaving at Derby and Melbourne. There are many tan-yards in various parts of the county, and several paper-mills. Connected with the iron trade are various manufactories, some of them very extensive. In the cast-iron works at Chesterfield, Butterley, &c. a large quantity of cannon, cannon-balls, &c. was cast during the war. Agricultural utensils are made in various parts of the county; scythes, sickles, hoes, and spades being made chiefly in the northern part between Chesterfield and Sheffield. Cutlery and other articles of steel are

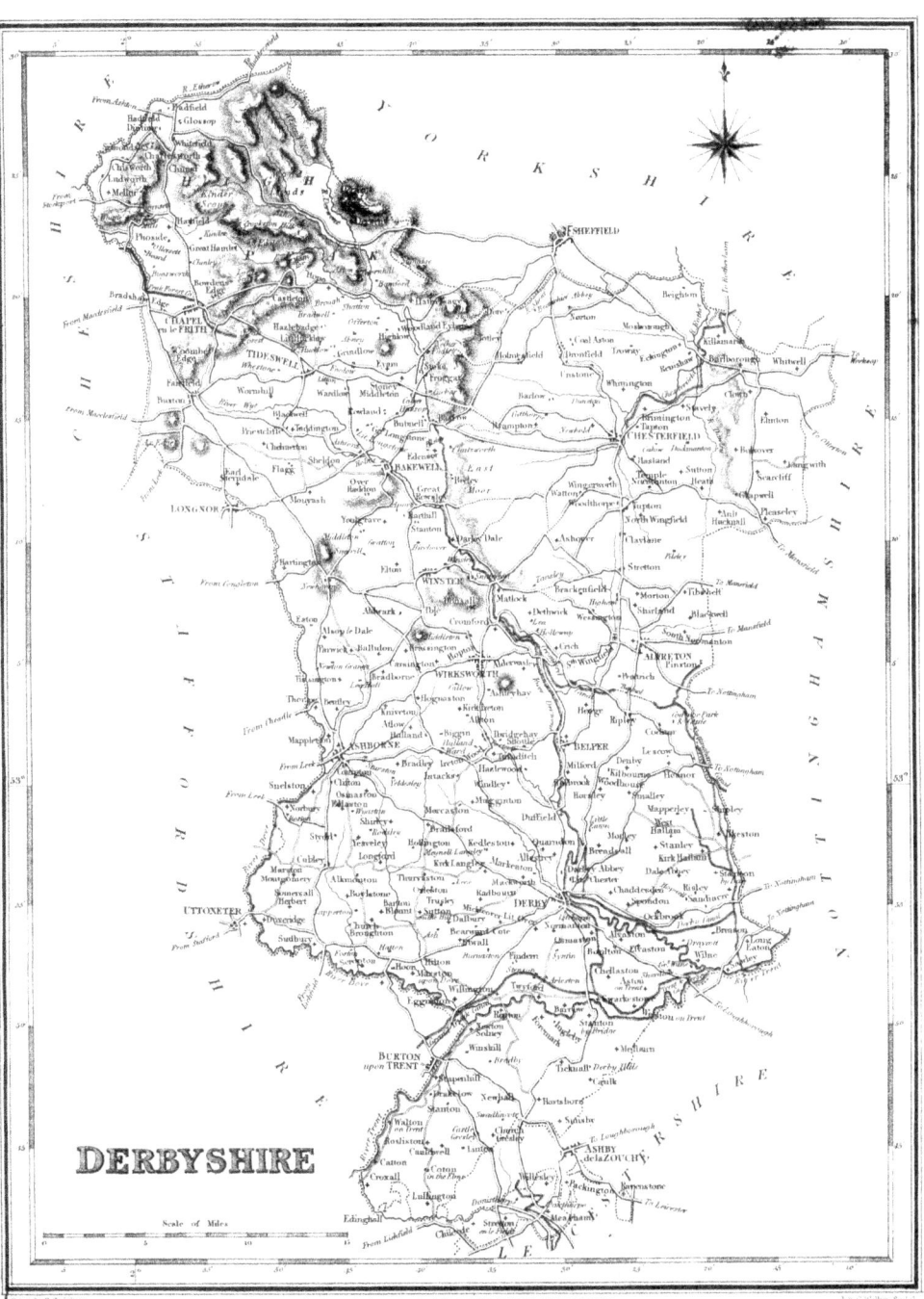

DERBYSHIRE

Scale of Miles

made at Derby and Chesterfield, and in the villages north of the latter. There are six chain-manufactories, principally in the northern part of the county, and nail-making is carried on to a considerable extent, chiefly in Belper and its neighbourhood. Whet-stones and hones are made in great quantities within a few miles north-east of Derby, and sent to the southern counties. There is a large manufactory for spar or fluor ornaments at Derby; and there are saw-mills, for marble and stone, at Bonsall, Lea-Bridge, and Wirksworth. There is a long established porcelain manufactory at Derby, and one of later establishment at Pinxton : there are also potteries at and near Chesterfield, Alfreton, Belper, Ilkeston, Gresley, Hartshorn, Tickenhall, &c. A great quantity of hats is made for exportation at Lea-Bridge, Chesterfield, &c.; and shoes are made for the wholesale trade at Chesterfield and other places.

The surface of the southern part of Derbyshire is for the most part tolerably level, containing nothing remarkable in its hills, and little that is picturesque in its scenery ; but in that part which lies north of Derby the hills begin gradually to rise ; and in the north-western part of the county some of them attain a considerable elevation, forming the commencement of that mountainous ridge which from this place divides the northern part of the island: the four highest points in Derbyshire are Kinderscout, Holme-Moss, near the north-western extremity of the county ; Ax-edge, about three miles south-west of Buxton ; and Lord's Seat, near Castleton ; the altitudes of which, according to observations made during the Trigonometrical survey, are, of the first, two thousand one hundred and fifty feet, of the second one thousand eight hundred and fifty-nine, and of the two latter, one thousand seven hundred and fifty-one. Some of the valleys in this tract are very beautiful, particularly those of Castleton, Monsall-dale, and Glossop ; but the most picturesque and remarkable scenery is composed of the great number and variety of smaller valleys or dales with which the limestone district abounds, the general characteristics of which are precipitous rocks of singular and striking forms, with mountain streams and rivulets winding through the lower parts, which are frequently well-wooded. The most celebrated of these are, Matlock-dale, on the river Derwent ; Monsall-dale, on the Wye ; Middleton-dale, Eyam-dale, and Dove-dale, the latter on the river Dove. Except in these valleys, however, the scenery is by no means beautiful or agreeable; it consists chiefly of uncultivated moors, on some parts of which large masses and groups of rock are seen projecting, some of them in very grotesque forms.

The southern and middle portions of the county are for the most part in cultivation. Extending northward from Ashover and Darley, through the parish of Bakewell and its chapelries, almost to the northern limit of the county, is the great East Moor, a considerable part of which lies waste. And in the northern part of the Peak, bordering on Yorkshire, in the parishes of Hope and Glossop, are most extensive sheep-walks, called the Woodlands, without any sort of fences to separate the different manors, parishes, or counties. A great quantity of excellent wheat and barley is cultivated in the southern and eastern parts of the county. The arable land in the Peak is chiefly tilled for oats, of which there is a great local consumption, oaten cakes being still, as they have long been, the principal species of bread eaten

by the poorer class. On an average, more corn is produced, of every sort, than is consumed in the county. The principal dairy district is the neighbourhood of Ashbourn : about two thousand tons of cheese are said to be annually sent from the wharfs at Derby, Shardlow, &c. The grass lands in the parishes of Beighton, Eckington, and Norton, chiefly supply the town of Sheffield with milk, which is carried thither in barrels slung on horses or asses. A considerable quantity of camomile is cultivated, for medicinal purposes, in the parishes of Ashover, Morton, Shirland, and North and South Winfield; this plant having been introduced into the county about the year 1740 : about eighty acres are now planted, the cultivation and gathering of which afford employment to a great number of women and children. Neat cattle, chiefly for the purposes of the dairy, form a principal feature in the economy of the Derbyshire farms, although the county possesses no original nor distinct breed, notwithstanding that some of the breeders call their stock the New Derbyshire Long-horned breed. The practice of making cheese from the new milk, and butter afterwards from the whey, is either entirely unknown, or very little practised in the greater part of England, though here well established and approved. The breeds of sheep now most prevalent are, the Woodland sheep, in the northern tract still called the Woodlands (though now nearly bare of wood), and the New Leicester, in the southern and eastern parts of the county. Derbyshire has long been celebrated, and ranks next to Leicestershire of all the English counties, for its stout, clean-legged breed of work horses, principally black. The number of asses kept in the county is considerable; they are chiefly employed in carrying coal from the pits in the vicinity of the towns, for the supply of the poor, and in hawking pottery. This being so considerable a dairy county, a great number of hogs is kept in it, though there is no particular or characteristic breed.

The soil consists chiefly of clay, loam, sand, and peat, very irregularly intermixed : the southern part, which has been distinguished by the name of the fertile district, consists principally of a red loam on various under soils. Peat mosses abound in the northern part of the county, denominated the High Peak. The sub-strata of the southern part, comprised within a line drawn east and west from Sandiacre to Ashbourn, consist of gravel, intermixed with large portions of red marl, of very irregular forms; in several parts of which are beds of gypsum of considerable extent ; the gravel occupies a tract of nearly seventy-seven thousand acres, and the red marl eighty-one thousand. The sub-strata of the other parts of Derbyshire are, limestone of various kinds, with toad-stone ; grit-stone, with shale ; and coal, with indurated clay ; all of which appear in the surface in certain parts, owing to their dipping in various directions. The lowermost of these is a stratum of limestone, the thickness of which has not been ascertained ; it occupies a narrow space on the western side of the county, extending southerly from the mountain called Mam Tor, to Hopton and Parwich, and nearly to Thorp, and contains forty-thousand five hundred acres: it abounds in caverns, of which several are of great extent, many are lined with incrustations of stalactite, and some have subterraneous streams running through them. Immediately above this stratum of limestone are three others of limestone, and three of toad-stone, in alternate layers, occupying nearly fifty-one thousand five hundred acres of the surface, and extending from Castleton, southward, to Hopton; and from Matlock, Youlgrave, Bakewell, and Stony-Middleton, on the eastern side, to Wormhill, and Chelmorton, on the western. The limestone is the true metalliferous rock of Derbyshire, and exclusively occupies the attention of the miner : there are few situations in the Peak where this rock does not contain numerous veins of lead-ore, or calamine. The several strata are also very abundant in corallines, shells, and various organic remains. In different parts the limestone is of so compact a quality as to be used as marble, particularly at Ashford, where it is black, and at Monyash, where it is of a mottled grey colour. The respective thicknesses of the six alternate strata of limestone and toad-stone, in a section between Grange Mill and Darley Moor, are stated by Mr. Whitehurst, in his "Inquiry into the Original State and Formation of the Earth," to be, "Of the first or uppermost limestone, fifty yards ; the first toad-stone, sixteen yards ; the second limestone, fifty yards ; the second toad-stone, forty-six yards ; the third limestone, sixty yards ; and the third toad-stone, twenty-two yards :" there are detached portions of these alternate strata in several parts of the county, but of no great extent. The strata which come next in succession above those of limestone and toad-stone, are millstone-grit and shale ; the former being, according to Farey's View, from one hundred and fifty to one hundred and seventy yards thick, and resting on the latter, which is about the same thickness. This district is surrounded by the grit-stone district, as it is called, though in several parts the grit-stone is wanting, only the shale appearing. There are many detached patches of the grit rock, under which, on all sides, the shale is conspicuous, both in the grit-stone and in the limestone district. Within this extensive stratum of 'shale are several masses of dark blue, or black limestone, one of which, immediately north of Fenny-Bentley, and another north-west of Bakewell, and south-west of Ashford, are of considerable extent. That portion of the county in which the grit-stone and shale strata appear, comprises one hundred and sixty thousand five hundred acres.

The coal strata, usually termed coal measures, occupy a large portion of the eastern side of the county, bounded on the north by a part of Yorkshire, on the west extending to Duffield ; on the south to Dale Abbey, and nearly to Sandiacre : the seams vary in thickness, and are separated by numerous strata of grit-stone and argillaceous earth, known by the names of 'bind, clunch, and shale. Several of the coal shales contain beds of iron-stone, and an abundance and variety of impressions of ferns and other plants. Part of the coal field, of which Ashby de la Zouch lies nearly in the centre, extends into this county, near its southern extremity, in the parishes of Hartshorn, Gresley, and Measham, being surrounded by the layer of red marl, to which it dips in every direction. There are also small veins of coal at Axe-edge, and Chinley hills. Mr. Farey computes the total extent of the coal measures at one hundred and ninety thousand acres. On the eastern side of the county is a stratum of yellow magnesian limestone, extending from Barlborough, southward, to Hardwick, and bounded on the west by Barlborough, Bolsover, and Hault-Hucknall, occupying about twenty-one thousand six hundred acres. In several parts of the county, more

especially in the coal district, the strata are broken and dislocated in various directions; and these fractures, some being of great extent, are, by the miners, called faults.

The chief subterraneous productions, as articles of commerce, are lead, iron, calamine, fluor, gypsum, coal, marble, and various sorts of stone. It has been satisfactorily ascertained that the Derbyshire lead mines were worked by the Romans, and probably by the Britons. They are chiefly in the hundreds of Wirksworth, and High Peak, so far north as Castleton : there are lead mines also in the parishes of Ashover and Crich. The whole number enumerated by Mr. Farey, in his View of the Minerals of this county, amounts to about two hundred and fifty, of which twenty-two are stated to produce an abundant supply of ore ; the latter are situated in the parishes or chapelries of Ashover, Matlock, Cromford, Wirksworth, Bonsall, Youlgrave, Elton, Winster, Hope, Eyam, Great Longstone, and Monyash. The annual quantity of lead raised in Derbyshire, about 1789, as stated by Pilkington, was between five and six thousand tons ; but of late years, not above half that quantity has been raised, many mines having ceased working on account of the reduced price of lead. The most productive mine, of late years, has been the Gang-mine, in the liberty of Cromford. The lead was originally smelted by wood fires, on hills in the open air ; but this inconvenient mode was succeeded by hearth-furnaces the last of which was pulled down about the year 1780, the improved cupola furnace, now in use, having been introduced from Wales. The smelting business has of late been on the decline, and there are now only nine cupolas at work in the county. A considerable quantity of lead is sent from Cromford to Derby, where it is used in making white lead, red lead, sheet-lead, pipes, and shot : the remainder is chiefly sent down the canal from Chesterfield to coasting vessels in the Trent, for the Hull and London markets. Several of the lead mines produce ores of zinc in considerable quantity; the more valuable of which, the calamine, or oxyde of zinc, is found in twenty-four mines, in the parishes of Matlock, Bonsall, Carsington, Castleton, Bakewell, Youlgrave, and Bradborne ; the most productive being the Whitlow mine, in the parish of Bonsall. The principal source of demand for this mineral is its utility in the composition of brass, first discovered about sixty years ago : the average annual quantity raised for the four or five years preceding 1817, was four hundred tons ; its price in 1817, in a crude state, was from £5 to £6. 10. per ton; and in a prepared state, from £14. 10. to £15. 10. per ton. A great quantity is sent to Sheffield, for the brass company at that place. The other species of zinc-ore is called blende, or black-jack, which is found in thirteen of the mines ; it is of inferior value, and less used. Fluors of various colours are found in several of the mines, being much used in the fusion of brittle and churlish ore : the more beautiful specimens, called Blue-john, are wrought into vases and various other ornamental articles, at the manufactory at Matlock.

Iron has been known as the produce of this county from a very early period : the district in which the iron-stone is found extends from the neighbourhood of Dale Abbey, northward, throughout the hundred of Scarsdale into Yorkshire. Mr. Farey ranks Derbyshire as the fourth county in England as to its produce of pig iron. Until about the year 1770, all the cast and bar iron in Derbyshire was made by small charcoal furnaces; the first furnace of the modern construction, heated with coke, or pit-coal, having been erected at Morley-Park. Of the eleven furnaces which were in full work in 1806, some have not, of late, been regularly worked, on account of the low price of British iron. There are eight forges in the county, in which bar iron is made from the pigs. The lead mines in the Peak, and in the hundred of Wirksworth, belonged at an early period to the crown. The dukes of Devonshire have long been lessees of those in the hundred of High Peak; and the lease of those in the hundred of Wirksworth having been sold under a decree of Chancery, is now vested in Richard Arkwright, Esq. The mines and miners of this county are governed by certain ancient customs and regulations, which were ascertained by a jury under a commission granted in the year 1287, but which vary in different manors. The mining concerns are under the superintendence of an officer, called a bar-master, who holds courts twice a year, at which all questions are decided respecting the duties payable to the crown or the lessee; all disputes are settled relative to working the mines, and punishments are inflicted for all aggressions upon mineral property. Debts incurred in working the mines are also cognizable in the bar-mote courts, which are held for the High Peak at Monyash, and for the hundred of Wirksworth at Wirksworth. One of the most remarkable of the ancient mining customs is that by which any adventurer who shall discover a vein of lead unoccupied, in the king's field, has a right to work it on the land of any person, without making any compensation to the proprietor: this custom is still in force, but it is understood that gardens, orchards, and highways, are excepted; it is the office of the bar-master, being applied to for that purpose, to put adventurers in possession of such veins by them discovered. The duties, or tolls payable to the crown, and to the lord of the manor, are of great antiquity, and vary much in different manors. Tithe is paid for lead-ore in the parishes of Eyam and Wirksworth. The brazen dish, by which the measure of the ore is regulated, and which appears from the inscription upon it to have been made in the year 1512, is kept at Wirksworth.

It is probable that some of the Derbyshire collieries were worked by the Romans: there is evidence of their having been known to the Saxons; and it is on record that those at Derby, which are still considered to produce some of the best coal in the county, were worked as early as 1306. The principal coal district is the same as that of the iron-stone, including the greater part of the hundred of Scarsdale, and extending, southward, on the eastern side of the county, as far as Dale Abbey. The coal exported is chiefly of the hard kind, being that which finds the readiest sale in the midland counties, to which the Derbyshire coal is sent. Gypsum, or alabaster, is obtained in considerable quantities, chiefly in the parish of Chellaston; the average annual quantity raised from the pit at that place was, about the year 1817, nearly one thousand tons. In its native state it is used for columns, chimney-pieces, and ornamental buildings, as also for tomb-stones and monumental effigies: in a calcined state it is applied, at the potteries and elsewhere, to all the uses of plaister of Paris; the inferior sort is used for plaister-floors. The limestone of this county forms an important article of its mineral produce. Mr. Farey enumerates forty-six quarries,

and sixty-three kilns, in which it is burned for sale, and from which great quantities are sold, chiefly for agricultural purposes, for the use of this and some of the neighbouring counties; the largest quarries are at Ashover, Buxton, Crich, and Calver, near Baslow: a considerable quantity of lime is sent from Calver into Yorkshire, and from the neighbourhood of Buxton into Cheshire and Staffordshire. A species of the Derbyshire limestone is in request as marble, for chimney-pieces, slabs, &c.: the quarries from which this sort of limestone, commonly called Derbyshire marble, is procured, are nineteen in number, and are situated in the parishes of Bakewell and Matlock. The number of stone quarries is one hundred and thirty-eight, some of which produce stone of a good and durable quality for building, which has been much used in the principal private and public edifices in the county, and is exported in large quantities, especially from the quarries in the parish of Wingerworth. Grindstones, of the millstone-grit, are obtained from nineteen quarries; they are in great request, and are extensively shipped by the canals to the south-eastern parts of England. Stones for whetting scythes are procured from thirteen quarries; finer whet-stones from seven others; and the finest, called hones, from quarries at Codnor Park and Woodthorp, near Wingerworth. Several of the mines produce ochres, and a few of them small quantities of china-clay, which has of late years been sent to the potteries in Staffordshire. Few counties exhibit a greater number or variety of extraneous fossils than this; the several strata of limestone, and some of those of grit-stone, containing an abundance of organic remains, both animal and vegetable.

The principal rivers are, the Trent, the Derwent, the Wye, the Dove, the Erwash, and the Rother. The Trent first becomes a boundary between Derbyshire and Staffordshire in the parish of Croxall, and so continues to Newton-Solney, a little beyond which village it enters the county, crossing it, from west to east, in a course of about twenty-four miles, and quitting at its junction with the Erwash, near Nottingham. Pursuant to an act of parliament procured by the Earl of Uxbridge, in 1699, the Trent was made navigable to Burton bridge; but, in the year 1805, the navigation from that bridge down to Shardlow was given up, by agreement with the proprietors of the Trent and Mersey canal, which runs by its side, and, as connected with Derbyshire, it is now navigable only from Shardlow to the mouth of the Erwash. The Derwent rises on the moors, at the northern extremity of the county; it flows by Hathersage, through Chatsworth park, Darley-dale, Matlock, Cromford, Belper, and Derby, and falls into the Trent about a mile beyond Little Wilne, after a course of about forty-six miles: this river was formerly navigable from Wilne ferry up to Derby, but the navigation was given up when the Derby canals were completed, in 1794. The Wye rises a little above Buxton, and, running through Monsall-dale, Ashford, and Bakewell, falls into the Derwent near Rowsley. The Dove, which rises in the same hill as the Wye, a few miles south of Buxton, is for many miles the boundary between Derbyshire and Staffordshire, and, passing through Dove-dale, falls into the Derwent near Newton-Solney. The Erwash rises on the skirts of Sherwood Forest, in Nottinghamshire, and is, during the greater part of its course, the boundary between that county and Derbyshire, passing by Pinxton, and near Ilkeston and Sandiacre, and falling into the Trent about a mile and a half east from Long Eaton. The Rother, rising near Padley, runs by Chesterfield, and enters Yorkshire, between Killamarsh and Beighton.

It having been found of great importance to procure the convenience of water-carriage for the produce of the numerous mines and quarries, and the goods of its manufactories, many canals have in consequence been projected, and several of them completed, some entirely within the county, and others commencing or terminating in it. The great undertaking of the Trent and Mersey, or Grand Trunk canal, which forms part of the grand communication between Liverpool, Hull, Bristol, and London, was begun in 1766, by the celebrated Mr. Brindley, and completed in 1777, under his successors, Mr. Smeaton and Mr. Rennie: it passes through Derbyshire, from Burton to its termination at Shardlow, following the course of the Trent: its chief utility, as relates to the produce of Derbyshire, is for the conveyance of cheese, malt, and gypsum. The Chesterfield canal was begun in 1771, by Mr. Brindley, and finished in 1776, by his brother-in-law, Mr. Henshall: it enters Derbyshire at Killamarsh, and terminates at Chesterfield. its objects, as connected with this county, are the exportation of coal, lead, cast iron, limestone, freestone, pottery-ware, &c.; and the importation of grain, deals, bar iron, &c. The Erwash canal, begun about 1777, has its line chiefly through Derbyshire, in the vale of the Erwash: it commences in the Trent navigation, and terminates at Langley Mill, where it joins the Cromford canal: it is chiefly serviceable in the exportation of coal, limestone, iron, lead, millstones, grind-stones, marble, freestone &c.; and the importation of corn, malt, deals, &c. The Cromford canal was begun about 1789, and completed about 1793: its line is wholly in Derbyshire, commencing at Langley Mill, and terminating at Cromford: its chief use is the same as that of the Erwash canal. At Butterley is a tunnel, about fifty-seven yards below the Derwent ridge, two thousand nine hundred and seventy-eight yards long, and nine feet wide; at Lea-Bridge near Cromford, the canal is carried over the river Derwent by an aqueduct, two hundred yards long, and thirty feet high, built in 1792; and over the Amber, at Bull bridge, is another aqueduct, of the same length, fifty feet high. The line of the Derby canal, which is forty-four feet wide, is wholly in the county; commencing in the Trent and Mersey canal, north of Swarkston, passing by Derby, with branches to Little Eaton, whence is a railway to the collieries at Horsley, Denby, &c.: its chief use is for supplying Derby with coal, building-stone, gypsum, &c.; and for exporting coal, manufactured goods, cheese, &c. The Nutbrook canal, constructed about 1793, for the exportation of coal, and the importation of lime-stone, commences in the Erwash canal, and terminates at Shipley wharf. The Ashby de la Zouch canal, begun about 1794, and completed in 1805, is connected with the southern part of Derbyshire, and by it coal and limestone are exported. The Peak Forest canal, begun about 1794, and completed in 1806, enters Derbyshire at Marple bridge, and terminates at Bugsworth: at Marple is an aqueduct over the river Mersey, nearly one hundred feet high, completed in 1797: the objects of this canal, as connected with Derbyshire, are, the exportation of lime-stone, building and paving-stones, and, at its north end,

coal, and the importation of deals, and pig iron; and, at its south end, coal. The great road from London to Manchester enters Derbyshire at Cavendish bridge, and, passing through Derby and Ashbourn, enters Staffordshire at Hanger bridge, about a mile and three quarters beyond the latter town. Another turnpike road to Manchester goes from Ashbourn, by way of Buxton, about six miles beyond which town, at Whaley bridge, it enters Cheshire. And a third road to Manchester passes from Derby through Matlock, Bakewell, and Chapel en le Frith, joining the last-mentioned road at Whaley bridge.

Derbyshire exhibits few British remains, except the numerous artificial formations of earth and stones, called *cairns*, which have been raised upon the moors, several of which, on being opened, have been found to contain human bones, and urns, with beads, rings, and other relics. The only Roman remains worthy of particular mention are, the altar preserved at Haddon hall, the inscribed blocks or pigs of lead found in different situations, and the silver plate found in Risley park: Roman coins have frequently been found in various parts of the county. One of the principal British roads, the Iknield-street, ran through the whole extent of the county, from south-west to north-east, from the borders of Staffordshire to those of Yorkshire. Derbyshire was also traversed in various directions by Roman roads; those most distinctly visible being that called the Bathom-gate, leading from Brough to Buxton; a second, leading from Buxton towards Little Chester; and a third, supposed to have come from Chesterton, near Newcastle, in Staffordshire, to Little Chester. The undoubted Roman stations in the county are, Little Chester, Brough, Melandra Castle, in the parish of Glossop, and Buxton. Many of the churches present considerable remains of early Norman architecture, the most remarkable specimens appearing in those of Repton and Melbourne, and the desecrated church of Steetley, in the parish of Whitwell. Prior to the Reformation, there were thirteen religious houses, including two preceptories of the Knights Hospitallers, and one of the brethren of St. Lazarus; there were two collegiate churches, and five ancient hospitals. Of the monastic buildings, the remains, all of inconsiderable magnitude, are those of Dale abbey, Beauchief abbey, Repton priory, and the preceptory at Yeveley, alias Stidd. The only ancient castles of which there are any considerable remains, are those of the Peak, Codnor, Horseley, and Melbourne. The most remarkable old mansion-houses are Haddon hall, Hardwick hall, and South Winfield manor-house, which last is in ruins. The custom of *rush-bearing* still prevails in the northern part of the county: the ceremony of strewing the church with rushes annually takes place on the festival of its tutelar saint, but in the Peak Forest is always held on Midsummer eve. The ancient custom of hanging up garlands of roses in the churches, with a pair of gloves cut out of white paper, which had been carried before the corpse of a young unmarried woman at her funeral, prevails in many of the parishes of the Peak. The most remarkable tepid springs in Derbyshire, are those of Buxton, Matlock, and Bakewell. There are different sulphureous springs, of which that at Kedleston is most used, and various chalybeate waters, the most celebrated being at Quarndon, two miles from Derby: there is an ebbing and flowing well, at the distance of two miles eastward from Chapel en el Frith.

DERBY HILLS, an extra-parochial liberty, in the hundred of REPTON and GRESLEY, county of DERBY, 9 miles (S.) from Derby, containing 76 inhabitants.

DERBY (WEST), a chapelry in the parish of WALTON on the HILL, hundred of WEST DERBY, county palatine of LANCASTER, 4½ miles (W.) from Prescot, containing 6304 inhabitants. The living is a perpetual curacy, in the archdeaconry and diocese of Chester, endowed with £800 private benefaction, £200 royal bounty, and £3000 parliamentary grant, and in the patronage of the Rector of Walton. The chapel is dedicated to St. Mary. West Derby is a very ancient place, having given name to the hundred. At the period of the Norman survey here was a decayed castle, which had belonged to Edward the Confessor.

DEREHAM (EAST), a market town and parish in the hundred of MITFORD, county of NORFOLK, 17 miles (W.N.W.) from Norwich, and 101 (N.E. by N.) from London, containing 3244 inhabitants, and, including the hamlet of Dillington, in the hundred of Launditch, 3273. This place, anciently called *Deerham*, from the number of deer by which it was frequented, and distinguished by its adjunct from a village of the same name, is of very remote antiquity. During the Heptarchy, Withburga, youngest daughter of Anna, King of the East Angles, founded a monastery here, of which she became prioress, and dying in 743, was buried in the church-yard; her remains, in 798, were removed into the conventual church, and after the destruction of the monastery by the Danes, were, in 974, translated to Ely, where they were enshrined with those of her sisters, in the cathedral church of that city. A spring, to which miraculous cures were attributed, is said to have risen up in that part of the church-yard where she was first interred, which is now a public bath; the Norman arch with which it was covered is still carefully preserved. In 1581, the town suffered severely from fire, and in 1679 the greater part of it was by a similar calamity reduced to ashes. It is pleasantly situated nearly in the centre of the county, and within the last century has been so materially improved by widening and levelling the streets, as to render it one of the handsomest market towns in Norfolk: it is paved with pebbles; the houses are in general neatly built, and of modern appearance, and the inhabitants are amply supplied with excellent water: in the centre of the town is a handsome obelisk, erected by Sir Edward Astley, Bart. The theatre, a small but neat building of brick, is opened every alternate year by a regular company of performers: a book club has been established under good regulations, and is patronised by the most respectable inhabitants of the town and neighbourhood; and on the site of the ancient market cross, a handsome assembly-room has been erected by subscription. The market is on Friday, for corn, general provisions, cattle, and pigs, for which last it is the most considerable mart in the county: the fairs are on the Thursday and Friday before Old Midsummer-day, and on the Thursday and Friday before Old Michaelmas-day, for cattle, sheep, and toys. The county magistrates hold a petty session for the division every alternate week; and a court baron and court leet are held annually by the lord of the manor.

The living is a vicarage with the perpetual curacy of Hoe, in the archdeaconry of Norfolk, and diocese of

Norwich, rated in the king's books at £17. 3. 4½., and in the patronage of the Crown: there is also a rectory, rated at £41. 3. 1½. The church, dedicated to St. Nicholas, formerly the conventual church of the monastery of St. Withburga, and made parochial in 798, is a spacious cruciform structure, partly in the Norman and partly in the early style of English architecture, with a tower rising from the intersection, and open for a considerable height to the interior of the church: connected with the transepts were the chapels of the Holy Cross, over which was the treasury of St. Withburga, St. Mary, and St. Edmund; in the chancel is an ancient eagle on a pedestal of brass, supported on three small lions. The roof on the north side is supported by clustered, and on the south by round massive, columns; the font is beautifully sculptured with representations of the four Evangelists, eight of the Apostles, the Crucifixion, and the Seven Sacraments of the Romish church: in the south transept is an antique chest of oak, richly carved, taken from Buckingham castle, in which are deposited the records of the church and parish. Among the monuments is a white marble tablet to the memory of Cowper the poet, who resided in this place for the last nine years of his life, and was interred in the church. The bells, which were supposed to endanger the tower, have been removed into a detached building called the New Clocher, erected for that purpose in the church-yard. There are places of worship for Baptists, Independents, and Wesleyan Methodists. A National school, for children of both sexes, is supported by subscription. Mr. Aaron Williamson, in 1710, left by will some houses and land for apprenticing two poor boys of the parish; and there are several charitable bequests for distribution among the poor. Bishop Bonner was rector of this parish from 1534 to the year 1540.

DEREHAM (WEST), a parish in the hundred of CLACKCLOSE, county of NORFOLK, 3¾ miles (W. by N.) from Stoke-Ferry, containing 520 inhabitants. The living is a perpetual curacy, in the archdeaconry of Norfolk, and diocese of Norwich, endowed with £33 per annum private benefaction, £400 royal bounty, and £500 parliamentary grant, and in the patronage of the Rev. C. L. Jenyns. The church, dedicated to St. Andrew has at the west end a large round tower, built of ragstone, upon which another of brick has been erected, of an octagonal form, embattled and coped. Another church, which was dedicated to St. Peter, formerly stood here, but no traces of it are discernible. An abbey for Premonstratensian canons was founded in 1188, to the honour of the Blessed Virgin Mary, by Hubert, Dean of York, and afterwards Archbishop of Canterbury; it was valued, in the 26th of Henry VIII., at £252. 12. 11. There are considerable remains of this once stately structure, particularly the gate-house, a lofty quadrangular pile of brick, embattled, from each angle of which rises an octagonal tower, groined with free-stone: over the arched entrance is a shield, bearing the arms of the abbey.

DERITEND, a chapelry in the parish of ASTON, Birmingham division of the hundred of HEMLINGFORD, county of WARWICK, 1 mile (S. E. by S.) from Birmingham. The population is returned with the parish. There is an extensive brewery of ale at this place.

DERSINGHAM, a parish in the Lynn division of the hundred of FREEBRIDGE county of NORFOLK, 4¼ miles (N. N. E.) from Castle-Rising, containing 534 inhabitants. The living is a vicarage, in the archdeaconry and diocese of Norwich, rated in the king's books at £5. 6. 8., and in the patronage of D. Hoste, Esq. The church, dedicated to St. Nicholas, is a large pile, composed of boulder and flint, and covered with lead; it has, at the west end, a strong quadrangular tower, crowned with a lantern and a small shaft. At the south-east side of the church-yard there is an ancient chapel in ruins.

DERTHORPE, a chapelry in the parish of WELL, Wold division of the hundred of CALCEWORTH, parts of LINDSEY, county of LINCOLN. The population is returned with the parish.

DESBOROUGH, a parish in the hundred of ROTH-WELL, county of NORTHAMPTON, 1¾ mile (N. N. W.) from Rothwell, containing 908 inhabitants. The living is a discharged vicarage, in the archdeaconry of Northampton, and diocese of Peterborough, rated in the king's books at £8, endowed with £10 per annum private benefaction, and £200 royal bounty. R. S. Cotton, Esq. was patron in 1800. The church is dedicated to St. Giles. Ferdinando Poulton, an eminent lawyer, who compiled the statutes at large, from Magna Charta to the 16th of James I., was born here; he died in 1617, and lies buried in the chancel, under a plain slab, with a latin inscription.

DESFORD, a parish in the hundred of SPARK-ENHOE, county of LEICESTER, 5 miles (E.) from Market-Bosworth, containing, with the hamlet of Barrons-Park, 872 inhabitants. The living is a discharged rectory, in the archdeaconry of Leicester, and diocese of Lincoln, rated in the king's books at £8. 9. 7., and in the patronage of the Crown. The church is dedicated to St. Martin.

DETCHANT, a township in that part of the parish of BELFORD which is in the northern division of BAM-BROUGH ward, county of NORTHUMBERLAND, 2¼ miles (N. W. by N.) from Belford, containing 128 inhabitants.

DETHWICK-LEA, a chapelry in that part of the parish of ASHOVER which is in the hundred of WIRKS-WORTH, county of DERBY, 2 miles (S. E. by E.) from Matlock, containing, with the hamlet of Holloway, 492 inhabitants. The living is a perpetual curacy with the rectory of Ashover, in the archdeaconry of Derby, and diocese of Lichfield and Coventry, endowed with £400 private benefaction, and £1000 royal bounty. The chapel, a small edifice with a handsome and lofty tower, was built in 1530, by Mr. Babington. Dethwick is in the honour of Tutbury, duchy of Lancaster, and within the jurisdiction of a court of pleas held at Tutbury every third Tuesday, for the recovery of debts under 40s.

DEUXHILL, a parish within the liberty of the borough of WENLOCK, though locally in the hundred of Stottesden, county of SALOP, 4 miles (S. by W.) from Bridgenorth, containing 49 inhabitants. The living is a discharged rectory, with Glazeley, consolidated in 1760 with the rectory of Chetton, in the archdeaconry of Salop, and diocese of Hereford, rated in the king's books at £4. 12. 3½. V. Vickers, Esq. was patron in 1822.

DEVEREUX (ST.), a parish in the hundred of WEBTREE, county of HEREFORD, 7¾ miles (S. W.) from Hereford, containing, with the hamlet of Didley, 208 inhabitants. The living is a rectory, in the archdeaconry and diocese of Hereford, rated in the king's

books at £6, 15. 7¼., and in the patronage of Edward Bolton Clive, Esq.

DEVERHILL (LONGBRIDGE), a parish in the southern division of the hundred of DAMERHAM, though locally in the hundred of Heytesbury, county of WILTS, 2½ miles (S.) from Warminster, containing 1349 inhabitants. The living is a vicarage, with the curacy of Monckton-Deverhill, in the archdeaconry and diocese of Salisbury, rated in the king's books at £12. The Marquis of Bath was patron in 1805. The church is dedicated to St. Peter and St. Paul. Deverhill derives its name from the rivulet Dever, which here has a subterranean course.

DEVERHILL (MONCKTON), a parish in the southern division of the hundred of DAMERHAM, though locally in the hundred of Mere, county of WILTS, 4¼ miles (N. E. by N.) from Mere, containing 181 inhabitants. The living is a perpetual curacy annexed to the vicarage of Longbridge-Deverhill, in the archdeaconry and diocese of Salisbury.

DEVIL'S-HOUSE, in the parish of WOOLWICH, hundred of BLACKHEATH, lathe of SUTTON at HONE, county of KENT, though locally in the hundred of Becontree, county of Essex, ½ a mile (N. by E.) from Woolwich, to and from which there is a regular ferry across the Thames. A chapel of ease formerly stood here, together with several houses, the foundations of which are still discernible; there is now only an inn, called the Devil's House, with about five hundred acres of marsh land attached.

DEVIZES, a borough and market town, having separate jurisdiction, locally in the hundred of Potterne and Cannings, county of WILTS, 22 miles (N. W. by N.) from Salisbury, 19 (E. by S.) from Bath, and 89 (W. by S.) from London, on the road from London to Bath, containing 4208 inhabitants. Amongst the early writers this town has received the several appellations of

Arms.

Devisæ, Divisæ, De vies, and *Divisio,* because it is said to have been divided between the King and the Bishop of Salisbury, &c. It appears to have had its origin in the erection of a spacious and strong castle, or fortress, by Roger, the celebrated and wealthy bishop of Salisbury, in the reign of Henry I., who, with his two nephews, Alexander, Bishop of Lincoln, and Nigel, Bishop of Ely, was subsequently sentenced to imprisonment within its walls by King Stephen, on a charge of disaffection. Before the order could be executed, Nigel escaped, and having fled to this fortress, garrisoned it with troops, and prepared to defend it, until the expected arrival of the Empress Matilda; but the king having besieged it and demanded immediate surrender, on the alternative of hanging the son of Bishop Roger on a gallows which had been erected in front of the castle, that prelate, to save the youth from an ignominious death, bound himself by a solemn oath to take no sustenance till the king should be put in possession. This oath being made known to the Bishop of Ely, effected the surrender of the castle at the end of three days, and that fortress, together with the bishop's treasures, amounting to the value of forty thousand marks, fell into the hands of Stephen. About three years after this event, the castle was seized by Robert Fitz-Hubert, on pretence of holding it for Matilda; on her arrival, however, he refused to give up possession, and was in consequence treated as a rebel by both the contending parties, and eventually hanged as a traitor. In 1233, Hubert de Burgh, formerly prime minister to Henry III., was imprisoned within the castle, but on the appointment of Peter de Rupibus, his avowed enemy, to the government of it, he prevailed on two of his guards to contrive his escape, and took sanctuary behind the high altar of the parish church, whence he was dragged, with the crucifix in his hand, and carried back to prison. This violation of ecclesiastical privileges produced a remonstrance to the king from several prelates, on which the prisoner was re-conveyed to the church, and the sheriff received orders from that monarch to blockade it, and compel Hubert, by famine, to surrender himself; but notwithstanding that precaution, he once more effected his escape, and fled into Wales. About the end of the reign of Edward III., the castle was dismantled, and part of its materials were subsequently used to erect a mansion at Bromeham, about three miles distant. In the reign of Henry VIII., the town, then called by Leland *The Vies*, (an appellation still retained by the Wiltshire peasantry,) was celebrated for its market, and chiefly inhabited by clothiers. During the parliamentary war, a battle was fought here between the parliamentarian and the royalist forces, under the Marquis of Hertford and Prince Maurice, who were pursued hither by Sir William Waller, on their retreat towards Oxford, after the battle of Lansdown; the town was intrenched, and the approaches to it barricadoed by Lord Ralph Hopton, and the Earl of Marlborough, and Sir William, having invested the town closely, constructed a battery upon a neighbouring height, fired upon the place, and made several unsuccessful attempts to penetrate into the interior; he likewise intercepted the approach of the Earl of Crawford with a supply of powder for the royalists, and having captured the whole convoy, summoned the besieged to surrender. A treaty for capitulation was begun, but at this juncture Sir William was obliged to withdraw his troops from before the town, in order to oppose Lord Wilmot, who had been despatched by the king from Oxford, with one thousand five hundred horse, and two pieces of artillery, to protect the infantry in their retreat to the main army. The parliamentarian general awaited the approach of Lord Wilmot on Roundaway Hill, where, encouraged by the small number of his antagonist's forces, he commenced the attack, which terminated in the total dispersion of his cavalry, the capture of his artillery, and the destruction of his infantry, who being attacked by the troops from Devizes, were most of them slain or taken prisoners. Sir William fled to Bristol, having sustained a loss of more than two thousand men, together with all his cannon, ammunition, baggage, and stores: the loss of the royalists on this occasion was comparatively inconsiderable.

The town, which is nearly in the centre of the county, stands on an elevation, and consists of several streets, which are paved, and lighted with gas; the houses, many of which are handsome, are for the most part irregularly built; the inhabitants are supplied with water from deep wells dug in the sand rock. The woollen manufacture, once the principal branch of business, is now extinct: the manufacture of silk has been recently introduced, and affords employment to upwards of four hundred persons, principally children; there are three manufactories in the town, and one about half a mile distant, for silk-throwing: the weaving of crape and sarsenet is on the increase. The malting business is carried on extensively; and a large snuff manufactory has been established for many years. The Kennet and Avon canal intersects the parish, which abounds with coal and Bath stone. The market is on Thursday, and is the largest in the West of England for corn, of which a great quantity is pitched in the market-place, besides what is sold by sample. There are fairs annually, on February 14th, for horses; Holy Thursday and April 20th, for cattle; and June 13th, July 5th, and October 2nd and 20th, for cattle, hops, cloth, &c.: those on the 20th of April and the 20th of October are held on the green, beyond the boundaries of the borough. A market-cross, erected in 1815, at the sole expense of Lord Sidmouth, many years recorder, and also a representative in parliament for this borough, is said to have cost nearly £2000.

Corporate Seal.

The first charter of incorporation, granted by the Empress Matilda, was suspended during the reign of Stephen, renewed by Henry II., and confirmed, together with the grant of additional privileges, by John, Henry III., and Edward III., which placed the burgesses upon an equality with the citizens of Winchester. Several immunities were added during subsequent reigns, until the time of Charles I., under whose charter the government is vested in a mayor, recorder, and thirty-four common council-men; twelve of whom, including the recorder and justice, are styled capital burgesses, from among whom the mayor is annually chosen by the common council, who also fill up vacancies in their own body, and have the power of electing an unlimited number of free burgesses. The mayor, recorder, and justice, (who is chosen by the corporation), are justices of the peace within the borough, and have power to hold a court of record, for the recovery of sums not exceeding £40, every Friday, at which either the mayor, recorder, or his deputy, must preside, assisted by any number of the capital burgesses, in all not less than four. The petty sessions for the Devizes division of the hundred of Potterne and Cannings are held here, as are also the quarter sessions for the county, in rotation with Salisbury, Warminster, and Marlborough. This borough returned members to all the parliaments of Edward I., to those of the 1st, 8th, and 19th of Edward II., and 4th of Edward III., since which its returns have been constant. The right of election is vested in the corporation, including a few honorary members: the mayor is the returning officer. Meetings for the nomination of county members and coroners are always held in this town. The town-hall is a handsome modern edifice, having a semicircular front, supported by Ionic columns on a rustic basement: it contains appropriate offices for public business, and a large room used for public meetings and assemblies;

F 2

on the ground floor a cheese market is held. A new gaol, constructed of brick and stone, was erected in 1810, about a mile north-westward from the town : it consists of the governor's house, which is polygonal in form, and occupies the centre, having an infirmary above it, and from the top commands a fine prospect towards Bath and Gloucester ; the cells, which in this part of the building are also polygonal, are separated from the boundary wall by a considerable space of ground, laid out in gardens : the front of the house and the whole boundary wall are very substantially built of hewn stone.

Devizes comprises the parishes of St. John and St. Mary the Virgin, the livings of which form a united rectory, not in charge, in the archdeaconry and diocese of Salisbury, and in the patronage of the Crown. St. John's church is a spacious structure, partly in the Norman style and partly in the later style of English architecture, with a square embattled tower, and consists of a nave and two aisles, transept, chancel, and two chantry chapels; the oldest portion, which comprises the chancel, transept, and tower, is supposed to have been built by Bishop Roger, about the same period as the castle : the chancel is arched with bold ribs springing from clustered capitals, and the tower is supported by two circular and two pointed arches, enriched with foliage and zigzag mouldings of different periods : it contains several marble monuments of the families of Heathcote and Sutton. St. Mary's, in the north-eastern part of the town, has evidently been erected at different periods : the chancel is the oldest portion, being in the early Norman style, and built probably soon after the Conquest; the south porch, having a pointed arch, with zigzag mouldings, is a fine specimen of the prevailing style in the reigns of Henry II. and Richard I. ; the rest of the edifice was rebuilt by William Smyth, who died in 1436 : the tower and body of the church are embattled and crowned with pinnacles : the nave and aisles are spacious and lofty, and the arches which separate them spring from octagonal columns : the architecture of the chancel resembles that of St. John's. At the eastern extremity of the town, and beyond the limits of the borough, is St. James' chapel, belonging to the vicarage of Bishop's Cannings. There are places of worship for Baptists, the Society of Friends, Independents, Presbyterians, and Wesleyan Methodists.

The Boar Club charity school, in which about forty boys are clothed, and, after three years' education, apprenticed, is supported by the donations and annual subscriptions of the members. A National school was erected at the expense of John Pearse, Esq. : there are likewise schools on the Lancasterian system, and infant schools. The site of the ancient castle, of which there are no vestiges, has been converted into pleasure grounds. Richard of Devizes, a Benedictine monk of the twelfth century, who wrote a chronicle of English History, was a native of this place. Mr. Joseph Allein, a non-conformist divine, and polemical writer of some celebrity, was born here in 1633. The late Sir Thomas Lawrence, the eminent portrait painter, and President of the Royal Society, passed much of the earlier part of his life in this town.

DEVONPORT, (formerly called Plymouth Dock,) a celebrated naval arsenal, in the parish of STOKE-DA-MERALL, hundred of ROBOROUGH, county of DEVON, 1¼ mile (W.) from Plymouth, and 218 (W. by S.) from London. The population is returned with the parish. In the reign of William III., a naval arsenal was established here under the name of Plymouth Dock, and to this event the town is indebted for its importance and present magnitude : in 1824, the appellation of Devonport was conferred upon it by royal permission. It was first fortified in the reign of George II., but the works have been much improved under an act of parliament passed in the 21st of George III. In the early part of the American war, Colonel Dixon, then commanding engineer at Plymouth, applied, on behalf of the troops in garrison at Dock, to the corporation of Plymouth, for supplies of water from a leat, a stream which had been conveyed to that borough by Sir Francis Drake; the application was refused for the alleged reason that this stream was insufficient to supply both places : various other plans were devised and proposed without success, till 1792, when Mr. Bryer, Messrs. Jones and Grey, and others, submitted a plan to the government, and also to the inhabitants, for supplying the latter with water on the same terms as those of Plymouth, and the government departments at a stipulated price ; which plan, under an act of parliament obtained in the same year, though not without strenuous opposition, was carried into effect by means of a stream brought from Dartmoor, in a circuitous line of thirty miles, to a reservoir on the north side of the town.

Devonport is situated on an eminence, bounded on the south and west by the mouth of the Tamar, which, expanding into an irregular æstuary, forms the capacious harbour at Hamoaze, and on the east by Stonehouse creek. The town is of an oblong figure, and the streets, which are regular and well built, nearly intersecting each other at right angles, are paved and lighted ; the footpaths, when washed by a shower, have a remarkably beautiful appearance, being paved with marble obtained on the manor, which receives a considerable polish from the action of the weather and the feet of passengers. The Fore-street, which crosses the upper part of the town in a direct line, is approached through a plain but handsome gateway on the east, where there is a fosse with a draw-bridge : the houses are in general respectable, and some of a superior order; the entire thoroughfare forming a good approach to the dock-yard. The town is protected on the north-east and south sides by a wall about twelve feet in height, called "the King's interior boundary wall ;" skirted on the west by the dock-yard and gun-wharf; and fortified on the sea side entrance by heavy batteries on Mount Wise: immediately south of the town are the houses of the Port Admiral and Governor, the telegraph, and grand parade. Without the wall is a line, or breastwork, with a fosse excavated in the solid rock, of from twelve to twenty feet in depth, planned by a Mr. Smelt, of the engineer department, and begun about the year 1756. In the lines are three barrier gates : the North Barrier, which leads to the passage across the Tamar; the Stoke Barrier, leading towards Tavistock, and the Stonehouse Barrier, conducting towards Stonehouse, Plymouth, &c. On the south side of the town, immediately above the sea-shore, is Richmond walk, raised under the direction of the Duke of Richmond, when master-general of the ordnance, for the accommodation of the inhabitants; it commands a fine view of Mount Edgecumbe, and forms a healthy and pleasant promenade. There is a small theatre in the southern part of the town : the public subscription library is ornamented with an Egyptian façade; and there is an elegant assembly-room at the royal hotel. Southward from the town are hot, cold, shower, vapour, and swimming-baths, with six convenient lodging-houses handsomely furnished. The commerce will be noticed in the account of Plymouth, of which port Devonport is a branch. The principal quays are at Mutton Cove, North Corner, and Morice Town. On the south is a ferry to Mount Edgecumbe, and another on the north-west, to Torpoint. The market days are Tuesday, Thursday, and Saturday, but the market is not chartered : the market-place is of recent erection, and for extent and accommodation, is inferior to none in the western part of England; it is well supplied with all kinds of provision, particularly with fish, but it is not a corn market.

The government of the town is vested in commissioners, among whom are the lord of the manor, who holds courts leet and baron at Michaelmas, the stewards of the manor, the rector of the parish, the commissioner of his majesty's dock-yard, the port admiral, the mayor, aldermen, and recorder of the boroughs of Plymouth and Saltash, the manorial lords of East Stonehouse, and of East and West Anthony, with the stewards of those manors : the affairs of the poor, the lighting, watching, and cleansing of the town, and the granting of licenses to porters and watermen, are all under their superintendence. The county magistrates hold petty sessions every Wednesday at the town-hall, for the despatch of business connected with the town and parish. The town-hall includes, in addition to its principal room, which is seventy-five feet by forty, a watch-house, temporary prison, engine-house, &c.; the front is decorated with a noble Athenian-Doric portico, finished with a horizontal blocking-course and tablet, instead of the usually adopted pediment ; near this edifice is a column erected to commemorate the naming of the town anew ; it is a fluted column of the Doric order, and from its summit, which is accessible by a spiral flight of one hundred and forty steps, there is a most splendid view. The port admiral's house is a new and elegant structure; the semaphore near it communicates with the flag-ship in the harbour, and is the first of thirty-two telegraphic stations connecting this place with the Admiralty in London. It is said that a communication has been conveyed to and from the metropolis in the short space of fifteen minutes. The dock-yard, one of the finest in the world, is bounded on the east by the town, from which it is separated by a wall, which is in some places thirty feet high, extending from north to south ; its water boundary forms a curve bending outwards in a westerly direction ; it occupies an area of seventy-two acres, including the projections of the jetties, and was extended to its present dimensions in 1768 : the land entrance is from Fore-street, having a carriage gate and a gate for foot passengers. Near this entrance is a chapel recently built by government, on the site of one erected in 1700, "by the generous and pious contributions of officers and seamen belonging to a squadron of men of war" under the superintendence of George St. Leo, Esq., at that time commissioner of the yard. In addition to a stipend from government, the chaplain receives twopence per

month from the pay of each of the officers and seamen belonging to ships laid up in ordinary. Opposite to this edifice are the military guard, and navy pay offices. To the south-west is a row of excellent houses occupied by the commissioner and other officers of the establishment, and fronted by a double row of lime trees, from which is a descent by a number of steps to two handsome buildings, one of which, the "Joiner's shop," is surmounted by a cupola. Facing these are the basin and dock, constructed in the reign of William III; the latter is sufficiently capacious for a seventy-four gun ship, being in length one hundred and ninety-seven feet three inches, in width sixty-five feet ten inches, and in depth twenty-three feet one inch : the basin is bounded on each side by jetty heads ; that on the south is named " the Master Attendant's stairs." Adjoining to this jetty is a handsome edifice of lime-stone, with the quoins and cornices of Portland-stone, four hundred and eighty feet in length, and three stories high, forming one side of a quadrangle, and called the " Rigging House :" over it is the sail loft ; and different store-houses complete the quadrangle, the area of which is the "Combustible Store-house," entirely composed of iron and stone, the geometrical staircase of which is greatly admired. To the southward is a slip for cleaning the bottoms of vessels, and beyond it the Camber, a canal seventy feet wide, terminating in a basin, which is bounded on the north by the boat-house : this was the boundary of the yard previously to 1768 ; all beyond, in a southerly direction, is called the New Ground. Here are the "Blacksmith's Shop," a building about two hundred and ten feet square, containing forty-eight forges, the fires of which annually consume one thousand three hundred chaldrons of coal, the anchor-wharf (the largest anchors made here weigh five tons), a boiling-house, mast-house, and pond, of which the last is enclosed from the sea by a strong wall ten feet thick, and three hundred and eighty long : it is supplied with water through two openings, of about forty feet wide, crossed by light wooden bridges.

Near the mast-house, in a southerly direction, is a small mount, called Bunker's hill, surmounted by a battery of five cannon (nine pounders), one of which is a beautiful brass piece, made at Paris : from this elevation the prospect is very fine and extensive. In the dock-yard are two lime-stone buildings, parallel to each other, two stories high, and one thousand two hundred feet long, called rope houses ; the largest cables made here are twenty-five inches in circumference, and one hundred fathoms long, weighing 116 cwt. 1 qr. 16 lb., and worth £ 404. 9. 3. ; a cable of this weight contains three thousand two hundred and forty yarns. Behind these buildings, in addition to dwellings and store-houses, is the Mould, or Model loft. On the north is the jetty, north stairs, and double dock, so called from being sufficiently large to contain two ships at a time: the gates form the segment of a circle, with their convex sides to the sea. The second dock, called the Union, or North dock, is two hundred and thirty-nine feet four inches, by eighty-six feet seven, and twenty-six feet ten in depth: it is constructed of blocks of granite, faced with Portland-stone, and was built in 1762. The New North dock, two hundred and fifty-nine feet nine inches, by eighty-five feet three, and twenty-seven feet eight inches deep, is said to be the largest in the kingdom ;

it was finished in 1789. Amongst the objects of prominent interest, is the Breakwater, erected for the security of the harbour, for an account of which see Plymouth. The immense roofs over the docks, being on the principle of an arch without a buttress, are extraordinary specimens of architectural skill; the square contents of one of them amount to one acre, thirty-nine poles, and two hundred feet. The buildings on the gun-wharf, which is separated from the northern part of the dock-yard by a branch of the town, were erected after designs by Sir John Vanburgh; the armouries, and the immense piles of ordnance in the yard, each marked with the name of the ship in Hamoaze bay to which it belongs, are worthy of especial notice. The barracks are calculated to accommodate three thousand troops. The harbour of Hamoaze is about four miles long, and half a mile broad: its greatest depth, at high water, is between eighteen and twenty fathoms, at low water, about fifteen : it is a grand repository for ships of war of all classes.

There are two episcopal chapels of ease: St. Aubyn's, a neat edifice with a portico and octagonal spire at the west end, erected by subscription in 1771; and St. John's chapel, also erected by subscription in 1799 : the inhabitants have also free access to the dock-yard chapel. There are places of worship for Baptists, Independents, Wesleyan Methodists, and Moravians; the chapel belonging to the Baptists has a front in the Hindoo style. A classical subscription school was erected by subscription, and opened in 1821 : about one hundred scholars are educated in it. The public school for boys adjoins St. John's chapel, and was erected, also by subscription, in 1809 ; over it is a school-room for girls, of whom there are about one hundred : the children are clothed and educated. The Baptists and Methodists have their respective schools. A public dispensary, for this and the adjoining town of East Stonehouse, was established in 1815 ; and a savings bank in 1829. The work-house, under the management of the commissioners, contains an excellent infirmary, and schools for children of both sexes.

DEVONSHIRE, a maritime county, bounded on the north by the Bristol channel, on the east by the counties of Somerset and Dorset, on the south by the English channel, and on the west by Cornwall, extending from 50° 12′ to 51° 17′ (N. Lat.), and from about 3° to 4½° (W. Lon.): it is about two hundred and eighty miles in circumference, of which one hundred and thirty miles embrace a line of sea coast; including, according to the ordnance survey, one million five hundred and nineteen thousand three hundred and sixty acres, or two thousand three hundred and seventy-four square miles. The population, in 1821, amounted to 439,040. This portion of the island was called by the Cornish Britons *Dunan*, (apparently from the inequality of its surface), of which name the Δαμνονιον, and *Damnonium* of the geographer Ptolemy, seem to be only the Greek and Latin modifications. The Welch called it *Deuffneynt*, which, according to Camden, signifies deep vallies, a denomination which, like the former, is descriptive of the surface of the county. A softening of this last word, with the addition of the word *scyre*, signifying a share or portion, appears to have produced the Anglo-Saxon *Devenascyre*, *Devnascyre*, and *Devenschire*, in modern English *Devonshire*. This territory was probably inhabited at a very remote period, and its inhabi-

tants, the Cimbri, are supposed to have had commercial transactions with the Phœnicians, the Greeks, and other foreign nations. The settlement of a portion of the Belgic invaders of Britain, in the south-eastern parts of Devon, compelled some of the aboriginal inhabitants to emigrate to Ireland, and confined the remainder within the north-western part of their ancient territory. Devonshire under the Romans formed an important part of Britannia Prima, and in the early period of the Saxon era it became part of the kingdom of the West Saxons, or Wessex. The numerous remains of fortresses indicate that it was, at a very remote period, the scene of frequent warfare; and it is probable that many of them were constructed by the aboriginal Britons, as means of defence against the Belgæ and other invaders: but the earliest military transaction authentically recorded, is the battle at *Beamdune*, now Bampton, in which Cynegils, King of the West Saxons, vanquished the Britons with great slaughter, about the year 614. According to Matthew of Westminster. Brien, the nephew of Cadwallo, the last British king, was besieged in Exeter, by Penda, King of Mercia, in 633; but Cadwallo himself having collected an army, repaired to the assistance of his nephew, and defeated the Saxon king. The Danes, at the commencement of their ravages in the south of England, wintered in Exeter in 876 and 877, and in the latter year were besieged there by King Alfred, who compelled them to enter into a truce. In the ensuing year, the Danish chief, Hubba, having landed on the northern coast, was defeated, with the loss of his famous standard of the raven. In 894, the Danes again landed in Devonshire, and besieged Exeter, but retreated to their ships on the approach of Alfred's army. About the year 926, Athelstan is supposed to have vanquished Howell, King of Cornwall, near Exeter, and to have expelled the Britons (who then inhabited that town in common with the Saxons) beyond the river Tamar. William of Malmesbury relates, that the Danes laid waste Devonshire, and burnt Exeter, in the reign of Ethelred, in which reign, in the year 997, they sailed up the Tamar, and ravaged the country as far as Lidford. In 1001, having landed at Exmouth, they marched to Exeter, and, after an ineffectual attack upon that city, plundered the surrounding country, and returned with great spoil to their ships. In 1003, having again landed at Exmouth, they gained possession of Exeter, and nearly destroyed it.

In 1067, Exeter held out against William the Conqueror, but was surrendered to that king in person ; and in the next year, the sons of Harold having landed in Somersetshire, made great ravages in the counties of Devon and Cornwall. In 1069, the disaffected Saxons having taken up arms in Devonshire, attempted to regain possession of Exeter, but the citizens refused to admit them, and the king sent some forces by which the insurgents were defeated with great slaughter. On the accession of William Rufus, Exeter was laid waste by Robert Fitz-Baldwin, who had taken up arms in behalf of Robert, Duke of Normandy; and soon after that of Stephen, the extensive manors of Baldwin de Rivers, Earl of Devon, were devastated, on account of his adherence to the Empress Matilda. The interval between this period and the middle of the fifteenth century is devoid of historical events, with the exception of some attacks made by

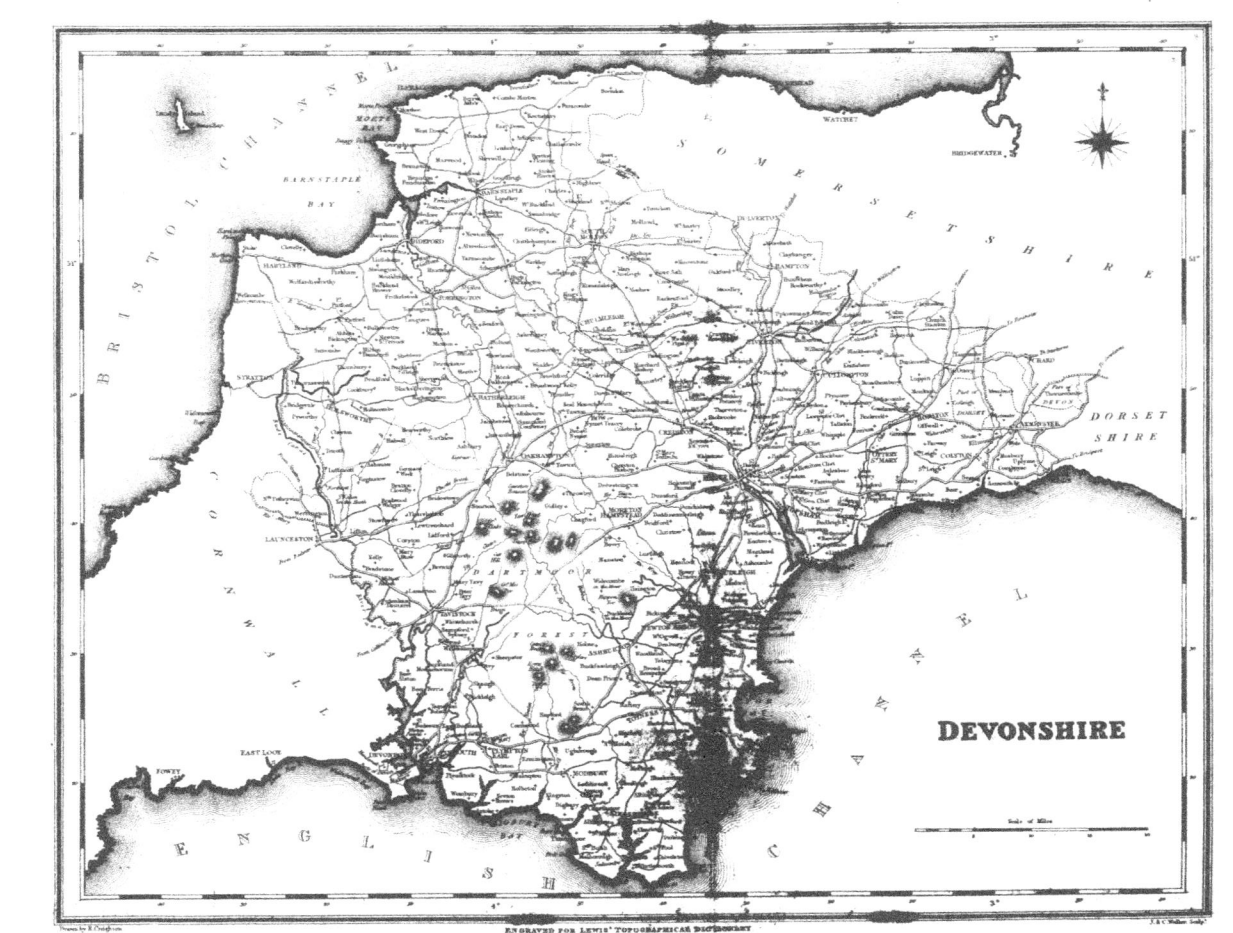

DEVONSHIRE

the French upon the maritime towns, in which Teignmouth, Plymouth, and others, were plundered and burnt. During the intestine wars between the houses of York and Lancaster, Devonshire was much divided : although no battle is recorded to have been fought within its limits, bloodshed sometimes occurred between the partizans of the two houses ; and in 1472, the Lancastrian forces from Cornwall and Devon, under Sir John Arundell and Sir Hugh Courtenay, mustered at Exeter, whence they marched to the field of Tewkesbury. In 1497, the Cornish rebels appeared before Exeter, but were repulsed by the citizens, and marched forward into Somersetshire. In the same year Exeter was besieged by Perkin Warbeck, when the siege was raised by Edward Courtenay, Earl of Devon, attended by several Devonshire knights, with the *posse comitatus*; upon which Warbeck and his followers proceeded towards Taunton. In 1549, some serious commotions took place in the county, occasioned by the change of religion, which broke out at Sampford-Courtenay on Whit-Monday, the day after the act for reforming the church service had been carried into execution. The disturbance was at first confined to some riotous proceedings among the lower orders, but assumed, by degrees, a more serious aspect; and the disaffected, amongst whom were several of the gentry, assembled all over this county and that of Cornwall. On the 2nd of July they laid siege to Exeter, having previously transmitted to the king certain articles, to which they demanded his assent. The council, on the 8th of July, drew up an answer, refusing to comply with their demands, but discussing the alleged grievances at considerable length, and exhorting them to return to their allegiance; this they sent to the rebels, but it failed to produce the desired effect. Lord Russell was then ordered down to suppress the rebellion : he marched into Devonshire with a considerable force, by way of Honiton, and after defeating the insurgents in several engagements, compelled them to raise the siege of Exeter, which had been reduced to the greatest distress, entering that city on the 6th of August, to the great joy of the inhabitants : most of the ringleaders were eventually taken and executed.

At the commencement of the protracted contest between Charles I. and the parliament, the whole of Devonshire was under the control of the committees ; and most of the inhabitants, especially in the northern part of the county, were attached to the parliament. Plymouth was fortified against the king by the townsmen ; Exeter was garrisoned by the parliament, in October, 1642; and about the beginning of 1643, Sir George Chudleigh, an active parliamentarian officer, was stationed at Tavistock with some troops of cavalry raised in the county. From this period until the final decline of the royal cause, the course of events was powerfully influenced by the operations of the royalist forces raised in Cornwall, and commonly called the Cornish army. After the defeat of the parliamentary troops at Bradock down, near Liskeard, on the 19th of January, 1643, the Cornish forces, having captured Saltash, quartered at Tavistock ; whence Sir John Berkeley made incursions into various parts of the county, dispersing the parliamentarians in all directions. In February, Sir Nicholas Slanning being intrenched at Modbury with two thousand men, was defeated by the Devonshire club-men. About this period a treaty of

pacification for the counties of Devon and Cornwall was set on foot, and a cessation of hostilities agreed on ; but the negociations were soon broken off. After the battle of Stratton, in May of the same year, the king's forces, under Sir Ralph Hopton, marched into Devonshire, established some small garrisons near Exeter, as a check upon that city, and advanced to Tiverton. Later in the summer, as Lord Clarendon informs us, the king had no force in this county, except a small garrison at Columbjohn, the seat of Sir John Acland. Sir John Berkeley was then sent into Devonshire with a regiment of horse, to take the command of the royalist troops, to recruit their numbers, and adopt measures for blockading Exeter, which was in consequence closely invested. About the same time, the parliament, which had a strong fort at Appledore, garrisoned Barnstaple and Bideford : its power being thus strengthened in the north of the county, Colonel John Digby was sent thither by the king, with a regiment of horse, and soon procured reinforcements from Cornwall : having defeated a considerable detachment from these garrisons, Appledore fort, Barnstaple, and Bideford, successively surrendered to him in the beginning of September. Exeter was surrendered to Prince Maurice on the 4th of the same month, and Dartmouth on the 4th of October. Plymouth was then the only important post in the county that remained in the possession of the parliament, and the siege, or blockade, of it was prosecuted for many months, with varied success. In July, 1644, the Earl of Essex arrived with his army, and fixed his quarters at Tiverton, upon which Barnstaple was once more secured for the parliament : and about the end of the same month the earl marched into Cornwall, the king's forces at the same time retiring from before Plymouth. The king having determined to follow Essex, entered the county by way of Honiton, on the 25th of July, came to Exeter on the 26th, and to Crediton on the 27th ; on the 30th he was with his army at Oakhampton, and on the 31st at Lifton, whence he passed into Cornwall by way of Polston bridge. On his return, the king was at Tavistock with his army on the 8th of September ; he then invested and summoned Plymouth, but the garrison refusing to surrender, the blockade was renewed. On the 14th he returned with his army to Tavistock ; on the 16th he marched thence to Oakhampton ; and on the 17th they arrived at Exeter, and the army was quartered about Bradninch, Crediton, &c.: on the 23rd they halted at Honiton on their route eastward. In October, Ilfracombe and Barnstaple surrendered to the royal forces. Whitelocke relates that in 1645 the club-men of Devon declared for the parliament. From this period the royal party sustained a series of reverses ; nor, observes Lord Clarendon, is it to be wondered at that these disasters should have been hastened by the cruelties and oppressions of Sir Richard Grenville, the licentious conduct of Lord Goring, and the dissensions among all the king's generals. In the midst of these dissensions, Sir Thomas Fairfax, commander in chief of the parliament's army, entered Devonshire, and pursued his victorious career till he had reduced every town and fortress in the county. Having reached Honiton on the 14th of October, he stormed the castle and church of Tiverton on the 19th ; on the 26th of December he held a rendezvous of his army at Cadbury fort, and on the 29th Ashburton surrendered to the parliament. Fairfax was there with his army on the 10th of January, 1646, about which time the blockade of Plymouth was finally abandoned. Dartmouth was stormed and taken by Fairfax on the 18th, assisted by the co-operation of the fleet under Admiral Batten. Fairfax then marched into the northern part of the county. Having held a rendezvous of his army at Ashreigny, on the morning of the 16th of February, he attacked Lord Hopton the same night in his quarters at Torrington, and totally defeated his army : a thanksgiving was appointed for this victory, which appears to have been the death-blow to the power of the royalists in the west. Exmouth fort was surrendered on the 15th of March. Exeter, which had been blockaded from the 9th of February, was surrendered upon articles by its governor, Sir John Berkeley, on the 9th of April ; and on the 11th Barnstaple surrendered to Fairfax in person, on nearly the same terms as Exeter ; which city he entered with his victorious army on the 14th, and stayed there four days. The last garrison in the county that held out for the king was Charles-fort, at Salcombe Regis, which was defended by Sir Edmund Fortescue until the beginning of June, when it was surrendered on honourable terms. In 1688, this county became memorable as having witnessed the first scene of the Revolution. The Prince of Orange landed at Torbay on the 5th of November, made a public entry into Exeter on the 8th, and remained there until the 21st, on which day he quitted it, accompanied by several gentlemen of Somerset and Devon, and proceeded to Axminster, where he remained four days. In 1690, Teignmouth was burned by the French, and in 1719, in consequence of their great preparations for the invasion of England, several regiments of horse and foot were sent into Devonshire, and there was an encampment on Clist heath. In 1779, the combined fleets having appeared off Plymouth, caused great alarm, especially on account of the dock-yard, and the numerous prisoners of war then collected at that port ; the prisoners were removed to the county bridewell at Exeter. During the expectation of a French invasion, in 1778, several regiments of volunteers were raised in the county ; and in the following year, ordnance was brought from Plymouth for the defence of Exeter, and a camp was formed on Woodbury down. These preparations were repeated in 1803.

This county is in the diocese of Exeter, and province of Canterbury, and is divided into the three archdeaconries of Barnstaple, Exeter, and Totness, comprising twenty-four deaneries, viz: in the archdeaconry of Barnstaple, the deaneries of Barum or Barnstaple, Chulmleigh, Hertland, Shirwell, South Molton, and Torrington ; in the archdeaconry of Exeter, those of Aylesbeare, Cadbury, Christianity or Exeter, Dunkeswell, Dunsford, Honiton, Kenne, Plymtree, and Tiverton; and in the archdeaconry of Totness, those of Holsworthy, Ipplepen, Moreton, Oakhampton, Plympton, Tamerton, Tavistock, Totton or Totness, and Woodleigh. The office of rural dean is, in this diocese, an efficient office, the deans being elected annually at the visitations. The number of parishes is four hundred and sixty-six, of which two hundred and fifty-one are rectories, one hundred and forty vicarages, and seventy-five perpetual curacies. For civil purposes, the county is divided into three districts, called the North, East, and South divisions, comprising thirty-three hundreds ; viz., in the North

division, the hundreds of Black-Torrington, Braunton, Fremington, Hartland, North Tawton with Winkley, Shebbear, Sherwill, South Molton, and Witheridge ; in the East division, those of Axminster, Bampton, Cliston, Colyton, East Budleigh, Halberton, Hayridge, Hemyock, Ottery-St. Mary, and Tiverton ; and in the South division, those of Coleridge, Crediton, Ermington, Exminster, Haytor, Lifton, Plympton, Roborough, Stanborough, Tavistock, Teingbridge, West Budleigh, and Wonford. It contains the city of Exeter, the borough and market towns of Ashburton, Barnstaple, Dartmouth, Honiton, Oakhampton, Plymouth, Plympton, Tavistock, Tiverton, and Totness ; the borough of Beer-Alston, which has no market, and the market towns of Axminster, Bampton, Bideford, South Brent, Brixham, Chagford, Chudleigh, Chulmleigh, Cullompton, Colyton, Crediton, Devonport, Hatherleigh, Holsworthy, Ilfracombe, Kingsbridge, Modbury, South Molton, Moreton-Hampstead, Newton-Abbot, Sidmouth, Stonehouse, East Teignmouth, Topsham, Torrington, and Uffculme. Of the above, eight are sea-ports, viz., Barnstaple, Bideford, Brixham, Dartmouth, Exeter, Ilfracombe, Kingsbridge, and Plymouth ; besides which, there are the ports of Axmouth, Comb-Martin, Hartland, Salcombe, Teignmouth (within the port of Exeter), and Torquay. Lundy island is also within the limits of this county. Twenty-six members are returned to parliament, viz., two knights for the shire, two representatives for the city of Exeter, and two for each of the boroughs : the county members are elected at Exeter : Devonshire is included in the western circuit : the assizes and quarter sessions for the county are held at Exeter : there are one hundred and sixty-seven acting magistrates. The stannary laws, which have been in force from an early period in the mining district, in the south-western part of the county, constitute the only peculiarity in the civil jurisdiction of Devonshire ; the stannary parliaments, the practice of holding which has long fallen into disuse, anciently met in the open air, on an elevated spot called Crokern-tor, in Dartmoor : the stannary towns are Ashburton, Chagford, Plympton, and Tavistock. The rates raised in the county for the year ending March 25th, 1827, amounted to £247,641. 8.; the expenditure to £244,887. 10., of which £213,538. 11. was applied to the relief of the poor.

The principal branch of manufacture is that of woollen cloth, which was made here so early as the reign of Edward I. ; but only frieze and plain coarse cloth were made in Devonshire until that of Edward IV., when the manufacture of Kersey was introduced. The Devonshire kersey had acquired celebrity, and was an important article of commerce to the Levant in the early part of the sixteenth century : the trade in that article experienced a still further increase in the succeeding century, towards the latter part of which it was at its greatest height. During the continental war, the woollen trade sustained a most serious decline in its foreign consumption, from which it has but partially recovered. More than two-thirds of the cloths now made in the county are for the East India Company, who purchase about one hundred and fifty thousand pieces annually. The principal manufacturing towns are Exeter, Crediton, Cullompton, Ashburton, and South Molton ; the secondary ones are Totness, Tavistock, Kingsbridge, Modbury, Brent, Chagford, and Barnstaple, and the villages of Buckfastleigh, Bishop's Morchard, and North Tawton. The general state of the woollen trade, as compared with the period of its greatest prosperity, may be ascertained from the entries at the custom-house at Exeter, from which city by far the greater part of the woollen goods manufactured in the county is exported. The years 1768 and 1787 are considered to have been the periods of the greatest prosperity of the trade ; in the former, three hundred and thirty thousand four hundred and fourteen pieces of cloth were exported from Exeter ; in the latter, two hundred and ninety-five thousand three hundred and eleven pieces : in 1820, the number was one hundred and twenty-seven thousand four hundred and fifty-nine. The principal foreign markets now are those of Spain and Portugal : and besides the trade with the East India Company, long ells are purchased for the private trade of India, and have been introduced into China by American and other foreign vessels. At some of the towns in which the clothing trade has been discontinued, the operative manufacturers are employed in preparing materials for the masters in other towns. The manufacture of bone-lace, at Honiton and Bradninch, introduced probably in the reign of Elizabeth, is now much on the decline. Large quantities of shoes, made at Ashburton, Kingsbridge, and Dartmouth, are sent to Newfoundland. The principal exports are woollen goods, fish, corn, malt, cider, timber and bark, silver, copper, tin and lead ores, antimony (from Cornwall), manganese, marble, granite, lime, pipe and potters' clay. The principal imports are coal, culm, dried fish from Newfoundland, hemp, tallow, deals, iron, wine, and grocery.

This county is more uniformly hilly than any other of the same or nearly the same extent in England, the proportion of level ground in it being extremely small. The Forest of Dartmoor is the highest ground in Devonshire, its mean height being estimated at one thousand seven hundred and eighty-two feet, and its extreme height at two thousand and ninety : the highest point of Exmoor, on the border of Somersetshire, is one thousand eight hundred and ninety feet ; and Sholsbury Castle, in the parish of High Bray, is one thousand five hundred feet high. The general character of a great proportion of the county is a continued succession of hills of the same height. This circumstance, and the lofty banks and hedges by which most of the high roads are shut in, render them tedious and unpleasant to the traveller. Nevertheless, the county possesses many remarkably fine distant views, particularly near the coast, and in many parts the scenery is beautifully picturesque, especially on the banks of some of the rivers. The soil is extremely various, but may in general be characterized according to the stratified substances which it covers, as aganitical, slaty, calcareous, arenaceous, argillaceous, gravelly, and loamy. The poorest of all these is the soil that covers the granite of Dartmoor, which has also the disadvantages of a cold wet climate ; that which lies on the slate district possesses greater or less degrees of fertility, and is fit for all the purposes of agriculture ; very extensive tracts of it, however, are of a thin staple; others are in contact with a cold bed of clay, and some are so elevated as to have a very low degree of temperature. In general, the more broken the surface is, the less it partakes of these defects, the broadest swells being the most barren. The portions of this soil most

distinguished for their fertility, appear to owe it to their contiguity to lime-stone or green-stone rocks, which occur frequently in the slate district, more especially in the South Hams. The red colour which characterizes the best soils, both in the South Hams and in the eastern division of the county, and which seems to be so closely connected with the principle of fertility, proceeds from an abundant mixture of iron in a highly oxydised state. This soil prevails in that part of the South Hams which is bounded by the rivers Dart and Erme : the hills and slopes are excellent corn and sheep lands ; the valleys are remarkably rich, and consist chiefly of orchards and irrigated meadows ; the former being noted for cider, the latter producing the finest hay, and the earliest grass. The soil of that part of the South Hams which lies between the river Dart and Torbay, is still more red and fertile, generally on a sub-stratum of marble-rock, and produces excellent pasturage for cattle. The other part of the South Hams, situated north-west of the river Erme, is nearly similar to those already described. There is also an abundance of rich meadow land in the vales of the Exe and the Otter. A considerable part of the county north of Hatherleigh and Holsworthy, and extending eastward to Chulmleigh, Bradninch, &c., is principally on clay. A large district, extending from Dartmoor, westward, to the Tamar, northward, to Hatherleigh and Holsworthy, and eastward, towards Newton-Bushell, is sandy or gravelly. North-east of the Taw the soil is light, on a sub-stratum of grey *wacke*, or, as it is called in Devonshire, *dunstone*. Towards Hartland Point there is much clay and moorland. The soil about Black-down and Holden is flinty. The rich red soil, which is of great depth, is sometimes used as a manure for the poorer lands. The principal manures are sea-sand, brought in great quantities from Bude, on the northern coast of Cornwall (for the conveyance of which a canal has been constructed), and lime. It has been estimated that the waste lands in the county amount to three hundred and twenty thousand acres, being a fifth of the whole surface. Of these, Dartmoor is computed to contain fifty-three thousand six hundred and forty-four, exclusively of the numerous and extensive commons which adjoin it. There are also very extensive commons adjoining Exmoor, as also near Bridestowe, besides Roborough-down, Black-down near Plymouth, Black-down on the borders of Somersetshire, Haldon, &c. Of the land in cultivation, somewhat the greater portion is pasture land ; in the South Hams, however, the arable predominates, in the proportion of at least three to one ; and in the northern parts of Devon the grazing land prevails in about the same proportion.

An abundance of corn grows in the neighbourhood of Hartland, Bideford, and Ilfracombe, and a considerable quantity of it is exported. The principal corn markets are those of Exeter, Tavistock, Totness, Barnstaple, Plymouth, and Kingsbridge. A large quantity of potatoes is produced in the South Hams : in 1820, ninety thousand four hundred and ninety-eight bushels were shipped from Dartmouth. Plymouth and its populous neighbourhood are entirely supplied from the tract south of Dartmoor. The cultivation of apples for the making of cider was first an object of general care about the commencement of the seventeenth century. A great quantity of cider is now made, in a productive year, for exportation, besides the vast quantity made for home consumption. In the year 1820, eleven thousand two hundred and sixty-five Devonshire hogsheads (each of sixty-three gallons) were sent from the ports of Exeter and Dartmouth (the former including Teignmouth, and the latter Salcombe), besides what was shipped by the growers, and therefore not liable to duty. There are orchards in almost every part of the county; but the cider of the South Hams is preferred; and it is there only, and in the neighbourhood of Exeter, that it is made for exportation: it is sent to London, Newcastle upon Tyne, Sunderland, Leith, Swansea, Liverpool, and from that place by the canals into Yorkshire. A considerable quantity of butter is sent from the neighbourhood of Honiton, Axminster, &c. to London. The number of cattle bred in the county is considerable: the breed most esteemed is the North Devon, which is most prevalent in that district, though in general request throughout the county, on account of its great superiority for the purposes of grazing or draught. The Devonshire cattle are for the most part sent in droves from various parts of the county, to the graziers in Somersetshire, Essex, &c., who fatten them for the London market. The native breeds of sheep are the Exmoor, the Dartmoor, and the Old Devonshire dim-faced nott sheep; the two former are the most prevalent, but the latter has been much improved by a cross with the New Leicester: the Dorsetshire breed prevails in that part of Devonshire which borders upon that county. The wool is the chief object of attention with the owners of the forest or moorland flocks, which are large and numerous. It is a remarkable circumstance, that the rot has never yet been known to have originated with sheep constantly depasturing upon either of the forests of Dartmoor or Exmoor. A small breed of horses, between the pack-horse and the larger cart-horse, is much in use in different parts of the county; but in the less hilly portions, where one and two horse carts are more commonly in use, a larger breed is preferred. In the southern and western parts of the county mules and asses are continually employed in carrying packs of sand from the sea-side to the distance of several miles inland. The native Devonshire hog grows to a large size, and is long in all its dimensions, but has been much improved by a cross with the Leicester breed, and a further cross with the Chinese, which have considerably reduced its size, and rendered it much more profitable.

Geologically considered, this county may be resolved into four grand divisions; the district of granite, and primitive argillaceous slate; that of transition slate, or grey *wacke*; that of red sand-stone; and that of green sand. The granite strata compose the greater part of the elevated tract in the south-western part of the county, known by the name of Dartmoor, which is closely surrounded on all sides by a district of argillaceous slate: the transition slate occupies the northern part of the county, including Exmoor; the red sand-stone occupies the least elevated portions of the county, and skirts the base of the last-mentioned district, extending north-eastward into Somersetshire, and westward as far as Hatherleigh: the green sand formation constitutes the largest portion of the hills in the south-eastern part of the county, and, being unfavourable to agriculture, its surface is generally marked by extensive tracts of common, the intermediate valleys being at the

same time extremely fertile, as they are composed principally of the red marl. It appears, from Strabo, Herodotus, &c., that the Phœnicians, and afterwards successively the Greeks and the Romans, traded for tin with the inhabitants of south-western Britain, and it is believed to have continued to be an article of commerce even in the middle ages. So early as the reign of Richard I., it constituted one of the principal sources of the revenue of the earldom of Cornwall; and in 1250, Henry III. granted a charter of protection to the tinners of Devon. There have been old tin mines in most of the parishes bordering on Dartmoor, and stream-works on most of the rivers in its neighbourhood. The average quantity of tin raised annually within the county, for six years ending at Michaelmas, 1820, was one thousand one hundred and seventy-one blocks, weighing 586 cwt. 9lb., and yielding a duty of £45. 17. 9. The tin was formerly smelted and coined in the county, but, on account of the great diminution in the produce of the mines, it is now taken to Cornwall to be smelted. Some copper mines were in operation early in the last century, but it was not till the commencement of the present that they were worked to much extent: the augmented price of the metal then stimulated the miners to greater exertions, and, from about the year 1800, the quantity of ore dug greatly increased. The average annual quantity of fine copper obtained from the Devonshire mines, which lie chiefly within a few miles of the town of Tavistock, for ten successive years, ending in 1820, was about four hundred tons: four hundred and sixty-three tons were raised in that year, which brought about £39,590.

The lead mines of this county, and of Cornwall, contain a greater proportion of silver than those in any other part of the kingdom. The mines of Beer-Alston and Beer-Ferrers are remarkable for the length of time for which at different periods they have been worked, and for the quantity of silver extracted from them, being in the proportion of from eighty to one hundred and twenty ounces from each ton of lead. The lead veins, or lodes, range from north to south, crossing the usual direction of the copper and tin mines. The greater part of the ore dug in the mines near Tavistock is shipped at Plymouth. Manganese has been found in great quantities in this county, and since about the year 1770, when it was first discovered, has been a considerable article of commerce. There are deep and extensive beds of pipe and potter's clay in the parishes of Hennock, Ilsington, Bovey-Tracey, Teigngrace, King's Teington, &c.; both of them being now obtained on Bovey Heathfield, and in the parish of King's Teington, and conveyed by the Stover canal to Teignmouth, whence about twenty thousand tons are annually shipped to most parts of the united kingdom. Several attempts have been made to procure coal, but without effect; and it is the opinion of the most scientific geologists, that coal does not subsist in the Devonshire strata. Various beautiful marbles occur in the lime-stone rocks in different parts of the county, from which also a vast quantity of lime is obtained; and so extensive is the use of this article as manure, that in addition to the immense quantity burnt in the county, there is a number of kilns on the northern coast, used for burning lime-stone imported from Wales. Granite of the best quality may be obtained to almost any extent from the Dartmoor rocks, but on account of the inconvenience of carriage it has never, until recently, been made an article of commerce. A rail-road has lately been constructed to convey it from Dartmoor to Plymouth; and another rail-road conveys it from the quarries at Heytor to the Stover canal, which communicates with the æstuary of the Teign near Newton-Abbots; the Heytor granite is said to be equal in quality to that of Aberdeen. There are quarries of good building-stone and slate. The soft sand-stone on the side of Blackdown is worked, while wet, into whetstones, which are sent to Bristol, Gloucester, Worcester, &c.

Salmon are caught in all the principal rivers; but the fishery has of late years declined: lampreys are found in the Exe and the Mole. The herring fishery on the northern coast has been, of late years, much less productive than it was formerly. The pilchard fishery, on the southern coast, is carried on chiefly in Bigbury bay, at Dartmouth, and at Brixham. In Torbay is the principal fishery for ·turbot, soles, whiting, mackarel, and other fish; the Bath and Exeter markets are supplied from it, and a great quantity is sent by sea to Portsmouth, whence the fish is conveyed by land-carriage to London. At Star-Cross are oyster beds, to which the oysters are brought from the Teign, from Weymouth, Pool, Saltash, &c., and having been fed for a while in these beds, are sent to the Exeter market. Young oysters from the Teign are also sent to be fed in the Thames for the London markets.

The rivers are very numerous; the principal are, the Axe, the Otter, the Exe, the Teign, the Dart, the Aven, the Erme, the Yealm, the Plym, the Tamar, the Tavy, the Torridge, and the Taw. The Exe from Tops-ham to Exmouth is on an average more than a mile broad, and is navigable for large vessels; from the former place barges reach Exeter by means of a canal. The Dart is navigable up to Totness. The Yealme is navigable for sloops and small briggs up to Kitley quay, and for barges and small boats half a mile higher. The Plym is navigable for vessels of war up to Catwater, and for ships of about fifty tons up to Crabtree. The Torridge is navigable for vessels of large burden up to Bideford, and for boats up to Wear-Gifford. The Taw is not usually navigated up to Barnstaple by vessels of more than eighty tons, though vessels of one hundred and forty tons sometimes come up to that port: for boats and barges it is navigable to New-bridge. The Tamar is navigable for vessels of one hundred and thirty tons up to New Quay, about twenty-four miles above Plymouth. The Stover, or Teingrace canal, from Bovey-Tracey to the river Teign, at Newton-Abbots, was completed about 1794, at the sole expense of James Templer, Esq. A canal was completed in 1817, from Morwellham quay to Tavistock, for the importation of coal, lime, &c., and the conveyance of ore from the mines of Morwellham down, &c., with a branch two miles long to the slate quarries at Mill-hill; on the line of this canal is a tunnel through the hills, nearly two miles long; goods are conveyed from the Tamar to this canal, being raised to the height of two hundred and forty feet by an inclined plane. In 1819, an act passed for making a canal from Bude, in Cornwall, to Thornbury, &c., in Devon. A short canal extends from the sea locks, about a mile south of Topsham, to Exeter.

The great road from London to Exeter and Plymouth enters the county between the ninth and tenth mile-stone from Bridport, and passes through Axminster, Honiton, Exeter, Ashburton, South Brent, and Plympton, to Plymouth; its course through the county being about seventy-seven miles. Another road from Exeter to Plymouth branches off at Alphington, and passes through Totness, its course being about forty-six miles. The great road from London to Falmouth and the Land's End branches off at Exeter, passes through Oakhampton, and quits the county at Polston bridge, forty miles from Exeter. Another road from Exeter to the Land's End passes over Dartmoor, and through Tavistock, entering Cornwall at New-bridge, thirty-five miles from Exeter.

Among British antiquities may be classed the remarkable circular enclosure formed by loose stones, called Grimspound, in the parish of Manaton; and the smaller ones found on many parts of Dartmoor, and in other similar situations; the large cromlech at Drewe's Teignton, and the several tumuli or barrows which occur on the downs in various parts of the county, especially in the north. Of the numerous ancient encampments, many are believed to be British; and it has been the opinion of some antiquaries, that the chain of strong posts on the eastern side of Devonshire was constructed by the Damnonii, to defend their frontier against the Morini: that several of these camps, however, were occupied, if not constructed, by the Romans, appears from the Roman coins that have been found in them. The following are the principal ancient roads still to be traced, in parts of their course through the county; the Iknield-way, which crosses the county from Dorsetshire into Cornwall, passing through Exeter; the Fosse-way, which fell into, or crossed the former near the eastern border of the county; and the Port-way, which led from the centre of Somersetshire towards Exeter, in the line of the present turnpike-road from Taunton. Of the many Roman stations, the only one, the situation of which has been fixed with certainty, is *Isca Damnoniorum*, near Exeter. Before the Reformation there were thirty-three religious houses, including a preceptory of the Knights Templars; but the relics of monastic buildings, except those of Tavistock abbey, are inconsiderable: there were also twelve collegiate churches, and one collegiate chapel, of which societies only that of the church of St. Peter, at Exeter, remains; the number of ancient hospitals was sixteen, of which seven are still in existence. In the ruins of ancient castles and castellated mansions there is little that is remarkable; those of Berry-Pomeroy castle are probably the most interesting.

In most parts of the cider district the custom still prevails of what was anciently called wassailing the apple-trees, the ceremony being performed, in some places, on Christmas-eve, in others on Twelfth-day eve, by drinking a health to one of the apple-trees in cider, with wishes for its fruitful bearing. The yule, or Christmas log, is still burned on Christmas-eve, in some parts of the county; in other parts they burn a large fagot of green ash. Wrestling is a favourite sport in the north of Devon, in the neighbourhood of Plymouth, and on the borders of Cornwall. Red deer, *feræ naturâ*, the remaining stock of those which inhabited the royal forest of Exmoor, still abound sufficiently in the Devonshire woods, south of the forest, to yield sport to the neighbouring nobility and gentry, and a stag hunt has been for many years kept up in the vicinity. Devonshire gives the title of duke to the family of Cavendish.

*

DEWCHURCH (LITTLE), a parish in the upper division of the hundred of WORMELOW, county of HEREFORD, 6 miles (S. by E.) from Hereford, containing 330 inhabitants. The living is a perpetual curacy, annexed to the vicarage of Lugwardine, in the archdeaconry and diocese of Hereford. The chapel is dedicated to St. David.

DEWCHURCH (MUCH), a parish in the upper division of the hundred of WORMELOW, county of HEREFORD, 6½ miles (S. W. by S.) from Hereford, containing 585 inhabitants. The living is a discharged vicarage, in the archdeaconry and diocese of Hereford, rated in the king's books at £9. 13. 4., and in the patronage of T. H. Symons, Esq. The church is dedicated to St. David.

DEWLISH, a parish and liberty in the Blandford (North) division of the county of DORSET, 9½ miles (S. W.) from Blandford-Forum, containing 386 inhabitants. The living is a vicarage, annexed to the vicarage of Milbourn St. Andrew, in the archdeaconry of Dorset, and diocese of Bristol, rated together at £13. 6. 8. The church is dedicated to All Saints.

DEWSALL, a parish in the upper division of the hundred of WORMELOW, county of HEREFORD, 5½ miles (S.W. by S.) from Hereford, containing 33 inhabitants. The living is a discharged vicarage, in the peculiar jurisdiction of the Dean of Hereford, rated in the king's books at £4, endowed with £200 royal bounty, and in the patronage of the Governors of Guy's Hospital, London. The church is dedicated to St. Michael.

DEWSBURY, a parish comprising the market town of Dewsbury, the chapelry of Ossett, and the townships of Soothill, in the lower division of the wapentake of AGBRIGG, and the chapelry of Clifton, and the township of Hartshead, in the wapentake of MORLEY, West riding of the county of YORK, containing 16,261 inhabitants, of which number, 6380 are in the town of Dewsbury, 34 miles (S. W.) from York, and 188 (N. N. W.) from London. This place is supposed to have derived its name from Dui, the tutelar deity of the Brigantes, to whom a votive altar, dedicated by Aurelianus, is still preserved at Bradley, said to have been called Duis burgh, or Duisborough, from which its present appellation is derived. It was a place of importance during the infancy of the Christian Church in Britain, and was the mother church in this part of the county. Edwine, King of Northumbria, had a royal mansion here, in which his queen Ethelburga, who had subscribed to the Christian faith, was attended by Paulinus, first Archbishop of York, by whom Edwine himself, and subsequently his whole court, were converted to Christianity, in the year 627 ; in memory of which a cross was erected, with the inscription *Paulinus Hic Prædicavit et celebravit*, which was many years since found buried in the ground about a foot from the surface ; a fac-simile within the last twenty years was made by order of the Rev. J Buckworth, and placed in the gardens of the vicarage, together with several Saxon and Norman antiquities, which that gentleman had collected. The town is pleasantly situated at the base of a hill rising from the river Calder, and consists of several good streets and well built houses ; it is lighted with gas, and well supplied with water. There is a public subscription library ; and a mechanics' institution has been established within the last five years. For some years Dewsbury has been

rising into importance for its manufacture of blankets, carpets, and woollen cloths, for which there are numerous factories (one of which is the largest in the kingdom), giving employment to more than five thousand persons in the town and neighbourhood : the water of the Calder is peculiarly favourable for the fulling of woollen goods. Abundance of coal of very superior quality is found in the neighbourhood. The river Calder and the canals afford a direct communication between the eastern and western seas, and with Liverpool, Manchester, Rochdale, Halifax, and Wakefield, to the Humber. The market is on Wednesday : the fairs are on the Wednesdays before Old May-day, and New Michaelmas-day, and October 6th. The living is a discharged vicarage, in the archdeaconry and diocese of York, rated in the king's books at £22. 13. 9., endowed with £200 private benefaction, and £200 royal bounty, and in the patronage of the Crown. The church, dedicated to All Saints, a very ancient structure, having given way in 1767, was rebuilt, with a due regard to the preservation of its ancient character : during the progress of the work, part of a Saxon tomb was found and removed to the parsonage-house. The church, at Dewsbury Moor, dedicated to St. John, and containing six hundred sittings, of which two hundred and forty-eight are free, was erected in 1827, at an expense of £5502. 16. 8., by grant from the parliamentary commissioners, who have built similar churches at Earl's-Heaton and Hanging-Heaton. There are places of worship for the Society of Friends, Independents, and Wesleyan and other Methodists. The charity school has an endowment of £108 per annum, arising from an estate purchased with donations of Mrs. Bedford, Mr. Thomas Bedford, and Mr. William Walker : a separate house for the master, with a large school-room, was built in 1810, at an expense of £1300, defrayed from the sale of coal on the estate ; there are one hundred boys instructed in this school by a master, whose salary is £80 per annum. A school-house has been recently built by a decree of Chancery, relating to the Wheelwright charity, at an expense of £600, in which one hundred boys and one hundred girls are instructed on the National system ; and an infant school has recently been established. Among the remains of antiquity discovered here were a spear-head of an unknown metal resembling gold, one hundred yards from the river Calder, on the premises of Mr. Halliley ; a Roman urn, and other relics.

DIBDEN, a parish in the liberty of New Forest (East) division of the county of SOUTHAMPTON, 3 miles (S. W.) from Southampton, containing 443 inhabitants. The living is a rectory, in the archdeaconry and diocese of Winchester, rated in the king's books at £5. 12. 11., and in the patronage of the Earl of Malmesbury. The parish is bounded on the east by the Southampton water.

DICKLEBURGH, a parish in the hundred of DISS, county of NORFOLK, 2 miles (N. N. E.) from Scole, containing, with the hamlet of Langmere, which is in the hundred of Earsham, 804 inhabitants. The living is a rectory in four portions, in the archdeaconry of Norfolk, and diocese of Norwich, rated in the king's books at £28, and in the patronage of the Master and Fellows of Trinity College, Cambridge : it was anciently divided into four portions, each having a rector of its own, who alternately performed divine service. The church is dedicated to All Saints. At the Conquest there was a large town within the parish, called Semere, now only a hamlet

DIDBROOK, a parish in the lower division of the hundred of KIFTSGATE, county of GLOUCESTER, 2¾ miles (N.E.) from Winchcombe, containing 291 inhabitants. The living is a discharged vicarage, with which the rectory of Pinnock is consolidated, in the archdeaconry and diocese of Gloucester, rated in the king's books at £7. 9. 10., endowed with £200 royal bounty, and in the patronage of C. Hanbury Tracy, Esq. The church, dedicated to St. George, appears from an inscription to have been built about 1470; it is in the later style of English architecture, with an embattled tower and some stained glass. There is a chapel of ease at Hayles, in this parish.

DIDDINGTON, a parish in the hundred of TOZE-LAND, county of HUNTINGDON, 3¾ miles (N.) from St. Neot's, containing 157 inhabitants. The living is a discharged vicarage, in the archdeaconry of Huntingdon, and diocese of Lincoln, rated in the king's books at £7. 4. 7½., and in the patronage of the Warden and Fellows of Merton College, Oxford. The church is dedicated to St. Lawrence. The river Ouse runs through this parish.

DIDDLEBURY, a parish in the hundred of MUNS-LOW, county of SALOP, comprising the townships of Diddlebury, Middlehope, Peaton, and Sutton, and containing 987 inhabitants, of which number, 434 are in the township of Diddlebury, 8½ miles (N.) from Ludlow. The living is a discharged vicarage, in the archdeaconry of Salop, and diocese of Hereford, rated in the king's books at £12. 1. 3., and in the patronage of the Dean and Chapter of Hereford. The church is dedicated to St. Peter. Here was formerly an Alien priory, which, with the patronage of the church, belonged to the abbot and convent of Sagium, or Seez, in Normandy, and was afterwards appropriated to the abbey of Shrewsbury.

DIDLING, a parish in the hundred of DUMPFORD, rape of CHICHESTER, county of SUSSEX, 4 miles (S.W. by W.) from Midhurst, containing 81 inhabitants. The living is a rectory with Trayford, in the archdeaconry and diocese of Chichester. The church is in the early style of English architecture.

DIDLINGTON, a tything in the parish of CHAL-BURY, hundred of BADBURY, Shaston (East) division of the county of DORSET, 1 mile (N.W.) from Chalbury, with which the population is returned. Here was anciently a chapel, the remains of which are still visible, having been converted into a farm-house: foundations of houses have often been discovered in a neighbouring field.

DIDLINGTON, a parish in the southern division of the hundred of GREENHOE, county of NORFOLK, 6 miles (E.S.E.) from Stoke-Ferry, containing 71 inhabitants. The living is a discharged vicarage with the rectory of Colveston, in the archdeaconry of Norfolk, and diocese of Norwich, rated in the king's books at £12. 14. 7. Robert Wilson, Esq. was patron in 1808. The church is a neat structure, and the windows are ornamented with various devices in stained glass.

DIDMARTON, a parish in the upper division of the hundred of GRUMBALD'S ASH, county of GLOUCESTER, 4¾ miles (S.W.) from Tetbury, containing 101 inhabitants. The living is a discharged rectory united to the rectory of Oldbury on the Hill, in the archdeaconry and diocese of Gloucester, rated in the king's books at £8. The church, dedicated to St. Lawrence, is a small building of a singular form, with a turret of wood.

DIDSBURY, a chapelry in the parish of MAN-CHESTER, hundred of SALFORD, county palatine of LANCASTER, 3 miles (W.) from Stockport, containing 933 inhabitants. The living is a perpetual curacy, in the archdeaconry and diocese of Chester, endowed with £400 private benefaction, and £600 royal bounty. The chapel is dedicated to St. John. There are fairs for cattle, held April 30th and October 22d. Sir Edward Moseley, in 1685, conveyed certain lands, which, with subsequent donations, produce £46 a year, for the maintenance of a schoolmaster, who teaches forty children in a school-room built by subscription.

DIGBY, a parish in the wapentake of FLAXWELL, parts of KESTEVEN, county of LINCOLN, 6 miles (N. by E.) from Sleaford, containing 277 inhabitants. The living is a discharged vicarage, united, in 1717, to rectory of Bloxham, in the archdeaconry and diocese of Lincoln, rated in the king's books at £5. 2. 11. The church is dedicated to St. Thomas à Becket.

DIGSWELL, a parish in the hundred of BROAD-WATER, county of HERTFORD, 1¼ mile (S.E. by S.) from Welwyn, containing 204 inhabitants. The living is a rectory, in the archdeaconry of Huntingdon, and diocese of Lincoln, rated in the king's books at £7. 4. 2. The Rev. J. J. Watson, D.D. was patron in 1811. The church, dedicated to St. John the Evangelist, has a chapel on the north side, and a square embattled tower at the west end; it contains many ancient effigies in brass, with various other sepulchral emblems. The parish is bounded on the north by the river Mimeram, and on the south by the Lea.

DILHAM, a parish in the hundred of TUNSTEAD, county of NORFOLK, 4¾ miles (S.E.) from North Walsham, containing 420 inhabitants. The living is a discharged vicarage with the vicarage of Honing united, in the archdeaconry of Norfolk, and diocese of Norwich, rated in the king's books at £5. 7. 11., and in the patronage of the Bishop of Ely. The church is dedicated to St. Nicholas.

DILHORNE, a parish in the northern division of the hundred of TOTMONSLOW, county of STAFFORD, 2¼ miles (W.) from Cheadle, containing, with the township of Forsbrook, 1409 inhabitants. The living is a discharged vicarage, in the archdeaconry of Stafford, and diocese of Lichfield and Coventry, rated in the king's books at £8. 13., and in the patronage of the Dean and Chapter of Lichfield and Coventry. The church, dedicated to All Saints, is a spacious structure; the body is modern, but the chancel and tower are very ancient, the latter being of an octagonal form, large, and unadorned, and esteemed the most perfect specimen of the Norman style to be found in England. Adjoining the church-yard is the free grammar school, said to have been founded by an earl of Huntingdon, in the reign of Henry VIII., and endowed by the inhabitants; the income is about £250 a year, which is applied to the maintenance of a schoolmaster, who instructs from fifty to sixty children, but they are not taught the classics. Dilhorne is in the honour of Tutbury, duchy of Lancaster, and within the jurisdiction of a court of pleas held at Tutbury every third Tuesday, for the recovery of debts under 40s.

DILLIKER, a township in that part of the parish of KENDAL which is in LONSDALE ward, county of WEST-

MORLAND, 8½ miles (N.E. by E.) from Kendal, containing 89 inhabitants. It is bounded on the east by the river Lune.

DILLINGTON, a hamlet in that part of the parish of EAST DEREHAM which is in the hundred of LAUNDITCH, county of NORFOLK, 2¼ miles (N.N.W.) from East Dereham, containing 29 inhabitants.

DILSTON, a township in the parish of CORBRIDGE, eastern division of TINDALE ward, county of NORTHUMBERLAND, 3 miles (E. by S.) from Hexham, containing 162 inhabitants. Its name, a corruption of Devilstone, is derived from its situation on a rivulet called Devil water, which, after flowing through a deep and gloomy dell, falls into the Tyne on the northern boundary of the parish. There is a tower remaining of the ancient baronial residence of the Devilstones, also a chapel formerly belonging to the mansion of the Ratcliffes, earls of Derwentwater, and which shared the fate of their other estates, on the attainder of the last earl, who was beheaded for high treason in 1716. Though the chapel is not used for divine service, it is kept in repair as a mark of respect for the unfortunate family, many of whom lie buried in a vault in it. Bede says that Oswald, armed with faith in Christ, killed Ceadwall, the British tyrant, at this place, which he calls *Devilesbourne*.

DILTON, a chapelry in the parish and hundred of WESTBURY, county of WILTS, 2¼ miles (S.S.W.) from Westbury, containing 2006 inhabitants. The chapel is dedicated to St. Mary. There is a fair for cattle, horses, and cheese, on the 24th of September.

DILWORTH, a township in that part of the parish of RIBCHESTER which is in the lower division of the hundred of BLACKBURN, county palatine of LANCASTER, 7 miles (N.E.) from Preston, containing 969 inhabitants.

DILWYN, a parish in the hundred of STRETFORD, county of HEREFORD, 2⅝ miles (N.E. by N.) from Weobley, containing 1026 inhabitants. The living is a vicarage, in the archdeaconry and diocese of Hereford, rated in the king's books at £6. 2. 6., and in the patronage of the Bishop of Hereford. The church is dedicated to St. Mary. A chapel formerly stood at Little Dilwyn. A school is endowed with a house, orchard and garden, given by Lacon Lambe, Esq., and with nine acres of land by Thomas Phillips, Esq., which, with annual donations of £2. 2. each from the vicar and Samuel Peploe, Esq., constitutes the master's salary. There are also a Sunday and a working school supported by voluntary donations and collections. Here is thought to have been formerly a monastic establishment to which were annexed certain lands, called College lands, previously belonging to the priory of Wormsley.

DINCHOPE, a township in the parish of BROMFIELD, hundred of MUNSLOW, county of SALOP, 7¾ miles (N.W. by N.) from Ludlow, containing 83 inhabitants.

DINDER, a parish in the hundred of WELLS-FORUM, county of SOMERSET, 2 miles (E. S. E.) from Wells, containing 175 inhabitants. The living is a rectory, in the peculiar jurisdiction of the Dean of Wells, rated in the king's books at £2. 10. 7½., endowed with £200 private benefaction, and £400 royal bounty, and in the patronage of the Bishop of Bath and Wells. The church is dedicated to St. Michael.

DINEDOR, a parish in the hundred of WEBTREE, county of HEREFORD, 4½ miles (S. E. by S.) from Here-

ford, containing 301 inhabitants. The living is a rectory, with the curacy of Rotherwas, in the peculiar jurisdiction of the Dean of Hereford, rated in the king's books at £8. 9. 7., and in the patronage of the Provost and Fellows of Worcester College, Oxford. The church is dedicated to St. Andrew.

DINGESTOW, a parish in the lower division of the hundred of RAGLAND, county of MONMOUTH, 4 miles (W. S. W.) from Monmouth, containing, with the extraparochial liberty of Grace-Dieu park, 174 inhabitants. The living is a discharged vicarage, with the chapelry of Tregare, in the archdeaconry and diocese of Llandaff, rated in the king's books at £4. 10., and in the patronage of the Archdeacon and Chapter of Llandaff. The church is dedicated to St. Mary. The river Trothey runs through the parish, and sometimes overflows the adjacent grounds.

DINGLEY, a parish in the hundred of CORBY, county of NORTHAMPTON, 2½ miles (E. by N.) from Market-Harborough, containing 150 inhabitants. The living is a rectory, in the archdeaconry of Northampton, and diocese of Peterborough, rated in the king's books at £9. 9. 4½., and in the patronage of H. H. Hungerford, Esq. The church is dedicated to All Saints. There is a Sunday school with a trifling endowment. The parish is bounded on the north-west by the river Welland, and is beautifully diversified with hill and dale. On the site of Dingley hall there was formerly a preceptory of the knights of St. John of Jerusalem; it was founded in the reign of Stephen, and at the dissolution possessed a revenue valued at £108. 13. 5. per annum : near the spot an ancient bead and a coin of Cunobeline have been found.

DINHAM, a hamlet in the parish of LANVAIR-DISCOED, upper division of the hundred of CALDICOTT, county of MONMOUTH, 5 miles (W. by S.) from Chepstow, containing 30 inhabitants. Here was formerly a chapel, but it has been demolished.

DINKLEY, a township in the parish and lower division of the hundred of BLACKBURN, county palatine of LANCASTER, 6¼ miles (N.) from Blackburn, containing 238 inhabitants.

DINMORE, an extra-parochial liberty, in the hundred of GRIMSWORTH, county of HEREFORD, 9 miles (N. by W.) from Hereford, containing 14 inhabitants. On Dinmore hill stood a commandery of the knights of St. John of Jerusalem, founded by a brother of the order, in the reign of Henry II.

DINMORE, an extra-parochial liberty, locally in the parish of Clungunford, hundred of PURSLOW, county of SALOP, containing 12 inhabitants.

DINNINGTON, a township in the parish of PONTELAND, western division of CASTLE ward, county of NORTHUMBERLAND, 6½ miles (N. by W.) from Newcastle upon Tyne, containing 205 inhabitants. A few years ago foundations and fragments of an ancient building, supposed to have been a chapel, and some human skulls, were discovered near the village.

DINNINGTON, a chapelry in the parish of SEAVINGTON-ST. MICHAEL, southern division of the hundred of PETHERTON, county of SOMERSET, 4 miles (N. W. by W.) from Crewkerne, containing 208 inhabitants. The chapel is dedicated to St. Nicholas.

DINNINGTON, a parish in the southern division of the wapentake of STRAFFORTH and TICKHILL, West riding of the county of YORK, 7 miles (N. W.) from Worksop, containing 189 inhabitants. The living is a discharged rectory, in the archdeaconry and diocese of York, rated in the king's books at £4, endowed with £200 royal bounty, and in the patronage of the Crown. The church is dedicated to St. Nicholas.

DINSDALE (LOW), a parish in the south-western division of STOCKTON ward, county palatine of DURHAM, 6 miles (S. E. by E.) from Darlington, containing 111 inhabitants. The living is a discharged rectory, in the archdeaconry and diocese of Durham, rated in the king's books at £4. 11. 5½., endowed with £200 private benefaction, and £200 royal bounty, and in the patronage of the Dean and Chapter of Durham. The church is dedicated to St. John. There is a trifling endowment for a school, left by Thomas Wivill, in 1675. A sulphureous well was discovered in 1789, at the depth of seventy-two feet from the surface; it has received the name of Dinsdale Spa, and has become a place of great resort since the recent erection of a commodious inn by Lord Durham, and an extensive suite of hot and cold baths, for the greater comfort of invalids: the water is serviceable in chronic and cutaneous cases: nearly surrounding the spa are beautiful plantations and walks. About two miles up the river Tees are the remains of an old bath, the water of which is of a saline quality; and below the village is a productive salmon-fishery, belonging to Lord Durham. Francis Place, the celebrated painter, was born here; he discovered a species of earth for making porcelain, and manufactured some at York, where he died in 1728.

DINSDALE (OVER), a township in that part of the parish of SOCKBURN which is in the wapentate of ALLERTONSHIRE, North riding of the county of YORK, 6½ miles (S. W. by W.) from Yarm, containing 66 inhabitants.

DINTING, a township in the parish of GLOSSOP, hundred of HIGH PEAK, county of DERBY, 9½ miles (N. by W.) from Chapel en le Frith, containing 152 inhabitants.

DINTON, a parish chiefly in the hundred of AYLESBURY, but comprising also the hamlet of Aston-Mollins in the hundred of ASHENDON, and the liberty of Moreton in the hundred of DESBOROUGH, county of BUCKINGHAM, 4 miles (W. S. W.) from Aylesbury, containing 817 inhabitants. The living is a vicarage, in the archdeaconry of Buckingham, and diocese of Lincoln, rated in the king's books at £17. 9. 7., and in the patronage of the Crown. The church, dedicated to St. Peter and St. Paul, has a small portion in the Norman style of architecture. The river Tame runs through the parish; and there is a petrifying spring, called Holywell. Fossils of the *cardium* and *buccinum genera* are found here in abundance.

DINTON, a parish in the hundred of WARMINSTER, though chiefly in the hundred of Dunworth, county of WILTS, 5 miles (W.) from Wilton, containing 517 inhabitants. The living is a vicarage, in the archdeaconry and diocese of Salisbury, rated in the king's books at £6, and in the patronage of the President and Fellows of Magdalene College, Oxford. The church is dedicated to St. Mary. At Great Teffont, in this parish, is a chapel of ease. There is a place of worship for dissenters, who have assumed no particular denomination. The celebrated lawyer, statesman, and historian, Edward Hyde, Earl of Clarendon, was born here in 1608.

DIPPENHALL, a tything in the parish and hundred of CRONDALL, Basingstoke division of the county of SOUTHAMPTON, 1¼ mile (W.) from Farnham, containing 312 inhabitants. Dippenhall is within the jurisdiction of the Cheyney Court held at Winchester every Thursday, for the recovery of debts to any amount.

DIPTFORD, a parish in the hundred of STANBOROUGH, county of DEVON, 5¾ miles (W. S. W.) from Totness, containing 653 inhabitants. The living is a rectory, in the archdeaconry of Totness, and diocese of Exeter, rated in the king's books at £29. 2. 1. Miss Taylor was patroness in 1817. The church is dedicated to St. Mary.

DIRHAM, a parish in the lower division of the hundred of GRUMBALD'S ASH, county of GLOUCESTER, 4 miles (W. N. W.) from Marshfield, containing, with the tything of Hinton, 526 inhabitants. The living is a rectory, in the archdeaconry and diocese of Gloucester, rated in the king's books at £14. 12. 6. W. Blaithwayt, Esq. was patron in 1828. The church, dedicated to St. Peter, is a handsome building, with portions in the early and later styles of English architecture. The Rev. W. Langton, in 1668, devised two-thirds of the proceeds of £600, now amounting to £60. 12. a year, for educating and apprenticing poor children of the parish. The Rev. Peter Grand, in 1791, bequeathed a house and an annuity of £10, producing together £42 per annum for the master; and £16 a year is paid to a schoolmistress at Hinton, for teaching twenty children. Several small springs rise in the parish, which unite and form the river Boyd. There are remains of huge ramparts, called Barhill camp, near which Ceawlin, the Saxon, in a most sanguinary battle, slew Commeail, Condidan, and Fariemeiol, petty kings of the Britons, and took possession of their country.

DISCOVE, a tything in the parish and hundred of BRUTON, county of SOMERSET, 1 mile (S. E. by S.) from Bruton, containing 43 inhabitants. At this place, called in Domesday-book Dinescove, were discovered, in 1711, some remains of a Roman tesselated pavement.

DISEWORTH, a parish in the western division of the hundred of GOSCOTE, county of LEICESTER, 6 miles (N. W. by W.) from Loughborough, containing 718 inhabitants. The living is a discharged vicarage, in the archdeaconry of Leicester, and diocese of Lincoln, rated in the king's books at £4, endowed with £200 private benefaction, and £200 royal bounty, and in the patronage of the Master and Wardens of the Haberdashers' Company. The church is dedicated to St. Michael. Diseworth is in the honour of Tutbury, duchy of Lancaster, and within the jurisdiction of a court of pleas held at Tutbury every third Tuesday, for the recovery of debts under 40s. William Lilly, the celebrated astrologer, was born here in 1602.

DISHFORTH, a chapelry in that part of the parish of TOPCLIFFE which is in the wapentake of HALLIKELD, North riding of the county of YORK, 4 miles (N. N. W.) from Boroughbridge, containing 340 inhabitants. The living is a perpetual curacy, in the peculiar jurisdiction of the Dean and Chapter of York, endowed with £1200 royal bounty, and in the patronage of the Vicar of Topcliffe. There is an endowment of £6 per annum, for teaching six children.

DISHLEY, a chapelry in the parish of THORPACRE, western division of the hundred of GOSCOTE, county of

LEICESTER, 1¾ mile (N.W.) from Loughborough, containing, with Thorpacre, 351 inhabitants. The chapel is dedicated to All Saints. The river Soar and the Loughborough canal pass through the parish.

DISS, a market town and parish in the hundred of DISS, county of NORFOLK, 22 miles (S.S.W.) from Norwich, and 92 (N.E.) from London, containing 2764 inhabitants. This place, formerly *Disce* or *Dice*, was held in royal demesne in the reign of Henry I., and in that of Edward I. became the property of Robert Fitzwalter, who obtained for it the privilege of a market. The town is pleasantly situated near the river Waveney, by which it is separated on the south from the county of Suffolk, and consists of several streets, of which the principal are spacious and well paved : the houses are in general well built, and have a neat and handsome appearance : the inhabitants are amply supplied with water ; and at the extremity of the town, and nearly in the centre of the parish, is a mere of seven acres in extent, which abounds with eels. The principal branch of manufacture is that of hempen cloth. The market is on Friday, which is also for the sale of yarn and linen cloth : the fair is on the 8th of November, for cattle and toys. The living is a rectory, in the archdeaconry of Norfolk, and diocese of Norwich, rated in the king's books at £33. 6. 8., and in the patronage of the Rev. W. Manning. The church, dedicated to St. Mary, is an ancient structure in the early and decorated styles of English architecture, with a square embattled tower : the nave is lighted by a fine range of double clerestory windows ; and the south porch has a semicircular-headed door-way, over which is a large window of stained glass : it was probably erected by some of the Fitz-Walters, about the close of the thirteenth or fourteenth century. There are places of worship for the Society of Friends and Independents. A charity school, originally endowed at Palgrave, in the county of Suffolk, was, in 1713, removed to this town, and kept in a building which was formerly the town-hall. Ralph de Diceto, Dean of St. Paul's in the reign of Henry II.; Walter, a Carmelite friar of Norwich, confessor to John of Gaunt, were natives of this parish; of which also, John Skelton, poet-laureat to Henry VIII., and styled by Erasmus " the light and ornament of English scholars," was rector.

DISSINGTON (NORTH), a township in that part of the parish of NEWBURN which is in the western division of CASTLE ward, county of NORTHUMBERLAND, 10 miles (N.W. by W.) from Newcastle upon Tyne, containing 65 inhabitants. There was formerly a chapel, subordinate to Tynemouth priory, every vestige of which has been long since obliterated. Admiral Sir Ralph Delaval was born here; he died in 1707.

DISSINGTON (SOUTH), a township in that part of the parish of NEWBURN which is in the western division of CASTLE ward, county of NORTHUMBERLAND, 9 miles (N.W. by W.) from Newcastle upon Tyne, containing 74 inhabitants.

DISTINGTON, a parish in ALLERDALE ward above Darwent, county of CUMBERLAND, 4¼ miles (N.E. by N.) from Whitehaven, containing 988 inhabitants. The living is a rectory, in the archdeaconry of Richmond, and diocese of Chester, rated in the king's books at £7. 1. 0½., and in the patronage of the Earl of Lonsdale. This parish stretches almost to the Irish sea, and contains coal pits, and quarries of excellent lime-stone, much

of which is burnt into lime : mill-stones, and grind-stones are also obtained. There are manufactures for linen-thread, hats, and edge tools. A school was erected in 1754, and is endowed with about £3 a year, arising from land then given by the parish. South of the village are the remains of Hayes castle, the ancient residence of the family of Moresby.

DISTLEY, a chapelry in the parish of STOCKPORT, hundred of MACCLESFIELD, county palatine of CHESTER, 6¾ miles (S.E.) from Stockport, containing 1533 inhabitants. The living is a perpetual curacy, in the archdeaconry and diocese of Chester, endowed with £8 per annum private benefaction, £400 royal bounty, and £1200 parliamentary grant, and in the patronage of Thomas Legh, Esq. The chapel, dedicated to All Saints, which was rebuilt in 1558, in the later style of English architecture, has an embattled tower; also windows of stained glass, exhibiting several portraits and armorial bearings. A school is endowed with £10. 5. per annum, the produce of divers benefactions. The Peak Forest canal passes through the parish.

DITCHAMPTON, a parish in the hundred of BRANCH and DOLE, county of WILTS, ¼ of a mile (N.) from Wilton, with which the population is returned. The living is a rectory united to the rectory of Wilton, in the archdeaconry and diocese of Salisbury, rated in the king's books at £10. The church, which was dedicated to St. Andrew, has been demolished.

DITCHBURN, (EAST and WEST), a township in the parish of ELLINGHAM, southern division of BAMBROUGH ward, county of NORTHUMBERLAND, containing 97 inhabitants : the former is 8½ miles (N.N.W.), and the latter 8 (N.W. by N.), from Alnwick. Within this township was a fortified tower with a place of safety for cattle during the border warfare.

DITCHEAT, a parish in the hundred of WHITESTONE, county of SOMERSET, 3¼ miles (N.N.W.) from Castle-Cary, containing 1223 inhabitants. The living is a rectory, in the archdeaconry of Wells, and diocese of Bath and Wells, rated in the king's books at £46. 5. Mrs. Leir and another were patrons in 1812. The church is dedicated to St. Mary Magdalene. The old Roman fosse-way bounds the parish on the northwest.

DITCHELLING, a parish in the hundred of STREET, rape of LEWES, county of SUSSEX, 3 miles (E.S.E.) from Hurst-Pierpoint, containing 844 inhabitants. The living is a discharged vicarage, in the archdeaconry of Lewes, and diocese of Chichester, rated in the king's books at £11, endowed with £210 private benefaction, and £200 royal bounty, and in the patronage of the Chancellor in the Cathedral Church of Chichester. The church, dedicated to St. Margaret, is mostly in the early style of English architecture, with some windows in the decorated style. There is a place of worship for Independents. Ditchelling was formerly a market town : a fair for sheep and hogs is held on the 5th of April, and one for pedlary on the 12th of October. In the neighbourhood there is an old quadrangular camp; and vestiges of a Roman road may be traced.

DITCHFORD, a parish in the Brails division of the hundred of KINGTON, county of WARWICK, 3 miles (S.W.) from Shipston upon Stour. The population is returned with Stretton on the Foss. The living is a rectory, annexed, in 1642, to the rectory of

Stretton on the Foss, in the archdeaconry of Gloucester, and diocese of Worcester, rated in the king's books at £6. The church, which was dedicated to St. Giles, has been demolished.

DITCHFORD, a hamlet in the parish of BLOCKLEY, upper division of the hundred of OSWALDSLOW, county of WORCESTER, though locally in the upper division of the hundred of Kiftsgate, county of Gloucester, 4¼ miles (S.W. by W.) from Shipston upon Stour, containing 46 inhabitants.

DITCHINGHAM, a parish in the hundred of LODDON, county of NORFOLK, 13½ miles (S.E. by S.) from Norwich, containing 761 inhabitants. The living is a rectory, in the archdeaconry of Norfolk, and diocese of Norwich, rated in the king's books at £16, and in the patronage of the Duke of Norfolk, who presents to a fellow of St. John's College, Cambridge. The church is dedicated to St. Mary.

DITTERIDGE, a parish in the hundred of CHIPPENHAM, county of WILTS, 7¾ miles (W. S. W.) from Chippenham, containing 86 inhabitants. The living is a discharged rectory, in the archdeaconry of Wilts, and diocese of Salisbury, rated in the king's books at £2. 8. 9., endowed with £200 royal bounty, and in the patronage of the Rev. E. Northey.

DITTISHAM, a parish in the hundred of COLERIDGE, county of DEVON, 5½ miles (N. by W.) from Dartmouth, containing 704 inhabitants. The living is a rectory, in the archdeaconry of Totness, and diocese of Exeter, rated in the king's books at £34. 15. Viscount Valletort was patron in 1827. The church, dedicated to St. George, has a richly sculptured stone pulpit. The parish, which is remarkable for the beauty of its scenery, is crossed by the navigable river Dart, over which there is a ferry.

DITTON, a chapelry in the parish of STOKE-POGES, hundred of STOKE, county of BUCKINGHAM, 1½ mile (W. N.W.) from Colnbrook. The population is returned with the parish. The chapel is dedicated to St. Mary.

DITTON, a parish in the hundred of LARKFIELD, lathe of AYLESFORD, county of KENT, 3½ miles (N.W. by W.) from Maidstone, containing 192 inhabitants. The living is a rectory, in the archdeaconry and diocese of Rochester, rated in the king's books at £11. 15. The Earl of Aylesford was patron in 1796. The church, dedicated to St. Peter, is a small building with a square tower at the west end.

DITTON, a township in the parish of PRESCOT, hundred of WEST DERBY, county palatine of LANCASTER, 5½ miles (S.S.E.) from Prescot, containing 455 inhabitants.

DITTON (FEN), a parish in the hundred of FLENDISH, county of CAMBRIDGE, 2¾ miles (N.E. by E.) from Cambridge, containing 461 inhabitants. The living is a rectory, rated in the king's books at £26. 12. 1., and in the peculiar jurisdiction and patronage of the Bishop of Ely. The church is dedicated to St. Mary. A market, now disused, was granted, in 1270, to one of the bishops of Ely, who resided at Bigging, in this parish. A charity school was founded, in 1729, by Elizabeth March, and endowed with the fifth part of an estate, now producing about £100 per annum. An almshouse for six poor widows was built by one of the Willys family, in 1665.

DITTON (LONG), a parish in the second division

of the hundred of KINGSTON, county of SURREY, 2¼ miles (S.S.W.) from Kingston upon Thames, containing, with the hamlet of Talworth, 595 inhabitants. The living is a rectory, in the archdeaconry of Surrey, and diocese of Winchester, rated in the king's books at £12. 0. 5., and in the patronage of the Warden and Fellows of New College, Oxford. The church is dedicated to St. Mary.

DITTON (PRIORS), a parish partly in the hundred of MUNSLOW, but chiefly within the liberty of the borough of WENLOCK, county of SALOP, 7¾ miles (W.S.W.) from Bridgenorth, containing, with the township of Ruthale with Ashfield, which is in Munslow hundred, 685 inhabitants. The living is a discharged vicarage, in the archdeaconry of Salop, and diocese of Hereford, rated in the king's books at £5. 15. 8. John Baxter, Esq. was patron in 1791. The church is dedicated to St. John the Baptist.

DITTON (THAMES), a parish comprising the manor of Cleygate, in the second division of the hundred of KINGSTON, and the hamlet of Ember with Weston, in the second division of the hundred of ELMBRIDGE, county of SURREY, 2¼ miles (S.W. by W.) from Kingston upon Thames, and containing 1592 inhabitants. The living is a perpetual curacy, in the archdeaconry of Surrey, and diocese of Winchester, and in the patronage of the Provost and Fellows of King's College, Cambridge. The church, dedicated to St. Nicholas, was formerly a chapel of ease to Kingston upon Thames, from which it was separated and made parochial, by act of parliament in 1769 : it is a small building near the bank of the Thames, with a low square tower and wooden spire at the west end, and formerly contained many ancient monuments and sepulchral brasses, which have been either taken away, or are now concealed by the pews. There is a place of worship for Independents. An almshouse for four poor widows, with a small endowment, was founded about 1630, by Elizabeth Hill; and, in 1720, Henry Bridges bequeathed a rent-charge of £30 to endow an almshouse containing tenements for six poor men or women. William Hatton, in 1703, left by will a rent-charge of £20 to the minister of Thames-Ditton, subject to the approval of a majority of the inhabitants, otherwise to poor housekeepers not receiving alms. There is also a considerable number of small benefactions, and the overseers have the .privilege of sending three patients annually to the Westminster Infirmary.

DITTON (WOOD), a parish in the hundred of CHEVELEY, county of CAMBRIDGE, 2¾ miles (S.S.E.) from Newmarket, containing 812 inhabitants. The living is a discharged vicarage, consolidated with the rectory of St. Mary, Newmarket, in the archdeaconry of Sudbury, and diocese of Norwich, rated in the king's books at £12. 16. 5½. The church is dedicated to St. Mary.

DIXON, or DICKLESTON, a hamlet in the parish of ALDERTON, upper division of the hundred of TEWKESBURY, county of GLOUCESTER, 4¼ miles (W.N.W.) from Winchcombe. The population is returned with the parish. This place in the reign of Edward III. was the seat of the Dicklestons ; near the mansion was formerly a chapel, dedicated to All Saints, but it has been long since desecrated. Vestiges of an ancient intrenchment are discernible in the neighbourhood.

DIXTON (HADNOCK), a hamlet in the parish of NEWTON-DIXTON, lower division of the hundred of

H

SKENFRETH, county of MONMOUTH, 1¾ mile (N.E.) from Monmouth, containing 360 inhabitants.

DIXTON (NEWTON), a parish in the lower division of the hundred of SKENFRETH, county of MONMOUTH, comprising the hamlets of Hadnock-Dixton and Newton-Dixton, and containing 565 inhabitants, of which number, 205 are in the hamlet of Newton-Dixton, 1½ mile (N.E.) from Monmouth. The living is a discharged vicarage, in the archdeaconry and diocese of Hereford, rated in the king's books at £7. 3. 1½., and endowed with £200 royal bounty. Lord Viscount Gage was patron in 1823. The church is dedicated to St. Peter.

DOBCROSS, a chapelry in that part of the parish of ROCHDALE which is in the upper division of the wapentake of AGBRIGG, West riding of the county of YORK, 13 miles (S.W.) from Huddersfield. The living is a perpetual curacy, in the archdeaconry and diocese of Chester, endowed with £200 private benefaction, £1000 royal bounty, and £2000 parliamentary grant, and in the patronage of certain Trustees.

DOCKER, a township in that part of the parish of KENDAL which is in KENDAL ward, county of WESTMORLAND, 4¼ miles (N.E. by E.) from Kendal, containing 89 inhabitants.

DOCKING, a parish in the hundred of SMITHDON, county of NORFOLK, 5¼ miles (S.W. by W.) from Burnham-Westgate, containing 1107 inhabitants. The living is a discharged vicarage, in the archdeaconry of Norfolk, and diocese of Norwich, rated in the king's books at £13. 6. 8., and in the patronage of the Provost and Fellows of Eton College, on the nomination of the Bishop of Norwich. The church is dedicated to St. Mary. There is a place of worship for Wesleyan Methodists. In the charter of endowment of Eton College, mention is made of the Alien priory of Dokkyng : the monks are supposed by Dr. Tanner to have belonged to the abbey de Ibreio in Normandy, to which this church was formerly appropriated. Summerfield House, about two miles north-westward, is a corruption of Suthmere, which at the period of the Norman survey, and later, was a town of some importance, with a church dedicated to All Saints, of which there are not at present any vestiges.

DOCKINGFIELD, a tything in that part of the parish of FRENSHAM which is in the hundred of ALTON, Alton (North) division of the county of SOUTHAMPTON, 4¾ miles (S. by W.) from Farnham, containing 169 inhabitants.

DOCKLOW, a parish in the hundred of WOLPHY, county of HEREFORD, 5½ miles (E. by S.) from Leominster, containing, with the township of Fencott, 191 inhabitants. The living is a perpetual curacy, annexed, with that of Stoke-Prior, to the vicarage of Leominster, in the archdeaconry and diocese of Hereford, endowed with £200 private benefaction, £400 royal bounty, and £200 parliamentary grant, and in the patronage of the Vicar of Leominster. The church is dedicated to St. Bartholomew.

DODBROKE, a market town and parish in the hundred of COLERIDGE, county of DEVON, ½ a mile (E.) from Kingsbridge, containing 885 inhabitants. This place derives its name from the Dod, a small stream by which it is separated from the town of Kingsbridge; it is a place of some antiquity, and in the time of Edward the Confessor was the property of Bric-

tric, sheriff for the county. It obtained, in the reign of Henry III., the grant of a weekly market, and an annual fair for two days on the festival of St. Mary Magdalene. The town, situated on the declivity of a hill, is indifferently built, but well supplied with water : it is noted for its white ale, a beverage peculiar to this part of Devonshire, which is ready for use on the day after it is brewed, and in this parish is subject to tithe, in lieu of which, the rector receives a commutation of ten-pence from each inn-keeper. The market, formerly held regularly, is now held only on the third Wednesday in every month : there is a cattle fair on the Wednesday before Palm-Sunday. The living is a discharged rectory, in the archdeaconry of Totness, and diocese of Exeter, rated in the king's books at £8. 11. 4., and in the patronage of the Rev. Dr. Owen. The church, dedicated to St. Thomas à Becket, is built on rising ground, at the extremity of the town ; it is an ancient structure, strengthened with buttresses, and embattled, and contains an ancient stone font in the early English style, and a wooden screen finely carved. Dr. Wolcott, the satirical poet, more generally known by the assumed name of Peter Pindar, was a native of this place.

DODCOT, a joint township with Wilkesley, partly in the parish of WRENBURY, but chiefly in that of AUDLEM, hundred of NANTWICH, county palatine of CHESTER, 4 miles (W. S. W.) from Audlem, containing 670 inhabitants. The chapel of Burley Dam, which is in the parish of Audlem, stands in this township ; it is a neat modern structure, founded by Sir Lynch Salusbury Cotton, Bart. In that part of the township which is in the parish of Wrenbury, Hugh de Malbanc, in 1133, founded the Cistercian monastery of Combermere, and dedicated it to St. Mary and St. Michael, the revenue of which, at the dissolution, was valued at £258. 6. 6. : the site and buildings were granted, in the 32nd of Henry VIII., to William Cotton, Esq., an ancestor of Lord Combermere, whose family seat, occupying the spot, is agreeably situated on the margin of the beautiful lake of Combermere, his lordship deriving the title of baron from this place.

DODDENHAM, a chapelry in the parish of KNIGHTWICK, lower division of the hundred of DODDINGTREE, county of WORCESTER, 7¼ miles (W. by N.) from Worcester, containing 252 inhabitants. The chapel is dedicated to St. Andrew.

DODDERHILL, a parish partly within the borough of DROITWICH, but chiefly in the upper division of the hundred of HALFSHIRE, county of WORCESTER, ½ a mile (N.) from Droitwich, containing, with the chapelry of Elmbridge, 1565 inhabitants. The living is a vicarage, in the archdeaconry and diocese of Worcester, rated in the king's books at £12. 12. 3½., and in the patronage of George Penrice, Esq. The church, dedicated to St. Augustine, is a curious edifice, which having been partly destroyed in the parliamentary war, and rebuilt, consists of the north transept of a Norman church, with a chancel of later date, and a tower in place of the south transept. A free chapel, or hospital, was founded in the 13th of Edward I., and dedicated to St. Mary, by William de Dovere, for a master and poor brethren, who were under the government of the prior of Worcester, and whose lands, at the suppression of free chapels in the reign of Edward VI., were valued at £21. 11. 8.

DODDERSHALL, a hamlet in the parish of QUAINTON, hundred of ASHENDON, county of BUCKINGHAM, 7½ miles (N.W. by W.) from Aylesbury. The population is returned with the parish.

DODDINGHURST, a parish in the hundred of BARSTABLE, county of ESSEX, 3½ miles (N.) from Brentwood, containing 356 inhabitants. The living is a rectory, in the archdeaconry and diocese of Exeter, rated in the king's books at £10. 3. 9. Jarvis Kenrick, Esq. was patron in 1813. The church is dedicated to All Saints.

DODDINGTON, a parish in the northern division of the hundred of WITCHFORD, ISLE of ELY, county of CAMBRIDGE, 4½ miles (S. by W.) from March, comprising the chapelries of Benwick and Marsh, and the hamlet of Wimblington, and containing 5899 inhabitants. The living is a rectory, in the peculiar jurisdiction of the Bishop of Ely, and in the patronage of Sir H. Peyton, Bart. The church is dedicated to St. Mary. The sum of £500, given in 1719, by Lionel Walden, Esq., a native of the parish, for the erection of a free school, having for many years remained unappropriated, has accumulated to £1800 three per cents., and £500 four per cents., and a school has been recently established, the master of which has a salary of £40 per annum and a house.

DODDINGTON, a township in the parish of WYBUNBURY, hundred of NANTWICH, county palatine of CHESTER, 5½ miles (S. E.) from Nantwich, containing 39 inhabitants. There is a mutilated tower, which formed part of Doddington castle, erected by Sir John Delves in 1364, where are preserved statues of Lord Audley and his four squires who fought under the Black Prince at Poictiers; near it stood the old hall, which was made a parliamentary garrison in the civil war, taken for the king by Lord Byron, in January 1644, and retaken for the parliament shortly after. Sir Thomas Delves, who died in 1727, gave by deed £1535 for the purchase of land, the income derived from which is applied for the support of schools at Doddington and Weston, in which twenty boys and ten girls of the parish of Wybunbury are educated.

DODDINGTON, a parish in the hundred of TEYNHAM, lathe of SCRAY, county of KENT, 4¾ miles (S. by E.) from Sittingbourne, containing 451 inhabitants. The living is a discharged vicarage, in the archdeaconry and diocese of Canterbury, rated in the king's books at £6. 13. 4., endowed with £400 royal bounty, and in the patronage of the Archdeacon of Canterbury. The church, dedicated to St. John the Baptist, is principally in the early style of English architecture. There is a place of worship for Wesleyan Methodists.

DODDINGTON, a parish in the lower division of the wapentake of BOOTHBY-GRAFFO, parts of KESTEVEN, county of LINCOLN, 6½ miles (W. by S.) from Lincoln, containing, with the chapelry of Whisby, 227 inhabitants. The living is a discharged rectory, in the archdeaconry and diocese of Lincoln, rated in the king's books at £7. 9. 6. The church is dedicated to St. Peter.

DODDINGTON, a parish in the eastern division of GLENDALE ward, county of NORTHUMBERLAND, comprising the townships of Doddington, Earl (otherwise Yeard) Hill, Ewart, Humbleton, and Nesbitt, and containing 865 inhabitants, of which number, 419 are in the township of Doddington, 3 miles (N. by E.) from

Wooler. The living is a perpetual curacy, in the archdeaconry of Northumberland, and diocese of Durham, and in the patronage of the Duke of Northumberland. Until 1725, this was a chapelry to the vicarage of Chatton. Coal is obtained in the parish; and there is a considerable spring near the village, which turns a cornmill. A school-room has been erected at the expense of the Earl of Tankerville.

DODDINGTON (DRY), a parish in the wapentake of LOVEDEN, parts of KESTEVEN, county of LINCOLN, 8 miles (N.N.W.) from Grantham, containing 227 inhabitants. The living is a vicarage united to a mediety of the rectory of Westborough, in the archdeaconry and diocese of Lincoln. The church is dedicated to St. James.

DODDINGTON (GREAT), a parish in the hundred of HAMFORDSHOE, county of NORTHAMPTON, 2½ miles (S. by W.) from Wellingborough, containing 442 inhabitants. The living is a discharged vicarage, in the archdeaconry of Northampton, and diocese of Peterborough, rated in the king's books at £8. 13. 4., and in the patronage of the Crown. The church is dedicated to St. Nicholas.

DODDISCOMBSLEIGH, a parish in the hundred of EXMINSTER, county of DEVON, 6 miles (S.W.) from Exeter, containing 356 inhabitants. The living is a rectory, in the archdeaconry and diocese of Exeter, rated in the king's books at £16. 6. 5½. The Rev. George Hole was patron in 1823. The church is dedicated to St. Michael. There was formerly a chapel at a place called Sheldon, in this parish. Here is a small endowed charity school.

DODDLESTON, a parish in the lower division of the hundred of BROXTON, county palatine of CHESTER, comprising the townships of Doddleston and Lower Kinnerton, and containing 351 inhabitants, of which number, 266 are in the township of Doddleston, 5 miles (S.W.) from Chester. The living is a rectory, in the archdeaconry and diocese of Chester, rated in the king's books at £7. 0. 2½., and in the patronage of the Dean and Chapter of Chester. The church, dedicated to St. Mary, contains the remains of Thomas Egerton, Baron Ellesmere, Viscount Brackley, Lord Keeper of the Great Seal to James I., and ancestor of the Earls of Bridgewater, who occasionally resided here; he died in London in 1617. A school is supported by charitable contributions. During the siege of Chester, in 1645, the old mansion-house was fortified and garrisoned by the parliamentary general, Sir William Brereton, who here fixed his head-quarters.

DODFORD, a parish in the hundred of FAWSLEY, county of NORTHAMPTON, 2½ miles (E.S.E) from Daventry, containing 247 inhabitants. The living is a vicarage, in the archdeaconry of Northampton, and diocese of Peterborough, rated in the king's books at £10. Robert Andrew, Esq. was patron in 1801. The church, dedicated to St. Mary, has portions in the early style of English architecture; the font is Norman. Joseph Cook, in 1779, bequeathed £500, the income arising from which is £25 a year, applied in educating and apprenticing poor children; thirty-five are taught by means of this charity. The Grand Junction canal passes along the east side of the parish.

DODINGTON, a parish in the lower division of the hundred of GRUMBALD'S ASH, county of GLOUCESTER,

H 2

2½ miles (S.E. by E.) from Chipping-Sodbury, containing 106 inhabitants. The living is a rectory, in the archdeaconry and diocese of Gloucester, rated in the king's books at £5. 6. 5½. C. Codrington, Esq. was patron in 1816. The church, dedicated to St. Mary, is a small building, with a low tower. The river Frome has its source in this parish. Urns, bones, and Roman coins, have been discovered in a place called Dodington Field.

DODINGTON, a township in the parish and hundred of WHITCHURCH, Bradford (North) division of the county of SALOP, ¼ of a mile (S.) from Whitchurch, with which the population is returned.

DODINGTON, a parish in the hundred of WILLITON and FREEMANNERS, county of SOMERSET, 9½ miles (W. N.W.) from Bridg-water, containing 113 inhabitants. The living is a discharged rectory, in the archdeaconry of Taunton, and diocese of Bath and Wells, rated in the king's books at £5. 6. 8. The Duke of Buckingham was patron in 1821.

DODNASH, in the parish of BENTLEY, hundred of SAMFORD, county of SUFFOLK, 7½ miles (S.W.) from Ipswich. A priory of Black canons, dedicated to St. Mary, was founded here, as it is said, by an ancestor of the Howard family, to which the patronage belonged from the time of Edward I. till the dissolution, when it contained a prior and three religious, whose revenue was valued at £42. 18. 8. per annum.

DODWORTH, a township in the parish of SILK-STONE, wapentake of STAINCROSS, West riding of the county of YORK, 2½ miles (W.S.W.) from Barnesley, containing 1227 inhabitants. The manufacture of linen is here carried on to a limited extent.

DOGDYKE, a township in the parish of BILLING-HAY, first division of the wapentake of LANGOE, parts of KESTEVEN, county of LINCOLN, 11 miles (E.N.E.) from Sleaford, containing 231 inhabitants.

DOGMERSFIELD, a parish in the hundred of ODIHAM, Basingstoke division of the county of SOUTH-AMPTON, 2 miles (E. by N.) from Odiham, containing 213 inhabitants. The living is a rectory, in the archdeaconry and diocese of Winchester, rated in the king's books at £9. 6. 8., and in the patronage of Lady Mild-may. The church is dedicated to All Saints. Foundations, supposed to be the remains of a palace of the archbishops of Canterbury, which stood here so early as the twelfth century, were discovered a few years since. The Basingstoke canal passes through the parish, which contains a lake covering thirty-six acres.

DOGS (ISLE of), or STEPNEY MARSH, in the parish of STEPNEY, Tower division of the hundred of OSSULSTONE, county of MIDDLESEX, 5 miles (E. S.E.) from St. Paul's Cathedral, London. The population is returned with the parish. The isle comprises about eight hundred and thirty-six acres of ground, and is thought to have received name from a kennel for the king's hounds having been anciently situated upon it. The site of a chapel, dedicated to St. Mary, is now occupied by a farm-house, sometimes called the Chapel House. There is a ship-canal across it, from Limehouse to Blackwall, to avoid a curve of the Thames between those two places. At the south-eastern part of it is a ferry over the Thames to Greenwich; and near it the Steam washing-Company have an establishment: there are also mills for extracting oil from lin-

seed, and for making oil-cake for feeding cattle; a manufactory for chain cables, and another for smelling-salts. There is a place of worship for Independents.

DOGSTHORPE, a chapelry in that part of the parish of ST. JOHN the BAPTIST, PETERBOROUGH, which is within the liberty of PETERBOROUGH, county of NORTHAMPTON, 1¾ mile (N.) from Peterborough, containing 379 inhabitants. The chapel is dedicated to St. Botolph.

DOLTON, a parish in the hundred of NORTH TAW-TON and WINKLEY, county of DEVON, 6 miles (N. N. E) from Hatherleigh, containing 748 inhabitants. The living is a rectory, in the archdeaconry of Barnstaple, and diocese of Exeter, rated in the king's books at £20. 16. 8. J. Cleveland, Esq. was patron in 1823. The church is dedicated to St. Edmund. There are two fairs for cattle, on the Wednesday before March 25th, and October 1st. There are donations amounting to about £7. 11. 6. per annum, for the instruction of children.

DOMINICK (ST.), a parish in the middle division of the hundred of EAST, county of CORNWALL, 2¾ miles (E. S. E) from Callington, containing 690 inhabitants. The living is a rectory, in the archdeaconry of Cornwall, and diocese of Exeter, rated in the king's books at £23. 11. 0½., and in the patronage of Mrs. Bluett. William Brent, in 1784, gave £5 per annum for teaching poor children. On the glebe estate are vestiges of a Roman intrenchment, called Berry, and the remains of an old monastery at Baber. The navigable river Tamar forms the eastern boundary of the parish. At Halton was born, in 1579, Francis Rous, a distinguished politician, speaker of the Little Parliament in the time of Cromwell, and provost of Eton College.

DONCASTER, a parish comprising the borough and market town of Doncaster, which has a separate jurisdiction, the townships of Balby with Hexthorp, and Long Sandal with Wheatley, in the soke of DONCASTER, and the township of Lang-thwaite with Tilts, in the northern division of the wapentake of STRAFFORTH and TICKHILL, West riding of the county of YORK, and containing 9117 inhabitants, of which number, 8544 are in the borough of Doncaster, 37 miles (S. by W.) from York, and 162 (N.N.W.) from London. This place, the *Danum* of Antoninus, a Roman station on the river Don, was by the Saxons called *Dona Ceaster*, from which its present name is derived. According to Camden, the town was entirely destroyed by lightning about the year 759, at which period the castle, of which the founder and the time of its foundation are unknown, is supposed to have been burnt. The town is pleasantly situated on the southern bank of the river Don, and the surrounding scenery, especially on the western side, is delightfully picturesque; it consists of several streets, of which the High-street, about a mile in length, is the principal, and is considered to be the best, for width and beauty, on the road from London to Edinburgh; they are well paved, and lighted with gas, at the expense of the corporation, who have ample revenues for the improvement of the town, and the inhabitants are supplied

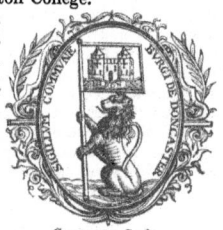

Corporate Seal.

with water by means of water-works near the Friar's bridge, from a reservoir at the top of the High-street, under the direction of the corporation, the expense being defrayed by a rate. An elegant cross, in the later style of English architecture, stands on an eminence called Hall-cross hill, and has superseded a rude and ancient structure of a similar kind, which was formerly placed in the centre of a road leading into the town, but removed in order to widen and improve the carriage-way. An agricultural society, established in 1803, holds an annual meeting in July or August. A very commodious suite of apartments was erected in 1821, for a public library and news-room, established by private subscription, to which a collection of old books, kept for many years in a room over the church porch, has been recently added : this institution is open to the use of all the inhabitants, though not members of the society.

The races, which for some years have been increasing in splendour and attraction, and are attended by nearly all the families of rank in the North of England, are generally held in the third week in September, and continue five days. About a mile from the town is the celebrated race-ground, on which a very elegant and commodious stand has been built at the expense of the corporation, who also have for many years given an annual plate, of the value £50, of and a subscription of £42 towards the stakes : in addition to these donations are His Majesty's plate of £105, and a gold cup of £105, given by the stewards. An elegant building of the Ionic order, called the Betting-room, was erected in 1826 : it is ninety feet in length, and twenty-two feet wide, lighted during the day by a handsome dome, and at night with gas introduced into three superb chandeliers. The theatre is a handsome building, also erected at the expense of the corporation, in 1774 ; the performances commence in the race week, and continue about six weeks. Doncaster has but little trade or manufacture. There are two or three cast-iron foundries, and a sacking and twist manufactory, but all on a very small scale. The river Don is crossed by two bridges : Friars' bridge was erected by the corporation in 1614, and subsequently widened and handsomely ornamented with iron balustrades : the mill bridge was rebuilt in 1782. A long causeway has been constructed from both the bridges, to obviate the danger arising to passengers from the overflow of the river, which, being navigable to Sheffield, supplies a ready means of conveyance for articles of commerce, which are sent to London, Hull, and other places, in small vessels of from thirty to fifty tons' burden : timber, deals, grocery, and other goods are returned. The market is held on Saturday : fairs are held, February 2d, April 5th, August 5th, for horned cattle, horses, sheep, and coarse woollen cloth, and November 16th, which is a statute fair for hiring servants. A wool market commences on the second Saturday in June, and continues every Saturday until the 6th of August. The market-places occupy nearly the centre of the town, consisting of that for holding the corn-market, a spacious area, adjoining which is the market for meat, or the new shambles, built by the corporation in 1756, the roof of which is slated, and supported on twenty-four columns : an octagonal building was also erected by them in the same year, for the sale of fowls, butter, eggs, &c., and for fish, vegetables, and fruit.

The government of the town, by charter of Richard I., confirmed by succeeding kings, and modified by James II., is vested in a mayor, recorder, twelve aldermen, twenty-four common council-men, assisted by a town clerk and other officers. The mayor is chosen from among the aldermen, who elect to vacancies in their own body from the members of the common council, in which vacancies are filled up by the mayor, aldermen, and the capital and free burgesses : the mayor may appoint one of the aldermen who has passed the chair as his deputy. The recorder, who must be an outer barrister at least, is elected by the mayor, aldermen, and common council-men. The mayor, and three senior aldermen, are justices of the peace within the borough and soke of Doncaster. The freedom is inherited by birth, or obtained by seven years' apprenticeship within the borough, or by purchase for £3. 6. 8. The corporation hold quarterly courts of session, for determining on offences not capital ; and a court of record, under the charter of Henry VIII., for the recovery of debts to any amount. A court of requests is held under commissioners appointed by an act passed in the 4th of George III., for the recovery of debts under 40s. within the borough and soke : the annual session for the wapentake of Strafforth and Tickhill is also held here, and the county magistrates hold a meeting every Saturday for the adjoining district. The mansion-house, which is an elegant structure, was completed in 1748, and furnished at an expense of more than £8000 : it was enlarged in 1800, and an attic raised above the columns to screen the roof. The principal room is decorated with a full length portrait of his late Majesty, George III., in his coronation robes ; also with portraits of the present Earl Fitzwilliam, and of the Marquis of Rockingham, in parliamentary robes, both presented to the corporation by the earl. Here the muniments of the corporation are preserved, the feasts of the corporate body held, and concerts and assemblies periodically take place. This town had a residence especially appropriated for its chief magistrate before either London or York. The town-hall, which occupies the site of a church dedicated to St. Mary Magdalene, was thoroughly repaired and beautified in 1784, and considerably enlarged and improved in 1828, and is now one of the most convenient court-rooms in the county. The corporation are about to remove the present gaol, built in 1778, and to erect a new one upon the radiating plan, adapted to receive four classes of prisoners, with distinct airing-courts to each, the gaoler's house to occupy the centre, and to command an entire inspection of the prisoners.

The living is a vicarage, in the archdeaconry and diocese of York, rated in the king's books at £32. 19. 9., and in the patronage of the Archbishop of York ; it is under lay impropriation to Miss Sharp, a lineal descendant of the archbishop of that name, and from this lady the vicar receives an annual stipend of £60. The church, dedicated to St. George, is a spacious cruciform structure, principally in the later style of English architecture, with a tower, of which the details are exquisitely rich. According to Leland, it was partially built with materials from the ruins of the old castle : the exact period of its original erection is uncertain, but a stone, discovered a few years since, during some repairs, with the date of 1071 upon it, strengthens the opinion that part of it was erected about the time of the Conquest : it has, however, undergone so many alterations that no part of the original structure now remains, though there are some traces of an earlier date. The building consists of a nave, aisles, and a transept, with a choir and side chapels, or chantries, extending north and south to the extremity of the transept. The roof of the nave is sustained by twelve massive octangular pillars, with plain capitals, whence spring ten obtusely pointed arches. The tower is 'supported by four ponderous octagonal columns, with richly decorated capitals, of a later date than the rest of the fabric; and from these rise four finely pointed arches, on each side of which and in the belfry are monograms, armorial ensigns, &c., commemorative of various benefactors. The height of the church is seventy-eight feet, breadth sixty-eight feet, and length one hundred and fifty-four feet; the height of the tower is one hundred and forty-one feet. In the interior is an ancient font, though probably not of such remote antiquity as the date 1061 upon it implies : a magnificent east window has been recently erected, containing figures of the Apostles and the Prophets, the gift of Mrs. Baker. Among the various monuments is that of Robin of Doncaster, placed just behind the reading-desk, and bearing a curious inscription with the date 1579 ; the tomb is an altar of free-stone near the north-west supporter of the tower; also the tomb of Ellis, founder of the hospital, and five times mayor of Doncaster. A new church, in the later style of English architecture, called Christ's church, has lately been erected, from a fund of £13,000, granted by John Jarratt, Esq., a native of Doncaster, and formerly an iron-master at Bowling, near Bradford : it consists of a nave and side aisles, is ninety-five feet long and fifty-two feet wide, separated by slender-shafted pillars, and the spire, which is one hundred and sixty feet in height, is remarkable for its lightness and elegance. There are places of worship for the Society of Friends, Independents, Presbyterians, and Wesleyan Methodists.

The grammar school, kept on the ground-floor of the town-hall, was founded for the sons of freemen, by the corporation, who appoint the master, and allow him a salary of £80 per annum : there is a scholarship of £10 per annum in Jesus College, Cambridge, belonging to this and the school at Arksey. A National school has been lately established, in which two hundred and twelve boys, and one hundred and eight girls are taught reading, writing, and arithmetic ; the girls being likewise instructed in needle-work : it is supported by voluntary contributions, including an annual gift of £20 by the corporation. Sunday schools were introduced here at their first institution. St. Thomas' Hospital was erected in 1588, by Thomas Ellis, whose tomb is in the church, for the support of six poor and decayed housekeepers ; the founder endowed it with an estate then let for £10 per annum, but which, from the increased value of land, now produces about £400 per annum, enabling the trustees, who are the mayor and vicar, with others, to give pensions to twelve poor persons not resident, but who are admitted as vacancies arise. A dispensary was established in 1792, and is supported by voluntary contributions, and an annual gift of £105 from the corporation, at whose expense the building was erected. The poor-house, situated in St. Sepulchre's gate, was erected in 1719 by

subscriptions of the more wealthy inhabitants; the annual rent of fifty-nine acres and sixteen perches of land, in a place called the Intacks, with a rate on the inhabitants, under the management of a select vestry, is paid to the master for the maintenance of the poor. Edward Fenwick, of London, bequeathed £100 for the benefit of the poor of Doncaster, at the disposal of the mayor and corporation; Thomas Martin gave £20, charged on lands at Stainforth and Tudwath, to apprentice three, four, or five poor boys, natives of, and resident in, Doncaster ; Mr. Quinston Kay, of Ludgate-hill, London, upholsterer, in 1804, gave to the corporation £2000 three per cent. Bank Annuities, and £6000 four per cent. Bank Annuities, producing £300 per annum, in trust, to apply the dividends as follows; viz., £2. 2. to the vicar, or curate, for a sermon on the first Sunday in September, and £5 to be distributed on that day in bread to the poor ; £60 to apprentice every year six poor children, of either sex, residing in the township, at the age of fourteen, to some useful mechanical business ; £3. 3. annually to the dispensary ; £10 to the town clerk, for his trouble in making payments, and keeping accounts; the residue of the dividends to be paid in sums of £1. 1. per month to poor reduced persons, of either sex, being resident, and not less than fifty years of age. John Jarratt, Esq., of Doncaster, invested £2200 with the corporation, for an annuity of £110 per annum, to be divided amongst six reduced housekeepers.

The ancient Roman road, Watling-street, on which the town stands, may be traced over Scawsby Lees, near Adwick le Street, and in many other places northward, towards *Legiolium*, now Castleford, near the confluence of the rivers Aire and Calder ; and some years since, a Roman votive altar was dug up in the cellar of a house belonging to John Jarratt, Esq., near St. Sepulchre's gate. Among the religious establishments anciently existing here, were the hospitals of St. James and St. Nicholas, founded for lepers in the reign of Henry III. ; a house of Grey friars, founded in 1315 ; and a house of Black friars, of which the founder and the date are unknown. John Lacy, an actor and writer of plays in the time of Charles II., was born here. Henry Heaton, chaplain to Archbishop Herring, one of the young academics who assisted the Yorkes in the production of the Athenian Letters ; and Dr. Edward Miller, who in 1804 published the "History of Doncaster," resided here. Doncaster gives the title of earl to the Duke of Buccleuch.

DONHEAD (ST. ANDREW), a parish in the hundred of DUNWORTH, county of WILTS, 5½ miles (S. by E.) from Hindon, containing 753 inhabitants. The living is a rectory, in the archdeaconry and diocese of Salisbury, rated in the king's books at £13. 6. 8. T. Warburton, Esq. was patron in 1820. The church has lately received an addition of one hundred and four free sittings, the Incorporated Society for the enlargement of churches and chapels having granted £130 toward defraying the expense. On the western side of the village, on the summit of Tittle-path hill, is an old earth-work, called Castle-ring, enclosing an area of fifteen acres and a half.

DONHEAD (ST. MARY), a parish in the hundred of DUNWORTH, county of WILTS, 5½ miles (S.) from Hindon, containing, with the chapelry of Charlton, and the tythings of Dognell and Haystone, 1361 inhabitants. The living is a rectory, in the archdeaconry and diocese of

Salisbury, rated in the king's books at £30. 14. 4½., and in the patronage of the Warden and Fellows of New College, Oxford.

DONINGTON, a market town and parish in the wapentake of KIRTON, parts of HOLLAND, county of LINCOLN, 32 miles (S. E. by S.) from Lincoln, and 108 (N.) from London, containing 1638 inhabitants. It 'is situated in the fen district, through which a wide rampart of earth has been made, forming a convenient road to Sempringham. Hemp is very extensively cultivated in the neighbourhood, for the manufacture of thread and cloth, and for the seed. Canals, called Blacksluice and Hammond-beck, pass through the parish; and there is a port for barges, by which goods are conveyed between Boston and the Washes. A market is held on Saturday; and fairs, May 16th and October 26th, for horses, cattle, flax, and hemp. The living is a vicarage, in the archdeaconry and diocese of Lincoln, rated in the king's books at £13. 17. 3½., and in the patronage of the Rev. John Wilson. The church is dedicated to St. Mary and the Holy Rood. There are places of worship for Baptists and Wesleyan Methodists. Here is a large endowed school, founded by Lord Cowley; and there are also other charities.

DONINGTON, a parish in the Shiffnall division of the hundred of BRIMSTREE, county of SALOP, 5¼ miles (E.S.E.) from Shiffnall, containing 330 inhabitants. The living is a rectory, in the archdeaconry of Salop, and diocese of Lichfield and Coventry, rated in the king's books at £13. 6. 8. The Marquis of Stafford was patron in 1773. The church is supposed to have been built early in the fourteenth century, and the additions and alterations, though made at intervals, harmonize with the more ancient parts of the structure: at the foot of the rocky eminence upon which it stands is a spring, formerly called St. Cutbeard's, or St. Cuthbert's well. A free grammar school was founded by Thomas Alcocke, in 1627, at Donnington, then described as being in the parish of Wroxeter; to the original endowment other donations were made in 1658: it is open to forty boys of Wroxeter and Uppington, but at present a few only are upon the foundation: two exhibitions at Christ Church College, Oxford, are appropriated to this school, of which the late Dr. Douglas, Bishop of Salisbury, was in early life the master, where Richard Baxter, the non-conformist divine, and Dr. Allertree, Provost of Eton, received the elementary part of their education. Adjoining the parish is the extra-parochial place, Boscobel and White Ladies; it is regarded as within the cure of souls of the minister, and pays six shillings and eightpence in lieu of tithes and offerings: though formerly populous, there is now only the house celebrated as having been the hiding-place of Charles II., within a few hundred yards of which stood the oak, whose branches concealed the king, September 6th, 1653; no vestiges of this tree remain, but there is another close to its site, produced from one of its acorns, and distinguished by the title of The Royal Oak, the brick wall for the protection of which was superseded ten years ago by a handsome and lofty iron railing that now surrounds it. The priory of white or Cistercian nuns, dedicated to St. Leonard, is supposed to have been founded either in the reign of Richard I., or in that of John; at the dissolution it contained six religious, and was valued at £31. 1 4.: the nave, choir, and transepts of the chapel still remain, with a handsome Saxon arch over one of the doors; the interior is used as a burial-place by the Roman Catholic families in the neighbourhood.

DONINGTON upon BAIN, a parish in the northern division of the wapentake of GARTREE, parts of LINDSEY, county of LINCOLN, 6¾ miles (S.W. by W.) from Louth, containing 269 inhabitants. The living is a discharged rectory, in the archdeaconry and diocese of Lincoln, rated in the king's books at £15. 12. 2. Lord Monson was patron in 1797. The church is dedicated to St. Andrew.

DONINGTON (CASTLE), a parish in the western division of the hundred of GOSCOTE, county of LEICESTER, 9½ miles (N. E.) from Ashby de la Zouch, containing 2560 inhabitants. The living is a discharged vicarage, in the archdeaconry of Leicester, and diocese of Lincoln, rated in the king's books at £8. 2. 3½., endowed with £200 private benefaction, and £200 royal bounty, and in the patronage of the Marquis of Hastings. The church is dedicated to St. Edward. There is a place of worship for Independents. The parish is bounded on the north-west by the river Trent. Fairs are held, March 18th, on Whit-Thursday, and September 29th. On an eminence are the remains of an old castle from which the parish derives its distinguishing prefix; and there are vestiges of an hospital, dedicated to St. John the Evangelist, supposed to have been founded by John Lacy, constable of Chester in the time of Henry II., for a master and thirteen brethren and sisters, who received a portion of the tithes of the parish, and whose revenue at the dissolution was valued at only £3. 13. 4. per annum. Castle-Donington is in the honour of Tutbury, duchy of Lancaster, and within the jurisdiction of a court of pleas held at Tutbury every third Tuesday, for the recovery of debts under 40s.

DONISTHORPE, a hamlet partly in the parish of NETHER SEAL, western division of the hundred of GOSCOTE, county of LEICESTER, and partly in the parish of CHURCH-GRESLEY, hundred of REPTON and GRESLEY, county of DERBY, 3½ miles (S.W.) from Ashby de la Zouch, containing, with the hamlet of Oakthorpe, 732 inhabitants. Donisthorpe is in the honour of Tutbury, duchy of Lancaster, and within the jurisdiction of a court of pleas held at Tutbury every third Tuesday, for the recovery of debts under 40s.

DONNINGTON, a tything in the parish of SHAW, hundred of FAIRCROSS, county of BERKS, 1 mile (N.) from Speenhamland. The population is returned with the parish. Donnington castle, built by Sir Richard de Abberbury, who was guardian to Richard II. in his minority, stood upon a declivity, at the foot of which runs the river Kennet: it was garrisoned for Charles I., and withstood two sieges during the civil war, in the first of which three of its towers were demolished, and in 1644 it was almost battered down by Colonel Dalbier, from whom a field in the vicinity, in which he planted his cannon, is still named: the only remains of this once impregnable fortress consist of a gateway flanked by two towers, a great portion of the ruins having been removed and appropriated for the erection of a house close by. A friary of the order of the Holy Trinity was also founded by Sir Richard de Abberbury, the revenue of which, at the dissolution, was valued at £20. 16. 6. per annum. An hospital, called God's House, is supposed to have been founded in 1392, by the same individual, who endowed it with lands for a minister and certain poor persons, whose revenue, at its suppression was valued at £19. 3. 10. : upon the petition of the Earl of Nottingham it was rebuilt, in 1570, and restored under the title of Queen Elizabeth's hospital, for a master and twelve poor brethren.

DONNINGTON, a hamlet in the parish of STOW on the WOLD, upper division of the hundred of SLAUGHTER, county of GLOUCESTER, 1½ mile (N.) from Stow on the Wold, containing 201 inhabitants. A battle was fought here in 1645, in which the royalists under Lord Aston were defeated by Colonel Morgan ; this victory occasioned the surrender of the king's garrison at Oxford, and hastened the termination of the protracted war.

DONNINGTON, a parish in the hundred of RADLOW, county of HEREFORD, 2¼ miles (S. by W.) from Ledbury, containing 103 inhabitants. The living is a discharged rectory, in the archdeaconry and diocese of Hereford, rated in the king's books at £3. 9. 9. The Rev. E. Freeman was patron in 1817. The church is dedicated to St. Mary.

DONNINGTON, a joint chapelry with Hugglescote, in the parish of IBSTOCK, hundred of SPARKENHOE, county of LEICESTER, 5½ miles (S.E. by E.) from Ashby de la Zouch, containing 683 inhabitants. The chapel is dedicated to St. Peter.

DONNINGTON, a parish in the hundred of Box and STOCKBRIDGE, rape of CHICHESTER, county of SUSSEX, 2 miles (S.S.W.) from Chichester, containing 267 inhabitants. The living is a vicarage, in the archdeaconry and diocese of Chichester, rated in the king's books at £9. 10. 5., and in the patronage of the Bishop of Chichester. The church is in the early style of English architecture. The Arundel and Portsmouth canal passes through the parish.

DONNINGTON-WOOD, a chapelry in the parish of LILLESHALL, Newport division of the hundred of BRADFORD (South), county of SALOP, 3¾ miles (E.N.E.) from Wellington. The population is returned with the parish. The living is a perpetual curacy, in the archdeaconry of Salop, and diocese of Lichfield and Coventry, endowed with £200 private benefaction, £800 royal bounty, and £300 parliamentary grant, and in the patronage of the Marquis of Stafford. The chapel is dedicated to St. George. There is a place of worship for Baptists.

DONYATT, a parish in the hundred of ABDICK and BULSTONE, county of SOMERSET, 2¼ miles (W.S.W.) from Ilminster, containing 518 inhabitants. The living is a rectory, in the archdeaconry of Taunton, and diocese of Bath and Wells, rated in the king's books at £15. 15. R. T. Combe, Esq. was patron in 1822. The church is dedicated to St. Mary. The river Isle runs through the parish, and over it are four bridges. At a place called Crockstreet there are three potteries. John Dunster, citizen and cloth-worker of London, founded, in 1625, an almshouse, with an endowment now producing £48 per annum, for three poor men and three women.

DONYLAND (EAST), a parish in the Colchester division of the hundred of LEXDEN, county of ESSEX, 3¼ miles (S.E. by S.) from Colchester, containing 562 inhabitants. The living is a rectory, in the archdeaconry of Colchester, and diocese of London, rated in the king's books at £10. The Rev. Charles Hewitt was patron in 1801. The church is dedicated to St. Lawrence. The

navigable river Colne forms the eastern boundary of the parish, and there receives the river Roman.

DONYLAND (WEST), county of ESSEX. See BERECHURCH.

DORCHESTER, a borough and market town, having separate jurisdiction, locally in the hundred of Uggscome, Dorchester division of the county of DORSET, on the southern bank of the river Frome, 120 miles (S. W. by W.) from London, containing 2743 inhabitants. The early existence of this town is evident from the etymology of its Roman names *Durnovaria* and

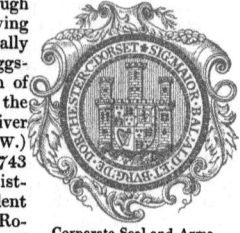

Corporate Seal and Arms.

Durinum, " a place on or near the *Varia*," which was the old British appellation of the Frome. Ptolemy describes it as the chief town of the Durotriges, and calls it *Dunium ;* it was named by the Saxons *Dornceaster*, whence the modern *Dorchester* is derived. In Athelstan's charter to Milton abbey, dated at this place, Dorchester, which then belonged to the crown, is called *Villa Regalis*, to distinguish it from Dorchester in Oxfordshire, which was styled *Villa Episcopalis*. The Roman station stood on the Via Iceniana, and the remains of its ancient walls, the several vicinal roads leading from it, and the discovery of coins and other relics of antiquity, evince it to have been a place of great importance. In the Saxon age, two mints were granted to this place by Athelstan. In 1003, it was besieged and burnt, and its walls thrown down, by Sweyn, King of Denmark, in revenge for the attempt of Ethelred to extirpate the Danes by a general massacre. In the reign of Elizabeth, several Roman Catholic priests were executed here ; and, in 1595, the ravages of the plague were very extensive. In 1613, a fire consumed several houses, together with the churches of the Holy Trinity and All Saints : the damage amounted to £200,000. A second conflagration took place in 1662, and a third in 1775. During the civil wars, according to Lord Clarendon, Dorchester was considered one of the strongest holds of the parliament : it was fortified for this purpose in 1642-3 ; but, on the approach of the Earl of Caernarvon, with two thousand men, the town was immediately relinquished, and the governor fled by sea to Southampton : the Earl of Essex afterwards took possession of it. In 1645, an action took place here between General Goring at the head of fifteen hundred cavalry, and about four thousand of the parliamentary troops under Cromwell, in which the latter sustained a defeat, but kept possession of the town. In 1685, on the occasion of the Duke of Monmouth's rebellion, the assizes were held here, before Judge Jefferies, when twenty-nine out of thirty persons tried in one day, were found guilty and condemned : on the following day, two hundred and ninety-two pleaded guilty and were condemned, of whom eighty were executed : on the morning of trial, Jefferies ordered the court to be hung with scarlet.

The town, is pleasantly situated on elevated ground, the river Frome, flowing on the north-western side ; it occupies an area of about eighty acres, and consists principally of three spacious streets, the union of which, in the centre of the town, where the corn-market is held, is called Cornhill : these streets severally terminate in the roads to London, Weymouth, and Exeter; and from West-street, in a northerly direction, is the road to Bath : they are kept remarkably clean, well paved, and lighted. A small theatre was erected in 1828 : races are held annually in September. The town is environed for two-thirds of its extent by a fine promenade, overshadowed with lofty trees; and the surrounding scenery, which consists of extensive downs, sloping hills, and fertile enclosures, watered by branches of the Frome, forms a picturesque and beautiful landscape. It is also surrounded by a tract called Fordington Field, partly meadow-land, and partly in tillage, without any enclosure, seven miles in circumference; it belongs to the duchy of Cornwall, and is held by the owners on lives, with a widowhood. Six hundred thousand sheep were formerly computed to have been constantly fed within a circuit of six miles, and that number is now exceeded : the high estimation of Dorchester mutton is attributable to the sweet herbage of the soil; and the water, which springs from a chalky bed, is particularly favourable for brewing beer, which is here made to a great extent, and of a superior quality. During the reigns of Elizabeth, Charles I., and James I., there was a flourishing cloth manufactory; but this branch of business has greatly declined, there being only a little blanketting and linsey now manufactured, in addition to the spinning of worsted-yarn. The principal market day is Saturday, and there is an inferior market on Wednesday. The fairs are on Candlemas-day, Trinity-Monday, St. John the Baptist's and St. James's days; the three last being principally for sheep and lambs.

Dorchester is a borough by prescription and charter, and, in the reign of Edward II., was under the government of two bailiffs and burgesses. In 1610, James I. appointed fifteen burgesses and two bailiffs, with power to choose a recorder and other officers. By charter of Charles I., the borough was incorporated under a mayor, two bailiffs, six aldermen, six capital burgesses, a governor, and twenty-four common council-men, with a recorder, town clerk, and other officers, of whom the mayor, the late mayor, the recorder, two bailiffs, and one capital burgess, are justices of the peace within the borough. The mayor and the two bailiffs are chosen annually by the corporate body, from among the capital burgesses, from whom the aldermen are also appointed by the same mode. A court of record is held " every Monday, from three weeks to three weeks," for the recovery of debts not amounting to £40. The town-hall was erected by the corporation in 1791; underneath is the market-house. The shire-hall is a plain and commodious edifice of Portland stone, containing court-rooms wherein the assizes and quarter sessions for the county are held : by a right vested in the corporation the sessions for the borough are also held in this edifice. The new county gaol was erected on the site of the old castle, between 1789 and 1795, at the expense of £16,179. 10. 6., on the plan of the benevolent Howard, and comprises the county gaol, penitentiary, and house of correction : the exterior is handsome, and the interior is divided into various departments for the classification of prisoners, having four wings, which, though detached, communicate with the central building by cast-iron bridges. This borough has returned two members to parliament from the 23rd of Edward I., who are elected by about four hundred

VOL. II.

voters : the franchise was formerly in the inhabitants paying scot and lot, but is now equally vested in non-residents having real estates within the borough, and paying church and poor rates, which arrangement has led to a very minute division of the portion of land so entitled, to feoffees in trust, in order to produce a preponderance in the number of electors. The primary title to this property has long been vested in the noble family of Cooper, Earls of Shaftesbury, whose influence is necessarily paramount. The ancient family of Williams has also considerable weight. The mayor is the returning officer. During the usurpation, Cromwell, in 1653, appointed one member for the borough.

The town is divided into three parishes, viz., All Saints', commonly called All Hallows, or the lower parish, St. Peter's, and the Holy Trinity, in the archdeaconry of Dorset and diocese of Bristol. The living of All Saints' is a discharged rectory, rated in the king's books at £4. 4. 7., endowed with £200 private benefaction, £400 royal bounty, and £400 parliamentary grant, and in the patronage of the Mayor and Corporation. The church was rebuilt after the great fire. The living of Trinity parish is a rectory, to which the rectory of St. Peter's was united by act of parliament in 1610, rated in the king's books at £17. 8. 6½., and in the patronage of the Mayor and Corporation. The church, erected nearly on the site of an ancient edifice pulled down in 1821, in consequence of its dilapidated state and its protruding so far into the street, is an elegant and commodious structure, ornamented with beautifully painted glass, and containing a marble tablet to the memory of Dr. Cuming, who, according to the epitaph, was buried in the church-yard, rather than in the church, " lest he who studied, while living, to promote the health of his fellow citizens, should prove detrimental to it when dead." The living of St. Peter's, formerly a rectory, has for ages been considered only a curacy to the rectory of the Holy Trinity parish, to which it was united by act of parliament in the 7th of James I., the church having been used as a chapel of ease since that period : St. Peter's is, however, for all legal purposes, a distinct parish, having its own officers, maintaining its own poor, and the inhabitants contributing only to the repairs of their own church : the living is now a perpetual curacy, having been endowed in 1823 with £1200 private benefaction, £1500 royal bounty, and £2000 parliamentary grant, under the provisions of an act passed in the sixth year of Queen Anne's reign. The church is ancient, spacious, and well built, and consists of a chancel, nave, and side aisles, and an embattled tower with pinnacles, ninety feet in height : it contains several ancient and curious monuments, one to the memory of Denzil, Lord Holles, of white marble, which represents that nobleman in a recumbent posture, and bears a Latin and English inscription ; also the handsome tomb of Sir John Williams, of Herringstone, Knt., and his lady. In the north aisle, on a stone coffin, lies the effigy of a knight, cross-legged, and completely armed in a coat of mail and helmet, with belt, spurs, and shield, but without armorial devices; there is a similar figure in the south window : they are supposed to represent two crusaders belonging to the family of the Chidiocks, founders of the neighbouring priory, and to have been removed hither on the demolition of the priory church. There are places of worship for Baptists, Independents, Wes-

I

leyan Methodists, and Unitarians. A free grammar school was founded and endowed in the year 1579, by Mr. Thomas Hardy, of Wyke, near Weymouth; the government is vested in trustees: it has a trifling exhibition of £5 per annum, arising from the profits of the markets, at any college in either University; in addition to which, there are two exhibitions, of £10 per annum each, at St. John's College, Cambridge, for scholars either from St. Paul's school, London, or from the free school of Dorchester. A second school was re-founded by the corporation, about 1623, having existed prior to the establishment of the grammar school, and intended as a subordinate institution: the master is appointed by the corporation, and instructs gratuitously five boys of their nomination, in reading, writing, and arithmetic. A handsome almshouse, called Napper's or Napier's Mite, adjoins the free school; it was founded by Sir Robert Napier, in 1615, for ten poor men: near the priory is another, founded and endowed previously to 1617, by Matthew Chubb, one of the representatives of this borough, for nine poor women; and in the vicinity of All Saints' church, are Whetstone's almshouses, for the maintenance of four persons, or four couple, at the discretion of the corporation. Dorchester hospital, erected in 1616, was originally a kind of work-house, and having been subsequently otherwise occupied, was again converted to its primary use, in 1744, for the poor of the three parishes: it is now used both as a workhouse and an hospital, each of the parishes appointing three guardians, and partly for the boys of the National school also.

This town, when in the possession of the Romans, was entirely surrounded by a wall and a fosse, having two exterior ramparts visible on the south and west; on which side there are still remains of the old wall, sixty-five paces in length, six feet thick, and, in some places, twelve feet high: its foundation is on the solid chalk-rock, and the wall is built of rag-stone, laid obliquely and covered with mortar; every second course, in the Roman manner, running the reverse way, and having occasional horizontal ones for binding, intermixed with flint. A great part of these fortifications was levelled and destroyed in making the walks which partially surround the town, particularly in 1764, when eighty-seven feet of wall were pulled down, and only sixty-seven feet left standing. A castle, probably of Roman origin, formerly stood here, the site of which is placed, by tradition, in a large field near the county prison, still called Castle Green; but there are not the slightest traces of the building. A priory of the Franciscan order was constructed from the materials, a little eastward from the castle, by a member of the Chidiock family, some time previously to the 4th of Edward III. The church was pulled down at the Reformation, and the house altered by Sir Francis Ashley for his own residence; it contains many of his armorial bearings and insignia. Here Denzil, the celebrated Lord Holles, died; after which the mansion was converted into a Presbyterian meeting-house, and so continued till 1722. Opposite to it, on the north, are the priory close and meadow. Several Danish burial places, or tumuli, are scattered round the town. In 1725, a large tesselated pavement was discovered, at the depth of three or four feet, in a garden near South-street; and, in 1747, a brazen image of some Roman deity, probably of Bacchus, was found at the depth of five feet. In preparing the foundations for the new gaol, a

great number of Roman coins were dug up, including those of Antoninus Pius, Vespasian, Constantine, Carausius, Valerian, Valens, and Gallienus. In the immediate vicinity of the town are some interesting remains of a supposed Roman amphitheatre, of the Roman camp of Poundbury, and of the Roman or British one of Maiden castle. Henry Pierpoint, Earl of Kingston, was created Marquis of Dorchester, March 25th 1645, but the title, after having been revived on the 23rd of December, 1706, finally became extinct on the death of Evelyn Pierpoint, the last duke of Kingston.

DORCHESTER, a parish (formerly a market town) in the hundred of DORCHESTER, county of OXFORD, 8¼ miles (S. E. by S.) from Oxford, and 49 (N. W.) from London, containing 854 inhabitants. The town is situated on the banks of the river Thame, over which there is a stone bridge, at a short distance to the north of its junction with the river Isis, or Thames. It is a place of great antiquity, supposed to have been a British town, and afterwards a Roman station, called by Richard of Cirencester *Dorocina*, being situated on the Roman road passing through the centre of the island, and Roman coins and medals having been frequently discovered here. Under the Saxons it flourished greatly, and Cynegils, King of Wessex, having been converted to Christianity, and baptized at Dorchester, by Birinus, an Italian priest, founded here a bishoprick, of which Birinus was the first bishop; and the see continued, with a short intermission, to be fixed here till after the Norman Conquest, when it was removed to Lincoln. King Athelstan held a council at Dorchester, in 958, when he granted a charter to the abbey of Malmesbury, in which this place is styled the celebrated city of Dornacestre. According to Leland, it suffered greatly from the incursions of the Danes. After the removal of the bishoprick it rapidly declined in importance, so that William of Malmesbury, who wrote about 1140, mentions it as small and thinly inhabited; and subsequently it fell into a state of greater decay. About the middle of the twelfth century, Alexander, Bishop of Lincoln, placed here a convent of Augustine canons, instead of the clergy who had belonged to the cathedral, whose revenue at the dissolution was £219. 12. The market has long been discontinued; but there is still an annual fair on Easter-Tuesday.

The living is a perpetual curacy, in the jurisdiction of the peculiar court of Dorchester, and in the patronage of the Trustees of Mr. Fettiplace. The church, which was formerly the cathedral, is dedicated to St. Peter and St. Paul: it is a large and very curious structure, with a tower at the west end, and exhibits in its various parts the different styles from the Norman to the later English. In the north aisle there is a remarkable Norman doorway; the windows of the chancel display much singularity in their ornamental tracery; some stone stalls have peculiarly rich canopies, and in the windows above them are remains of fine stained glass. There is a very ancient leaden font, with Norman arches and figures in relief on the sides of it; and among the sepulchral monuments are some which appear to be extremely ancient. Leland mentions three parish churches, but there are no traces of two of them. A grammar school, founded in 1656, by John Fettiplace, has an endowment of £10 per annum, for the education of six boys. In the church-yard is still standing a part of the conventual buildings, now used for the free grammar school. On the west side of the town is a double intrenchment, called Dike hills, supposed to be of Roman origin.

DORE, a chapelry in the parish of DRONFIELD, hundred of SCARSDALE, county of DERBY, 5 miles (N.W. by W.) from Dronfield, containing 476 inhabitants. The living is a perpetual curacy, in the archdeaconry of Derby, and diocese of Lichfield and Coventry, endowed with £400 private benefaction, £400 royal bounty, and £800 parliamentary grant. Earl Fitzwilliam was patron in 1807. A new chapel has been erected upon a more convenient site than that of the ancient one. The Rev. Robert Turie, in 1720, gave £40 towards endowing a school, in aid of which, the Duke of Devonshire, and other benefactors, have, by various bequests and donations, raised the income to £37. 18. per annum, this sum being applied to the education of thirty children, in a school-room recently erected by subscription.

DORE-ABBEY, a parish in the hundred of WEBTREE, county of HEREFORD, 12 miles (S.W. by W.) from Hereford, containing 523 inhabitants. The living is a rectory, in the archdeaconry and diocese of Hereford, rated in the king's books at £8, and in the patronage of John Hickford, Esq. The church is dedicated to the Holy Trinity and St. Mary. An abbey of white monks, in honour of the Blessed Virgin Mary, was founded in the reign of Stephen, by Robert, son of Harold, lord of Ewyas, which consisted of an abbot and eight religious, whose revenue at the dissolution was valued at £118. 2.

DORKING, a market town and parish in the second division of the hundred of WOTTON, county of SURREY, 12 miles (E.) from Guildford, and 23 (S.S.W.) from London, on the road through Epsom to Worthing, Bognor, and Brighton, containing 3812 inhabitants. This place, anciently called *Dorchinges*, appears to have derived its name from its situation in a valley abounding with springs of water. It was probably founded by the Saxons, and, after its destruction by the Danes, was rebuilt, and had become a town of some importance prior to the Norman Conquest, at which period it was held in royal demesne, and had a church and three mills. In the reign of Edward I., it obtained the grant of a weekly market and an annual fair, and was endowed with many privileges. In a survey of the manor in 1649, the town is stated to have considerably improved, and to have been paved : the summer assizes for the county were held here in 1699, but from what particular cause does not appear ; the quarter sessions were also held here occasionally. The town is situated in a sandy vale, and towards the south side of it, on a stratum of sandrock, in which excellent cellars are excavated : a small stream flowing into the river Mole, intersects the vale, which is sheltered on the north by a ridge of chalky downs, extending from Farnham on the western side of the county into Kent, and abounding with picturesque scenery : the soil is luxuriantly fertile, and the heights command extensive and magnificent views, embracing the metropolis on one side, and the British channel on the other. In the environs are several handsome villas and stately mansions, of which Shrub Hill deserves notice on account of its fine hanging gardens. Box Hill, about a mile from the town, a picturesque eminence planted with box trees, in the reign of Charles I., by the Earl of Arundel, from which circumstance it takes its name, commands an extensive view of the surrounding country, and is a place of resort for summer excursions from London. Betchworth castle, occupying the site of an ancient fortress of that name, on the western bank of the river Mole, is beautifully situated in an extensive park, celebrated for the stateliness of its fine chesnut trees, some of which are seven yards in girth, and produce fruit equal to the Spanish tree. There were also two other ancient fortresses in the parish, called Benham and Ewtons castles, which are stated to have been demolished by the Danes : vestiges of the moat that surrounded each are still apparent, and the former has given name to a meadow in which it stood. The vale beneath Box Hill, called Holmward or Holmdale, was for several ages the retreat of the ancient Britons, in their conflicts with the Romans, and afterwards that of the Saxons, when the county was harassed by the Danes, on which account it has become the subject of a distich declaratory of the unconquerableness of the dale : in the reign of Charles II. it was celebrated for red deer, which the Duke of York, afterwards James II., preserved for his own sport : it was subsequently noted for the production of immense quantities of strawberries, which were conveyed to market in horse-loads, but is now overgrown with furze. The streets are spacious, and the foot-paths have been recently paved ; the houses, though mostly of ancient date, are in general well built, and of neat appearance : the town is lighted with oil by subscription, and supplied with water brought from a spring by water-works, the property of a private individual, who has constructed baths adjoining them for the public accommodation. A book society has been formed under the patronage of the gentry resident in the neighbourhood ; a reading society is principally supported by the inhabitants of the town ; and a circulating library has been established by a number of subscribers, who pay an annual subscription of £2. 2. in advance. The trade is principally in meal and lime, the latter being considered superior in quality to any produced elsewhere ; poultry (of which a particular species, having five claws, stated to have been brought hither by the Romans, is known among the poulterers as Dorking fowls,) is sold in large quantities for the supply of the London market. The county magistrates hold petty sessions here for the division ; and a court leet and court baron are held in October, under the lord of the manor. The custom of Borough English prevails in this parish, which is divided into the several districts of Eastborough, including West Betchworth and part of the town; Chipping borough, including the remainder of the town; Holmwood borough, including the northern and southern suburbs; Milton borough, including the hamlet of Milton-street ; and Westcote borough, so called from a hamlet about a mile and a half west of the town.

The living is a vicarage, in the archdeaconry of Surrey, and diocese of Winchester, rated in the king's books at £14.13.11½., and in the patronage of the Co-heirs of the Duke of Norfolk. The church, dedicated to St. Martin, is a spacious cruciform structure, principally in the later style of English architecture, with a low embattled tower rising from the centre ; the upper part of the tower was rebuilt in 1672, and the church extensively repaired, but it still retains much of its original character; a flight of steps leads down from the church-yard, the ground of which has been raised to a considerable height above the level of the foundation of the church : the interior is lighted with several fine windows, in which is some good tracery; and in the south transept, near the chancel, is an elegant tablet, erected by public subscription to the memory of the Right Hon. the Earl of Rothes, who died suddenly, in 1817, while hunting in Betchworth park. There are places of worship for the Society of Friends and Independents. A National school for boys and girls, and an infant school, established in 1829, in which are one hundred and fifty children, are supported by subscription. An alms-house, containing eighteen apartments, was founded on Cotmandean common, and endowed by Mrs. Susannah Smith, with land producing £40. 10. per annum. The rents of an estate, purchased with a sum of money left for that purpose, by Mrs. Margaret Fenwicke, producing £52. 10. per annum, are distributed in marriage-portions to servant maids, and apprentice-fees to poor children; and there are several other charitable bequests for the relief of the poor of the parish. Traces of the Roman Stane-street, which passed through Dorking, are frequently discovered in digging the ground in the church-yard; and on the summit of a hill, three miles and a half from the town, is Anstie Bury, a Roman encampment, enclosing more than eleven acres, defended by a triple intrenchment, and having the entrance on the east side, where the works have been levelled by the plough. On Winterfield farm, near this camp, a wooden box was dis-covered in 1817, about ten or twelve inches below the sur-face of the ground, containing seven hundred Anglo-Saxon coins, of which the uppermost were firmly ce-mented together by an incrustation formed by the de-composition of the metal used as an alloy to the silver; these coins were purchased on the spot by Robert Bar-clay and George Dawdney, Esqrs., who presented them to the trustees of the British Museum, in order that they might select such as might be found requisite to com-plete their series : many curious fossils have been found in the chalk-pits; and within two miles of the town is Mag's well, the water of which is slightly impregnated with sulphate of magnesia and iron; it closely resembles the Malvern water, and is used as an alterative. Jeremiah Markland, a learned critic, who resided here, and died in 1763, and Abraham Tucker, Esq., author of the "Light of Nature," who resided at Betchworth castle, were bu-ried in the chancel of the church; and John Hoole, translator of Tasso and Ariosto, was interred in the church-yard : the Rev. John Mason, author of a Trea-tise on Self-Knowledge, lived for several years in this town.

DORMINGTON, a parish in the hundred of GREY-TREE, county of HEREFORD, 5½ miles (E. by S.) from Hereford, containing, with the chapelry of Bartestree, 172 inhabitants. The living is a discharged vicarage, in the archdeaconry and diocese of Hereford, rated in the king's books at £4. 6. 8., endowed with £200 private benefaction, and £200 royal bounty, and in the patron-age of E. T. Foley, Esq. The church is dedicated to St. Peter.

DORMSDEN, a chapelry in the parish of BARKING, hundred of BOSMERE and CLAYDON, county of SUF-FOLK, 2 miles (S. by E.) from Needham, containing 74 inhabitants. The chapel is dedicated to St. Andrew.

The Stow-Market and Ipswich navigation bounds the parish on the north-east.

DORMSTON, a parish in the upper division of the hundred of PERSHORE, though locally in the middle division of the hundred of Oswaldslow, county of WOR-CESTER, 7 miles (W. by N.) from Alcester, containing 113 inhabitants. The living is a perpetual curacy ex-onerated, in the archdeaconry and diocese of Worcester, endowed with £400 royal bounty, and £400 parliamen-tary grant, and in the patronage of Thomas Taylor Vernon, Esq.

DORNE, a hamlet in the parish of BLOCKLEY, upper division of the hundred of OSWALDSLOW, county of WORCESTER, though locally in the upper division of the hundred of Kiftsgate, county of Gloucester, 1½ mile (N.) from Moreton in the Marsh, containing 45 inha-bitants. Tradition relates that Dorne was once a city of some importance; and this is confirmed by the disco-very, from time to time, of ancient foundations, with some Roman and British coins.

DORNEY, a parish in the hundred of BURNHAM, county of BUCKINGHAM, 2¼ miles (W. N. W.) from Eton, containing 279 inhabitants. The living is a discharged vicarage, in the archdeaconry of Buckingham, and diocese of Lincoln, rated in the king's books at £8. 10. 5, en-dowed with £200 private benefaction, and £200 royal bounty, and in the patronage of Sir Charles Harcourt Palmer, Bart. The church, dedicated to St. James, has a handsome tower. The parish is bounded on the west and south by the Thames.

DORNFORD, a hamlet in the parish of CHESTER-TON, hundred of NORMAN-CROSS, county of HUNTING-DON, 5½ miles (N. N. W.) from Stilton. The population is returned with the parish. This was the Durobrivæ of Antoninus, implying the passage of the river, and is now, in the same sense, called Dornford, to which the Roman road leads straight from Huntingdon; there are evident traces of the ruined city, besides many ancient coins which have been found on its site.

DORRINGTON, a parish in the wapentake of FLAX-WELL, parts of KESTEVEN, county of LINCOLN, 4¾ miles (N.) from Sleaford, containing 284 inhabitants. The living is a discharged vicarage, in the archdeaconry and diocese of Lincoln, rated in the king's books at £6. 3. 9., and endowed with £200 royal bounty. Sir G. Heath-cote, Bart. was patron in 1823. The church is dedicated to St. James.

DORRINGTON, a township in that part of the parish of MUCKLESTON which is in the Drayton divi-sion of the hundred of BRADFORD (North), county of SALOP, 5¾ miles (N. E. by N.) from Drayton in Hales, containing 185 inhabitants.

DORSETSHIRE, a maritime county, bounded on the north by the counties of Somerset and Wilts; on the east by the county of Southampton; on the west by the county of Devon, and part of that of Somerset; and on the south by the British channel : it extends from 50° 30' to 51° 6' (N. Lat.), and from 1° 58¼' to 3° 18' (W. Lon.), comprising about seven hundred and seventy-five thousand acres, or one thousand two hun-dred and eleven square miles. The population, in 1821, amounted to one hundred and forty-seven thousand four hundred.

Prior to the landing of Cæsar, Dorsetshire was in-habited by the Durotriges, and Morini, two tribes of the

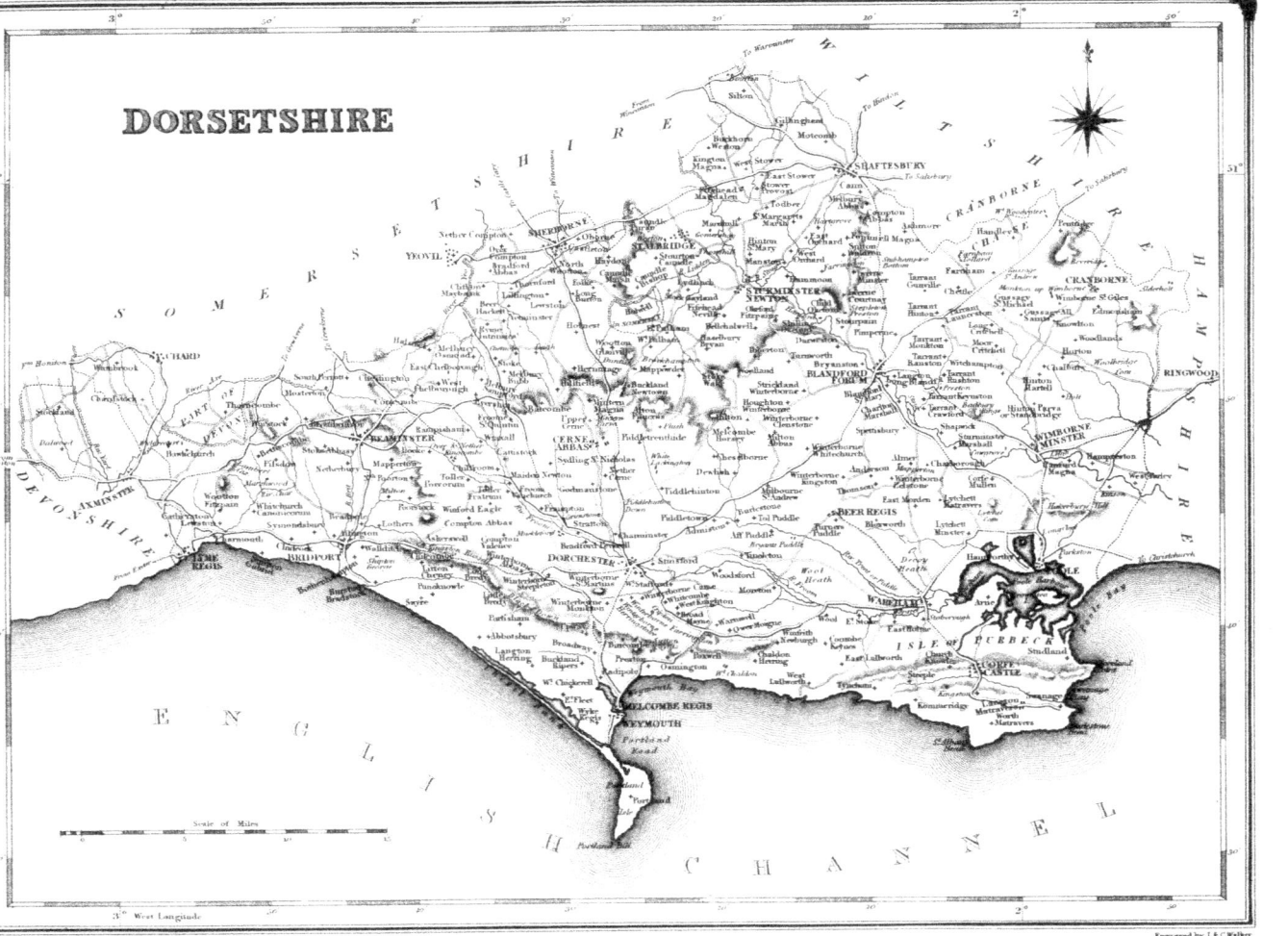

DORSETSHIRE

Drawn by R.Creighton.

Engraved by J.& C.Walker.

Scale of Miles

Britons, whose names signify dwellers on the sea-shore. By the Saxons it was styled *Dor satta*, which is of similar meaning, signifying the dwellers by the water. The Romans included it in the division called Britannia Prima, and the Saxons in the kingdom of Wessex. Of the early history of this county there are but few authentic memorials. On the departure of the Romans, the Saxons, notwithstanding the vigorous opposition they met with from King Arthur, obtained possession of this and most of the other western counties; and Cerdic, who landed in the year 495, completed his conquest of these parts in 530, by the capture of the Isle of Wight; and, having founded the kingdom of Wessex, was crowned at Winchester in the following year: several memorials of his name are preserved near the southern coast of Dorsetshire. This kingdom became at length the most considerable of the heptarchal states. In 1002, Sweyn, King of Denmark, having landed at Exeter to revenge the massacre of the Danes, in his march from that city to Wilton, destroyed Dorchester, Clifton, Sherborne, and Shaston (now Shaftesbury); this having been the first instance in which Dorsetshire endured, to an extent worthy of being recorded, the miseries inflicted by that people. During the Norman times, history does not furnish us with any material events as having occurred in this county. There is an account indeed of a dreadful plague which broke out in Dorsetshire in 1348, so terrible that in many of the villages all the inhabitants died, the houses fell down, and were never again inhabited. In 1588, great preparations were made to fortify the southern coast, on the approach of the Spanish Armada; and Portland, in particular, was strongly fortified and garrisoned. During the parliamentary war the most considerable of the higher orders were attached to the king; but the people, where the clothing trade was carried on, which was the case in several parts of the county, were chiefly disaffected. Lyme and Poole were constantly garrisoned by the parliament. Wareham, Melcombe-Regis, Weymouth, Bridport, Dorchester, Shaftesbury, Blandford, and Sherborne, being open and generally unguarded, were alternately occupied as each party was master of the field. Sherborne castle, Corfe Castle, Chidiock castle, and the isle and castle of Portland, were garrisoned by the king; but except the sieges of Lyme, Corfe Castle, and Sherborne castle, the rising of the club-men, and a few casual skirmishes, nothing very remarkable happened within this county. In 1685, the Duke of Monmouth landed at Lyme, and thence marched into Somersetshire, which was the seat of the rebellion at that time. An action took place at Bridport; and the duke was taken in an enclosure called the Island, in the midst of the heath, in the parish of Horton, having concealed himself in a ditch, where is still to be seen an ash-tree, bearing on its sides the initials of the numerous persons who have visited it. Many of his followers were tried at Dorchester, where several were executed, as also in various other places within this county. On the 5th of November, 1688, the Prince of Orange landed with his forces at Lyme, Torbay, and the adjacent parts of the coast, without any opposition, and encamped about Exeter. In 1756, a camp of six regiments of foot and two of dragoons was formed on Pimperne down, near Blandford; and in the following year another near Dorchester.

This county was successively under the episcopal jurisdiction of the see of Dorchester in Oxfordshire, of that of Winchester, and of that of Sherborne; and when the last was united to that of Sarum, it remained part of that diocese till the 31st of Henry VIII., when it became part of the newly constituted bishoprick of Bristol, by patent, June 4th, 1542. Of the six deaneries into which that diocese is divided, five are within this county, *viz.*, those of Bridport, Dorchester, Pimperne, Shaston, and Whitchurch, comprising two hundred and fifty-eight parishes, of which one hundred and sixty-three are rectories, sixty-two vicarages, and thirty-three perpetual curacies. The archdeaconry of Dorset is co-extensive with the diocese of Bristol, and comprises the whole of this county. The bishop holds his triennial, and the archdeacon his yearly, visitation, at Bridport, Dorchester, Blandford, Shaftesbury, Cerne-Abbas, or Whitchurch. For civil purposes it is separated into the following divisions: Blandford (North and South), Bridport, Cerne (sub-division), Dorchester, Shaston (East and West), Sherborne, and Sturminster. Blandford North division contains the hundreds of Coombs-Ditch, Pimperne, and Rushmore, and the liberty of Dewlish: Blandford South division contains the hundreds of Corfe-Castle, Beer-Regis, Hundredsbarrow, Hasilor, Rowbarrow, and Winfrith, and the liberties of Bindon, Owermoigne, and Stoborough. Bridport division contains the hundreds of Beaminster-Forum and Redhone, Eggerton, Godder-Thorne, and Whitchurch-Canonicorum, and the liberties of Broadwinsor, Frampton, Lothers and Bothenhampton, and Poorstock. Cerne sub-division contains the hundreds of Buckland-Newton, Cerne, Totcombe and Modbury, and Whiteway, and the liberties of Alton-Pancras, Piddletrenthide, and Sydling-St. Nicholas. Dorchester division contains the hundreds of Culliford-Tree, George, Piddletown, Tollerford, and Uggscombe, and the liberties of Fordington, Isle of Portland, Piddlehinton, Sutton-Pointz, Wayhouse, and Wyke Regis and Etwall. Shaston East division contains the hundreds of Badbury, Cogdean, Knowlton, Loosebarrow, Monckton-up-Wimbourne, and Wimbourne-St. Giles, with parts of the hundreds of Cranborne and Sixpenny-Handley. Shaston West division contains the remaining parts of the hundreds of Cranborne and Sixpenny-Handley: and the liberties of Alcester and Gillingham. Sherborne division contains the hundreds of Sherborne and Yetminster, and the liberties of Halstock and Ryme-Intrinsica; and Sturminster division contains the hundreds of Brownshall, Redlane, and Sturminster-Newton-Castle, and the liberty of Stower-Provost. Dorsetshire contains the town and county of the town of Poole, the borough and market towns of Bridport, Dorchester, Lyme-Regis, Shaftesbury, Wareham, and the united boroughs of Weymouth and Melcombe-Regis. The borough of Corfe-Castle, which is not a market town, and the market towns of Beaminster, Blandford-Forum, Cerne-Abbas, Sherborne, Sturminster-Newton, and Wimbourne-Minster. Bridport, Lyme-Regis, Poole, Wareham, and Weymouth are ports also. Two knights are returned to parliament for the shire, and two representatives for each of the nine boroughs: the county members are elected at Dorchester. Dorsetshire is included in the western circuit; the assizes were anciently held, sometimes at Sherborne, and sometimes, though very rarely, at Shaftesbury; but generally, in latter times, and now always, at Dorchester, where the shire-hall and county gaol have long been. The Epiphany quarter sessions are held at Blandford ; the Easter, at Sherborne ; the Midsummer, at Shaftesbury ; and the Michaelmas, at Bridport. There are sixty-three acting magistrates. The rates raised in the county for the year ending March 25th, 1827, amounted to £120,455. 7., the expenditure to £115,453. 12., of which £99,108. 17., was applied to the relief of the poor.

The surface of the county is hilly, and a considerable portion of it consists of open downs, affording pasturage to numerous flocks of sheep, of which, however, more are fed in the vicinity of Dorchester than in any other part of the county, though great numbers of both sheep and oxen are fattened in the vale of Blackmore, which is celebrated as rich pasture land, containing upwards of one hundred and seventy thousand acres. There are also in this district several large apple orchards, producing excellent cider. On the south-western side are many vales of great luxuriance; but on the south-eastern, there is much waste land, dreary and barren, scarcely supporting, even in the summer months, a few sheep and cattle, and supplying the neighbouring villages with turf for fuel. Even in this part, however, cultivation is advancing, and detached portions have been improved. The soil of these downs is principally a light chalk, covered with a turf remarkably fine, producing hay, in the enclosed parts, of an excellent quality. About Bridport the lower lands are mostly a deep rich loam, intermixed with flint, well adapted to the growth of beech trees. To the north of Sherborne, where is some of the best arable land in the county, it is a stone brack, which is the case in the isles of Portland and Purbeck : in the centre of the county the soil is good, and the land well managed. Dorsetshire is not a well-wooded county, and, in general, native timber is scarce and dear. In some spots, where the land is cold and wet, such as Duncliff, in the vale of Blackmore, Heycombe wood, in the vale of Sherborne, and others of a similar nature, some plantations may be seen. The climate is noted for its mildness and salubrity; and this, added to the beauty of its scenery, has procured this county the appellation of the Garden of England. Weymouth has long been celebrated as a fashionable watering-place ; and, owing to the general calmness of the sea there, its pleasant situation, and its commodiousness for bathing, has, through the repeated visits of the royal family, risen to a place of consequence.

The principal articles of produce are corn, cattle, butter, sheep, wool, timber, flax, and hemp. Of the different kinds of grain, barley affords the best returns, and from ten to twelve thousand bushels of malt are made annually : the strong beer is in high repute ; the ale also is particularly celebrated, and in some respects unequalled. The sheep have long been celebrated, and it is supposed that not fewer than eight hundred thousand are constantly kept in the county, of which number more than one hundred and fifty thousand are sold annually, and sent out of it. They are highly esteemed for the fineness, shortness, and close texture of their wool, which is much used in the manufacture of broad cloth; the aggregate quantity annually sold being estimated at ninety thousand weighs, of thirty-one pounds each. The Dorsetshire sheep are horned, white-faced, with long,

small, white legs, the carcass being rather long and thin; the mutton is fine-grained and of good flavour, weighing, in wethers of three years and a half old, from sixteen to twenty pounds per quarter. Many of the ewes are bought by the farmers within forty miles of London, for the sake of their lambs, which come earlier than most others, and are fattened for the London market. But besides the peculiar Dorsetshire breed, there is a very small kind in the isles of Portland and Purbeck, and the neighbouring coast, inferior in size to the Welch sheep, weighing, when full fed, not more than eight or nine pounds per quarter. Little regard is paid in this county to the breed of horses : oxen are frequently used in agriculture, and those are mostly the red Devonshire ox, with a mixture of the Hampshire and Wiltshire : the pigs are of a light colour, and not equal to those of Hampshire and some other species. Butter is the chief article of produce, though some cheese is also made. The mackarel fishery is of considerable consequence : vast quantities are taken near Abbotsbury, and along the shore from Portland to Bridport : they are generally caught from the middle of March, if the season be not too cold, till Midsummer, and sometimes later. The fishery, however, has not been so productive of late years as formerly, and the exposed situation of the coast renders it very uncertain, even in the best of seasons.

The principal articles of manufacture are rope-yarn, ropes, and sail-cloth, which are chiefly carried on in the neighbourhood of Bridport and Beaminster. A manufacture of the same kind, but on a smaller scale, has been established in the Isle of Purbeck. At Shaftesbury is a manufactory for making all kinds of shirt buttons, which affords employment to a great number of women and children. A sort of flannel, or coarse white woollen cloth, is likewise made at this town, called swanskin, but the chief trade in this latter article is carried on at Sturminster. There is a large manufactory for shirt buttons at Blandford. At Stalbridge is a manufactory for spinning silk, and at Sherborne is another on a larger scale. At Wimbourne considerable business is transacted in the worsted trade, and more than one thousand women and children are employed in knitting stockings. Though neither coal nor metallic ores have ever been obtained in Dorsetshire, the stone quarries of Purbeck and Portland have long been celebrated. Purbeck, though called an island, is more properly a peninsula, of an irregular oval form, about twelve miles in length and seven in breadth. The soil is altogether calcareous, and, for the most part, a continued mass of either white or brownish limestone, the latter having a mixture of sea-shells. The quarries on the south side of the isle afford an inexhaustible fund of natural curiosities. The best quarries are at Kingston, Worth, Langston, and Swanwich; the stone got in the last of these is white, full of shells, susceptible of a good polish, and not unlike alabaster. About Wareham and Morden is found a stone of an iron colour, called fire-stone. Near Dunshay, marble of various colours, blue, red, grey, and spotted, is obtained, but all of a coarse grain. Much of the stone of this district was used in the building of St. Paul's cathedral, Westminster bridge, and Ramsgate pier, and may be discovered in many of our ancient cathedral churches, as also in grave-stones and monuments. The rocks in the Isle of Portland rise frequently to the height of one hundred, or one hundred and fifty feet, and large masses lie scattered on the shore. These are composed of calcareous grit, containing moulds, or larox, of various shells, and emitting, when rubbed with steel, a bituminous smell. The grit is cemented together by a calcareous paste. The quarries are scattered among these rocks, more or less, in every part of the isle, but those of most repute are at Kingston. At this place is a pier, where upwards of six thousand tons of stone, on an average, are supposed to be shipped annually. The first stratum in these quarries is about one foot of blackish or reddish earth ; then six feet of stone not fit for exportation : below this is the bed of good stone, ten or twelve feet deep, and beneath it flint or clay. The stratum of stone that is worked for sale lies nearly parallel with the upper surface of the island, and without much earth or rubbish on it. When the beds are cleared, the quarry-men proceed to cross-cut the large flats, which is done with wedges. The beds being cut into distinct lumps, are squared by the hammer to the largest size which they will admit, and blocks are thus formed from half a ton to six or eight tons' weight. The colour of the Portland-stone, or freestone, as it is sometimes called, from the freedom with which it may be broken into any shape, is well known, as almost white, and as composing the materials of the most splendid erections in London, as well as in other parts of the British empire.

The principal rivers are the Frome, the Stour, the Piddle, and the Ivel. The Frome rises in the north-western part of the county, near Evershot, and passing by Dorchester, falls into Poole bay. The Stour enters this county from Wiltshire, near Gillingham, and pursuing a southern and south-eastern direction, runs into Hampshire. The Piddle rises in the north, and flowing to the south-east, unites with Poole bay. The Ivel, anciently the Yoo, has its origin from several springs near Horethorn, in a little hill north-east of Sherborne, from which town it flows into Somersetshire, and falls into the Parrett. The Dorset and Somerset canal passes through a portion of this county : it has its commencement in the Kennet and Avon canal at Widbrook, near Bradford, and terminates in the river Stour, near Gainscross in Shillingstone-Okeford : the principal objects of this canal are to supply the manufacturing towns and districts through which it passes with coal, and to open an inland communication between the Bristol channel, the Severn, the Thames, and the southern coast of the island. The navigation is continued from Gainscross by means of the river Stour, which has been made navigable across the county, and terminates at Christchurch harbour, in Hampshire. The road from London to Lyme-Regis enters the county near Woodyates Inn, and passes through Blandford-Forum, Dorchester, and Bridport, to Lyme. In the north-eastern part of the county are several ditches and valla, which Dr. Stukeley supposes to have been successively made by the Belgæ, in their progressive conquest of this part of Britain. Several Roman stations and roads have been traced in this county ; of the former, the principal is the Via Iceniana, or Icening way, which enters Dorsetshire from Wiltshire, near Woodyates, and passes through Dorchester, to the west of which it takes the name of the Ridge-way, and quits the county in its course towards Seaton in Devonshire, being distinctly visible in different parts of its line. The Roman stations, according to the best authorities, are Londinis, or Lyme-Regis, Canca Arixa, or Charmouth, Durnovaria, or Dorchester, Vindagladia, or Wimbourne-Minster, Clavinio, or Weymouth, Morino, or Wareham, and Bolclaunio, or Poole. Among these, in various directions, numerous barrows are dispersed, as well as other memorials of our British ancestors. Near Dorchester are the remains of a Roman amphitheatre, which is computed to have held near thirteen thousand spectators. A large circular intrenchment may be traced on Woodbury Hill, supposed to have been the Castra Statica of the Romans. On Hambledon Hill is another encampment, also the remains of what has been thought a labyrinth. The relics of ancient castles are numerous in Dorsetshire, of which, the most considerable were those of Corfe, Brownsea, and Portland. Numerous barrows, or tumuli, are dispersed over the county, especially the more open part of it.

Before the Reformation there were in this county twenty-nine religious houses (including one preceptory of the Knights Hospitallers) and eight ancient hospitals. The monasteries, the ruins of which may yet be discerned, are those of the monastery of Benedictines at Cranborne, a part of which now forms the parish church, one of the oldest in the county ; Cerne abbey, said to have been founded by St. Augustine, the few remains of which are interesting ; Milton abbey, whose church is now used as a private chapel ; the monastery of Shaftesbury, the ruins of which are discernible near the mansion of Sir Thomas Arundel ; some parts of the cloister and domestic buildings of the abbey of Sherborne, now occupied by silk machinery ; besides considerable remains of several more. The church of Fordington is partly in the Saxon style : those of Dorchester, Sherborne, Milbourne, Rapisham, Weymouth, and Shaftesbury, are venerable buildings, but this county cannot boast of many ancient ecclesiastical edifices. Mr. Hutchins remarks of the mineral waters, that "they are chalybeate at Farrington, Aylwood, and Corfe ; sulphureous at Sherford, Morden, Nottington, and Sherborne ; saline at Chilcomb ; and petrifying at Sherborne and Bothenwood, near Wimbourne-Minster." The "pebbly desert," called the Chesil Bank, is, as Dr. Maton remarks, one of the most extraordinary ridges or shelves of pebbles in Europe, and perhaps the longest, except that of Memel in Polish Prussia : its length is supposed to be about seventeen miles, and its breadth in some places nearly a quarter of a mile. Dorset gives the title of duke to the family of Sackville.

DORSINGTON, a parish in the upper division of the hundred of KIFTSGATE, county of GLOUCESTER, 8 miles (N. by W.) from Chipping-Campden, containing 121 inhabitants. The living is a rectory, in the archdeaconry and diocese of Gloucester, rated in the king's books at £12. 19. 2. W. Rawlins, Esq. was patron in 1816. The church, dedicated to St. Peter, was burnt down in 1754, and rebuilt with brick in 1758. The greater part of the village was destroyed in the same conflagration.

DORSINGTON (LITTLE), a hamlet in that part of the parish of WELFORD which is in the Stratford division of the hundred of BARLICHWAY, county of WARWICK, 6½ miles (S. E. by S.) from Alcester, containing, with Bickmersh, 61 inhabitants.

DORSTONE, a parish in the hundred of WEBTREE,

county of HEREFORD, 8 miles (E. by S.) from Hay, comprising the townships of Lower Dorstone and Upper Dorstone, and containing 591 inhabitants, exclusively of a part of the township of Vowmine, which is in this parish, of whieh number, 402 are in Lower, and 189 in Upper Dorstone. The living is a discharged vicarage, in the archdeaconry and diocese of Hereford, rated in the king's books at £7. 11. 10., and in the patronage of the Rev. Thomas Prosser. The church is dedicated to St. Peter. There are four fairs for horned cattle, horses, sheep, and pigs, on April 27th, May 18th, September 27th, and November 18th. A castle formerly stood within the parish.

DORTON, a parish in the hundred of ASHENDON, county of BUCKINGHAM, 5½ miles (N. N.W.) from Thame, containing 133 inhabitants. The living is a perpetual curacy in the archdeaconry of Buckingham, and diocese of Lincoln, endowed with £8 per annum private benefaction, and £200 royal bounty, and in the patronage of the Dean and Canons of Christ Church, Oxford. The church is dedicated to St. John the Baptist.

DOSTHILL, a hamlet in the chapelry of WILNE-COTE, in that part of the parish of TAMWORTH which is in the Tamworth division of the hundred of HEMLING-FORD, county of WARWICK, 3 miles (S.) from Tamworth, containing 653 inhabitants.

DOTTON, an extra-parochial liberty, in the eastern division of the hundred of BUDLEIGH, county of DEVON, containing 13 inhabitants.

DOUGHTON, a joint parish with Dunton, in the hundred of GALLOW, county of NORFOLK, 2 miles (W.) from Fakenham. The living is a discharged vicarage, consolidated with that of Dunton, with which the population is returned.

DOUGLAS, a chapelry in the parish of ECCLESTON, hundred of LEYLAND, county palatine of LANCASTER, 5½ miles (E. by N.) from Ormskirk. The population is returned with the parish. The living is a perpetual curacy, in the archdeaconry and diocese of Chester, endowed with £400 private benefaction, and £600 royal bounty, and in the patronage of the Rector of Eccleston.

DOULTING, a parish in the hundred of WHITE-STONE, county of SOMERSET, 2 miles (E.) from Shepton-Mallet, containing 633 inhabitants. The living is a vicarage, with East and West Cranmore, Downhead, and Stoke Lane annexed, in the archdeaconry of Wells, and diocese of Bath and Wells, rated in the king's boobs at £29. 12. 6. James Fussell, Esq. was patron in 1823. The church, dedicated to St. Aldelme, is a spacious cruciform structure, with an octagonal tower and spire rising from the intersection, and stands on the site of a chapel, or oratory, erected by the monks of Glastonbury, in honour of that saint, who was distinguished for his learning and piety, and died bishop of Sherborne in 709. In the church-yard is a singularly perfect cross, upon which are carved all the emblems of the Crucifixion, the cross, ladder, crown of thorns, reed, &c. In digging the foundations of the parsonage-house, a number of skeletons was discovered, indicating its having been the cemetery belonging to the ancient chapel. Extensive quarries of freestone are wrought here, whence it is said the materials were obtained for the erection of Wells cathedral.

DOVENBY, a township in the parish of BRIDE-KIRK, ALLERDALE ward below Darwent, county of CUMBERLAND, 2¾ miles (N.W.) from Cockermouth, containing 214 inhabitants. Sir Thomas Lamplugh, in 1609, endowed an hospital for four poor widows, with the tithes of Redmain, now worth £50 per annum, £4 of which, for reading prayers at the hospital, are paid to the master of the grammar school, founded by the same individual, with an endowment consisting of land producing £33 a year : the school was built in 1708, by voluntary contributions.

DOVER-COURT, in the county of ESSEX. See HARWICH.

DOVERDALE, a parish in the upper division of the hundred of HALFSHIRE, county of WORCESTER, 3¼ miles (N.W. by W.) from Droitwich, containing 60 inhabitants. The living is a discharged rectory, in the archdeaconry and diocese of Worcester, rated in the king's books at £5. 3. 6½., endowed with £200 private benefaction, and £200 royal bounty. The Rev. George Thomas was patron in 1807. The church is dedicated to St. Mary.

DOVERIDGE, a parish in the hundred of APPLE-TREE, county of DERBY, 1¾ mile (E. by N.) from Uttoxeter, containing 843 inhabitants. The living is a vicarage, in the archdeaconry of Derby, and diocese of Lichfield and Coventry, rated in the king's books at £12. 2. 1. The Duke of Devonshire was patron in 1785. The church, dedicated to St. Cuthbert, has considerable portions in the early style of English architecture. Isaac Dance, in 1786, bequeathed 40s. a year towards the support of a school, which annuity is vested in Lord Waterpark, by whose further contributions twenty-five children are taught in a school-room built by subscription in 1787, at which time a house for the master was also erected. Doveridge is in the honour of Tutbury, duchy of Lancaster, and within the jurisdiction of a court of pleas held at Tutbury every third Tuesday, for the recovery of debts under 40s. A market formerly held at this place was granted to the prior of Tutbury in 1275, but it has been long disused.

DOVOR, or DOVER, one of the cinque ports, a borough and market town, having separate jurisdiction, locally in the lathe of St. Augustine, eastern division of the county of KENT, 16 miles (S.E. by S.) from Canterbury, and 72 (E.S.E.) from London, containing 10,327 inhabitants. The ancient British name of the town was *Dwyr*, derived from *Dwfyrrha*, a steep place.

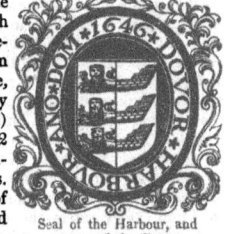

Seal of the Harbour, and Arms of the Town.

By the Romans it was called *Dubris*, and by the Saxons *Dofra*, and *Dofris*, which in Domesday-book are softened into *Dovere*. In the time of the Romans Dovor was a sea-port, and at one period was surrounded by walls having ten gates. This is supposed to be the place at which Julius Cæsar first endeavoured to effect a landing ; but finding the coast dangerous, and the cliffs covered with warriors, he landed about eight miles to the eastward. The Romans attached considerable importance to this position, and the celebrated Roman road Watling-street, which passed over Barham-downs to

Canterbury, in its course towards the western parts of the kingdom, commenced here. At a very early period the Saxon invaders made themselves masters of the castle, and constructed works which are yet in existence. Edward the Confessor granted to Dover a charter of privileges, and in his reign the institution of the cinque-ports is supposed to have taken place, and Dovor to have been made one of them. Earl Godwin was governor of the castle, and considerably strengthened its fortifications. After the battle of Hastings, many of the natives fled to Dovor castle, as an impregnable fortress, which was however taken by the Conqueror, who put the governor to death, and destroyed the town by fire. According to Domesday-book, Dovor equipped twenty vessels annually for the king's service, in consideration of being exempt from all tolls and taxes, and of various other privileges. Some authors have supposed that the house of the Knights Templars, in this place, was the scene of King John's humiliating surrender of his crown to Pandulph, the pope's legate, when he bound himself as a feudatory vassal of the see of Rome; but it is more probable that this ceremony took place at St. John's, in the adjoining parish of Swingfield, where there was a preceptory of Knights Templars, founded previously to 1190. In 1216, Lewis the Dauphin having landed at Stonar, near Sandwich, and captured several strong places, besieged Dovor castle, but was unable to take it; and in the reign of Edward I. a great part of the town, with some religious houses, was burnt by the French, who were nevertheless soon driven back to their ships. According to the town records, Dovor, in the reign of Edward II., was divided into twenty-one wards, each of which was compelled to provide, at its own charge, a ship for the king's service, and in return the town had the exclusive privilege of a license for a packet boat, to convey passengers to and from France. In 1382, Anne, daughter of the Emperor Charles IV., and afterwards consort of Richard II., arrived here. When the Emperor Sigismund disembarked at Dovor, in 1416, on a visit to his cousin, Henry V., he was formally met at the water's edge by the Duke of Gloucester and several of the nobility, with drawn swords, in order to oppose his landing, should the object of his visit prove to be of a hostile nature. In 1520, the Emperor Charles V. was met here by Henry VIII., whence both monarchs proceeded to Canterbury, and there kept the festival of Whitsuntide. Henry, aware of the importance of Dovor, then called "the key to the kingdom," contributed £80,000 towards the erection of a pier, which was completed in the reign of Elizabeth, at which period the harbour likewise was constantly undergoing improvements. Its more effectual preservation is to be ascribed to the charter of James I., under which were appointed eleven commissioners (the lord warden of the cinque-ports, the lieutenant of the castle, and the mayor of Dovor, being always the principal), as special conservators of the port, incorporated under the title of "Warden and Assistants of the Port and Harbour of the Port of Dovor;" and their powers have been repeatedly enlarged by acts passed in subsequent reigns. In 1814, on the restoration of Louis XVIII. to the French throne, his Majesty George IV. (then Prince Regent,) accompanied that sovereign to Dovor; and, in the same year, Alexander, Emperor of Russia, and Frederic William, King of Prussia, with the veteran Blucher, and other distinguished foreigners in their train, embarked at Boulogne on board his

majesty's ship the impregnable, bearing the flag of his Royal Highness the Duke of Clarence, as admiral of the fleet, and landed here on a visit to the Prince Regent.

The town, which is built in a semicircular form, is seated in a beautiful valley, between stupendous cliffs of chalk-stone, from the summits of which the view of the sea in front, with the opposite coast of France, is grand and beautiful. It is well built, many of the houses being excellent, and most of them modern; it has one principal street, more than a mile long, and several inferior ones, which are well paved, and lighted with gas, under an act passed in the 3rd of George IV. A theatre and assembly-rooms were erected in 1790. On the parade are warm, cold, and shower baths of salt water, with every accommodation for sea-bathing; also good libraries and reading-rooms. The many respectable families which frequent the town during the summer, have rendered it a watering-place of great celebrity. The environs are delightfully picturesque, and there are several fine views in the neighbourhood.

The castle is of very ancient foundation, being attributed by the vulgar to Julius Cæsar, but by respectable antiquaries to Claudius. It is situated on a lofty eminence, about half a mile northward from the town, is approached by a bold ascent, occupies a site of thirty acres of land, and consists at the present time of two courts, defended by wide ditches, and communicating with the towers within, by means of subterraneous passages. The lower court, excepting on the side next the sea, is surrounded by an irregular wall, called the curtain, and flanked at unequal distances by numerous towers of different shapes and ages. During the lapse of years they have all undergone very considerable alterations. That which Godwin erected, in the time of Canute, has long been removed, nor was its site known for ages, until recently discovered in making a new road; Chilham or Caldescot tower is the third from the edge of the cliff, and at the back of it was a postern upon the vallum which joined the Roman and Saxon works, with a subterraneous passage into the castle, through which Stephen Pincester is said to have led the reinforcement that enabled Hubert de Burgh successfully to withstand the Dauphin, in the reign of John. This tower was built by Fulbert de Lucy, whose family came over with the Conqueror, and originally named after the manor of Chilham, the possessors of which are still bound to keep it in repair; but Caldescot having succeeded to the command, it subsequently went by his name. In the front of this building is a house for an officer, called the Bodar of the castle, under the lord warden of the cinque-ports, who has power to take within his jurisdiction, and keep in custody in this tower, crown and other debtors. Fiennes, or New-gate tower, called also the Constable's tower, has been used ever since the Conquest as the governor's apartments; it stands upon the site of a more ancient tower, said to have been built after a design by Gundulph, Bishop of Rochester, who was employed by the Conqueror in making designs for castles, and superintending their erection. Crevignor, Craville, or Earl of Norfolk's tower is opposite the north entrance of the quadrangle of the keep, and near it is a subterraneous passage leading to a vault, which is sufficiently capacious to contain a large garrison, and is protected by a draw-bridge, moat, and round tower: the tower in the ditch, and the adjoining subterraneous works are supposed to have been constructed in the reign of John, by Hubert de Burgh, then constable of the castle, who bravely defended it, in 1216, against the aggressions of the French. Fitzwilliam's, or St. John's tower is the next in order; it was named after Adam Fitzwilliam, who accompanied the Conqueror to England and received from that monarch the scarf from off his own arm at the battle of Hastings, as a reward for his distinguished bravery. Avianches, or Maunsel's tower stands in an angle formed by the curtain wall, and is one of the noblest relics of the Norman towers; it was named after two constables, or governors, the latter of whom was lord warden in the reign of Henry III.: the first floor was a kind of vault, arched with stone, and open in front, and in the wall, which is very thick, is a gallery, or passage, ascended by stone steps, where archers could range one above another, and, through small apertures, command the ditch on either side, as also the approaches to it from the curtain. Through the gallery is an ascent to a platform over the top of the vault, partly surrounded by a wall, and having a spiral stone staircase, which leads to the top of the tower. Near the entrance denominated the Palace Gate is a stately fabric, named, in the reign of Edward IV., Suffolk tower, from de la Pole, Duke of Suffolk; adjoining which is the old arsenal tower, and farther on were formerly the king's kitchen and other offices. All this side of the castle presents. a modern appearance, the back part having been cased over, and the front being hid by barracks erected in 1745. The keep, or palace tower, built after a design by Gundulph, stands near the centre of this court: the entrance, originally on the east, is now on the south side; it opened by a grand portal, now walled up, into the state apartments, in general lofty and spacious, which, as was usual in castles in earlier days, were on the third story. The staircase has two vestibules, and was guarded at different heights by three strong gates. Ascending by the vestibule on the right hand, is a room apparently designed for the warden of the first gate, and opposite is another, probably the chapel, adorned on every side with beautiful arches, richly embellished with zigzag and other work. Above this is a third, similarly ornamented, and under the chapel and the first vestibule is the dungeon, in which at different times persons of distinction have been confined. In the walls of the keep are galleries with holes, through which an enemy might be fired at, but so constructed as to protect the defenders. The second floor was intended for the use of the garrison, and the ground-floor for stores. Part of the castle is used for a gaol. In the north angle a well, for ages arched over, has been recently found, and is probably that which Harold, before his accession to the throne, promised on oath to deliver up to William, Duke of Normandy; there are also four other wells, each three hundred and seventy feet deep, within the Saxon lines of defence. The more recent works are, batteries mounted with heavy ordnance, casemates in the chalk rock, magazines, covered ways, and subterraneous passages, with accommodations therein for two thousand men, light and air being admitted through holes cut in the chalk and other apertures, extending to the front of the cliff. The old road to Deal having become so hollow as to afford protection to an enemy approaching the castle from the town, a new one has been constructed under the direction of the board

of ordnance, to the top of the hill, which is completely commanded by the batteries. Near the edge of the cliff is a curious piece of brass ordnance, twenty-four feet in length, cast at Utrecht, in 1544, and called Queen Elizabeth's pocket pistol, having been presented to her majesty by the States of Holland: it carries a twelve-pound shot, and it has been affirmed that, if loaded well and kept clean, it would carry a shot to the French shore. Dovor castle was formerly extra-judicial, but as several of the franchises are lost or in disuse, the civil authorities have of late years exercised a jurisdiction within its limits, independently of the lord warden: it is still extra-parochial. During the late war with France, the western heights of this town were strongly fortified upon the modern system: the works are so admirably arranged, and the position so advantageous, that, whilst a small garrison would suffice for its defence, a large army can be disposed of within the walls. There are three entrances to the heights, one by Archcliff fort, another by the New Military road, and the third from the head of the town, by a staircase of very peculiar construction, called the Grand Military Shaft. The immediate entrance to the harbour is protected by Archcliff fort, at the extremity of the pier, and Amhurst battery at the north pier head. A new military road has been constructed to the fortifications of the western heights, the lines which connect these extending from the eastern redoubt to the sally-port west of Archcliff fort. Thus the whole line of defence round the town is complete, from the castle to Shakspeare's cliff, so called from the sublime but somewhat exaggerated description given by the great dramatist, in his tragedy of King Lear. There is a military hospital of recent erection at the west side of the town. An hospital of ancient foundation, called the *Maison Dieu*, was converted into a victualling office in 1555.

As a port, Dovor derives its chief importance from its proximity to the continent, and, at a large annual expenditure on the harbour, receives and protects ships not exceeding five hundred tons' burden: this expenditure is defrayed out of an annual revenue applicable to the reparation and improvement of the harbour, arising from land granted by royal charter, or devised by will, and let on lease, and from the duty paid on tonnage, &c. During the war this port was famous for privateers, and supplied the service with many cutters and some transports: the docks are well constructed, and there are several good store-houses, and a custom-house. The passage to and from the continent, especially Calais and Boulogne, is a very lucrative source of employment to the inhabitants: steam packets sail daily to Calais and Boulogne. The foreign trade is very trifling, but the coasting somewhat considerable, and many vessels are employed in the fisheries. The number of vessels which entered inwards from foreign parts, in 1826, was six hundred and ninety-one British, and three hundred and eight foreign; and that which cleared outwards, seven hundred and fifty-one British, and three hundred and seventy-six foreign. In 1828, one hundred and twelve ships belonged to the port, of which, thirteen were upwards of one hundred tons' burden. A large quantity of grain is shipped at this port for the London market, and there are several corn mills in the vicinity. At Buckland and River, near the town, are paper-mills, and some business is done in the tanning of leather. The market days are Wednesday and Saturday, and there is an annual fair on the 23rd of November.

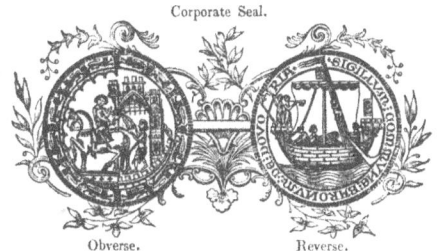

Corporate Seal.

Obverse. Reverse.

The first charter of incorporation was granted by Edward I.; another was offered by Charles II., but not accepted. The old charter was probably surrendered to Charles II., and, in 1684, a new one was granted, according to the provisions of which the town is now governed, though the charter is lost The corporation consists of a mayor, twelve jurats, thirty-six common council-men, with a recorder, town clerk, and other officers. The mayor, who is coroner for Dovor and its liberties, is chosen on the 8th of September. The borough was formerly divided into twenty-one wards, but now comprises only thirteen. It returns two members to parliament : the right of election is vested in the freemen by birth, marriage, apprenticeship, purchase, and gift, the number of whom, resident and non-resident, is upwards of two thousand three hundred : the mayor is the returning officer. A court of record of unlimited extent was granted by charter of confirmation in the 20th of Charles II., to Dovor, as well as to the rest of the cinque-ports : the judges of this court are the mayor and jurats; the town clerk issues the processes. Sessions for the town and liberties, which latter comprise the parishes of St. Mary the Virgin, St. James the Apostle, Hougham, or Huffam, and Charlton, in Dovor; the parishes of St. John the Baptist, St. Peter the Apostle, Birchington, and the vill of Wood, in the Isle of Thanet; and Ringswould, near Dovor, twice a year, or oftener if occasion require, in the town-hall over the market-house. A court of requests was established by an act passed in the 24th of George III., for the recovery of debts not amounting to forty shillings, and upwards of two shillings, the jurisdiction of which extends over the town and port of Dovor, including also the parishes of Charlton, Buckland, River, Ewell, Lydden, Coldred, East Langdon, West Langdon, Ringwould, St. Margaret's at Cliff, Whitfield, otherwise Beansfield, Guston, Hougham, or Huffam, Caple le Fern, Alkham, and the liberty of Dovor castle.

Dovor formerly consisted of the parishes of St. James the Apostle, St. John, St. Martin the Greater, St. Martin the Less, St. Mary the Virgin, St. Nicholas, and St. Peter, the churches of all which have been demolished, and the parishes themselves merged into those of St. James and St. Mary. The living of St. Mary's is a perpetual curacy, in the peculiar jurisdiction of the Archbishop of Canterbury, and in the patronage of the Parishioners : the church was built by the prior and convent of St. Martin's, in this town, and has some portions in the Norman style of architecture. The living of St. James is a discharged rectory, in the peculiar jurisdiction and patronage of the Archbishop of Canterbury, rated in the king's books at £4. 17. 6., and

endowed with £400 private benefaction, and £400 royal bounty : the church belonged to the castle, and to this day the courts of Chancery and Admiralty for all the cinque-ports and their members are held in it. According to tradition, Lucius, the first Christian British king, built a church within the castle, and endowed it with the duties of the port ; of this edifice, the chapel is demolished, but the steeple, in which several Roman bricks are visible, and the principal parts of the external walls, forming the body of the church, are yet standing; it was dedicated to St. Mary, and subsequently called "the Lady of Pity's chapel :" there is still a chapel in the castle for the garrison. There are places of worship for General and Particular Baptists, the Society of Friends, Independents, Wesleyan Methodists, Unitarians, and Roman Catholics. A charity school for the maintenance and education of forty-five boys and thirty-four girls was founded in 1789, and is supported by voluntary contributions, in addition to an endowment of £900 five per cent. stock, producing together on an average about £220 per annum : a new building was erected for it in 1820, sufficiently spacious to accommodate two hundred boys and two hundred girls, together with a house for the master and mistress. A school of industry for girls was established in 1819; and there are likewise an infant school, a dispensary, and a savings-bank. A priory of secular canons was founded here in the seventh century, which in 1140 was changed into a Benedictine priory, the revenue of which, at the dissolution, was £232. 1. 5¼. The remains of a preceptory of the Knights Templars at Swingfield, near Dovor, and of their successors, the Knights of St. John, are now a farm-house ; the eastern or oldest part was the chapel, the east wall of which has three windows of early English architecture, and three Norman ones above them : various other fragments of the original edifice are still apparent, and the remains of foundations to a considerable extent may yet be traced in different parts of the farm-yard.   Dr. White Kennet, Bishop of Peterborough, who died in 1728 ; and Earl Hardwicke, Lord High Chancellor of England, who died in 1764, were natives of this town.

The CINQUE-PORTS, or five havens, viz., Hastings, Sandwich, Dovor, Romney, and Hythe, so named from their supremacy over the other ports opposite the coast of France, still retain that designation, although two other ports, viz., Rye and Winchelsea, have been added. They are not mentioned collectively in Domesday-book, but Dovor, Sandwich, and Romney, only as privileged ports, whence it has been inferred, that at that period there was no community in these ports ; yet John, in his charter to the cinque-ports, expressly refers to charters in the possession of the barons, granted to them by various kings, from the time of Edward the Confessor. Hastings, which, together with Hythe, was added by William the Conqueror, has always been esteemed the first port in precedency; Rye and Winchelsea were added after the Conquest, but more in the character of appendages than equal ports. The members of Hastings are Seaford, Pevensey, Hidney, Rye, Winchelsea, Beaksbourn, Bulverheath, and Grange; those of Sandwich, are Fordwich, Reculver, Sarre, Walmer, Ramsgate, and Deal; of Dovor, Faversham, St. Peter's, Woodchurch, Goresend, Kingsdown, Birchington, Margate, Ringwould, and Folkestone; of Romney, Lydd, Promehill, Oswarstone, Dangemarsh, and Old Romney;

of Hythe, West Hythe: Tenterden is a member of Rye, and Winchelsea has no member. Most of the coast from the north side of the Isle of Thanet to Hastings is within the jurisdiction of the cinque-ports. Anciently they were all safe and commodious harbours, but great alterations have taken place in some of them : the harbours of Hastings, Romney, and Hythe, are entirely destroyed, and the rivers Rother and Stour are becoming gradually more difficult of navigation. Dovor harbour, by the annual expenditure of a large sum, is rendered capable of admitting ships of moderate burden, and will probably survive all the other ports. By an inquisition taken at the court of admiralty held near the sea-side at Dovor, in June 1682, it was found that the jurisdiction of the admiralty of the cinque-ports extended from Shore-beacon, in Essex, to Red cliff, near Seaford, in Sussex. The offices of lord warden of the cinque-ports and constable of Dovor castle are now invariably united. The lord warden has a right of warren over a very extensive tract, called the Warren, and appoints warreners to preserve the game. The freemen of the cinque-ports are styled "Barons," and in former times enjoyed great dignity, being ranked amongst the nobility of the kingdom. Before the formation of two houses of parliament, the members were called over in the following order, viz., on the first day the lower class, as burgesses and citizens ; on the second, the knights ; and on the third, the barons of the cinque-ports and the peers ; whence it may be concluded that the barons ranked with the peers, and above the knights, and that these two superior orders, previously to the investiture of knights and citizens with legislative authority, composed the national council. The barons of the cinque-ports have the honour of bearing the canopies over the king and queen at the coronation, where none but noblemen (except certain of the royal domestics) and privileged individuals form part of the procession, and at the feast after the coronation, they dine at a table on the right hand of the king. In the 34th of Henry VI., the perquisites for this service were at a brotherhood allotted to each of the cinque-ports alternately ; and in the 25th of Henry VIII. it was decreed that the canopies should be taken by the ports in this order,—Dovor and Romney; Rye, Sandwich, and Hythe; Hastings and Winchelsea. In some of the ports the resident freemen have a voice in the election of the canopy bearers, but those of Dovor are chosen by the mayor, jurats, and common council-men. Although the services rendered by the cinque-ports have ceased with the alteration in naval affairs, yet for a long period they were eminently useful. During several reigns they fitted out fleets which formed a great portion of the royal navy, and were engaged in many renowned actions. By their aid, John, who had been obliged to flee to the Isle of Wight, recovered his kingdom, and soon afterwards Hubert de Burgh, with "forty tall ships" belonging to the cinque-ports, defeated a French fleet of eighty ships, carrying reinforcements for Louis the Dauphin. In the reign of Edward III., the shipping of the cinque-ports conveyed the armies of that warlike prince to France, and guarded our coasts ; and in the reigns of Henry VII. and Henry VIII., the "Ports' Navy" was frequently employed on similar services. The records which mention the number of vessels that were, or ought to have been, furnished by the cinque-ports and their append-

ant members, vary ; but the general number (before large ships were introduced into the navy) which these ports furnished was fifty-seven, manned and equipped at their own cost, for the space of fifteen days, and if their services were needed longer, they were victualled and paid by the king. Hastings provided twenty-one ships, armed and manned with twenty-one men each, besides a boy; Dovor the same number ; Sandwich, five ships ; New Romney, five ships, and Hythe, five ships, all equipped as above, making the whole number of mariners one thousand two hundred and fifty-four. The last charter granted to the cinque-ports was in the 20th of Charles II., who not only confirmed the preceding charters, but conferred on the freemen additional privileges. This was confirmed by James II., and under it the ports are now governed. The arms of the cinque-ports collectively are the same as those of Dovor, and each of the other ports separately.

DOWDESWELL, a parish in the hundred of BRADLEY, county of GLOUCESTER, 4¼ miles (S.E. by E.) from Cheltenham, containing 181 inhabitants. The living is a rectory, rated in the king's books at £13.6.8., in the peculiar jurisdiction of the Rector of Withington, who does not however exercise any authority. Miss Rogers was patroness in 1826. The church, dedicated to St. Michael, is a cruciform structure, built in 1577, with a tower and spire rising from the intersection. There are remains of several ancient fortifications, and some leaden coffins have been found within the parish. Near Andover's Ford a battle was fought between Charles I. and the parliamentary forces.

DOWLAND, a parish in the hundred of NORTH TAWTON with WINKLEY, county of DEVON, 5 miles (N. N. E.) from Hatherleigh, containing 196 inhabitants. The living is a perpetual curacy, in the archdeaconry of Barnstaple, and diocese of Exeter, endowed with £400 private benefaction, and £400 royal bounty. Sir S. H. Northcote, Bart. was patron in 1797.

DOWLES, a parish in the hundred of STOTTESDEN, county of SALOP, 1¼ mile (N. by W.) from Bewdley, containing 61 inhabitants. The living is a discharged rectory, in the archdeaconry of Salop, and diocese of Hereford, rated in the king's books at £4. William Burton and another were patrons in 1818. The church is dedicated to St. Andrew.

DOWLISH (WEST), a parish in the hundred of ABDICK and BULSTONE, county of SOMERSET, 1 mile (S.E. by S.) from Ilminster, containing 32 inhabitants. The living is a rectory, in the archdeaconry of Taunton, and diocese of Bath and Wells, rated in the king's books at £3. 7. 6. W. Speke, Esq. was patron in 1827. The church, which was dedicated to St. John the Baptist, has been demolished, and the inhabitants attend the church of Dowlish-Wake.

DOWLISH-WAKE, a parish in the southern division of the hundred of PETHERTON, county of SOMERSET, 1¼ mile (S.E. by S.) from Ilminster, containing 319 inhabitants. The living is a discharged rectory, in the archdeaconry of Taunton, and diocese of Bath and Wells, rated in the king's books at £8. 9. 9½. W. Speke, Esq. was patron in 1827. The church is dedicated to St. Andrew.

DOWN, a parish in the hundred of RUXLEY, lathe of SUTTON at HONE, county of KENT, 6 miles (S.S.E.) from Bromley, containing 340 inhabitants. The living is a perpetual curacy, annexed to the vicarage of Orpington, in the peculiar jurisdiction of the Archbishop of Canterbury. The church contains various sepulchral memorials of the Petlees, lords of the manor from Edward III. to Henry VIII., whose once sumptuous mansion has been converted into a farm-house. There is a place of worship for Baptists. George Phillips, Esq., in 1771, bequeathed £100, the interest of which is paid to a schoolmistress for teaching eight children.

DOWN (EAST), a parish in the hundred of BRAUNTON, county of DEVON, 6¾ miles (N. N. E.) from Barnstaple, containing 422 inhabitants. The living is a rectory, in the archdeaconry of Barnstaple, and diocese of Exeter, rated in the king's books at £18. 3. 9. The Rev. J. P. Coffin was patron in 1800. The church is dedicated to St. John the Baptist. At a place called Nortcote are several stones, probably commemorative of some British heroes slain in battle.

DOWN (ST. MARY), a parish in the hundred of NORTH TAWTON with WINKLEY, county of DEVON, 2¾ miles (N. E.) from Bow, containing 400 inhabitants. The living is a rectory, in the archdeaconry and diocese of Exeter, rated in the king's books at £12. 13. 4. Miss Wyvill was patroness in 1812. The church has a Norman door-way, and contains some curiously carved oak seats, and ancient tiles in the same style. The river Yeo passes through the parish.

DOWN (WEST), a parish in the hundred of BRAUNTON, county of DEVON, 4 miles (S.) from Ilfracombe, containing 562 inhabitants. The living is a discharged vicarage, in the archdeaconry of Barnstaple, and diocese of Exeter, rated in the king's books at £8. 14. 9., and in the patronage of the Bishop of Exeter. The church, dedicated to the Holy Trinity, contains a monument to the memory of Sir J. Stowford, a justice of the common pleas in 1343, for the welfare of whose soul the prior of Wells founded a chantry, and endowed it with a stipend for the maintenance of a priest.

DOWNHAM, a parish in the hundred and Isle of ELY, county of CAMBRIDGE, 3 miles (N.N.W.) from Ely, containing 1350 inhabitants. The living is a rectory, rated in the king's books at £17. 2. 1., and in the peculiar jurisdiction and patronage of the Bishop of Ely. The church is dedicated to St. Leonard. A palace at this place was formerly one of the principal residences of the diocesans, but since the arrest of Bishop Wren, by order of parliament, in 1642, it has gone to decay; there are still considerable remains, the offices having been converted into a farm-house.

DOWNHAM, a parish in the hundred of BARSTABLE, county of ESSEX, 4¼ miles (E. by N.) from Billericay, containing 315 inhabitants. The living is a rectory, in the archdeaconry of Essex, and diocese of London, rated in the king's books at £12. 2. 8½. R. B. De Beauvoir, Esq. was patron in 1827. The church is dedicated to St. Margaret.

DOWNHAM, a chapelry in that part of the parish of WHALLEY which is in the higher division of the hundred of BLACKBURN, county palatine of LANCASTER, 3 miles (E.N.E.) from Clitheroe, containing 620 inhabitants. The living is a perpetual curacy, in the archdeaconry and diocese of Chester, endowed with £10 per annum and £200 private benefaction, and £400 royal bounty. Earl Howe was patron in 1818. The chapel is dedicated to St. Peter. Ralph Assheton, by will without

date, gave £110 to be laid out in land for the support of a school, the income arising from which is £26 a year; of this sum, £21 is appropriated to the instruction of fifteen children, and the rest is retained for repairs: adjoining the school-room are apartments for the master.

DOWNHAM, a township in the parish of WYMONDHAM, hundred of FOREHOE, county of NORFOLK, 1½ mile (N. E. by N.) from Wymondham, containing 935 inhabitants.

DOWNHAM-MARKET, a market town and parish in the hundred of CLACKCLOSE, county of NORFOLK, 42½ miles (W.) from Norwich, and 85 (N. by E.) from London, containing 2044 inhabitants. This place, which, from its situation near a navigable river, is called in ancient records *Downham Port*, derives its name from the Saxon *Dune*, a hill, and *Ham*, a residence. In the reign of Edgar, the town was granted to the abbey of Ramsey, in Huntingdonshire, and the abbot, in the reign of Edward the Confessor, obtained for it the grant of a weekly market, and in that of John, the privilege of an annual fair. Near the foot of the bridge was an ancient hermitage, and adjoining the church was anciently a Benedictine priory, a cell to the abbey of Ramsey, to the abbots of which Henry III. granted very extensive privileges, among which was the power to try, condemn, and execute felons at their gallows of Downham. The town is pleasantly situated on the declivity of an eminence, about a mile to the eastward of the river Ouse, commanding an extensive view to the west of the fens, with which it is connected by an ancient wooden bridge. It consists of three streets, well paved by subscription, and is amply supplied with water from springs. Here is an extensive foundry for casting church bells; and within a mile of the town is a considerable manufactory for mustard, and for the preparation of linseed oil, the machinery of which is propelled by steam. Downham has for ages been celebrated for its butter, of which immense quantities were sent by the navigable river Ouse to Cambridge, and being afterwards forwarded from that town by land carriage to London, it erroneously obtained the name of Cambridge butter. The market, which is amply supplied with wild fowl and fish from the fens, is on Saturday: the fairs are, March 3rd (one of the largest for horses in the kingdom), May 8th for cattle, and November 13th for toys; statute fairs are also held in the week preceding, and in the week following, old Michaelmas-day. The county magistrates hold here a petty session for the division weekly; and a court baron is held quarterly by the lord of the manor.

The living is a discharged rectory, in the archdeaconry of Norfolk, and diocese of Norwich, rated in the king's books at £6. 13. 4. Miss Franks was patroness in 1811. The church, dedicated to St. Edmund, is a venerable structure in the ancient style of English architecture, with a low square embattled tower, strengthened with buttresses, and surmounted by a small spire: the interior is remarkable for the dissimilarity of the arches which support the roof: the font, which is octagonal, has at each of the angles a shield, on which are sculptured the arms of St. Edmund. The church-yard, occupying the summit of the eminence on which the town is built, is ascended by a flight of steps on the north-west, and is approached from the south by a fine avenue of lime-trees. There are places of worship for Particular Baptists, the Society of Friends, and Independents. A charity school, in which sixty-five boys are taught reading, writing, and arithmetic, on the Lancasterian system was founded in 1808, by the late Mr. Zachary Clarke, and is supported by his widow; and a National school for seventy girls is supported by subscription.

DOWNHAM-SANTON, a parish in the hundred of LACKFORD, county of SUFFOLK, 2¾ miles (E.N.E.) from Brandon-Ferry, containing 79 inhabitants. The living is a perpetual curacy, in the archdeaconry of Sudbury, and diocese of Norwich, endowed with £200 private benefaction, and £1200 royal bounty. The Earl of Cadogan was patron in 1815. The church is dedicated to St. Mary. The navigable river Ouse flows on the northern side of this parish, which suffered greatly in the seventeenth century by the sands that overspread the neighbourhood.

DOWNHEAD, a hamlet in the parish of WEST CAMEL, hundred of SOMERTON, county of SOMERSET, 3¼ miles (N.E. by E.) from Ilchester. The population is returned with the parish. Here was formerly a chapel, but it has been demolished.

DOWNHEAD, a chapelry in the parish of DOULTING, hundred of WHITESTONE, county of SOMERSET, 5½ miles (E.N.E.) from Shepton-Mallet, containing 208 inhabitants. The living is a perpetual curacy, annexed to the vicarage of Doulting, in the archdeaconry of Wells, and diocese of Bath and Wells. The chapel is dedicated to All Saints.

DOWNHOLME, a parish in the western division of the wapentake of HANG, North riding of the county of YORK, comprising the townships of Downholme, Ellerton-Abbey, Stainton, and Walburn, and containing 251 inhabitants, of which number, 113 are in the township of Downholme, 4¾ miles (S. W. by W.) from Richmond. The living is a vicarage, in the archdeaconry of Richmond, and diocese of Chester, rated in the king's books at £5. 15. 10., endowed with £600 private benefaction, and £600 royal bounty. John Hutton, Esq. was patron in 1808. The church is dedicated to St. Michael. In a fertile part of this parish, near the river Swale, are situated the ruins of Ellerton nunnery, consisting principally of the shell of the chapel. Tradition refers its foundation to a person of the name of Wymer, or Wymor, in the reign of Henry II., for nuns of the Cistercian order: at the dissolution, its annual revenue was estimated only at £8.

DOWNSIDE, a tything in the parish of MIDSUMMER-NORTON, hundred of CHEWTON, county of SOMERSET, containing 442 inhabitants.

DOWNTON, a parish in the hundred of WIGMORE, county of HEREFORD, 5½ miles (W. by S.) from Ludlow, containing 111 inhabitants. The living is a discharged vicarage, in the archdeaconry of Salop, and diocese of Hereford, rated in the king's books at £4.10., and in the patronage of the Crown. The church is dedicated to St. Giles.

DOWNTON, a borough town and parish, in the hundred of DOWNTON, county of WILTS, 6¼ miles (S.S.E.) from Salisbury, and 88 (S. W.) from London, containing 3114 inhabitants. The town consists principally of one long irregular street, neither lighted nor paved, extending from east to west, in the course of which there are three bridges over the Upper Avon, which is here divided into three channels. It appears to have been anciently a place of importance, having given

name to the hundred in which it is situated. Here was a castle, the intrenchments of which may still be traced at the south-east extremity of the town; and in the centre of them is a large conical mount, upon which the keep is supposed to have been erected. King John is said to have had a palace at this place: and in taking down part of an old building, called the Court House, or King John's Stables, were found two wooden busts, imagined to be representatives of that prince and his consort. Downton is a borough by prescription: it first sent members to parliament in the 23rd of Edward I., and continued to exercise that privilege till the 38th of Edward III., after which there was only one return (in the 1st of Henry V.) until the 20th of Henry VI., since which they have been regularly continued. The right of election is vested in persons having a freehold interest in burgage tenements holden by a certain rent, fealty and suit of court to the Bishop of Winchester, who is lord of the borough, and paying reliefs on descent and fines on alienation. The number of voters is about twenty: the twenty established burgage tenements, which are all numbered, were sometimes divided at contested elections, so as to make the number of voters amount to one hundred or more; but after repeated contests, the late Lord Radnor obtained, by purchase, the entire patronage of the borough; and the deputy steward of the lessee of the hundred, who is chosen at the court leet, and commonly styled mayor, is the returning officer. On the Avon are several paper and grist-mills; and there is a large tan-yard: malting is carried on to some extent, and several persons are engaged in a branch of the silk manufacture, and in making straw-plat. A market was formerly held on Friday, which has been discontinued. There is a fair on April 23d, for cattle, and another on October 2nd, for sheep and horses.

The living is a vicarage, in the archdeaconry and diocese of Salisbury, rated in the king's books at £20, and in the patronage of the Warden and Fellows of Winchester College. The church, dedicated to St. Lawrence, is a spacious edifice, consisting of a nave, aisles, transept, and chancel, with a central tower, which in 1791 was raised thirty feet higher, at the expense of the late Earl of Radnor, who also largely contributed to the cost of some subsequent repairs in the body of the church; and, more recently, a neat organ and gallery have been erected by subscription. There is a chapel of ease at Nunton, in this parish. There are places of worship for General and Particular Baptists, and Wesleyan Methodists. A free school was founded in 1679, by Joseph Ashe, for the instruction of twelve poor boys, the sons of free burgage holders, or in default of such, the children of other inhabitants of the borough, and endowed with a school-house, the rent of the ground on which the fairs are held, and the interest of £130 in the funds. In 1784, Mrs. Emma Noyes left by will £200 to the vicar and churchwardens, to be placed in the funds, and the interest to be applied in payment of a schoolmistress, for teaching six or eight children to read and work, and for the support of a similar school at East Downton. A parochial school is supported by voluntary contributions, for which a school-room has been erected through the exertions of the present incumbent of the parish, the Rev. Liscombe Clarke, Archdeacon of Salisbury. In 1627, William Stockman gave Chadwell farm, in Whiteparish, now producing between £40 and £50 per annum, for the benefit of poor persons of Downton, "surcharged with children." Here is an ancient cross, called the borough cross, as being the place for elections, except when a poll is demanded : in 1797, it was repaired at the expense of the burgesses. About two miles from Downton is Standlinch, or Trafalgar House, bestowed by the nation, as a token of gratitude for distinguished services, on Admiral Lord Nelson.

DOWSBY, a parish in the wapentake of AVELAND, parts of KESTEVEN, county of LINCOLN, 6 miles (N. by E.) from Bourne, containing 201 inhabitants. The living is a rectory, in the archdeaconry and diocese of Lincoln, rated in the king's books at £11. 19. 2. The Rev. T. Forster was patron in 1807. The church is dedicated to St. Andrew.

DOXFORD, a township in the parish of ELLINGHAM, southern division of BAMBROUGH ward, county of NORTHUMBERLAND, 7½ miles (N.) from Alnwick, containing 54 inhabitants.

DOYNTON, a parish in the upper division of the hundred of LANGLEY and SWINEHEAD, though locally in the hundred of Pucklechurch, county of GLOUCESTER, 7 miles (S. by W.) from Chipping-Sodbury, containing 415 inhabitants. The living is a rectory, in the archdeaconry and diocese of Gloucester, rated in the king's books at £14. 11. 3., and in the patronage of the Crown. The church is dedicated to the Holy Trinity ; the chancel was rebuilt about 1768. On the summit of some lofty rocks, between which runs the river Boyd, are intrenchments, supposed to be Roman. Veins of lead-ore are found here, but they are not sufficiently productive to pay the expense of working. The Rev. William Langton, about 1666, gave certain money in trust for the purchase of lands, now producing £30. 6. 2. a year ; this bequest has been consolidated with two smaller legacies amounting to £6 per annum, making together £36. 6. 2., of which income, £14 is paid to a schoolmistress for teaching children, and the residue is laid out in books, &c. for the school, and in apprentice fees, according to the directions of the testator.

DRAKELOW, a township in the parish of CHURCH-GRESLEY, hundred of REPTON and GRESLEY, county of DERBY, 3 miles (S. S. W.) from Burton upon Trent, containing 84 inhabitants. It is in the honour of Tutbury, duchy of Lancaster, and within the jurisdiction of a court of pleas held at Tutbury every third Tuesday, for the recovery of debts under 40s. Here is one of the depôts on the line of the Chesterfield and Trent canal, which at this place passes through a tunnel two hundred and fifty yards long.

DRAUGHTON, a parish in the hundred of ROTHWELL, county of NORTHAMPTON, 7½ miles (W. by S.) from Kettering, containing 170 inhabitants. The living is a rectory, in the archdeaconry of Northampton, and diocese of Peterborough, rated in the king's books at £12. 2. 11. J. P. Hungerford, Esq. was patron in 1790. The church is dedicated to St. Catherine. There are quarries of good freestone in the parish.

DRAUGHTON, a township in that part of the parish of SKIPTON which is in the eastern division of the wapentake of STAINCLIFFE and EWCROSS, West riding of the county of YORK, 3½ miles (E. by N.) from Skipton, containing 279 inhabitants.

DRAX, a parish in the lower division of the wapentake of BARKSTONE-ASH, West riding of the county

of YORK, comprising the townships of Camblesforth, Drax, Long Drax, and Newland, and containing 1083 inhabitants, of which number, 370 are in the township of Drax, 4 miles (N. N. E.) from Snaith. The living is a discharged vicarage, in the archdeaconry and diocese of York, rated in the king's books at £4, endowed with £600 royal bounty, and £1600 parliamentary grant, and in the patronage of the Crown. The church is dedicated to St. Peter. The free grammar school was erected in 1669, by Charles Reed, Esq., and endowed by him with £2000, for teaching all the poor children of the parish, and for occasionally putting out apprentices ; he farther directed, should any be found capable, that they were to be sent to one of the Universities. He also erected six almshouses, to be kept in repair from the same fund, for three aged persons of each sex. This benefactor, when an infant, was discovered lying among some reeds, and was, from that circumstance, named Reed ; having been brought up by the parish, he was put to the sea service at the age of sixteen, and after fifty years' absence returned opulent, and testified his gratitude to his preservers by the above benevolent acts.

DRAX (LONG), a township in the parish of DRAX, lower division of the wapentake of BARKSTONE-ASH, West riding of the county of YORK, 4¾ miles (N. E. by N.) from Snaith, containing 187 inhabitants. A priory of Black canons was founded in the time of Henry I., by William Paynell, to the honour of St. Nicholas, the annual revenue of which, at the dissolution, was valued at £121. 18. 3.

DRAYCOT-CERNE, a parish in the hundred of MALMESBURY, county of WILTS, 4 miles (N. by E.) from Chippenham, containing 169 inhabitants. The living is a rectory, in the archdeaconry of Wilts, and diocese of Salisbury, rated in the king's books at £6. 7. 11., and in the patronage of the Hon. W. T. L. P. Wellesley. The church is dedicated to St. Peter. Dr. Buckeridge, successively Bishop of Rochester and Ely, was born here, about 1562 ; he died in 1631.

DRAYCOT-FOLIATT, a parish in the hundred of KINGSBRIDGE, county of WILTS, 4½ miles (S. S. E.) from Swindon, containing 24 inhabitants. The living is a rectory, in the archdeaconry of Wilts, and diocese of Salisbury, rated in the king's books at £6. 6. 8. A. Godderd, Esq. was patron in 1817. The church has long since been demolished.

DRAYCOT-FOLIATT, a chapelry in the parish of WILCOT, hundred of SWANBOROUGH, county of WILTS, 2¼ miles (N.) from Pewsey. The population is returned with the parish.

DRAYCOTT, a joint liberty and chapelry with Wilne, in the parish of SAWLEY, hundred of MORLESTON and LITCHURCH, county of DERBY, 6½ miles (E. S. E.) from Derby, containing, with Wilne, 1102 inhabitants.

DRAYCOTT, a tything in the parish of LIMINGTON, hundred of STONE, county of SOMERSET, containing 31 inhabitants.

DRAYCOTT, a hamlet partly in the parish of CHEDDER, and partly in that of RODNEY-STOKE, hundred of WINTERSTOKE, county of SOMERSET, 6 miles (N. W. by W.) from Wells.

DRAYCOTT, a township in the parish of HANBURY, northern division of the hundred of OFFLOW, county of STAFFORD, 6 miles (S. E. by E.) from Uttoxeter, containing 321 inhabitants.

DRAYCOTT, a hamlet in the parish of BLOCKLEY, upper division of the hundred of OSWALDSLOW, county of WORCESTER, though locally in the upper division of the hundred of Kiftsgate, county of Gloucester, $3\frac{1}{2}$ miles (N. N. W.) from Moreton in the Marsh, containing 197 inhabitants.

DRAYCOTT in the MOORS, a parish in the southern division of the hundred of TOTMONSLOW, county of STAFFORD, $2\frac{1}{4}$ miles (S. W.) from Cheadle, containing 579 inhabitants. The living is a rectory, in the archdeaconry of Stafford, and diocese of Lichfield and Coventry, rated in the king's books at £9. 6. 8., and in the patronage of the Dowager Lady Stourton. The church, dedicated to St. Peter, contains some fine old monuments of the Draycot family: in the church-yard is a pyramidal stone, similar to those with which the Danes marked the depository of their deceased heroes. There is a place of worship for Roman Catholics. The parish, through which runs the river Blythe, is in the honour of Tutbury, duchy of Lancaster, and within the jurisdiction of a court of pleas held at Tutbury every third Tuesday, for the recovery of debts under 40s. Near the village is the hamlet of Totmonslow, which gives name to the hundred; it contains but a few houses, though it is supposed to have been anciently a place of some importance.

DRAYTON, a parish in the hundred of OCK, county of BERKS, $2\frac{1}{4}$ miles (S. W. by S.) from Abingdon, containing 498 inhabitants. The living is a perpetual curacy annexed to the vicarage of St. Helen's, Abingdon, in the archdeaconry of Berks, and diocese of Salisbury. The chapel is dedicated to St. Peter. The Wilts and Berks canal passes through this chapelry. In 1780, a dreadful fire which raged in the village destroyed more than thirty houses.

DRAYTON, a township in the parish of BRINGHURST, hundred of GARTREE, county of LEICESTER, $2\frac{3}{4}$ miles (W.) from Rockingham, containing 104 inhabitants. Here was formerly a chapel, which was dedicated to St. James, now desecrated. There is a small endowed free school. George Fox, founder of the sect called the Society of Friends, was born at this place in 1624.

DRAYTON, a parish in the hundred of TAVERHAM, county of NORFOLK, $4\frac{1}{2}$ miles (N. W.) from Norwich, containing 283 inhabitants. The living is a discharged rectory united with that of Hellesden, in the archdeaconry and diocese of Norwich, rated in the king's books at £6. 2. 9., and in the patronage of the Bishop of Norwich. The church is dedicated to St. Margaret.

DRAYTON, a hamlet in the parish of DAVENTRY, hundred of FAWSLEY, county of NORTHAMPTON, $\frac{3}{4}$ of a mile (N. W. by W.) from Daventry, with which the population is returned. A Roman pavement was discovered near this place in 1736.

DRAYTON, a parish in the hundred of BLOXHAM, county of OXFORD, 2 miles (N. W. by W.) from Banbury, containing 185 inhabitants. The living is a rectory, in the archdeaconry and diocese of Oxford, rated in the king's books at £12. 16. 0½., and in the patronage of the Earls of Guildford, Plymouth, and Delawarr, as coheirs of the late Duchess of Dorset. The church is dedicated to St. Peter.

DRAYTON, a parish in the hundred of DORCHESTER, county of OXFORD, 5 miles (N.) from Wallingford, containing 343 inhabitants. The living is a perpetual cu-

racy, within the jurisdiction of the peculiar court of Dorchester, endowed with £400 private benefaction, and £400 royal bounty, and in the patronage of the Dean and Canons of Christ Church, Oxford. The church is dedicated to St. Leonard.

DRAYTON, a parish in the hundred of ABDICK and BULSTONE, county of SOMERSET, 2 miles (S. W.) from Langport, containing, with the tything of Middleney, 469 inhabitants. The living is a perpetual curacy, in the archdeaconry of Taunton, and diocese of Bath and Wells, endowed with £600 private benefaction, and £600 royal bounty. R. T. Combe, Esq. was patron in 1816. The church, dedicated to St. Catherine, is an ancient structure, with an embattled tower at the west end, and a fine south porch of Norman architecture.

DRAYTON, a township in that part of the parish of PENKRIDGE which is in the eastern division of the hundred of CUTTLESTONE, county of STAFFORD, $1\frac{1}{4}$ mile (N. by E.) from Penkridge. The population is returned with the township of Penkridge.

DRAYTON, a township in the parish of OLD STRATFORD, Stratford division of the hundred of BARLICHWAY, county of WARWICK, $2\frac{1}{4}$ miles (W.) from Stratford upon Avon. The population is returned with the parish.

DRAYTON (DRY), a parish in the hundred of CHESTERTON, county of CAMBRIDGE, 5 miles (W.N.W.) from Cambridge, containing 420 inhabitants. The living is a rectory, in the archdeaconry and diocese of Ely, rated in the king's books at £21. 1. 3., and in the patronage of the Dean of Christ Church, Oxford. The church is dedicated to St. Peter and St. Paul. There is a school supported by donations from the Rev. Richard Haslop, in 1729, and Elizabeth Hetherington, in 1777, producing about £7. 17. 6. per annum.

DRAYTON (EAST), a parish in the South-clay division of the wapentake of BASSETLAW, county of NOTTINGHAM, 4 miles (N.E.) from Tuxford, containing 266 inhabitants. The living is a vicarage, rated in the king's books at £9. 3. 4., and in the peculiar jurisdiction and patronage of the Dean and Chapter of York. The church is dedicated to St. Peter. There are chapels of ease at Askham and Stokeham, in this parish. Here is a free school endowed with £25 per annum.

DRAYTON (FEN), a parish in the hundred of PAPWORTH, county of CAMBRIDGE, $3\frac{3}{4}$ miles (S.E. by S.) from St. Ives, containing 325 inhabitants. The living is a perpetual curacy, in the archdeaconry and diocese of Ely, and in the patronage of the Master and Fellows of Christ College, Cambridge. The inhabitants have the right of sending four boys to the free school of Fen-Stanton, in Huntingdonshire.

DRAYTON (FENNY), a parish in the hundred of SPARKENHOE, county of LEICESTER, 6 miles (W.N.W.) from Hinckley, containing 118 inhabitants. The living is a rectory, in the archdeaconry of Leicester, and diocese of Lincoln, rated in the king's books at £11. 1. 5½., and in the patronage of the Rev. Samuel Bracebridge Heming. The church is dedicated to St. Michael.

DRAYTON (WEST), a parish in the hundred of ELTHORNE, county of MIDDLESEX, $3\frac{1}{4}$ miles (N.E.) from Colnbrook, containing 608 inhabitants. The living is a discharged vicarage, united to that of Harmondsworth, in the peculiar jurisdiction of the Dean and Chapter of St. Paul's, London, rated in the king's books at £13. 6. 8., and endowed with £200 private benefaction, and £200 royal bounty. The church, dedicated to St. Martin, has an embattled tower at the west end, and contains a font curiously sculptured in compartments. The Grand Junction canal passes through the parish.

DRAYTON (WEST), a chapelry in the parish of EAST MARKHAM, South-clay division of the wapentake of BASSETLAW, county of NOTTINGHAM, 3 miles (N.W. by N.) from Tuxford, containing 117 inhabitants. Henry Walter, in 1688, directed a house to be built, and bequeathed an annual rent-charge of £25 towards the maintenance of a schoolmaster, for teaching all the poor boys of this place, of Bothamsall, Haughton, Elksley, Gamston, Milton, and Bevercotes.

DRAYTON-BASSETT, a parish in the southern division of the hundred of OFFLOW, county of STAFFORD, 2¾ miles (S.S.W.) from Tamworth, containing 468 inhabitants. The living is a rectory, in the archdeaconry of Stafford, and diocese of Lichfield and Coventry, rated in the king's books at £7. 8. 4., and in the patronage of the Crown. The church is dedicated to St. Peter. The Birmingham and Fazeley canal passes through the parish.

DRAYTON-BEAUCHAMP, a parish in the hundred of COTTESLOE, county of BUCKINGHAM, 2 miles (W. by N.) from Tring, containing 272 inhabitants. The living is a rectory, in the archdeaconry of Buckingham, and diocese of Lincoln, rated in the king's books at £11. 9. 7. Lady R. Manners was patroness in 1808. The church is dedicated to St. Mary. A school has been established on the British system.

DRAYTON in HALES, or MARKET-DRAYTON, a parish comprising the market town of Drayton in Hales, Drayton division of the hundred of BRADFORD (North), county of SALOP; and the townships of Almington, Bloore in Tyrley, and Hales, in the northern division of the hundred of PIREHILL, county of STAFFORD, and containing 4426 inhabitants, of which number, 3700 are in the town of Drayton in Hales (including the hamlet of Little Drayton), 19¼ miles (N. E. by N.) from Shrewsbury, and 159½ (N. W. by N.) from London. Nennius endeavours to identify this with the Caer Draithon of the Britons, enumerating it as one of the principal cities belonging to that people; and the correctness of his opinion has not been arraigned by any succeeding writer. It is evident, from the discovery of the foundations of several houses in the adjoining fields, that the town anciently occupied a more extended site than it does at present. In the record of Domesday it is mentioned by the name Draitune. The manor was successively in the possession of the abbot of St. Ebrulph, in Normandy, and the abbot of Combermere, in Cheshire; the latter, in 1246, received the grant of a market to be held at Drayton, on Wednesday, and a fair on the eve, day, and morrow, of the nativity of the Virgin Mary. At Bloreheath, about two miles from the town, but in the county of Stafford, a sanguinary encounter occurred, on the 23rd of September, 1459, between five thousand Yorkists under the command of Richard Neville, Earl of Salisbury, and ten thousand Lancastrians under that of James Touchet, Lord Audley; although the numbers were thus disproportionate, the latter were defeated, and their general and two thousand four hundred men slain: after this the earl proceeded to join the Duke of York at Ludlow, whither he was hastening when interrupted by the opposite party. During the parliamentary war, this neighbourhood was the scene of a skirmish, on the 25th of January, 1643, when Prince Rupert routed the enemy, who were commanded by Sir Thomas Fairfax. The town stands on the north-western bank of the river Tern; it is clean and moderately well paved, and the houses present a neat appearance. There are manufactories for paper, and for hair-cloth for chair-bottoms, and some business is done in malting; but the trade, which was formerly very considerable, has declined, in consequence of the construction of the Grand Trunk canal. The market, formerly of greater repute than at present, is on Wednesday. Fairs, for horned cattle, horses, sheep, pigs, and hempen and woollen cloth, are held on the Wednesday before Palm-Sunday, Wednesday before June 22nd, September 19th, and October 24th. The petty sessions for the Drayton division of the hundred are held here.

The living is a vicarage, in the archdeaconry of Salop (except that portion of the parish lying in the county of Stafford, which is within the peculiar jurisdiction of the courts leet and baron of the manor of Tyrley), and diocese of Lichfield and Coventry, rated in the king's books at £12. 10. 7½., and in the patronage of Richard Corbet, Esq. The church, dedicated to St. Mary, was built, with the exception probably of the steeple, in the reign of Stephen; it consists of a nave, aisles, a chancel, and a square tower supported by buttresses and adorned with battlements and pinnacles: the whole of the building, except the tower, was thoroughly repaired in 1787; and it has lately received an addition of one hundred and fifty sittings, one hundred of which are free, the Incorporated Society for the enlargement of churches and chapels having granted £100 towards defraying the expense. Here are places of worship for Baptists, Independents, and Wesleyan Methodists. A free grammar school was founded in 1554, and endowed with a rent-charge of £22 per annum by Sir Rowland Hill, and £10 per annum by Lady Lake, for a master and an usher, whose offices were consolidated by a decree of the court of Chancery in 1816, and the master's salary fixed at £25 per annum; the school is open to all the boys of the parish, the usual number of scholars being about sixty. In 1730, the Rev. Richard Price left property producing £8. 14. per annum, for teaching children, and other purposes; and John Bill bequeathed £240, for teaching and apprenticing ten boys. There are also various smaller benefactions, for apprenticing poor children, and other charitable purposes.

DRAYTON-PARSLOW, a parish in the hundred of COTTESLOE, county of BUCKINGHAM, 5¼ miles (E. by N.) from Winslow, containing 372 inhabitants. The living is a rectory, in the archdeaconry of Buckingham, and diocese of Lincoln, rated in the king's books at £12. The Rev. J. Lord, D.D., was patron in 1817. The church is dedicated to the Holy Trinity.

DREGG, a parish in ALLERDALE ward above Darwent, county of CUMBERLAND, comprising the townships of Carleton and Dregg, and containing 433 inhabitants, of which number, 289 are in the township of Dregg, 3 miles (N. W. by N.) from Ravenglass. The living is a perpetual curacy, in the archdeaconry of

Richmond, and diocese of Chester. endowed with £800 royal bounty, and in the patronage of Lord Muncaster. The church is dedicated to St. Peter. Joseph Walker, in 1727, gave £260, now producing £11. 14. per annum, for the education of the children of such of the parishioners as had previously contributed towards the erection of a school-house. A school-room was built in 1828, by the Rev. William Thompson, a native of the parish, the master of which is to teach eight children, for 1s. entrance, and 1s. per quarter each; and he is allowed to admit others upon his own terms: the superintendence is vested in seven trustees, one of whom, the Bishop of Chester, is appointed visitor. The parish anciently abounded with oaks, from which it seems to have derived its name, *Derigh* or *Dergh* signifying, in the Celtic tongue, oak; it is intersected by the river Irt, bounded on the south by the Mite, and on the west by the Irish sea, near the shore of which there is a powerful chalybeate spring.

DREWSTEINGTON, county of DEVON. See TEINGTON (DREW).

DREWTON, a joint township with Everthorp, in the parish of NORTH CAVE, Hunsley-Beacon division of the wapentake of HARTHILL, East riding of the county of YORK, 1½ mile (N. by W.) from South Cave, containing 177 inhabitants.

DRIBY, a parish in the Wold division of the wapentake of CANDLESHOE, parts of LINDSEY, county of LINCOLN, 4¾ miles (W. by S.) from Alford, containing 82 inhabitants. The living is a discharged vicarage, united in 1774 to the rectory of South Ormsby, in the archdeaconry and diocese of Lincoln, rated in the king's books at £8. 19. 4. B. Massingberd, Esq. was patron in 1825. The church is dedicated to St. Michael.

DRIFFIELD, a parish in the hundred of CROWTHORNE and MINETY, county of GLOUCESTER, 4½ miles (E. S. E.) from Cirencester, containing 144 inhabitants. The living is a vicarage, in the archdeaconry and diocese of Gloucester, rated in the king's books at £8. 2. 3½., and in the patronage of T. Smith, Esq. The church is dedicated to St. Mary. A free school was founded in 1825, by Arthur Vansittart, Esq. and Susannah Cumberland, the former granting a messuage and garden, and the latter bestowing £300, the interest of which, together with other voluntary contributions, is applied to the instruction of about twenty children on the National system.

DRIFFIELD (GREAT), a parish partly within the liberty of ST. PETER of YORK, but chiefly in the Bainton-Beacon division of the wapentake of HARTHILL, East riding of the county of YORK, comprising the market town of Great Driffield, the chapelry of Little Driffield, and the township of Emswell with Kelleythorpe, and containing 2471 inhabitants, of which number, 2303 are in the town of Great Driffield, 29 miles (E. by N.) from York, and 193 (N.) from London. The town is agreeably situated at the foot of the Wolds, near the source of one of the streams which being united form the river Hull. It consists principally of a long street, extending from north to south, parallel to which runs the brook, which at the southern extremity of the town is enlarged into a navigable canal, joining the Hull below Frodingham bridge, after a course of three miles. The soil is particularly adapted to the production of corn, the trade in which has greatly increased within the last fifty years, owing partly to the facility for water carriage afforded by the canal. The market is on Thursday, when the quantity of grain brought for sale is often very considerable. The living is a discharged vicarage, rated in the king's books at £7. 10. 2½., endowed with £100 private benefaction, and £200 royal bounty, and in the peculiar jurisdiction and patronage of the Precentor in the Cathedral Church of York, as Prebendary of Driffield. The church, dedicated to All Saints, is an ancient structure, with a steeple in the later English style, built by one of the Hotham family. Here are places of worship for Baptists, Independents, and Primitive and Wesleyan Methodists. A dispensary is supported by voluntary contributions; also a National school for one hundred children, established in 1816. At Danes Hill, a hamlet in this parish, is a great number of tumuli, called "Danes' Graves," supposed to be the monuments of Danish chiefs who fell in some engagement in the vicinity.

DRIFFIELD (LITTLE), a chapelry in the parish of GREAT DRIFFIELD, partly within the liberty of ST. PETER of YORK, and partly in the Bainton-Beacon division of the wapentake of HARTHILL, East riding of the county of YORK, 1 mile (W.) from Great Driffield, containing 75 inhabitants. The living is a perpetual curacy, rated in the king's books at £5. 3. 4., endowed with £100 private benefaction, and £700 parliamentary grant, and in the peculiar jurisdiction and patronage of the Precentor in the Cathedral Church of York, as Prebendary of Driffield. The church, dedicated to St. Peter, was taken down and rebuilt in 1807: the ancient structure was celebrated as the burial-place of Alfred, King of Northumberland, who died in 705, to whose memory an inscription is still preserved against the south wall of the chancel. There is a place of worship for Wesleyan Methodists. Fairs are held on Easter-Monday, Whit-Monday, August 26th, and September 19th, for horses, cattle, and sheep.

DRIGHLINGTON, a chapelry in the parish of BIRSTALL, wapentake of MORLEY, West riding of the county of YORK, 5 miles (S. E. by E.) from Bradford, containing 1719 inhabitants. The living is a perpetual curacy, in the archdeaconry and diocese of York, endowed with £200 private benefaction, and £2300 parliamentary grant, and in the patronage of J. Birstall, Esq. This was the birthplace of Dr. James Margetson, Archbishop of Armagh, who built here a school and endowed it, in 1678, with a rent-charge of £60 per annum. In the reign of William and Mary, Sir John Tempest and eight others were constituted a body corporate, with a common seal, to act as governors of the foundation, upon which twelve children are educated, as free scholars, and are taught Latin if required.

DRINGHOE, a joint township with Upton and Brough, in the parish of SKIPSEA, northern division of the wapentake of HOLDERNESS, East riding of the county of YORK, 11 miles (E. by S.) from Great Driffield, containing 164 inhabitants.

DRINGHOUSES, a township partly in the parish of the HOLY TRINITY, MICKLEGATE, YORK, partly in the parish of ACOMB, ainsty of the city of YORK, but chiefly in the parish of ST. MARY BISHOPSHILL, SENIOR, liberty of St. PETER of YORK, East riding of the county of YORK, 1½ mile (S. W.) from York, containing 156 inhabitants.

DRINKSTONE, a parish in the hundred of THED-WESTRY, county of SUFFOLK, 6½ miles (W. N.W.) from Stow-Market, containing 456 inhabitants. The living is a rectory, in the archdeaconry of Sudbury, and diocese of Norwich, rated in the king's books at £16. 17. 1. J. Edgar Rust, Esq. was patron in 1824. The church is dedicated to All Saints. John Moseley, Esq., in 1804, bequeathed £700, which was vested in the funds, for the support of a day and Sunday school, the proceeds of which, in 1828, amounted to £114. 4. 7. There is also a bequest by Thomas Cranborne, in 1692, for supplying the poor with work, consisting of land producing £46 a year, which is now applied to apprenticing poor children.

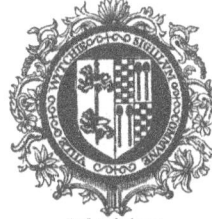

Seal and Arms.

DROITWICH, a borough and market town, having exclusive jurisdiction, though locally in the upper division of the hundred of Half-shire, county of WORCES-TER, 6¾ miles (N. E. by N.) from Worcester, and 118 (N.W.) from London, and containing 2176 inhabitants. This place was anciently denominated *Wich*, or *Wiche*, from the wiches, or salt springs, with which the neighbourhood abounds; and the prefix *Droit*, right or legal, is supposed to refer to some exclusive privilege for the manufacture of salt, obtained by the inhabitants. Droitwich appears to have been a town of the ancient Britons, called by Richard of Cirencester *Salinæ*, from its saline springs; having been situated on a British road, called the Saltway. There is no evidence of its having ever been occupied by the Romans; but under the Saxon government it rose to importance, and seems to have given name to their province of *Wiccia*, of which Worcestershire constituted the principal part. During the war between Charles I. and the parliament, the inhabitants adhered steadily to the royal cause, and subsequently received a letter from that unfortunate monarch, acknowledging a due sense of their loyalty. The town is situated on the river Salwarp, upon which there are several corn-mills. The manufacture of salt is probably coeval with the town itself; but it was not until the year 1725, that the strong brine, for which it is now famous, was discovered. Its purity is considered superior to that of any salt obtained elsewhere; and the quantity produced amounts to about seven hundred thousand bushels a year. Various acts of parliament have passed for the better regulation of this branch of manufacture. By charter of James I. the exclusive privilege of sinking brine pits within the borough was given to the corporation, who granted licenses to others; but this was overthrown about 1690, by a legal decision in favour of an enterprising individual, who, by a breach of this supposed right, successfully encountered the opposition of the party claiming it. Pits then became numerous, and the trade was thrown open to competition, to the great advantage of the community. At the distance of from thirty to forty feet from the surface of the ground is a hard bed of talc, or gypsum, generally about one hundred and fifty feet thick. A small hole is bored through this to the river of brine, which is in depth about twenty-two inches, and beneath which is a hard rock of salt. The water, which rises rapidly through this aper-ture, is pumped into a capacious reservoir, whence it is conveyed into iron boilers and heated. This produces evaporation, and the salt, which sinks to the bottom, is collected, dried, and made ready for the market. Previously to 1610, wood alone was used in boiling it; but owing to a scarcity in this article of fuel, coal was then adopted, and has since been continued. Of the brine obtained, one-fourth part is salt, whilst in that of North-wich, in Cheshire, the proportion of salt is only one-sixth. The want of conveyance by water for a long time operated as an impediment to the extension of the trade, but in 1655 a project was formed for making the Salwarp navigable, though not then undertaken. However, soon after the Restoration, the design was renewed, and operations commenced: but, when five out of the six locks which were considered necessary for the purpose were completed, the attempt was abandoned, from a conviction of its inefficacy. An act of parliament was then obtained, in 1767, for cutting a canal from this town to the Severn: it was consequently begun in 1768, and completed in 1771, under the direction of Brindley, the celebrated engineer, at an expense of £25,000. The canal is navigable for vessels of sixty tons' burden, and the junction takes place at Hawford. A building, called the Exchequer-house, where the payments from the persons who held licenses to make salt, and the other profits derived by the corporation from the brine pits, were made weekly, was erected about the year 1581, but it was taken down about the year 1826, and new court-rooms have been built near the spot on which it stood. At the same time an old market-house was taken down, and a new one formed under the court-rooms; also two good prisons. The malting trade is carried on to a limited extent. The market is on Friday; and fairs are held on the Thursday before the 20th of June, and the Wednesday before St. Thomas' day; during which a court of pie-powder is held.

The town was originally incorporated by a charter from John, conferring on the inhabitants various privileges, which have been confirmed and increased by succeeding monarchs. By the charter of the 22nd of James I., which refers to prior charters, the body corporate consists of two bailiffs, a recorder, two justices, a town clerk, burgesses, &c. The bailiffs, the recorder, and the bailiffs for the preceding year, are justices of the peace: the bailiffs are also clerks of the market, and coroners for the borough. A court of record is held every Thursday before the bailiffs and town-clerk, for the recovery of debts under £10. A court of session is held quarterly by the bailiffs, recorder, &c.; and a court leet twice a year before the town clerk. The bailiffs and burgesses have the power of enacting bye-laws, and in all cases exercise exclusive jurisdiction. The borough returned two burgesses to the parliaments of Edward I., and to those held in the 2nd and 4th of Edward II., from which period the privilege ceased until its renewal in 1554. The right of election, according to a decision of the house of commons in 1690, is vested in the burgesses of the corporation of the salt-springs: the number of voters is about forty, and the bailiffs are the returning officers. The heir apparent, or the adopted heir to a deceased burgess, is entitled to the freedom of the borough; and an heiress communicates the same privilege to her husband; but if a burgess die, leaving daughters, without having adopted either of them as the successor to his burgage tenure, his burgess-ship becomes extinct. The freedom may also be obtained by gift of the corporation at large. Each person made free must possess, at least, a quarter of a plat of inheritance. The parliamentary influence is possessed by Lord Foley, who nominates both members.

The borough comprises the greater part of the united parishes of St. Andrew and St. Mary de Witton, those of St. Peter de Witton and St. Nicholas, and a small portion of that of St. Augustine de Wich, or Dodderhill; all in the archdeaconry and diocese of Worcester. The parishes of St. Andrew and St. Mary were united by letters patent of Edward VI., dated 4th of June, in the second year of his reign, which union was confirmed by an act obtained in the 13th of Charles II. The living is a discharged rectory, rated in the king's books at £7. 12. 1., and in the patronage of the Crown. The church, which was rebuilt after having been destroyed by a casual fire in 1293, has some fine portions in the early English style, with additions of later date : the southern entrance, which still remains, appears to be Saxon. The living of St. Peter's is a discharged vicarage, rated in the king's books at £6, and in the patronage of Earl Somers. The church has a tower in the later English style, some fine decorated windows, and a small quantity of ancient stained glass. A chapel of ease to this church formerly stood on the bridge, but it was taken down and a new one built in 1763, on a different site. The living of St. Nicholas' is a rectory, rated in the king's books at £4. 9. 7., and in the patronage of the Crown. The church was greatly injured during the parliamentary war, and only about half of the tower remains. Here are places of worship for Independents and Wesleyan Methodists. The hospital of St. Mary, in the parish of St. Augustine, was founded for a master and brethren, by Walter de Dovere, in the reign of Edward I., under the patronage of the prior and convent at Worcester: part of the building still remains near Chapel bridge. The Coventry charity hospital, which is situated in St. Peter's parish, comprises nineteen tenements occupied by thirty-eight old men and women above sixty years of age : it was founded in consequence of a bequest from Henry Coventry, Esq., who, in 1686, left £1000, to erect a workhouse, or hospital, and £240 for its support. Here is a charity school for forty boys and forty girls, who are educated, clothed, and, on leaving school, apprenticed. Richard de Wich, Bishop of Chichester, was born here : he was a man of extensive erudition for those times, and was canonized by Urban IV., in 1262, nine years after his death. The inhabitants of the borough held his fame in great estimation, and were wont to celebrate an annual festival, with games, &c., in honour thereof. Serjeant Wilde, an eminent republican lawyer, who was made Lord Chief Baron of the Exchequer, under the Protectorship of Cromwell, was also a native of Droitwich.

DRONFIELD, a parish in the hundred of SCARSDALE, county of DERBY, 6 miles (N. W. by N.) from Chesterfield, comprising the chapelries of Dore and Holmesfield, the townships of Coal-Aston and Unstone, and the hamlet of Totley, and containing (exclusively of part of the township of Barlow which is in this parish) 3680 inhabitants. The living is a discharged

vicarage, in the archdeaconry of Derby, and diocese of Lichfield and Coventry, rated in the king's books at £10. 2. 1., endowed with £600 private benefaction, £200 royal bounty, and £600 parliamentary grant, and in the patronage of the Crown. The church, dedicated to St. John the Baptist, has a tower and spire at the west end, opposite to which there was once a chantry chapel, now converted into an inn. There are places of worship for the Society of Friends, Independents, and Wesleyan Methodists. Dronfield, in Domesday-book called Dranefield, had formerly the privilege of a market, but on account of its proximity to Chesterfield and Sheffield, it has been long discontinued. There is a fair for cattle and cheese on April 25th, and another fair on August 11th. Scythes, sickles, and edge-tools, are manufactured here; and there are manufactories for cast ware, various articles in cutlery, and saddlers' ironmongery, also for spindles for cotton works. A great quantity of coal is obtained in the neighbourhood. The grammar school was erected in 1579, by Thomas Fanshawe, Esq., in pursuance of the will of his father, dated in 1567, by which it is endowed with lands now producing an annual income of £200. Queen Elizabeth, by letters patent, empowered the above-named executor to make the necessary statutes for its government, and ordained that the vicar and churchwardens, or in default, six wise and honest men, to be chosen by his heirs, should be constituted a body corporate, by the name of "The governors of the grammar school of Henry Fanshawe, Esq." The master's salary is £130, the usher's £66, besides which they have each a dwelling-house ; one hundred and thirty children are educated upon this foundation. There are two other free schools in the parish, one at Dore, and another at Holmesfield. At Cawley is a sulphureous spring, with a bath annexed. About two miles from the town are the remains of Beauchief abbey, founded in 1183, for Premonstratensian, or White canons, by Robert Fitz-Ranulph, Lord of Alfreton, one of the executioners of Thomas à Becket, to whom it was dedicated; on its dissolution, in the 26th of Henry VIII., the revenue was valued at £157. 10. 2.

DROXFORD, a parish in that part of the hundred of BISHOP'S WALTHAM which is in the Portsdown division of the county of SOUTHAMPTON, 3¼ miles (E. by N.) from Bishop's Waltham, containing 1410 inhabitants. The living is a rectory, in the peculiar jurisdiction of the Incumbent, rated in the king's books at £17. 19. 4½., and in the patronage of the Bishop of Winchester. The church, dedicated to St. Mary and All Saints, is a curious specimen of early Norman architecture. The parish is within the jurisdiction of the Cheyney Court held at Winchester every Thursday, for the recovery of debts to any amount.

DROYLSDEN, a township in the parish of MANCHESTER, hundred of SALFORD, county palatine of LANCASTER, 4 miles (E.) from Manchester, containing 2855 inhabitants. The cotton manufacture is carried on here.

DRUMBURGH, a township in the parish of Bowness, ward and county of CUMBERLAND, 9¼ miles (W. by N.) from Carlisle, containing 418 inhabitants. Here was formerly a chapel, but it has been demolished. This was the station *Gabrosentum*, garrisoned by the *Cohors Secunda Thracum*; the ramparts are still very high, and the deep ditch encloses an area of about one hundred and ten yards square, which has been converted into a garden to Drumburgh castle, built out of the ruins of the fort, and with part of the remains of Adrian's wall, which terminated a little to the westward. Two draw-wells, cased with fine ashlar work, were discovered about 1780.

DRURIDGE, a hamlet in the parish of WOODHORN, eastern division of MORPETH ward, county of NORTHUMBERLAND, 9¼ miles (N.E. by N.) from Morpeth. The population is returned with the parish. It is situated on the shore of a bay of the same name in the North sea.

DRYBECK, a township in the parish of ST. LAWRENCE, APPLEBY, EAST ward, county of WESTMORLAND, 3 miles (S. S. W.) from Appleby, containing 100 inhabitants.

DRYPOOL, a parish in the middle division of the wapentake of HOLDERNESS, East riding of the county of YORK, comprising the townships of Drypool and Southcoates, and containing 2207 inhabitants, of which number, 1409 are in the township of Drypool, ½ a mile (E.) from Kingston upon Hull. The living is a perpetual curacy, in the archdeaconry of the East riding, and diocese, of York, endowed with £600 royal bounty, and £1000 parliamentary grant. W. Wilberforce, Esq. was patron in 1826. The church, dedicated to St. Peter, has been lately rebuilt in the style of the ancient structure, and has received an addition of eight hundred and fourteen sittings, of which five hundred and sixty-two are free, the Incorporated Society for the enlargement of churches and chapels having granted £500 toward defraying the expense. There is a place of worship for Wesleyan Methodists. The parish is bounded on the east by the river Hull, and the village is deemed a part of the town of Kingston upon Hull, being contiguous thereto. Near this place was situated the village of Frisneck, which was swallowed up by inundations of the Humber.

DUCKINGTON, a township in the parish of MALPAS, higher division of the hundred of BROXTON, county palatine of CHESTER, 3½ miles (N.) from Malpas, containing 81 inhabitants.

DUCKLINGTON, a parish in the hundred of BAMPTON, county of OXFORD, 1¾ mile (S.) from Witney, containing, with the hamlet of Hardwicke, 497 inhabitants. The living is a rectory, in the archdeaconry and diocese of Oxford, rated in the king's books at £24.10.5., and in the patronage of the President and Fellows of Magdalene College, Oxford. The church is dedicated to St. Bartholomew.

DUCKMANTON, a parish in the hundred of SCARSDALE, county of DERBY, 3¾ miles (E.) from Chesterfield, containing, with Sutton, 685 inhabitants. The living is a discharged vicarage annexed to the rectory of Sutton in the Dale, in the archdeaconry of Derby, and diocese of Lichfield and Coventry. The church, which was dedicated to St. Peter and St. Paul, has been demolished. There is a place of worship for Independents. A charity school is endowed with £20 per annum, for teaching twenty children. Iron-ore and coal are obtained at works called the Adelphi.

DUDCOTE, a parish in the hundred of MORETON, county of BERKS, 6 miles (W. by N.) from Wallingford, containing 197 inhabitants. The living is a rectory, in the archdeaconry of Berks, and diocese of Salisbury,

rated in the king's books at £20. 12. 6., and in the patronage of the Principal and Fellows of Brasenose College, Oxford. The church is dedicated to All Saints.

DUDDEN, a township in that part of the parish of TARVIN which is in the second division of the hundred of EDDISBURY, county palatine of CHESTER, 3 miles (N. W. by W.) from Tarporley, containing 243 inhabitants.

DUDDINGTON, a parish in the hundred of WILLYBROOK, county of NORTHAMPTON, 6 miles (W. by N.) from Wandsford, containing 352 inhabitants. The living is a perpetual curacy annexed to the vicarage of Gretton, in the peculiar jurisdiction and patronage of the Prebendary of Gretton in the Cathedral Church of Lincoln. The church is dedicated to St. Mary. There is a place of worship for Independents. Here is a free school for twelve poor children, endowed with £10 per annum under the will of Mr. Jackson.

DUDDO, a township in the parish of NORHAM, otherwise Norhamshire, county palatine of DURHAM, though situated to the northward of the county of Northumberland, 13 miles (N.N.W.) from Wooler, containing 285 inhabitants. On the summit of Grindon Rigg are the remains of Duddo tower, and near it six rude stones, set up in commemoration of the victory gained by the English over the Scots, in 1558.

DUDDO, a township in the northern division of the parish of STANNINGTON, western division of CASTLE ward, county of NORTHUMBERLAND, 4¾ miles (S.S.W.) from Morpeth. The population is returned with the parish.

DUDLEY, a market town and parish, in the lower division of the hundred of HALFSHIRE, county of WORCESTER, though locally in the southern division of the hundred of Offlow, county of Stafford, 26 miles (N. N. E.) from Worcester, and 127 (N. W. by N.) from London, containing 18,211 inhabitants. This place derives its name from Dodo, or Dudo, a Saxon prince, to whom it belonged at the time of the Heptarchy, and who built a castle here about the year 700, which was afterwards, during the contest between Stephen and the Empress Matilda, garrisoned for the latter, by Gervase Paganell, to whom the barony at that time belonged. Gervase having subsequently taken part in the rebellion of Prince Henry against his father, Henry II., his castle was demolished in the 20th year of that monarch's reign. Roger de Somery having obtained possession of the barony, began to convert his mansion into a castle, and for his firm adherence to Henry III., in his wars with the barons, was permitted by his sovereign to complete the fortifications. In the early part of the parliamentary war the castle was garrisoned by the royalists, and in 1644 defended by Colonel Beaumont with great bravery against the parliamentarians, who were compelled to raise the siege by the arrival of a detachment from Worcester; it does not appear to have been repaired after the damage it sustained during the siege, and an accidental fire, which occurred in 1750, is said to have completed its demolition. The castle was built on an extensive and elevated limestone rock, the summit and acclivities of which are richly wooded; the remains, which are extensive and highly interesting, consist of the gateway-tower leading into the outer court, the keep, of ponderous strength, situated on a lofty mount of artificial elevation, part of the postern tower, the walls and windows of the state apartments, the kitchens, and other offices: the site is extra-parochial. The prevailing character is that of the early decorated style of English architecture, of which there are several fine portions remaining, intermixed with others of the later English style. The grounds are very extensive, and have been beautifully laid out in shrubberies and walks, affording a succession of different views of this highly picturesque ruin. About half a mile from the town was a monastery of Cluniac monks, founded about the year 1161, by Gervase Paganell, and dedicated to St. James, as a cell to the abbey at Wenlock, the revenue of which, at the dissolution, was £36. 3.: there are still considerable remains, forming an interesting feature in the view from the castle hill; and near them, the Earl of Dudley has erected within the last few years a handsome building, which, from its proximity to the ruins, is called the priory, in the later style of English architecture, as a residence for his mining agent.

The town is pleasantly situated in a tract of country, the surface of which is finely varied, though in several places disfigured by mining operations, which are extensively prosecuted in the vicinity; the principal street is spacious, and the whole town is well paved, and lighted with gas; the houses are in general neat and well built, and many of them are large and elegant; the inhabitants are supplied with water from wells of considerable depth; and the environs, besides the castle hill, which is a favourite place of resort, abound with pleasant walks and rides. A public subscription library, established in 1805, contains an extensive collection of books: assemblies are held occasionally at the hotel. The trade arises chiefly from the geological character of the neighbourhood, which is remarkable for the variety and extent of its mines of coal and iron-stone, lying on each side of a line of basaltic rock and limestone. Among the beds of coal is one vein of excellent quality and extraordinary thickness, called the "Ten-Yard coal," which is supposed to be now nearly exhausted: other strata, but much thinner, have been found at a greater depth from the surface within the last twenty years, and many other mines have been discovered in the neighbourhood, which supply the great consumption of the surrounding iron-works and manufacturing places: the produce, by means of the canals, is also conveyed to several of the inland counties. The iron manufacture is carried on to a very considerable extent; a large quantity of ore is smelted in the neighbourhood, and the metal is not only formed into pigs, bars, sheets, and rods, but in extensive foundries cast into every kind of article for use or ornament, and manufactured into implements of agriculture, and tools of every description: the vicinity, for a circuit of several miles, abounds with nail-manufacturers. The limestone is used for various purposes: exclusively of what is consumed in the iron-works, a considerable quantity is burnt for agricultural uses, and some is manufactured into chimney-pieces, which are much admired for the beauty and variety of the fossils with which the stone abounds. The basalt is chiefly obtained in the adjoining parish of Rowley, and is well adapted to the purpose of making and repairing roads, being little, if at all, inferior to granite. The manufacture of flint-glass is carried on extensively, and there are several cutting-mills. Here is a brewery; and the business done

in malting is very considerable. A tunnel, one mile and three quarters in length, thirteen feet high, and nine feet wide, has been cut through the rock on which the castle is built, for the conveyance of the limestone from the caverns under the castle hill, in which it is procured, to the kilns; it is in some places more than twenty yards below the surface, and forms a communication with the Birmingham and Stourbridge canals. The market is on Saturday: the fairs are on May 8th, for cattle, cheese, and wool; August 5th, for lambs; and October 2nd, for horses, cattle, cheese, and wool.

The town, though formerly a borough, having returned two members to parliament in the 23d of Edward I., is within the jurisdiction of the county magistrates; a mayor, bailiff, and other officers are appointed annually at the court leet of the lord of the manor, but exercise no magisterial authority. An application is at present being made for the renewal of certain privileges, under an ancient charter which is said to have been granted to the town. Dudley formerly comprised the parishes of St. Thomas and St. Edmund, now united, the church of the former being parochial, and that of the latter used as a chapel of ease. The living is a vicarage, in the archdeaconry and diocese of Worcester, rated in the king's books £7. 18. 6½., and in the patronage of the Earl of Dudley. The church of St. Thomas was rebuilt in 1819, at an expense of £23,000, of which sum, £7600, including £2000 contributed by the Earl of Dudley, was raised by subscription, and the remainder by a rate; it is a handsome structure in the later style of English architecture, with an elegant and lofty spire, and is not only an ornament to the town, but from its elevated situation forms a fine feature in the landscape. The church of St. Edmund having been demolished during the parliamentary war, was afterwards rebuilt, chiefly at the expense of two brothers of the name of Bradley, assisted by a subscription among the parishioners, about the commencement of the last century. At Netherton another large chapel of ease, dedicated to St. Andrew, has recently been erected, by grant from the parliamentary commissioners, the site having been given by the Earl of Dudley. There are three places of worship for the Primitive, one for the Kilhamites, and two for the Wesleyan, Methodists, and one each for Baptists, the Society of Friends, Independents, and Unitarians. The free grammar school was founded in 1562, by Thomas Wattewood, clothier, of Stafford, and Mark Bysmor, of London, still-worker, and endowed by letters patent of Queen Elizabeth, with land, the present annual rental of which is from £300 to £400: out of this the master receives a salary of about £200: the average number of scholars is from thirty to forty, who are admitted by the master as soon as they can read, and may remain until fit for the University. Besides the classics, they are taught mathematics, history, geography, French, Italian, &c., the course of study being varied according to circumstances. Under the superintendence of the present master, the school has much improved. A charity school, for clothing and educating forty girls, and another charity, for clothing seven poor men, were established on the 3rd, and enrolled in Chancery on the 19th, of June, 1819, by Mrs. Cartwright, in consequence of a legacy bequeathed for that purpose by the Rev. Henry Antrobus, formerly minister of St. Edmund's, who died about forty years ago : the girls are taught to read, knit, and sew, and are brought up in the principles of the established church. A school, for clothing and instructing fifty boys was founded in 1732, and endowed with land, by Messrs Robert and Samuel, and Mrs. Ann, Baylis : the school-room has been recently rebuilt, and, exclusively of those on the foundation, about two hundred other boys are now educated, the funds having much increased, from the improvement of the land, &c. : the school is now under the care of the Unitarians. The Blue-coat school was founded in 1708, in which there are now about two hundred and thirty boys ; part of the funds is applied to the support of an infant school recently established. A school of industry has been established, in which two hundred and twenty girls are educated and taught to work. The Unitarians also support a similar school for girls, the number at present being about eighty. In Lady-wood is a valuable spring, called the Spa Well, in high estimation for its efficacy in cutaneous disorders, and complaints arising from indigestion. There are also several chalybeate springs. In the lime quarries a fossil, called the Dudley locust, is found in great numbers and variety of size, and supposed to be a petrifaction of an extinct species of the monoculus. About a quarter of a mile from the town is a tract of country, comprising about twenty acres, vulgarly called the Fiery Holes, from which smoke continually issues, and sometimes flame ; veins of coal underneath are supposed to have been set on fire by some accident, and to have continued burning ever since. Richard Baxter, the celebrated non-conformist divine in the reign of Charles II., was for some time master of one of the schools in this parish. Dudley confers the title of earl on the family of Ward.

DUDLESTON, a chapelry in the parish of ELLESMERE, hundred of PIMHILL, county of SALOP, 4¾ miles (N.W. by W.) from Ellesmere, with which the population is returned. The living is a perpetual curacy, in the archdeaconry of Salop, and diocese of Lichfield and Coventry, endowed with £510 private benefaction, and £400 royal bounty, and in the patronage of the Vicar of Ellesmere. The chapel, dedicated to St. Mary, has lately received an addition of one hundred and eighty free sittings, the Incorporated Society for the enlargement of churches and chapels having granted £200 toward defraying the expense. There is a trifling endowment for the education of children.

DUESHILL, a township in the parochial chapelry of HALLYSTONE, hundred of COQUETDALE ward, county of NORTHUMBERLAND, 7½ miles (W.) from Rothbury, containing 41 inhabitants. At Harehaugh is the site of a strong triple intrenchment, thrown up by the Saxons.

DUFFIELD, a parish in the hundred of APPLETREE, county of DERBY, 4¼ miles (N.) from Derby, comprising the chapelries of Belper, Heage, Holbrook, and Turnditch, and the townships of Hazlewood, Shottle with Postern, and Windley, and containing 13,896 inhabitants. The living is a discharged vicarage, in the archdeaconry of Derby, and diocese of Lichfield and Coventry, rated in the king's books at £8. 4., endowed with £400 private benefaction, £400 royal bounty, and £300 parliamentary grant, and in the patronage of the Bishop of Lichfield and Coventry. The church is dedicated to St. Alkmund. There are places of worship

for General Baptists, Wesleyan Methodists, and Unitarians. In Domesday-book it is called *Dunelle*, and is described as having " a church, a priest, and two mills ;" it afterwards formed part of the demesne of Henry de Ferrars, who, in 1096, possessed a castle on an eminence north-west of the village, the site of which is now called Castle-Orchard. This fortress was held by several of the turbulent descendants of that powerful baron, of whom William, for rebellion in the reign of Henry II., lost his estates by confiscation, but, in 1199, they were restored by King John to his son William, with the title of Earl of Derby. Earl Robert joined in Simon de Montford's rebellion, and garrisoned his castle of Duffield against Henry III., but was defeated and taken prisoner at Chesterfield, by Henry de Almaine, upon which the king sent his son, afterwards Edward I., into the county of Derby, to ravage with fire and sword the lands of the earl, and take revenge for his disloyalty, and under that order the castle was dismantled, and the demesne fell to the crown. In 1330, Henry, Earl of Lancaster, claimed seven parks in Duffield Frith, and, in the reign of Elizabeth, frequent mention is made of the extent and importance of the royal possessions at Duffield, the appointments of stewards, rangers, and various other officers, and of great leets, and three weeks' courts held there, it being then a portion of the duchy of Lancaster, and so it continued till the reign of Charles I., when it was granted to several persons. The village, pleasantly situated on a fine plain, through which flows the river Derwent, contains many good houses, and is very respectable. There are cattle fairs on the Thursday following New Year's day, and on March 1st. William Gilbert, in the 7th of Elizabeth, surrendered a cottage and lands for the maintenance of a school, towards which Joseph Webster, in 1685, bequeathed an annuity of £10 ; the annual income of the schoolmaster is £124. 9. 10., with a house and garden : twenty-four children are educated upon this foundation. An almshouse was built by Mr. Anthony Bradshaw, who died in 1614 ; it is endowed with a rent-charge upon an estate at Holbrook, and with £100, the gift of William Potterell, in 1735 ; the inmates are two old men and two old women, who have each two apartments, with allowances of 1s. per week, and 5s. a year for fuel. There were formerly other almshouses, erected in 1676, but they were taken down in 1810.

DUFFIELD (NORTH), a township in the parish of SKIPWITH, wapentake of OUZE and DERWENT, East riding of the county of YORK, 5½ miles (N.E.) from Selby, containing 433 inhabitants.

DUFFIELD (SOUTH), a township in the parish of HEMINGBROUGH, wapentake of OUZE and DERWENT, East riding of the county of YORK, 5 miles (E.N.E.) from Selby, containing 181 inhabitants. There is a place of worship for Wesleyan Methodists.

DUFFRIN, a hamlet in that part of the parish of BASSALEG which is in the upper division of the hundred of WENTLLOOG, county of MONMOUTH, containing 228 inhabitants.

DUFTON, a parish in EAST ward, county of WESTMORLAND, 3¼ miles (N.) from Appleby, containing 151 inhabitants. The living is a discharged rectory, in the archdeaconry and diocese of Carlisle, rated in the king's books at £19. 2. 6., and in the patronage of the Earl of Thanet. The church, dedicated to St. Cuthbert, was rebuilt about 1775; it is a plain structure, situated half a mile north of the village. A place of worship for Wesleyan Methodists was erected in 1820. There are considerable lead mines in the parish, worked by the London Lead Company, producing about one hundred and forty-four stone of pig lead per week: the ore is smelted at a mill about a mile from the village. The free school, founded in 1670 by Christopher Walker, was rebuilt by subscription in 1824, and is principally supported by a yearly rent-charge, the bequest of Michael Todd, in 1692. Dufton-pike, Knock-pike, and Merton-pike, each about one thousand feet in height, uniform, and of easy ascent, are supposed to be artificial mounds raised over the relics of ancient British heroes of rank, or for some religious purpose.

DUGGLEBY, a township in the parish of KIRBY-GRINDALYTH, wapentake of BUCKROSE, East riding of the county of YORK, 6¾ miles (E. S. E.) from New Malton, containing 154 inhabitants.

DUKESHAGG, a township in the parish of OVINGHAM, eastern division of TINDALE ward, county of NORTHUMBERLAND, 13 miles (W. S.W.) from Newcastle upon Tyne, containing 9 inhabitants. This township, called also Ducashagg, and Dukershagg, consists of only a farm-house and farm.

DUKINFIELD, a chapelry in the parish of STOCKPORT, hundred of MACCLESFIELD, county palatine of CHESTER, 6½ miles (N. E. by N.) from Stockport, containing 5096 inhabitants. The village, called by the Saxons Dockenveldt, is seated upon a pleasant eminence, at the foot of which, to the northward, runs the rapid river Tame, separating the township from the town of Ashton under Lyne, in Lancashire, as it did the kingdoms of Northumberland and Mercia during the Heptarchy, when strong fortifications for the protection of each at this point were constructed, on opposite banks of the stream, some vestiges of which are still discernible. Thirty years ago the inhabitants of Dukinfield consisted of only a few farmers and day-labourers, but since the introduction of the cotton trade it has become an extensive and flourishing place; there are several cotton factories, worked by eleven steam-engines, equal in power to two hundred and fifty-five horses, which put in motion one thousand four hundred and seventy-five power-looms, and turn one hundred and thirteen thousand one hundred and fifty-four spindles. The mines and quarries wrought in the township yield a considerable profit to the proprietors: there are also extensive collieries, the shafts of some of them being sunk to the depth of one hundred and twenty feet. Iron-ore is abundant, and a furnace has been recently erected for smelting it, an operation that seems to have been carried on in remote times, from the otherwise unaccountable breaks which are frequently met with in the strata of the ore of one particular mine, and the large quantity of scoriæ found in the vicinity. Fire-bricks are made here in great perfection. Many advantages are derived from the Peak Forest and the Huddersfield canals, which pass through the township. One of the wings of Dukinfield hall, an ancient mansion, contains a chapel, founded in 1398, as an oratory, which has been since used as a chapel of ease to Stockport. Independents, Wesleyan Methodists, Moravians, and Unitarians, have each a place of worship, and the three last have established schools; that of the Methodists being sufficiently commodious to contain one thousand children; there is also a Roman Catholic chapel. A Sunday school, for children of all denominations, is kept in a neat brick building, erected by subscription, upon land given by the late F. D. Astley, Esq., and containing a well selected library for the use of the inhabitants. Lieutenant-Colonel Robert Duckenfield, a distinguished parliamentary officer, and a member of Cromwell's council of state in 1653, was born here.

DULAS, a parish in the hundred of WEBTREE, county of HEREFORD, 13½ miles (S.W. by W.) from Hereford, containing 60 inhabitants. The living is a perpetual curacy, in the archdeaconry of Brecon, and diocese of St. David, endowed with £200 private benefaction, £600 royal bounty, and £200 parliamentary grant, and in the patronage of the Bishop of Gloucester. The church is dedicated to St. Michael.

DULLINGHAM, a parish in the hundred of RADFIELD, county of CAMBRIDGE, 3¾ miles (S. by W.) from Newmarket, containing 625 inhabitants. The living is a discharged vicarage, in the archdeaconry and diocese of Ely, rated in the king's books at £12. 15. 5. Mrs. Pigott was patroness in 1828. The church is dedicated to St. Mary. There is a school with an endowment of about £4 per annum, the gift of Borradill Millicent, in 1678.

DULOE, a parish in WEST hundred, county of CORNWALL, 3¾ miles (N. N. W.) from West Looe, containing 779 inhabitants. The living is a vicarage and a rectory consolidated, in the archdeaconry of Cornwall, and diocese of Exeter, rated together in the king's books at £30. 15. 2½., and in the patronage of the Master and Fellows of Balliol College, Oxford. The church, dedicated to St. Cuby, contains an altar-tomb with sculptured ornaments, upon which is a recumbent figure of an armed knight, with an inscription in memory of Sir John Colshull, who died in 1483. The Looe navigation bounds the parish on the east. A silver and lead mine was opened several years ago, but being unprofitable it was soon afterwards neglected.

DULVERTON, a market town and parish in the hundred of WILLITON and FREEMANNERS, county of SOMERSET, 13 miles (W.) from Wiveliscombe, and 163 (W. by S.) from London, containing 1127 inhabitants. This place probably derives its name from being situated in a deep valley, and upon a ford on the river Barle, which rises in Exmoor Forest, and, after flowing through the town under a stone bridge of five arches, falls into the river Ex, near Brushford. Dulverton, probably from the remoteness of its situation from any of the great public thoroughfares, is but little connected with events of historical importance, of which the only circumstance upon record is the execution in the market-place of several individuals who were concerned in the rebellion of 1745. The town consists principally of two streets, the houses are in general well built, and the inhabitants amply supplied with water. There is a great number of forest deer in the vicinity, which are preserved in the adjoining woods. A silk-manufactory has recently been established, in which several children are employed. The market (originally granted by Philip and Mary to twelve trustees, who were to apply the profits to the improvement of the town, and to the benefit of the poor not receiving parochial aid,) is on Friday, and is well supplied with corn and the produce of the dairy: the fairs are, July 10th and November 8th.

Courts leet and baron are held annually, at the former of which, two constables, two tythingmen, two ale-tasters, two surveyors of weights and measures, and other officers, are chosen and sworn into office before the steward of the manor. The living is a vicarage, in the archdeaconry of Taunton, and diocese of Bath and Wells, rated in the king's books at £21. 10. 10., and in the patronage of the Dean and Chapter of Wells The church, dedicated to All Saints, is a neat edifice in the ancient style of English architecture, with a square embattled tower. A charity school was founded in 1736, by Mrs. Elizabeth Dyke, of Pixton, who endowed it for thirty poor children of the parish, with a tenement producing £12 per annum; the endowment was subsequently increased with a legacy of £150 bequeathed by Humphrey Sydenham, Esq. in 1764; with £40 left by Mrs. Penelope Sydenham; and, in 1769, with a legacy of £100 by the Rev. Lawrence Jackson; producing in the whole about £30 per annum, by means of which, and partly by subscription, the school is now conducted upon the National system. About a mile and a half west-north-west of the town is Bury castle, an ancient en-campment. In the neighbourhood is a mineral spring, the water of which is impregnated with iron, but it is not now used medicinally: there is also a spring, called Holy well, to which, on Holy Thursday, it is still the custom to carry persons afflicted with disease.

DULWICH, a hamlet in the parish of CAMBER-WELL, eastern division of the hundred of BRIXTON, county of SURREY, 4½ miles (S.) from London. The population is returned with the parish. The village is pleasantly situated in a small vale, sheltered by rising grounds in the immediate vicinity, and by the Surrey hills in the distance: the houses are irregularly built, but of handsome and respectable appearance: the en-virons abound with elegant villas, which, from their proximity to the metropolis, have become the residence of many opulent families. The village is lighted by subscription among the inhabitants, and is within the limits of the new police establishment under Mr. Peel's act. A fair for toys is held on the Monday after Trinity Monday: a court leet is held annually. At the east-ern extremity is God's Gift College, founded in 1619, by Edward Alleyn, Esq., who endowed it with the ma-nor of Dulwich, and tenements in the parishes of St. Botolph, Bishopsgate, in London, and St. Luke's, in the county of Middlesex, producing at present an annual re-venue of £14,000, for a master (who must bear the same name as the founder), warden, four fellows, six poor brethren, six poor sisters, twelve poor scholars, six assistants, and thirty non-resident members, to be chosen from the parishes of St. Botolph, St. Saviour (Southwark), St. Luke, and St. Giles, Camberwell. Of the four fellows, three must be in holy orders, and graduates of Oxford or Cambridge, and the fourth well skilled in music; the two senior fellows are to officiate in the chapel of the college, the third to be master of the grammar school, and the fourth, who officiates as organist and choir-master, to be the usher. In addition to the twelve scholars on the foundation, the sons of inhabitants of Dulwich are entitled to gratuitous instruction, and strangers are admitted on payment of such sum to the master and usher as shall be appointed by the mas-ter and the warden of the college; according to whose discretion, certain sums may be allowed as exhibitions

to either of the Universities. Scholars sent from this school, and taking the degree of Master of Arts, receive a farther sum, and obtain a preference in election to any of the offices in the college. The poor brethren and sisters have apartments in the college, with every thing requisite supplied them, and a very considerable pecu-niary allowance. The buildings, chiefly in the Elizabethan style, occupy three sides of a quadrangle, of which the chapel constitutes one: the east wing was handsome-ly rebuilt of red brick ornamented with stone, in 1740, and contains the school-room and apartments for the fellows; the opposite wing comprises the library and apartments for the scholars. The chapel has been en-larged by the addition of an aisle and a gallery, for the accommodation of the inhabitants; divine service is performed regularly in the morning and afternoon: the altar-piece is ornamented with a fine painting of the Ascension, presented to the college by Mr. Hall; and in front of the chancel is a black marble slab, covering the tomb of the founder, who was buried in the chapel. An extensive collection of pictures was bequeathed to the college by Sir Francis Bourgeois, in 1811, for the recep-tion of which a handsome gallery has been erected at the south end of the college: the building, which is well calculated to display the pictures, is divided into five rooms, in each of which are many specimens of the first masters, of the Italian, Flemish, and English schools. The collection is open to the public under certain re-gulations, and attracts numerous visitors, particularly during the summer months. A free school was founded in 1741, by James Alleyn, Esq., Master of God's Gift College, who endowed it with lands and messuages in the parish of Kennington, now producing a rental of more than £200 per annum, for the instruction of poor chil-dren of both sexes, of the hamlet of Dulwich, or within a mile of it; there are sixty boys and sixty girls in the school, of which number twelve boys and twenty girls are clothed by subscription. The school-house, a hand-some building facing the college, containing two distinct school-rooms, and residences for the master and mis-tress, was given for that purpose by the master and warden of the college. There are several medicinal springs in the immediate neighbourhood, the water of which is similar in its properties to that of Sydenham.

DUMBLETON, a parish in the lower division of the hundred of KIFTSGATE, county of GLOUCESTER, 6 miles (N. by W.) from Winchcombe, containing 374 in-habitants. The living is a rectory, in the archdeaconry and diocese of Gloucester, rated in the king's books at £18. 16. 8. The church, dedicated to St. Peter, has an embattled tower at the west end. A rivulet, called the Isborn, runs through the parish; and on the side of a hill a mineral spring rises. Dorothy Cocks, in 1754, bequeathed £2 per annum for teaching children to read; and Richard Cocks, in 1728, gave an estate at Tainton, worth £21 per annum, part for apprenticing a boy, and the remainder to the poor not receiving alms.

DUMMER, a parish in the hundred of BERMOND-SPIT, Basingstoke division of the county of SOUTHAMPTON, 5 miles (S.W.) from Basingstoke, containing 393 inha-bitants. The living is a rectory, in the archdeaconry and diocese of Winchester, rated in the king's books at £14. 12. 3½. Thomas Terry, Esq. was patron in 1826. The church, dedicated to All Saints, has a tower of wood. John Millingate, in 1610, gave a house and a rent-charge of £4 a year, for teaching six poor children ; subsequent bequests have increased the income to £15. 5. which is paid to a schoolmaster for the free education of twenty boys.

DUMMER-ANDREWS-SWATHLING, an extra-parochial liberty, in the hundred of MANSBRIDGE, Fawley division of the county of SOUTHAMPTON, 3 miles (N. N. E.) from Southampton. The population is returned with the parish of South Stoneham.

DUNCHIDEOCK, a parish in the hundred of EXMINSTER, county of DEVON, 4½ miles (S.W. by W.) from Exeter, containing 200 inhabitants. The living is a rectory, in the archdeaconry and diocese of Exeter, rated in the king's books at £14. 17. 1. Sir L. V. Palk, Bart. was patron in 1793. The church, dedicated to the Holy Trinity, contains a handsome monument to the memory of General L. Lawrence, Commander-in-chief in India about the middle of the last century. Here is a house for the poor to live in, capable of receiving eighty persons.

DUNCHURCH, a parish in the Rugby division of the hundred of KNIGHTLOW, county of WARWICK, 15 miles (E.N.E.) from Warwick, containing, with the hamlets of Toft and Thurlaston, 1251 inhabitants. The living is a vicarage, in the archdeaconry of Coventry, and diocese of Lichfield and Coventry, rated in the king's books at £14. 1. 10½., and in the patronage of the Bishop of Lichfield and Coventry. The church, dedicated to St. Peter, is a handsome and curious edifice, with a square embattled tower ; the western porch has a fine Norman arch, ornamented with heads and zigzag mouldings ; the chancel is of early English architecture, with some windows in the decorated style ; the nave is also decorated, and the door-ways of the aisles are ornamented with remarkably rich mouldings : the tower is in the later English style, much enriched, but mutilated. Here is a free grammar school, founded in 1707, and endowed by a bequest from Francis Boughton, of twenty-seven acres of land and a house for the master, who must be a clergyman : the same benefactor left twenty-four acres of land, directing the produce to be applied in apprenticing poor boys : both charities are vested in eight trustees. In 1695, Thomas Newcombe, printer to the kings Charles II., James II., and William III., bequeathed property for erecting and endowing six almshouses, for three poor men and three poor widows, which were rebuilt in 1818. The village of Dunchurch, being a thoroughfare on the great north road, contains some good inns, and several respectable houses, presenting the appearance of a small market town ; at its northern extremity is an obelisk, where stood an ancient cross. A court of requests is held here every three weeks.

DUNCTON, a parish in the hundred of ROTHERBRIDGE, rape of ARUNDEL, county of SUSSEX, 3½ miles (S. by W.) from Petworth, containing 246 inhabitants. The living is a rectory not in charge, in the archdeaconry and diocese of Chichester. The Earl of Egremont was patron in 1815. Duncton once formed part of the parish of Petworth.

DUNDRAW, a township in that part of the parish of BROOMFIELD which is in CUMBERLAND ward, county of CUMBERLAND, 3 miles (W.N.W.) from Wigton, containing 316 inhabitants. This township lies within a curvature of the river Waver.

DUNDRY, a parish in the hundred of CHEW, county

of SOMERSET, 5½ miles (N. W. by W.) from Pensford, containing 454 inhabitants. The living is a perpetual curacy, annexed to the vicarage of Chew Magna, in the archdeaconry of Bath, and diocese of Bath and Wells. The church, dedicated to St. Michael, stands on a lofty hill, and has at the west end a fine embattled tower, ornamented with clustered pinnacles. On the same hill is a rude building, supposed to have been intended for a beacon. There is a trifling endowment, the gift of Benjamin Symes, in 1778, for teaching two poor boys ; and another, the bequest of Joseph Hellier, for seven girls. A fair for cattle and sheep is held on the 12th of September.

DUNHAM, a township in the parish of THORNTON, second division of the hundred of EDDISBURY, county palatine of CHESTER, 5 miles (S. W.) from Frodsham, containing 306 inhabitants. The Duke of Bridgewater's canal passes near this place. There is a trifling bequest for the education of children.

DUNHAM, a parish in the South-clay division of the wapentake of BASSETLAW, county of NOTTINGHAM, 5¾ miles (N. E. by E.) from Tuxford, containing, with the chapelry of Ragnall, 415 inhabitants. The living is a discharged vicarage, rated in the king's books at £4. 13. 4., and in the peculiar jurisdiction and patronage of the Prebendary of Dunham in the Collegiate Church of Southwell. The church is dedicated to St. Oswald. There is a chapel of ease at Darlton, in this parish. Dunham once enjoyed the privilege of a market, which is now disused ; but there is a fair for cattle and merchandise on the 12th of August. The river Trent runs through the parish, and frequently inundates the village, sometimes to the depth of ten feet, causing considerable damage to the buildings ; the inhabitants on such occasions communicate with each other and carry on their traffic through the streets by means of boats, almost every house having one attached to it for the purpose.

DUNHAM (GREAT), a parish in the hundred of LAUNDITCH, county of NORFOLK, 5¼ miles (N.E.) from Swaffham, containing 468 inhabitants. The living comprises the consolidated discharged rectories of St. Andrew and St. Mary, in the archdeaconry and diocese of Norwich, rated in the king's books at £12. 1. 10½. John Peele, Esq. and another were patrons in 1788.

DUNHAM (LITTLE), a parish in the hundred of LAUNDITCH, county of NORFOLK, 4 miles (N.E. by E.) from Swaffham, containing 307 inhabitants. The living is a discharged rectory, in the archdeaconry and diocese of Norwich, rated in the king's books at £9. 16. E. Parry, Esq. was patron in 1792. The church is dedicated to St. Margaret. Here is a free school.

DUNHAM-MASSEY, a township in the parish of BOWDON, hundred of BUCKLOW, county palatine of CHESTER, 3½ miles (W. by S.) from Altrincham, containing 1090 inhabitants. Here is a free school. The village of Donehame is mentioned in Domesday-book, and the Norman barons of Dunham had a castle here, which was defended by its owner, Hamo de Massey, in a rebellion against Henry II., in 1173, but not a relic of it now remains, nor can its site be ascertained. A court of pleas formerly held here, for the recovery of debts under £10, is now in disuse. A school is supported by the produce of various small donations. The Duke of Bridgewater's canal passes near this place ;

and in the neighbouring park are vestiges of an old military road, and several tumuli, near which urns have been found. The Earl of Stamford and Warrington has the title of Baron Delamere, of Dunham-Massey.

DUNHOLM, a parish in the wapentake of LAWRESS, parts of LINDSEY, county of LINCOLN, 6 miles (N.N.E.) from Lincoln, containing 220 inhabitants. The living is a discharged vicarage, in the peculiar jurisdiction of the Dean and Chapter of Lincoln, rated in the king's books at £4. 6. 8., endowed with £200 royal bounty, and in the patronage of the Bishop of Lincoln. The church is dedicated to St. Chad. A bead court is held twice a year, when ten shillings and a coat each are given to six poor men.

DUNKERTON, a parish in the hundred of WELLOW, county of SOMERSET, 5 miles (S. W. by S.) from Bath, containing 365 inhabitants. The living is a rectory, in the archdeaconry of Wells, and diocese of Bath and Wells, rated in the king's books at £10. 4. 7., and in the patronage of Sir George Bampfylde, Bart. The church is dedicated to All Saints. The old fosse road, the Radford canal, and the Kennet and Avon canal, pass through the parish.

DUNKESWELL, a parish in the hundred of HEMYOCK, county of DEVON, 5½ miles (N. by W.) from Honiton, containing 441 inhabitants. The living is a donative, endowed with £400 private benefaction, and £400 royal bounty, and in the patronage of Miss Graves. The church is dedicated to St. Nicholas. Dunkeswell, which anciently belonged to a Jew named Amadio, was purchased by William Briwere, who founded, in 1201, an abbey for White monks, to the honour of the Virgin Mary; the annual revenue of which, at the dissolution, was estimated at £298. 11. 10.

DUNKESWITH, a township in that part of the parish of HAREWOOD which is in the upper division of the wapentake of CLARO, West riding of the county of YORK, 6½ miles (W. by S.) from Wetherby, containing 257 inhabitants. It is in the Forest division of the honour of Knaresborough, and within the jurisdiction of the peculiar court thereof.

DUNKIRK-VILLE, an extra-parochial liberty, in the hundred of WESTGATE, lathe of ST. AUGUSTINE, county of KENT, 5 miles (W. by N.) from Canterbury, containing 543 inhabitants. This was anciently the royal forest of Bleane; it consists of a large tract, containing about five thousand acres, mostly covered with coppices, interspersed with farm-houses and cottages.

DUNMOW (GREAT), a parish (formerly a market town) in the hundred of DUNMOW, county of ESSEX, 12½ miles (N. N.W.) from Chelmsford, and 37½ (N.E. by N.) from London, containing 2409 inhabitants. It is supposed by Bishop Gibson to have been the site of the Roman station *Cæsaromagus*, and this conjecture has been adopted by some other antiquaries : Roman coins have been discovered at several places near the town, and the road leading from it to Colchester, which was probably *Camalodunum*, displays some indications of Roman construction. At the time of the Norman survey it was the principal place in the hundred to which it gives name; and in 1253 it was made a market town. It is agreeably situated near the river Chalmer, and consists of two principal streets, which are paved and lighted : and the inhabitants are supplied with water from springs. The town obtained a charter of incorpo-

ration from Philip and Mary, which was confirmed by Elizabeth, under which the government is vested in a recorder, bailiff, and twelve burgesses; but at present they do not possess magisterial authority, and the only function they exercise, is the appointment of a constable, bread-weighers and leather-sealers, which takes place annually on the Tuesday after Michaelmas-day. The petty sessions for the division are held here : a court leet for the manor is also held occasionally. Formerly the manufacture of baize and blankets was carried on very extensively, but at present there is only a small establishment for making sacking and coarse cloth. The market, which was on Saturday, has been discontinued; but there are fairs on May 6th and November 8th, for cattle. The living is a vicarage, in the archdeaconry of Middlesex, and diocese of London, rated in the king's books at £18. 13. 4., and in the patronage of the Bishop of London. The church, dedicated to St. Mary, is a spacious edifice in the decorated and later styles of English architecture, consisting of a nave, aisles, and chancel, with a fine east window : it has lately received an addition of two hundred and thirty sittings, of which two hundred are free, the Incorporated Society for the enlargement of churches and chapels having granted £50 towards defraying :the expense. Here are places of worship for Baptists, the Society of Friends, and Independents. There is an almshouse for six poor persons : a charity school for fifty boys, and another for twenty girls, are supported by voluntary contributions.

DUNMOW (LITTLE), a parish in the hundred of DUNMOW, county of ESSEX, 2¼ miles (E. S. E.) from Great Dunmow, containing 342 inhabitants. The living is a perpetual curacy, in the archdeaconry of Middlesex, and diocese of London, endowed with £200 private benefaction, £600 royal bounty, and £200 parliamentary grant. N. R. Toke, Esq. was patron in 1824. The church, dedicated to St. Mary, consists only of the south aisle and part of the nave of a church which belonged to a priory of Augustine canons, founded in 1104, the revenue of which, at the dissolution, was £173. 2. 4. Under an arched recess in the south wall is a coffin-shaped tomb, supposed to be that of Lady Juga, sister of Ralph Baynard, foundress of the priory; near it is a monument, with the figures of an armed knight and a lady, said to have been erected for Sir Walter Fitz-Walter, who died in 1198; and on the opposite side of the church, a monument with a female figure in alabaster, said to represent Matilda Fitz-Walter, famous in legendary story as the wife or mistress of Robin Hood, and the object of the illicit passion of King John, who is stated to have caused her to be poisoned, in revenge for her having rejected his addresses. There is an ancient custom connected with the manor of Little Dunmow, of delivering a gammon, or flitch of bacon, on demand, to any couple, who, after having been married a year and a day, will swear that neither party has repented, and that no cause of quarrel or complaint has arisen between them. Before the Reformation, the oath used to be administered, and the bacon given by the prior of the convent; and since, the ceremony has been occasionally performed at a court baron before the steward of the manor. The institution of this custom is supposed to have taken place soon after the Norman Conquest, but the earliest instance on record of the delivery of the bacon is in the 23rd of Henry VI., and the latest in

M 2

1751; and the whole number of successful claimants is said to have been but six couple.

DUNNERDALE, a chapelry in the parish of KIRK-BY-IRELETH, hundred of LONSDALE, north of the sands, county palatine of LANCASTER, 8¼ miles (W. by S.) from Hawkeshead, containing 143 inhabitants. There is a trifling sum for the education of children.

DUNNINGTON, a township in the parish of BEE-FORD, northern division of the wapentake of HOLDER-NESS, East riding of the county of YORK, 10 miles (E.S.E.) from Great Driffield, containing 76 inhabitants.

DUNNINGTON, a parish partly in the wapentake of OUZE and DERWENT, but chiefly within the liberty of ST. PETER of YORK, East riding of the county of YORK, 4½ miles (E. by N.) from York, containing, with the township of Grimston, 623 inhabitants. The living is a rectory, in the archdeaconry of Cleveland, and diocese of York, rated in the king's books at £19, and in the patronage of the Trustees of the late Earl of Bridge-water. The church is dedicated to St. Nicholas. There is a place of worship for Wesleyan Methodists. The high road here separates the East from the North riding.

DUNNINGWORTH, a hamlet in the parish of TUNSTALL, hundred of PLOMESGATE, county of SUF-FOLK, 5½ miles (E. by N.) from Wickham-Market. The population is returned with the parish. This was formerly a distinct parish, but the living, a discharged rectory, has been united to that of Tunstall; and the church, which was dedicated to St. Mary, has fallen into ruins.

DUNNOCKSHAW, a township in that part of the parish of WHALLEY which is in the higher division of the hundred of BLACKBURN, county palatine of LAN-CASTER, 3½ miles (S.S.W.) from Burnley, containing 76 inhabitants.

DUNSBY, a parish in the wapentake of AVELAND, parts of KESTEVEN, county of LINCOLN, 4 miles (N. by E.) from Bourne, containing 190 inhabitants. The living is a rectory, in the archdeaconry and diocese of Lincoln, rated in the king's books at £12. 14. 7., and in the patronage of the Governors of the Charter-house, London. The church, dedicated to All Saints, is partly in the early and partly in the decorated style of English architecture; the tower is a handsome specimen of the latter.

DUNSBY, a parish in the wapentake of FLAX-WELL, parts of KESTEVEN, county of LINCOLN, 4 miles (N.N.W.) from Sleaford. The population is returned with Brauncewell. The living is a discharged rectory, united to the rectory of Brauncewell, in the archdea-conry and diocese of Lincoln. The church is dedicated to St. Andrew.

DUNSCROFT, a hamlet in the parish of HATFIELD, southern division of the wapentake of STRAFFORTH and TICKHILL, West riding of the county of YORK, 3¼ miles (S.W.) from Thorne. The population is returned with the parish. Here was formerly a small cell to the ab-bey of Roche.

DUNSDEN, a joint liberty with Eye, in that part of the parish of SONNING which is in the hundred of BINFIELD, county of OXFORD, 5 miles (S.S.W.) from Henley upon Thames, containing 845 inhabitants.

DUNSFOLD, a parish in the first division of the hundred of BLACKHEATH, county of SURREY, 5¾ miles

(S.S.E.) from Godalming, containing 578 inhabitants. The living is a rectory, in the archdeaconry of Surrey, and diocese of Winchester, rated in the king's books at £12. 0. 7½., and in the patronage of the Crown. The church, dedicated to St. Mary, has portions in the deco-rated style of architecture. The Arun and Wey Junc-tion canal passes through the parish.

DUNSFORD, a parish in the hundred of WON-FORD, county of DEVON, 7 miles (W. by S.) from Exeter, containing 819 inhabitants. The living is a vicarage, in the archdeaconry and diocese of Exeter, rated in the king's books at £19. 10., and in the patronage of Bald-win Fulford, Esq. The church, dedicated to St. Mary, has a plain Norman door-way. Seven poor children are educated for about £3 per ann., the bequests of Agnes Harrison, in 1750, and others. In the parliamentary war, the manor-house, erected in the time of Elizabeth, was garrisoned by Colonel Sir Francis Fulford, its owner, for the king; but the garrison surrendered to Fairfax, in 1645.

DUNSFORTH (LOW), a chapelry in that part of the parish of ALDBOROUGH which is in the upper division of the wapentake of CLARO, West riding of the county of YORK, 2¼ miles (E.S.E.) from Aldborough, containing 115 inhabitants. The living is a perpetual curacy, en-dowed with £400 royal bounty, and £200 parliamentary grant, and in the peculiar jurisdiction and patronage of the Dean and Chapter of York. The chapel is dedicated to St. Mary.

DUNSFORTH (UPPER), a joint township with Branton-Green, in that part of the parish of ALD-BOROUGH which is in the upper division of the wapen-take of CLARO, West riding of the county of YORK, 3½ miles (S.E. by E.) from Aldborough, containing 156 in-habitants.

DUNSLEY, a joint township with Newholm, in the parish of WHITBY, liberty of WHITBY-STRAND, North riding of the county of YORK, 3 miles (W.) from Whitby, containing 259 inhabitants. From this place a Roman road, now called Wade's causeway, runs for many miles over the moors to York; it is paved with flints, and has been traced twelve feet wide and three high, with a defaced milliary on it.

DUNSTABLE, a market town and parish in the hundred of MANSHEAD, county of BEDFORD, 18 miles (S. by W.) from Bedford, and 33¾ (N.W. by N.) from London, containing 1831 inhabitants. The origin of this town may be traced to the time of the ancient Bri-tons, who are supposed to have had a settlement here, which they named Maes Gwyn, or "White Field," as de-scriptive of the chalky soil of the vicinity: it is thought to have been the Magiovinium of Antoninus, a name of similar import. That it was a place of great im-portance at this period is evident from its situation at the very point of contact between the Watling and Iknield-streets, as also from immense adjacent ramparts of earth which mark the ancient circular fortifications. Its modern appellation was bestowed after the Danes had desolated the town, and, according to Hearne and Bishop Gibson, was derived from Dunum, or Dun, a hill, and Staple, a commercial mart; by others it is considered to have been taken from Dun, the name of a notorious robber in the time of Henry I., who with his associates became so much an object of terror, that the destruc-tion of the neighbouring forest was resorted to as the only effectual means of their dispersion. This object being accomplished, Henry erected a royal residence at Kingsbury, rebuilt the town of Dunstable, and having invited settlers, constituted it a borough, endowing it with a grant of lands at a trifling nominal rent, and investing the inhabitants with various privileges, among which was an exemption from the jurisdiction of justices itinerant at any place throughout the realm, except within their own town and liberty. During this reign markets were held weekly on Sunday and Wednesday, and a fair on St. Peter's day. The priory of Black canons, near the royal palace, founded by Henry, under the authority of Pope Eugenius III., was extensively endowed, and enjoyed many privileges; the priors had a gaol, possessed the power of life and death, and usually sat as judges at Dunstable, with the king's justices itinerant. These circumstances gave occasion to the exercise of great tyranny, and the townsmen became entirely subject to the monks; hence arose dissatisfaction and tumults, so that in the reign of Richard II. the inhabitants revolted against the prior, and extorted a charter of liberties from him, which he soon afterwards revoked. In 1204, King John conferred his palace on the prior, on condition that royal visitors should be freely entitled to the hospitality of the priory; and many English sovereigns have been entertained here. In 1290, the corpse of Queen Eleanor, consort of Edward I., rested at the market-place, on being conveyed through the town, and a handsome cross, erected in commemoration of that event, was demolished in the reign of Charles I., as a relic of popery. In the chapel of our Lady, at the priory, the sentence of divorce between Henry VIII. and Catherine of Arragon was pronounced, by Archbishop Cranmer; and Gervase Markham, who was the last prior, having assisted to effect that measure, was in consequence treated with comparative liberality.

The town is pleasantly situated near the Chiltern hills, and consists of four principal streets, which intersect each other at right angles, and correspond exactly with the four cardinal points. They are neither paved nor lighted: the inhabitants were formerly supplied with water from public reservoirs, of which there was one in each street; but it is now obtained from wells, which, from the chalky nature of the sub-stratum are sunk to a great depth. The manufacture of articles in straw, both useful and ornamental, is extensively carried on, particularly in the well known "Dunstable hats;" and there is one of the largest manufactories for whiting in the kingdom, from which most of the manufacturing towns are supplied. This town was also formerly distinguished for the number of its inns, and is still proverbially famed for larks. The market is on Wednesday: fairs are held on Ash-Wednesday, May 22nd, August 12th, and November 12th, the last being the largest fair for sheep in the county. Dunstable was once under the government of a mayor, but it has now only the ordinary parochial authorities. The King is lord of the manor, and the Duke of Bedford, as his lessee, holds courts leet and baron, but at no stated periods.

The living is a rectory not in charge, in the archdeaconry of Bedford, and diocese of Lincoln, endowed with £200 private benefaction, and in the patronage of the Crown. The church, which, with some rooms having vaulted and groined stone roofs, forms the only remains of the ancient priory, is dedicated to St. Peter

and St. Paul, and was originally a magnificent and extensive cruciform structure, with a tower rising from the intersection: Henry VIII. having abandoned his design of making it a cathedral, a considerable part of the edifice was demolished. The remains consist of the west front, nave, and two aisles; each of the latter extends from the western doors to the entrance to what was once the choir, being about one hundred and twenty feet long: at the north-west angle is a tower embellished with a double row of niches, which formerly contained statues. The architecture combines some portions in the Norman, with others in the early and later English styles. The windows are of comparatively modern date; the eastern end terminates in a flat wall, the two arches adjoining which form the present choir: the roof is of finely carved oak in the decorated style, the beams being supported by figures representing angels: the western entrance is surmounted by an elegant stone rood-loft of four pointed arches and clustered columns. Over the communion-table is a painting of the Lord's Supper, by Sir James Thornhill. The ancient altar-cloth, (which is now in the possession of John Miller, Esq., of Bedford, or his representatives), is a fabric of the richest crimson and gold brocade, so exquisitely wrought, that it has hitherto been impossible to discover the mode in which it was manufactured; and, though upwards of three hundred years old, it still retains its original freshness and beauty. Amongst the various monuments in the church are several to the Chew family, who were great benefactors to the town. On the eastern side of the church, stone coffins and various relics of antiquity have been dug up. There are two places of worship for Baptists, and one for Wesleyan Methodists.

A charity school, founded by the direction of Mr. William Chew, was built in 1727, and is endowed by various benefactors, with land at Caddington, Luton, Houghton-Regis, Hamstidde, Totternhoe, and Whipsnade, producing an annual income of more than £300: forty boys and fifteen girls are clothed, educated, and apprenticed, and the master has a salary of £40 per annum: a donation by Mark Brown, Esq. supplies an additional apprenticeship every third year. The boys are admitted at the age of seven, and apprenticed at fourteen. Adjoining the school are six almshouses, founded and endowed by Mrs. Cart, for the residence and maintenance of as many poor widows: and in West-street are six others, founded and endowed by Mrs. Ashton for a similar purpose. Nearly opposite the church are six houses founded by Mrs. Blandina Marsh, in 1713, and designated "The Maidens' Lodge," for six unmarried gentlewomen, whose income has been increased by a benefaction fom another lady, to £120 per annum. A workhouse has existed for many years, in which the poor are employed in the straw-plat manufacture. In 1770, a great quantity of coins of Antoninus and Constantine, with ornaments of bridles and armour, was dug up on an adjacent down. The first dramatic representations in England, called Mysteries, are said to have taken place here under the direction of a priest, or friar. Elkanah Settle, a dramatist and political writer of notoriety in the reign of Charles II., was a native of this place: he was the opponent of Dryden, and during the violence of party feeling his works were very popular, but have been long since utterly forgotten.

DUNSTALL, a township in the parish of TATEN-

HILL, northern division of the hundred of OFFLOW, county of STAFFORD, 4½ miles (W. S.W.) from Burton upon Trent, containing 184 inhabitants.

DUNSTALL, a township in that part of the parish of TAMWORTH which is in the southern division of the hundred of OFFLOW, county of STAFFORD, 1¾ mile (W.) from Tamworth, with which the population is returned. Dunstall is in the honour of Tutbury, duchy of Lancaster, and within the jurisdiction of a court of pleas held at Tutbury every third Tuesday, for the recovery of debts under 40s.

DUNSTAN (ST.), a parish in the hundred of WESTGATE, lathe of ST. AUGUSTINE, county of KENT, ¼ of a mile (N.W.) from Canterbury, containing 719 inhabitants. The living is a discharged vicarage, in the archdeaconry and diocese of Canterbury, rated in the king's books at £5, and in the patronage of the Archbishop of Canterbury. Here is a National school.

DUNSTER, a market town and parish in the hundred of CARHAMPTON, county of SOMERSET, 38 miles (W.N.W.) from Somerton, and 158 (W. by S.) from London, containing 895 inhabitants. The town, which is called *Torre* in Domesday-book, owes its origin to a baronial castle built here by William de Mohun, a Norman baron, on whom William the Conqueror bestowed large estates in this part of the kingdom. He also founded a priory of Benedictine monks, as a cell to the abbey at Bath, the revenue of which, at the dissolution, was £37. 4. 9½. The castle, which was held by the family of Mohun till the reign of Edward III., was the scene of hostilities during the civil wars which took place in the reigns of Stephen and John, and in the contests between the houses of York and Lancaster; and the Marquis of Hertford took possession of it for Charles I., during the war with the parliament. The castle has been the residence of the family of Luttrell since the time of Edward III.: the present structure, which is comparatively of recent erection, stands in a commanding situation at the southern extremity of the principal street, embracing fine views of the Bristol channel, and the Welch and Gloucestershire hills. The town is situated on a gentle eminence, about a mile to the south of the Bristol channel, and the surrounding country is beautifully diversified with hill and dale, through which flows a rapid stream, formed by springs rising at Dunkery hill, which passes on the south and east sides of the town, and after turning several mills, runs under a stone bridge of three arches, and falls into the sea. It is small, and of little importance at present, having materially suffered from the loss of its wool trade, which formerly afforded employment to a considerable part of the population of this and the surrounding parishes. There are but two principal streets, one of which has been much improved by the removal of some unsightly old shambles that stood in the centre. An ancient market-house is still standing. The market is on Friday; and a fair is held on Whit-Monday. Considerable advantage is anticipated from the recent construction of a new line of road from this place to Dulverton, which will afford great facility for the conveyance of commodities to the market. This town sent members to a parliament in the 34th of Edward III., and at present it enjoys the elective franchise in conjunction with Minehead, the right of election for that place being vested, by a resolution of the House

of Commons, February 24th, 1717, in the parishioners of Dunster and Minehead, being housekeepers in the borough of Minehead, and not receiving alms.

The living, formerly a vicarage, is now a perpetual curacy, in the archdeaconry of Taunton, and diocese of Bath and Wells, rated in the king's books at £4. 13. 4., endowed with £1200 private benefaction, £800 royal bounty, and £1200 parliamentary grant, and in the patronage of John Fownes Luttrell, Esq. The church, dedicated to St. George, is a very spacious edifice in the later style of English architecture, having been erected by Henry VII., in acknowledgment of the assistance afforded him by the men of Dunster, in the battle of Bosworth Field: it consists of a nave, aisles, and chancel, with a central tower, ornamented with battlements and pinnacles; beyond which, to the east, is a kind of chapel, formerly the conventual church of the priory: this part of the building was also used by the incumbent of the parish, for the performance of divine service until the year 1499, when a dispute arising between the monks and the parishioners, the matter was referred to arbitrators, who decided that the latter should have a choir separate from that of the convent: it contains many fine sepulchral monuments belonging to the families of Mohun and Luttrell, which, as well as the chapel itself, are hastening to decay. Here is a charity school.

DUNSTEW, a parish in the hundred of WOOTTON, county of OXFORD, 2½ miles (S. S. W.) from Deddington, containing 460 inhabitants. The living is a vicarage, in the archdeaconry and diocese of Oxford, rated in the king's books at £8. 2. 8¼. Sir H.W. Dashwood, Bart. was patron in 1794. The church is dedicated to St. Mary.

DUNSTON, a parish in the second division of the wapentake of LANGOE, parts of KESTEVEN, county of LINCOLN, 8¼ miles (S.E.) from Lincoln, containing 406 inhabitants. The living is a vicarage, in the archdeaconry and diocese of Lincoln, rated in the king's books at £7. 0. 10., endowed with £200 private benefaction, £200 royal bounty, and in the patronage of the Bishop of Lincoln. The church is dedicated to St. Peter. Here was an hospital for lepers in the reign of Henry III. Dunston pillar, a pyramidal shaft ninety-two feet high, crowned with a gallery and lantern, was erected in 1751, by F. Dashwood, Esq., as a land-mark to guide the traveller over the then surrounding waste, which has been since enclosed.

DUNSTON, a parish in the hundred of HUMBLEYARD, county of NORFOLK, 4 miles (S.) from Norwich, containing 111 inhabitants. The living is a perpetual curacy, in the archdeaconry of Norfolk, and diocese of Norwich, endowed with £400 royal bounty, and in the patronage of the Misses S. and S. Long. The church is dedicated to St. Remigius.

DUNSTON, a township in the parish of EMBLETON, southern division of BAMBROUGH ward, county of NORTHUMBERLAND 6¼ miles (N.E.) from Alnwick, containing 213 inhabitants.

DUNSTON, a chapelry in that part of the parish of PENKRIDGE which is in the eastern division of the hundred of CUTTLESTONE, county of STAFFORD, 2½ miles (N. by E.) from Penkridge, containing 234 inhabitants. The living is a perpetual curacy, within the jurisdiction of the peculiar court of Penkridge, endowed with £1200 royal bounty, and in the patronage of E. J. Littleton, Esq. The chapel is dedicated to St. Leonard.

DUNTERTON, a parish in the hundred of LIFTON, county of DEVON, 5 miles (S.E. by S.) from Launceston, containing 126 inhabitants. The living is a rectory, in the archdeaconry of Totness, and diocese of Exeter, rated in the king's books at £8. 7. 1. The Rev. W. Royce was patron in 1800. The church, dedicated to All Saints, is small, but the tower is handsome. At a place called Chapel Field formerly stood a chantry chapel, the remains of which have been converted into a cow-house.

DUNTISH, a tything in the parish and hundred of BUCKLAND-NEWTON, Cerne sub-division of the county of DORSET, 11½ miles (N. by W.) from Dorchester, containing 101 inhabitants. There is a circular camp of ten acres, in which arms and Roman coins have been discovered.

DUNTON, a parish in the hundred of BIGGLESWADE, county of BEDFORD, 3½ miles (E. by S.) from Biggleswade, containing, with Millo, 332 inhabitants. The living is a discharged vicarage, in the archdeaconry of Bedford, and diocese of Lincoln, rated in the king's books at £10. Earl Spencer was patron in 1806. The church is dedicated to St. Mary.

DUNTON, a parish in the hundred of COTTESLOE, county of BUCKINGHAM, 5 miles (S.E. by E.) from Winslow, containing 98 inhabitants. The living is a rectory, in the archdeaconry of Buckingham, and diocese of Lincoln, rated in the king's books at £9. 9. 7. Earl Spencer was patron in 1817. The church is dedicated to St. Martin.

DUNTON, a parish in the hundred of BARSTABLE, county of ESSEX, 3½ miles (N.N.W.) from Horndon on the Hill, containing 33 inhabitants. The living is a rectory, in the archdeaconry of Essex, and diocese of London, rated in the king's books at £14. 13. 4., and in the patronage of the Provost and Fellows of King's College, Cambridge. The church is dedicated to St. Mary.

DUNTON, a joint parish with Doughton, in the hundred of GALLOW, county of NORFOLK, 3 miles (W. by N.) from Fakenham, containing 124 inhabitants. The living is a discharged vicarage, in the archdeaconry of Norfolk, and diocese of Norwich, rated in the king's books at £5. 6. 8. T. W. Coke, Esq. was patron in 1800. The church is dedicated to St. Mary.

DUNTON-BASSETT, a parish in the hundred of GUTHLAXTON, county of LEICESTER, 3¾ miles (N.) from Lutterworth, containing 460 inhabitants. The living is a discharged vicarage, in the archdeaconry of Leicester, and diocese of Lincoln, rated in the king's books at £6. 0. 10. George Payne, Esq. was patron in 1802. The church is dedicated to All Saints. There is a medicinal spring in this parish.

DUNTSBOURN (ABBOT'S), a parish partly in the hundred of RAPSGATE, comprising the township of Duntsbourn-Leer, but chiefly in the hundred of CROWTHORNE and MINETY, county of GLOUCESTER, 5 miles (N.W. by N.) from Cirencester, containing 256 inhabitants. The living is a rectory, in the archdeaconry and diocese of Gloucester, rated in the king's books at £13. D. Mesman, Esq. was patron in 1794. The church is dedicated to St. Peter. The Roman road Ermin-street passes through this parish.

DUNTSBOURN-LEER, a township in that part of the parish of ABBOT'S DUNTSBOURN which is in the hundred of RAPSGATE, county of GLOUCESTER, 5½ miles (N. by W.) from Cirencester, containing 85 inhabitants.

DUNTSBOURN-ROUSE, a parish in the hundred of CROWTHORNE and MINETY, county of GLOUCESTER, 3¾ miles (N.W. by N.) from Cirencester, containing 100 inhabitants. The living is a rectory, in the archdeaconry and diocese of Gloucester, rated in the king's books at £8. 14. 9½., and in the patronage of the President and Fellows of Corpus Christi College, Oxford. The church is dedicated to St. Michael. The Roman road Ermin-street crosses this parish.

DUNWICH, a sea-port, borough, (formerly a market town), and parish, having separate jurisdiction, locally in the hundred of Blything, county of SUFFOLK, 29 miles (N.E.) from Ipswich, and 98 (N.E.) from London, containing 200 inhabitants. It is supposed by some to have been a town of the Britons, or a Roman station; this opinion having been chiefly grounded on the discovery of some Roman coins. During the Heptarchy it was a place of great importance, having been the metropolis of East Anglia, and the seat of a bishop's see. By the Saxons it was called Dommoc-ceaster, or Donmoc, whence is derived its present appellation. Sigebert, King of the East Angles, having been converted to Christianity in 630, founded a bishoprick at Dunwich, which was held by Felix, a Burgundian, and a succession of prelates till about the middle of the ninth century, when this part of the country was devastated by the Danes. At the time of the Norman survey it was a place of considerable importance, having an extensive herring fishery, as the king received from the burgesses annually £50, and sixty thousand herrings. The town had anciently a mint; and William of Newburgh, who wrote in the reign of Henry II., styles it a wealthy and famous sea-port. In the reign of Richard I., a fine of one thousand and sixty marks was levied on the town, because the inhabitants had supplied the king's enemies with corn; and Ipswich and Yarmouth were fined two hundred marks each for the same offence; whence an estimate may be formed of the relative importance of this place. During the wars of the barons with King John, it was fortified with a ditch and a rampart; and that monarch bestowed on the town a charter of incorporation, and a grant of sea-wreck. In the reign of Edward I. it maintained eleven ships of war; and in 1359 it furnished six ships, and one hundred and two mariners, for the siege of Calais. Such was the ancient prosperity and importance of this place that it contained more than fifty religious foundations, including churches, chapels, priories, and hospitals, but being situated on a hill composed of loam and loose sand, it has yielded to the successive encroachments of the sea, which has demolished its churches and convents, ruined its haven, swallowed up its streets, and reduced it to an insignificant village.

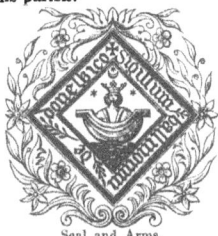

Seal and Arms.

The borough, as originally established by John, was governed by a mayor; but the charter having been renewed by Edward II., the corporation now consists of a recorder, two bailiffs, two assistant justices, twelve capital burgesses, a coroner, town clerk, and serjeant at mace, with other inferior officers, who are all elected annually on the 29th of August, and sworn into office on the 29th of September. The bailiffs and assistant justices (who are the bailiffs for the preceding year), are magistrates for the borough, exercising exclusive jurisdiction. The corporation are empowered to hold courts of assize and session, the yearly sessions being held in October. There is an admiralty court, at which the bailiffs and assistant justices preside; also a court of requests for the recovery of debts under 40s. within the borough. The freedom of the borough is inherited by the eldest sons of freemen, born while their fathers possessed that privilege, or it may be obtained by gift of the freemen at large. The borough has sent members to parliament ever since the 23rd of Edward I. The right of election is vested in the resident freemen not receiving alms: the number of voters is fourteen. The bailiffs are the returning officers. The market, which was held on Monday, has been discontinued; but there is an annual fair on the 25th of July. Several small boats are employed in the herring fishery, and there are fish-houses, where herrings and sprats are dried, and prepared for sale.

Dunwich anciently contained six parish churches, but they have all been entirely destroyed, except that of All Saints, of which only the walls and a square tower remain: it is now reduced to a single parish, the living of which is a perpetual curacy, in the archdeaconry of Suffolk, and diocese of Norwich, and in the patronage of Lord Huntingfield and Colonel Baine. The old church, dedicated to All Saints, being dilapidated, the erection of a new one was commenced in 1826: it is built of white brick, with an octagonal tower, the expense having been defrayed by subscription among the inhabitants. An hospital for lepers, dedicated to St. James, was founded here so early as the reign of Richard I., and richly endowed: the revenue was reduced to £26 per annum, but is now £80, which is divided among a few of the indigent poor. There was another ancient hospital, called Maison Dieu, a great part of the property belonging to which having been lost, through the encroachment of the sea, it has been united to the other charity. A convent of Franciscan friars was founded here in the reign of Henry III., of which there are remains of the walls and two gateways; and there were also a Dominican convent, and a house of the Knights Templars, long since entirely destroyed. Dunwich gives the title of viscount to the Earl of Stradbroke.

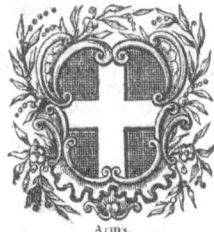

Arms.

DURHAM, a city, the capital of the county palatine of DURHAM, 67 miles (E. S. E.) from Carlisle, 87 (N. E.) from Lancaster, 67 (W. N. W.) from York, and 259 (N. by W.) from London; containing 9822 inhabitants, exclusively of those in Easington ward. The name is probably derived from the Saxon words, Dun, a hill, and Holme, a river island, being descriptive of its situation on a rocky eminence partially surrounded by the river Wear. The Normans called it Duresme, whence more immediately is deduced its present appellation. The earliest account of this place is in 995, when the monks of Lindisfarne, or Holy Island, who had removed to Chester le Street, and afterwards to Ripon, for sanctuary from the violence of Danish aggression, were returning to their church at Chester le Street, after an absence of four months, with the disinterred body of St. Cuthbert, which had been buried at Lindisfarne, in 687; according to the superstitious legend, on their arrival at the spot where Durham now stands, a miraculous interposition rendered the carriage which conveyed the body, and other relics, immoveable, and this incident they construed into a divine prohibition against the return of the saint's remains to their former resting-place. They likewise interpreted some other circumstances into an intimation that Dunholme was destined to receive the sacred relics; and there are still some emblematic devices on the west corner tower of the east transept of the cathedral, designed to commemorate this occurrence. They forthwith proceeded to construct a sort of ark, or tabernacle, of wicker-work, wherein they deposited the saint's body; they subsequently erected a more appropriate edifice, called the White Church, and, three years after their arrival, a stone church was built by Bishop Aldun, and dedicated to St. Cuthbert, whose remains were then removed and enshrined in it. Determined on permanent residence, these strangers cleared away the trees which skirted the hill, and began to build substantial houses; thus arose the Saxon town of Dunholme, about the commencement of the eleventh century; the increase of which, both in buildings and population, was so rapid, that in 1040, being then partially fortified, Duncan of Scotland besieged it, but his forces were totally vanquished, and the heads of the Scottish leaders, who were slain or captured, were fixed on poles around the market-place. At the Conquest, many of the Anglo-Saxon malcontents assembled here, erected a castle and other fortifications, and made a temporary defence, but being disappointed in not receiving assistance, they fled; and William the Conqueror entered the city, and granted many privileges to the inhabitants. In 1069, Robert Comyn, Earl of Northumberland, being appointed governor, entered Durham with a Norman guard of seven hundred soldiers, and such were the enormities they committed, that the enraged populace of the adjacent country, taking advantage of the inaction to which the forces were reduced by drunkenness and revelling, burst into the city, set fire to the governor's house, and put them all to the sword, except one man, who was wounded, but made his escape. In revenge for this carnage, William, desolating in his progress the whole country between York and Durham, advanced upon the city, on which the whole of the inhabitants fled, and the monks left their convent; but on the departure of the troops, the fugitives returned from the neighbouring mountains, where they had taken shelter, after an absence of four months. A dreadful famine and consequent mortality were the result, and the people were under the necessity of eating horses, dogs, and cats, and even human bodies. The whole of the district through which the Norman had passed remained without culture for nine years, infested by robbers and beasts of prey; and many of the inhabitants who escaped the sword, starved in the fields. During this calamity, the bones of St. Cuthbert were removed, after a repose of seventy-five years, to Lindisfarne, on which occasion it is superstitiously related that the sea retired, and allowed the wanderers who accompanied the holy relics to pass over to the island dry-shod. At length tranquillity was restored, and the body was replaced in the shrine at Durham ; but the bishop having been detected in a rebellion against the Conqueror, was imprisoned till his death. The king, on his return from an expedition against Malcolm of Scotland, in 1072, appointed Walcher, a Norman, to the bishoprick, and ordered a fortress to be erected here, to overawe the inhabitants, and form a barrier to the northern territories. This prelate purchased the earldom of Northumberland, assumed the title of Count Palatine, and, by uniting temporal and ecclesiastical power, excited an insurrection, in which he was slain. During the protracted warfare which followed this outrage, Carilepho, who had succeeded to the see, took part with Malcolm, against William, and at its termination fled to Normandy. William Rufus seized on the temporalties, and appointed John de Tailbois and Ernesius de Burone, governors of the castle and palatinate : in 1091, the bishop was restored. The shrine of St. Cuthbert having been greatly enriched under the six prelates who preceded Carilepho, that bishop, having brought from Normandy the plan of a new church, pulled down the old one, and began the present edifice, the foundation of which was laid by King Malcolm, Carilepho, and Turgot the prior, on the 11th of August, 1093, the building having taken upwards of thirty years in its completion. Bishop Ralph Flambard conveyed St. Cuthbert's remains to the new church, erected a splendid shrine near the choir for their reception, improved the fortifications of the city and castle, and built Framwell-gate bridge. During his episcopacy, Durham sustained considerable injury from fire. In 1139, the Empress Queen, Maud, daughter of Henry I., and Prince Henry, son of David, King of Scotland, with the members of congress, were entertained by the citizens, on the negociation of peace between England and Scotland. During the reign of Henry II., Bishop Pudsey having incurred the royal displeasure, that monarch took possession of the city and castle, and at the bishop's death, the officers of the crown having seized the keys, the see was for a long time vacant. To this bishop the city was indebted for several improvements, particularly for the erection of Elvet bridge, and the extension of the city wall from Northgate to Southgate. King John resided here in 1213, as also did Henry III. for a short time during the prelacy of Bishop Farnham ; and the latter monarch deprived the shrine of St. Cuthbert of a considerable treasure, which he never restored. Edward I. held a council here, to dispose of the estates of some Scottish barons, after the victory of Falkirk ; and in 1300, he again visited Durham, as a mediator between the bishop and his convent. In 1313, the suburbs were reduced to ashes by a numerous body of Scottish invaders ; and in 1316, they also destroyed the seat of the prior at Beaurepaire, now Bear park : about this time Bishop Beaumont repaired the city walls, and put them into a state of defence. In 1327, this city was for some time the head-quarters of Edward III. and his army: in 1333, that monarch rested here, on his march to Hallidown, when he was splendidly entertained by Bishop Bury ; and in 1356 he again visited Durham,

issuing from it his summons for the military tenants to attend him on a northern expedition. In 1404, two peers and two knights were executed here for engaging in a conspiracy against Henry IV. On the liberation and marriage of James I. of Scotland, in 1424, Durham was crowded with the nobility : the hostages were received here, and the King and Queen of Scotland remained in the city a considerable time. About this period the plague commenced, and continued to rage for five years ; during which, the assizes and all public assemblies were suspended, and several thousands of the inhabitants of the city and its vicinity fell victims to it. During the episcopacy of Neville, the English and Scottish delegates held several meetings here : in 1448, Henry VI. came on a pilgrimage to the shrine of St. Cuthbert : in 1463, Lord Montague and his army were quartered at Durham, previously to the battle of Hedgeley Moor ; and in 1503, Bishop Fox entertained Margaret, daughter of Henry VII., with other distinguished personages, in the great hall of his palace, on her way to Scotland, where she was married to James IV. At the close of the rebellion under the Nevilles, in the reign of Elizabeth, sixty-six persons were executed in the city ; and from 1589 to 1597, with some slight intermission, the plague again raged in it. In 1603, James I. was presented by the mayor with a gold cup on entering the city ; and in 1633, Bishop Morton entertained Charles I. and his retinue during his residence here, at the daily expense of £1500. After the battle of Newburn, in 1640, when the Scottish army entered England, the city of Durham became almost utterly depopulated.

The city is about one mile in length, and as much in breadth, and from the peculiar course of the river, which environs it in the form of a horse-shoe, it is peninsular, occupying a considerable eminence, which is surmounted by the cathedral and the remains of the ancient castle, now used as the bishop's palace, together with other ecclesiastical residences. These are immediately surrounded by the streets called the North and South Baileys, enclosed within the remains of the old city walls, and skirted by sloping gardens, which descend to the brink of the river, on each side of which are public walks of extreme beauty, called the Banks, formed along the winding margin of the river, and approached by an avenue from Palace Green, a large open area before the cathedral. Framwell-gate bridge, situated at the northern extremity of the city, having one pier and two elliptic and finely proportioned arches of ninety feet span, adapted to the low shores on each side, was erected by Bishop Flambard, about 1120 : a large tower gateway, which formerly stood at the end of this bridge, next the city, was taken down in 1760. Elvet bridge, of eight arches, was built about 1170 by Bishop Pudsey, and afterwards repaired by Bishop Fox, who granted an indulgence to all contributors ; in 1806, it was improved and widened to twice its former breadth. The New bridge, which crosses the river nearly opposite the only remaining city gate, at the extremity of the South Bailey, is an elegant structure, erected between 1772 and 1777, consisting of three semicircular arches, with a balustraded battlement : an old bridge, which stood higher up the river, was carried away by a flood in 1771. The castle, now used as the occasional residence of the bishop, stands northward of the cathedral. The original edifice is attributed to William the Conqueror, in 1072 : it has undergone various alterations and additions at different periods : the oldest portion of it is the keep, now a mere shell, in the form of an irregular octagon, occupying the summit of an artificial mount, around which are three terraces, commanding a beautiful view of the city and its environs. The great north gateway was used as a county gaol till 1820, when it was removed, and its site occupied, on the west side, by a subscription library and news-room, and on the east by shops, with a spacious assembly-room over them. The habitable part consists of a large mass of buildings of almost every date from the Norman to the present time. The late Bishop Barrington has thrown open some fine inner Norman doors, previously concealed, but the interior in general is fitted up in a style subsequent to the reign of Elizabeth. The town is paved, flagged, lighted with gas, and watched under the direction of commissioners appointed under acts of parliament passed in the 30th of George III. and the 3rd of George IV. The pant, or public fountain, stands in the centre of the market-place, and is surmounted by a statue of Neptune riding on a dolphin, which was placed there in 1729 : the reservoir is of an octagonal form. In the year 1450, an excellent spring of water, situated in his manor of Sidgate, was granted to the city for ever, by Thomas Bellingham, Esq., whence the water is conveyed through pipes into the reservoir. There is a theatre in Sadler-street, built in 1791 ; and in this street is also a mechanics' library, established in 1825 : the race-ground is near Old Elvet, where the races are held in May, and continue four days : they appear to have been established in the reign of Charles II.

The trade of Durham was formerly much more extensive than it is at present ; a cotton manufactory, which existed previously to 1804, was in that year destroyed by fire. Here are manufactories for stuffs and carpets, for spinning and combing wool, a brass-foundry, and two iron-foundries ; and on the north side of Elvet bridge is a manufactory for hats, formerly the house of correction, erected in 1632. A market for corn and provisions is held on Saturday, under a piazza at the bottom of the market square, where the corn is pitched. Fairs for horned cattle, sheep, and horses, are annually held on the 29th, 30th, and 31st of March, Whit-Tuesday, Saturday before May 13th, September 15th, and Saturday before November 23d : the March fair is an object of peculiar attraction to the principal horse dealers from the south, on account of the excellent breed of horses in the adjacent district, which are then brought for sale. A court of pie-powder is held during each fair, by the corporation.

The government, in the earliest times, was vested in a bailiff appointed by the bishop. About 1440, the title of the principal civil officer was changed from " bailiff of the borough," to " bailiff of the city ;" and in 1171 the first charter was granted by Bishop Pudsey to the burgesses, by which they were exempted from the payment of tolls and other feudal exactions, granting also " all such free customs as the burgesses of Newcastle en-

Corporate Seal.

joyed." From this period to the Reformation, the city was governed by a bailiff, but an officer was then appointed under the statute of Edward III. and other laws, who, under the title of marshal, or clerk of the markets, kept the alnage seal both for the city and province. In 1377, Bishop Hatfield granted a charter imposing certain duties on wares coming into the city, as a fund for keeping the walls and pavement in repair. A charter of incorporation was granted in 1565, by Bishop Pilkington, vesting the government in an alderman and twelve burgesses, and authorising a weekly market and three annual fairs : in 1602, Bishop Matthew granted a new charter, whereby the body politic and corporate was made to consist of a mayor, twelve aldermen, and a common council, with divers privileges, power to purchase lands, and a common seal. This was confirmed by James I., and several charters were subsequently obtained. The charter of 1602 continued in force till 1684, when Bishop Crewe granted a new one, which, owing to some informality, was set aside, when the former being restored, subsisted till 1761, when the corporation was dissolved, in consequence of irregularities in the election of the mayor and other members ; the city was then placed under the government of a bailiff, till Bishop Egerton granted a new charter in 1780, which is still in force. This charter ordains that the corporation shall consist of a mayor, twelve aldermen, twenty-four common council-men, with a recorder, town clerk, two serjeants at mace, and other inferior officers, under the designation of " The Mayor, Aldermen, and Commonalty of Durham and Framwellgate." The election of the mayor takes place annually on the first Monday after the Feast of St. Michael, and for common council-men on the following Monday ; the latter are chosen from thirteen incorporated companies : there are also three more incorporated companies, but they have not a representative in the common council. Neither the mayor nor any other member of the corporation possesses magisterial authority, the county magistrates exercising jurisdiction within the city. The corporation hold a court leet and a court baron, as lessees of the manor, under the Bishop of Durham, for the recovery of debts under 40s. A court of pleas for the county palatine is held by prescription every three weeks, with trials twice a year before the judges travelling the northern circuit ; it is a superior court of record, in which sums to any amount are recoverable : the assizes for the county are also held here. In the market-place is the guildhall, erected by Bishop Tunstall, in 1555, and repaired by George Bowes, Esq., in 1752 ; in the back room of which edifice are portraits of Charles II. and Bishop Crewe ; in the front room, which was built in 1754, public meetings are held. The exchequer, built in 1450, by Bishop Neville, is on the Palace Green ; within it are offices for the auditor, cursitor, prothonotary, treasurer, and clerk of the county, registrar, &c. In 1809, extensive buildings, comprising a house of correction, county courts, and a new gaol, were erected at the expense of £120,000. : the prisoners are divided into thirteen classes ; and there are forty-eight wards, three work-rooms, eighteen day-rooms, and thirteen airing-yards, besides a chapel, school-room, &c. : a tread-mill has been erected, but the prisoners are employed chiefly in weaving woollen and linen cloth. The elective franchise was conferred by act of parliament, in 1673, since which time the city has returned two members : the freedom is acquired by birth for *all the sons* of freemen of two incorporated companies, and for the *eldest sons only* of freemen belonging to the remaining eleven, and by servitude : the right of election belongs to the members of the corporation and the freemen, resident and non-resident, amounting to about twelve hundred; the mayor is the returning officer.

The bishoprick of Durham is one of the most wealthy in the kingdom : it includes the county of Durham, and all Northumberland (excepting those parishes which are within the peculiar jurisdiction of Hexham), and the parishes of Alston-Moor, in Cumberland, and Craike and Howden, in Yorkshire, making a total of one hundred and thirty-five parishes,

Arms of the Bishoprick.

whereof eighty-seven are impropriate ; there are two archdeaconries, and nine deaneries. This see has given eight saints and one cardinal to the church of Rome ; one lord chief justice, five lord chancellors, three lord treasurers, one principal secretary of state, one chancellor to the University of Oxford, and two masters of the rolls, to the British nation. The Bishop of Durham is a secular prince, and as Earl of Sadberg, and Count Palatine of Durham, he is *Custos Rotulorum* of the county: before the abridgment of his privileges by Henry VIII., he had power to create barons, to appoint judges, convoke parliaments, raise taxes, and coin money ; the courts of justice were held in his name, and he could grant pardons for offences and felonies of all kinds ; he granted markets and fairs, was lord admiral within the county palatine, and a great part of the lands was held of him *in capite*. The judges and officers of the court still receive their ancient salaries from the bishop, who even now exercises the right of presiding at the assizes, attired in purple robes, with the judges on the circuit ; he also appoints the high sheriff, who accounts to the bishop, without being responsible to His Majesty's exchequer.

The cathedral is situated on an eminence partly clothed with plantations and gardens, and almost encircled by the river; near it is the bishop's palace, constructed from the remains of the ancient castle, the deanery and other ecclesiastical residences : the general aspect of this mass of building is at every point of view peculiarly grand and impressive. The north front faces an open space between the venerable cathedral and the castle ; on the south and east it is so surrounded as to prevent a complete view, but from the opposite bank of the river the western front is visible, under that advantage of distance which is favourable to the concealment of the more modern alterations in detail, which have taken place during the various repairs it has undergone : the plan exhibits a Galilee at the west front, a nave, aisles, and transept, with a choir and aisles, and the chapel of nine altars (extending beyond the north and south walls of the building) assuming the appearance of a second transept. The length of the edifice is four hundred and twenty feet ; the interior of the Galilee seventy-eight

by fifty; the height of the central tower two hundred and twelve, and that of the western towers each one hundred and forty-three. The general character of the largest portion of this cathedral is Norman, of a very bold character, with insertions in all the English styles. The foundation was laid on the 2nd of August, 1093, by Bishop Carilepho ; and the chapel of Galilee, or the Lady chapel, at the western end, was built by Bishop Pudsey, who had previously commenced the erection of a chapel at the eastern end of the edifice, for the devotional exercises of females, which was discontinued in consequence of the prevailing superstition of those times. The north aisle was for a long time used as a depository for wills, where also the register-office was kept prior to the erection of the present building in 1822; but it has been re-united to the fabric, and divine service is performed in it every Sunday evening during the summer months. The eastern portion of the choir, called the Chapel of the Nine Altars, is in the early English style, having a large decorated window at the north end : the large west window, and that of the north transept, are also of the decorated character, with rich composition ; and in various parts of the cathedral are many windows of a similar style, with fine tracery inserted in the openings, of earlier date. The two western towers are Norman below, the upper portions English, with an intermixture of semicircular and pointed arches ; to these have been added, during the late repair, pinnacles and a pierced battlement. The great central tower is very lofty ; of later English architecture above the nave, with Norman piers and arches below; and the upper story is short in comparison with the base : this tower has recently undergone an entire repair. The nave is magnificent in its proportions, and very bold in its details. The central tower is open to a great height, and although in other parts the effect is diminished, owing to the situation of the church not permitting a western entrance, and the division between the Galilee and the nave, this portion is exceedingly fine. The organ-screen, elaborately carved in oak, is of Italian character, which by no means harmonises with that of the cathedral, and, being almost black with age, and contrasted with the whiteness of the nave, abruptly terminates the view. Behind the screen is the chapel called the Feretory, where stood the gorgeous shrine of St. Cuthbert, erected over the place where his bones were deposited : during the progress of some alterations immediately behind this shrine, on the 17th of May, 1827, the vault, supposed to contain the holy relics, was opened, when a chest, apparently of oak, was discovered, in which lay the perfect skeleton of the saint, in vestments of linen and silk, which, having lain for inspection for some time, was carefully covered over, and the vault closed. The eastern arch of the choir is in the early English style ; and the altar-screen, in tabernacle-work of the later style, corresponds with the screen-work of the bishop's throne, which is erected over the magnificent tomb of Bishop Hatfield. The groins of the nave and choir are also in the early English style, the latter being of somewhat later character. The Norman portions of the cathedral, particularly several very curious door-ways, deserve great attention. The cathedral library contains five books of Ecclesiastical History, written by Bede, and a copy of the Bible, both in manuscript, supposed to be six hundred years old.

At the time of the dissolution, Hugh Whitehead held the priory, which was then rated at about £1600 per annum; and on the 12th of May, 1541, Henry VIII. granted his foundation charter to this church, altering its dedication from St. Mary and St. Cuthbert, to that of Christ and St. Mary. He instituted a dean and twelve prebendaries as a body corporate, and granted them the site of the monastery, with its ancient rights. The duties of the cathedral are now performed by a bishop, dean, twelve prebendaries, eight minor canons, eight singing men, an organist and choristers, and two bell-ringers, a master and under master of the grammar school, and eighteen scholars, besides servants; and eight poor men are supported by the establishment. The school in connexion with the cathedral has four exhibitions for sons of clergymen, of £25 per annum each at school, and £50 each per annum, at either of the Universities, given by the Dean and Chapter, who are trustees of the institution: it has also five scholarships, of £10 per annum each, at Peter House, Cambridge, founded by John Cosins, D. D., Bishop of Durham; one scholarship, of £16 per annum, at Emanuel College, Cambridge, founded by the Rev. Dr. Michael Smith, jointly with the school at Newcastle upon Tyne, for which also, and for this school, Dr. Hartwell bequeathed £20 per annum, to be divided between two exhibitioners at either University, and tenable for five years. In addition to the eighteen boys on the foundation, there are about sixty who pay a regular quarterage.

The city comprises the following parishes, all in the archdeaconry and diocese of Durham, viz., St Giles', or Gillegate, a perpetual curacy, endowed with £400 private benefaction, £400 royal bounty, and £1000 parliamentary grant, and in the patronage of the Marquis of Londonderry: the church has various portions in the Norman style of architecture, but the general style resembles the Galilee chapel of the cathedral. St. Mary's le Bow, North Bailey, a rectory not in charge, endowed with £400 private benefaction, £200 royal bounty, and £1100 parliamentary grant, and in the patronage of the Archdeacon of Northumberland: the church, which was rebuilt in 1685, is supposed to occupy the site of the chapel in which St. Cuthbert's remains were originally deposited; the bishop's and archdeacon's visitations are now held in it. St. Mary's the Less, South Bailey, a rectory not in charge, endowed with £200 private benefaction, and £600 royal bounty, and in the patronage of the Crown: the church is an ancient edifice, with modern alterations, and has only a mean appearance. St. Nicholas', a perpetual curacy, endowed with £400 private benefaction, £400 royal bounty, and £1200 parliamentary grant, and in the patronage of the Marquis of Londonderry: the church is a building of considerable antiquity, which, in 1768, was repaired, with the addition of an east window; it is that attended by the corporation. St. Oswald's, or Elvet, a vicarage, rated in the king's books at £16, and in the patronage of the Dean and Chapter of Durham: the church is a large and handsome edifice, the lower part of which is in the early English style, the windows and other portions decorated, and the tower and upper part of the building later English, with a vaulted wooden roof, supposed to have been constructed by William Catton, vicar, in the beginning of the fifteenth century. St. Margaret's, or Crossgate, is a perpetual curacy to the vicarage of St.

Oswald, endowed with £40 per annum private benefaction, and £400 royal bounty, and in the patronage of the Dean and Chapter of Durham: the church, an ancient Norman structure, with a low square tower, has undergone much alteration at different periods. There are places of worship for the Society of Friends, Independents, Primitive and Wesleyan Methodists, and Roman Catholics, the last having erected a handsome edifice in 1826, which has a stained window representing Christ in the garden of Gethsemane.

In addition to the cathedral grammar school abovementioned, are the united Blue-coat and Sunday schools, situated on the north side of Clay-path, erected by public subscription, and opened in 1812. To this institution Bishop Barrington subscribed £309. 17., being the purchase money of the ground on which it was erected. There are infant schools in which about one hundred and seventy children are instructed; a charity school in Gravel-lane, Hallgarth-street, endowed by Dr. Cox with £20 per annum, for educating the poor children of St. Oswald's parish, and Sunday schools attached to some of the religious communities: it is calculated that, altogether, the total number of children receiving gratuitous instruction in this city and its suburbs is one thousand and seventy-two. The infirmary is a spacious building in Allergate, erected by subscription in 1792, on a piece of ground given by Thomas Wilkinson, Esq., of Coxhoe: the average annual expenditure is about £800: it is supported by annual subscriptions and donations. Almshouses on Palace Green were founded in 1668, by Bishop Cosins, for four poor men and four poor women, who receive an annuity of £70, arising out of lands at Great Chilton, which is equally divided amongst the inmates by quarterly payments: the almspeople are appointed by the bishop, part to be natives of Durham, and part of Branspeth. Some school-houses attached were endowed by Bishop Langley, with a rent-charge of £16. 13. 4., arising out of the manor of Kaverdley, in Lancashire; but this charity has been transferred to the Blue-coat schools, and Bishop Cosins' school-houses converted into tenements. There is a long list of benefactors to the poor, among whom is Henry Smith, who in 1598 bequeathed his coal mines and personal estate to supply a fund for apprenticing poor boys, which property now produces £130 per annum. In addition to the above are several charitable associations and benefit societies, especially that of the Free Masons, who in 1810 erected a neat brick building in Old Elvet, called "Granby Lodge." An agricultural society holds its anniversary at the Waterloo Inn: there is a savings' bank in the town-hall. About three quarters of a mile eastward from the city is Old Durham, a spot supposed by some to have been occupied by the Saxons, before the foundation of the present city, and by others to have been a Roman station: it still exhibits a few traces of antiquity. Opposite to it, on the southern bank of the Wear, is the site of a fortification with more probability ascribed to the Romans, called Maiden Castle; and some remains of the Iknield-street, or Roman way, are discernible in the neighbourhood. Within one mile north-east of Durham, on the banks of the Wear, are the few remains of Kepier hospital, a monastic institution, founded in 1112, by Bishop Flambard, for the maintenance of a master and twelve brethren, valued at the dissolution

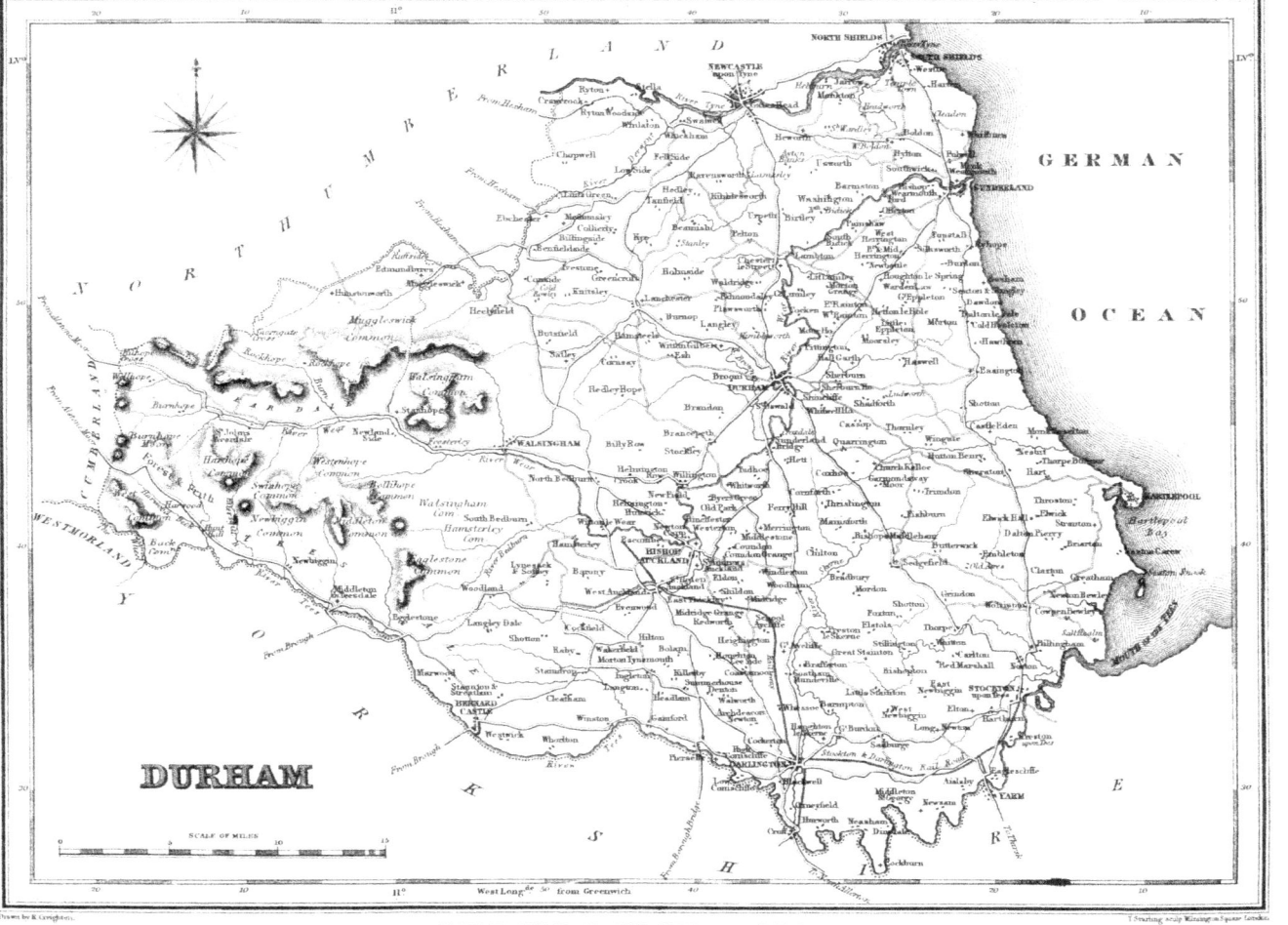

DURHAM

Drawn by R. Creighton.

DRAWN AND ENGRAVED FOR LEWIS TOPOGRAPHICAL DICTIONARY.

J. Starling sculp. Wilmington Square London.

SCALE OF MILES

West Long.ᵗʰᵉ 50' from Greenwich

at £186. 0. 10 : they consist of a gateway with pointed arches. The manor-house of Houghall, built by Prior Hotoun, is about a mile from the city ; and two miles distant is Beautrove, now Butterby, remarkable for its beauty and natural curiosities. In the moat surrounding the old mansion, a coat of mail was discovered, and in an adjoining field, the supposed site of an ancient hospital, several stone coffins and jars have been dug up. Here are saline, sulphureous, and chalybeate springs, the former of which are much frequented by persons who drink the waters medicinally. A mile westward from the city is the fragment of a once beautiful cross, called Nevill's cross, erected by Ralph, Lord Nevill, in commemoration of a battle in 1346, in which David Bruce, King of Scotland, was taken prisoner. The following literary persons were natives of Durham, Robert Hegg, author of the legend of St. Cuthbert, &c.; John Hall, a celebrated English poet of the seventeenth century, who, besides a volume of poems published a translation of Eugenius ; Dr. Richard Grey, author of the Memoria Technica, and several other works, born in 1693 ; William Eden, Lord Auckland, a distinguished statesman and diplomatist. Durham gives the title of baron to the Lambton family, the present representative of which was raised to the peerage by this title in January, 1828.

DURHAM (COUNTY of), a maritime county and a county palatine, bounded on the north by the county of Northumberland, on the east by the German ocean, on the south by the county of York, and on the west by the counties of Westmorland and Cumberland : it extends from 54° 29′ to 55° 3′ (N. Lat.), and from 1° 12′ to 2° 20′ (W. Lon.), and includes, without the detached portions, about six hundred and ten thousand acres, or nine hundred and fifty-three square miles. The population, in 1821, amounted to 207,673. That portion of the present county palatine of Durham which lies between the rivers Tees and Tyne, formed part of the extensive territories held by the powerful British tribe, whom the Romans denominated Brigantes. The districts of Norham, Holy Island, and Bedlington, were included in the possessions of the Ottadini, who occupied the eastern coast from the Tyne to the Frith of Forth. In the Roman division of Britain, these districts were all included in *Maxima Cæsariensis* ; and in the time of the Heptarchy they constituted part of the Anglo-Saxon kingdom of Northumberland. That kingdom itself was generally sub-divided into the two petty states of *Bernicia*, including the northern, and *Deira*, the southern portion, Durham appearing to have formed part of the latter. Although Christianity had been embraced by Edwin, King of Northumberland, yet its general introduction into that country, and the consequent origin of the see of Lindisfarne, from which that of Durham is derived, cannot be dated earlier than the reign of the Northumbrian king, Oswald. Aidan, a Scottish monk, who, after Oswald had embraced Christianity, had voluntarily undertaken the task of converting the rest of the Northumbrian nation, chose for the residence of himself and his brethren, the small island of Lindisfarne, separated twice each day from the coast of Northumberland by the influx of the tide, and situated within view of the town of Bambrough, at that time the residence of the Northumbrian kings. Finan, the successor of Aidan, is said to have erected a church in Lindisfarne,

built of timber, and covered with reeds, after the manner of those in Scotland. At this period the Scottish church had not acknowledged the ecclesiastical superiority claimed by the bishops of the Romish church; for, at a synod held in the abbey of Whitby, in 664, in the presence of Oswy, King of Northumberland, Colman, the successor of Finan, defended the regulations and the independence of his own church, against Wilfrid, afterwards Archbishop of York, who contended for the supremacy of Rome : the decision of the assembly, however, was in favour of the latter ; the observance of the Romish rites was established, and Colman, in consequence, relinquished the see, and returned into Scotland : he was succeeded by Tuda, who died within the same year, and was the last of the Scottish bishops of Lindisfarne ; his successors in the Northumbrian diocese fixing their residence at York. On pretence, however, of the inconvenient extent of that diocese, Theodore, Archbishop of Canterbury, erected Lindisfarne into a separate see, bestowing on it the spiritual jurisdiction of the province of Bernicia, and confining that of the see of York to the southern province of Deira. The Danish conquests and devastations in that part of England, about the close of the eighth century, occasioned the cathedral and monastery of Lindisfarne to be abandoned, and when the exertions of Alfred had triumphed over the invaders, Chester le Street, as being more securely situated, was chosen for the future residence of the ecclesiastics, and the whole county between the Tees and the Tyne was added to the patrimony of St. Cuthbert, who had been the second bishop of the new diocese of Lindisfarne, and who, having been for his great sanctity canonized after his death, was now regarded as the patron saint of the diocese : it was at the same time provided, that whatever lands should thereafter accrue to the see by purchase or benefaction, should be held by the successors of St. Cuthbert, discharged of every temporal service. The Danish invasions in the reign of Ethelred compelled the bishop and his ecclesiastics, in 995, to desert Chester le Street, and take shelter in the monastery of Ripon ; and on the return of peace the see was again removed from Chester to a place called Dunholme, still more strongly and securely situated. The gifts and oblations of the wealthy here flowed in profusely; and this was the origin of the present city of Durham. At the same time the patrimony of St. Cuthbert also received large accessions of territory from the donations of two individuals. The Danish sovereign, Canute, visited the shrine of St. Cuthbert, and made munificent donations of territory to the bishoprick. In the twentieth year of Bishop Eadmund, the Scots made an irruption as far as Durham, where they lost most of their troops.

At the time of the Norman Conquest, Bishop Egelwin, together with the Earls Edwin and Morcar, submitted to William, and swore allegiance to him at York. The possession of the northern portion of the Northumbrian province, however, was considered as very insecure, and the task of its entire subjugation was soon after entrusted by the Conqueror to Robert Comyn, a Norman nobleman, who, in carrying the design into execution, was met on the confines of the bishoprick by Egelwin, who is said to have warned him of the turbulent state of the people, notwithstanding which he persisted in marching to Durham with seven hundred troops, where, after a series of oppressive and cruel acts and continued licentiousness, he and his followers were massacred in an insurrection of the inhabitants. William, enraged at this, marched northward in person, and devastated the whole country, devoting the inhabitants to military execution. The royal troops were scarcely withdrawn when Malcolm, King of Scotland, at the head of a marauding army, penetrated through Cumberland into Cleveland and the bishoprick, ravaged Teesdale, and burned the towns and monasteries of Hartlepool and Wearmouth. Under the Norman yoke, the patrimony of the church was obliged, equally with the possessions of the laity, to provide soldiers and military aids; and Bishop Egelwin, having once more engaged in the enterprise of the Earls Edwin and Morcar, was taken, through treachery, with the other heads of his party, in the Isle of Ely, and sent prisoner to Abingdon, where he died in confinement. Shortly afterwards occurred the remarkable insurrection, in which the prelate Walcher, who had been appointed by the Conqueror to succeed the last mentioned bishop, was put to death by the insurgents at Gateshead. A second plundering of the bishoprick ensued, no less dreadful than the first; the Norman army being led by Eudes, or Odo, the military bishop of Baieux. After the permanent establishment of the Norman rule over all the provinces of England, the calamities which for several centuries most seriously afflicted this county, to whose devastations it was exposed by its vicinity to the border; hence the military transactions within the county during that long period, including the various marches of the English forces through this territory in their operations against the Scots, are much too numerous to recount; the most remarkable of them seems to have been the battle of Nevill's Cross, fought on Red hills, on the 17th of October, 1346, between David, King of Scotland, and Philippa, Queen of Edward III., assisted by Ralph, Lord Nevill, in which the Scottish king was taken prisoner, with the loss of from fifteen to twenty thousand men.

During the parliamentary war, the Scottish army, under Lesley, passed the Tyne at Newburn, on the 28th of August, 1640, after defeating the king's troops under Lord Conway, stationed there to oppose them; and the next morning the latter abandoned Newcastle, and pursued their march through this county into Yorkshire, to join the main body of the royal army, which was advancing under Lord Strafford. The Scots, entering Newcastle the same day, thus obtained possession of Northumberland and Durham; and the people, panic-struck and deserted by the regular troops, seem to have offered no farther opposition. In the accommodation which was soon after entered into with Scotland, the first preliminary article was, that the counties of Durham and Northumberland, and the town of Newcastle, should be charged with the sum of £850 per day, by weekly payments, for the maintenance of the Scottish army; under which burden the two counties continued until the conclusion of the definitive treaty with Scotland, on the 7th of August, 1641, when the British government was indebted to the bishoprick of Durham in a balance of £25,663. 13. 10. The day after the defeat at Newburn, Bishop Morton fled from Durham to his castle at Stockton, and from that place, soon after, to York and London, whence he never again returned to his diocese. At the same time nearly the whole of

the clergy deserted the cathedral, and the see and episcopal government of Durham were now virtually dissolved; the whole revenue of the former was seized by the Scots, the bishop's officers fled or were displaced, and the administration of the county passed entirely into the hands of the invaders, who, not long after, were succeeded by the parliamentary commissioners for treating with the second Scottish army, under David Lesley. In November, 1642, the Earl of Newcastle formed the counties of Northumberland, Durham, Cumberland, and Westmorland, and the town of Newcastle, into an association for the king's service: in the month of December, having been ordered to lead his forces towards York, he began his march from Newcastle, and the next day, after a skirmish of several hours with Captain Hotham, passed the Tyne at Pier's bridge. This county was not subsequently the scene of any action of importance until the second entry of the Scottish army into England, which crossed the Tyne on the 28th of February, 1644, at the three fords of Ovingham, Bywell, and Eltringham, and entered Sunderland on the 4th of March. The Marquis of Newcastle, with the Yorkshire cavalry under Sir George Lucas, being in possession of the city of Durham, kept them in check until the disasters of the royal party in Yorkshire occasioned the recal of the marquis from the north, and his departure from this county, by way of Pier's bridge, on the 14th of April. On the 20th, Lesley joined the parliament's forces under Fairfax at Tadcaster. The capture of Newcastle on the 19th of October following, placed the bishoprick of Durham entirely under the power of the parliament; and from that time it was, in effect, governed by Sir William Armine, and the rest of the parliamentary commissioners, and by the noted family of Lilburne, and Sir Arthur Haslerigg, whose extensive purchases of lands belonging to the see, sold by order of parliament, acquired him the nickname of the Bishop of Durham. In 1646, when the Scots had determined on delivering up King Charles to the English parliament, he was removed on the 3rd of February from Newcastle to Durham, on the 4th to Auckland, and on the 5th to Richmond, on his way to Holdenby House. This was one of the seven northern counties which, in 1648, when a last attempt was made by the royalists in the north to seize some of the strong places, was ordered by parliament to be associated forthwith, and put in a posture of defence. In 1651 and 1652, two acts were passed for the sale of the estates of several royalist gentlemen in the bishoprick, who had refused to compound for them. In 1653, the county of Durham, or a committee so styling themselves, presented an address to the Lord General Cromwell and his council of officers, expressing their adherence to his person and government, but it was signed by only one person of considerable family or connexions in the county; which, indeed, was one of those to which the restoration of royalty gave the greatest satisfaction.

This county lies within the diocese of Durham, and province of York, and forms an archdeaconry, comprising the deaneries of Chester le Street, Darlington, Easington, and Stockton, and containing seventy-five parishes, of which thirty-two are rectories, twenty-three vicarages, and twenty perpetual curacies: there are also twenty-four dependent chapels. For civil purposes it is divided into the four wards of Chester, Darlington, Easington, and Stockton. It rose gradually out of the ancient province of Northumberland, together with the increasing patrimony of the church of St. Cuthbert, and besides its principal portion, lying between the rivers Tyne, Tees, and Darwent, includes several scattered members of that patrimony, *viz.*, Norhamshire and Islandshire, including Holy Island and the Farne Isles, and a portion of the mainland, extending from the Tweed on the north and north-west, to the sea on the east, and separated from Northumberland on the south, partly by the course of the Till, and partly by an imaginary line; and Bedlingtonshire, lying in the heart of Northumberland, betwixt the rivers Blyth and Wansbeck : these are usually termed the north bishoprick, and are included in Chester ward besides the insulated territory of Craike, locally in the wapentake of Bulmer, in Yorkshire. The county contains the city of Durham, and the market towns of Barnard-Castle, Bishop-Auckland, Sunderland, Darlington, Gateshead, Hartlepool, Sedgefield, South Shields, Staindrop, Stanhope, Stockton upon Tees, and Walsingham, of which number, Hartlepool, South Shields, Stockton upon Tees, and Sunderland, are sea-ports. Two knights are returned to parliament for the county palatine, and two representatives for the city of Durham. The county members are elected at Durham. This county is included in the northern circuit : the assizes and the quarter sessions are held at Durham, where stands the county gaol and house of correction. There are seventy-four acting magistrates. The rates raised in the county for the year ending March 25th, 1827, amounted to £94,417. 13., the expenditure to £94,181. 6., of which £76,702. 17., was applied to the relief of the poor.

Although the present county of Durham is considered to be a county palatine by prescription, yet the first prelate who is known to have exercised the palatine jurisdiction was Bishop Walcher, who, soon after his elevation to this see, received also from the Conqueror the earldom of Northumberland, vacant by the wellknown deposition and death of the Saxon earl, Waltheof : it is probable that either then, or at some period very soon after, by grant, or tacit permission, the palatine powers were assumed by Walcher to the same extent in which they were constantly exercised by his successors. For the extent of these powers at that period, the situation of Durham as a border county, and the general disaffection of the Northumbrian province to the Norman government, appears sufficiently to account. From this time owning, within the limits of the palatinate, no earthly superior, the successive prelates continued for four centuries to exercise every right attached to a distinct and independent sovereignty. These rights included the paramount seignorial property of all lands ; the supreme jurisdiction, as well civil as military, the former exercised by the establishment of courts of law and equity, the appointment of officers, and the levying of taxes and subsidies, the latter by the power of array ; together with a jurisdiction of admiralty, as well along the coast as in the navigable and other waters ; and the privilege of coining money. These privileges continued unabridged until the passing of the statute of resumption in the 27th of Henry VIII., the most important provisions of which were as follows : the bishop was deprived of the privilege of pardoning treason, murder, manslaughter, felony, reversing out-

lawries, and of the appointment of the justices of the peace and of assize : all writs were directed to run in the king's name, and the ancient form of indictment, " *Contra pacem Episcopi*," was altered to the usual one, " Against the King's peace ;" and all sheriffs, bailiffs, and other officers, were made amenable to the general laws of the realm. The right of altering all processes within the franchise was reserved to the bishop, and it was directed that the bishop and his temporal chancellor should be always, *ipso facto*, two of the justices of the peace. The next invasion of the rights of the bishoprick was in the following reign, by the contrivance of Dudley, Duke of Northumberland, when, on the 21st of March, 1553, a bill was read for suppressing the bishoprick of Durham ; and "for the better preaching of God's Holy Word in those parts," it was proposed that two bishopricks should be endowed in that diocese, one at Durham, with a revenue of two thousand marks, the other at Newcastle, with a revenue of one thousand marks ; and by a patent, dated in May of the same year, the duke was appointed steward of all the remaining revenues of the bishoprick. On the accession of Mary, the bishoprick of Durham was restored by act of parliament ; but the influence of its bishop, Tunstall, was successfully exerted in screening the objects of religious persecution, so that no person suffered for heresy within the limits of his extensive diocese. In consequence of the ordinance for the total abolition of episcopacy, which passed both houses of parliament on the 9th of October, 1646, followed by an order for the sale of bishops' lands for the use of the commonwealth, the palatinate of Durham was dissolved, and from that year a sheriff for the county was annually appointed by parliament, who accounted to the public treasury : the ancient palatine courts of law and equity were suspended, and commissioners appointed to sit on gaol deliveries : a seneschal was also appointed for the court of halmote, who acted as such in the name of the different persons by whom the copyhold manors of the see had been purchased. The county, which, owing to its palatine privileges, had never before sent knights or burgesses to parliament, was represented in Cromwell's three parliaments of 1653, 1654, and 1656. The Restoration produced the restitution of the temporalties and privileges of the see, on the 14th of December, 1660. In the reign of Charles II., a bill was passed to enable the county palatine and city of Durham to send knights and burgesses to parliament, the first elections in pursuance of which took place in 1675.

The general aspect of the coast is bare and dreary; but between the swells of country lie numerous deep and narrow dells, the scenery of which is of a more pleasing character. Every brook which falls into the sea has its banks adorned with a profusion of romantic objects : the vales commencing imperceptibly together with the course of their streamlets, sometimes contract into narrow glens, scarcely affording a single rugged foot-path; sometimes open into irregular amphitheatres of rock, covered with native ash or hazel, or deepen into ravines resembling the bed of a rapid river, terminating on the coast, either in wide sandy bays, or in narrow outlets, where the stream mines its way under crags of the wildest and most grotesque appearance. In a district extending from the sea coast nearly to the top of Cross Fell, which is the highest land in England, (being three thousand four hundred feet above the level of the sea), and in which the rise is tolerably uniform from the coast to the western mountains, there is necessarily a considerable variety of climate.

The soil varies by such imperceptible degrees, as to render it difficult to describe all its diversities; clay, loam, and peat, may, however, be considered as the principal heads of classification. The south-eastern part of the county, from the mouth of the Tees to a few miles west of Stockton, and thence by Redmarshall, Wolviston, Elwick, and as far north as Hart, consists of a strong, fertile, clayey loam, which produces good crops of wheat, beans, and clover, and has rich old grazing pastures. Westward from this, as far as Sedgefield, Trimdon, and Eppleton, and northward nearly to Sunderland, the soil is chiefly a stubborn unprofitable clay, which produces thin crops of corn, and, when suffered to remain in grass, yields a herbage which scarcely any kind of stock will eat, except when compelled by hunger. A clayey soil, of an intermediate quality exists in numerous parts of the county. The deep, dry, fertile loams are generally found in the vicinity of rivers, as in the vales of Tees, Skern, Tyne, and their tributary streams; those on the Wear are of a more sandy nature: dry fertile loams are also found in small patches in many other parts of the county. The limestone district, extending from near Sunderland, by Houghton le Spring, Kelloe, Coxhoe, Ferry-Hill, and to Merrington, is mostly a dry, but not a productive loam, being very different from that which covers the limestone in the western parts of the county, where there are some of the most fertile soils and best grazing lands in the north of England. A moist soft loam, lying on a yellow ochreous clay, impervious to water and unfavourable to vegetation, is very extensively distributed through many parts of the county, and is known by the provincial epithet of "water-shaken:" it is generally thin, and the water being kept so near the surface occasions the plants to be thrown out by frost. The peaty soil is most prevalent in the western parts of the county, the greater portion of the moors which have been enclosed being of that description; it is generally accompanied with sub-strata of yellow ochreous clay, or white sand, in both cases unproductive. With respect to the agricultural peculiarities of this county, it may be mentioned that rye is very rarely cultivated alone, as the proportion of sandy soil suitable to the growth of that species of grain, is very small; but a mixture of rye and wheat, provincially termed maslin, or mislen is very generally produced. Mustard was formerly much cultivated in the county, and the "Durham mustard" was proverbial for its excellence, but the practice has almost wholly declined. The old meadow lands are nearly all upland meadows: the best old grazing pastures are on Skernside, and at Binchester, Stanhope, Billingham, Staindrop, Barnard-Castle, and a few other places. The climate is not favourable for orchards, so that the fruit produced is not nearly equal to the consumption, a considerable quantity being imported. The best wooded part is the vale of Derwent, the soil of which is peculiarly favourable to the growth of wood, especially of oak; in this vale is also a considerable quantity of underwood, particularly hazels. Within the last eighty years plantations have been made to a great extent, especially in the vicinity of gentlemen's seats. The cattle bred here for a great number of years have

been of the short-horned kind, the best variety of which having been long found on both sides of the river Tees, has for a considerable period been known by the appellation of "the Tees-water breed." The lower parts of the county were formerly famed for having the largest breed of sheep in the kingdom, many of them weighing from fifty pounds to sixty pounds a quarter; but of late years, the introduction of the Leicestershire breed has reduced the size of the Durham sheep, and improved the quality of their mutton: the rot is a malady in this animal very extensively felt over a large portion of the county. The south-eastern part of Durham, like the adjoining part of Yorkshire, has long been celebrated for a valuable breed of draught horses, with well-formed carcases, and strong, sinewy, light legs, known by the name of "Cleveland bays." The most prevailing breeds of swine are, the Berkshire black and white, which are large-boned, and a small white sort, bred in Leicestershire and Norfolk, which have a great propensity to fatten, and have very little offal. The wastes, with very few exceptions, consist of heathy moors; they are all situated in the western and mountainous part of the county, and are almost invariably covered with the common heath, or ling: the use of the greater part is in depasturing sheep of the black-faced kind. The improvable moors, fells, or commons, have chiefly been divided and enclosed. The principal embankment is that of Saltholm and Billingham marsh, near the mouth of the Tees, extending four miles, and enclosing one thousand four hundred acres.

The first agricultural society established in the county was at Darlington, in 1783, and was denominated the Agricultural Society for the county of Durham; they had four general meetings annually; two at Durham, and two at Darlington. In 1802, an agricultural society was formed at Barnard-Castle, and, in 1806, another at Walsingham; and, between that year and 1810, another at Shiney-Row, near Chester le Street. In 1805, one was established by a number of gentlemen on both sides of the Tyne; and, being limited to that district, was called the Tyne-side Society. Besides these, a society for agricultural experiments was formed in 1803, and agreed to meet four times a year at Rusheyford.

Coal is found throughout a considerable portion of the county; it is of the caking kind, burns into excellent cinders, and leaves few ashes: that in the western part of the county is of the best quality. The coal district is chiefly bounded on the east by the collieries of Jarrow, Penshaw, Rainton, Crowtrees, and Ferry Hill; on the west, by Wylam, Consit, Thornley, West Pits, and Woodlands; on the north by the river Tyne; and on the south by Ferry Hill, Brusleton, Cockfield, and Woodlands; including a space twenty-two miles long, eleven miles and a half broad, and comprising one hundred and sixty thousand acres, of which the water-sale collieries are about one-third, and the land-sale collieries two-thirds. In this space are found various strata, or seams of coal, differing in thickness and quality. Many of the collieries in the northern parts of the county are wrought for exportation, but those in the south and west are worked for land sale only. In 1810, there were employed in the coal trade upon the river Wear, six hundred and thirty-four keels, and one thousand two hundred and fifty-seven men: at the same time, the number of men employed in the same trade on the Tyne, was about two thousand. The coal trade also affords employment to a great number of workmen of various descriptions, such as carpenters, masons, smiths, founders, rope-makers, ship-builders, &c. Of the land-sale collieries the most valuable are those on the south side of the county, from which the southern part of Durham, and the northern parts of Yorkshire, are supplied. The quantity of coal obtained in the county annually, has been estimated to be, in the water-sale collieries, one million three hundred and thirty-three thousand chaldrons, of thirty-six bushels, affording employment to seven thousand and eleven pitmen; and in the land-sale collieries, one hundred and forty-seven thousand and eighty chaldrons, employing three hundred and eighty-two pitmen : the total number of men employed, including the keelmen, &c., on the two rivers, was ten thousand six hundred and fifty. The coal was formerly drawn out of the pits by horses, eight being frequently employed for that purpose where the shafts were deep; but within the last thirty years, machines have been erected for drawing them by steam, which are now in general use. The lead mines are situated in the western part of the county, and begin a little westward of the line where the coal district terminates. The number of lead mines in operation in 1809 was, in Tees dale, forty-eight; in Wear dale, thirty-eight; and in the vale of Derwent four : from many of these little ore was obtained, and some were being worked at a considerable loss. The ore is wrought by the bing of eight hundred weight, and four bings of clean ore generally produce a ton of lead. The rent paid to the proprietors of lead mines is usually one-fifth of the ore : the total number of smelting-mills, in the same year, was ten. Iron-ore is found in abundance in the western parts of the coal district, and great quantities have been smelted at some remote period, as is evident from the immense heaps of iron slag found in various places on the commons of Lanchester, Tanfield, Hamsterley, Evenwood, &c., and traditionally said to have been works of the Danes. Freestone for building, and grey slate for roofing, are met with in various parts of the county. In the south-eastern part is a limestone district bounded by Pierse-Bridge, Consley, Umby, Denton, Killerby, Langton, and Morton : farther north is another, on the ridge extending from Houghton, by Heighington, to Aykley; and farther still is a third, forming that hilly tract which extends from Merrington, by Ferry Hill, Bishop-Middleham, Coxhoe, Sherburn, Ellemore, Houghton le Spring, Pallion, Boldon, and Cleadon, and thence southward along the coast, to near Hartlepool. Limestone of the best quality abounds also in the lead-mining district; and in Wear dale, near Frosterley, is a vein which, from the stone being variegated, and taking a fine polish, is denominated marble, and is used for chimney-pieces and tomb-stones. Whin-stone is got in different parts of the Cockfield Fell dyke, and in many other similar places, for repairing roads, for which purpose it is superior to any other material yet discovered. The manufactures are various : Darlington has long been noted for that of linen, which is also carried on at Bishop-Auckland, Stanhope, and Stockton. Carpets are made at Barnard-Castle and Durham. The worsted manufacture is considerable at Durham and Darlington, and, to a limited extent, at Bishop-Auck-

land. There are iron manufactories at Darlington, Stockton, and Sunderland, and several for nails at each of these towns, and at Durham ; spades and edge-tools are made at Walsingham. Paper is made to a considerable extent at Durham ; glass, including crown and flint-glass, and glass bottles, at Sunderland and South. Shields ; and earthenware, both for home sale and exportation, on Gateshead Fell. Ship-building is also extensively carried on at Sunderland and South Shields, which, with Stockton, are the chief ports. The principal articles of exportation are the mineral and manufacturing produce of the county; the imports are timber, deals, flax, hemp, hides, bar iron, linseed, oak-bark, and linen-yarn.

The principal rivers are, the Tees, the Tyne, and the Wear. The Tees, rising in Cumberland, forms the whole south and south-western boundary of this county, separating it from Westmorland and Yorkshire : it flows by Barnard-Castle, and near Darlington, and falls into the German ocean a few miles below Stockton, being navigable to some distance above Yarm. Among the more striking features of the romantic scenery for which Tees dale is distinguished, are several very picturesque waterfalls. The Tyne forms the northern limit of the county, separating it from Northumberland, from about two miles above Ryton to its mouth, a little below South Shields, and is navigable up to a little above Newcastle. The Wear is formed by the junction of several small streams in the north-western part of the county, and runs from west to east, with a circuitous course, through the centre of it, passing by Stanhope, Walsingham, Bishop-Auckland, Durham, and Chester le Street, and falling into the German ocean at Sunderland : it is navigable nearly as far as Chester le Street. The Derwent is formed by the junction of several streams near Hunstonworth, and constitutes the northern limit of the county to about three miles below Ebchester, then crossing a portion of it, it falls into the Tyne about a mile below the village of Swalwell. The Skerne, rising near Kelloe, in Easington ward, flows southward by Bishop-Middleham and Darlington, and falls into the Tees opposite the village of Croft, in York shire. The fish in these rivers are, salmon, trout, eels, chevins, dace, pike (especially in the Skerne), and sparlings (in the Tees). The Darlington and Stockton railway was constructed pursuant to an act obtained in 1821, and completed in September, 1825, at an expense of £125,000, advanced by sixty shareholders; the entire length of the main line, from Witton Park colliery to Stockton, is twenty-five miles, and it has various branches diverging from it : coal, lime, and mineralogical productions are conveyed along it at the rate of three halfpence per ton per mile, and merchandise at three-pence per ton ; coaches drawn by horses are charged at the rate of threepence per mile ; the line is worked by two fixed locomotive engines, working four inclined planes half a mile in length. The great road from London to Berwick enters the county from Croft, in Yorkshire, and passing through Darlington, Durham, and Chester le Street, quits it at the passage of the Tyne, for Newcastle.

The Roman stations are, Lanchester, where numerous remains of that people have been found, and where Horsley places the *Glannibanta* of the Notitia; Binchester, the *Vinovium* of Antoninus; Ebchester and Cunscliffe, which Horsley identifies with the *Magæ* of the Notitia, and where numerous Roman coins, &c., have been found. Considerable remains of the Watling-street, and of other Roman roads connecting the different stations, are yet visible. The principal ancient encampment is Maiden Castle. The chief specimens of ancient ecclesiastical architecture are to be seen in the magnificent cathedral church of Durham, and in the churches of Chester le Street, Brancepeth, Darlington, Hartlepool, and Bishop-Wearmouth. Before the Reformation, the religious houses in this county were, six monasteries, six colleges, and five hospitals, of which the most interesting remains are those of Jarrow and Finchale monasteries, and of St. Edmund's hospital at Gateshead. Of ancient castles, the most remarkable remains are those of Barnard-Castle, and of the castles of Brancepeth, Durham, and Norham. The finest specimens of old castellated mansions are seen in Raby, Lumley, Hilton, and Auckland castles. The most remarkable mineral springs are at Dinsdale, Croft, Butterby, and Chester le Street, and of the saline springs the principal is at Birtley, from which about eleven hundred tons of salt are made annually.

DURLEIGH, a parish in the hundred of ANDERS-FIELD, county of SOMERSET, 1½ mile (W. S.W.) from Bridg-water, containing 127 inhabitants. The living is a perpetual curacy, in the archdeaconry of Taunton, and diocese of Bath and Wells, endowed with £200 royal bounty, and in the patronage of Wyndham Goodden, Esq.

DURLEY, a chapelry in the parish of UPHAM, in that part of the hundred of BISHOP'S WALTHAM which is in the Portsdown division of the county of SOUTH-AMPTON, 3¾ miles (W. by S.) from Bishop's Waltham, containing 319 inhabitants. It is within the jurisdiction of the Cheyney Court held at Winchester every Thursday, for the recovery of debts to any amount.

DURLEY, a tything in the parish of ELING, hundred of REDBRIDGE, New Forest (East) division of the county of SOUTHAMPTON. The population is returned with the parish.

DURNFORD, a parish in the hundred of AMES-BURY, though locally in the hundred of Underditch, county of WILTS, 2¼ miles (S.S.W.) from Amesbury, containing, with Little Durnford, Netton, Newtown, and Salterton, 472 inhabitants. The living is a vicarage, in the peculiar jurisdiction and patronage of the Prebendary of Durnford in the Cathedral Church of Salisbury, rated in the king's books at £9. The church, dedicated to St. Andrew, is a very ancient structure. Here is a school endowed with about £12 per annum. On the brow of a hill in this parish is an extensive earth-work, called Ogbury camp, supposed to have been a British settlement: it has no fosse, and is intersected by a number of small banks in different directions.

DURRINGTON, a chapelry in the parish of TAR-RING, hundred of BRIGHTFORD, rape of BRAMBER, county of SUSSEX, 3½ miles (N. W.) from Worthing, containing 194 inhabitants. The chapel is in ruins, and the inhabitants attend divine service at Tarring.

DURRINGTON, a parish in the hundred of AMES-BURY, county of WILTS, 3 miles (N.) from Amesbury, containing 370 inhabitants. The living is a perpetual curacy, in the archdeaconry and diocese of Salisbury, endowed with £200 royal bounty, and in the patronage

of the Dean and Chapter of Winchester. At a short distance from this place are the remains of an extensive British town, called Durrington Walls, or Long Walls.

DURSLEY, a market town and parish in the upper division of the hundred of BERKELEY, county of GLOU-CESTER, 15 miles (S. W. by S.) from Gloucester, and 108 (W. by N.) from London, containing 3186 inhabitants. It is an irregularly built town, situated at the foot of a steep hill, clothed with a wood chiefly of beech trees. A baronial castle of the Berkeleys, once lords of the manor, built as early as the reign of Edward the Confessor, stood here previously to the reign of Queen Mary I., when it was entirely destroyed: the site is now an orchard, at the north-western extremity of the town, the fields adjacent to which are called Castle Fields. The town contains several respectable and some handsome houses, and a few which have the appearance of considerable antiquity: the principal streets are paved. Near the centre of it is a market-house, built at the expense of the lord of the manor, about 1738. At its east end is a statue of Queen Anne. On the south-east side of the church-yard, springs of water rise so copiously as, at the distance of one hundred yards, to set in motion a fulling-mill; and on the banks of the stream are several cloth manufactories. This fountain is supposed to have occasioned the town to be called Dursley, from the British *Dwr*, water, and *Lega*, lea or pasture land. The market, held under a charter granted by Edward IV., in 1471, is on Thursday; and there are fairs, May 6th and December 4th, for the sale of cattle and pedlary. Dursley was one of the five boroughs in Gloucestershire which sent members to parliament in the reign of Edward I.; but it has long since lost that privilege. A bailiff and four constables are elected annually at the court of the manor, but the power of the bailiff only extends to the examination of weights and measures, and the superintendence of the police. Contiguous to the town are the remains of a rock of tufa, or puff-stone, which cuts easily when first raised, but is extremely durable. This stone is said to have been used in constructing the walls of Berkeley castle, part of the churches of Dursley and Cam, and the vaulted roof of the choir of Gloucester cathedral.

The benefice is a rectory, in the archdeaconry and diocese of Gloucester, rated in the king's books at £10. 14. 4½., and annexed to the archdeaconry of Gloucester, which is in the patronage of the Bishop. The church, dedicated to St. James, is a noble structure, consisting of a spacious nave, aisles, and chancel, with a tower at the west end. All the windows are pointed, and on the south side of the building is a handsome entrance porch, above which are three canopied niches. The whole south aisle, as well as the porch, is ornamented with battlements, pierced in quatrefoils, and other decorations in the style of the fifteenth century. The aisles are separated from the nave by a lofty arcade. On the timber roof are carved the arms of Berkeley and Fitzharding, and the device of Thomas Tanner, who, in the reign of Henry VI., erected a chantry chapel at the end of the south aisle, in which is a monumental figure of a skeleton beneath a canopy. The spire fell in 1699, and was rebuilt the next year, at the expense of £1000. The chancel likewise was re-erected in 1738. There are places of worship for Independents and Wesleyan Methodists. A school for poor children is endowed with £7. 4. per annum, the produce of an acre of garden-ground, the bequest of John Arundell, in 1703. In 1811, Richard Jones bequeathed £1900 in trust to the rector and churchwardens, of which £450 was ordered to be laid out in ornamenting and improving the church; £300 to be appropriated to the support of a Sunday school for boys; £300 to another for girls; and the residue for the benefit of friendly societies, and other charitable purposes. There is a charity school for poor children of Protestant dissenters, for the support of which Joseph Twemlow, in 1739, gave a school-house, for the residence of the master, who has a salary of £35 per annum, for instructing about thirty boys, the school having been benefitted by subsequent endowments. Almshouses existed here prior to 1617, which becoming ruinous, the ground whereon they stood was let, in 1821, on a building lease for ninety-nine years, at £8. 5. per annum, which is applied in aid of the church rate. The present poor-house occupies the site of a house called the Church-house, for which a consideration of £45 per annum is paid out of the rates, to be applied to the repairs of the church.. Hugh Smith, of Dursley, left by will, in 1637, three tenements for the use of the poor, the site of which is let on a building lease, for ninety-nine years, at £4. 5. per annum, which is distributed at the discretion of the churchwardens. In 1642, Sir Thomas Estcourt bequeathed property at Tetbury for charitable purposes, from which is paid a rent-charge of £10 to the poor of Dursley. In 1663, Throgmorton Trotman, merchant of London, left £2000 in trust to the Haberdashers' Company, out of the produce of which £15 per annum is paid for preaching a lecture at Dursley every market-day. This is the birthplace of Edward Fox, Bishop of Hereford, and almoner to Henry VIII., who has been reckoned among the reformers. Dursley gives the title of viscount to the Earl of Berkeley.

DURSTON, a parish in the northern division of the hundred of PETHERTON, county of SOMERSET, 4¾ miles (N.E. by E.) from Taunton, containing 211 inhabitants. The living is a perpetual curacy, in the archdeaconry of Taunton, and diocese of Bath and Wells. The Rev. R. Gray was patron in 1823. The church, which has been lately enlarged, is dedicated to St. John. At Minchin-Buckland, or Buckland-Sororum, in this parish, a priory of canons regular of the order of St. Augustine was founded about 1167, which being suppressed, the house and estates were given to the Knights Hospitallers, for the establishment of a nunnery of their own order. Subsequently there was a priory of canonesses of St. Augustine, and a preceptory of Knights Hospitallers, the former of which, at the dissolution, had a revenue amounting to £223. 7. 4½.

DURWESTON, a parish in the hundred of PIMPERNE, Blandford (North) division of the county of DORSET, 3 miles (N.W.) from Blandford-Forum, containing 454 inhabitants. The living is a consolidated rectory with Bryanston, in the archdeaconry of Dorset, and diocese of Bristol, rated in the king's books at £13. 11. 3., and in the patronage of E. B. Portman, Esq. The church is dedicated to St. Nicholas. Knighton, formerly a distinct parish, has long since been consolidated with Durweston. The river Stour is here navi-

gable, and is crossed by a bridge on the east of the village.

DUSTON, a parish in the hundred of NOBOTTLE-GROVE, county of NORTHAMPTON, 1¾ mile (W. by N.) from Northampton, containing 484 inhabitants. The living is a discharged vicarage, in the archdeaconry of Northampton, and diocese of Peterborough, rated in the king's books at £6. 8. 10., endowed with £200 private benefaction, and £400 royal bounty, and in the patronage of Lord Viscount Melbourne. The church is dedicated to St. Mary. The parish is bounded on the south-east and north-east by branches of the river Nine, or Nen. There are remains of St. James's abbey for Black canons, founded about 1112, by William Peverel, natural son of William the Conqueror, the revenue of which, at the dissolution, amounted to £175. 8. 2.

DUTTON, a township in that part of the parish of GREAT BUDWORTH which is in the hundred of BUCKLOW, county palatine of CHESTER, 5¼ miles (E.) from Frodsham, containing 325 inhabitants. This place, called in Domesday-book Duntune, was the seat of the ancient family of Dutton, who exercised peculiar authority over the musicians and minstrels of the county, requiring them to pay suit and service at a court held before the lord of Dutton, or his deputy, at Chester, every year on Midsummer-day, and to take out a license for the exercise of their calling. Though the right is still reserved to the proprietors of the manor of Dutton, no court has been held since 1756. One side of Dutton Hall, erected in 1542, is still standing, furnishing a remarkably rich relic of the domestic architecture of that period. The Grand Trunk canal passes through the parish. Dutton gives the title of baron to the family of Douglas, Dukes of Hamilton.

DUTTON, a township in that part of the parish of RIBCHESTER which is in the lower division of the hundred of BLACKBURN, county palatine of LANCASTER, 7 miles (N. by W.) from Blackburn, containing 521 inhabitants.

DUXBURY, a township in the parish of STANDISH, hundred of LEYLAND, county palatine of LANCASTER, 2 miles (S. by E.) from Chorley, containing 312 inhabitants.

DUXFORD, comprising the parishes of Duxford-St. Peter and Duxford-St. John, in the hundred of WHITTLESFORD, county of CAMBRIDGE, 6¼ miles (W.) from Linton, containing 605 inhabitants. The living of St. Peter's is a rectory, rated in the king's books at £21. 6. 8., endowed with £200 private benefaction, and £300 parliamentary grant, and in the patronage of the Master and Fellows of Corpus Christi College, Cambridge. That of St. John's is a discharged vicarage, rated in the king's books at £13.3.4., and in the patronage of the Master and Fellows of Clare Hall, Cambridge; they are in the archdeaconry and diocese of Ely. The boundaries of each parish not being accurately known, the two are assessed as one. Here is a school under the direction of nine feoffees, founded pursuant to the will of the Rev. Richard King, in 1649, and endowed with £27 per annum; also the remains of an ancient hospital, the chapel of which is now used as a barn.

DYKE, a hamlet in the parish of BOURNE, wapentake of AVELAND, parts of KESTEVEN, county of LINCOLN, 2 miles (N.N.E.) from Bourne, containing 144 inhabitants.

DYMCHURCH, a parish in the liberty of ROMNEY-MARSH, locally in the hundred of Worth, lathe of SHEPWAY, county of KENT, 4 miles (N. E. by N.) from New Romney, containing 543 inhabitants. The living is a rectory, in the archdeaconry and diocese of Canterbury, rated in the king's books at £7. 2. 8½., and in the patronage of the Crown. The church is dedicated to St. Peter and St. Paul. There is a place of worship for Wesleyan Methodists. This parish lies wholly on the level of Romney-Marsh, adjoining the sea, and is distinguished for its strong artificial wall, made to resist the encroaches of that element: this wall is about three miles long, more than twenty feet high, and the width at the top permits the high road to run along it: it has three grand sluices, for the general draining of the marsh; and the expense of repair, which amounts to £5000 per annum, is defrayed by *scot* payments levied on the whole district.

DYMOCK, a parish in the hundred of BOTLOE, county of GLOUCESTER, 3¾ miles (N. N. W.)˙ from Newent, containing 1558 inhabitants. The living is a vicarage, in the archdeaconry of Hereford, and diocese of Gloucester, rated in the king's books at £9. 13. 9., endowed with £800 parliamentary grant. A. Thompson, Esq. was patron in 1827. The church is dedicated to St. Mary. This place, supposed to derive its name from the Saxon *dim*, dark, and *Ac*, oak, was formerly of considerable extent and importance; as, in the reign of Henry III., it had the privilege of a market and three fairs, all long since disused. In the parliamentary war it was garrisoned for the king. A considerable quantity of cider and perry is made here. The Herefordshire and Gloucestershire canal, and the river Leden, pass through the parish. Two school-rooms for fifty boys and fifty girls, with residences for the master and mistress, were erected in 1825, at an expense of £1200, being a portion of the produce of a bequest in 1779, by Mrs. Ann Carn, the remaining sum (nearly £3000), being invested in the Bank three per cent. annuities, and the interest of it applied to the purposes of the charity: the school is conducted on the National plan, and, so far as the funds will allow, the children are provided with clothing. A rent-charge of £3 per annum was bequeathed in 1734, by William Hooper, which is also applied to the support of this school. Ten men and ten women are clothed annually from a bequest by Mr. Wintour, made about a century ago. This is the birth-place of John Kyrle, the benevolent original of Pope's "Man of Ross."

E.

EACHWICK, a township in the parish of HEDDON on the WALL, partly in the western division of Castle ward, but chiefly in the eastern division of TINDALE ward, county of NORTHUMBERLAND, 10½ miles (N. W. by W.) from Newcastle upon Tyne, containing 169 inhabitants. This was anciently a place of considerable importance. In making a road through an old intrenchment near the village, several hand mill-stones, a sacrificing knife, and a flint axe, were discovered.

EAGLE, a parish partly in the higher, but chiefly in the lower, division of the wapentake of BOOTHBY-GRAFFO, parts of KESTEVEN, county of LINCOLN, 7½

miles (W. S. W.) from Lincoln, containing, with the hamlet of Eagle-Hall, 353 inhabitants. The living is a discharged vicarage, in the archdeaconry and diocese of Lincoln, rated in the king's books at £3. 5. 10., endowed with £200 private benefaction, and £1000 royal bounty. Mrs. Buckworth was patroness in 1800. The church is dedicated to All Saints. There is a place of worship for Wesleyan Methodists. A school is endowed with a small sum, and a house for the master. Here was a commandery of the Knights Templars, which, on the suppression of their order, was transferred to the hospitallers: at the dissolution its revenue amounted to £144. 18. 10.

EAGLE-HALL, a hamlet in that part of the parish of EAGLE which is in the higher division of the wapentake of BOOTHBY-GRAFFO, parts of KESTEVEN, county of LINCOLN, 9 miles (W. S. W.) from Lincoln, containing 45 inhabitants.

EAGLE-WOODHOUSE, an extra-parochial liberty, in the lower division of the wapentake of BOOTHBY-GRAFFO, parts of KESTEVEN, county of LINCOLN, containing 10 inhabitants.

EAGLESCLIFFE, a parish in the south-western division of STOCKTON ward, county palatine of DURHAM, comprising the townships of Aislaby, Eaglescliffe, and Newsam, and containing 542 inhabitants, of which number, 332 are in the township of Eaglescliffe, ½ a mile (N. N. E.) from Yarm. The living is a vicarage, in the archdeaconry and diocese of Durham, rated in the king's books at £28. 17. 1., and in the patronage of the Bishop of Durham. The church is dedicated to St. John the Baptist. The river Tees, which is here navigable, is crossed by a cast-iron bridge of one arch, from which there is a railway that, at a short distance, joins the Stockton and Darlington railway.

EAGLESFIELD, a township in the parish of BRIGHAM, ALLERDALE ward above Darwent, county of CUMBERLAND, 2¾ miles (S. W. by W.) from Cockermouth, containing 405 inhabitants. It is one of the "five towns" annexed to the honour of Cockermouth. On the enclosure of Eaglesfield and Blindbothel commons, about 1814, twenty acres of land were set apart for the establishment of a school, in which all the poor children of those two townships may be educated, on payment of a small quarterage. The township abounds with excellent limestone, and some years since a Roman paved way was discovered in it.

EAKLEY, a hamlet, formerly a parish, now united to Stoke-Goldington, in the hundred of NEWPORT, county of BUCKINGHAM. The population is returned with Stoke-Goldington. The church has been demolished.

EAKRING, a parish in the South-clay division of the wapentake of BASSETLAW, county of NOTTINGHAM, 3¾ miles (S.S.E.) from Ollerton, containing 564 inhabitants. The living is a rectory, in the archdeaconry of Nottingham, and diocese of York, rated in the king's books at £9. 16. 0½., and in the patronage of Earl Manvers, and——Savile, Esq. alternately.

EALING, a parish in the Kensington division of the hundred of OSSULSTONE, county of MIDDLESEX, 6¼ miles (W.) from London, containing, with Old Brentford, 6608 inhabitants. This village, from its situation near the western parts of the metropolis, has become a favourite residence, and contains several handsome villas and pleasant seats. A pleasure fair is annually held on the 24th of June, and the two following days. The living is a vicarage, in the archdeaconry of Middlesex, and diocese of London, rated in the king's books at £13. 6. 8., and in the patronage of the Bishop of London. The church, dedicated to St. Mary, was erected in 1735; it is a brick building, with a square tower and cupola. A lectureship was founded here in 1629, and endowed with £40 per annum, by the Rev. John Bowman, Chancellor of St. Paul's Cathedral, who also left £20 per annum to the poor. A chapel of ease was built at Old Brentford in 1770, by subscription. There is a place of worship for Independents. A charity school for boys, for which a new school-room was built in 1817, is endowed with the twelfth part of an estate in Kent, given by Lady Capel, with £500 by Jonathan Gurnell, Esq., and with other benefactions: more than one hundred and twenty boys, of whom twenty are clothed, are instructed on the National system in this establishment. A charity school for girls was founded in 1712, by Lady Jane Rawlinson, who bequeathed £500 for that purpose: Peter Francis le Courayer left £200 for the purchase of land, to which £50 was added by Mrs. Frances Cole, besides several similar benefactions: seventy girls, of whom twenty-five are clothed, are taught on the National system: the school-room was built in 1819. In a stratum of gravel, near Old Brentford, have been found bones and teeth of the hippopotamus, the elephant, and the bullock; and in the sub-stratum, which is of calcareous earth, are found the bones and horns of deer: below this is a bed of blue clay, abounding with shells of the nautilus and other marine animals. Among the distinguished persons that have been inhabitants of Ealing may be enumerated, Dr. John Owen, a learned non-conformist divine, and a very voluminous writer, who died in 1683; Serjeant Maynard, an eminent lawyer, who died here in 1690, and was buried in the church; Sir Frederick Morton Eden, Bart., author of an elaborate history of the labouring class in England; and Robert Orme, author of Historical Fragments of the Mogul Empire, who died in 1801. John Horne Tooke, author of the Diversions of Purley; and the celebrated Mrs. Trimmer; were interred in the church-yard.

EAMONT-BRIDGE, a joint township with Yanwath, in the parish of BARTON, WEST ward, county of WESTMORLAND, 1¼ mile (S.S.E.) from Penrith, containing 244 inhabitants. A school is endowed with about £100 per annum, for children of both townships. On the southern bank of the river Eamont, in this township, is an intrenched amphitheatre, called King Arthur's Round Table, in ancient times used as a tilting ground; and near it is another relic of antiquity, named Mayburgh, which is supposed to have been the Gymnasium, where the wrestlers, racers, and others of the humbler class performed their exercises.

EARDINGTON, a township in that part of the parish of QUATFORD which is in the hundred of STOTTESDEN, county of SALOP, 2 miles (S. by E.) from Bridgenorth, containing 306 inhabitants. Iron-works have been established here.

EARDISLAND, a parish in the hundred of STRETFORD, county of HEREFORD, 5 miles (W.) from Leominster, containing 791 inhabitants. The living is a discharged vicarage, in the archdeaconry and diocese of Hereford, rated in the king's books at £4. 9. 7., endowed with £200 royal bounty, and in the patronage of the Bishop of Hereford. The church is dedicated to St. Mary. Here is an endowed free school, partly conducted on the Madras system. A court leet is held annually in the village, which is situated on the river Arrow, the rail-road from Kington to Leominster passing through it. A house still exists, called the Nun House, and part of the glebe land is denominated the Monks' Court; from which it is inferred that a place called Staick house was once a religious establishment, a supposition strengthened by its peculiar appearance, and contiguity to the Monks' Court. The Roman Watling-street is supposed to have passed through this parish, on the line of the road now leading to Street Court.

EARDISLEY, a parish in the hundred of HUNTINGTON, county of HEREFORD, 6¼ miles (S. by W.) from Kington, containing 683 inhabitants. The living is a vicarage, in the archdeaconry and diocese of Hereford, rated in the king's books at £7. 12. 6., and in the patronage of Thomas Perry, Esq. The church is dedicated to St. Mary Magdalene. Here is a National school. Courts leet and baron are held occasionally; and fairs for cattle, cheese, and butter, are on May 15th and October 18th. The Brecon and Kington rail-road passes at the south end of the village. Several helmets have been dug up; and there are slight remains of a castle. Half a mile hence is a remarkable oak tree, held in great respect by the poor inhabitants, and supposed to be four hundred years old. Some of its branches average about two feet in diameter; its girth at the bottom is sixty feet, and it covers a surface of three hundred and twenty-four feet in circular extent.

EARDLEY-END, a township in the parish of AUDLEY, northern division of the hundred of PIREHILL, county of STAFFORD, 5 miles (N.W.) from Newcastle under Line, containing 192 inhabitants.

EARESBY, a chapelry in the parish of SPILSBY, eastern division of the soke of BOLINGBROKE, parts of LINDSEY, county of LINCOLN, ½ a mile (W.S.W.) from Spilsby, with which the population is returned.

EARITH, a chapelry in the parish of BLUNTISHAM, hundred of HURSTINGSTONE, county of HUNTINGDON, 3 miles (S.E.) from Somersham, containing 674 inhabitants. The chapel, which was dedicated to St. James, has been demolished. A school is endowed with about £50 per annum. Cattle fairs are held, May 4th, July 25th, and November 1st.

EARL (otherwise YEARD) HILL, a township in the parish of DODDINGTON, eastern division of GLENDALE ward, county of NORTHUMBERLAND, 1¼ mile (S. by W.) from Wooler, containing 60 inhabitants. A few years since an urn, containing bones and a thin piece of flint, was found on the summit of a hill at this place.

EARL-SHILTON, a chapelry in the parish of KIRKBY-MALLORY, hundred of SPARKENHOE, county of LEICESTER, 3¾ miles (N. E.) from Hinckley, containing 1771 inhabitants. The chapel is dedicated to St. Peter. There is a place of worship for Independents. This place was formerly distinguished by its Norman castle, now entirely destroyed, the site being denoted only by a mount, and a place called the Castle-yard, or Hall-yard.

EARL-STOKE, a chapelry in the parish and hundred of MELKSHAM, county of WILTS, 3¾ miles (W.)

from East Lavington, containing 875 inhabitants. The chapel is dedicated to St. Mary.

EARLHAM (ST. MARY).—See NORWICH.

EARLY, a liberty in that part of the parish of Son-NING which is in the hundred of CHARLTON, county of BERKS, 2½ miles (S.E. by E.) from Reading, containing 447 inhabitants.

EARNLEY, a parish in the hundred of MANHOOD, rape of CHICHESTER, county of SUSSEX, 6½ miles (S.W. by S.) from Chichester, containing, with Almodington, 148 inhabitants. The living is a rectory, united in 1524 to the rectory of Almodington, in the archdeaconry and diocese of Chichester, rated in the king's books at £7. 6. 0½. Almodington was formerly in the patronage of the Earl of Arundel, and Earnley in that of the Bishop of Chichester; but since the union of the two benefices the Bishop has two turns, and the Duke of Norfolk one. The church of Earnley has been long ince demolished.

EARNSFORD, a liberty in the parish of BINLEY, Kirby division of the hundred of KNIGHTLOW, county of WARWICK, 3¼ miles (E.S.E.) from Coventry. The population is returned with the parish.

EARNSHILL, a parish in the hundred of ABDICK and BULSTONE, county of SOMERSET, 5 miles (S.W. by S.) from Langport, containing 13 inhabitants. The living is a rectory, in the archdeaconry of Taunton, and diocese of Bath and Wells, rated in the king's books at £2. 1. 0½. R. T. Combe, Esq. was patron in 1821. The church has been demolished.

EARSDON, a parish in the eastern division of CASTLE ward, county of NORTHUMBERLAND, comprising the townships of Blackworth, South Blyth with Newsham, Brierdean, Earsdon, Hartley, Holywell, Seaton-Delaval, and Sighill, and containing 4644 inhabitants, of which number, 271 are in the township of Earsdon, 4 miles (N.W. by N.) from North Shields. The living is a perpetual curacy, in the archdeaconry of Northumberland, and diocese of Durham, endowed with £800 royal bounty, and £1200 parliamentary grant, and in the patronage of the proprietors of land. The church, dedicated to St. Alban, is an ancient building, which in 1097 belonged to Tynemouth abbey, and has lately received an addition of four hundred and five free sittings; the Incorporated Society for the enlargement of churches and chapels having granted £300 towards defraying the expense. This is a fertile district, abounding also with excellent coal and stone. The village, seated upon a rocky eminence, is pleasant and well built.

EARSDON, a township in the parish of HEBBURN, western division of MORPETH ward, county of NORTHUMBERLAND, 5½ miles (N.) from Morpeth, containing 94 inhabitants.

EARSDON-FOREST, a township in the parish of HEBBURN, western division of MORPETH ward, county of NORTHUMBERLAND, 6 miles (N. by W.) from Morpeth, containing 34 inhabitants.

EARSHAM, a parish in the hundred of EARSHAM, county of NORFOLK, 1 mile (S.W. by W.) from Bungay, containing 750 inhabitants. The living is a rectory, in the archdeaconry of Norfolk, and diocese of Norwich, rated in the king's books at £15. Sir W. Dalling, Bart. was patron in 1812. The church is dedicated to All Saints.

EARSWICK, a township partly in the parish of STRENSALL, within the liberty of ST. PETER of YORK, but chiefly in the parish of HUNTINGTON, wapentake of BULMER, North riding of the county of YORK, 3¼ miles (N.N.E.) from York, containing 113 inhabitants, exclusively of those which are within the liberty of St. Peter

EARTHAM, a parish in the hundred of Box and STOCKBRIDGE, rape of CHICHESTER, county of SUSSEX, 5¾ miles (N.E. by E.) from Chichester, containing 105 inhabitants. The living is a vicarage, in the archdeaconry and diocese of Chichester, rated in the king's books at £7. 5. 2½., and in the patronage of the Prebendary of Eartham in the Cathedral Church of Chichester.

EARTHCOTT-GAUNTS, a tything in that part of the parish of ALMONDSBURY which is in the lower division of the hundred of BERKELEY, county of GLOUCESTER, 5¾ miles (S. by E.) from Thornbury. The population is returned with the parish.

EASBY, a township in the parish of BRAMPTON, ESKDALE ward, county of CUMBERLAND, 1½ mile (N.N.E.) from Brampton, containing 96 inhabitants. At Coathill, in this neighbourhood, is a chalybeate spring.

EASBY, a parish comprising the townships of Aske, Easby, and Skeeby, in the western, and the township of Brompton on Swale, in the eastern, division of the wapentake of GILLING, North riding of the county of YORK, and containing 765 inhabitants, of which number, 105 are in the township of Easby, 1½ mile (E.S.E.) from Richmond. The living is a vicarage, in the archdeaconry of Richmond, and diocese of Chester, rated in the king's books at £2. 13. 4., endowed with £600 royal bounty, and £600 parliamentary grant, and in the patronage of the Crown. The church, dedicated to St. Agatha, stands at a considerable distance from the village, and existed prior to 1152. In this village, pleasantly situated on the banks of the Swale, was an abbey for Premonstratensian canons, founded about 1152, by Roald, constable of Richmond castle, and valued at the dissolution at £111 per annum: the remains are extensive, and rich in architectural decoration. Here is an hospital for four persons.

EASBY, a township in the parish of STOKESLEY, western division of the liberty of LANGBAURGH, North riding of the county of YORK, 3 miles (E. by N.) from Stokesley, containing 124 inhabitants.

EASEBOURNE, a parish (formerly a market town) in the hundred of EASEBOURNE, rape of CHICHESTER, county of SUSSEX, 1 mile (N.E.) from Midhurst, containing, with the chapelry of Lodsworth Liberty, 1290 inhabitants. The living is a vicarage, in the archdeaconry and diocese of Chichester, rated in the king's books at £6. 6. 8., endowed with £200 private benefaction, and £1900 parliamentary grant, and in the patronage of Lord Montague. The church is dedicated to St. Margaret. In this parish, to the south of which the Rother, or Arundel navigation, passes, is a school founded in 1674 by John Locke, and endowed by him with £5 per annum. In the latter part of the reign of Henry III., John Bohun, of Midhurst, founded here a small Benedictine nunnery, the revenue of which at the dissolution was valued at £29 per annum.

EASENHALL, a hamlet in the parish of MONKS-KIRBY, Kirby division of the hundred of KNIGHTLOW, county of WARWICK, 4 miles (N. W.) from Rugby, containing 164 inhabitants.

EASHING, a tything in the parish and first division of the hundred of GODALMING, county of SURREY, 1¾ mile (W.) from Godalming, with which the population is returned. The river Wey runs through the tything.

EASINGTON, a hamlet in the parish of CHILTON, hundred of ASHENDON, county of BUCKINGHAM, 3½ miles (N. N. W.) from Thame. The population is returned with the parish. Here was formerly a chapel, but it has been long since demolished.

EASINGTON, a parish in the southern division of EASINGTON ward, county palatine of DURHAM, comprising the townships of Easington, Haswell, Hawthorn, and Shotton, and containing 1112 inhabitants, of which number, 593 are in the township of Easington, 9½ miles (E.) from Durham. The living is a rectory, not in charge, annexed, in 1255, to the archdeaconry, and in the diocese of Durham. The church, dedicated to St. Mary, is a lofty building, serving, from its situation on an eminence, as a land-mark for mariners. There is a place of worship for Wesleyan Methodists. In 1814, Archdeacon Prosser erected a school-room, which, by means of his own and other contributions, now affords education, on Dr. Bell's system, to about fifty boys and thirty girls. Dr. Gabriel Clarke, by will dated in 1662, bequeathed the sum of £60 to purchase a rent-charge of £10 per annum for the school-master. The village, which is of considerable extent and on an elevated situation, was the ancient head of the ward, deanery, and parish, to which it gives name. A halmote court is held twice a year, for the recoveryof debts under 40s.

EASINGTON, a township in that part of the parish of BELFORD which is in the northern division of BAMBROUGH ward, county of NORTHUMBERLAND, 1¼ mile (N. E. by E.) from Belford, containing 186 inhabitants.

EASINGTON, a parish in the hundred of EWELME, county of OXFORD, 4 miles (S. W. by S.) from Tetsworth, containing 25 inhabitants. The living is a discharged rectory, in the archdeaconry and diocese of Oxford, rated in the king's books at £4. 12. 6., and in the patronage of the Bishop of Lincoln. The church is dedicated to St. Peter.

EASINGTON, a parish in the southern division of the wapentake of HOLDERNESS, East riding of the county of YORK, comprising the townships of Easington and Out-Newton, and containing 557 inhabitants, of which number, 488 are in the township of Easington, 6½ miles (E. S. E.) from Patrington. The living is a discharged vicarage, in the archdeaconry of the East riding, and diocese of York, rated in the king's books at £10, and in the patronage of the Archbishop of York. The church, dedicated to All Saints, is a very ancient structure in the early style of English architecture. Twenty boys and girls are instructed by means of an annuity of £10, the gift of Mr. Robert Pattinson, in 1811.

EASINGTON, a parish in the eastern division of the liberty of LANGBAURGH, North riding of the county of YORK, 9½ miles (E. by N.) from Guilsbrough, containing 507 inhabitants. The living is a rectory, in the archdeaconry of Cleveland, and diocese of York, rated in the king's books at £14. 8. 6½., and in the patronage of the Crown. The church is dedicated to All Saints.

EASINGTON, a township in the parish of SLAID-

BURN, western division of the wapentake of STAINCLIFFE and EWCROSS; West riding of the county of YORK, 7½ miles (N. N. W.) from Clitheroe, containing 501 inhabitants. Here is a free school.

EASINGTON-GRANGE, a township in that part of the parish of BELFORD which is in the northern division of BAMBROUGH ward, county of NORTHUMBERLAND, 1½ mile (N. E.) from Belford, containing 54 inhabitants.

EASINGWOULD, a parish in the wapentake of BULMER, North riding of the county of YORK, comprising the market town of Easingwould, and the chapelry of Raskelf, and containing 2352 inhabitants, of which number, 1912 are in the town of Easingwould, 13 miles (N. N. W.) from York, and 208 (N. N. W.) from London. The town, which is irregularly built, is, from its inland situation, and the want of navigable conveyance, precluded from the advantages of trade. Considerable quantities of bacon and butter are sent from this place to York, whence the articles are forwarded to London by water; and the town derives some benefit from its being a thoroughfare on the high road from London to Edinburgh. The market is on Friday: the fairs are, July 6th and September 26th, for cattle and sheep. The living is a discharged vicarage, in the archdeaconry of Cleveland, and diocese of York, rated in the king's books at £12. 11. 0½., and in the patronage of the Bishop of Chester. The church, dedicated to All Saints, is situated on an eminence above the town, and commands an extensive view of the ancient forest of Galtres, and the vale of Mowbray. There are places of worship for Independents, and Primitive and Wesleyan Methodists. A free school was founded in 1781, by Mrs. Eleanor Westerman, who endowed it with £2500 reduced annuities, for the instruction of boys in English grammar, Latin, writing, arithmetic, and book-keeping; and of girls, in reading, writing, and arithmetic: there are thirty boys and girls in this school, who are nominated by the vicar, churchwardens, and overseers of the parish, as trustees. There is another school, with a small endowment, for ten boys; and Sunday schools are supported by subscription. In the neighbourhood are some small chalybeate springs issuing from the high grounds, and indicating the existence of coal or iron-stone, but none has yet been discovered of sufficient consequence to encourage any enterprise: the principal of these springs supplies a small bathing-house.

EAST BOURNE, county of SUSSEX. See BOURNE (EAST.)

EASTBRIDGE, an extra-parochial liberty, in the hundred of WESTGATE, lathe of ST. AUGUSTINE, county of KENT, containing 34 inhabitants. For an account of Eastbridge Hospital, see CANTERBURY.

EASTBRIDGE, a parish within the liberty of ROMNEY MARSH, locally in the hundred of Worth, lathe of SHEPWAY, county of KENT, 5 miles (N. by E.) from New Romney, containing 18 inhabitants. The living is a rectory, in the archdeaconry and diocese of Canterbury, rated in the king's books at £5. 6. 8., and in the patronage of the Archbishop of Canterbury. The church has been demolished.

EASTBURN, a township in the parish of KIRKBURN, Bainton-Beacon division of the wapentake of HARTHILL, East riding of the county of YORK, 3 miles (S. W.) from Great Driffield, containing 12 inhabitants.

EASTBURN, a joint township with Steeton, in the parish of KILDWICK, eastern division of the wapentake of STAINCLIFFE and EWCROSS, West riding of the county of YORK, 4 miles (N.W.) from Keighley, containing 753 inhabitants.

EASTBURY, a tything in the parish and hundred of LAMBOURN, county of BERKS, 2 miles (S. E. by E.) from Lambourn, containing, with Bockhampton, 398 inhabitants. Here was formerly a chapel, which was dedicated to St. James, but it has been demolished. There is a place of worship for Wesleyan Methodists.

EASTBY, a joint township with Embsay, in that part of the parish of SKIPTON which is in the eastern division of the wapentake of STAINCLIFFE and EWCROSS, West riding of the county of YORK, 3 miles (N. E.) from Skipton, containing 861 inhabitants. There is a place of worship for Wesleyan Methodists.

EAST-CHURCH, a parish in the liberty of the ISLE of SHEPPEY, lathe of SCRAY, county of KENT, 5 miles (E. by S.) from Queenborough, containing 705 inhabitants. The living is a vicarage, in the archdeaconry and diocese of Canterbury, rated in the king's books at £13. 6. 8., and in the patronage of Miles Barton, Esq. The church, which is dedicated to All Saints, is a spacious and handsome embattled edifice, formerly belonging to the convent of Boxley. There is a place of worship for Wesleyan Methodists. East-Church takes its name from being situated to the east of the parish of Minster. There is a free school, with a small endowment : a fair for toys is held on Holy-Thursday. Many petrified fossils, supposed to be antediluvian, have been found upon the sea-shore.

EASTCOTT, a tything in the parish of URCHFONT, hundred of SWANBOROUGH, county of WILTS, 1½ mile (N. E.) from East Lavington, containing 123 inhabitants.

EASTCOTTS, a chapelry in the parish of CARDING-TON, hundred of WIXAMTREE, county of BEDFORD, 3½ miles (S. E.) from Bedford, containing, with Cotton-End, Harrowden, and Fenlake, 588 inhabitants.

EASTCOURT, a tything in the parish of CRUD-WELL, hundred of MALMESBURY, county of WILTS, 4½ miles (N. E. by N.) from Malmesbury, containing 157 inhabitants.

EASTER (GOOD), a parish in the hundred of DUN-MOW, county of ESSEX, 7 miles (N. W. by W.) from Chelmsford, containing 478 inhabitants. The living is a discharged vicarage, with which the vicarage of High Easter was consolidated in 1771, in the peculiar jurisdiction of the Bishop of London, rated in the king's books at £8, and in the patronage of the Dean and Chapter of St. Paul's, London. The church is dedicated to St. Andrew. There is a strong chalybeate spring in the parish.

EASTER (HIGH), a parish in the hundred of DUN-MOW, county of ESSEX, 5 miles (S. by W.) from Great Dunmow, containing 819 inhabitants. The living is a vicarage, consolidated with that of Good Easter, in the archdeaconry of Middlesex, and diocese of London, rated in the king's books at £14. 14. 7. The church is dedicated to St. Mary.

EASTERGATE, a parish in the hundred of AVIS-FORD, rape of ARUNDEL, county of SUSSEX, 5¼ miles (W. by S.) from Arundel, containing 166 inhabitants. The living is a rectory, in the archdeaconry and diocese of Chichester, rated in the king's books at £7. 19. 9½.,

and in the patronage of the Dean and Chapter of Chichester. The church, dedicated to St. George, is a small rude building of rough stone.

EASTERTON, a tything in the parish of EAST LA-VINGTON, hundred of SWANBOROUGH, county of WILTS, 1 mile (N. E.) from East Lavington, containing 377 inhabitants. There is a small school for the education of the poor.

EASTFIELD, a hamlet in that part of the parish of ST. JOHN the BAPTIST, PETERBOROUGH, which is in the liberty of PETERBOROUGH, county of NORTHAMPTON, ¾ of a mile (N.N.E.) from Peterborough, containing, with Newark, 247 inhabitants.

EASTGATE, a hamlet in the parish of STANHOPE, north-western division of DARLINGTON ward, county palatine of DURHAM, 8¼ miles (W. by N.) from Walsingham. The population is returned with the parish. About one hundred children are educated at a National school built by the late Bishop of Durham : where divine service is performed every Sunday afternoon. There is a place of worship for Wesleyan Methodists.

EASTHAM, a parish in the higher division of the hundred of WIRRALL, county palatine of CHESTER, comprising the townships of Eastham, Hooton, Nether Pool, Over Pool, Great Sutton, Little Sutton, Thornton-Childer, and a part of that of Whitby, and containing 1430 inhabitants, of which number, 368 are in the township of Eastham, 5 miles (E. N. E.) from Great Neston. The living is a discharged vicarage, in the archdeaconry and diocese of Chester, rated in the king's books at £12. 13., and in the patronage of the Dean and Chapter of Chester. The church is dedicated to St. Mary. About a mile from the village is a ferry on the Mersey, called Eastham ferry ; and at the ferry-house is usually held the yearly meeting of the Wirrall Agricultural Society. There are two or three small bequests for the education of poor children.

EASTHAM, a parish in the upper division of the hundred of DODDINGTREE, county of WORCESTER, 4¼ miles (E.) from Tenbury, comprising the chapelries of Child-Hanley and Orleton, and containing 677 inhabitants. The living is a rectory with that of Hanley-William, in the archdeaconry of Salop, and diocese of Hereford, rated in the king's books at £28. 15. 10. The church, dedicated to St. Peter and St. Paul, has lately received an addition of eighty free sittings, the Incorporated Society for the enlargement of churches and chapels having granted £40 towards defraying the expense.

EASTHOPE, a parish in the hundred of MUNSLOW, county of SALOP, 4¾ miles (S.W.) from Much Wenlock, containing 93 inhabitants. The living is a discharged rectory, in the archdeaconry of Salop, and diocese of Hereford, rated in the king's books at £3. 3. 1½., and endowed with £200 royal bounty. R. Benson, Esq. was patron in 1825. The church is dedicated to St. Peter.

EASTHORPE, a parish in the Colchester division of the hundred of LEXDEN, county of ESSEX, 4¼ miles (E. by S.) from Great Coggeshall, containing 175 inhabitants. The living is a rectory, in the archdeaconry of Colchester, and diocese of London, rated in the king's books at £12. The Hon. Colonel and Mrs. Onslow were patrons in 1826. The church is dedicated to St. Mary.

EASTINGTON, a chapelry in that part of the parish of NAUNTON which is in the hundred of BRADLEY, county of GLOUCESTER, 1½ mile (S.E.) from North Leach, containing 220 inhabitants. The chapel is dedicated to St. Mary Magdalene.

EASTINGTON, a parish in the lower division of the hundred of WHITSTONE, county of GLOUCESTER, comprising the tythings of Alkerton and Eastington, and containing 1681 inhabitants, of which number, 718 are in the tything of Eastington, 5½ miles (W. by N.) from Stroud. The living is a rectory, in the archdeaconry and diocese of Gloucester, rated in the king's books at £32. 14. 9½. The Rev. R. Huntley was patron in 1817. The church is dedicated to St. Michael. There is a place of worship for Wesleyan Methodists. A free school ror about seventy children was established by subscription in 1764. During the civil war this place was garrisoned for the parliament.

EAST-LEACH-MARTIN, otherwise BURTHORPE, a parish in the hundred of BRIGHTWELLS-BARROW, county of GLOUCESTER, 4 miles (N.) from Lechlade, containing 231 inhabitants. The living is a rectory, in the archdeaconry and diocese of Gloucester, rated in the king's books at £10, and in the patronage of the Crown. The church is dedicated to St. Mary.

EAST-LEACH-TURVILLE, a parish in the hundred of BRIGHTWELLS-BARROW, county of GLOUCESTER, 4 miles (N. by E.) from Lechlade, containing 333 inhabitants. The living is a perpetual curacy, in the archdeaconry and diocese of Gloucester, endowed with £9 per annum private benefaction, and £600 royal bounty, and in the patronage of the Dean and Chapter of Gloucester. The church, an extremely small building, is dedicated to St. Andrew. The Roman Iknield-street enters this parish on the east from Oxfordshire, and joins the fosse-way at Cirencester. In Church-lane is a mineral spring, which is strongly cathartic.

EASTLEY, a tything in the parish of SOUTH STONE-HAM, hundred of MANSBRIDGE, Fawley division of the county of SOUTHAMPTON, 5 miles (N.N.E.) from Southampton. The population is returned with the parish.

EASTLING, a parish in the hundred of FAVERSHAM, lathe of SCRAY, county of KENT, 5 miles (S.W.) from Faversham, containing 406 inhabitants. The living is a rectory, in the archdeaconry and diocese of Canterbury, rated in the king's books at £16, and in the patronage of the Earl of Winchelsea. The church is dedicated to St. Mary. A fair is held on the 14th of September.

EASTMOORE, a hamlet in the parish of BARTON-BENDISH, hundred of CLACKCLOSE, county of NORFOLK, 2¾ miles (N.E. by N.) from Stoke-Ferry. The population is returned with the parish. Here was formerly a chapel, now demolished.

EASTNOR, a parish in the hundred of RADLOW, county of HEREFORD, 2¼ miles (S.E. by E.) from Ledbury, containing 475 inhabitants. The living is a discharged rectory, in the archdeaconry and diocese of Hereford, rated in the king's books at £7. 19. 5., and in the patronage of Earl Somers. The church, dedicated to St. John the Baptist, contains several handsome monuments of marble. The substratum of this parish is a grey limestone, in which shells are found thickly imbedded; it exists in large masses, and being susceptible of a high polish, is much used for chimney-pieces. There are some ancient intrenchments in the parish. Eastnor Castle, the splendid residence of Earl Somers, has been recently rebuilt, at an immense expense, on

the plan of the ancient baronial castles. On an eminence in the park is an obelisk, on which are recorded the public acts of Lord Chancellor Somers, as well as a tributary inscription to the memory of the present earl's eldest son, who was slain in the peninsular war.

EASTOFT, a chapelry in the parish of CROWLE, western division of the wapentake of MANLEY, parts of LINDSEY, county of LINCOLN, 3 miles (N.E.) from Crowle, containing 232 inhabitants.

EASTOFT, a joint township with Haldenby, in the parish of ADLINGFLEET, lower division of the wapentake of OSGOLDCROSS, West riding of the county of YORK, 10 miles (S.S.E.) from Howden, containing 69 inhabitants.

EASTON, a parish in the hundred of LEIGHTON-STONE, county of HUNTINGDON, 3¼ miles (N.E.) from Kimbolton, containing 172 inhabitants. The living is a vicarage not in charge, in the peculiar jurisdiction and patronage of the Prebendary of Longstow in the Cathedral Church of Lincoln, endowed with £200 royal bounty. The church is dedicated to St. Peter.

EASTON, a hamlet in that part of the parish of SOUTH STOKE which is in the soke of GRANTHAM, parts of KESTEVEN, county of LINCOLN, 1½ mile (N.) from Colsterworth, containing 206 inhabitants. The chapel has fallen into ruins.

EASTON, a parish in the hundred of FOREHOE, county of NORFOLK, 6¾ miles (W.N.W.) from Norwich, containing 165 inhabitants. The living is a discharged vicarage, in the archdeaconry of Norfolk, and diocese of Norwich, rated in the king's books at £7. 11. 10½., endowed with £200 private benefaction, and £200 royal bounty. E. R. Fellowes, Esq. was patron in 1809. The church is dedicated to St. Peter. There is a place of worship for Baptists at Easton Row.

EASTON, a parish in the hundred of WILLYBROOK, county of NORTHAMPTON, 2½ miles (S.W. by S.) from Stamford, containing 689 inhabitants. The living is a rectory, in the archdeaconry of Northampton, and diocese of Peterborough, rated in the king's books at £19. 8. 9. The Marquis of Exeter was patron in 1805. The church is dedicated to All Saints. Here is a free school endowed with about £50 per annum.

EASTON, a parish in the hundred of FAWLEY, Fawley division of the county of SOUTHAMPTON, 2¼ miles (N.E. by N.) from Winchester, containing 427 inhabitants. The living is a rectory, in the peculiar jurisdiction of the incumbent, rated in the king's books at £26. 6. 8., and in the patronage of the Bishop of Winchester. The church is dedicated to St. Mary. There is a trifling endowment for the education of poor children. Easton is within the jurisdiction of the Cheyney Court held at Winchester every Thursday, for the recovery of debts to any amount.

EASTON, a parish in the hundred of LOES, county of SUFFOLK, 2½ miles (N.N.W.) from Wickham-Market, containing 371 inhabitants. The living is a discharged rectory, in the archdeaconry of Suffolk, and diocese of Norwich, rated in the king's books at £10. 18. 6½., endowed with £200 private benefaction, and £200 royal bounty. The Earl of Rochford was patron in 1817. The church is dedicated to All Saints.

EASTON, a parish in the hundred of KINWARD-STONE, county of WILTS, 3¼ miles (E. by N.) from Pewsey, containing 447 inhabitants. The living is a perpetual curacy, in the archdeaconry of Wilts, and diocese of Salisbury, and in the patronage of the Marquis of Ailesbury. The church, which was dedicated to the Holy Trinity, has been demolished. Here is a small endowed free school. In the reign of Henry III. there was an hospital or priory at this place, for canons of the Trinitarian order, for the redemption of captives, said by some to have been founded by Stephen, Archdeacon of Salisbury: its revenue, at the time of the dissolution, amounted to £55. 14. 4.

EASTON, a hamlet in the parish of BRIDLINGTON, wapentake of DICKERING, East riding of the county of YORK, 1¼ mile (W.) from Bridlington, containing 21 inhabitants.

EASTON (GREAT), a parish in the hundred of DUNMOW, county of ESSEX, 2½ miles (N.N.W.) from Great Dunmow, containing 755 inhabitants. The living is a rectory, in the archdeaconry of Middlesex, and diocese of London, rated in the king's books at £18.13.4., and in the patronage of R. Saumarez, Esq. and Lord Viscount Maynard alternately. The church is dedicated to St. John. In 1759, Rebecca Mead bequeathed tenements and land, now producing £38 per annum, for clothing and teaching ten girls; and in 1761, Charles, Lord Maynard, endowed a school for six boys of this parish, and six of Little Easton. There is a small sum for apprenticing children.

EASTON (GREY), a parish in a detached portion of the hundred of CHIPPENHAM, county of WILTS, 3½ miles (W.) from Malmesbury, containing 151 inhabitants. The living is a discharged rectory, in the archdeaconry of Wilts, and diocese of Salisbury, rated in the king's books at £6. 0. 5., and in the patronage of John Howes, Esq. A branch of the Lower Avon passes through this parish. There is a trifling sum for the education of children: and an almshouse for six women is endowed with £50 per annum.

EASTON (LITTLE), a parish in the hundred of DUNMOW, county of ESSEX, 2½ miles (N.W.)from Great Dunmow, containing 303 inhabitants. The living is a rectory, in the archdeaconry of Middlesex, and diocese of London, rated in the king's books at £10. Lord Viscount Maynard was patron in 1815. Charles Lord Maynard, in 1761, endowed a school for six boys of this parish, and six of Great Easton, and by his will founded an almshouse for four poor widows.

EASTON (MAGNA), a chapelry in the parish of BRINGHURST, hundred of GARTREE, county of LEICESTER, 8¼ miles (E.N.E.) from Market-Harborough, containing 529 inhabitants. The chapel is dedicated to St. Andrew.

EASTON in GORDANO, a parish in the hundred of PORTBURY, county of SOMERSET, 7¼ miles (W. N. W.) from Bristol, containing 2109 inhabitants. The living is a discharged vicarage, in the peculiar jurisdiction and patronage of the Prebendary of Easton in the Cathedral Church of Wells, rated in the king's books at £5. 9. 4½., endowed with £200 private benefaction, and £200 royal bounty. The church is dedicated to St. George. There is a place of worship for Wesleyan Methodists. The river Avon, which is navigable along the north-east boundary of the parish, falls into the Bristol channel on the north of it. At the south-eastern extremity there was anciently a chapel, the site of which is still called Chapel Pill.

EASTON-BAVENTS, a parish in the hundred of BLYTHING, county of SUFFOLK, 2 miles (N.N.E.) from Southwold, containing 24 inhabitants. The living is a discharged rectory, annexed to that of Benacre, in the archdeaconry of Suffolk, and diocese of Norwich, rated in the king's books at £6, and endowed with £200 royal bounty. The church, which was dedicated to St. Nicholas, has fallen to ruin.

EASTON-MAUDIT, a parish in the hundred of HIGHAM-FERRERS, county of NORTHAMPTON, 6½ miles (S.) from Wellingborough, containing 178 inhabitants. The living is a discharged vicarage, in the archdeaconry of Northampton, and diocese of Peterborough, rated in the king's books at £6, endowed with £200 private benefaction, and £200 royal bounty, and in the patronage of the Dean and Canons of Christ Church, Oxford. The church is dedicated to St. Peter and St. Paul.

EASTON-NESTON, a parish in the hundred of CLELEY, county of NORTHAMPTON, 1¼ mile (E.) from Towcester, containing, with the hamlet of Hulcote, 137 inhabitants. The living is a vicarage, in the archdeaconry of Northampton, and diocese of Peterborough, rated in the king's books at £8. The Earl of Pomfret was patron in 1825. The church is dedicated to St. Mary. The children of this parish are instructed by a schoolmistress for £10 per annum, paid out of the church estate, and from the same fund £10 are annually contributed in aid of a Sunday school.

EASTON-PERCEY, a tything in the parish of KINGTON-ST. MICHAEL, northern division of the hundred of DAMERHAM, county of WILTS, containing 29 inhabitants. John Aubrey, a distinguised antiquary, was born here in 1629.

EASTRIDGE, a tything in the parish and hundred of RAMSBURY, county of WILTS, 6 miles (N.W. by N.) from Hungerford, containing 254 inhabitants.

EASTRINGTON, a parish in the wapentake of HOWDENSHIRE, East riding of the county of YORK, comprising the townships of Bellasize, Eastrington, Gilberdike, Newport-Wallingfen, and Portingten with Cavil, and containing 1649 inhabitants, of which number, 375 are in the township of Eastrington, 3¼ miles (E.N.E.) from Howden. The living is a discharged vicarage, within the jurisdiction of the peculiar court of Howdenshire, rated in the king's books at £12. 9. 7., and in the patronage of the Crown. The church is dedicated to St. Michael. There is a place of worship for Wesleyan Methodists. In 1726, Joseph Hewley gave a house and land, now producing £28 a year, for the use of a school, in which about thirty children are educated.

EASTRIP, an extra-parochial liberty, in the hundred of BRUTON, county of SOMERSET, 2 miles from Bruton, containing 17 inhabitants.

EASTROP, a parish in the hundred of BASINGSTOKE, Basingstoke division of the county of SOUTHAMPTON, ½ a mile (N.) from Basingstoke, containing 67 inhabitants. The living is a discharged rectory, in the archdeaconry and diocese of Winchester, rated in the king's books at £2, endowed with £200 royal bounty, and in the patronage of T. Terry, Esq.

EASTRY, a parish partly in the hundred of WINGHAM, but chiefly in that of EASTRY, lathe of ST. AUGUSTINE, county of KENT, 2¾ miles S. W. by S.) from Sandwich, containing 1062 inhabitants. The living is a vicarage with the curacy of Worth, rated in the king's books at £19. 12. 1., and in the peculiar jurisdiction and patronage of the Archbishop of Canterbury. The church, dedicated to St. Mary, is a spacious edifice. Wesleyan Methodists have a place of worship here. There is a trifling sum for the education of children. A fair is held for cattle, pedlary, and toys, on the 2nd of October. This village contains a spacious handsome building, appropriated as a workhouse for this and twelve other parishes.

EAST-VILLE, a township in the eastern division of the soke of BOLINGBROKE, parts of LINDSEY, county of LINCOLN, containing 118 inhabitants. There is a chapel in the East Fen belonging to the townships of East-Ville and Mid-Ville. This township, with six òthers, was made such by act of parliament in 1812, on the occasion of a very extensive drainage of fen lands, and is not dependent on any parish.

EASTWELL, a parish in the hundred of WYE, lathe of SCRAY, county of KENT, 3¾ miles (N.) from Ashford, containing 134 inhabitants. The living is a discharged rectory, in the archdeaconry and diocese of Canterbury, rated in the king's books at £9. 16. 8., and in the patronage of the Earl of Winchelsea and Nottingham. The church is an ancient structure, dedicated to St. Mary. The register of this parish is said to have contained the entry of the burial of Richard Plantagenet, natural son to King Richard III., who, having fled hither after the battle of Bosworth, was protected by Sir Thomas Moyle, lord of the manor, and died in 1550, at a small house erected by his permission, at the age of 81.

EASTWELL, a parish in the hundred of FRAMLAND, county of LEICESTER, 7 miles (N. by E.) from Melton-Mowbray, containing 109 inhabitants. The living is a rectory, in the archdeaconry of Leicester, and diocese of Lincoln, rated in the king's books at £9. 12. 1., and in the alternate patronage of the Crown and the Governors of St. James's Hospital, Leicester. The church is dedicated to St. Michael.

EASTWICK, a parish in the hundred of BRAUGHIN, county of HERTFORD, 4 miles (S.W. by W.) from Sawbridgeworth, containing 212 inhabitants. The living is a rectory, in the archdeaconry of Middlesex, and diocese of London, rated in the king's books at £7. 11. 8. Mrs. Plumer was patroness in 1825. The church is dedicated to St. Botolph.

EASTWOOD, a parish in the hundred of ROCHFORD, county of ESSEX, 1½ mile (S.W. by S.) from Rochford, containing 530 inhabitants. The living is a vicarage, in the archdeaconry of Essex, and diocese of London, rated in the king's books at £12, and in the patronage of the Crown. The church is dedicated to St. Lawrence and All Saints.

EASTWOOD, a parish in the southern division of the wapentake of BROXTOW, county of NOTTINGHAM, 9 miles (N.W. by W.) from Nottingham, containing 1206 inhabitants. The living is a discharged rectory, in the archdeaconry of Nottingham, and diocese of York, rated in the king's books at £4. 13. 1½. J. Plumptre, Esq. was patron in 1819. The church is dedicated to St. Mary. There is a place of worship for Wesleyan Methodists. Here are extensive coal-works. The Nottingham canal crosses the parish, and another runs parallel with it to the extent of about one mile and a half, communicating with the river that bounds this county on the Derbyshire side.

EATINGTON, a parish in two divisions, Lower and Upper, in the Kington division of the hundred of KINGTON, county of WARWICK, containing 641 inhabitants. Lower Eatington is 6¾ miles (S.W. by W.), and Upper Eatington 5¼ (W.S.W.), from Kington. The living is a discharged vicarage, in the archdeaconry and diocese of Worcester, rated in the king's books at £12. 0. 7½., and in the patronage of Evelyn John Shirley, Esq. The church, which is in Lower Eatington, is dedicated to St. Thomas à Becket. A chapel, dedicated to St. Mary, which stood in Upper Eatington, was pulled down about thirty years since, and rebuilt at Lower Eatington, which contains the greater part of the population. There is a place of worship for Baptists. In 1807, Sarah Roberts bequeathed a sum of £200, directing the interest to be applied to the education of poor children; about fifty are instructed. On the south-west, this parish is bounded by the river Stour.

EATON, a township in the parish of APPLETON, hundred of OCK, county of BERKS, 5¾ miles (N.W. by N.) from Abingdon, containing 85 inhabitants.

EATON, a township in the parish of ECCLESTON, lower division of the hundred of BROXTON, county palatine of CHESTER, 3¾ miles (S.) from Chester, containing 66 inhabitants. It is situated on the river Dee, near which stands Eaton Abbey, the princely residence of Earl Grosvenor, which within the last eight years has been considerably enlarged and beautified.

EATON, a township in the parish of TARPORLEY, first division of the hundred of EDDISBURY, county palatine of CHESTER, 1½ mile (E.N.E.) from Tarporley, containing 477 inhabitants.

EATON, a township in the parish of PRESTBURY, hundred of MACCLESFIELD, county palatine of CHESTER, 2 miles (N.N.E.) from Congleton, containing 327 inhabitants.

EATON, a township in the parish of DAVENHAM, hundred of NORTHWICH, county palatine of CHESTER, 2¾ miles (S. by W.) from Northwich, containing 18 inhabitants.

EATON, a township in that part of the parish of ASHBOURN which is in the hundred of WIRKSWORTH, county of DERBY, 7 miles (N.N.W.) from Ashbourn, containing, with the chapelry of Alsop le Dale, 61 inhabitants. This township is in the honour of Tutbury, duchy of Lancaster, and within the jurisdiction of a court of pleas held at Tutbury every third Tuesday, for the recovery of debts under 40s.

EATON, a parish in the hundred of FRAMLAND, county of LEICESTER, 8 miles (N.N.E.) from Melton-Mowbray, containing 284 inhabitants. The living is a discharged vicarage, in the archdeaconry of Leicester, and diocese of Lincoln, rated in the king's books at £7. 11. 3., endowed with £200 royal bounty, and in the patronage of the Crown. The church is dedicated to St. Denis. The Wesleyan Methodists have a place of worship here. There is a small sum for the education of children.

EATON, a parish in the South-clay division of the wapentake of BASSETLAW, county of NOTTINGHAM, 2¼ miles (S.) from East Retford, containing 215 inhabitants. The living is a discharged vicarage, in the peculiar jurisdiction of the Chapter of the Collegiate Church of Southwelrated l, in the king's books at £4. 13. 4., and in the patronage of the Prebendary of Eaton in the Collegiate Church of Southwell. The church is dedicated to All Saints. This parish is in the honour of Tutbury, duchy of Lancaster, and within the jurisdiction of a court of pleas held at Tutbury every third Tuesday, for the recovery of debts under 40s.

EATON, a township in the parish of STOKE upon TERN, Drayton division of the hundred of BRADFORD (North), county of SALOP, 6 miles (N.W.) from Newport, containing 123 inhabitants.

EATON, a parish within the liberty of the borough of WENLOCK, county of SALOP, 4¼ miles (S.E. by E.) from Church-Stretton, containing 566 inhabitants. The living is a discharged vicarage, in the archdeaconry of Salop, and diocese of Hereford, rated in the king's books at £5. H. and W. Lloyd, Esqrs. were patrons in 1810. The church is dedicated to St. Edith.

EATON (BISHOP), a parish in the hundred of WEBTREE, county of HEREFORD, 5 miles (W.) from Hereford, containing 452 inhabitants. The living is a discharged rectory, in the peculiar jurisdiction of the Dean of Hereford, rated in the king's books at £13, and in the patronage of the Bishop of Hereford. The church is dedicated to St. Michael.

EATON (BRAY), a parish in the hundred of MANSHEAD, county of BEDFORD, 3½ miles (W. by S.) from Dunstable, containing 816 inhabitants. The living is a vicarage, in the archdeaconry of Bedford, and diocese of Lincoln, rated in the king's books at £12. 16. 3., and in the patronage of the Master and Fellows of Trinity College, Cambridge. The church is dedicated to St. Mary. There is a place of worship for Wesleyan Methodists. Here was anciently a castle, built by Cantilupe, Baron of Abergavenny, in 1221, of which nothing remains.

EATON (CHURCH), a parish in the western division of the hundred of CUTTLESTONE, county of STAFFORD, 5½ miles (W.N.W.) from Penkridge, containing, with the townships of Marston, High Own, and Little Own, and the hamlets of Oslow and Wood-Eaton, 829 inhabitants. The living is a rectory, in the archdeaconry of Stafford, and diocese of Lichfield and Coventry, rated in the king's books at £14. 19. 9½., and in the patronage of Earl Talbot. The church is dedicated to St. Edith. There is an endowed grammar school, in which about twenty-five boys, and the same number of girls, are gratuitously educated.

EATON (LITTLE), a chapelry in that part of the parish of ST. ALKMUND, DERBY, which is in the hundred of MORLESTON and LITCHURCH, county of DERBY, 3¼ miles (N.N.E.) from Derby, containing 547 inhabitants. The living is a perpetual curacy, in the peculiar jurisdiction of the Dean and Chapter of Lichfield, endowed with £800 royal bounty, and £1400 parliamentary grant, and in the patronage of Sir J. Kaye, Bart.

EATON (LONG), a chapelry in the parish of SAWLEY, hundred of MORLESTON and LITCHURCH, county of DERBY, 6¼ miles (N.) from Kegworth, containing 682 inhabitants. It is within the peculiar jurisdiction of the Prebendary of Sawley in the Cathedral Church of Lichfield. The chapel is dedicated to St. Lawrence. There is a place of worship for Wesleyan Methodists.

EATON-CONSTANTINE, a parish in the Wellington division of the hundred of BRADFORD (South), county of SALOP, 5¼ miles (N.N.W.) from Much Wenlock, containing 251 inhabitants. The living is a rectory not in charge, in the archdeaconry of Salop, and

diocese of Lichfield and Coventry. The Marquis of Cleveland was patron in 1823. The church is dedicated to St. Mary. The inhabitants bury at Leighton. This place is bounded by the river Severn on the south-west.

EATON-HASTINGS, a parish in the hundred of SHRIVENHAM, county of BERKS, 3¼ miles (N.W. by N.) from Great Farringdon, containing 178 inhabitants. The living is a rectory, in the archdeaconry of Berks, and diocese of Salisbury, rated in the king's books at £18. 7. 1. The Rev. R. Rice was patron in 1784. The church is dedicated to St. Michael.

EATON-SOCON, a parish in the hundred of BARFORD, county of BEDFORD, 1½ mile (S.W.) from St. Neot's, containing, with Wyboston, 2039 inhabitants. The living is a discharged vicarage, in the archdeaconry of Bedford, and diocese of Lincoln, rated in the king's books at £20. 13. 9. The Duke of Bedford was patron in 1808. The church is dedicated to St. Mary. Here was anciently a castle, the residence of a branch of the family of Beauchamps; also a priory for Augustine friars, founded by Sir Oliver Beauchamp and his son Hugh, the only remaining portion of which is the refectory, now converted into stables. The river Ouse is navigable along the eastern boundary of the parish.

EATON-TREGOES, a township in the parish of FOY, upper division of the hundred of WORMELOW, though locally in the hundred of Greytree, county of HEREFORD, 2¾ miles (N. by E.) from Ross. The population is returned with the parish.

EAVES, a township in the parish of STOKE upon TRENT, northern division of the hundred of PIREHILL, county of STAFFORD, 5¼ miles (E.N.E.) from Newcastle under Line. The population is returned with the parish.

EAVESTONE, a township in that part of the parish of RIPON which is in the liberty of RIPON, West riding of the county of YORK, 6¼ miles (W.S.W.) from Ripon, containing 73 inhabitants.

EBBERSTON, a parish in PICKERING lythe, North riding of the county of YORK, 5¾ miles (E.) from Pickering, containing 505 inhabitants. The living is a discharged vicarage, in the peculiar jurisdiction and patronage of the Dean of York, rated in the king's books at £5. 17. 3½., and endowed with £400 parliamentary grant. The church is dedicated to St. Mary. There is a place of worship for Wesleyan Methodists.

EBBESBORNE-WAKE, a parish in the hundred of CHALK, county of WILTS, 8½ miles (S.W. by W.) from Wilton, containing 239 inhabitants. The living is a rectory, in the archdeaconry and diocese of Salisbury, rated in the king's books at £19. 14. 2., and in the patronage of the Succentor in the Cathedral Church of Salisbury. The church is dedicated to St. John the Baptist. There is a place of worship for Independents.

EBBS-FLEET, a hamlet in the parish of MINSTER, hundred of RINGSLOW, or ISLE of THANET, lathe of ST. AUGUSTINE, county of KENT, 3½ miles (S.W. by W.) from Ramsgate. The population is returned with the parish. Hengist and Horsa, the Saxon generals, landed here with their forces about 449, also St. Augustine, in 596.

EBCHESTER, a chapelry in that part of the parish of LANCHESTER which is in the western division of CHESTER ward, county palatine of DURHAM, 14 miles (N.W. by W.) from Durham, containing 200 inhabitants. The living is a perpetual curacy, in the archdeaconry and diocese of Durham, endowed with £200 private benefaction, and £200 royal bounty, and in the patronage of the Bishop of Durham. The church is a small ancient structure, dedicated to St. Ebba, daughter of Ethelfrid, King of Northumberland, who, before 660, founded a monastery upon the banks of the Derwent, which was subsequently destroyed by the Danes, and the royal foundress became abbess of Coldingham. Five hundred years afterwards, Ebchester is described as "the place of anchorets." The church and a few cottages occupy the site of a Roman station, two hundred yards square, with extensive outworks, supposed to be the *Vindomora* of Antoninus, traces of which are still discernible. Sepulchral and other monuments found upon the spot have been built up in the walls of the houses, and some are deposited in the library at Durham, with an urn of an uncommon size and shape, having a small cup in the centre, as a lachrymatory, or patera. The Roman road from Lanchester and Corbridge leads to Ebchester, where Gale places Ptolemy's *Epiacum*, but Horsley states it to be at Hexham. David II., King of Scotland, in his unfortunate invasion, is said to have entered the county by this road, which may still be traced where it crossed the Derwent, by a ford near the present foot-bridge.

EBONY, a chapelry in the parish of APPLEDORE, partly in the hundred of TENTERDEN, lathe of SCRAY, but chiefly in the hundred of OXNEY, lathe of SHEPWAY, county of KENT, 4¼ miles (S.E.) from Tenterden, containing 151 inhabitants. The chapel, dedicated to St. Mary, stands on the site of a larger and more ancient edifice, which was destroyed by lightning early in the reign of Elizabeth. The Grand Military canal passes through that part of the chapelry which is in the lathe of Scray, and the river Rother runs along the southern boundary.

EBRINGTON, a parish in the upper division of the hundred of KIFTSGATE, county of GLOUCESTER, 1¾ mile (E. by N.) from Chipping-Campden, containing, with Charingcoat and Hitcoat-Boyce, 535 inhabitants. The living is a discharged vicarage, united to the vicarage of Mickleton, in the archdeaconry and diocese of Gloucester, rated in the king's books at £9. 9. 4., endowed with £200 royal bounty, and in the patronage of the Crown. The church, dedicated to St. Edburgh, is a large and handsome structure, the east window of which is ornamented with stained glass, representing portions of the history of the patriarch Joseph : in the chancel is a monument, erected in 1677, to Sir John Fortescue, Lord Chancellor in the reign of Henry VI. Ebrington gives the title of viscount to Earl Fortescue.

ECCHINSWELL, a chapelry in that part of the parish of KINGSCLERE which is in the hundred of EVINGAR, Kingsclere division of the county of SOUTHAMPTON, 9 miles (N.N.E.) from Whitchurch, containing 399 inhabitants. The chapel is dedicated to St. Lawrence.

ECCLES, a parish in the hundred of SALFORD, county palatine of LANCASTER, 4 miles (W.) from Manchester, comprising the chapelries of Pendleton and Worsley, and the townships of Barton, Clifton, and Pendlebury, and containing 23,331 inhabitants. The living is a discharged vicarage, in the archdeaconry and diocese of Chester, rated in the king's books at £6. 8., and in the patronage of the Crown. The church, dedicated to St. Mary de Eccles, is in the later style of English architecture, and belonged to Whalley abbey,

but at the dissolution it was made parochial. Independents, Wesleyan Methodists, and Roman Catholics, have each a place of worship, with a school attached. There are manufactories for silk, nankeen, gingham, and linen cloth ; also a large cotton-mill, which affords employment to about four hundred people. A school-room in the church-yard was rebuilt by subscription in 1816, and is partly supported by a bequest from James Bradshaw, in 1800, of £8. 8. per annum, and partly from the parish fund of benefactions ; five hundred and thirty children are taught at this school. The Manchester and Liverpool rail-road passes close to the village. The abbot and convent of Whalley established a small settlement of monks at this place ; a small portion of the building remains, and forms part of a farm-house, bearing the name of Monks' Hall. Robert Ainsworth, author of the Latin and English Dictionary, was born here in 1660.

ECCLES, a parish in the hundred of HAPPING, county of NORFOLK, 9½ miles (E. by S.) from North Walsham, containing, with Hemstead, 212 inhabitants. The living is a discharged rectory, consolidated with that of Hemstead, in the archdeaconry of Norfolk, and diocese of Norwich, rated in the king's books at £8. E. Lombe, Esq. was patron in 1815. The church, dedicated to St. Mary, was swallowed up by the sea in 1605. The coast is defended by a ridge of sand hills, thrown up by the wind and surge, which seems to oppose a sufficient barrier to any future encroachment of the sea, though at the period when the church disappeared, the village was reduced from eighty to fourteen houses, and the land in the parish from one thousand three hundred to three hundred acres, by a terrible inundation, and in the time of Charles I. only one hundred acres remained after a similar calamity.

ECCLES, a parish in the hundred of SHROPHAM, county of NORFOLK, 2½ miles (N.E.) from East Harling, containing 122 inhabitants. The living is a rectory, in the archdeaconry of Norfolk, and diocese of Norwich, rated in the king's books at £14, endowed with £400 royal bounty. The Rev. C. Miller and another were patrons in 1800. The church is dedicated to St. Mary.

ECCLESALL-BIERLOW, a chapelry in that part of the parish of SHEFFIELD which is in the southern division of the wapentake of STRAFFORTH and TICKHILL, West riding of the county of YORK, 3½ miles (S.W.) from Sheffield, containing 9113 inhabitants. The living is a perpetual curacy, in the archdeaconry and diocese of York, endowed with £200 private benefaction, £400 royal bounty, and £1700 parliamentary grant, and in the patronage of the Vicar of Sheffield. Here is a free school endowed with £11 per annum.

ECCLESFIELD, a parish in the northern division of the wapentake of STRAFFORTH and TICKHILL, West riding of the county of YORK, comprising the chapelry of Bradfield, and the townships of Aldward and Ecclesfield, and containing 12,496 inhabitants, of which number, 7163 are in the township of Ecclesfield, 5½ miles (N.) from Sheffield. The living is a vicarage, in the archdeaconry and diocese of York, rated in the king's books at £19. 3. 4., and in the patronage of Earl Fitzwilliam. The church, dedicated to St. John the Baptist, is in the later style of English architecture, and has lately received an addition of three hundred and ninety-seven sittings, of which two hundred are free, the Incorporated Society for the enlargement of churches and chapels having granted £200 toward defraying the expense. There is a place of worship for Wesleyan Methodists. The manufacture of hardware, similar to that at Sheffield, is carried on at this place. There are several endowed schools; that at Ecclesfield is supported out of the feoffee estate of this extensive parish, with £21 per annum, for teaching eighteen poor children. Sylvester's hospital, for seven poor persons, was founded and endowed by Edward Sylvester, in 1693; the income, aided by a bequest of £200 from Ann Reresby, in 1801, amounts to about £100 per annum, which, after providing for repairs, &c., is divided among the inmates. Barnes Hall hospital, for six poor people, was erected in the 15th of Charles I., by Richard Watts, to whom Sir Richard Scott, in 1668, devised certain estates for the purpose. An almshouse, for three poor persons of Ecclesfield and three of Owleston, was erected by George Bamforth, and is kept in repair by the parish. There was formerly an Alien priory of Benedictine monks to the abbey of St. Wandragisilius, in Normandy, which, at their suppression, was granted by Richard II. to the Carthusian monastery of St. Anne, near Coventry. In the neighbourhood are vestiges of a Roman intrenchment, termed Devil's Ditch.

ECCLESHALL, a parish in the northern division of the hundred of PIREHILL, county of STAFFORD, comprising the market town of Eccleshall, the chapelries of Broughton and Chorlton, and the townships of Aspley, Bromley, Charnes, Chatcull, Chorlton-Hill, Coldmeece, Cotes, Croxton, Horseley, Mitmeece, Pershall, Podmore, Slindon, Great Sugnall, Little Sugnall, Three-Farms, Walton, and Wootton, and containing 4227 inhabitants, of which number, 1254 are in the town of Eccleshall, 7¼ miles (N.W. by W.) from Stafford, and 149 (N.W.) from London. This place, which is supposed to be of very remote antiquity, belonged at the time of the Conquest to the bishops of Lichfield, Bishop Durdent having procured for it, in 1160, the grant of a weekly market and an annual fair; and about the year 1200 Bishop Muschamp obtained from King John license to embattle the episcopal residence, and to empark the adjoining grounds. The castle was extensively repaired or entirely rebuilt by Bishop Langton, in 1310: during the parliamentary war, it sustained so much damage in a siege, prior to its being taken by the parliamentarians, as to be unfit for the residence of the bishops, until Bishop Lloyd, in 1695, rebuilt the south part, and connected it with the remaining old buildings, then occupied as a farm-house; since which time it has continued to be the episcopal palace of the see of Lichfield and Coventry, and has received repeated additional improvements. Bishop Hough planted the gorse, which has been since beautifully laid out in shrubberies and plantations; and Dr. Cornwallis, the late bishop, by draining the grounds, added greatly to the salubrity of the situation. The environs are pleasant, and the woods belonging to the palace are extensive. The town, which is pleasantly situated on the river Sow, contains some good houses, and is amply supplied with water. The market is on Friday: the fairs are on the Thursday before Mid-Lent, Holy-Thursday, August 16th, and the first Friday in November, for cattle, sheep, and horses. Two constables and four headboroughs are appointed at the court leet of the Bishop of Lichfield and Coventry, who is lord of the manor.

The living is a discharged vicarage, in the peculiar jurisdiction of the Prebendary of Eccleshall in the Cathedral Church of Lichfield, rated in the king's books at £7. 14. 4., endowed with £400 private benefaction, £200 royal bounty, and £700 parliamentary grant, and in the patronage of the Bishop of Lichfield and Coventry. The church, dedicated to the Holy Trinity, was the sanctuary of Queen Margaret, after Lord Audley's defeat by the Earl of Salisbury, at Blore Heath: it is a spacious structure in the ancient style of English architecture, and contains several monuments. There is a place of worship for Independents. A charity school, which is supported by the parishioners, has a trifling endowment; and a National school, in which nearly one thousand children are instructed, is supported by subscription. About a mile to the north of the town is a paved vicinal way; and about a mile to the east of it are some ancient remains.

ECCLESHILL, a township in the parish of BLACKBURN, lower division of the hundred of BLACKBURN, county palatine of LANCASTER, 3¼ miles (S.S.E.) from Blackburn, containing 456 inhabitants.

ECCLESHILL, a township in the parish of BRADFORD, wapentake of MORLEY, West riding of the county of YORK, 3¼ miles (N.E. by N.) from Bradford, containing 2176 inhabitants. Wesleyan Methodists and Independents have each a place of worship here. There are several scribbling and worsted-mills in the township.

ECCLESTON, a parish in the lower division of the hundred of BROXTON, county palatine of CHESTER, comprising the townships of Eaton and Eccleston, and containing 358 inhabitants, of which number, 292 are in the township of Eccleston, 2¾ miles (S.) from Chester. The living is a rectory, in the archdeaconry and diocese of Chester, rated in the king's books at £15. 13. 11½., and in the patronage of Earl Grosvenor, at whose expense the church, dedicated to St. Mary, and the burial-place of the family, was rebuilt in 1808: it is an elegant structure of red stone, with an embattled tower crowned with pinnacles; over the altar is a painting, by Caravaggio, of the Nativity. The village is situated on the river Dee, where is a free school, established by Earl Grosvenor. Eccleston was occupied by Sir William Brereton's army, during the siege of Chester, in 1645. The old Watling-street passes through the parish, and near the church is a tumulus.

ECCLESTON, a parish in the hundred of LEYLAND, county palatine of LANCASTER, comprising the townships of Eccleston, Hisken, Parbold, and Wrightington, and containing 2801 inhabitants, of which number, 727 are in the township of Eccleston, 5 miles (W.) from Chorley. The living is a rectory, in the archdeaconry and diocese of Chester, rated in the king's books at £28. 16. 0½., and in the patronage of the Rev. W. Yates. The church, an ancient edifice dedicated to St. Mary, has lately received an addition of forty free sittings, the Incorporated Society for the enlargement of churches and chapels having granted £40 towards defraying the expense. A market and fairs were formerly held here. A Sunday school was built by subscription in 1814. The free grammar school at Hesken was founded in 1597, by Sir James Pemberton. The river Yarrow, the Douglas, and the Leeds and Liverpool canal, pass through the parish. There are coal mines and stone quarries; and the dairies produce excellent cheese. Parbold hill commands an extensive prospect, including the Isle of Man and the mountains of Cumberland and Wales.

ECCLESTON, a township in the parish of PRESCOT, hundred of WEST DERBY, county palatine of LANCASTER, 2 miles (N. N. E.) from Prescot, containing 1931 inhabitants. The manufacture of crown glass and earthenware is considerable; and in the neighbourhood are stone quarries and mines of coal.

ECCLESTON (GREAT), a township in the parish of ST. MICHAEL, hundred of AMOUNDERNESS, county palatine of LANCASTER, 6 miles (N.) from Kirkham, containing 648 inhabitants. Several of the inhabitants are employed in cutting and preparing rushes for tallow-chandlers. There are fairs on April 14th, Trinity-Monday, and November 4th. A school, in which about eighty children are educated, is chiefly supported by the benefactions of William Fyld and William Gualter, the present income being £50 per annum.

ECCLESTON (LITTLE), a joint township with Larbrick, in the parish of KIRKHAM, hundred of AMOUNDERNESS, county palatine of LANCASTER, 6¼ miles (N. by E.) from Kirkham, containing 224 inhabitants.

ECCLESWELL, a hamlet in the parish of LINTON, hundred of GREYTREE, county of HEREFORD, 4¼ miles (E. by S.) from Ross. The population is returned with the parish. Here was formerly a chapel, but it has long since been demolished.

ECCUP, a joint township with Addle, in the parish of ADDLE, upper division of the wapentake of SKYRACK, West riding of the county of YORK, 7 miles (N. by W.) from Leeds, containing, with Brearey and Cookridge, 699 inhabitants. This is supposed to have been the site of the *Burgodunum* of the Romans. In 1742, upwards of five hundred coins, chiefly of Valerianus, Gallienus, Tetricus Victorinus, and Claudius Gothicus, were discovered.

ECKINGTON, a parish in the hundred of SCARSDALE, county of DERBY, comprising the townships of Eckington, Mosborough, Renishaw, and Troway, and containing 3598 inhabitants, of which number, 1013 are in the township of Eckington, 7 miles (N.E. by N.) from Chesterfield. The living is a rectory with Killamarsh in the archdeaconry of Derby, and diocese of Lichfield and Coventry, rated in the king's books at £40. 13. 4., and in the patronage of the Crown. The church is dedicated to St. Peter and St. Paul. There is a chapel of ease at Killmarsh. The Wesleyan Methodists have two places of worship, and there is a Roman Catholic chapel within the parish. Here are several manufactories for scythes and sickles, the produce of which, besides being transmitted to all parts of England, is exported to America, Russia, Poland, Scotland, Ireland, &c.: a considerable quantity of nails is made in the parish. A statute fair for the hiring of servants is held on the 5th of November. The Chesterfield canal passes through the parish. Thomas Cam, in 1704, gave lands for the endowment of a free school; in 1717, George Sitwell gave a school-house; and in 1719, Lady Trechville bequeathed £100 in furtherance of this charity, the present annual income of which is about £70: the school is partly conducted on the National plan. A school for girls, which is also a Sunday school, is supported entirely by Lady Sitwell. There are also endowed schools at Mosborough, Renishaw, and Ridgeway. There are several benefactions for the relief of the poor.

ECKINGTON, a parish in the upper division of the hundred of PERSHORE, county of WORCESTER, 4 miles (S. S. W.) from Pershore, containing 668 inhabitants. The living is a discharged vicarage, in the archdeaconry and diocese of Worcester, rated in the king's books at £5. 1. 8., endowed with £6 per annum and £100 private benefaction, and £200 royal bounty, and in the patronage of the Dean and Chapter of Westminster. The church is dedicated to the Holy Trinity. There is a stone bridge over the Avon, which is here navigable.

ECTON, a parish in the hundred of HAMFORDSHOE, county of NORTHAMPTON, 5 miles (S. W. by W.) from Wellingborough, containing 566 inhabitants. The living is a rectory, in the archdeaconry of Northampton, and diocese of Peterborough, rated in the king's books at £21. 8. 1½. The Rev. T. Whalley was patron in 1803. The church is dedicated to St. Mary Magdalene. There is a place of worship for Wesleyan Methodists. Here is a small free school.

EDALE, a chapelry in the parish of CASTLETON, hundred of HIGH PEAK, county of DERBY, 5¾ miles (N. E. by E.) from Chapel en le Frith, containing 435 inhabitants. The living is a perpetual curacy, in the archdeaconry of Derby, and diocese of Lichfield and Coventry, endowed with £8 per annum and £200 private benefaction, £400 royal bounty, and £600 parliamentary grant, and in the patronage of certain Trustees. The chapel is dedicated to the Holy Trinity. There is a place of worship for Wesleyan Methodists. A free school, rebuilt in 1819, by Mrs. Bowden, has sundry small endowments. Edale is in the honour of Tutbury, duchy of Lancaster, and within the jurisdiction of a court of pleas held at Chapel en le Frith, for the recovery of debts under 40s.

EDBURTON, a parish comprising the hamlet of Fulking, in the hundred of POYNINGS, rape of LEWES, and partly in the hundred of BURBEACH, rape of BRAMBER, county of SUSSEX, 4 miles (E.) from Steyning, and containing 269 inhabitants. The living is a rectory, in the peculiar jurisdiction and patronage of the Archbishop of Canterbury, rated in the king's books at £16. The church, dedicated to St. Andrew, is in the early style of English architecture, with later insertions.

EDDINGTON, a joint tything with Hiddon, in the parish of HUNGERFORD, hundred of KINTBURY-EAGLE, county of BERKS, 1 mile (N. E. by E.) from Hungerford, containing 421 inhabitants. It is most probable that this was the *Ethandune* of the Saxon Chronicle, where Alfred is recorded to have obtained a decisive victory over the Danes, in 878, though Camden and others have fixed the scene of that contest at Eddington, near Westbury, in Wiltshire. Roman moulds, for coining, some of them enclosing the metal itself, have been found here, and are deposited in the Ashmolean Museum: they have the impressions only of Severus and Caracalla, and their empresses, Julia and Plantilla. Near the spot was also discovered a tesselated pavement.

EDDINSHALL, a township in that part of the parish of ST. OSWALD, CHESTER, which is in the first division of the hundred of EDDISBURY, county palatine of CHESTER, containing 25 inhabitants.

EDDISBURY, a township in the parish of DELAMERE, first division of the hundred of EDDISBURY, county palatine of CHESTER, containing 72 inhabitants.

EDDLESBOROUGH, a parish in the hundred of

COTTESLOE, county of BUCKINGHAM, 3 miles (N.E.) from Ivinghoe, comprising the chapelry of Dagnell, and the hamlets of Hudnall and Northall, and containing 1378 inhabitants. The living is a discharged vicarage, in the archdeaconry of Buckingham, and diocese of Lincoln, rated in the king's books at £13. 17., endowed with £8 per annum private benefaction, and £200 royal bounty, and in the patronage of the Trustees of the late Earl of Bridgewater. The church, dedicated to St. Mary, is a handsome edifice, situated on an isolated hill, which has much the appearance of an ancient fortress. At Dagnell there was formerly a chantry chapel, dedicated to All Saints.

EDDLESTON, a township in the parish of ACTON, hundred of NANTWICH, county palatine of CHESTER, 2 miles (S.W. by W.) from Nantwich, containing 95 inhabitants.

EDDLETHORP, a township in the parish of WESTOW, wapentake of BUCKROSE, East riding of the county of YORK, 3½ miles (S.) from New Malton, containing 62 inhabitants.

EDECLIFT, a township in the parish of CLUN, hundred of PURSLOW, county of SALOP, containing 419 inhabitants.

EDEN (CASTLE), a parish in the southern division of EASINGTON ward, county palatine of DURHAM, 10½ miles (E. by S.) from Durham, containing 281 inhabitants. The living is a perpetual curacy, in the archdeaconry and diocese of Durham, endowed with £200 private benefaction, and £200 royal bounty, and in the patronage of Rowland Burdon, Esq. The church, dedicated to St. James, was rebuilt in 1764, at the expense of Rowland Burdon, Esq., whose son and successor enlarged it by the addition of two aisles. The petty sessions for the division are held here. This was a place of some note anterior to the Conquest. Robert de Brus, by charter, granted the chapel of Eden, which he had founded here, to the monks of St. Cuthbert, directing that a chapel should be built by the prior, within four years afterwards, which was probably the origin of the present parochial edifice. The ancient castle has long fallen to ruins, and has been succeeded by a modern mansion. The Dene, a narrow glen about four miles in length, through which runs the Eden rivulet, abounds with scenery of a wild and romantic description. The skeleton of a human figure, and a curious glass-vase, were found in 1775, beneath a cairn, about a hundred yards northward from the bridge, but they were not then removed: the cairn having been subsequently re-opened, the former, from exposure to the atmosphere, had mouldered into dust, and the latter was then taken away.

EDENBRIDGE, a parish in the hundred of WESTERHAM, lathe of SUTTON at HONE, county of KENT, 5½ miles (S.) from Westerham, containing 1454 inhabitants. The living is a vicarage, annexed to the perpetual curacy of Westerham, in the archdeaconry and diocese of Rochester. The church, dedicated to St. Peter and St. Paul, has a tower surmounted by a spire at the west end; in it are the remains of a rood loft, in which was formerly placed the image of our Saviour's Crucifixion, and the windows exhibit some interesting specimens of painted glass. There are fairs for cattle and toys on May 6th and October 16th. The river Eden, tributary to the Medway, passes through the parish,

and is here crossed by a bridge, which in the *Textus Roffensis* is called *Eddelnesbrege*.

EDENFIELD, a chapelry in the parish of BURY, hundred of SALFORD, county palatine of LANCASTER, 6 miles (N. by W.) from Bury, with which the population is returned. The living is a perpetual curacy, in the archdeaconry and diocese of Chester, endowed with £400 private benefaction, £600 royal bounty, and £500 parliamentary grant, and in the patronage of the Rector of Bury. The manufacture of cotton is here carried on to a considerable extent. A new road has lately been made to Blackburn.

EDENHALL, a parish in LEATH ward, county of CUMBERLAND, comprising the chapelry of Langwathby, and the township of Edenhall, and containing 501 inhabitants, of which number, 251 are in the township of Edenhall, 3½ miles (E.N.E.) from Penrith. The living is a discharged vicarage, in the archdeaconry and diocese of Carlisle, rated in the king's books at £17. 12. 1., and in the patronage of the Dean and Chapter of Carlisle. The church, dedicated to St. Cuthbert, is a singular and beautiful structure, with a low tower; it contains several monuments to the Musgraves. There is a neat private chapel at Eden Hall, which is a large, handsome edifice, built in the style which prevailed in the earlier part of the seventeenth century, and the residence of the ancient family of the Musgraves. The village is situated on the western bank of the river Eden. The proceeds of £75, bequeathed by Sir Philip Musgrave in 1759, are applied to the education of children.

EDENHAM, a parish in the wapentake of BELTISLOE, parts of KESTEVEN, county of LINCOLN, 3¼ miles (W.N.W.) from Bourne, containing, with the hamlets of Grinsthorpe, Ellsthorp, and Scottlesthorp, 657 inhabitants. The living is a perpetual curacy, in the archdeaconry and diocese of Lincoln, and in the patronage of Lord Gwydir and Lady Willoughby D'Eresby. The church, dedicated to St. Michael, has a Norman door-way.

EDENSOR, a parish in the hundred of HIGH PEAK, county of DERBY, 2¼ miles (E.N.E.) from Bakewell, containing, with Chatsworth and the hamlet of Pilsley, 752 inhabitants. The living, formerly a vicarage, rated in the king's books at £4. 13. 4., is now a perpetual curacy, in the archdeaconry of Derby, and diocese of Lichfield and Coventry, and in the patronage of the Duke of Devonshire. The church, dedicated to St. Peter, contains several monuments of the noble family of Cavendish. The village is situated entirely within Chatsworth Park. The Duke of Devonshire contributes £30 a year in aid of a school, which sum, with £5. 12. per annum arising from an enclosure of waste land, and the interest of £50, the gift of John Phillips in 1734, is appropriated for the instruction of sixty children.

EDGBASTON, a parish in the Birmingham division of the hundred of HEMLINGFORD, county of WARWICK, 1½ mile (S.W.) from Birmingham, containing 2117 inhabitants. The living is a perpetual curacy, in the peculiar jurisdiction of the Dean and Chapter of Lichfield, endowed with £200 private benefaction, and £200 royal bounty. Lord Calthorpe was patron in 1795. The church is dedicated to St. Bartholomew. The village has within the last few years become an extensive and handsome appendage to the town of Birmingham, and consists of several spacious streets well lighted with gas, containing many respectable houses, exclusively of several substantial mansions in detached situations, and numerous villas inhabited chiefly by proprietors of factories in the town, by the more opulent manufacturers, and private families : the buildings are chiefly of stone and brick, coated with Roman cement, and exhibit a great variety of architectural style. Of the few ancient buildings which existed previously to the erection of the modern town, the hall, which was garrisoned for the parliament in the reign of Charles I., and a private house called the Monument, from the erection of a very high octagonal tower of brick, near which passes the Roman Iknield-street, are the principal now remaining. The subscription bowling-green and pleasure-grounds are beautifully laid out and well attended. The reservoir of the Birmingham canal, which passes through the parish, an extensive sheet of water covering nineteen acres, and excavated to the depth of twenty feet, derives from the rich foliage on its banks all the beauty of a small lake. The church, an ancient structure, has been recently enlarged, and carefully restored, with a due regard to the preservation of its original character. The asylum for the deaf and dumb, on the borders of the canal, is a commodious edifice, resembling in some degree the ancient style of English architecture.

EDGBOLTON, a township in that part of the parish of SHAWBURY which is in the Whitchurch division of the hundred of BRADFORD (North), county of SALOP, 8 miles (N.E. by N.) from Shrewsbury, containing, with Muckleston and Great Witchford, 457 inhabitants.

EDGCOTT, a parish in the hundred of CHIPPING-WARDEN, county of NORTHAMPTON, 6¼ miles (N.E. by N.) from Banbury, containing 62 inhabitants. The living is a rectory, in the archdeaconry of Northampton, and diocese of Peterborough, rated in the king's books at £12. Thomas Carter, Esq. was patron in 1827. The church is dedicated to St. James. In a vale called Danes-moor, south of the village, a battle was fought between the Saxons and the Danes ; and in the time of Edward IV. a conflict took place between the houses of York and Lancaster, when the former having been defeated, the Earl of Pembroke and his two brothers were made prisoners and beheaded ; there are three small mounds in a triangular position upon the spot. In 1642, Charles I., with his two sons and a part of his army, encamped here previously to the battle of Edge-Hill, and returned the following day.

EDGE, a township in the parish of MALPAS, higher division of the hundred of BROXTON, county palatine of CHESTER, 3 miles (N. by E.) from Malpas, containing 298 inhabitants.

EDGE, a tything in the parish of PAINSWICK, hundred of BISLEY, county of GLOUCESTER, containing 1627 inhabitants.

EDGE, a township in the parish of PONTESBURY, hundred of FORD, county of SALOP, containing 372 inhabitants.

EDGECOTT, a parish in the hundred and county of BUCKINGHAM, 8 miles (S.W. by W.) from Winslow, containing 160 inhabitants. The living is a rectory, in the archdeaconry of Buckingham, and diocese of Lincoln, rated in the king's books at £11. 12. 8½. John Coker, Esq.

Esq. was patron in 1814. The church is dedicated to St. Michael.

EDGEFIELD, a parish in the hundred of HOLT, county of NORFOLK, 2¾ miles (S.) from Holt, containing 680 inhabitants. The living is a rectory, in the archdeaconry and diocese of Norwich, rated in the king's books at £11. 6. 8. John Marcon, Esq. was patron in 1764. The church is dedicated to St. Peter.

EDGE-HILL, a chapelry in the parish of WALTON on the HILL, hundred of WEST DERBY, county palatine of LANCASTER, 1 mile (S.E.) from Liverpool. The population is returned with the parish. The living is a perpetual curacy, in the archdeaconry and diocese of Chester. E. Mason, Esq. was patron in 1823. This is a pleasant village, situated on rising ground on the road to Wavertree and Childwell : the Liverpool Botanic Garden is in the vale beneath, and at a short distance from it. A chapel, dedicated to St. Mary, has been recently erected. There is a place of worship for Baptists.

EDGE-HILL, a joint township with Burntwood and Woodhouse, in that part of the parish of ST. MICHAEL, LICHFIELD, which is in the southern division of the hundred of OFFLOW, county of STAFFORD, 2¼ miles (W.S.W.) from Lichfield, containing 675 inhabitants.

EDGERLEY, a township in that part of the parish of ALDFORD which is in the lower division of the hundred of BROXTON, county palatine of CHESTER, containing 4 inhabitants.

EDGMOND, a parish in the Newport division of the hundred of BRADFORD (South), county of SALOP, 1¾ mile (W.) from Newport, comprising the chapelries of Church-Aston and Tibberton, and the townships of Cherrington and Chetwynd-Aston, and containing 2163 inhabitants. The living is a rectory, in the archdeaconry of Salop, and diocese of Lichfield and Coventry, rated in the king's books at £46. 8. 1½. J. K. Powell, Esq. and others were patrons in 1811. The church is dedicated to St. Peter. The Rev. Dryden Piggott, in 1734, gave £200, the income arising from which is applied for the clothing and education of poor children.

EDGTON, a parish in the hundred of PURSLOW, county of SALOP, 4½ miles (E.S.E.) from Bishop's Castle, containing, with the township of Brunslow, and the extra-parochial liberty of Harderlea, 220 inhabitants. The living is a perpetual curacy, annexed to the vicarage of Clun, in the archdeaconry of Salop, and diocese of Hereford. The church is dedicated to St. Michael. The river Ouny runs through the parish.

EDGWARE, a parish (formerly a market town) in the hundred of GORE, county of MIDDLESEX, 8 miles (N.W. by W.) from London, containing 551 inhabitants. This place, from its situation within a pleasant distance of the metropolis, and the excellence of the road leading to it through an almost uninterrupted succession of elegant villas and agreeable scenery, has become the residence of numerous opulent and respectable families. The Roman Watling-street, leading to the ancient city of *Verulam*, passes over a bridge near the entrance to the village, which consists of one principal street, of which the western side is in the parish of Little Stanmore, or Whitchurch, where, in the early part of the eighteenth century, James, Duke of Chandos, at an expense of £250,000, erected the magnificent palace of Canons, the walls of which were twelve feet in thickness at the base, and nine feet thick in the upper part; the pillars of the hall and the steps of the grand staircase were of the most beautiful marble, and the locks and hinges of the doors were of silver; the internal decorations were of the most splendid description, and the grounds were adorned with a profusion of statuary; the household establishment was in every respect equal to the splendour of this sumptuous mansion; the chapel was of like elegance, and richly embellished with paintings of the Italian school: the most eminent composers were employed in the arrangement, and the most eminent masters in the vocal and instrumental performance of the musical services. After the death of the duke, this noble mansion was taken down and sold piecemeal: the columns formed part of the portico of Wanstead-house; the marble staircase was put up in the Earl of Chesterfield's residence in Mayfair, London; and the celebrated equestrian statue of George I. at present decorates the area of Leicester-square. The village contains several respectable houses, and is supplied with water from a well dug in 1822, by public subscription. The market, formerly on Thursday, has been discontinued, but an annual fair is still held on the first Wednesday, Thursday, and Friday, in August, for cattle and toys: on the two last days races are held, which are in general well attended. Edgware is within the jurisdiction of a court of requests held at Brentford and Uxbridge, for the recovery of debts under 40s. There are courts baron and leet annually on the 1st of May; and the petty sessions for the division are held in that part of the village which is in the parish of Little Stanmore. Sir William Blackstone mentions a singular ancient custom as existing here, for the lord of the manor to provide a minstrel or piper to play for the amusement of the tenants, and there is in the parish a small field still called Piper's Green. The living is a perpetual curacy, but having been from time immemorial endowed with the vicarial tithes, it may be considered a vicarage not in charge; it has been further endowed with the rent of three houses in Hosier-lane, London, by Mr. John Jones; it is in the archdeaconry of Middlesex, and diocese of London, and in the patronage of John Lee, L.L.D. The church, dedicated to St. Margaret, with the exception of its square embattled tower, which is of flint and stone, was rebuilt of brick in 1763, and the interior was thoroughly repaired in 1822. An almshouse, containing four tenements, with a garden to each, was founded for four aged women, in 1680, by Samuel Atkinson, Esq., who endowed it with lands at Oakley, in the county of Buckingham, to which has been added a small bequest of land at Kenton, in Middlesex, by Thomas Napier, Esq., producing together, exclusively of the rents of Harrod's Green, given by Mr. Watts to the parish, and appropriated to this charity, an annual income of £32. 10. Charles Day, Esq., in 1828, founded almshouses for eight aged persons, five of Edgware, and three of Little Stanmore, and endowed them with £100 per annum: the premises, situated at the northern extremity of the village, are handsomely built, at an expense of £2000, in the later style of English architecture, fronted with stone brought from Eadley in Yorkshire, and have a clock in the centre.

EDGEWORTH, a parish in the hundred of BISLEY,

county of GLOUCESTER, 6½ miles (N.W. by W.) from Cirencester, containing 134 inhabitants. The living is a rectory, in the archdeaconry and diocese of Gloucester, rated in the king's books at £8, and in the patronage of Mrs. Westfaling. The church, dedicated to St. Mary, has some portions in the Norman style, and some of later date. There is a bequest of £5. 5. per annum, by Mrs. Joan Ridler, for teaching poor children.

EDGWORTH, a township in the parish of BOLTON, hundred of SALFORD, county palatine of LANCASTER, 5½ miles (N.N.E.) from Bolton, containing 1729 inhabitants. The Independents have a place of worship here. There are several establishments in the neighbourhood, for spinning and printing cotton. A school-room for the education of poor children, and a dwelling-house for the master, were erected in 1804, by subscriptions amounting to £500.

EDINGHALL, otherwise EDINGALE, a parish partly in the northern division of the hundred of OFFLOW, county of STAFFORD, and partly in the hundred of REPTON and GRESLEY, county of DERBY, 6 miles (N. by W.) from Tamworth. That part of the parish which is in Staffordshire contains 224 inhabitants, and the population of that part which is in Derbyshire is returned with the parish of Croxall. The living is a perpetual curacy, in the peculiar jurisdiction of the Prebendary of Alrewas and Weeford in the Cathedral Church of Lichfield, endowed with £200 private benefaction, and £300 royal bounty, and in the patronage of the Crown. The church is dedicated to the Holy Trinity. An ancient raised way, in the direction of Lullington in Derbyshire, passes through the parish, near which there is a tumulus. Edinghall is in the honour of Tutbury, duchy of Lancaster, and within the jurisdiction of a court of pleas held at Tutbury every third Tuesday, for the recovery of debts under 40s.

EDINGLY, a parish within the liberty of SOUTH WELL and SCROOBY, though locally in the wapentake of Thurgarton, county of NOTTINGHAM, 2¼ miles (W.N.W.) from Southwell, containing 344 inhabitants. The living is a discharged vicarage, rated in the king's books at £4, endowed with £800 royal bounty, and in the peculiar jurisdiction and patronage of the Chapter of the Collegiate Church of Southwell. The church is dedicated to St. Giles. A school is endowed with a house, garden, and a few acres of land, partly the gift of Samuel Wright, in 1731, and partly allotted in 1767 by the commissioners for enclosing common lands, for teaching poor children.

EDINGTHORPE, a parish in the hundred of TUNSTEAD, county of NORFOLK, 3 miles (N.E. by E.) from North Walsham, containing 175 inhabitants. The living is a discharged rectory, in the archdeaconry of Norfolk, and diocese of Norwich, rated in the king's books at £5. 5. 2½., and in the patronage of the King, as Duke of Lancaster. The church is dedicated to All Saints.

EDINGTON, a township in that part of the parish of MITFORD which is in the western division of CASTLE ward, county of NORTHUMBERLAND, 4¼ miles (S.W. by W.) from Morpeth, containing 44 inhabitants.

EDINGTON, a chapelry in the parish of MOORLINCH, hundred of WHITLEY, county of SOMERSET, 6½ miles (E.N.E.) from Bridg-water, containing 341 inhabitants. Near the chapel is a medicinal spring impregnated with sulphur and steel, said to be efficacious in scorbutic disorders. A tesselated pavement and other Roman antiquities have been discovered.

EDINGTON, a parish in the hundred of WHORWELSDOWN, county of WILTS, comprising the tythings of Baynton with West Coulston, Edington, and Tinhead, and containing 1099 inhabitants, of which number, 549 are in the tything of Edington, 3¾ miles (E.N.E.) from Westbury. The living is a perpetual curacy, in the archdeaconry and diocese of Salisbury, endowed with £200 royal bounty, and £1200 parliamentary grant. G. W. Taylor, Esq. was patron in 1826. The church, dedicated to All Saints, is a handsome cruciform structure with a tower rising from the intersection. William de Edington, a native of this place, and successively Bishop of Winchester, Lord High Treasurer, Chancellor of the Order of the Garter, and Lord High Chancellor, in the reign of Edward III., besides partly rebuilding the church, founded, about 1347, in honour of the Blessed Virgin Mary, St. Catherine, and All Saints, a college, consisting of a dean and twelve ministers, of whom some were prebendaries; for these were substituted, at the desire of the Black Prince, in 1358, a reformed order of Augustine friars, called Bonhommes, under the government of a rector: its yearly revenue at the suppression was estimated at £521. 12. 5. The bishops of Salisbury had a palace here, which was plundered and destroyed during the rebellion of Jack Cade, in 1450, when Bishop Ayscough was dragged from the altar of his chapel, where he was officiating at mass, and stoned to death on a neighbouring hill. On an eminence about two miles from the village is a strong irregular intrenchment, called Bratton Castle, enclosing an area of twenty-three acres; and on the south-western declivity of the same hill, a remarkable figure of a white horse, in a walking posture, is cut out, measuring one hundred feet both in length and height.

EDINGWORTH, a hamlet partly in the parish of EAST BRENT, and partly in the parish of LYMPSHAM, hundred of BRENT with WRINGTON, county of SOMERSET, 5½ miles (W. by S.) from Axbridge. The population is returned with the respective parishes. Here was formerly an alien priory of Benedictine monks, a cell to the abbey of St. Sever, in Normandy, which was granted in the 7th of Edward IV. to Eton College.

EDITH-WESTON, a parish in the hundred of MARTINSLEY, county of RUTLAND, 5¾ miles (E. S. E.) from Oakham, containing 301 inhabitants. The living is a rectory, in the archdeaconry of Northampton, and diocese of Peterborough, rated in the king's books at £14. 7. 6., and in the patronage of B. Lucas, Esq. The church is dedicated to St. Mary. Here was formerly an alien priory of Benedictine monks, a cell to the abbey of St. George, at Banguervill, in Normandy, to which it was given by William de Tankerville, chamberlain to Henry I.; at the suppression, in the reign of Richard II., it was conveyed to the 'Carthusians of Coventry, and as part of their possessions was granted, in the 4th of Edward VI., to the Marquis of Northampton.

EDLASTON, a parish in the hundred of APPLETREE, county of DERBY, 2½ miles (S.) from Ashbourn, containing, with Wyaston, 277 inhabitants. The living is a discharged rectory, in the archdeaconry of Derby, and diocese of Lichfield and Coventry, rated in the

king's books at £3. 18. 4., and in the patronage of the Dean of Lincoln. The church is dedicated to St. James.

EDLINGHAM, a parish in the northern division of COQUETDALE ward, county of NORTHUMBERLAND, comprising the chapelry of Bolton, and the townships of Abberwick, Broom-Park, Edlingham, Learchild, and Lemmington, and containing 666 inhabitants, of which number, 201 are in the township of Edlingham, 6 miles (S. W. by W.) from Alnwick. The living is a discharged vicarage, in the archdeaconry of Northumberland, and diocese of Durham, rated in the king's books at £6. 14. 4., and in the patronage of the Dean and Chapter of Durham. The church is dedicated to St. John the Baptist. The river Aln runs through the parish, in which are parochial and Sunday schools. There are some remains of Edlingham castle, built prior to the reign of Henry II.

EDLINGTON, a parish in the northern division of the wapentake of GARTREE, parts of LINDSEY, county of LINCOLN, 3½ miles (N. W.) from Horncastle, containing 263 inhabitants. The living is a discharged vicarage, in the archdeaconry and diocese of Lincoln, rated in the king's books at £8. 4. 7., and in the patronage of the Crown. The church is dedicated to St. Helen.

EDLINGTON, a parish in the southern division of the wapentake of STRAFFORTH and TICKHILL, West riding of the county of YORK, 5¼ miles (S. W. by S.) from Doncaster, containing 141 inhabitants. The living is a discharged rectory, in the archdeaconry and diocese of York, rated in the king's books at £9. Lord Molesworth was patron in 1818. The church is dedicated to St. Peter.

EDMONDBYERS, a parish in the western division of CHESTER ward, county palatine of DURHAM, comprising the chapelry of Hunstonworth, and the township of Edmondbyers, and containing 769 inhabitants, of which number, 358 are in the township of Edmondbyers, 12 miles (N. N. W.) from Wolsingham. The living is a discharged rectory, in the archdeaconry and diocese of Durham, rated in the king's books at £6. 11. 4., endowed with £200 royal bounty, and in the patronage of the Dean and Chapter of Durham. The church is dedicated to St. Edmund. The village, situated on the southern bank of the Derwent, is irregularly built. There is a smelting-mill, erected by the London Lead Company, the neighbouring parish abounding with lead-ore. A school-room was built in 1825, at the joint expense of the Dean and Chapter of Durham, and the trustees of Lord Crewe.

EDMONDSLEY, a township in that part of the parish of CHESTER le STREET which is in the middle division of CHESTER ward, county palatine of DURHAM, 5¼ miles (N. W. by N.) from Durham, containing 205 inhabitants.

EDMONDSTRIP-BENHAM, a tything in that part of the parish of KINGSCLERE which is in the hundred of KINGSCLERE, Kingsclere division of the county of SOUTHAMPTON, 1½ mile (N.) from Kingsclere, with which the population is returned.

EDMONDSTRIP-LANCES, a tything in that part of the parish of KINGSCLERE which is in the hundred of KINGSCLERE, Kingsclere division of the county of SOUTHAMPTON, 1½ mile (N.) from Kingsclere, with which the population is returned.

Q 2

EDMONDTHORPE, a parish in the hundred of FRAMLAND, county of LEICESTER, 7 miles (E. by S.) from Melton-Mowbray, containing 148 inhabitants. The living is a rectory, in the archdeaconry of Leicester, and diocese of Lincoln, rated in the king's books at £14. 12. 8½., and in the patronage of the Crown. The church is dedicated to St. Michael.

EDMONSHAM, a parish in that part of the hundred of CRANBORNE which is in the Shaston (East) division of the county of DORSET, 1½ mile (S. by E.) from Cranborne, containing 262 inhabitants. The living is a rectory, in the archdeaconry of Dorset, and diocese of Bristol, rated in the king's books at £6. 5. The Earl of Shaftesbury was patron in 1826. The church is dedicated to St. Nicholas. There is a chalybeate spring in the parish.

EDMONTON, a parish in the hundred of EDMONTON, county of MIDDLESEX, 7 miles (N.) from London, containing 7900 inhabitants. This place, which had risen into some consideration prior to the Conquest, is in Domesday-book called Ædelmeton, probably as having been the residence of some distinguished personage during the Heptarchy. The extensive forest in the neighbourhood, of which Enfield Chase formed a part, made it the resort of many individuals who occasionally retired hither to enjoy the diversion of hunting, and from its convenient distance from the metropolis, it became the residence of many opulent families. The village is pleasantly situated on the high road to Hertford, along which it extends for more than a mile, containing, exclusively of small dwellings, several ranges of respectable, houses, and, in detached situations, many elegant mansions and handsome villas ; it is well lighted with gas, and amply supplied with water : the New River winds through several parts of the parish, producing a pleasing and picturesque effect in the pleasure grounds and meadows through which it runs. A considerable coach manufactory has been established here within the last thirty years, which affords employment to more than sixty persons; and an extensive trade in timber is carried on by means of the Lea river navigation, which passes within three quarters of a mile of the village. Fairs are held annually on St. Giles' and Ascension days, on a part of Enfield Chase, near Southgate, in this parish, under letters patent of James I., chiefly for pleasure. The petty sessions for the division are held at the Angel Inn every alternate Friday. The jurisdiction of a court of requests at Enfield, for the recovery of debts under 40s., extends to this parish; and a court leet and court baron are held on the Tuesday in Whitsun-week.

The parish comprises the divisions of Church-Street, Fore-Street, Bury-Street, and Southgate-Street. The living is a vicarage, in the archdeaconry of Middlesex, and diocese of London, rated in the king's books at £18, and in the patronage of the Dean and Chapter of St. Paul's, London. The church, dedicated to All Saints, is a spacious modern brick structure with an old embattled tower ; the nave was rebuilt of brick in 1772. The chapel in Southgate-Street was erected and endowed in 1615, by Sir John Weld, Knt.; and another chapel in Winchmore Hill, dedicated to St. Paul, in the later style of English architecture, was erected in 1828, at an expense of nearly £5000, defrayed by subscription among the inhabitants, aided by a grant of £3500 from the parliamentary commissioners. There are places of worship for

Baptists, the Society of Friends, Independents, and Wesleyan Methodists. A charity school for boys was founded in 1624, by Mr. Edward Latymer, who bequeathed a messuage at Edmonton, and lands at Hammersmith, for clothing and educating eight poor boys, for which purpose also Mr. Thomas Styles, in 1679, bequeathed £20 per annum ; several similar benefactions have been consolidated, producing about £550 per annum, which is appropriated to the instruction of more than one hundred boys, of which number sixty are clothed : the school-room was built in 1811, pursuant to the will of Mrs. Ann Wyatt, who bequeathed £500 five per cent. Navy annuities for that purpose, and £100 to keep it in repair. A charity school for girls was established by subscription in 1778, since which period donations and legacies to the amount of £5000 have been given for its support ; the endowment arising from these sums is augmented by annual subscription, and appropriated to the clothing and instruction of more than seventy girls : the present school-house was built by subscription in 1818. There is a National school, in which nearly three hundred children are instructed. A fund arising from several bequests is appropriated to the apprenticing of poor children. Mr. John Wild, in 1662, built three almshouses, which he endowed with £4 per annum; and Mr. Thomas Styles erected twelve, which he endowed with £36. 16. per annum ; to the poor in the latter, Mr. John Lewitt, in 1771, bequeathed £800 ; and for the poor in both almshouses, Mr. George Stanbridge, in 1780, left £500; Mrs. Sarah Huxley, in 1800, bequeathed £1000; and other benefactors have contributed various sums for their support. On Bush Hill, in this parish, are remains of a large circular encampment, supposed to have been the site of a British town, near which Sir Hugh Myddelton had a residence. Bury hall, the seat of President Bradshaw, retains many of its original features. Peter Fabell, a learned man of eccentric character, who obtained the reputation of being a conjuror, is said to have been born in this parish, which became noted by the production of a drama about the year 1490, founded upon some of his alleged exploits, and called the "Merry Devil of Edmonton :" the place also gave rise to a tragedy founded on the history of an unfortunate woman who was condemned and executed on a charge of witchcraft, in 1621 ; and it has been lastly celebrated as the scene of Cowper's popular ballad of "John Gilpin," in allusion to which there is a painting in front of the Bell Inn. Dr. Brook Taylor, secretary to the Royal Society, and author of an ingenious treatie on Perspective, was born here in 1685; and Archbishop Tillotson resided here constantly while Dean of St. Paul's, and occasionally after his translation to the primacy.

EDSTASTON, a chapelry in that part of the parish of WEM which is in the Whitchurch division of the hundred of BRADFORD (North), county of SALOP, 1¼ mile (N. by E.) from Wem, containing 397 inhabitants.

EDSTON, a hamlet in the parish of WOOTTON-WAVEN, Henley division of the hundred of BARLICHWAY, county of WARWICK, 4¾ miles (S.E. by S.) from Henley in Arden. The population is returned with the parish. Somerville, the poet, was born here in 1692.

EDSTON (GREAT), a parish in the wapentake of RYEDALE, North riding of the county of YORK, 6½ miles (W. by S.) from Pickering, containing 156 inhabitants. The living is a discharged vicarage, in the archdeaconry of Cleveland, and diocese of York, rated in the king's books at £7. 10., and in the patronage of the Marquis of Salisbury.

EDSTON (LITTLE), a township in that part of the parish of SINNINGTON which is in the wapentake of RYEDALE, North riding of the county of YORK, 6¼ miles (W.) from Pickering, containing 16 inhabitants.

EDVIN-LOACH, a parish in the upper division of the hundred of DODDINGTREE, county of WORCESTER, though locally in the hundred of Broxash, county of Hereford, 3 miles (N. by E.) from Bromyard, containing 63 inhabitants. The living is a discharged rectory, with which the rectory of Tedstone-Wafer is united, in the archdeaconry of Salop, and diocese of Hereford, rated in the king's books at £2. 1. 10½. Mr. Higginson was patron in 1811.

EDWALTON, a parish in the northern division of the wapentake of RUSHCLIFFE, county of NOTTING-HAM, 3½ miles (S. S. E.) from Nottingham, containing 119 inhabitants. The living is a perpetual curacy, in the archdeaconry of Nottingham, and diocese of York, endowed with £600 royal bounty, and in the patronage of John Musters, Esq. The church is dedicated to the Holy Rood. Edwalton is in the honour of Tutbury, duchy of Lancaster, and within the jurisdiction of a court of pleas held at Tutbury every third Tuesday, for the recovery of debts under 40s.

EDWARDSTONE, a parish in the hundred of BABERGH, county of SUFFOLK, 1¾ mile (N. W.) from Boxford, containing 416 inhabitants. The living is a discharged vicarage, in the archdeaconry of Sudbury, and diocese of Norwich, rated in the king's books at £4. 13. 4. Charles Dawson, Esq. was patron in 1817. The church, dedicated to St. Mary, was given with the tithes and other appurtenances to the monastery of Abingdon, by Hubert Munchesni, lord of the manor, in 1114, when a society of Black monks was placed here; but in 1160 they were removed to the priory of Colne, to which the parish church became appropriated and belonged till the dissolution. There is a fair for cattle, horses, and pigs, on the 24th of December.

EDWIN-RALPH, a parish in the hundred of WOLPHY, though locally in the hundred of Broxash, county of HEREFORD, 2 miles (N.) from Bromyard, containing, with Butterley, 157 inhabitants. The living is a discharged rectory, in the archdeaconry and diocese of Hereford, rated in the king's books at £6. 6. 10¼., and in the patronage of Mrs. Pytts. Limestone is obtained in the parish.

EDWINSTOW, a parish in the Hatfield division of the wapentake of BASSETLAW, county of NOTTING-HAM, 2 miles (W. by S.) from Ollerton, comprising the chapelries of Carburton, Ollerton, and Perlethorpe, and the townships of Budby and Clipstone, and containing 1753 inhabitants. The living is a vicarage, in the archdeaconry of Nottingham, and diocese of York, rated in the king's books at £14., and in the patronage of the Dean of Lincoln. The church, dedicated to St. Mary, is a large ancient building. There is a place of worship for Wesleyan Methodists. John Bellamy, in 1719, bequeathed a school-house and land for the instruction of eight children: in 1824 it was taken down and a new house built on the site, at the expense of Earl Manvers: the income is £10 a

year, and the school is free for all the poor children of the parish. The principal object of note is the last remnant of the ancient Forest of Sherwood, celebrated in ballad story as the scene of the exploits of Robin Hood and his faithful band of archers, extending for the distance of three miles and a half from east to north, and two from north to south.

EDWORTH, a parish in the hundred of BIGGLES-WADE, county of BEDFORD, 3¾ miles (S. E. by S.) from Biggleswade, containing 87 inhabitants. The living is a rectory, in the archdeaconry of Bedford, and diocese of Lincoln, rated in the king's books at £15. 16. 3., and in the patronage of the Dean and Chapter of Lincoln. The church is dedicated to St. George.

EFFINGHAM, a parish in the hundred of EFFING-HAM, county of SURREY, 3¾ miles (S. W. by W.) from Leatherhead, containing 499 inhabitants. The living is a discharged vicarage, in the archdeaconry of Surrey, and diocese of Winchester, rated in the king's books at £7. 18. 9., endowed with £200 private benefaction, and £200 royal bounty, and in the patronage of the Crown. The church, dedicated to St. Lawrence, contains several old stalls and monuments. There are evident proofs of the village having been formerly much larger than it is at present; cavities similar to cellars have been frequently discovered in the adjacent fields and woods.

EGBROUGH, a township in the parish of KELLING-TON, lower division of the wapentake of OSGOLDCROSS, West riding of the county of YORK, 5¼ miles (W. by N.) from Snaith, containing 215 inhabitants.

EGDEAN, a parish in the hundred of ROTHER-BRIDGE, rape of ARUNDEL, county of SUSSEX, 2 miles (S. E.) from Petworth, containing 66 inhabitants. The living is a discharged rectory, in the archdeaconry and diocese of Chichester, rated in the king's books at £1.9.2. The Earl of Egremont was patron in 1788. The church is dedicated to St. Bartholomew. There are fairs on May 1st and September 4th, for horses and horned cattle. The Rother or Arundel navigation passes by the southern boundary of the parish.

EGERTON, a township in the parish of MALPAS, higher division of the hundred of BROXTON, county palatine of CHESTER, 5 miles (N. E. by N.) from Malpas, containing 115 inhabitants. There was formerly a chapel attached to an ancient manor-house which stood here; its remains have been converted into a barn.

EGERTON, a parish in the hundred of CALEHILL, lathe of SCRAY, county of KENT, 3¾ miles (W. S. W.) from Charing, containing 890 inhabitants. The living is a perpetual curacy, in the archdeaconry and diocese of Canterbury, endowed with £15 per annum private benefaction, and £1700 parliamentary grant, and in the patronage of the Dean and Chapter of St. Paul's, London. The church is dedicated to St. James. A fair is held on the 5th of August. There is a petrifying spring in the parish.

EGG-BUCKLAND, county of DEVON. See BUCK-LAND (EGG).

EGGESFORD, a parish in the hundred of NORTH TAWTON with WINKLEY, county of DEVON, 2½ miles (S.) from Chulmleigh, containing 144 inhabitants. The living is a discharged rectory, in the archdeaconry of Barnstaple, and diocese of Essex, rated in the king's books at £7. 18. 9., endowed with £200 private benefaction, and £200 royal bounty, and in the patronage of the Hon. Newton Fellowes. Here was formerly an hospital founded by Ibote Reigny.

EGGINGTON, a chapelry in the parish of LEIGH-TON-BUZZARD, hundred of MANSHEAD, county of BEDFORD, 2¾ miles (E.) from Leighton-Buzzard, containing 302 inhabitants. The living is a perpetual curacy, endowed with £200 parliamentary grant, and in the peculiar jurisdiction and patronage of the Prebendary of Leighton-Buzzard in the Cathedral Church of Lincoln.

EGGINTON, a parish in the hundred of MORLESTON and LITCHURCH, county of DERBY, 4¼ miles (N.N.E.) from Burton upon Trent, containing 319 inhabitants. The living is a rectory, in the archdeaconry of Derby, and diocese of Lichfield and Coventry, rated in the king's books at £8. 2. 8½., and in the patronage of Sir C. Eveny, Bart., C. Pole, and Joseph Leigh, Esqrs., the two former having each two presentations, and the latter one. The church, dedicated to St. Wilfrid, is a small ancient building with a low tower. The rivers Dove and Trent and the Grand Trunk canal pass through the parish. At the Norman survey *Eghintune* was described as having a church, a priest, a mill, and six farmers. In March, 1644, a battle was fought on Egginton Heath, in which the royalists were defeated by the parliamentarians under Sir John Gell.

EGGLESTON-ABBEY, a township in the parish of ROKEBY, western division of the wapentake of GILLING, North riding of the county of YORK, 1½ mile (S.E. by S.) from Barnard-Castle, containing 82 inhabitants. An abbey for Premonstratensian canons, dedicated to St. Mary and St. John the Baptist, was founded about 1189, by Ralph de Multon; it was re-founded in 1537, and at the dissolution its revenue was estimated at £36. 8. 3. per annum: there are still considerable remains of the buildings, part of which has been converted into cottages: the abbey church, a cruciform structure, is almost entire.

EGGLESTONE, a chapelry in the parish of MIDDLETON in TEESDALE, south-western division of DARLINGTON ward, county palatine of DURHAM, 6½ miles (N.W. by N.) from Barnard-Castle, containing 464 inhabitants. The living is a perpetual curacy, in the archdeaconry and diocese of Durham, endowed with £800 royal bounty, and in the patronage of the Rector of Middleton. There are lead-mines in the parish, said to have been in operation since the time of Henry VI., and which, from the discovery of ancient excavations and tools therein, are supposed to have been known to the Romans. The London Lead Company have a smelting-mill here. About a mile to the northward of the village, near a rivulet, is a circle of rough stones, with an inner trench enclosing a cairn; and close by the brook is a tumulus, intersected by a row of stones.

EGGLETON, a township in the parish of BISHOP'S FROOME, hundred of RADLOW, county of HEREFORD, 9¼ miles (E.N.E.) from Hereford, containing 172 inhabitants.

EGHAM, a parish in the second division of the hundred of GODLEY, county of SURREY, 20 miles (W. by S.) from London, containing 3616 inhabitants. The village is pleasantly situated on the banks of the river Thames, which here separates the counties of Surrey and Middlesex, and is intersected by the Roman road from Silchester, commencing at the Belvidere, in Shrub's park, and directing its course to the town, east of Virginia Water: it be-

comes conspicuous on the rising grounds, where it is remarkable for the almost entire preservation of its original form; and whence it may be traced, with some intervals, to Ashford, in Middlesex. In this parish are the plains of Runymede, appointed by King John for holding a conference with the barons, who had confederated for the preservation of their liberty, and celebrated as the spot on which, after a debate of a few days, the king consented to grant the privileges and exemptions contained in "Magna Charta," which he afterwards signed in a small island near the opposite bank of the Thames, still called Magna Charta island. The village, neatly built, and containing many respectable houses, is connected with the market town of Staines by a neat bridge, and another is now being erected in a more direct line with the London road. Cooper's Hill, within the parish, was first celebrated by the muse of Denham, who resided here, and afterwards by Pope and Somerville. Camomile Hill obtained its appellation from the luxuriant growth of that herb, with which it is covered, and which appears to be indigenous to the soil. Races are held annually in September, on Runymede, and are well attended. The only trade in this place is that arising from its situation as a great public thoroughfare. An annual fair is held on the 29th of May and the two following days. The parish is divided into four tythings, and courts baron for the manors of Egham and Mitton are held annually.

The living is a vicarage, in the archdeaconry of Surrey, and diocese of Winchester, rated in the king's books at £11. 9. 7., and in the patronage of Mrs. Gostling. The church, dedicated to St. John the Baptist, is a modern edifice of brick, ornamented with stone, and was built by subscription, his late Majesty, George III., having been a liberal contributor. There is a place of worship for Wesleyan Methodists. A charity school was founded in 1703, by Henry Strode, Esq., who bequeathed £6000 to the Coopers' Company in London, in trust for that purpose, and also for the foundation and endowment of almshouses for six aged men and six aged women; fifty boys are instructed in reading, writing, and arithmetic, on the National system. sixteen girls are also taught reading, writing, arithmetic, and needlework, by part of a legacy of £360, left by Mrs. Barker, for teaching children of the parishes of Egham, New Windsor, and Yately. This parish has also the privilege of sending boys for education to the foundation by Sir William Perkins, at Chertsey. Edmond Lee, Esq., in 1705, bequeathed £1000 to be laid out in land, the produce to be applied in apprenticing four boys, or girls, yearly. Twelve almshouses, containing each an upper and a lower room, have been erected in pursuance of Mr. Strode's will, and are tenanted by twelve aged persons appointed by the Coopers' Company; the income arising from this endowment is nearly £800 per annum. Five almshouses were founded in 1627, by Sir John Denham, who endowed them with a rent-charge of £30, and with tenements producing a rental of £8. 8. per annum, for five aged women of this parish. Viscountess Warren Bulkeley bequeathed £1000 for the benefit of the poor, in addition to which there are several other charitable bequests.

EGLETON, a chapelry in the parish and soke of OAKHAM, county of RUTLAND, 2 miles (S.E.) from Oakham, containing 131 inhabitants.

EGLINGHAM, a parish in the northern division of COQUETDALE ward, county of NORTHUMBERLAND, comprising the townships of Bassington, Beanly, New Bewick, Old Bewick, Brandon, Branton, Crawley, Eglingham, Hareup, Hedgeley, East Lilburn, West Lilburn, Titlington, and Wooperton, and containing 1440 inhabitants, of which number, 184 are in the township of Eglingham, 7½ miles (N.W.) from Alnwick. The living is a vicarage, in the archdeaconry of Northumberland and diocese of Durham, rated in the king's books at £23. 3. 1½., and in the patronage of the Bishop of Durham. The church is dedicated to St. Maurice. The river Bremish and several bournes rise in the Cheviot hills, and run through the parish. There is a lake covering ten acres, called Kimmer loch; also a spring of strong vitriolic water. In the eastern and southern parts of the parish are extensive moor lands. Coal, limestone, and freestone are obtained here. There are British and Roman encampments, and the ruins of an old border tower, in the parish. Percy's cross, on the road between Whittingham and Wooler, was erected on the spot where Sir Ralph Percy fell, in the battle of Hedgeley Moor, in 1463; at some distance from which is Percy's leap, where two stones commemorate an extraordinary leap which he took when closely pursued by the enemy.

EGLOSHAYLE, a parish in the hundred of TRIGG, county of CORNWALL, ¾ of a mile (S.E.) from Wade-Bridge, containing 1174 inhabitants. The living is a vicarage, in the peculiar jurisdiction and patronage of the Bishop of Exeter, rated in the king's books at £16. The church contains an ancient and curious stone pulpit; its lofty tower was built some centuries since, by the then vicar, named Lovibond, who left land producing about £20 a year for the support of a noble bridge of sixteen arches, erected by public contribution in the reign of Edward IV., across the Camel at Wade-Bridge, which river, at flood tides, is navigable for barges to and from Padstow. National schools, for children of both sexes, are supported by subscription. At Burnere or Brenere, the bishops of Exeter had formerly a seat. In the neighbourhood are the remains of an ancient treble intrenchment, called Castle Killibury.

EGLOSKERRY, a parish in the northern division of the hundred of EAST, county of CORNWALL, 3¾ miles (W.N.W.) from Launceston, containing 436 inhabitants. The living is a perpetual curacy, in the archdeaconry of Cornwall, and diocese of Exeter, endowed with £200 royal bounty, and £800 parliamentary grant, and in the patronage of F. H. Rudd, Esq. and others, as Trustees. The church is dedicated to St. Petrock. There is a place of worship at Tregeare for Wesleyan Methodists.

EGMANTON, a parish in the South-clay division of the wapentake of BASSETLAW, county of NOTTINGHAM, 1¼ mile (S.) from Tuxford, containing 320 inhabitants. The living is a discharged vicarage, in the archdeaconry of Nottingham, and diocese of York, rated in the king's books at £4.6.0½., endowed with £200 private benefaction, and £200 royal bounty. P. Barry, Esq. was patron in 1816. The church is dedicated to St. Mary. There is a place of worship for Wesleyan Methodists.

EGMERE, a parish in the northern division of the hundred of GREENHOE, county of NORFOLK, 2½ miles (W. by N.) from Little Walsingham, containing 47 inhabitants. The living is a rectory annexed to the vicarage of Holkham, in the archdeaconry and diocese of Norwich, rated in the king's books at £8, and in the patronage of T. W. Coke, Esq. The church, which was dedicated to St. Edmund, is desecrated. The two parishes are separated by Quarles farm, which is extraparochial.

EGREMONT, a market town and parish in ALLERDALE ward above Darwent, county of CUMBERLAND, 42½ miles (S. W. by S.) from Carlisle, and 293 (N. W. by N.) from London, containing 1741 inhabitants. This place is of great antiquity, and the neighbourhood is supposed to have been the scene of various conflicts between the Saxons and the Danes. At the time of the Conquest, Ranulph de Meschines, to whom William had granted the whole county of Cumberland, gave the great barony of Copeland (now called the barony of Egremont,) to his brother, William de Meschines, who erected his baronial castle on the site of an ancient Danish fort. The remains of this fortress, to the north-west of the town, though not extensive, exhibit traces of antiquity and strength: they consist chiefly of the gateway-tower and vaulted entrance, of circular arches in the Norman style; portions of the outer wall, enclosing a quadrangular area; the postern, and three narrow gateways, communicating with the outworks, which are of later date. The town is situated within less than three miles of the Irish sea, and consists principally of one spacious street: the houses are in general ancient, but many improvements have been recently effected, and a new bridge has been built over the river. The clothing business appears to have been anciently carried on here: the principal articles of manufacture at present are checks, linen, canvas, sail-cloth, and paper; the tanning and dressing of leather prevails to a limited extent, and in the parish are mines of iron-stone, from which about one hundred tons of ore are raised per day, and shipped at Whitehaven, for the supply of the iron-foundries of South Wales; limestone and red freestone are found in the neighbourhood, and a considerable quantity of lime is burnt. The market is on Saturday, and is well supplied with corn: the fairs are, February 18th for horses, the third Friday in May, and September 18th for horned cattle, sheep &c; on the three days following the last fair, a festival is celebrated, during which the inhabitants are allowed to sell ale without a license: statute fairs for hiring servants are held at Whitsuntide and Martinmas. The town was anciently a borough, and returned members to parliament in the 23rd of Edward I., but was, on its own petition, disfranchised, in the 24th of the same reign; the burgesses possessed many other privileges, of which all records are lost: there are about one hundred and twenty burgage tenements in the borough. A borough serjeant, two bailiffs, four constables, two hedge and corn-viewers, and assessors of damages, are annually appointed at the court leet of the lord of the manor, held in April, at which time a customary court is also held: a court baron is held every third Friday, under the Earl of Egremont, for the recovery of debts under 40s.: these courts are held, by adjournment from the castle, at the King's Arms Inn, the ancient court-house in the castle having gone to decay.

The living is a discharged rectory, in the archdeaconry of Richmond, and diocese of Chester, rated in the king's books at £7. 12. 1., and in the patronage of the Earl of Egremont. The church, dedicated to St. Michael, is an ancient structure, of which the east end is in the early style of English architecture, and the remainder chiefly Norman : it has a low tower. There is a place of worship for Wesleyan Methodists. A National school is supported by subscription, to which £4 per annum, arising from a bequest by Mr. John Nicholson, for apprenticing children, and another trifling sum, have been added. Near the ruins of the castle is a cairn of stones, called Woful Bank, which seems to have some reference to a battle fought prior to the Conquest. Egremont gives the title of earl to the family of Wyndham.

EGTON, a chapelry in the parish of ULVERSTONE, hundred of LONSDALE, north of the sands, county palatine of LANCASTER, 3 miles (N.N.E.) from Ulverstone, containing 470 inhabitants. The living is a perpetual curacy, in the archdeaconry of Richmond, and diocese of Chester, endowed with £400 royal bounty, and £1200 parliamentary grant. Mr. and Mrs. Machell were patrons in 1792. The chapel is dedicated to the Blessed Virgin Mary. Iron-ore obtained here is considered the richest hitherto found in the kingdom, and a large furnace for smelting it has been established for centuries. At Greenodd, a creek within the limits of the port of Lancaster, a considerable quantity of iron, in bars, copper-ore, slate, hoops, tanned leather, gunpowder, pyroligneous acid, and other articles of merchandise, are shipped for Liverpool, Glasgow, and Whitehaven. Henry Lindow, in 1735, gave certain property, now producing about £6 per annum, for the support of a school, for which eight children receive instruction.

EGTON, a parish in the eastern division of the liberty of LANGBAURGH, North riding of the county of YORK, 6¼ miles (W. S.W.) from Whitby, containing 1037 inhabitants. The living is a perpetual curacy, in the archdeaconry of Cleveland, and diocese of York, endowed with £200 royal bounty, and in the patronage of the Archbishop of York. The church, dedicated to St. Hilda, which is situated about half a mile from the town, was consecrated by the Bishop of Damascus, in 1349. There is a Roman Catholic chapel; and a Sunday school is supported by contributions. Egton received a charter for a market and four annual fairs from William III.; the former is now only held from the Tuesday before Palm-Sunday to Midsummer, weekly, and on the Tuesday before old Michaelmas for cattle : the fairs are on the Tuesday before February 15th, Tuesday before May 11th, September 4th, and Tuesday before November 22nd, for horned cattle, boots, and shoes. There is a fine spring, called Cold Keld well, much resorted to for strengthening weakly children.

EISEY, a parish in the hundred of HIGHWORTH, CRICKLADE, and STAPLE, county of WILTS, 1 mile (N. N. E.) from Cricklade, containing, with the township of Water-Eaton, 194 inhabitants. The living is a discharged vicarage, annexed to the vicarage of Latton, in the archdeaconry of Wilts, and diocese of Salisbury, rated in the king's books at £11. 14. 4., and in the patronage of the Earl of St. German's. The church is dedicated to St. Mary. The Thames and Severn canal passes through the parish.

ELBERTON, a parish in the lower division of the hundred of BERKELEY, county of GLOUCESTER, 2½ miles (S. W.) from Thornbury, containing 203 inhabit-

ants. The living is a discharged vicarage, consolidated in 1767 with the vicarage of Olveston, in the peculiar jurisdiction of the Bishop of Bristol, rated in the king's books at £6. 12. 6., endowed with £200 royal bounty, and in the patronage of the Dean and Chapter of Bristol, and the Bishop of Bristol, the former having two turns, and the latter one. The church, dedicated to St. Mary, has a central tower with a spire, and was probably erected in the thirteenth century. East of the village are some remains of a Roman intrenched camp, supposed to have been constructed for the protection of the *trajectus*, or ferry, at Aust; it was a regular parallelogram, enclosing two acres.

ELDEN, a parish in the hundred of KING'S SOMBOURN, Andover division of the county of SOUTHAMPTON, 4½ miles (S.E.) from Stockbridge. The living is a rectory, in the archdeaconry and diocese of Winchester, rated in the king's books at £2, and in the patronage of John Hussey, Esq. The church, dedicated to St. John the Baptist, is dilapidated, and unfit for service. The parish contains only one house, occupied by a farmer.

ELDERSFIELD, a parish forming, with the parishes of Chaseley and Staunton, a distinct portion of the lower division of the hundred of PERSHORE, county of WORCESTER, 7 miles (W. by S.) from Tewkesbury, containing 743 inhabitants. The living is a discharged vicarage, in the archdeaconry and diocese of Worcester, rated in the king's books at £8. 16. 8., and in the patronage of Sir Anthony Lechmere, Bart. The church, dedicated to St. John the Baptist, has a handsome spire. There is a place of worship for dissenters, also a charity school, supported by subscription.

ELDON, a township in that part of the parish of ST. ANDREW, AUCKLAND, which is in the south-eastern division of DARLINGTON ward, county palatine of DURHAM, 3½ miles (S. E. by E.) from Bishop-Auckland, containing 94 inhabitants. John Scott, Earl of Eldon, late Lord High Chancellor of England, was elevated to the peerage by the title of Baron Eldon, on the 18th of July, 1799, having also been raised to the dignities of Viscount Encombe and Earl of Eldon, July 7th, 1821.

ELDROTH, a hamlet in the parish of CLAPHAM, western division of the wapentake of STAINCLIFFE and EWCROSS, West riding of the county of YORK, 4¼ miles (W. by N.) from Settle. The population is returned with the parish. An ancient chapel of ease has been converted into a school, which is endowed with land and certain bequests for the education of children.

ELFORD, a township in the parish of BAMBROUGH, northern division of BAMBROUGH ward, county of NORTHUMBERLAND, 7 miles (E.S.E.) from Belford, containing 131 inhabitants.

ELFORD, a parish in the southern division of the hundred of OFFLOW, county of STAFFORD, 4½ miles (N. by W.) from Tamworth, containing 424 inhabitants. The living is a rectory, in the archdeaconry of Stafford, and diocese of Lichfield and Coventry, rated in the king's books at £13. 6. 8., and in the patronage of the Hon. F. G. Howard. The church is dedicated to St. Peter. A school was founded in the reign of James I., by the Rev. John Hill, which is supported by a moiety of the produce of various bequests subsequently made, amounting to about £15 per annum, and applied to the education of eighty children on the National system. The river Tame bounds the parish on the south-west.

ELHAM, a parish in the hundred of LONINGBO-ROUGH, lathe of SHEPWAY, county of KENT, 7 miles (N. W. by N.) from Folkestone, containing 1168 inhabitants. This place, which was anciently of greater importance, and contained several handsome structures, of which there are scarcely any vestiges, was, at the time of the Conquest, in the possession of the Norman earl Ewe, a near relation of the Conqueror's, who obtained for it many valuable privileges: in the reign of Henry III. it belonged to Prince Edward, who procured for it the grant of a weekly market, which, though for some time disused, is held occasionally in the market-house, every five or six years, in order to preserve the right. The village is situated on the smaller river Stour, and contains many houses neatly built of brick, and of modern appearance. Elham park, of which notice occurs in the time of Henry III., is now overgrown with wood. Fairs are held annually on Palm-Monday, Easter-Monday, and Whit-Monday, and October 20th, for horses, cattle, and pedlary. The county magistrates hold a petty session for the division monthly; and the parish is within the jurisdiction of a court of requests held at Folkestone, for the recovery of debts above 2s. and not exceeding 40s.: manorial courts are held on the Thursday in Easter week, and on the Thursday after the 20th of October. The living is a vicarage, in the archdeaconry and diocese of Canterbury, rated in the king's books at £20, and in the patronage of the Warden and Fellows of Merton College, Oxford, on the nomination of the Archbishop of Canterbury. The church, dedicated to St. Mary, is a spacious and handsome structure in the early style of English architecture, with a massive square embattled tower; over the west door is a fine window of three lights, in the decorated style, which has been subsequently inserted; the ancient timber roof is still preserved in the nave and aisles. There is a place of worship for Wesleyan Methodists. A school was founded here in 1725, by Sir John Williams, Knt., who endowed it with a house and lands now producing upwards of £60 per annum, for the clothing and instruction of six poor boys, of whom one is placed out apprentice. A house of industry for this and several adjoining parishes has been recently erected.

ELING, a parish in the hundred of REDBRIDGE, New Forest (East) division of the county of SOUTHAMPTON, 5 miles (W. by N.) from Southampton, containing, with Wigley, and a portion of Cadnam, 4314 inhabitants. The living is a vicarage, in the archdeaconry and diocese of Winchester, rated in the king's books at £11. 18. 1½. William Phillips, Esq. was patron in 1802. The church, dedicated to St. Mary, has been enlarged at different periods, as is evident from the variety in its architecture. Domesday-book records that at the Norman survey Eling had a church, two mills, a fishery, and a saltern. It is situated at the upper end of Southampton water, and a considerable trade in coal, timber, and corn, is carried on, there being depth sufficient for vessels of three hundred tons' burden, to load or unload at the quay, by the side of which numerous granaries and warehouses have been erected, for storing the several articles of merchandise. There are docks for ship-building, from which, of late years, several West Indiamen have been launched, and where vessels are frequently repaired, the proximity of the New Forest rendering timber plentiful, and the expense moderate.

There is a fair for toys on the 5th of July. At Marchwood, about two miles east from Eling, is a magazine of gunpowder, for the supply of Portsmouth garrison, with proper accommodations for the detachment of troops stationed for its protection. Tatchbury Mount is supposed to have been anciently a military station, and tradition records it as the site of a royal hunting seat; the trenches may still be traced from the terrace that surrounds it. The mansion and manor of Bury farm is held of the crown, on presenting to the king a brace of white greyhounds in silver couples, whenever His Majesty visits the New Forest, which tenure was last discharged in 1789, by the late Rev. Sir C. Mill, Bart., to George III. on his alighting from the royal carriage at Lyndhurst. The tythings of Ower, Wade, and Wigley, in this parish, are entitled to partake of the benefit schools founded by John Nowes, at Romsey and Yeovil, for teaching and clothing poor boys.

ELISHAW, a hamlet in the parish of ELSDON, southern division of COQUETDALE ward, county of NORTHUMBERLAND, 9 miles (N. by E.) from Bellingham. The population is returned with the parish. Here was formerly an hospital, the ruins of which are still remaining.

ELKINGTON, a parish in the hundred of GUILSBOROUGH, county of NORTHAMPTON, 11 miles (N.N.E.) from Daventry, containing 56 inhabitants. The church has been entirely demolished, but at what period neither history nor tradition informs us: it belonged to the monastery of Daventry, and afterwards to that of Pipewell, the rectory being valued in the return of the impropriations of the latter: there is now no living appointed to, the inhabitants being obliged to resort to the neighbouring parochial churches.

ELKINGTON (NORTH), a parish in the Wold division of the hundred of LOUTH-ESKE, parts of LINDSEY, county of LINCOLN, 4¼ miles (N.W.) from Louth, containing 74 inhabitants. The living is a discharged vicarage, in the archdeaconry and diocese of Lincoln, rated in the king's books at £4. 19. 4½., and endowed with £600 royal bounty. The Rev. William Smyth, Jun. was patron in 1818. The church is dedicated to St. Helen.

ELKINGTON (SOUTH), a parish in the Wold division of the hundred of LOUTH-ESKE, parts of LINDSEY, county of LINCOLN, 2¼ miles (W.N.W.) from Louth, containing 268 inhabitants. The living is a discharged vicarage, in the archdeaconry and diocese of Lincoln, rated in the king's books at £5. 7. 6. The Rev. William Smyth, Jun. was patron in 1822. The church is dedicated to All Saints.

ELKSLEY, a parish in the Hatfield division of the wapentake of BASSETLAW, county of NOTTINGHAM, 4 miles (N. W.) from Tuxford, containing 347 inhabitants. The living is a discharged vicarage, in the archdeaconry of Nottingham, and diocese of York, rated in the king's books at £3. 16. 0½., endowed with £200 royal bounty, and in the patronage of the Duke of Newcastle. The church is dedicated to St. Giles.

ELKSTONE, a parish in the hundred of RAPSGATE, county of GLOUCESTER, 7½ miles (N.N.W.) from Cirencester, containing 296 inhabitants. The living is a rectory, in the archdeaconry and diocese of Gloucester, rated in the king's books at £12. 9. 2., and in the patronage of the Hon. B. Craven. The church, dedicated to

St. John the Evangelist, is an ancient, though small edifice, affording a fine specimen of Norman architecture in the ornamented south porch, the east window, and the interior of the chancel; it has at the west end a square embattled tower in the later English style, erected in the reign of Richard II. The old Ermin-street traces the western boundary of the parish. A kind of stone is obtained here, which is easily cut when raised from the quarry, but becomes exceedingly hard by exposure to the air.

ELKSTONE, a chapelry comprising the townships of Lower Elkstone and Upper Elkstone, in the parish of ALLSTONEFIELD, northern division of the hundred of TOTMONSLOW, county of STAFFORD, 5½ miles (E. N. E.) from Leek, and containing 259 inhabitants, of which number, 108 are in Lower Elkstone, and 151 in Upper Elkstone. The living is a perpetual curacy, in the archdeaconry of Stafford, and diocese of Lichfield and Coventry, endowed with £1400 royal bounty, and in the patronage of certain Trustees. The chapel is dedicated to St. John the Baptist.

ELLA (KIRK), a parish in the county of the town of KINGSTON upon HULL, locally in the East riding of the county of YORK, comprising the townships of Kirk-Ella and West Ella, and a portion of the townships of Anlaby and Willerby, and containing, with the whole of Anlaby, which is partly in the parish of Hessle, 875 inhabitants, of which number, 246 are in the township of Kirk-Ella, 5 miles (W. by N.) from Kingston upon Hull, and 122 in the adjoining township of West Ella. The living is a discharged vicarage, in the archdeaconry and diocese of York, rated in the king's books at £13. 2. 8½. N. Sykes, Esq. was patron in 1813. The church, dedicated to St. Andrew, is a very ancient structure. Some of the merchants of Hull have elegant residences here. A school-room, with a house for the master, has been erected.

ELLAND, a chapelry in the parish of HALIFAX, wapentake of MORLEY, West riding of the county of YORK, 3 miles (S. S. E.) from Halifax, containing, with Greetland, 5088 inhabitants. The living is a perpetual curacy, in the archdeaconry and diocese of York, endowed with £200 private benefaction, £200 royal bounty, and £400 parliamentary grant, and in the patronage of the Vicar of Halifax. The chapel is dedicated to St. Mary. There are four places of worship for dissenters. Elland is a very ancient village, situated on the river Calder. Woollen cloths are manufactured, and there are mines of coal and stone quarries in the neighbourhood. It had formerly a market, by charter of Edward II., which has been long disused. Grace Ramsden, in 1734, bequeathed an estate at Bingley, now producing about £63. 10. a year, for erecting a school-house, and for the free education of poor boys of this chapelry. There is a dwelling-house for the master, whose salary is £20 per annum; also a recently erected school-room, in which thirty boys receive instruction in reading, writing, and arithmetic. A part of the funds of this charity was applied to the purchase of a cottage, in which ten girls are taught to read, knit, and sew, the mistress receiving £22 a year, and the minister £8 for catechising them, from a bequest by Frances Thornhill, in 1718. There is also a school for the children of dissenters, about forty being taught on the Lancasterian plan, by the minister of the Unitarian congregation, who receives £90 per annum

arising from bequests in 1712 and 1756, by James Brooksbank, and his grandson of the same name, and from Lady Hewley's charity, the greater part of which was given as an endowment upon the chapel.

ELLASTONE, a parish in the southern division of the hundred of TOTMONSLOW, county of STAFFORD, 4½ miles (W. S. W.) from Ashbourn, comprising the townships of Calwick, Prestwood, Ramshorn, Stanton, and Wootton, and containing 1328 inhabitants. The living is a discharged vicarage, in the archdeaconry of Stafford, and diocese of Lichfield and Coventry, rated in the king's books at £4. 9. 2., endowed with £200 private benefaction, and £200 royal bounty, and in the patronage of D. Davenport, Esq. The church, dedicated to St. Peter, was built in 1388, and contains memorials of the Fleetwoods, the ancient owners of a great part of the parish: it has lately received an addition of two hundred sittings, of which one hundred and fifty are free, the Incorporated Society for the enlargement of churches and chapels having granted £160 towards defraying the expense. The village, which is of considerable size, is situated on the river Dove, in a neighbourhood abounding with fine scenery, and enjoying a salubrious atmosphere. A National school-room was erected by subscription in 1812, which will accommodate two hundred children. The petty sessions for the division are held here. There are mines of copper and lead near Stanton, and in the fields and lanes are found many rare plants. On the top of the Weaver hill are several barrows, from which have been dug some ancient coins: there are also vestiges of a Roman encampment. Gilbert Sheldon, Archbishop of Canterbury, was born in this parish; he died in 1677.

ELLEL, a chapelry in the parish of COCKERHAM, hundred of LONSDALE, south of the sands, county palatine of LANCASTER, 4 miles (S. by E.) from Lancaster, containing 1851 inhabitants. The living is a perpetual curacy, in the archdeaconry of Richmond, and diocese of Chester, endowed with £200 private benefaction, and £600 royal bounty, and in the patronage of the Vicar of Cockerham. The chapel was built in 1802, at the expense of the inhabitants. Here are two silk-mills, in which about four hundred persons are employed. A school with a small endowment was established in 1753.

ELLENBOROUGH, a township in the parish of DEARHAM, ALLERDALE ward below Darwent, county of CUMBERLAND, 1 mile (E. S. E.) from Maryport, containing, with Unerigg, 621 inhabitants. It partakes in the benefit of the school at Unerigg, founded in 1718 by Ewan Christian, Esq. Coal is obtained near the village. This was an important Roman station, which Camden and Baxter consider to have been *Volantium*, Horsley, *Virosidum*, and others, *Olenacum*. Camden says that the first band of the Dalmatians was quartered here. There is, perhaps, no station in Britain where a greater number of altars and inscribed tablets has been found, many of which are preserved in the adjoining mansion and grounds of Netherhall. The Rt. Hon. Sir Edward Law, late Lord Chief Justice of the Court of King's Bench, derived his title from this place, having been created Baron Ellenborough in 1802, which title is now enjoyed by his eldest son.

ELLENHALL, a parish in the southern division of the hundred of PIREHILL, county of STAFFORD, 2¼ miles (S. by E.) from Eccleshall, containing 287 inhabitants. The living is a perpetual curacy, in the archdeaconry of Stafford, and diocese of Lichfield and Coventry, endowed with £200 private benefaction, and £600 royal bounty, and in the patronage of Viscount Anson. The church is dedicated to St. Mary. There is a trifling endowment, the gift of William Morteboys, in 1733, for teaching six poor children.

ELLERBECK, a township in the parish of Osmotherley, wapentake of Allertonshire, North riding of the county of York, 5½ miles (E.N.E.) from North Allerton, containing 81 inhabitants.

ELLERBURN, a parish in Pickering lythe, North riding of the county of York, 3¼ miles (E. by N.) from Pickering, comprising the chapelry of Witton, and containing 203 inhabitants, exclusively of a portion of the township of Farmanby, which is in this parish. The living is a discharged vicarage, rated in the king's books at £7. 4. 9½., endowed with £200 royal bounty, and in the peculiar jurisdiction and patronage of the Dean of York. The church is dedicated to St. Hilda.

ELLERBY, a township in that part of the parish of Swine which is in the middle division of the wapentake of Holderness, East riding of the county of York, 7¾ miles (N.E. by N.) from Kingston upon Hull, containing 233 inhabitants.

ELLERBY, a township in the parish of Lythe, eastern division of the liberty of Langbaurgh, North riding of the county of York, 7½ miles (W.N.W.) from Whitby, containing 80 inhabitants.

ELLERKER, a chapelry in that part of the parish of Brantingham which is in the wapentake of Howdenshire, East riding of the county of York, 1¼ mile (S. by W.) from South Cave, containing 249 inhabitants. It is within the jurisdiction of the peculiar court of Howdenshire. There is a place of worship for Wesleyan Methodists.

ELLERTON-ABBEY, a township in the parish of Downholme, western division of the wapentake of Hang, North riding of the county of York, 7 miles (W.S.W.) from Richmond, containing 47 inhabitants. Here was a small priory of Cistercian nuns, thought to have been founded by Warnerius, dapifer to the Earl of Richmond, in the time of Henry II., which, at the dissolution, was valued at £15. 10. 6.

ELLERTON-PRIORY, a parish in the Holme-Beacon division of the wapentake of Harthill, East riding of the county of York, 9 miles (N.N.W.) from Howden, containing 318 inhabitants. The living is a perpetual curacy, in the archdeaconry of the East riding, and diocese of York, endowed with £210 private benefaction, and £400 royal bounty. John Bethell, Esq. was patron in 1814. The church is dedicated to St. Mary. There is a place of worship for Wesleyan Methodists. There are three almshouses for six poor persons. William Fitz-Piers, before 1212, founded here a priory of the Sempringham order, who were obliged to maintain thirteen poor people : at the dissolution the establishment consisted of a prior and about nine religious, whose revenue was valued at £78. 0. 10.

ELLERTON upon SWALE, a township in that part of the parish of Catterick which is in the eastern division of the wapentake of Gilling, North riding of the county of York, 1¼ mile (E. by S.) from Catterick, containing 140 inhabitants. Henry Jenkins, who lived to the extraordinary age of one hundred and sixty-nine years, was born here; he died on the 8th of December,

1670, at this place, and a monument, with a suitable epitaph, was erected to his memory in the church of Bolton upon Swale, in 1743, where he was interred.

ELLESBOROUGH, a parish in the hundred of Aylesbury, county of Buckingham, 2½ miles (W. by S.) from Wendover, containing 581 inhabitants. The living is a rectory, in the archdeaconry of Buckingham, and diocese of Lincoln, rated in the king's books at £11. 9. 7. R. G. Russell, Esq. was patron in 1825. The church is dedicated to St. Peter and St. Paul : near it, on a circular eminence, is an ancient fortification, called Belinus' Castle, where tradition relates Belin resided ; above it is a high hill, still retaining the name of Belinesbury. There are almshouses for four poor widowers and four widows.

ELLESMERE, a market town and parish in the hundred of Pimhill, county of Salop, 16¼ miles (N.N.W.) from Shrewsbury, and 178½ (N.W.) from London, containing, with the chapelries of Cockshut, Dudlaston, and Penley (the last of which, is in the county of Flint), 6056 inhabitants. This place takes its name from an adjoining lake, or mere, which, being more extensive than some others in the neighbourhood, was, by way of pre-eminence, called Al, or Aelsmere, from which its present appellation is derived. The lake comprises more than one hundred acres, and is bordered on one side by the town, and on the other by Oatley park, in which are some of the finest elm trees to be found in any part of the country. The town consists of some tolerably well paved streets ; the houses are in general well built, and have a respectable appearance, and the inhabitants are amply supplied with water. On the elevated site of an ancient castle, which was alternately in the possession of the princes of North Wales and of the English monarchs, (having been a frontier fortress of considerable note during the unsettled period which preceded the final subjugation of Wales,) and which was probably demolished after the parliamentary war, is a very fine bowling-green, commanding a pleasing view, where an annual festival, called the meeting of Ellesmere club, is celebrated at Midsummer. The trade is principally in malt, which is carried on to a very great extent, and in leather ; and many of the labouring class are employed in the spinning of flax, and in the manufacture of stockings. The Ellesmere canal passes to the south of the town, and, with its different branches, forms a connexion between the Severn, the Dee, and the Mersey, being a line of navigation from Liverpool to Bristol, and a communication with North Wales. The market, granted to Sir Edward Kynaston, Knt., in 1598, is on Tuesday, and is noted for corn : the fairs are on the Tuesday after February 2nd, the third Tuesday in April, Whit-Tuesday, August 26th, and November 14th, for horses, cattle, and sheep. Ellesmere formerly gave name to a hundred, which, with its dependencies, was annexed to the hundred of Pimhill, in the 27th of Henry VIII.; a hundred court is held for the recovery of debts under 40s.

The living is a vicarage, in the archdeaconry of Salop, and diocese of Lichfield and Coventry, rated in the king's books at £17. 18. 1½., and in the patronage of the Trustees of the late Earl of Bridgewater. The church, dedicated to St. Mary, is an ancient structure in the decorated style of English architecture, with a square embattled tower crowned with pinnacles ; the east window is a remarkably fine composition in the later style. The livings of the chapelries in this parish are perpetual curacies, in the patronage of the Vicar. A National school is supported by subscription; and near the margin of the lake, at a short distance from the town, is the house of industry, for the reception of the poor of five adjoining parishes.

ELLINGHAM, a parish in the hundred of CLAVERING, county of NORFOLK, 2¾ miles (N.E. by E.) from Bungay, containing 339 inhabitants. The living is a rectory, in the archdeaconry of Norfolk, and diocese of Norwich, rated in the king's books at £12. The patronage is annexed to the Mastership of Magdalene College, Cambridge. The church is dedicated to St. Mary.

ELLINGHAM, a parish in the southern division of BAMBROUGH ward, county of NORTHUMBERLAND, comprising the townships of North Charlton, South Charlton, Chathill, East Ditchburn, West Ditchburn, Doxford, Ellingham, Preston, and Shipley, and containing 1027 inhabitants, of which number, 257 are in the township of Ellingham, 8½ miles (N.) from Alnwick. The living is a vicarage, in the archdeaconry of Northumberland, and diocese of Durham, rated in the king's books at £6. 5. 5., and in the patronage of the Dean and Chapter of Durham. The church, dedicated to St. Maurice, which stands at a short distance from the village, was founded by Ranulph de Guagy, in the twelfth century, and rebuilt a few years ago, A free school was erected by subscription on the glebe land, in 1821 : the master receives £5 a year from the trustees of Lord Crewe, which is augmented to £20 by voluntary contributions. Coal and limestone are obtained in the parish.

ELLINGHAM, a parish in the hundred of FORDINGBRIDGE, New Forest (West) division of the county of SOUTHAMPTON, 2¼ miles (N. by W.) from Ringwood, containing 397 inhabitants. The living is a discharged vicarage, in the archdeaconry and diocese of Winchester, rated in the king's books at £8. 4. 9½., endowed with £200 private benefaction, and £200 royal bounty, in the patronage of the Provost and Fellows of Eton College. The church is dedicated to St. Mary. In the church-yard is a plain stone commemorating the execution of Alicia Lisle, in her old age, pursuant to a sentence passed by Judge Jeffreys, on a charge of harbouring known rebels in her mansion of Moyle's Court, which sentence was reversed at the Revolution. The navigable river Avon runs through the parish.

ELLINGHAM (GREAT), a parish in the hundred of SHROPHAM, county of NORFOLK, 2 miles (N.W. by W.) from Attleburgh, containing 760 inhabitants. The living is a discharged vicarage, with which the rectory of Little Ellingham is united, in the archdeaconry and diocese of Norwich, rated in the king's books at £6. 5. 10., endowed with £200 private benefaction, and £200 royal bounty. Dover Colby, Esq. was patron in 1814. The church is dedicated to St. James. There is a place of worship for Baptists.

ELLINGHAM (LITTLE), a parish in the hundred of WAYLAND, county of NORFOLK, 3¼ miles (N.W.) from Attleburgh, containing 240 inhabitants. The living is a discharged rectory united to the vicarage of Great Ellingham, in the archdeaconry and diocese of Norwich, rated in the king's books at £7. 1. 10½., endowed with £200 private benefaction, and £200 royal

bounty. The church, dedicated to St. Peter, has a quadrangular tower on the south side. At the time of the Conquest this place, though now only an inconsiderable village, is said to have been three miles long.

ELLINGSTRING, a township in the parish of MASHAM, partly within the liberty of ST. PETER of YORK, but chiefly in the eastern division of the wapentake of HANG, North riding of the county of YORK, 4¼ miles (N. W. by W.) from Masham, containing 204 inhabitants. There is a place of worship for Wesleyan Methodists.

ELLINGTON, a parish in the hundred of LEIGHTONSTONE, county of HUNTINGDON, 5½ miles (W. by N.) from Huntingdon, containing 344 inhabitants. The living is a vicarage, in the archdeaconry of Huntingdon, and diocese of Lincoln, rated in the king's books at £20, endowed with £200 private benefaction, £400 royal bounty, and £300 parliamentary grant, and in the patronage of the Master and Fellows of Peter-House, Cambridge. The church is dedicated to All Saints.

ELLINGTON, a township in the parish of WOODHORN, eastern division of MORPETH ward, county of NORTHUMBERLAND, 7 miles (N.E. by E.) from Morpeth, containing 255 inhabitants. It is situated on the north side of the river Line, across which there is a stone bridge.

ELLINGTON (NETHER and OVER), a township in the parish of MASHAM, partly within the liberty of ST. PETER of YORK, but chiefly in the eastern division of the wapentake of HANG, North riding of the county of YORK, containing 152 inhabitants. Nether Ellington is 2¼ miles (N. W.) and Over Ellington 2½ miles (N. W. by W.) from Masham.

ELLISFIELD, a parish in the hundred of BERMONDSPIT, Basingstoke division of the county of SOUTHAMPTON, 4 miles (S.) from Basingstoke, containing 218 inhabitants. The living is a rectory, in the archdeaconry and diocese of Winchester, rated in the king's books at £8. 3. 6½., endowed with £200 royal bounty, and in the patronage of Bernard Brocas and Thomas Terry, Esqrs., alternately. The church is dedicated to St. Martin. There are two churches prior to the reign of Edward III., when that dedicated to All Saints was taken down, by consent of the two patrons and the diocesan. There is an endowment of £3 a year, the gift of Stephen Terry, Esq., in 1737, for teaching six poor children. The name of this parish seems to be a corruption of Ella's field, from the Saxon king, Ella. A field of about three acres, encompassed by a deep moat, is supposed to be the site of an ancient castle; and in other parts of the parish are various intrenchments.

ELLOUGH, a parish in the hundred of WANGFORD, county of SUFFOLK, 3 miles (S. E. by S.) from Beccles, containing 155 inhabitants. The living is a discharged rectory, in the archdeaconry and diocese of Norwich, rated in the king's books at £12. The Earl of Gosford was patron in 1811. The church is dedicated to All Saints.

ELLOUGHTON, a parish partly within the liberty of ST. PETER of YORK, but chiefly in the Hunsley-Beacon division of the wapentake of HARTHILL, East riding of the county of YORK, 2½ miles (S.E. by S.) from South Cave, containing, with Brough, 383 inhabitants. The living is a discharged vicarage, rated in the king's books at £5. 0. 5., and in the patronage of the

Prebendary of Wetwang in the Cathedral Church of York. The church, dedicated to St. Mary, is a very ancient structure. There are places of worship for Calvinists and Wesleyan Methodists.

ELLSTHORP, a hamlet in the parish of EDENHAM, wapentake of BELTISLOE, parts of KESTEVEN, county of LINCOLN, containing 58 inhabitants.

ELM, a parish in the hundred of WISBEACH, Isle of ELY, county of CAMBRIDGE, 2 miles (S. S. E.) from Wisbeach, containing 1368 inhabitants. The living is a vicarage to which the curacy of Emneth is annexed, in the peculiar jurisdiction of the Bishop of Ely, rated in the king's books at £14. 15. 10., and in the patronage of the Rector of Elm with Emneth; the rectory is a sinecure, rated in the king's books at £17, and in the patronage of the Bishop of Ely. The church is dedicated to All Saints. Thomas Squire, in 1689, bequeathed a school-room with a house and lands, now producing about £50 a year, for teaching poor children.

ELM, a parish in the hundred of FROME, county of SOMERSET, 2¼ miles (N.W. by W.) from Frome, comprising the hamlets of Great Elm and Little Elm, and containing 449 inhabitants. The living is a discharged rectory, in the archdeaconry of Wells, and diocese of Bath and Wells, rated in the king's books at £9. 13. 6½., endowed with £50 per annum private benefaction, and £200 royal bounty, and in the patronage of the Rev. Charles Griffith, D. D. The church is dedicated to St. Mary. The river Frome, which runs through the parish, has extensive iron-works and manufactories for agricultural implements on its banks. Near the northern bank of a rivulet, and on the edge of a precipice, are the remains of a Roman intrenchment called Tedbury, in which a vessel containing coins of the Lower Empire was found in 1691.

ELMBRIDGE, a chapelry in that part of the parish of DODDERHILL which is in the upper division of hundred of HALFSHIRE, county of WORCESTER, 2¾ miles (N.) from Droitwich, containing 336 inhabitants. The chapel is dedicated to St. Mary.

ELMDON, a parish in the hundred of UTTLESFORD, county of ESSEX, 5½ miles (W. by N.) from Saffron-Walden, containing 601 inhabitants. The living is a vicarage, to which is annexed the rectory of Wendon-Lofts, in the archdeaconry of Colchester, and diocese of London, rated in the king's books at £19. J. Wilkes, Esq. was patron in 1814. The church is dedicated to St. Nicholas. There is a charity school, supported by donations amounting to about £14 per annum.

ELMDON, a parish in the Solihull division of the hundred of HEMLINGFORD, county of WARWICK, 4¾ miles (S.W. by S.) from Coleshill, containing 146 inhabitants. The living is a discharged rectory, in the archdeaconry of Coventry, and diocese of Lichfield and Coventry, rated in the king's books at £3. 8. 1½., in the patronage of Abraham Lillington Spooner, Esq. The church, dedicated to St. Peter, which stands on an eminence and has a tower at the west end, was built in 1781, at the expense of Abraham Spooner, Esq., and cost £3000. This place is supplied with water by a self-acting engine, situated a short distance from Elmdon hall.

ELMER, a joint township with Crakehall, in that part of the parish of TOPCLIFFE which is in the

wapentake of BIRDFORTH, North riding of the county of YORK, 7 miles (N. by E.) from Boroughbridge, containing 78 inhabitants.

ELMHAM (NORTH), a parish in the hundred of LAUNDITCH, county of NORFOLK, 5¼ miles (N.) from East Dereham, containing 1046 inhabitants. The living is a discharged vicarage, in the archdeaconry of Norfolk, and diocese of Norwich, rated in the king's books at £13. 15., and in the patronage of R. Mills, Esq. The church, dedicated to St. Mary, has at the west end a quadrangular tower with a slender spire one hundred and nineteen feet high. The kingdom of the East Angles, which from its first conversion by Felix had been under one bishop, was, about 673, divided into two dioceses, when one of the episcopal seats was fixed at Dunwich, and the other in this ancient town, which had a succession of ten bishops, till the martyrdom of Humbert by the Danes, in 870. The two sees were again united about 950, and the episcopal chair transferred to Thetford in 1075, and soon afterwards to Norwich. The site of the cathedral is still discernible, and near it are some old wells. Herbert, first bishop of Norwich, rebuilt the parish church, but the present seems to be of later date : from the altar ran a subterranean passage to the palace, situated on a neighbouring hill, which Bishop Spencer, in the turbulent reign of Richard II., converted into a castle, and surrounded with a double intrenchment, the inner moat enclosing the keep ; its remains are now almost obscured by thorns and briars. Not far from the village, numerous Roman urns and coins were discovered in 1710; and in a field called Broomclose, urns of various sizes and colours, containing bones, ashes, glass, divers brass instruments, and a silver seal-ring with an eagle holding a thunderbolt, have been found.

ELMHAM (SOUTH) ALL SAINTS, a parish in the hundred of WANGFORD, county of SUFFOLK, 5 miles (N.W.) from Halesworth, containing 239 inhabitants. The living is a discharged rectory, with that of St. Nicholas annexed, in the archdeaconry of Suffolk, and diocese of Norwich, rated in the king's books at £8, and in the patronage of Alexander Adair, Esq.

ELMHAM (SOUTH) ST. CROSS, or SANDCROFT, a parish in the hundred of WANGFORD, county of SUFFOLK, 4 miles (E. by N.) from Harleston, containing 233 inhabitants. The living is a discharged rectory, annexed to the rectory of Homersfield, in the archdeaconry of Suffolk, and diocese of Norwich, rated in the king's books at £10, and in the patronage of Alexander Adair, Esq. The church is dedicated to St. George.

ELMHAM (SOUTH) ST. JAMES, a parish in the hundred of WANGFORD, county of SUFFOLK, 5½ miles (N.W. by W.) from Halesworth, containing 351 inhabitants. The living is a discharged rectory, in the archdeaconry of Suffolk, and diocese of Norwich, rated in the king's books at £8, and in the patronage of Alexander Adair, Esq.

ELMHAM (SOUTH) ST. MARGARET, a parish in the hundred of WANGFORD, county of SUFFOLK, 6¼ miles (N.W.) from Halesworth, containing 181 inhabitants. The living is a discharged rectory, with that of St. Peter annexed, in the archdeaconry of Suffolk, and diocese of Norwich, rated in the king's books at £6. 2. 11., and in the patronage of Alexander Adair, Esq.

ELMHAM (SOUTH) ST. MICHAEL, a parish in the hundred of WANGFORD, county of SUFFOLK, 6 miles (N. N. W.) from Halesworth, containing 128 inhabitants. The living is a discharged rectory, with the perpetual curacy of Rumburgh annexed, in the archdeaconry of Suffolk, and diocese of Norwich, rated in the king's books at £4. 17. 11., endowed with £800 royal bounty, and in the patronage of Mrs. Athill.

ELMHAM (SOUTH) ST. NICHOLAS, a parish in the hundred of WANGFORD, county of SUFFOLK, 6¼ miles (N. W.) from Halesworth, containing 91 inhabitants. The living is a discharged rectory, annexed to the rectory of All Saints, in the archdeaconry of Suffolk, and diocese of Norwich, rated in the king's books at £6. The church has been long since demolished.

ELMHAM (SOUTH) ST. PETER, a parish in the hundred of WANGFORD, county of SUFFOLK, 3¾ miles (S.) from Bungay, containing 139 inhabitants. The living is a discharged rectory, annexed to that of St. Margaret, in the archdeaconry of Suffolk, and diocese of Norwich, rated in the king's books at £8.

ELMHURST, a joint township with Curborough, in that part of the parish of ST. CHAD which is in the northern division of the hundred of OFFLOW, county of STAFFORD, 1¾ mile (N. by W.) from Lichfield, containing 250 inhabitants.

ELMINGTON, a hamlet in the parish of OUNDLE, hundred of POLEBROOK, though locally in the hundred of Willybrook, county of NORTHAMPTON, 1½ mile (N. E. by N.) from Oundle, with which the population is returned. Here was formerly a chapel.

ELMLEY CASTLE, a parish in the middle division of the hundred of OSWALDSLOW, county of WORCESTER, 4¾ miles (W. S. W.) from Evesham, containing 316 inhabitants. The living is a discharged vicarage, in the archdeaconry and diocese of Worcester, rated in the king's books at £5. 6. 5½., endowed with £200 private benefaction, and £400 royal bounty, and in the patronage of the Bishop of Worcester. The church, dedicated to St. Mary, contains some handsome monuments. On one of the Breedon hills a strong castle was erected, in the reign of William the Conqueror, and destroyed in that of Henry III.: a college, or chantry, for eight priests was founded in it by Guy Beauchamp, Earl of Warwick, in honour of the Blessed Virgin: the site and surrounding moat are still discernible. Henry III. granted to this place a weekly market and an annual fair on St. Lawrence's day. Here are quarries of stone, one kind of which is blue, used for the flooring of kitchens. A small stone cross stands within the parish.

ELMLEY (ISLE OF), a parish in the liberty of the Isle of SHEPPY, lathe of SCRAY, county of KENT, 3½ miles (S. E. by S.) from Queenborough, containing 23 inhabitants. The living is a rectory, in the archdeaconry and diocese of Canterbury, rated in the king's books at £5, and in the patronage of the Warden and Fellows of All Souls' College, Oxford. The church, dedicated to St. James, is dilapidated, and only used on the induction of a new rector. This small island, adjoining that of Sheppy, is in length about three miles, and in breadth two, a small tract on the northern side being within the bounds of the parish of East Church. It has a ferry across the Swale to Milton, and consists principally of rich pastures, affording herbage for numerous flocks of sheep.

ELMLEY-LOVETT, a parish in the lower division of the hundred of HALFSHIRE, county of WORCESTER, 4 miles (E. by S.) from Stourport, containing 447 inhabitants. The living is a rectory, in the archdeaconry and diocese of Worcester, rated in the king's books at £17. 2. 6., and in the patronage of John Lynes, Esq. The church is dedicated to St. Michael. There are two schools, endowed with part of the profits of an estate bequeathed, at a very early period, by an individual now unknown, for the benefit of the church and the poor of the parish. This place gives the title of viscount to the Lygon family.

ELMORE, a hamlet in the parish of MOTCOMB, liberty of GILLINGHAM, Shaston (West) division of the county of DORSET, ½ a mile (N.) from Shaftesbury. On Elmore Green are several wells, from which the town of Shaftesbury is supplied with water, and as an acknowledgment for the benefit derived therefrom, a particular custom is annually kept up, by ancient agreement between the lord of the manor and the mayor and burgesses, who, on the Monday before Holy Thursday, go in procession to the wells, with what is termed a prize besom, richly ornamented with plate and peacocks' feathers, carrying also a raw calf's head and a pair of gloves, all which are presented to the steward, who returns the former, when it is brought back to the town with great formality.

ELMORE, a parish in the middle division of the hundred of DUDSTONE and KING'S BARTON, county of GLOUCESTER, 6½ miles (W. S. W.) from Gloucester, containing 355 inhabitants. The living is a perpetual curacy, in the archdeaconry and diocese of Gloucester, endowed with £200 private benefaction, and £800 royal bounty, and in the patronage of Sir Berkeley William Guise, Bart. The church, dedicated to St. John the Baptist, has an embattled tower at the west end. The waters in the neighbourhood abound with eels, from which Elmore probably derived its name. The river Severn is navigable on the west of the parish; but, owing to a rock extending nearly across the stream there is only a narrow channel for vessels of light draught, except at high water. There are a day and Sunday schools, supported by Sir B. W. Guise.

ELMSALL (NORTH), a township in the parish of SOUTH KIRKBY, upper division of the wapentake of Os-GOLDCROSS, West riding of the county of YORK, 6¾ miles (S. by E.) from Pontefract, containing 113 inhabitants.

ELMSALL (SOUTH), a township in the parish of SOUTH KIRKBY, upper division of the wapentake of OSGOLDCROSS, West riding of the county of YORK, 7¾ miles (S. by E.) from Pontefract, containing 453 inhabitants.

ELMSETT, a parish in the hundred of COSFORD, county of SUFFOLK, 4 miles (N. E. by N.) from Hadleigh, containing 371 inhabitants. The living is a rectory, in the archdeaconry of Sudbury, and diocese of Norwich, rated in the king's books at £13. 7. 1., and in the patronage of the Master, Fellows, and Scholars of Clare Hall, Cambridge. The church, dedicated to St. Peter, is built of flint and stone, and the parsonage-house is surrounded by a moat. There is a fair for toys on Whit-Thursday. On the declivity of a hill is a cold mineral spring, called the Dropping Well, issuing out of limestone rock, and producing fibrous chrystallizations.

ELMSTEAD, a parish in the hundred of TENDRING, county of ESSEX, 4½ miles (E. by N.) from Colchester, containing 693 inhabitants. The living is a discharged vicarage, in the archdeaconry of Colchester, and diocese of London, rated in the king's books at £8, endowed with £200 private benefaction, and £200 royal bounty, and in the patronage of the Master and Fellows of Jesus College, Cambridge. The church is dedicated to St. Anne. There is a place of worship for Wesleyan Methodists. The river Coln forms a boundary to the parish, which is crossed by a Roman road, called Stone-street. There is a fair for toys on the 15th of May.

ELMSTED, a parish in the hundred of STOUTING, lathe of SHEPWAY, county of KENT, 8 miles (E. by N.) from Ashford, containing 454 inhabitants. The living is a discharged vicarage, in the archdeaconry and diocese of Canterbury, rated in the king's books at £6. 13. 4., and in the patronage of the Archbishop of Canterbury. The church is dedicated to St. James. There is a fair on the 25th of July.

ELMSTHORPE, a parish in the hundred of SPARKENHOE, county of LEICESTER, 3 miles (N. E. by E.) from Hinckley, containing 46 inhabitants. The living is a rectory, annexed to the rectory of Barwell, in the archdeaconry of Leicester, and diocese of Lincoln, rated in the king's books at £6. 13. 4. The church is desecrated, the ruins having been converted into a barn.

ELMSTONE, a parish in the hundred of PRESTON, lathe of St. AUGUSTINE, county of KENT, 2¼ miles (N. E. by N.) from Wingham, containing 76 inhabitants. The living is a rectory, in the archdeaconry and diocese of Canterbury, rated in the king's books at £6. 7. 8½., and in the patronage of Thomas Delmar, Esq. There is a school endowed with donations amounting to about £3 per annum.

ELMSTONE-HARDWICKE, a parish partly in the lower division of the hundred of DEERHURST, but chiefly in the lower division of the hundred of WESTMINSTER, county of GLOUCESTER, 3¾ miles (N. N. W.) from Cheltenham, containing, with the chapelry of Uckington (which is in Deerhurst hundred), 357 inhabitants. The living is a discharged vicarage, in the archdeaconry and diocese of Gloucester, rated in the king's books at £9. 2. 3½., and in the patronage of the Crown. The church is dedicated to St. Mary Magdalene.

ELMSWELL, a parish in the hundred of BLACKBOURN, county of SUFFOLK, 5¾ miles (N.W.) from Stow-Market, containing 628 inhabitants. The living is a rectory, in the archdeaconry of Sudbury, and diocese of Norwich, rated in the king's books at £11. 7. 11., and in the patronage of Sir Robert Gardiner. The church is dedicated to St. John the Evangelist. There is a place of worship for Wesleyan Methodists. An almshouse was founded and endowed with lands by Sir Robert Gardiner, in the 12th of James I., for six poor widows.

ELMTON, a parish in the hundred of SCARSDALE, county of DERBY, 9 miles (E. by N.) from Chesterfield, containing 352 inhabitants. The living is a discharged vicarage, in the archdeaconry of Derby, and diocese of Lichfield and Coventry, rated in the king's books at £5. 1. 3., endowed with £200 private benefaction, £400 royal bounty, and £300 parliamentary grant, and in the patronage of the Rev. C. H. R. Rhodes. The church is dedicated to St. Peter. Limestone abounds in the parish. The extraordinary arithmetical calculator, Jedediah Bux-

ton, was born at this place in 1707; he died in 1772, and was buried here.

ELSDON, a parish in the southern division of COQUETDALE ward, county of NORTHUMBERLAND, comprising the townships of Elsdon ward, Monkridge ward, Otterburn ward, Rochester ward, Troughend ward, and Woodside ward, and containing 1848 inhabitants, of which number, 299 are in the township of Elsdon ward, 18½ miles (W. N. W) from Morpeth. The living is a rectory, in the archdeaconry of Northumberland, and diocese of Durham, rated in the king's books at £20, and in the patronage of the Duke of Northumberland. The church, dedicated to St. Cuthbert, is a large cruciform structure. A few years since, in clearing away the earth against the north transept, upwards of one hundred skeletons were discovered, lying in double rows alternately between the legs of each other. The river Reed and the new Edinburgh road intersect the parish. There are some fine seams of coal, which, with limestone and iron-stone, is obtained in abundance. A fair for cattle, sheep, linen and woollen cloth, is held on the 26th of August. Elsdon is supposed to have been a Roman town, and the first of a chain of forts between Watling-street and the Devil's causeway. North-east of the village is an ancient intrenchment, called Moat-hill, which, from the relics discovered in it, seems to have been used as a place of sepulture by the Romans. About two miles to the north-west is Tod-law, an eminence upon which are three large columns of stone, in a triangular position, said to have been set up to the memory of some distinguished Danish leaders. Elsdon castle was erected by David, King of Scotland; it is a strong tower building, now the rectory-house, the lower story of which is spanned by a single arch, having in front the armorial bearings of Umfraville, Lord of Prudhoe, who died about 1325.

ELSENHAM, a parish in the hundred of UTTLESFORD, county of ESSEX, 2 miles (N. E.) from Stansted-Mountfitchet, containing 434 inhabitants. The living is a vicarage, in the archdeaconry of Colchester, and diocese of London, rated in the king's books at £11. 10., and in the patronage of the Bishop of London. The church is dedicated to St. Mary. There is a small endowment for teaching two poor children.

ELSFIELD, a parish in the hundred of BULLINGTON, county of OXFORD, 3¼ miles (N. E. by N.) from Oxford, containing 188 inhabitants. The living is a vicarage, in the archdeaconry and diocese of Oxford, rated in the king's books at £6. 8. 1½., and endowed with £200 royal bounty. The Earl of Guildford was patron in 1804. The church is dedicated to St. Thomas à Becket.

ELSHAM, a parish in the northern division of the wapentake of YARBOROUGH, parts of LINDSEY, county of LINCOLN, 5 miles (N. E. by N.) from Glandford-Bridge, containing 383 inhabitants. The living is a discharged vicarage, in the archdeaconry and diocese of Lincoln, rated in the king's books at £7. 18. 4. W. T. Corbett, Esq. was patron in 1801. The church, dedicated to All Saints, is a neat structure in the early style of English architecture, with a handsome western porch. An hospital, or priory of Augustine canons, was founded early in the twelfth century, by Beatrix de Amundevill, and dedicated to St. Mary and St. Edmund, the annual revenue of which, at the dissolution, amounted to £83. 17. 10.

ELSING, a parish in the hundred of EYNSFORD, county of NORFOLK, 5 miles (N. E. by E.) from East Dereham, containing 374 inhabitants. The living is a discharged rectory, in the archdeaconry of Norfolk, and diocese of Norwich, rated in the king's books at £5.11.8. The Rev. R. Browne was patron in 1820.

ELSLACK, a joint township with Broughton, in the parish of BROUGHTON in AREDALE, eastern division of the wapentake of STAINCLIFFE and EWCROSS, West riding of the county of YORK, 4¾ miles (W.S.W.) from Skipton, containing 427 inhabitants.

ELSTEAD, a parish in the hundred of FARNHAM, county of SURREY, 4¾ miles (W.) from Godalming, containing 608 inhabitants. The living is a perpetual curacy, in the archdeaconry of Surrey, and diocese of Winchester, endowed with £200 royal bounty, and £1400 parliamentary grant, and in the patronage of Robert Colmer, Esq. The church is dedicated to St. James. The navigable river Wey runs through the parish.

ELSTEAD, a parish in the hundred of DUMPFORD, rape of CHICHESTER, county of SUSSEX, 4½ miles (W. by S.) from Midhurst, containing 190 inhabitants. The living is a rectory, in the archdeaconry and diocese of Chichester, rated in the king's books at £11. 13. 4. Lord Selsey was patron in 1822. The church has portions in the Norman style of architecture.

ELSTOB, a township in the parish of STAINTON, north-eastern division of STOCKTON ward, county palatine of DURHAM, 9 miles (N. E. by N.) from Darlington, containing 28 inhabitants.

ELSTON, a township in the parish of PRESTON, hundred of AMOUNDERNESS, county palatine of LANCASTER, 4¾ miles (E.N.E.) from Preston, containing 76 inhabitants.

ELSTON, a parish in the southern division of the wapentake of NEWARK, county of NOTTINGHAM, 5½ miles (S.W. by S.) from Newark, containing 446 inhabitants. The living is a rectory, in the archdeaconry of Nottingham, and diocese of York, rated in the king's books at £9. 8. 9. W. B. Darwin, Esq. was patron in 1819. The church, dedicated to All Saints, contains several monuments to the Darwin family. A commodious school-house was erected in 1812, at the expense of Robert Waring Darwin, Esq., which is endowed with land allotted in 1801 by the commissioners for enclosing the open fields of Elston, in lieu of that bequeathed in 1652 by the Rev. Robert Pendleton, and other land purchased with £100, the legacy of Elizabeth Darwin, in 1784 : there are also a dwelling-house, garden, and orchard, for the master, who gratuitously teaches nine poor children. An almshouse, for four poor widows, was built in 1744, in pursuance of the will of Ann Darwin, in 1722.

ELSTON, a chapelry in the parish of EAST STOKE, southern division of the wapentake of NEWARK, county of NOTTINGHAM, 5½ miles (S.W. by S.) from Newark. The population is returned with the parish. The chapel, a small neat edifice, stands contiguous to the parish of Elston, and the two villages are so intermingled as not to be distinguishable from each other. There is a place of worship for Wesleyan Methodists.

ELSTON, a tything in the parish of ORCHESTON-ST. GEORGE, hundred of HEYTESBURY, county of WILTS, 7 miles (N. W. by W.) from Amesbury. The population is returned with the parish.

ELSTON-COMBE, a hamlet in the parish of YEOVIL, hundred of STONE, county of SOMERSET. The population is returned with the parish. Here was formerly a chapel, now demolished.

ELSTOW, a parish in the hundred of REDBORNESTOKE, county of BEDFORD, 1¼ mile (S. by W.) from Bedford, containing 548 inhabitants. The living is a discharged vicarage, in the archdeaconry of Bedford, and diocese of Lincoln, rated in the king's books at £7. 9., endowed with £800 royal bounty, and in the patronage of William Henry Whitbread, Esq. The church, dedicated to St. Mary and St. Helen, a fine old structure in the Norman style, was formerly the conventual church, and is now, with its detached tower to the north-west, the only remains, of an abbey of Benedictine nuns, founded in the reign of William the Conqueror, by his niece, Judith, Countess of Huntingdon, to the honour of the Holy Trinity, St. Mary, and St. Helen ; at the dissolution it contained an abbess and twenty-one nuns, whose annual revenue amounted to £325. 2. 1. There are fairs for all sorts of cattle on May 14th and 15th, and November 5th and 6th. John Bunyan, author of the Pilgrim's Progress, was born here.

ELSTREE, or IDLESTREE, a parish in the hundred of CASHIO, or liberty of ST. ALBAN'S, county of HERTFORD, 3 miles (N. by W.) from Edgware, containing 309 inhabitants. The living is a discharged rectory, in the archdeaconry of St. Alban's, and diocese of London, rated in the king's books at £8, and in the patronage of the Crown. The church, dedicated to St. Nicholas, was enlarged and new seated in 1824, and received an addition of one hundred and ninety sittings, of which one hundred and sixty-four are free, at an expense of more than £900, of which sum, £250 was granted by the Incorporated Society for enlarging churches and chapels : it is said to have been first erected out of the ruins of the ancient city Sulloniacim, the site and foundations of which are still visible about one mile to the southward. The village stands upon the spot where the old Watling-street crosses from Middlesex into Hertfordshire, and is partly in four parishes, viz. Aldenham, Edgware, Elstree, and Whitchurch. There is a bequest of £5 a year from Robert Warren, for apprenticing one poor child. A National school was established in 1813.

ELSTRONWICK, a chapelry in the parish of HUMBLETON, middle division of the wapentake of HOLDERNESS, East riding of the county of YORK, 9¾ miles (E.N.E.) from Kingston upon Hull, containing 154 inhabitants. The chapel is of great antiquity. There is a small endowed school.

ELSWICK, a township in the parish of ST. MICHAEL, hundred of AMOUNDERNESS, county palatine of LANCASTER, 5½ miles (N.) from Kirkham, containing 290 inhabitants.

ELSWICKE, a township in that part of the parish of ST. JOHN, NEWCASTLE, which is in the western division of CASTLE ward, county of NORTHUMBERLAND, 1 mile (W.) from Newcastle, containing 464 inhabitants. Elswicke adjoins the town of Newcastle on the west, and extends along the northern bank of the Tyne : it contains many good houses, and various manufactories, particularly a shot tower, which was erected in 1796, rising to the height of one hundred and seventy-five feet. There are extensive coal-works in the neighbourhood, and in a place termed the Quarry field large quantities of stone are obtained for building.

ELSWORTH, a parish in the hundred of PAPWORTH, county of CAMBRIDGE, 4½ miles (N.N.E.) from Caxton, containing 773 inhabitants. The living is a rectory, in the archdeaconry and diocese of Ely, rated in the king's books at £14. 6. 0½. The church is dedicated to the Holy Trinity. There is a trifling endowment for a school. Dr. Franklin, in 1695, bequeathed £400 for building and endowing three almshouses for poor widows.

ELTHAM, a parish in the hundred of BLACKHEATH, lathe of SUTTON at HONE, county of KENT, 8½ miles (S. E. by S.) from London, containing, with the hamlet of Mottingham, part of which is in the parish of Chiselhurst, 1977 inhabitants. This place, in Domesday-book called *Alteham*, from which its present appellation is deduced, is supposed to have derived its name from the Saxon *Eald*, old, and *Ham*, a dwelling. It formed part of the royal demesne in the reign of Edward the Elder, by whom it was given to Odo, Archbishop of Canterbury, and at a very early period became a favourite retreat of the English kings. Henry III. kept a grand festival in 1270, attended by his queen and the whole court, in the palace, which was enlarged by Anthony Beck, Bishop of Durham, about the close of the thirteenth century.` Edward II. resided here for some time, where also his son was born (and from this circumstance called John of Eltham), and the palace, erroneously, King John's palace. Edward III. held parliaments here in 1329 and 1375, and in 1364 sumptuously entertained his prisoner, King John, of France, in the palace. Richard II. here celebrated the festival of Christmas, in 1384 and 1386; and Henry IV. in 1405, on which occasion the Duke of York was accused of an attempt to surprise and murder the king. Edward IV. repaired the palace and enclosed one of the parks; Henry VII. built a front to it, and otherwise improved it, and it continued to be the occasional residence of the kings of England till the reign of Henry VIII., who celebrated two splendid festivals in it, after which time it began to yield in importance to Greenwich, which, in the reign of Elizabeth, obtained the ascendancy. During the civil war in the reign of Charles I., Eltham was occupied by the Earl of Essex, the parliamentary general, who died here in 1646. Of the extent of this once magnificent pile, some idea may be formed from the parliamentary survey, in which it is described as having "one fair chapel, one great hall, forty-six rooms and offices below stairs, with two large cellars; and above stairs, seventeen lodging-rooms on the king's side, twelve on the queen's side, and nine on the princes' side, thirty-five bayes of building, or seventy-eight rooms in the offices round the court-yard, which contained one acre of ground." Of these, the only remains are, the great hall, being one hundred feet long, and thirty-six wide, having ten windows on each side, and a finely ornamented roof, which has for many years been used as a barn, but is now being restored, with a view to its preservation; two ancient stone bridges, portions of the walls, subterranean passages, and parts of the inferior offices converted into modern buildings, and, with the surrounding lands, constituting what is called the Court Farm: the area is enclosed by a stone wall of great thickness, and from eighteen to twenty feet

VOL. II.

in height: the moat by which it was surrounded was from seventy to eighty feet in breadth, and from fourteen to fifteen in depth; it is quite dry, and though converted into a garden, its original form may be distinctly traced; the principal bridge has two pointed arches finely groined.

The village is irregularly built, but contains many handsome houses, and the environs abound with noble mansions and elegant seats; Shooter's hill, so named from its having been anciently used for the practice of archery, and on which a singular triangular tower has been erected, by his lady, to the memory of Sir William Daines, Bart., is celebrated for the beauty of its situation, and the extent and variety of its prospects; on its summit has been erected one of the telegraphs communicating between London and Dover. The parish is within the jurisdiction of the court of requests held weekly at Greenwich, under an act passed in the 47th of George III., for the recovery of debts not exceeding £5. The living is a discharged vicarage, in the archdeaconry and diocese of Rochester, rated in the king's books at £3. 2. 6., endowed with £400 private benefaction, and £400 royal bounty. Sir Gregory Page Turner, Bart. was patron in 1783. The church, dedicated to St. John the Baptist, is a plain edifice, with a spire: in it were interred the remains of Dr. Horne, Bishop of Norwich, who died in 1792; and in the church-yard, those of Sir William Daines, Bart., and Dogget, the comedian, partner with Wilks and Cibber, and who left a coat and badge to be rowed for annually on the 1st of August. There is a place of worship for Independents. A free school was built in 1634, and endowed in 1714, by Mrs. Elizabeth Leggatt, with lands producing more than £30 per annum; there are sixteen boys at present taught in this school. An almshouse was founded, in 1680, by Mr. Thomas Phillipot, for six aged persons, four of this parish, and two of the parish of Chiselhurst, and endowed with lands producing upwards of £30 per annum. This parish has the privilege of sending three of the pensioners to Queen Elizabeth's hospital at Greenwich. Among the benefactions to the poor are a grant of land by Henry VII., in 1492, and another in 1509, by Mr. John Passey. On the summit of a hill south by east from the town, are the remains of a Roman camp. Dr. William Sherard, the celebrated botanist, resided here in the early part of the eighteenth century, and cultivated a botanical garden, assisted by the German botanist, Dillarius, who published a catalogue of the plants in two volumes, folio, under the title of Hortus Elthamensis, in 1732. The learned herald and Kentish historian, John Phillipot, was either a native of this place, or resided here. Frederick, Prince of Wales, was created Earl of Eltham in 1726, which title is still borne by the King of England.

ELTISLEY, a parish in the hundred of LONGSTOW, county of CAMBRIDGE, 3 miles (N.W. by W.) from Caxton, containing 319 inhabitants. The living is a discharged vicarage, in the archdeaconry and diocese of Ely, rated in the king's books at £7. 16. 8., endowed with £600 royal bounty, and £200 parliamentary grant, and in the patronage of the Crown. The church, dedicated to St. Pandiana and St. John the Baptist, is partly in the early style of English architecture, with later insertions. A school has been lately erected by Sir

S

G. W. Leeds, and an annual donation of £6 is appropriated towards teaching poor children. A nunnery formerly stood near the vicarage-house, where St. Pandiania, the daughter of a king of Scotland, is said to have been buried: it was destroyed about the time of the Conquest.

ELTON, a township in the parish of THORNTON, second division of the hundred of EDDISBURY, county palatine of CHESTER, 5¼ miles (W.S.W.) from Frodsham, containing 179 inhabitants. The Grand Trunk canal passes through this parish.

ELTON, a township in the parish of WARMINGHAM, hundred of NORTHWICH, county palatine of CHESTER, 2¼ miles (W. by S.) from Sandbach, containing 379 inhabitants.

ELTON, a chapelry in that part of the parish of YOULGRAVE which is in the hundred of WIRKSWORTH, county of DERBY, 1¼ mile (W.) from Winster, containing 548 inhabitants. The living is a perpetual curacy, in the archdeaconry of Derby, and diocese of Lichfield and Coventry, endowed with £200 private benefaction, £200 royal bounty, and £200 parliamentary grant, and in the patronage of the Inhabitants. The chapel is dedicated to All Saints. This chapelry is in the honour of Tutbury, duchy of Lancaster, and within the jurisdiction of a court of pleas held at Tutbury every third Tuesday, for the recovery of debts under 40*s*.

ELTON, a parish in the south-western division of STOCKTON ward, county palatine of DURHAM, 3¼ miles (W.S.W.) from Stockton upon Tees, containing 105 inhabitants. The living is a discharged rectory, in the archdeaconry and diocese of Durham, rated in the king's books at £7. 1. 5½., and in the patronage of R. E. D. Shafto, and — Hogg, Esqrs., the former having two, and the latter one turn in the presentation.

ELTON, a parish in the hundred of WIGMORE, county of HEREFORD, 4¾ miles (S.W. by W.) from Ludlow, containing 93 inhabitants. The living is a perpetual curacy, united with Yarpole to the rectory of Croft, in the archdeaconry and diocese of Hereford, endowed with £800 royal bounty. The church is dedicated to St. Mary.

ELTON, a parish in the hundred of NORMAN-CROSS, county of HUNTINGDON, 4¾ miles (N.E.) from Oundle, containing 785 inhabitants. The living is a rectory, in the archdeaconry of Huntingdon, and diocese of Lincoln, rated in the king's books at £23. 9. 2., and in the patronage of the Master and Fellows of University College, Oxford. The church, dedicated to All Saints, has portions in the decorated, with insertions in the later, English style. There is a place of worship for Wesleyan Methodists. A free school is endowed with between £40 and £50 per annum.

ELTON, a township in that part of the parish of BURY which is in the hundred of SALFORD, county palatine of LANCASTER, 2¾ miles (W. by N.) from Bury, containing 2897 inhabitants.

ELTON, a parish in the northern division of the wapentake of BINGHAM, county of NOTTINGHAM, 4¼ miles (E. by S.) from Bingham, containing 93 inhabitants. The living is a rectory, in the archdeaconry of Nottingham, and diocese of York, rated in the king's books at £8. 0. 5. W. F. N. Newton, Esq. was patron in 1813. The church is dedicated to St. Michael. This parish is in the honour of Tutbury, duchy of Lancaster, and within the jurisdiction of a court of pleas held at Tutbury every third Tuesday, for the recovery of debts under 40*s*.

ELTRINGHAM, a township in the parish of OVINGHAM, eastern division of TINDALE ward, county of NORTHUMBERLAND, 13½ miles (W. by S.) from Newcastle, containing 52 inhabitants.

ELVASTON, a parish in the hundred of MORLESTON and LITCHURCH, county of DERBY, 5 miles (S.E. by E.) from Derby, containing 493 inhabitants. The living is a discharged vicarage, in the archdeaconry of Derby, and diocese of Lichfield and Coventry, rated in the king's books at £5. 3. 9., endowed with £400 private benefaction, and £400 royal bounty, and in the patronage of the Earl of Harrington. The church is dedicated to St. Bartholomew. In January, 1643, Elvaston hall, the seat of Lady Stanhope, was plundered by the parliamentarian troops under Sir John Gell. The river Derwent runs through this parish. Earl Stanhope enjoys the inferior title of Baron Stanhope of Elvaston.

ELVEDON, otherwise ELDEN, a parish in the hundred of LACKFORD, county of SUFFOLK, 3½ miles (S.W. by W.) from Thetford, containing 277 inhabitants. The living is a rectory, in the archdeaconry of Sudbury, and diocese of Norwich, rated in the king's books at £12. 17. 6. ——Newton, Esq. was patron in 1796. The church is dedicated to St. Andrew.

ELVETHAM, a parish in the hundred of ODIHAM, Basingstoke division of the county of SOUTHAMPTON, 1¼ mile (S.S.E.) from Hartford-Bridge, containing 497 inhabitants. The living is a rectory, in the archdeaconry and diocese of Winchester, rated in the king's books at £9, and in the patronage of Lord Calthorpe. The water near Hartford-Bridge, in this parish, is strongly impregnated with iron. Here was formerly a splendid mansion belonging to the Earls of Hertford, where Queen Elizabeth, in 1591, was sumptuously entertained for four days.

ELVINGTON, a parish in the wapentake of OUZE and DERWENT, East riding of the county of YORK, 7 miles (E.S.E.) from York, containing 405 inhabitants. The living is a discharged rectory, in the archdeaconry of Cleveland, and diocese of York, rated in the king's books at £5. 17. 3½., and in the patronage of the Crown. The church, dedicated to the Holy Trinity, is a neat building, erected in 1801, by the Rev. A. Cheap, L.L.B., rector. There is a place of worship for Wesleyan Methodists. A school is supported by subscription, to the master of which £20 per annum is paid, for the instruction of twenty poor boys.

ELWICK, a township in the parish of HART, north-eastern division of STOCKTON ward, county palatine of DURHAM, 9¼ miles (N. by E.) from Stockton upon Tees, containing 213 inhabitants.

ELWICK, a township in that part of the parish of BELFORD which is in the northern division of BAMBROUGH ward, county of NORTHUMBERLAND, 2¼ miles (N.E. by N.) from Belford, containing 73 inhabitants.

ELWICK-HALL, a parish in the north-eastern division of STOCKTON ward, county palatine of DURHAM, 9 miles (N. by E.) from Stockton upon Tees, containing 176 inhabitants. The living is a rectory, in the archdeaconry and diocese of Durham, rated in the king's books at £20. 18. 1½., and in the patronage of the Bishop of Durham. The church, dedicated to

St. Peter, stands on a remarkable elevation at the east end of the parish, and is approached on one side by a great number of steps, rising from the dell which separates this place from the village of Elwick. A little to the north-west of the church is an eminence called Beacon hill, which had formerly a beacon on its summit.

ELWORTHY, a parish in the hundred of WILLITON and FREEMANNERS, county of SOMERSET, 5¼ miles. (N.) from Wiveliscombe, containing 187 inhabitants. The living is a rectory, in the archdeaconry of Taunton, and diocese of Bath and Wells, rated in the king's books at £6. 6. 8., and in the patronage of William Locke, Esq. The church is dedicated to St. Martin.

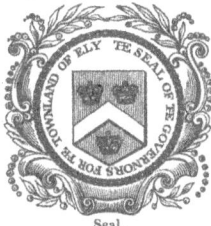

Seal.

ELY, a city in the Isle of ELY, county of CAMBRIDGE, 16 miles (N. N. E.) from Cambridge, and 67 (N. by E.) from London, containing 5079 inhabitants. This place, which is the capital of an extensive district in the fens, comprising the greater part of the northern division of Cambridgeshire, derived its Saxon name *Elig*, either from the British *Helyg*, a willow, with which tree, from the marshy nature of the soil, it especially abounded, or, according to Bede, from *Elge*, an eel, for which fish, from the same cause, it was equally remarkable. Ethelreda, daughter of Anna, King of the East Angles, founded a monastery here in 673, for monks and nuns, which she dedicated to the Blessed Virgin Mary, and, though married to Egfrid, King of Northumberland, devoted herself to a monastic life, and became its first abbess. This monastery, which was destroyed by the Danes in 870, was, a few years afterwards, partially restored by some of the monks who had escaped the massacre, and established themselves as secular priests under the government of provosts for nearly a century. In 970, Ethelwold, Bishop of Winchester, having purchased from Edgar the whole of the Isle of Ely, rebuilt the monastery, which he munificently endowed, and placed in it an abbot and regular monks, to whom Edgar granted the secular jurisdiction of two hundreds within and five hundreds without the fens, with many important privileges, which were subsequently confirmed by Canute, and increased by Edward the Confessor, who here received part of his education. Soon after the Conquest, many of the English nobility, unable to brook the tyranny of William, retired to this place in 1071, where, under the conduct of Edwin, Earl of Chester, and Egelwyn, Bishop of Durham, they ravaged the adjacent country, headed by Hereward, an English nobleman, who built a castle of wood in the marshes, and made a vigorous stand against that monarch, who besieged the island, constructed roads through the marshes, built bridges over the streams, and erected a castle at Wiseberum; by these means, with the exception of Hereward and his followers, compelling his opponents to submit to his authority. The camp occupied by William upon this occasion, and which Dr. Stukeley affirms to have been a Roman camp repaired by his engineers, is still visible, in a field which in some records of the time of Henry III. is called Belasis, probably from one of William's generals, who was quartered on the monastery, of which

on his conquest of the isle, he took possession, but suffered the monks to remain with certain restrictions under an abbot of his own appointment, at whose intercession he subsequently restored the privileges they previously enjoyed. Richard, the tenth and last abbot, a short time prior to his death, obtained from Henry I. permission to establish an episcopal see at Ely, which in 1107 was carried into effect, and Hervey, who has been driven by the Welch from his own see of Bangor, was made first bishop. To him and his successors Henry I. gave for a diocese, the county of Cambridge, which had previously belonged to the bishop of Lincoln, and invested them with sovereign powers in the isle. On the accession of Hervey, who was to supersede the abbot, a new division of lands belonging to the abbey took place, between the bishop and the prior and monks; the bishop's share was, in the 26th of Henry VIII., valued at £2134. 18. 6., and that of the prior and monks at £1301. 8. 2. The bishop granted a fair, to continue for seven days, commencing on the 20th of June, the anniversary of Ethelreda's death. A castle was built here, by Bishop Nigel, in the reign of Stephen, of which there are no remains, its probable site being only distinguishable by a mount to the south of the church. In 1216, during the contest between John and his barons, William Bunk, with a party of Brabanters, taking advantage of a frost, together with the Earl of Salisbury and others, entered the Isle of Ely, plundered the churches, and committed dreadful ravages, compelling the inhabitants to pay large sums of money for the ransom of their lives, and the prior two hundred marks to save the cathedral from being burnt.

The city is situated on elevated ground nearly at the southern extremity of the isle, and on the river Ouse, which is navigable from Lynn for barges: it consists of one long street, partially paved, with smaller streets diverging from it, both in the upper and lower parts of the town, in the centre of which is a spacious market-place: the houses in general are of indifferent appearance, and, with the exception of the cathedral and ecclesiastical buildings, the town has few claims to architectural notice. The ground in the vicinity, though flat and marshy, is extremely fertile, producing excellent herbage, and a considerable portion of it is cultivated by market gardeners, who supply the neighbouring towns with vegetables: great quantities of fruit and butter are also sent to the London market, and the strawberries and asparagus produced are remarkably fine. There is a considerable manufactory for earthenware and tobacco-pipes; and there are numerous mills in the isle for the preparation of oil from flax, hemp, and cole-seed. The market is on Thursday, for corn and cattle: the fairs are on Ascension-day and the eight following days, and October 29th for horses, cattle, hops, and Cottenham cheese.

The charter of privileges granted to the monastery by Edgar, in the 13th of his reign, enlarged and confirmed by Edward the Confessor, William the Conqueror, and Henry I., who granted to the bishop *jura regalia* within the isle, has always been regarded as the foundation of that temporal jurisdiction which the abbot continued to exercise from the time of the re-establishment of the monastery till the erection of the see, and which from that time has been vested in, and is at present exercised by, the bishops of the diocese. The royal franchise of

S 2

Ely, in several statutes, was designated the county palatine of Ely, till the 27th of Henry VIII., when, by act of parliament, the justices of oyer and terminer and gaol delivery, and justices of the peace for the Isle of Ely, were ordered to be appointed by letters patent under the great seal, and all writs to be issued in the king's name. Exclusive jurisdiction, both in civil and criminal matters, is vested in the bishops, who, with their "temporal steward" of the isle, are by the same act justices of the peace, and hold a general assize of oyer and terminer and gaol delivery twice in the year, and a court of pleas for the trial of civil actions to any amount, the proceedings in which are similar to those in the Nisi Prius court at Westminster, and quarterly courts of session alternately here and at Wisbeach: the bishop is also *Custos Rotulorum* of the isle, which includes the three hundreds of Ely, Wisbeach, and Witchford. A court of requests, under an act passed in the 18th of George III., is held monthly at Ely, March, Wisbeach, and Whittlesea, for the recovery of debts under 40s. The municipal government of the city is vested in magistrates appointed by the bishop, who are justices of the peace within the isle; of these, the chief bailiff, called in the act of the 27th of Hen. VIII. "the temporal steward," exercises the functions of high sheriff, his appointment being for life; he summons the juries, both in civil and criminal cases, from the inhabitants of the isle only, who are exempt from serving on juries for the county, and also from all contributions to the public rates for that part of the county which is beyond the limits of the isle. The court-house is a neat and commodious building, consisting of a centre, erected in 1821, containing apartments for holding the several courts, in front of which is a handsome portico of four columns; and two wings, of which the north is an infirmary, and the south a chapel. The common gaol, adjoining it, comprises four divisions for the classification of prisoners, one general day-room, and one airing-yard. The house of correction, situated behind the court-house, and erected at the same time, comprises the governor's house in the centre, on each side of which are eight cells for male felons, and on the east side of the quadrangle, wards for females and prisoners confined for small debts: it is well adapted to the classification of prisoners, and contains two work-rooms, four day-rooms, and four airing-yards.

At the dissolution of the monastery, which was dedicated to St. Peter and St. Ethelreda, Henry VIII. altered the ecclesiastical establishment of the see, and by charter converted the conventual into a cathedral church, which was dedicated to the Holy Trinity; he endowed it with the site and a portion of the revenue of the dissolved priory; and

Arms of the Bishoprick.

under his charter, re-modelled by Charles II., the establishment consists of a dean, eight canons, or prebendaries, five minor canons, eight lay-clerks, eight choristers, a schoolmaster, usher, and twenty-four king's scholars. The cathedral, begun in 1081, and not entirely completed till 1534, is a splendid cruciform structure, displaying, through almost imperceptible gradations, the various changes which have characterised the progress of ecclesiastical architecture, from the earliest times of the Norman to the latest period of the English style. The plan differs from that of other cathedrals in the length of the nave, which is continued through an extended range of twelve arches, and in the shortness of the transepts, which have only a projection of three arches: the west front, though incomplete from the want of the south wing of the façade, is strikingly magnificent; in the lower part it is in the Norman style, with a handsome octagonal turret at the southern extremity, a projecting porch of early English architecture, and a lofty, massive, and highly enriched tower, with angular turrets, of Norman character in the lower stages, and in the upper, of early English, formerly surmounted by a lofty spire, which has been taken down; from the intersection of the nave and transepts rises a noble octagonal lantern, which is considered one of the finest compositions in the decorated style of English architecture, and equally admirable for the excellence of its details and the beauty of its arrangement: it is eighty feet in diameter, and rests on piers which supported a tower, that fell down in 1322. The interior of the cathedral is singularly elegant, and derives a simple grandeur of effect from the judicious arrangement by which the various styles of its architecture are made to harmonise: the nave and transepts are in the Norman style; the choir, partly in the early and partly in the decorated style of English architecture, is separated from the nave by three of the western arches, which were originally part of it, and now form an ante-choir: the eastern part, or present choir, consisting of a range of six arches, is lighted by a double range of windows, and forms one of the richest specimens of the early English style extant; the roof is beautifully groined, and the intersections embellished with flowers and foliage of elegant design; the east window is ornamented with a fine painting of St. Peter: the three western arches forming the ante-choir, are of the decorated character, and assimilate with the beautiful lantern, by which the style of the nave and transepts is finely contrasted. The lady chapel is an elegant edifice in the later decorated style; the groining of the roof, and the series of niches surrounding the interior, are of exquisite beauty: the chapels of Bishops Alcock and West are elaborately decorated with a profusion of architectural embellishments, but inferior in general effect to other portions of this beautiful structure. There are many interesting monuments, among which is the tomb and effigies of Bishop Alcock, under an arch of stone on the north side of his chapel; the monuments of several bishops, and the tomb of Tiptoft, Earl of Worcester, and his two wives, erected in the time of Richard III. The length of the cathedral is five hundred and thirty-five feet from east to west, and the breadth one hundred and ninety from the north to the south transept. Of the cloisters and chapter-house there are scarcely any remains, and the refectory has been converted into a residence for the dean: the prebendal houses retain many vestiges of ancient architecture, of which some are supposed to be of Saxon origin: among these buildings, a chapel, erected by Prior Craunden, is a curious and valuable composition in the decorated style of English architecture, of excellent design, and abounding with interest; the floor is of Mosaic pavement, still in a very perfect state, representing some of the earlier subjects of Scripture history. At some distance from the cathedral is the gate of the ancient monastery, in the later style of English architecture.

The city, exclusively of the liberty of the college, which is extra-parochial, comprises the parishes of St. Mary and the Holy Trinity, in the peculiar jurisdiction and patronage of the Dean and Chapter. The living of St. Mary's is a perpetual curacy, endowed with £200 royal bounty, and £800 parliamentary grant. The church is an interesting structure, partly in the Norman, and partly in the early style of English architecture, with a handsome tower surmounted by a spire; the nave is in the Norman style, with clerestory windows of later English architecture; the chancel is in the early English style, with insertions of a later date, and contains some remains of the ancient stalls; the north porch and door are of the early English style. The living of Holy Trinity parish is also a perpetual curacy, endowed with £200 private benefaction, £200 royal bounty, and £400 parliamentary grant. The church was formerly the lady chapel of the cathedral, now fitted up for the parishioners. There are places of worship for Baptists, those in the Countess of Huntingdon's connexion, Independents, and Wesleyan Methodists. The king's grammar school was founded in 1541, by Henry VIII., on the establishment of the cathedral: it is under the control of the Dean and Chapter, who appoint the master. Jeremiah Bentham, the celebrated political writer, received the rudiments of his education in this school, which at present is not attended by any scholars. A charity school was founded in 1730, by Mrs. Catherine Needham, who endowed it with lands and tenements producing nearly £400 per annum, for the instruction and clothing of thirty boys, with each of whom an apprentice fee of £20 is given, for which latter purpose, Bishop Laney, in 1674, bequeathed lands and tenements. A National school for boys and girls is supported by subscription; the boys are taught in that part of the abbey called the Gallery, formerly used as the grammar school. There are several charitable bequests.

ELYAUGH, a township in that part of the parish of FELTON which is in the eastern division of COQUETDALE ward, county of NORTHUMBERLAND, 9 miles (S.S.W.) from Alnwick, containing 13 inhabitants.

EMBER, a hamlet in that part of the parish of THAMES-DITTON which is in the second division of the hundred of ELMBRIDGE, county of SURREY, containing, with Weston, 1033 inhabitants.

EMBERTON, a parish in the hundred of NEWPORT, county of BUCKINGHAM, 1½ mile (S.) from Olney, containing, with the parish of Okeney cum Petsoe, 549 inhabitants. The living is a rectory, in the archdeaconry of Buckingham, and diocese of Lincoln, rated in the king's books at £15. 2. 11. The Rev. Thomas Fry was patron in 1804. The church is dedicated to All Saints.

EMBLETON, a chapelry in the parish of BRIGHAM, ALLERDALE ward above Darwent, county of CUMBERLAND, 2¾ miles (E. by S.) from Cockermouth, containing 391 inhabitants. The living is a perpetual curacy, in the archdeaconry of Richmond, and diocese of Chester, and in the patronage of the Earl of Lonsdale. The chapel, dedicated to St. Cuthbert, is a neat edifice, rebuilt in 1816.

EMBLETON, a chapelry in the parish of SEDGEFIELD, north-eastern division of STOCKTON ward, county palatine of DURHAM, 8½ miles (N. by W.) from Stockton upon Tees, containing 102 inhabitants.

EMBLETON, a parish in the southern division of BAMBROUGH ward, county of NORTHUMBERLAND, comprising the chapelries of Renington and Rock, and the townships of Brocksfield, High Bruton, Low Bruton, Craster, Dunston, Embleton, Fallowdon, Newton, and Stamford, and containing 1806 inhabitants, of which number, 413 are in the township of Embleton, 7¼ miles (N. E. by N.) from Alnwick. The living is a vicarage, in the archdeaconry of Northumberland, and diocese of Durham, rated in the king's books at £11. 3. 4., endowed with £600 royal bounty, and £200 parliamentary grant, and in the patronage of the Warden and Fellows of Merton College, Oxford. The church is dedicated to St. Mary. A free school is endowed with £20 per annum.

EMBLEY, a tything in the parish of EASTWELLOW, hundred of THORNGATE, Andover division of the county of SOUTHAMPTON, 2¼ miles (W.) from Romsey. The population is returned with the parish.

EMBORROW (IN and OUT), a parish in the hundred of CHEWTON, county of SOMERSET, 5½ miles (N.E.) from Wells, containing, with the tything of Whitnell, 250 inhabitants. The living is a perpetual curacy annexed to the vicarage of Chewton-Mendip, in the archdeaconry of Wells, and diocese of Bath and Wells. The church is dedicated to St. Mary. By the road side is a lake covering about ten acres, with a thick wood behind, and some pleasant walks, the whole presenting a very agreeable appearance. There were formerly mines of coal and lapis calaminaris, the working of which has been discontinued between forty and fifty years.

EMBSAY, a joint township with Eastby, in that part of the parish of SKIPTON which is in the eastern division of the wapentake of STAINCLIFFE and EWCROSS, West riding of the county of YORK, 2 miles (N.E. by N.) from Skipton, containing 861 inhabitants. William de Meschines, and Cecilia de Romili, his wife, founded a monastery here in 1120, for canons regular of the order of St. Augustine, which about thirty years after was translated, by their daughter Adeliza, to Bolton in Craven: a chapel was continued long after its translation. There is a spring in the township still bearing the name of St. Cuthbert's well.

EMLEY, a parish in the lower division of the wapentake of AGBRIGG, West riding of the county of YORK, 7½ miles (E. S. E.) from Huddersfield, containing, with a portion of the township of Skelmanthorpe, 1351 inhabitants. The living is a rectory, in the archdeaconry and diocese of York, rated in the king's books at £14. 0. 7½.., and in the patronage of the Hon. and Rev. Lumley Savile. The church is dedicated to St. Michael. There is a trifling endowment for the education of children.

EMMINGTON, a parish in the hundred of LEWKNOR, county of OXFORD, 3¼ miles (S.E.) from Thame, containing 77 inhabitants. The living is a rectory, in the archdeaconry and diocese of Oxford, rated in the king's books at £11. 0. 2½, and in the patronage of P. T. Wykeham, Esq. The church is dedicated to St. Nicholas.

EMNETH, a parish in the Marshland division of the hundred of FREEBRIDGE, county of NORFOLK, 2½ miles (S. E. by E.) from Wisbeach, containing 970 inhabitants. The living is a perpetual curacy, annexed to the rectory and vicarage of Elm, in the peculiar jurisdiction of the Bishop of Ely. The church is dedicated to St. Edmund.

EMPINGHAM, a parish in the hundred of EAST, county of RUTLAND, 6¼ miles (E. by S.) from Oakham, containing 759 inhabitants. The living is a discharged vicarage, rated in the king's books at £7. 14. 9½., endowed with £200 private benefaction, and £200 royal bounty, and in the peculiar jurisdiction and patronage of the Prebendary of Empingham in the Cathedral Church of Lincoln. The church, dedicated to St. Peter, is a handsome edifice, principally in the early English style, with some later insertions. There is a free school.

EMPSHOT, a parish in the hundred of SELBORNE, ALTON (North) division of the county of SOUTHAMPTON, 5 miles (N.) from Petersfield, containing 139 inhabitants. The living is a discharged vicarage, in the archdeaconry and diocese of Winchester, rated in the king's books at £5. 16. 5½., endowed with £400 private benefaction, and £400 royal bounty, and in the patronage of Mrs. Butler. The church is dedicated to the Holy Rood.

EMSWELL, a joint township with Kelleythorpe, in that part of the parish of DRIFFIELD which is in the Bainton-Beacon division of the wapentake of HARTHILL, East riding of the county of YORK, 2 miles (W.) from Great Driffield, containing 93 inhabitants.

EMSWORTH, a tything in the parish of WARBLINGTON, hundred of BOSMERE, Portsdown division of the county of SOUTHAMPTON, 2 miles (E. by S.) from Havant. The population is returned with the parish. This place lies upon the Sussex border, at the head of Emsworth channel, which is navigable along Hayling island to the English channel. Fairs for the sale of toys, &c. are held, April 15th and July 18th.

ENBORNE, a parish in the hundred of KINTBURY-EAGLE, county of BERKS, 2¼ miles (W. S. W.) from Newbury, containing 349 inhabitants. The living is a rectory, in the archdeaconry of Berks, and diocese of Salisbury, rated in the king's books at £10, and in the patronage of the Earl of Craven. The church is dedicated to St. Michael. The Kennet and Avon canal passes through the parish. The custom of free bench prevails in the manor of East and West Enborne, whereby the widow of a tenant is entitled to an estate in copyhold, for her dower, while she continues single and chaste, in default of which she forfeits her lands, unless she choose to demand them by riding into court backwards on a black ram, and repeating a piece of loose doggrel rhyme.

ENDELLION, a parish in the hundred of TRIGG, county of CORNWALL, 5¼ miles (N.) from Wade-bridge, containing 1149 inhabitants. The living is a rectory, in the archdeaconry of Cornwall, and diocese of Exeter, rated in the king's books at £10, and in the patronage of the Crown. The church, dedicated to St. Edelienta, stands on high ground, its tower being visible as a land-mark at a great distance; it is collegiate, containing three prebends, which are sinecures, exclusively of the rectory: the king's prebend is in the patronage of the Crown; that of Trehaverock is in the patronage of the Hon. Mr. Agar, as representative of the family of Robartes, Earl of Radnor; and that of Heredum-

Marney is in the patronage of Richardson Gray, Esq. In this parish is Port Isaac, which has a considerable pilchard fishery, and a small market on Friday, for butchers' meat. The principal export of the place, which is bounded on the north by the British channel, consists of pilchards, and slate from the Delabole quarries: coal is imported from Wales. In the parish also is Port Guin, formerly a large fishing town. At Port Isaac is a charity school, established about 1804, and supported by voluntary subscriptions.

ENDERBY, a parish in the hundred of SPARKENHOE, county of LEICESTER, 4½ miles (S. W.) from Leicester, containing 1143 inhabitants. The living is a discharged vicarage, in the archdeaconry of Leicester, and diocese of Lincoln, rated in the king's books at £10. 8. 9. C. L. Smith, Esq. was patron in 1824. The church is dedicated to St. John the Baptist. There is a chapel of ease at Whetstone, in this parish. A school for thirty poor children was endowed with a house and £20 per annum, by Richard Smith, Esq., in 1762. Towards the south-east, the parish is bounded by the river Soar.

ENDERBY (BAG), a parish in the hundred of HILL, parts of LINDSEY, county of LINCOLN, 5½ miles (N. W. by N.) from Spilsby, containing 107 inhabitants. The living is a discharged rectory, in the archdeaconry and diocese of Lincoln, rated in the king's books at £6. 18. 1½. R. Burton, Esq. was patron in 1816. The church is dedicated to St. Margaret.

ENDERBY (MAVIS), a parish in the eastern division of the soke of BOLINGBROKE, parts of LINDSEY, county of LINCOLN, 1¼ mile (W. by N.) from Spilsby, containing 189 inhabitants. The living is a discharged rectory, in the archdeaconry and diocese of Lincoln, rated in the king's books at £12. 11. 3. The Rev. C. Semple was patron in 1803. The church is dedicated to St. Michael.

ENDERBY (WOOD), a parish in the soke of HORNCASTLE, parts of LINDSEY, county of LINCOLN, 4 miles (S. by E.) from Horncastle, containing 183 inhabitants. The living is a perpetual curacy, in the archdeaconry and diocese of Lincoln, endowed with £1000 royal bounty, and in the patronage of the Bishop of Carlisle. The church is dedicated to St. Benedict.

ENDFORD, a parish in the hundred of ELSTUB and EVERLEY, county of WILTS, 8¼ miles (W. by N.) from Ludgershall, containing, with the tything of Fyfield, 901 inhabitants. The living is a vicarage, in the archdeaconry and diocese of Salisbury, rated in the king's books at £19. 4. 9½., and in the patronage of the Governors of Christ's Hospital, London. The church is dedicated to All Saints.

ENDON, a chapelry in that part of the parish of LEEK which is in the northern division of the hundred of TOTMONSLOW, county of STAFFORD, 4½ miles (S. W. by W.) from Leek, containing 445 inhabitants. The living is a perpetual curacy, in the archdeaconry of Stafford, and diocese of Lichfield and Coventry, endowed with £400 private benefaction, £400 royal bounty, and in the patronage of the Earl of Macclesfield. The Caldon Branch canal passes through this parish. There are two trifling bequests for the education of the poor.

ENFIELD, a parish (formerly a market town) in the hundred of EDMONTON, county of MIDDLESEX, 10 miles (N. by E.) from London, containing 8227 inhabitants. This place is in Domesday-book called Ene-

felde, from which its present name, denoting its situation among fields, or in the felled part of the forest, is derived. The Chase formerly extended to the river Lea, in the neighbourhood of which, for the facility of its conveyance, the timber growing in this extensive tract, would probably be felled prior to that in any other part of the parish. Richard II. granted the inhabitants exemption from tolls, and various privileges, which were confirmed by succeeding monarchs. Edward VI. had a palace here, in which he kept his court for a considerable time; and in 1557, the princess, afterwards Queen Elizabeth, spent some days in the palace, when, with great pomp, she came to hunt in Enfield Chase, which was well stocked with deer. In the earlier part of her reign the queen made this her principal residence, where she held her court previously to its removal to London. James I., who had a palace at Theobald's, made frequent excursions to this forest, to enjoy the diversion of the chase; and Charles II. here had a hunting seat, where he occasionally resided. During the great civil war, the parliamentarian army destroyed the game, and cut down the trees; and a considerable part of the land was divided into small farms: it continued in this state till after the Restoration, when it was re-planted and stocked with deer. In 1777, it was finally disafforested by act of parliament, and allotments assigned to such parishes and individuals as claimed a right of common: the Chase, on admeasurement, was found to contain eight thousand three hundred and fifty acres, of which the greater part is now in tillage. Of the ancient palace, which was probably repaired during the reigns of Edward VI. and Elizabeth, but of which the major part was taken down in 1792, only one of the principal rooms on the ground floor is remaining; it is still in its original state, with oak panels and a richly ornamented ceiling: the chimney-piece of freestone, which is embellished with finely sculptured birds and foliage, is supported by columns of the Corinthian and Ionic orders, and decorated with the rose and portcullis crowned, and with the arms of England and France quartered, having for supporters a lion and dragon, and the motto " *Sola salus servire Deo ; sunt cætera fraudes :* " part of a similar chimney-piece, removed from one of the upper rooms, has been placed on the wainscot over the door. A fine cedar of Libanus was planted in the garden of the palace in 1666, the girth of which at a short distance from the ground is nineteen feet three inches. A knife and fork, and a gilt silver spoon, were found in taking down part of the ancient building in 1789, and among the ruins another silver spoon, apparently of the date of Elizabeth, which is in the possession of the present occupier of the premises, a sixpence of the reign of Elizabeth, and a gold coin of that of Charles I.

The town, which is situated to the west of the road from London to Ware, consists of two streets, in which are several handsome houses, and is well supplied with water from springs. A royal manufactory for small arms, previously carried on at the Tower and at Lewisham, was, in 1816, established partly in this parish and partly at Waltham Abbey: there are a corn-mill, and a mill for dressing skins, a brewery, and an extensive tannery; and at Ponder's End, in the parish, is a large manufactory for finishing crape, which affords employment to one hundred and fifty persons. The New River

runs through the town, and the Lea navigation passes through part of the parish. The market on Monday, granted by charter of Edward I. in 1304, and another on Saturday, by charter of James I., are both discontinued; but fairs are still held on September 23d, which is a statute fair, and November 30th, for horses, cows, and cheese. Near the market-house, a handsome stone cross, in the ancient style of English architecture, was erected in 1826, by subscription. The county magistrates hold here a petty session for the division every alternate Wednesday: courts leet and baron are held on the Wednesday in Whitsun-week; and a court of requests is held for the hundred, for the recovery of debts under 40s. Enfield is a liberty belonging to the duchy of Lancaster, and the inhabitants appoint their own coroner. The parish comprises the town, the Chase, Bull's cross, Baker street, and Green-street, with Ponder's End.

The living is a vicarage, in the archdeaconry of Middlesex, and diocese of London, rated in the king's books at £26, and in the patronage of the Master and Fellows of Trinity College, Cambridge. A lectureship was established in 1631, by Mr. Henry Loft, who endowed it with £4 per annum. The church, dedicated to St. Andrew, is an ancient structure in the decorated and later styles of English architecture, with a low square embattled tower; the nave is separated from the aisles by clustered columns and pointed arches: it contains many ancient, and several splendid monuments, among which are the tomb and effigies of Sir Nicholas Raynton and his lady; an altar-tomb to the memory of Joyce, Lady Tiftoft, mother of the talented Earl of Worcester; a handsome monument of Italian veined marble to Thomas Stringer, Esq., and various others. In enlarging the arch which separates the chancel from the nave, a rude painting of the Resurrection in six compartments was removed; and in opening a vault in 1829, some coffins in the shape of the human frame were discovered. A chapel of ease is about to be built in the division of Green-street and Ponder's End, at an estimated expense of £4800, to be defrayed partly by a grant from the parliamentary commissioners, and partly by subscription. There are places of worship for Independents, Wesleyan Methodists, and Presbyterians.

The free grammar school was originally endowed with funds arising from a bequest by Mr. Robert Blossom, in 1418, of land and premises in the parish of South Bemfleet, for the establishment of a chantry in that place, which after the dissolution was granted to trustees for the payment of a schoolmaster for the instruction of poor children of the parish of Enfield, with remainder, after paying the expenses of repairs, &c., for distribution among the poor: the produce arising from this and subsequent benefactions, and from the sale of timber, is at present nearly £400 per annum: there are about one hundred and seventy boys in the school, who are taught reading, writing, arithmetic, the mathematics, and the classics. Mrs. Mary Turpin, in 1775, bequeathed £200 to be vested in the three per cent. consols., for the instruction of three poor girls. A school of industry, in which forty-five girls are clothed and instructed, established in 1800; a similar school, in which forty girls are clothed and instructed, established by the dissenting congregations in 1806; and an infant school, instituted in 1825, are supported by subscrip tion : an infant school was also established at Ponder's End in 1830. Sir Nicholas Raynton, in 1646, bequeathed £10 per annum in trust to the Haberdashers' Company, for apprenticing children of this parish, to which the churchwardens have added £3 per annum, being the dividend on £100 stock, purchased with a sum of £70 returned to them by the company, who for thirty-five years had deducted £2 per annum for the land tax. Henry Dixon, Esq., in 1693, left considerable estates in the parishes of Bennington and Munden, in the county of Herts; of Enfield in the county of Middlesex; and of St. Mildred's in the Poultry, London, in trust to the Drapers' Company, for apprenticing boys of these parishes above the age of fifteen ; such as bear his christian and surname, wherever born, are to be preferred, and to receive a premium of £5, and £5 on the expiration of their indenture : those who bear only his surname receive a premium of £4, the sons of tenants of any of his lands, wherever born, £3, and any who are nominated by the court of assistants of the Drapers' Company, £4. Mrs. Anne Crowe, in 1763, endowed almshouses for four aged persons, with £500 reduced Bank Annuities. Thomas Wilson, Esq., in 1590, bequeathed the rents of three houses in Whitechapel, London, producing £162. 14. 6. per annum, for distribution among six aged men of this parish; one of these houses was sold by act of parliament and the money vested in the purchase of £2091 three per cent. consols., the interest of which, with £150, the rental of the two remaining houses, amounts to about £212 per annum. John David, Esq. bequeathed the rents of tenements on Enfield-green, producing £50. per annum, to be divided among four aged widows. King James I. gave £500 for the purchase of three hundred and thirty-five acres of land, a part of Enfield Chase, with which sum the churchwardens bought an estate at North Mimms, in Hertfordshire, afterwards exchanged for another at Eastwood, in Essex, which is distributed among aged widows : there are several other bequests for charitable purposes. A charity for the relief of lying-in women was established in 1797, and is supported by subscription.

The Ermin-street led through part of the Chase to Hertford ; and in a meadow called Old Bury, about half a mile to the east of the church, is the site of an ancient mansion, surrounded by a wide and deep moat, with high intrenchments, including a quadrilateral area of ninety-six yards in length, and forty in breadth ; at the north-west angle is an eminence having the appearance of the keep of a castle, probably the manorial residence of Humphrey de Bohun. To the south-west of the town, and about a mile from Old Bury, is a smaller moat, on the estate of John Clayton, Esq. ; and to the south of Goulsdown-lane is another, separating two square fields, in the first of which are the remains of out-buildings belonging to a mansion in which Judge Jeffreys is said to have resided, and near the entrance a deep well, called King's Ring, the water of which is deemed efficacious in diseases of the eye : a celt was dug up in 1793, at the depth of twelve feet from the surface. In 1816, several Roman urns and coins were found in a gravel pit in the vicinity ; and in Windmill field, large painted tiles have been frequently discovered by the plough; and recently part of a coffin and some urns, in one of which were bones, and in another three

pieces of gold. In September, 1820, several Roman coins of silver and brass were ploughed up in a field near Clay Hill ; they were of the reigns of Domitian, Nerva, Trajan, Aurelius, Hadrian, Antoninus Pius, and one with the head of the Empress Sabina, and several others, about seventy in number, many of which are in the possession of Dr. May and C. P. Meyer, Esq. William Pitt, Earl of Chatham, was an inhabitant of Enfield for several years, and Richard Gough, the antiquary, resided here till his decease in 1809. Enfield gives the title of baron to the Earl of Rochford.

ENGLEFIELD, a parish in the hundred of THEALE, county of BERKS, 6 miles (W.) from Reading, containing 343 inhabitants. The living is a rectory, in the archdeaconry of Berks, and diocese of Salisbury, rated in the king's books at £11. 12. 8½., and in the patronage of R. P. W. Benyon de Beauvoir, Esq. The church has some portions in the early English style, but has been much modernised : it contains several interesting monuments to the memory of the ancestors of the Marquis of Winchester. This parish, which is not unfrequently called Inglefield, derives its name from the Saxon word Ingle, a fire or beacon light, and probably had its origin about the middle of the ninth century, at which time the Danes, having made themselves masters of Reading, sent out a detachment from their army to attack the Saxons, who were encamped at this place, and who drove them back with great loss. Elias Ashmole, the herald and antiquary, retired to this place in 1647, where he pursued his researches.

ENHAM (KING'S), a hamlet in the parish and hundred of ANDOVER, Andover division of the county of SOUTHAMPTON, 2 miles (N.) from Andover, with which the population is returned. This place is within the jurisdiction of the Cheyney Court held at Winchester every Thursday, for the recovery of debts to any amount.

ENHAM (KNIGHTS'), a parish in the hundred of ANDOVER, Andover division of the county of SOUTHAMPTON, 1¾ mile (N.) from Andover, containing 77 inhabitants. The living is a rectory, in the archdeaconry and diocese of Winchester, rated in the king's books at £10, and in the patronage of the Provost and Fellows of Queen's College, Oxford. The church is dedicated to St. Michael. Here is a charity school, endowed with £25 per annum.

ENMORE, a parish in the hundred of ANDERSFIELD, county of SOMERSET, 4 miles (W.S.W.) from Bridg-water, containing 287 inhabitants. The living is a rectory, in the archdeaconry of Taunton, and diocese of Bath and Wells, rated in the king's books at £8. 4. 2., endowed with £200 private benefaction, and £300 parliamentary grant, and in the patronage of the Earl of Egmont. The church is dedicated to St. Michael. The Earl of Egmont enjoys the inferior title of Lord Lovel and Holland, of Enmore.

ENNERDALE, a parochial chapelry in that part of the parish of ST. BEES which is in ALLERDALE ward above Darwent, county of CUMBERLAND, 5 miles (N. E.) from Egremont, containing 209 inhabitants. The living is a perpetual curacy, in the archdeaconry of Richmond, and diocese of Chester, endowed with £1000 royal bounty, and £1200 parliamentary grant, and in the patronage of H. C. Curwen, Esq. The chapel is a small neat edifice, which was repaired in 1786, and in 1825 the thorn hedge which enclosed the burial-ground, was removed, and a stone wall built in its stead. A school-room has been built by subscription among the inhabitants. On the second Tuesday in September a sheep fair is held in the village. The Earl of Lonsdale, as lord of the manor, holds a court here at Michaelmas.

ENODER (ST.), a parish in the hundred of PYDER, county of CORNWALL, 2¾ miles (N.E.) from St. Michael, containing, with a part of the borough of St. Michael's, or Midshall, 833 inhabitants. The living is a vicarage, in the archdeaconry of Cornwall, and diocese of Exeter, rated in the king's books at £26. 13. 4., and in the patronage of the Bishop of Exeter. In the church is a curious Norman font. At Summer Court, in this parish, are large fairs for horses, bullocks, sheep, &c., on the 28th of July and 25th of September.

ENODOCK (ST.), a chapelry in the parish of ST. MINVER, hundred of TRIGG, county of CORNWALL, 2½ miles (N.E.) from Padstow. The population is returned with the parish.

ENSHAM, a parish in the hundred of WOOTTON, county of OXFORD, 5½ miles (E. by S.) from Witney, containing 1705 inhabitants. The living is a discharged vicarage, in the archdeaconry and diocese of Oxford, rated in the king's books at £15. 14., endowed with £200 private benefaction, and £200 royal bounty. The church, holds a handsome edifice, is dedicated to St. Leonard. There is a place of worship for Independents. In 1700, John Bartholomew gave £350, to be applied to the education and apprenticing of ten poor boys: in the year following the school was built by subscription, and fourteen boys are now instructed. This place derives its name from the Saxon Egonesham, and was formerly a Saxon frontier town. King Ethelred held a council at Ensham, on the advice of Alphege and Wulstan, Archbishops of York and Canterbury, at which many ecclesiastical and civil decrees were enacted. At one period it was famous for its abbey, founded by Ethelware, Earl of Cornwall, in the reign of Ethelred, who confirmed the charter in 1005: its revenue, at the dissolution, was valued at £441; there are no remains. Here is a paper-mill of high repute. The river Thames and the Oxford canal pass in the vicinity. There are some Roman, Saxon, and Danish encampments.

ENSON, a joint township with Salt, in that part of the parish of ST. MARY, LICHFIELD, which is in the southern division of the hundred of PIREHILL, county of STAFFORD, 4 miles (N. by E.) from Stafford, containing 439 inhabitants.

ENSTONE (CHURCH), a parish in the hundred of CHADLINGTON, county of OXFORD, comprising the hamlets of Cleveley, Church-Enstone, Neat-Enstone, Gagingwell, Lidstone, and Radford, and containing 1077 inhabitants, of which number, 254 are in the hamlet of Church-Enstone, ¾ of a mile (N. by E.) from Neat-Enstone, and 326 in Neat-Enstone, 15 miles (N. W. by N.) from Oxford. The living is a discharged vicarage, in the archdeaconry and diocese of Oxford, rated in the king's books at £9. 14. 4., endowed with £800 parliamentary grant, and in the patronage of C. D. Lee, Esq. The church is dedicated to St. Kenelm. There is a place of worship for Wesleyan Methodists.

ENTWISLE, a township in the parish of BOLTON, hundred of SALFORD, county palatine of LANCASTER, 6½ miles (N. by E.) from Great Bolton, containing 677 inhabitants.

VOL. II.

ENVILLE, a parish in the southern division of the hundred of SEISDON, county of STAFFORD, 5 miles (W. N. W.) from Stourbridge, containing 842 inhabitants. The living is a rectory, in the archdeaconry of Stafford, and diocese of Lichfield and Coventry, rated in the king's books at £27. 2. 11., and in the patronage of the Earl of Stamford and Warrington. The church is dedicated to St. Mary. In 1654, Edward Gravenor bequeathed a small endowment for the education of six poor children; and in 1755, and 1757, Lady Dorothy Grey gave two annuities of £50 and £20, for clothing, maintaining, and educating twelve poor girls: subsequent bequests have raised the income to £101. 2. 10. per annum, but at present only four children receive the benefits of the charity.

EPPERSTONE, a parish in the southern division of the wapentake of THURGARTON, county of NOTTINGHAM, 6 miles (S. W.) from Southwell, containing 513 inhabitants. The living is a rectory, in the archdeaconry of Nottingham, and diocese of York, rated in the king's books at £13. 1. 8. E. White, Esq. was patron in 1822. The church is dedicated to the Holy Cross. There is a place of worship for Wesleyan Methodists.

EPPING, a parish comprising the market-town of Epping, and the chapelry of Epping-Upland, in the hundred of WALTHAM, and the hamlet of Ryhill, in the hundred of HARLOW, county of ESSEX, and containing 2146 inhabitants, of which number, 1688 are in the town of Epping, 17½ miles (W. by S.) from Chelmsford, and 16¾ (N. E. by N.) from London, on the road to Newmarket. This place, which is of some antiquity, was given by Henry II. to the monks of Waltham abbey, but reverting to the crown, it became afterwards a part of the duchy of Lancaster. The town is pleasantly situated near the extensive forest to which it gives name, and consists of two parts, one near the church, called Epping-Upland, and the other nearly a mile and a half to the south-east of it, called Epping-Street, in which the market is held: the latter is a spacious street, nearly a mile in length, having at the west end a newly-erected chapel, and in the centre a range of shambles, which are much decayed and of mean appearance; the houses are irregularly built, but the town being, from its situation, a great thoroughfare and place of traffic, it possesses some good inns. Epping is celebrated for its butter, of which large quantities are sent for the supply of the London market, where, from the excellence of its quality, it maintains a superiority in price: the pork and sausages of this place are also in high estimation. The market is on Friday: the fairs are on the Tuesday in Whitsun-week, which is but thinly attended; November 13th, a very considerable fair for the sale of stock; and on the 11th of October, a statute fair for hiring servants. Courts leet and baron are held annually under the lord of the manor.

The living is a vicarage, in the peculiar jurisdiction of the court of the Commissary of London concurrently with the Consistorial Episcopal Court, rated in the king's books at £17. 13. 4., endowed with £600 parliamentary grant, and in the patronage of Henry John Conyers, Esq. The church is dedicated to All Saints. A small chapel of ease has been recently erected. There are places of worship for the Society of Friends and Independents; the former, though bordering on the town, is in an adjoining parish. A National school

T

and a Sunday school, are supported by subscription. Adjoining the town is Epping Forest, a royal chase, comprehending an extensive tract, anciently called the Forest of Essex, subsequently Waltham Forest, and at present deriving its name from the town. Its original limits have been gradually contracted, many thousand acres having been thrown into cultivation, and numerous handsome villas erected: among these, Copped Hall, the seat of John Conyers, Esq., built on the site of an ancient structure raised by the monks of Waltham abbey, when they had possession of the manor, is a noble edifice, and one of the chief ornaments of the county; it is situated in the centre of a fine park, of nearly four thousand acres, planted with every kind of forest trees, among which is a cedar of Libanus of extraordinary beauty. The forest is under the jurisdiction of a lord warden, whose office is hereditary in the family of the late Sir James Tilney Long, Bart., and four verdurers, who are elected by the freeholders of the county, and retain their office for life: the forest rights vary according to the particular tenure prevailing in the different manors included in the district. Though so near the metropolis, wild stags are still found here, and one is annually turned out on Easter-Monday for the Epping Hunt, which has been long established, and is still well supported: the kennel for the hounds, and other buildings connected with the hunt, have been recently re-erected at an expense of several thousand pounds. On that part near Barking, called Hainault Forest, where a society for the revival of archery established their meetings, was an oak of extraordinary dimensions, called Fairlop Oak, the girth of which, at the height of three feet from the ground, was thirty-six feet, the branches extending over an area of three hundred feet in circumference. Round this tree a fair has for many years been held, on the first Friday in July, and is still numerously attended: it originated in the annual visit of an individual from London to dine with a select party of his friends under the shade of the Fairlop Oak, from the trunk of which he distributed a supply of beans and bacon to many poor persons who were attracted to the spot. On the forest was found a small earthen figure of a child, which was shewn to the Antiquarian Society in 1721.

EPPLEBY, a township in that part of the parish of GILLING which is in the western division of the wapentake of GILLING, North riding of the county of York, 8 miles (N. by E.) from Richmond, containing 157 inhabitants.

EPPLETON (GREAT), a township in the parish of HOUGHTON le SPRING, northern division of EASINGTON ward, county palatine of DURHAM, 7¼ miles (N. E. by E.) from Durham, containing 43 inhabitants.

EPPLETON (LITTLE), a township in the parish of HOUGHTON le SPRING, northern division of EASINGTON ward, county palatine of DURHAM, 6¼ miles (E. N. E.) from Durham, containing 32 inhabitants.

EPSOM, a parish in the first division of the hundred of COPTHORNE, county of SURREY, 16 miles (E. N. E.) from Guildford, and 15 (S. W. by S.) from London, on the road to Worthing, containing, with the hamlet of Horton, 2890 inhabitants. This place was by the Saxons called *Ebbisham*, from which its present name is derived. It is delightfully situated on the western verge of Banstead downs, and from the

salubrity of the air and the estimation in which its medicinal waters were formerly held, it became the resort of many families, and rapidly increased in the number of its buildings and the extent of its population. In the centre of the town is a large sheet of water : the houses are in general handsome and well built, and the inhabitants are tolerably supplied with water. The environs, which are exceedingly pleasant, abound with handsome villas; and on the downs, which command an extensive and interesting view of the surrounding country, is an excellent course, on which races are held annually, commencing on the Tuesday and continuing till the end of the week preceding Whitsuntide; the Derby stakes are run for on Thursday, which is the principal day, and the Oaks on Friday. The grand stand, a handsome and commodious edifice, was erected in 1829-30, the expense being estimated at £13,890, raised in one thousand £20 shares; the interior comprises several rooms for refreshment, and a saloon, one hundred and one feet in length, and thirty-eight feet wide; the whole length of the building is one hundred and twenty-six feet, arranged for the accommodation of five thousand persons, with seats on the roof for two thousand five hundred: a second meeting also takes place in October: much of the support of the town arises from the great influx of strangers at the time of the races. The market, formerly on Friday, has been discontinued; but it is in contemplation to erect a market-house for the renewal of the market, with a room over it for holding the sessions, on the site of an old watch-house, which is about to be taken down : a fair is held annually on the 5th of August for toys. The medicinal springs, though less frequented than formerly, still retain their efficacy. The county magistrates hold here a petty session for the division on the first Monday in every month; and the town is within the jurisdiction of a court held at Kingston, for the recovery of debts to any amount : a court baron is held in April, and a court leet in October.

The living is a discharged vicarage, in the archdeaconry of Surrey, and diocese of Winchester, rated in the king's books at £8. 9. 9½., and in the patronage of — Speirs, Esq. The church, dedicated to St. Martin, was rebuilt at an expense of £7000 in 1825, when it received an addition of five hundred and forty-seven sittings, three hundred and thirty-nine of them free, towards defraying the expense of which, the Incorporated Society for the enlargement of churches and chapels granted £500 : in the modern edifice the architectural style of the ancient structure has in most instances been carefully preserved. There is a place of worship for Independents. In 1694, John Brayne, Esq. bequeathed £300, to be invested in the purchase of land, of which the rents were to be applied to the instruction of poor children, from which fund, augmented with other benefactions, arises an annual income of more than £70, by which, and by annual subscriptions, all the children of the parish are instructed on the National system : the school-rooms were built in 1828, by subscription. An almshouse for twelve aged widows was erected by the parishioners, on land given for that purpose by Mr. John Livingstone, about the year 1703. Samuel Cane, Esq., in 1786, bequeathed £500 three per cent. consols.; and in 1814, Langley Brackenbury, Esq. left by will £300 in the same funds, to be distributed in bread and coal to the inmates of the almshouse. There are also charitable bequests for the relief of the poor generally. On the south-east side of the parish is an irregularly intermitting spring.

EPWELL, a chapelry in that part of the parish of SWALCLIFFE which is in the hundred of BANBURY, county of OXFORD, 7 miles (W.) from Banbury, containing 355 inhabitants.

EPWORTH, a market town and parish in the western division of the wapentake of MANLEY, parts of LINDSEY, county of LINCOLN, 28¾ miles (N.W. by N.) from Lincoln, and 157¾ (N. by W.) from London, containing 1763 inhabitants. This place, which is the principal town in the Isle of Axholme, a district occupying the north-west part of the county, was anciently the residence of the Howard family, who had a castellated mansion, of which there are no remains except the site, where within the last half century were dug up some of the cannon belonging to the fortifications. The town is of considerable extent, but irregularly built; the adjacent lands are flat, and, previously to the introduction of a more efficient method of draining, were subject to frequent inundation. The principal branch of trade is the dressing of flax and hemp, a great quantity of which grows in the neighbourhood; and the manufacture of sacking and canvas is carried on to a considerable extent. The market is on Tuesday: the fairs are on the first Thursday after May 1st, and September 29th, for cattle, hemp, and flax. A court leet is held twice in the year by the lord of the manor, in a building erected for that purpose in the market-place. The living is a rectory, in the archdeaconry of Stow, and diocese of Lincoln, rated in the king's books at £28. 16. 8., in the patronage of the Crown. The church is dedicated to St. Andrew. There are places of worship for Baptists, the Society of Friends, the Old and the New Connexion of Methodists, and Primitive Methodists. A school for the instruction of children of this parish was founded in 1711, and endowed with a house and a small portion of land by subscription: there are some charitable bequests for the relief of the poor. A Carthusian monastery was founded here in the reign of Richard II., by Thomas Mowbray, Earl of Nottingham, and Earl Marshal of England, the revenue of which at the dissolution was £290. 11. 7.; the remains have been converted into a private mansion. The Rev. John Wesley, founder of the sect of Methodists, was born in this parish, in 1703, during the incumbency of his father, who was rector for fifty-nine years; and Mr. Alexander Kilham, founder of a class of seceders from that sect, called Kilhamites, was also a native of this place.

ERCALL (CHILD'S), a parish in the Drayton division of the hundred of BRADFORD (North), county of SALOP, 7 miles (N.W.) from Newport, containing 389 inhabitants. The living is a perpetual curacy, in the archdeaconry of Salop, and diocese of Lichfield and Coventry, endowed with £400 private benefaction, and £800 royal bounty. Sir Andrew Corbett, Bart. was patron in 1801. The church is dedicated to St. Michael.

ERCALL (MAGNA), a parish in the Wellington division of the hundred of BRADFORD (South), county of SALOP, 6 miles (N.W.) from Wellington, containing 1952 inhabitants. The living is a discharged vicarage, in the archdeaconry of Salop, and diocese of Lichfield and Coventry, rated in the king's books at £17. 6. 8.

H. Pulteney, Esq. was patron in 1795. The church is dedicated to St. Michael. In this parish is a free school for the education of poor boys, and an hospital for the maintenance of eight decayed householders.

ERISWELL, a parish in the hundred of LACKFORD, county of SUFFOLK, 3 miles (N. by E.) from Mildenhall, containing 346 inhabitants. The living is a rectory, in the archdeaconry of Sudbury, and diocese of Norwich, rated in the king's books at £16. 6. 8. T. B. Evans, Esq. was patron in 1815. The church is dedicated to St. Peter.

ERITH, a parish in the hundred of LESSNESS, lathe of SUTTON at HONE, county of KENT, 2¼ miles (N.) from Crayford, containing 1363 inhabitants. The living is a vicarage, in the archdeaconry and diocese of Rochester, rated in the king's books at £9. 12. 6. S. Dashwood, Esq. was patron in 1804. The church, dedicated to St. John the Baptist, is an ancient structure, almost wholly overgrown with ivy. There is a small sum for the education of poor children. This is a decayed market town, which at one period was incorporated, situated on the banks of the Thames; it had formerly fairs on Holy-Thursday, Michaelmas-day, and Whit-Tuesday. The Thames forms a haven here, and there is a branch establishment in connexion with the custom-house. The East India ships which frequently anchor opposite this place, in their passage up the river, occasion a considerable traffic. An abbey for Canons Regular was founded here in 1180.

ERME (ST.), a parish in the western division of the hundred of POWDER, county of CORNWALL, 3¼ miles (N. by E.) from Truro, containing 561 inhabitants. The living is a rectory, in the archdeaconry of Cornwall, and diocese of Exeter, rated in the king's books at £22. 13. 4., and in the patronage of E. W. Wynne Pendarves, Esq. The church was taken down in 1819, and rebuilt on a handsomer and more uniform plan.

ERMINGTON, a parish in the hundred of ERMINGTON, county of DEVON, 3 miles (N. W.) from Modbury, containing 1370 inhabitants. The living comprises a vicarage and a mediety rectory, in the archdeaconry of Totness, and diocese of Exeter: the vicarage is rated in the king's books at £33. 11. 3., and the rectory at £24. The patronage is vested in the Crown and the Rev. W. Cholwich alternately. The church is dedicated to St. Peter. A market was formerly held here: two small cattle fairs are now held on February 2d and June 23d. In 1513, an almshouse and a charity school were endowed with lands by Alice Hatch.

ERNEY (ST.), a chapelry in the parish of LANDRAKE, southern division of the hundred of EAST, county of CORNWALL, 2 miles (N. by E.) from St. Germans. The population is returned with the parish. The river Lynher is navigable on the east, and the St. Germans on the west of this chapelry; on the south they unite.

ERPINGHAM, a parish in the southern division of the hundred of ERPINGHAM, county of NORFOLK, 3 miles (N. by E.) from Aylsham, containing 349 inhabitants.· The living is a discharged rectory, in the archdeaconry and diocese of Norwich, rated in the king's books at £9. 18. 9., and in the patronage of the Bishop of Norwich and Lord Suffield alternately. The church is dedicated to St. Mary.

ERRINGDEN, a chapelry in the parish of HALIFAX, wapentake of MORLEY, West riding of the county of YORK, 7 miles (W.) from Halifax, containing 1471 inhabitants. The living is a perpetual curacy, in the archdeaconry and diocese of York, endowed with £1600 parliamentary grant, and in the patronage of the Vicar of Halifax. The chapel is dedicated to St. John.

ERTH (ST.), a parish in the hundred of PENWITH, county of CORNWALL, 4 miles (N.E. by N.) from Marazion, containing 1604 inhabitants. The living is a vicarage, in the archdeaconry of Cornwall, and diocese of Exeter, rated in the king's books at £14. 1. 0½., and in the patronage of the Dean and Chapter of Exeter. Here is a place of worship for Wesleyan Methodists. There is a small sum for the education of children. Near the church is a bridge over the river Hayter, and a little lower down a causeway and bridge, built by subscription, for the convenience of persons going to Penzance, who formerly had to wait for the tide. A bridge, it is supposed, was built about the middle of the fourteenth century, under which ships of large burden sailed till the haven was choaked up by the sands. Some stone coffins have been lately dug up in this parish. Near the vicarage-house is a double circular intrenchment, called Carhangives, supposed to have been the site of a baronial castle. Pieces of tin have also been found, with inscriptions partly in Greek and partly in Latin, which may be translated, " Near this well was a Roman fort."

ERVAN (ST.), a parish in the hundred of PYDER, county of CORNWALL, 4 miles (S.S.W.) from Padstow, containing 422 inhabitants. The living is a rectory, in the peculiar jurisdiction of the Bishop of Exeter, rated in the king's books at £18. 6. 8. Sir W. Molesworth, Bart. was patron in 1817.

ERWARTON, a parish in the hundred of SAMFORD, county of SUFFOLK, 8¼ miles (S.S.E.) from Ipswich, containing 157 inhabitants. The living is a rectory, in the archdeaconry of Suffolk, and diocese of Norwich, rated in the king's books at £10. 13. 4., and in the patronage of Lady M. Chedworth. The church is dedicated to St. Mary.

ERYHOLME, a chapelry in that part of the parish of GILLING which is in the eastern division of the wapentake of GILLING, North riding of the county of YORK, 4¼ miles (S.E. by S.) from Darlington, containing 177 inhabitants. The living is a perpetual curacy, in the archdeaconry of Richmond, and diocese of Chester, endowed with £200 royal bounty, and in the patronage of the Vicar of Gilling. The chapel is dedicated to St. Mary.

ESCOMBE, a parochial chapelry in the north-western division of DARLINGTON ward, county palatine of DURHAM, 1¾ mile (W.) from Bishop-Auckland, containing 232 inhabitants. The living is a perpetual curacy, in the archdeaconry and diocese of Durham, endowed with £200 private benefaction, and £400 royal bounty, and in the patronage of the Bishop of Durham. There is an extensive colliery at Etherley-lane, a hamlet in this chapelry.

ESCRICK, a parish in the wapentake of OUZE and DERWENT, East riding of the county of YORK, comprising the townships of Deighton and Escrick, and containing 716 inhabitants, of which number, 548 are in the township of Escrick, 6 miles (S. by E.) from York. The living is a rectory, in the archdeaconry of Cleveland, and diocese of York, rated in the king's books at £23. 3. 9. Henry Gale, Esq. was patron in 1827. The church, dedicated to St. Helen, is a handsome structure, built about fifty years ago by Beilby Thompson, Esq., on the site of the prior edifice.

ESH, or ASH, a chapelry in that part of the parish of LANCHESTER which is in the western division of CHESTER ward, county palatine of DURHAM, 5 miles (W.N.W. from Durham, containing 470 inhabitants. The living is a perpetual curacy, in the archdeaconry and diocese of Durham, endowed with £800 royal bounty, and in the patronage of the Perpetual Curate of Lanchester. The church, dedicated to St. Michael, is a small structure without a tower. There is a Roman Catholic chapel in the village, and at a short distance to the east of it is a Catholic seminary, called Ushaw College, a handsome and extensive building in the form of a square, sufficiently capacious to accommodate one hundred and fifty students, besides apartments for the professors, &c.: it is conducted by the ecclesiastics of the ancient English Catholic college of Douay, in French Flanders, who made their escape from the Republican army during the French Revolution, and arriving in England in 1794, the greater part of them established a seminary at Crook Hall. This, however, soon became too small for their growing institution; by the liberal support of the Catholic clergy and laity, they were enabled to raise the present ample edifice on the Ushaw estate, which was purchased by them for that purpose. The estate is subject to a rent-charge of £20 per annum for the education of children of this chapelry.

ESHAM, a hamlet in the parish of SYLEHAM, hundred of HOXNE, county of SUFFOLK. The population is returned with the parish. Here was formerly a chapel, which has been long since demolished.

ESHER, a parish partly in the hundred of KINGSTON, but chiefly in the second division of the hundred of ELMBRIDGE, county of SURREY, 13½ miles (N.E.) from Guildford, containing 1108 inhabitants. The living is a rectory, in the archdeaconry of Surrey, and diocese of Winchester, rated in the king's books at £9. 18. 4., and in the patronage of the Warden and Fellows of Wadham College, Oxford. The church is dedicated to St. George. In 1789, George Nathaniel Petre bequeathed £850 three per cents., towards improving and supporting the Sunday school: between twenty and thirty children are educated in it. Three poor children are also educated for the sum of £6 a year, the gift of John Winkins in 1779. In this parish are situated the mansions of Claremont and Esher Place; the former well known as the residence of the Princess Charlotte of Wales, and the latter as the seat of Cardinal Wolsey. The scenery is highly interesting, being enriched with mansions and seats of the first order. Adjoining Esher common, an hospital, or priory, was founded in the reign of Henry II., the site of which is now called Sandon Farm. There is a fair for horses on the 4th of September.

ESHOLT, a township in that part of the parish of OTLEY which is in the upper division of the wapentake of SKYRACK, West riding of the county of YORK, 4¼ miles (S.S.W.) from Otley, containing 355 inhabitants. Simon de Ward founded a nunnery here in the middle of the twelfth century, of which a few pointed arches may still be seen; at the dissolution it was valued at £19.

ESHOTT, a township in that part of the parish of FELTON which is in the eastern division of MORPETH ward, county of NORTHUMBERLAND, 9¾ miles (N.) from Morpeth, containing 114 inhabitants. There is a seam of coal in this township, but the colliery was abandoned many years since.

ESHTON, a township in the parish of GARGRAVE, eastern division of the wapentake of STAINCLIFFE and EWCROSS, West riding of the county of YORK, 5½ miles (N.W.) from Skipton, containing 69 inhabitants.

ESKDALE, a joint chapelry with Wasdale, in that part of the parish of ST. BEES which is in ALLERDALE ward above Darwent, county of CUMBERLAND, 7 miles (N.E. by E.) from Ravenglass, containing, with the township of Wasdale-head, 296 inhabitants. The living is a perpetual curacy, in the archdeaconry of Richmond, and diocese of Chester, endowed with £400 private benefaction, and £800 royal bounty. G. E. Stanley, Esq. was patron in 1814. The chapel is dedicated to St. Catherine. There is a small sum for the education of children.

ESKDALE-SIDE, a chapelry in the parish of WHITBY, liberty of WHITBY-STRAND, North riding of the county of YORK, 5½ miles (S.W.) from Whitby, containing 395 inhabitants. The living is a perpetual curacy, in the archdeaconry of Cleveland, and diocese of York, endowed with £24. 13. 4. per annum and £1400 private benefaction, £800 royal bounty, and £1800 parliamentary grant, and in the patronage of the Rev. William Walker. The old chapel being ruinous, a new and very elegant one on a different site was built, in 1767, at the expense of Robert Bower, Esq., Tabitha, his wife, and Mrs. Gertrude Burdett, her sister: they likewise built the parsonage-house, and endowed the living. The ancient chapel is said to have been erected more than five hundred years before, by Roger, abbot of Whitby. Eskdale-side is situated on the river Esk, and composes one side of a fine valley; the ground rises gradually from the river, the higher land forming part of some of the highest moors in Yorkshire. There are large quarries of freestone, besides an abundance of alum rock, which was once extensively worked: there are also numerous springs, most of them containing alum and iron. In the reign of John a small priory was founded at this place.

ESKE, a township in that part of the parish of ST. JOHN, BEVERLEY, which is in the northern division of the wapentake of HOLDERNESS, East riding of the county of YORK, 3¼ miles (N.E. by N.) from Beverley, containing 18 inhabitants.

ESP-GREEN, a hamlet in that part of the parish of LANCHESTER which is in the western division of CHESTER ward, county palatine of DURHAM, 9¾ miles (N.W. by W.) from Durham. The population is returned with the parish. There was anciently a chapel at this place.

ESPERSHIELDS, a joint township with Millshields, in the parish of BYWELL-ST. PETER, eastern division of TINDALE ward, county of NORTHUMBERLAND, 11½ miles (S.S.E.) from Hexham, containing 180 inhabitants. At Winnis Hill, a little westward, is a meeting-house for the Society of Friends, built in 1775, on land given by Sir Thomas Clavering. Near it is a place called

Hare Town, where it is supposed there was formerly a collection of houses. The country between Espershields and Newbiggin, in the county of Durham, was anciently covered by a thick wood, which is said to have been burnt down by the owner, well known by the appellation of "Mad Maddison," who was afterwards hanged at Durham.

ESSENDINE, a chapelry in the parish of RYALL, EAST hundred, county of RUTLAND, 4¼ miles (N. by E.) from Stamford, containing 175 inhabitants. The chapel, dedicated to St. Mary, has portions in the Norman and early English styles of architecture: the Norman south door is much enriched.

ESSENDON, a parish in the hundred and county of HERTFORD, 3½ miles (E.) from Bishop's Hatfield, containing 595 inhabitants. The living is a rectory, with Bayford, in the archdeaconry of Huntingdon, and diocese of Lincoln, rated in the king's books at £18. The Marquis of Salisbury was patron in 1790. The church is dedicated to St. Mary. There is a National school supported by subscription, in which thirty boys and twenty-six girls are instructed; also an infant school on the National plan, for boys and girls, supported in the same manner. A branch of the river Lea bounds the north side of the parish.

ESSEX, a maritime county, bounded on the north by the counties of Suffolk and Cambridge; on the west by those of Hertford and Middlesex; on the south by the river Thames, which separates it from Kent; and on the east by the German ocean: it extends from 51° 30' to 52° 7' (N. Lat.), and from 0° 3' to 1° 12' (E. Lon.), and includes one thousand five hundred and thirty-two square miles, or nine hundred and eighty thousand four hundred and eighty statute acres. The population in 1821 amounted to 289,424. At the time of Cæsar's invasion this part of Britain was inhabited by the Trinobantes; and in the subdivision of the island by Constantine the Great, the present county of Essex formed part of Flavia Cæsariensis. The origin of its name is coeval with the establishment of the kingdom of the East Saxons, of which London was the metropolis, and of which the tract now comprised within the limits of this county formed a very important part. The foundation of that kingdom took place about the year 530, and it was called East Seaxa, meaning land of the Eastern Saxons, from its relative position to the other Saxon kingdoms. The conversion of Sabert, King of the East Saxons, to Christianity, took place in 604. At the time of the dissolution of the Anglo-Saxon octarchy, it was subjugated by Egbert, in the year 823. From 787 until the period of the division of England between Canute and Edmund, Essex was dreadfully harassed by the frequent descents and depredations of the Danes. The most memorable events which took place within its limits during that disastrous period were, the recovery of Colchester from the Danes by Edward the Elder, in 921, and the decisive battle between Canute and Edmund Ironside, which is believed to have been fought at Ashingdon, in this county. The next historical event of importance which appears to have had a particular reference to Essex, is the great rebellion of the commons, headed by Wat Tyler and Jack Straw, in the reign of Richard II. The Norman Conquest had in this, as in all the other counties of England, occasioned a great revolution of property, which brought large and valuable domains here into the possession of the distinguished family of Bohun, Earls of Hereford, Essex, and Northampton; which, in 1421, were divided between King Henry V. and Anne, Countess of Stafford, the two co-heirs of that family. By act of parliament, in 1414, that portion of the honours, castles, manors, and other estates, once belonging to the Bohun family, and which descended to Henry V., was severed from the crown of England, and annexed for ever to the duchy of Lancaster. In 1588, Queen Elizabeth reviewed at Tilbury the forces assembled to oppose the Spanish invasion. In 1642, at the commencement of the civil war, the popular feeling appears to have displayed itself in the cause of the parliament, the people having assembled in large bodies, and done considerable damage to the houses of different royalists. In the same year this county united with those of Suffolk, Norfolk, Cambridge, Hertford, the Isle of Ely, and the city of Norwich, in an association for preserving the peace of each. The siege and capture of Colchester, and the military execution of its defenders, Sir Charles Lucas and Sir George Lisle, is one of the most remarkable occurrences which took place in Essex during the war. The last important transaction connected with the history of this county was the sea-fight off Harwich, on the 3rd of June, 1665, in which the Dutch fleet was defeated by the Duke of York, the Dutch admiral's vessel being blown up, fourteen others destroyed, and eighteen captured.

This county is in the diocese of London, and province of Canterbury, and comprises the archdeaconries of Essex and Colchester, and part of that of Middlesex. The archdeaconry of Essex contains the deaneries of Barstaple, Barking, Chafford, Chelmsford, Dengie, Ongar, and Rochford; that of Colchester, the deaneries of Colchester, Lexden, Newport, Sampford, Tendring, and Witham; and that portion of the archdeaconry of Middlesex which is in this county, those of Dunmow, Harlow, and Hedingham. The number of parishes is four hundred, of which two hundred and fifty are rectories, one hundred and thirty-four vicarages, and the remainder perpetual curacies. For civil purposes it is divided into the fourteen hundreds of Barstable, Becontree, Chafford, Chelmsford, Clavering, Dengie, Dunmow, Freshwell, Harlow, Hinckford, Lexden, Ongar, Rochford, Tendring, Thurstable, Uttlesford, Waltham, Winstree, and Witham, and the royal liberty of Havering-atte-Bower. It contains the borough and market towns of Colchester and Maldon; the borough, market town, and port of Harwich; and the market towns of Barking, Billericay, Braintree, Brentwood, Chelmsford, Chipping-Ongar, Coggeshall, Dunmow, Epping, Grays-Thurrock, Halstead, Malden, Manningtree, Rayleigh, Rochford, Romford, Thaxted, Saffron-Walden, Waltham-Abbey, and Witham. Two knights are returned to parliament for the shire, and two representatives for each of the three boroughs: the county members are elected at Chelmsford. This county is in the home circuit: the assizes and quarter sessions are held at Chelmsford, where stands the old county gaol and house of correction; the new county gaol is at Springfield: there are one hundred and eighty-eight acting magistrates. The rates raised in the county for the year ending the 25th of March, 1827, amounted to £306,430. 2., the expenditure to £306,794. 16., of which £261,278. 2. was applied to the relief of the poor.

Several small islands in the German ocean and the æstuary of the Thames are included within the limits of this county: the first and most valuable, to the south-east, is the island of Mersea, eight or ten miles south of Colchester, between the mouths of the rivers Colne and Blackwater, a rich and fertile spot, about five miles from east to west, and two from north to south. The islands towards the south, in the hundred of Rochford, are, Foulness, Wallasea, Potten, Havengore, and New England, lying contiguous to each other, and bounded to the north by the Crouch river; to the east and south-east by the German ocean; and to the west by the continental part of the hundred of Rochford; being about four or five miles from the town of Rochford. The remaining island, towards the south-west, is Canvey Isle, which is in nine several parishes; it is surrounded by branches of the river Thames, and situated nearly at its mouth. The most beautiful part of Essex, without the addition of a river, is in the liberty of Havering-atte-Bower. From Romford to Brentwood is a fine country; but the more striking scenes are not within view of the road. From Thorndon to Epping is all nearly of the same description, exhibiting a perpetual variety of hill and dale, thickly wooded, with gentlemen's houses interspersed in every direction. Between Hockley and Rayleigh there is a beautiful view of a richly cultivated and well wooded vale, terminated by high grounds in the distance. Langdon Hills command the most extensive and the finest prospect in the county: the Thames is distinctly seen for several miles, and the distant hills of Kent bound the view with an interesting outline. Danbury is the highest ground in the county, and commands a striking view, but not equal to that from Langdon Hills. The high lands at Purfleet, formed by a chalk cliff projecting toward the Thames, without the intervention of marsh, present an animating scene not common on the Essex side of that river; the bustle of the shipping being agreeably relieved by the rural features of the landscape. The vale on the northern verge of the county, through which the river Stour flows, has great variety in breadth and features; and the bounding hills offer in all directions rich scenes of cultivation. The climate is generally mild; but part of the eastern and southern limits of the county, for ten or twelve miles from the sea and the river Thames, in the hundreds of Thurstable, Dengie, Rochford, Barstable, and Chafford, are subject, during the autumnal months, to thick and noisome fogs, which are often productive of quartan agues. The draining of marshes and the highly improved cultivation of the lands, however, have greatly abated this evil.

With regard to the soil, every species of loam, from the most stubborn to the most congenial, is to be found: the county has also a portion of light gravelly sand, and a good share of meadow and marsh ground, the major part of which, with management adapted to its different qualities, is very productive. The late Mr. Arthur Young, Secretary of the Board of Agriculture, has divided these soils into eight districts, viz., the crop and fallow district of strong loam; the maritime district of fertile loam; three districts of strong loam not peculiar in management; the turnip land district; the chalk district and the district of miscellaneous loams. The first of these, called also the district of the Roothings, or Rodings, from six or seven parishes which are named

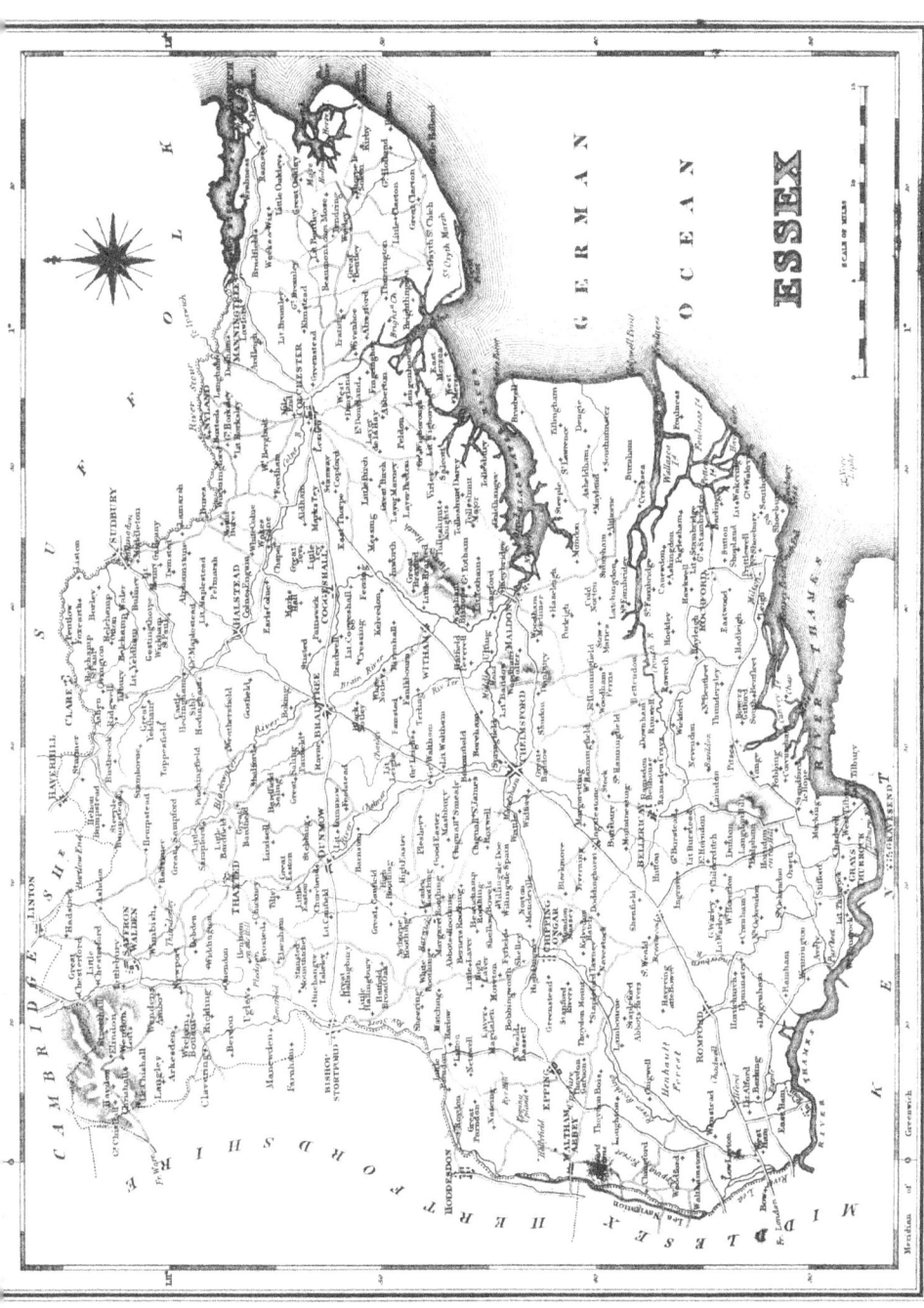

ESSEX

SCALE OF MILES

from the river Roding, is, with respect to similarity of soil and husbandry, much more extensive than the limits of those parishes: it lies in the north-western part of the county, verging towards the borders of Hertfordshire and Cambridgeshire; extending nearly twenty miles from south to north, from the neighbourhood of Chipping-Ongar to that of Saffron-Walden, and averaging about nine miles in breadth, having the town of Great Dunmow nearly in the centre. It is a hilly tract, in which the surface loam in the vales is dryer and better than on the hills, and in some cases forms a very good soil; but the general feature is a wet loam on a clay marl bottom. The second district extends, with an average breadth of about three miles, along the whole southern and eastern border of the county, along the margin of the Thames and on the sea-coast, environing the æstuaries of the rivers Crouch and Blackwater, and including the islands before mentioned: the soil of Foulness island is the richest in the whole county. Of the strong wet land, or clay districts, one is situated in the north-western part of the county, on the borders of Suffolk and Cambridgeshire, its length being about twelve miles from east to west, and its average breadth about seven; another is a small tract, about six miles long, and four broad, adjoining the marshes on the north side of the Blackwater: of the third, the western boundary, commencing near Malden, runs in a south-westerly direction by South Hanningfield, Great Burstead, and Langdon Clay, to Vange, and on every other side it is bounded by the marsh district. The turnip loam district lies in the north-eastern part of the county, on the banks of the rivers Colne and Stour, being bounded on the north by the latter river; on the east by the marsh district; and extending about twelve miles from east to west, and nine from north to south. Considerable tracts near Colchester, which is situated in this district, are in the occupation of gardeners, who, besides supplying that town with vegetables, raise a considerable quantity of garden seeds for the country. The chalk district is of small extent, its length being about twelve miles, and its average breadth about four; it lies at the north-western extremity of the county, and is a continuation of the chalk districts of Hertfordshire and Cambridgeshire. The district of miscellaneous loams extends the whole length of the county, from the marshes on the banks of the Thames to the border of Suffolk; and, commencing on the borders of Middlesex and Hertfordshire, occupies nearly two-thirds of its breadth towards the German ocean, excepting the two intervening districts of clay, and the one of chalk, already mentioned, in the north-western part of the county. The extent of these several districts in square miles is as follows: that of the Roodings, one hundred and fifty-six; the maritime district, two hundred and fifty-five; the three districts of strong loam, or clay, two hundred and twenty-two; the turnip land, one hundred and fourteen; the chalk, forty-five; and the miscellaneous district, six hundred and eighty-one.

Essex has for several centuries been an enclosed county: it possesses rich marshes, extending a hundred miles in length, but the leading feature is its arable land, the fertility of which, and the good husbandry practised upon it, enable Essex to occupy a prominent station among the agricultural counties of England. Part of the plan of the Essex farmers in the tillage of their lands,

is, to keep the soil clean by the interposition of a fallow, or a fallow crop between every two of white corn: there is, however, no regular course of crops throughout the whole county. The average produce of wheat per acre, is estimated at twenty-four bushels, two pecks; of barley, four quarters, six bushels, and three pecks; of oats, five quarters, five bushels, and half a peck; of beans, twenty-seven bushels; and of peas, twenty bushels and a quarter. Potatoes are extensively cultivated in Essex, which circumstance is chiefly attributable to its proximity to London, which it largely supplies with that vegetable. The culture of hops is confined to a small number of parishes. In the islands of Foulness, Wallasea, &c., and in the embanked marshes, white or brown mustard seed is sown, the average produce of which is twenty-four bushels per acre. Some of the extensive marsh lands are very valuable, and the district of Epping feeds considerable herds of cattle; but, excepting these, the grass lands are of inferior consideration. The annual quantity of grain sent to London is estimated at about two hundred and fifty thousand quarters of wheat, and one hundred and fifty thousand quarters of malt; besides a vast quantity of oats, peas, and beans. An agricultural society, holding its meetings at Chelmsford, was established in this county about the year 1792.

There are many cherry orchards at Burnham, Southminster, &c. The natural woods of Essex have been much diminished both in number and extent within the last seventy years: the principal remains of them are the curtailed forests of Epping and Hainault. The Forest of Epping was formerly called the Forest of Essex, and comprehended the whole county: by a charter of King John, dated the 25th of March, in the fifth year of his reign, and confirmed in the 8th of Edward IV., all that part of the forest which lay to the north of the highway from Stortford to Colchester, was disafforested. The forest was further reduced by a perambulation made in the 29th of Edward I., in pursuance of the *Charta de Forestâ*; but the metes and bounds of it were finally settled by an inquisition and perambulation on the 8th of September, 1640, by virtue of a commission under the great seal of England, in pursuance of the act of the 16th of Charles I., for settling the bounds of the forests. The boundaries fixed by that perambulation comprehend twelve parishes lying wholly within the forest, and parts of nine other parishes: the former are Wanstead, Layton, Walthamstow, Woodford, Loughton, Chigwell, Lambourn, Stapleford-Abbots, Waltham Holy Cross, Epping, Nazeing, and Chingford. The whole forest contains about sixty thousand statute acres, of which about forty-eight thousand are estimated to be enclosed private property, and the remaining twelve thousand the amount of the unenclosed woods and wastes. The crown has in this, as in other forests, an unlimited right to keep deer in all the unenclosed woods and wastes within its bounds; and the owners and occupiers of land have a common right of pasturage for horses and cows; no other cattle being commonable in the forest. Those within the parishes of Stapleford, Lambourn Chigwell, Barking, and Dagenham, and at Woodford Bridge turn in their cattle on the part called Hainault Forest. The cattle are sent in as early in the spring, and remain as late in the winter, as the owners choose; but the forest is constantly cleared of them during the fence month : they are marked by the reeves of the respective parishes, with a particular forest mark for each parish.

Essex has never been famous for its live stock, having no breed of its own; the general object of the farmers being to keep cows for suckling calves, and to fatten cattle in the marshes. The dairy district is not considerable ; the largest dairy farms are at or in the neighbourhood of Epping, so deservedly famous for the richness of its cream and butter : there is no particular choice or preference as to breed or stock of cows. Skimmed milk is usually applied to the purpose of feeding small pigs for the London market. The sheep generally preferred are the Norfolk and Cambridgeshire breed, with a cross of the west country and Hertfordshire : in the marsh districts the rot is unknown, but agues are very prevalent. The favourite breed of hogs in the southern part of the county is the Berkshire ; in the northern there is every variety. The breed of horses most esteemed is the Suffolk. This county producing no coal, wood is much used for fuel by the poor. In the Blackwater river is a considerable oyster fishery ; and West Mersea is one of the principal stations of the dredgers : the number of vessels engaged is about two hundred, varying in burden from eight tons' to fifty, and employing from four hundred to five hundred men and boys. The principal breeding rivers are the Crouch, the Blackwater, and the Coln : the oysters are sent to London, Hamburgh, Bremen, and in time of peace to Holland, Flanders, and France. The quantity annually obtained is estimated at from twelve thousand to fifteen thousand bushels. In Foulness island are salt water stews for various sorts of sea fish, which are well contrived, and answer the purpose completely. Among the manufactures, from time immemorial, until of late years, the woollen manufacture was the principal ; and although it has long been declining, a considerable quantity of woollen cloth of various kinds is still sent to the metropolis, or exported to foreign countries, from Bocking, Braintree, Halstead, Coggeshall, and Colchester.

The greater part of Essex is well watered by the many rivers and brooks which run through its vales. The principal rivers are, the Thames, the Lea, the Crouch, the Chelmer, the Blackwater, the Coln, and the Stort. The Thames forms the southern boundary of the county in the whole of its course along it, from the influx of the Lea to the German ocean, except a space of about two miles, where a slip of land on the Essex side of the river, forming part of the parish of Woolwich, is included in the county of Kent; in the whole of this course the Thames is navigable for merchant vessels of the largest burden. The Lea, coming from Hertfordshire, forms the western boundary of the county, from its junction with the Stort to its confluence with the Thames, separating it from Hertfordshire and Middlesex, and is navigable in all this part of its course. The Crouch rises from two springs in the parishes of Little Burstead and Langdon, flows eastward, and after forming a long and narrow æstuary, falls into the German ocean between Foulness island and the opposite marshes. The Chelmer, the Blackwater, and the Coln, rise among the hills in the north-western part of the county ; the Chelmer flowing south-eastward by Chelmsford, and the Blackwater by Braintree and Coggeshall, and near Wi-

tham, unite near Malden, and form the broad æstuary of the Blackwater, which joins the sea twelve miles below, and the navigation of which, by the Chelmer, is continued up to Chelmsford. The Coln, flowing eastward by Halstead and Colchester, falls into the German ocean opposite Mersea island, and near the mouth of the Blackwater. The Stort, rising near Haverhill, on the border of Suffolk, becomes near Sturmer the boundary between this county and Suffolk, and so continues for the remainder of its course, passing by Manningtree, then forming a long and wide æstuary, which, contracting at its mouth, unites with the German ocean at Harwich ; it is navigable up to Sudbury. The Roding rises in the north-western part of the county, and running southward through the district called the Rodings, by Chipping-Ongar, through Epping Forest, and by Barking, falls into the Thames about two miles below the latter town. The London and Cambridge canal passes along the north-western verge of the county.

The great road from London to Norwich, through Ipswich, enters the county at Bow bridge, and passing through Stratford, Romford, Brentwood, Ingatestone, Chelmsford, Witham, and Colchester, enters Suffolk at Stratford on the river Stort. The road from London to Norwich, through Sudbury, branches off from the latter at Chelmsford, and passing through Braintree, Halstead, and Sudbury, quits the county at the last place. The road from London to Norwich, through Newmarket, enters Essex at Lea bridge, passes through Walthamstow, Epping, and Harlow, a mile beyond which it crosses the Lea into Hertfordshire, but re-entering the county near the thirtieth mile-stone, passes through Saffron-Walden, and quits Essex for Cambridgeshire about forty-seven miles from London. The road from London to Harwich branches off from the Norwich road at Colchester, and passes through Manningtree.

Under the Roman government this territory was very early and thoroughly explored ; one great road ran the whole length of it, another skirted its northern borders, and many vicinal ways crossed it in different places. In it was established the first Roman colony in Britain, with several other stations and towns in different parts of it : the following are the names of such of them as are mentioned in the Itinerary of Antoninus ; *Ad Ansam*, of undetermined locality ; *Camalodunum*, at Colchester, or Malden ; *Canonium*, near Kelvedon ; *Cæsaromagum*, at Chelmsford, or Writtle ; and *Durositum*, below Brentwood. Camden, and all subsequent antiquaries, testify that both the ancient roads and stations throughout this county are more obliterated and difficult to settle than in any other county of England ; owing, probably, in part to the nature of the soil, and in part to the general extent of its tillage. The great battle between Suetonius and Boadicea was fought somewhere between Epping and Waltham, near which a fine camp remains. The principal Roman remains have been discovered at Colchester, in great abundance : among the rest, upwards of thirteen hundred Roman and British coins were collected by Morant, the historian and antiquary, in a period of thirty years, during which he resided in that town. There are also Roman remains at Leyton, Wanstead, Great Burstead, Tolleshunt-Knights, West Mersey, Harwich, and other places ; and tumuli, or barrows, at Lexden, Bures ad Montem, West Mersey, and Wigborough. The remarkably large tumuli, called Bartlow Hills, are in this county, though taking their name from the neighbouring village of Bartlow, in Suffolk. Of the ancient castles, or castellated mansions, which were twelve in number, the castle of Colchester is the only one which is not either utterly demolished, or extremely ruinous. Before the Reformation there were forty-seven religious houses, viz., two mitred and six other abbeys, twenty-two priories, three nunneries, nine hospitals, three colleges, and two preceptories of the Knights Templars. The most remarkable monastic remains are those of St. Botolph's priory, Colchester, of St. Osyth's abbey, and of Waltham Abbey church. Greenstead church, with its nave of timber, is one of the most ancient and curious in the kingdom; and that of Little Maplestead is one of the very few now remaining that are built on the model of the Holy Sepulchre. Fossils are found in various parts of the county, but no where so abundantly as in Harwich cliff. Essex gives the title of earl to the family of Capel.

ESSINGTON, a township in that part of the parish of BUSHBURY which is in the eastern division of the hundred of CUTTLESTONE, county of STAFFORD, 5¼ miles (N.E.) from Wolverhampton, containing 605 inhabitants.

ESTON, a hamlet partly in the parish of ARTHURET, and partly in that of KIRK-ANDREWS, ESKDALE ward, county of CUMBERLAND. The population is returned with the parish. Eston was anciently a distinct parish.

ESTON, a chapelry in that part of the parish of ORMSBY which is in the eastern division of the liberty of LANGBAURGH, North riding of the county of YORK, 5½ miles (W.N.W.) from Guisbrough, containing 272 inhabitants. The living is a perpetual curacy, in the archdeaconry of Cleveland, and diocese of York, endowed with £400 royal bounty. The chapel is a very ancient edifice. The village lies at the base of a detached hill of considerable elevation, called Barnaby, or Eston Moor, the summit of which terminates in a bold point or promontory, called Eston Nab, where a telegraphic beacon, or watch-house, has been lately erected. On the summit of the promontory is an ancient encampment, conjectured to be of Saxon origin, of the date 492, and coeval with the battle of Badon Hill, which was fought in this neighbourhood.

ETALL, a township in the parish of FORD, western division of Northumberland, county of NORTHUMBERLAND, 10½ miles (N.N.W.) from Wooler. The population is returned with the parish. A castle was built at this place in the 1st of Edward I., by Sir Robert Manners, which James IV., before the battle of Flodden, captured and destroyed.

ETCHELLS, a township partly in the parish of NORTHEN, or NORTHENDEN, and partly in that of STOCKPORT, hundred of MACCLESFIELD, county palatine of CHESTER, 3¾ miles (W. S.W.) from Stockport, containing 1525 inhabitants. There is a small free school.

ETCHILHAMPTON, a chapelry in the parish of ALLCANNINGS, hundred of SWANBOROUGH, county of WILTS, 3 miles (E.S.E.) from Devizes, containing 252 inhabitants. The chapel is dedicated to St. Andrew.

ETCHINGHAM, a parish in the hundred of HENHURST, rape of HASTINGS, county of SUSSEX, 6¾ miles

(S.E.) from Wadhurst, containing 625 inhabitants. The living is a rectory, in the archdeaconry of Lewes, and diocese of Chichester, rated in the king's books at £11. Mrs. A. Lade was patroness in 1792. The church is partly in the decorated and partly in the later English style, with a central tower.

ETLOE, a tything in the parish of AWRE, hundred of BLIDESLOE, county of GLOUCESTER, 1¼ mile (S.) from Blakeney. The population is returned with the parish.

ETON, a parish in the hundred of STOKE, county of BUCKINGHAM, 1 mile (N.) from Windsor, and 23 (W. by S.) from London, containing 2475 inhabitants. This place, which is chiefly distinguished for its public school, is pleasantly situated in a valley on the north bank of the river Thames, by which it is separated from Windsor, and over which is a neat iron bridge, supported on piers of stone. The village consists principally of one street well paved and lighted by means of a highway rate, and is supplied with water by a company whose works also supply the town and castle of Windsor : the houses are in general neatly built, and there are several boarding-houses for the accommodation of those students who do not reside in the college. The site on which the college stands is said to be extra-parochial, but the usual rites and ceremonies of the church were formerly performed, for the benefit of the parishioners, in the collegiate church. The college was originally founded by Henry VI., in 1440, for a provost, ten priests, six clerks, six choristers, twenty-five poor grammar scholars, with a master to instruct them, and twenty-five almsmen, and directed to be called " The College Roiall of our Ladie of Eton, beside Windesor ; " and though deprived of part of its endowment by Edward IV., it was especially exempted in the act of dissolution, at which time its revenue was estimated at £1101. 13. 7. The present establishment consists of a provost, vice-provost, six fellows, two masters, with assistants, seven clerks, seventy king's scholars, ten choristers, and inferior officers and servants. The number of independent scholars, the sons of noblemen and gentlemen, is generally from three to four hundred. Scholars on the foundation are entitled to fellowships and scholarships in King's College, Cambridge, for which purpose there is an annual election, but they are not removed till vacancies occur, to which they succeed according to seniority, and on three years' residence at the college are entitled to a fellowship. For those who do not succeed in obtaining an election to King's College, there are two scholarships founded in Merton College, Oxford, in 1582, by the Rev. John Chamber, and augmented in 1754, by the Rev. George Vernon, of which one is in the patronage of the Provost of Eton, and the other in that of the Provost of King's College ; three exhibitions, of £20 each per annum, founded in Pembroke College, Oxford, by the Rev. Francis Rouse, Provost of Eton, with preference to his relatives; two scholarships, one of £48, and one of £42, for superannuated collegers, in the patronage of the Provost ; and one of £42 per annum for an actual scholar of King's College, in the patronage of the Head Master of Eton, founded by Provost Davies; three exhibitions, founded in Exeter College, by the Rev. Dr. John Reynolds, in the patronage of the Provost and Fellows of Eton; one by-fellowship and one scholarship, of £6 per annum each, founded in Catherine Hall, Cambridge, for scholars of Eton, or Merchant Taylors' school. The Rev. Mr. Chamberlayne, Fellow of Eton, bequeathed an estate in Norfolk, producing £87 per annum, for founding scholarships for superannuated collegers; and Mr. Bryant bequeathed £30 per annum, for one or more additional scholarships, at the discretion of the provost. The buildings comprise two spacious quadrangles, communicating by an ancient tower-gateway of great beauty; in the centre of the outer quadrangle is a bronze statue of the royal founder; on the south side are an elegant chapel in the later style of English architecture, strengthened with enriched buttresses, and ornamented with a pierced parapet and pinnacles, and the school, divided into the upper and lower school (each of which is subdivided into three classes), besides lodgings for the masters and scholars on the foundation: the inner quadrangle contains apartments for the provost and fellows, and the library, a handsome building, containing one of the best collections in Europe, having been augmented with numerous magnificent contributions from various benefactors; some very valuable paintings, drawings, and oriental manuscripts, enrich this depository of rare and curious productions. In the provost's apartments is a portrait, on panel, of Jane Shore, which is said to be an original. The grounds for recreation and exercise, on the north-west side of the college, are extensive, and beautifully shaded by a lengthened avenue of stately trees; and the bounds of the college are marked by stones set up in various places. To mention the many eminent characters which this noble institution has produced, would be to enumerate a very considerable portion of the most distinguished names which history has recorded in the proud list of British heroes, statesmen, scholars, and divines. A custom, designated the Montem, is triennially observed by the scholars on Whit-Tuesday, which, though its origin is involved in obscurity, has certainly existed from the reign of Elizabeth, and, most probably, from the very foundation of the college, as it is included in the list presented to the queen, when on a visit here, " of the ceremonies observed from its foundation." The chief object of this ceremony is to collect " salt money," and by the procession advancing to a small tumulus, on the south side of the Bath road, the spot has acquired the name of Salt Hill, which is celebrated for its extensive posting inns. The scholars appointed to collect the money are called " salt-bearers," and are arrayed in silk, of various colours, assisted by " scouts," also dressed in silk, of less striking appearance. Immense numbers of people assemble to witness the procession, and scholars are placed on all the neighbouring roads to levy " salt money," which, as the custom is viewed as an innocent diversion, attended with a positive benefit, nearly the whole neighbourhood make a point of offering. George III. and his royal consort, with characteristic condescension, almost invariably participated in this juvenile festivity, by offering their contributions; and his present Majesty George IV. has, with equal beneficence, contributed £100 at each Montem. Every contributor on these occasions is furnished with a ticket, exempting him from any further demand. The sum collected has frequently exceeded £1000, which, after deducting the necessary expenses of the day, is given to the senior scholar, called the Captain of the school, on his removal to Cambridge, and usually forms an ample provision for him while at the University. There is not any particular branch of trade carried on: a fair is held annually on Ash-Wednesday, for horses and cattle.

The living is a rectory, in the peculiar jurisdiction and incumbency of the Provost of Eton College. The church, dedicated to St. Mary and St. Nicholas, is collegiate, and was frequented by the parishioners prior to the erection of a neat chapel in the centre of the town, by Mr. Hetherington, late fellow of the college, for the accommodation of the inhabitants. A charity school was founded by Mark Anthony, formerly French master at Eton College, who endowed it with funds for the instruction of sixty boys and thirty girls. An almshouse for ten poor widows was founded by Dr. Godolphin, formerly provost of Eton College; and an annual income of about £120 is appropriated to the apprenticing of children: there are also other charitable bequests for the benefit of the poor. William Oughtred, an eminent mathematician, is stated to have been born here in 1573.

ETRURIA, a hamlet formerly in the parish of Stoke upon Trent, now in the parish of Shelton, which has been recently separated from Stoke by act of parliament, northern division of the hundred of Pirehill, county of Stafford, 1½ mile (N.E.) from Newcastle under Line. The population is returned with the parish. There is a place of worship for Wesleyan Methodists. Here are the celebrated potteries of Wedgewood and Co., where the ware, commonly called Wedgewood ware is manufactured.

ETTERBY, a township in that part of the parish of Stanwix which is in Eskdale ward, county of Cumberland, 1¼ mile (N.W.) from Carlisle, containing 67 inhabitants. It is said that the British King Arthur was entertained here in 550, when carrying his victorious arms against the Danes and Norwegians.

ETTON, a parish in the liberty of Peterborough, county of Northampton, 7 miles (N.W. by N.) from Peterborough, containing, with the hamlet of Woodcroft, 125 inhabitants. The living is a rectory, in the archdeaconry of Northampton, and diocese of Peterborough, rated in the king's books at £9. 9. 9½., and in the patronage of Earl Fitzwilliam. The church is dedicated to St. Stephen.

ETTON, a parish in the Hunsley-Beacon division of the wapentake of Harthill, East riding of the county of York, 4¼ miles (N.W. by W.) from Beverley, containing 380 inhabitants. The living is a rectory, in the archdeaconry of the East riding, and diocese of York, rated in the king's books at £20. 9. 4½., and in the patronage of the Archbishop of York. The church is dedicated to St. Mary.

ETWALL, a parish in the hundred of Appletree, county of Derby, comprising the townships of Etwall and Bearward-Cote, and the hamlet of Burnaston, and containing 593 inhabitants, of which number, 445 are in the townships of Etwall and Bearward-Cote, 6 miles (W. S. W.) from Derby. The living is a vicarage, in the archdeaconry of Derby, and diocese of Lichfield and Coventry, rated in the king's books at £8, and in the patronage of the Rev. Mr. Cokburne. The church is dedicated to St. Helen. In 1566, Sir John Port, Knt., devised lands for the foundation and endowment of an almshouse at this place, and a grammar school at Repton. By charter, in the nineteenth year of James I., this establishment was incorporated, and special governors appointed: there are at present fifteen persons in the almshouse; the income of the estate is about £2700.

EUSTON, a parish in the hundred of BLACKBOURN, county of SUFFOLK, 3½ miles (S. E. by S.) from Thetford, containing 164 inhabitants. The living is a rectory, with Fakenham (Parva), and Barnham (St. Gregory and St. Martin), in the archdeaconry of Sudbury, and diocese of Norwich, rated in the king's books at £13. 7. 11. The church is dedicated to St. Genevieve. The Duke of Grafton enjoys the inferior title of Earl of Euston.

EUXTON, a chapelry in the parish and hundred of LEYLAND, county palatine of LANCASTER, 2½ miles (W. N. W.) from Chorley, containing 1360 inhabitants. The living is a perpetual curacy, in the archdeaconry and diocese of Chester, endowed with £400 private benefaction, and £400 royal bounty. The Rev. J. Armetriding was patron in 1799. A free school, under the management of trustees, is endowed with about £30 per annum.

EVAL (ST.), a parish in the hundred of PYDER, county of CORNWALL, 5½ miles (N.W. by N.) from St. Columb Major, containing 323 inhabitants. The living is a vicarage, in the peculiar jurisdiction and patronage of the Bishop of Exeter, rated in the king's books at £6. 13. 4. The church is dedicated to St. Eval: the tower having fallen, it was rebuilt from the foundation, and finished in 1727: the expense, nearly £400, was defrayed by contributions, including a donation from the merchants of Bristol, to whose vessels it serves as a conspicuous land-mark. The parish lies on the shore of the Bristol channel.

EVEDON, a parish in the wapentake of ASWARDHURN, parts of KESTEVEN, county of LINCOLN, 2½ miles (N. E. by E.) from Sleaford, containing 89 inhabitants. The living is a rectory, in the archdeaconry and diocese of Lincoln, rated in the king's books at £9. 8. 1½., and in the patronage of Mrs. Nesbett. The church is dedicated to St. Mary.

EVENLEY, a parish in the hundred of KING's SUTTON, county of NORTHAMPTON, 1 mile (S. by W.) from Brackley, containing 468 inhabitants. The living is a discharged vicarage, in the archdeaconry of Northampton, and diocese of Peterborough, rated in the king's books at £7, endowed with £400 private benefaction, and £400 royal bounty, and in the patronage of the President and Fellows of Magdalene College, Oxford. The church is dedicated to St. George.

EVENLOAD, a parish in the upper division of the hundred of OSWALDSLOW, county of WORCESTER, though locally in the upper division of the hundred of Westminster, county of Gloucester, 3 miles (S.E.) from Moreton in the Marsh, containing 297 inhabitants. The living is a rectory, in the archdeaconry of Gloucester, and diocese of Worcester, rated in the king's books at £11. 11. 8., and in the patronage of Joseph Pitt, Esq. The church is dedicated to St. Edward.

EVENWOOD, a township in that part of the parish of ST. ANDREW AUCKLAND which is in the north-western division of DARLINGTON ward, county palatine of DURHAM, 5¼ miles (S. W.) from Bishop-Auckland, containing 306 inhabitants. The village is pleasantly situated on the summit of a steep bank to the south of the Gaunless, and contains a place of worship for Wes-

leyan Methodists. Here was formerly a castle, which has now totally disappeared, the site being occupied by a farm-house; the moat may still be traced.

EVERCREECH, a parish in the hundred of WELLS-FORUM, county of SOMERSET, 3¾ miles (S.E. by S.) from Shepton-Mallet, containing, with Chesterblade, 1253 inhabitants. The living is a vicarage, in the peculiar jurisdiction of the Dean of Wells, rated in the king's books at £16. 19., and in the patronage of —— Talbot, Esq. The church, dedicated to St. Peter, is a large and noble edifice, with a tower in the decorated style of English architecture, one hundred and thirty feet high, terminated with elegant pinnacles. The Wesleyan Methodists have a place of worship here. There is an endowed school for ten boys. The manufacture of silk is carried on to a considerable extent, furnishing employment to several hundred persons. In this parish are a Roman encampment, and a spring strongly impregnated with salt.

EVERDON, a parish in the hundred of FAWSLEY, county of NORTHAMPTON, 4¼ miles (S.S.E.) from Daventry, containing 640 inhabitants. The living is a rectory, in the archdeaconry of Northampton, and diocese of Peterborough, rated in the king's books at £24. 2. 11., and in the patronage of the Provost and Fellows of Eton College. The church, dedicated to St. Mary, has a beautiful door in the decorated style of English architecture. There is a place of worship for Independents. The interest of £500, the bequest of William Folwell in 1813, is applied to the instruction of children; and the Sunday schools receive, towards their support, the dividends of about £200, bequeathed by the Rev. Sir John Knightley.

EVERINGHAM, a parish in the Holme-Beacon division of the wapentake of HARTHILL, East riding of the county of YORK, 5 miles (W. by N.) from Market-Weighton, containing 271 inhabitants. The living is a discharged rectory, in the archdeaconry of the East riding, and diocese of York, rated in the king's books at £8. 6. 8. The Rev. W. Alderson was patron in 1809. The church, a neat modern edifice, is dedicated to the Blessed Virgin Mary. There is also a Roman Catholic chapel.

EVERLEY, a parish in the hundred of ELSTUB and EVERLEY, county of WILTS, 4¼ miles (W. N. W.) from Ludgershall, containing 316 inhabitants. The living is a rectory, in the archdeaconry of Wilts, and diocese of Salisbury, rated in the king's books at £16. 4. 4½., and in the patronage of Sir J. D. Astley, Bart. The church, dedicated to St. Peter, is a chaste and elegant edifice, erected in 1813, at the sole expense of Francis Dugdale Astley, Esq. This was anciently a market town, and a place of considerable note. Ina, King of the West Saxons, had a palace here, in which he frequently resided; and, in 1603, it was visited by James I. About two miles to the south is the fortified camp of *Chidbury*, to which there appears to have been a covered way from Everley.

EVERLEY, a joint township with Suffield, in the parish of HACKNESS, liberty of WHITBY-STRAND, North riding of the county of YORK, 4¼ miles (W. by N.) from Scarborough. The population is returned with Suffield.

EVERSAW, a hamlet in the parish of BIDDSDNOLE, hundred and county of BUCKINGHAM, 5¼ miles (N.W by W.) from Buckingham. The population is returned with the parish. Here was anciently a chapel dedicated to St. Nicholas.

EVERSDEN (GREAT), a parish in the hundred of LONGSTOW, county of CAMBRIDGE, 7 miles (S. E. by E.) from Caxton, containing 268 inhabitants. The living is a discharged vicarage, in the archdeaconry and diocese of Ely, rated in the king's books at £6. 14. 2., endowed with £200 royal bounty, and £200 parliamentary grant, and in the patronage of the Crown. The church is dedicated to St. Mary.

EVERSDEN (LITTLE), a parish in the hundred of LONGSTOW, county of CAMBRIDGE, 7¾ miles (S.E. by E.) from Caxton, containing 232 inhabitants. The living is a rectory, in the archdeaconry and diocese of Ely, rated in the king's books at £5. 2. 6., and in the patronage of the President and Fellows of Queen's College, Cambridge. The church is dedicated to St. Helen.

EVERSHOLT, a parish in the hundred of MANSHEAD, county of BEDFORD, 2½ miles (E. by S.) from Woburn, containing 870 inhabitants. The living is a rectory, in the archdeaconry of Bedford, and diocese of Lincoln, rated in the king's books at £16. 11. 8., and in the patronage of the Marquis of Downshire. The church is dedicated to St. John the Baptist. There is a small sum for the education of children.

EVERSHOT, a chapelry in the parish of FROME ST. QUINTIN, hundred of TOLLERFORD, Dorchester division of the county of DORSET, 7¼ miles (E. by N.) from Beaminster, containing 567 inhabitants. The chapel is dedicated to St. Osmond. A market formerly held here on Saturday has been discontinued : a fair for bullocks and toys is held on the 12th of May. There is a free grammar school, with an endowment of about £145 per annum.

EVERSLEY, a parish in the hundred of HOLDSHOTT, Basingstoke division of the county of SOUTHAMPTON, 2 miles (N.) from Hartford-Bridge, containing, with the tythings of Great Bramshill and Little Bramshill, 767 inhabitants. The living is a rectory, in the archdeaconry and diocese of Winchester, rated in the king's books at £11. 8. 9., and in the patronage of Sir John Cope, Bart. Cattle fairs are held on May 16th and October 18th.

EVERTHORP, a joint township with Drewton, in the parish of NORTH CAVE, Hunsley-Beacon division of the wapentake of HARTHILL, East riding of the county of YORK, 1½ mile (W. N. W.) from South Cave, containing 177 inhabitants.

EVERTON, a parish in the hundred of BIGGLESWADE, county of BEDFORD, 4¾ miles (N. by E.) from Biggleswade, containing, with Tetworth, 334 inhabitants. The living is a vicarage with that of Tetworth united to it, in the archdeaconry of Bedford, and diocese of Lincoln, rated in the king's books at £6. 13. 9., and in the patronage of the Master and Fellows of Clare Hall, Cambridge. The church, which stands in the county of Huntingdon, is dedicated to St. Mary.

EVERTON, a chapelry in the parish of WALTON on the HILL, hundred of WEST DERBY, county palatine of LANCASTER, 1 mile (N. N. E.) from Liverpool, containing 2109 inhabitants. The living is a perpetual curacy, in the archdeaconry and diocese of Chester, and in the patronage of the Rector of Walton. The chapel was consecrated in 1814. This is a neat and agreeable village, situated on a bold eminence, opposite to the bay of Bootle : its proximity to Liverpool, and the salubrity of the air, have rendered it the residence of several genteel families. A new church, dedicated to St. George, has lately been erected. Here was an ancient beacon, supposed to have been erected in 1220, by Ranulph de Blundeville, Earl of Chester, which was blown down in 1803.

EVERTON, a parish in the liberty of SOUTHWELL and SCROOBY, though locally in the wapentake of Bassetlaw, county of NOTTINGHAM, 2¾ miles (S. E. by E.) from Bawtry, containing, with the township of Scaftworth, 741 inhabitants. The living is a discharged vicarage, in the archdeaconry of Nottingham, and diocese of York, rated in the king's books at £7. 2. 2., and in the patronage of the Duke of Devonshire. The church is dedicated to the Holy Trinity. There is a small sum for the education of children. The Chesterfield canal passes through the parish on the southeast.

EVESBATCH, a parish in the hundred of RADLOW, county of HEREFORD, 5½ miles (S. E. by S.) from Bromyard, containing 87 inhabitants. The living is a discharged rectory, in the archdeaconry and diocese of Hereford, rated in the king's books at £1. 16. 10½. R. Yate, Esq. was patron in 1812. The church is dedicated to St. Andrew.

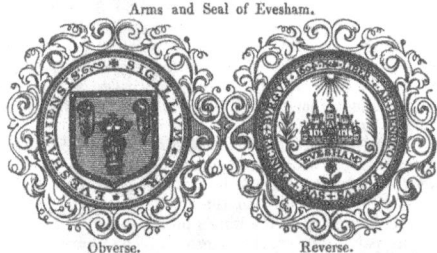

Arms and Seal of Evesham.

Obverse.   Reverse.

EVESHAM, a borough and market town, having separate jurisdiction, locally in the lower division of the hundred of Blackenhurst, county of WORCESTER, 15 miles (S. E.) from Worcester, 13 (N. E.) from Tewkesbury, and 96 (N. W. by W.) from London, containing, exclusively of the parish of Bengworth, 2634 inhabitants. This place has at different times been called Homme, Chronuchomme, Hatholm, Hethelhomme, and Æthommo, all originating in the Saxon holm, a river island, and sometimes a hill, or rising ground, in either sense applicable to its situation. The appellation Evvesholme, or Evvesham, is said to be derived from Evves, a swineherd in the service of Egwin, third bishop of Huicca, a Saxon province and bishoprick, the greater part of which now forms the diocese of Worcester. Evves is superstitiously said to have had an interview with the Virgin Mary on this spot, and to this circumstance is attributed the erection of an abbey for Benedictine monks, the foundation of which was laid in 702 and the building completed in 709, when the charter, was confirmed : it was consecrated in 712, and dedicated to the Virgin Mary in 714, by Egwin, who retired hither after he had been unjustly dispossessed of the bishoprick of Worcester by the pope. To this establishment the town owes its origin and subsequent participation in the varied fortunes of the former. The abbot and convent received several grants of land, manorial privileges, and ecclesiastical property, from the Anglo-Saxon kings and nobility, as well as from other benefactors, both before and after the Conquest: its possessions were ample, and its privileges numerous; the abbots sat in parliament as spiritual barons. It shared the fate of similar institutions, having been suppressed on the 17th of November, 1539, at which time the annual revenue amounted to £1268. 9. 10. The buildings and site were then alienated by the King; the former, with the church, were demolished, and the materials sold: an arch, or gateway, on the northern side of the present church-yard, probably leading to the cloisters, and a few fragments visible in some out-buildings, are the only remains of this edifice, which appears to have been of the decorated style of English architecture, and highly enriched with sculpture. The handsome isolated tower, which is so great an ornament to the town, was erected by Clement Lichfield, the last abbot but one; it is a beautiful specimen of the later English style, strengthened with panelled buttresses, and crowned with open battlements and pinnacles; but it does not appear to have been connected with the monastic buildings. From recent excavations, the old tower appears to have stood at the north side of the west entrance to the great cathedral. At the general demolition, the present tower was purchased by the inhabitants: it is one hundred and ten feet high, and about twenty-eight feet square at the base; the north side is plain, the other three sides adorned with tracery. In 1745, a clock with chimes was put up in the tower, by Edward Rudge, Esq. Several abbots and monks have been interred here, among whom was abbot Lichfield, whose tomb was opened in 1817; but so complete has been the destruction of this once magnificent pile, that the exact place of their interment cannot be ascertained. The most memorable occurrence in the history of the town is the decisive battle which was fought here, on the 4th of August, 1265, between Prince Edward and Simon Montfort, Earl of Leicester, by whom Henry III. was detained a prisoner. The combat was characterised by savage ferocity; and of those who fell victims were the earl and his son, about one hundred and sixty knights, and four thousand of their followers. The bodies of the Earl and his son, with those of Henry and Hugh le Despenser, were interred in the abbey church, before the high altar, the king himself assisting solemnly at the earl's funeral. The issue of this contest, by releasing the captive monarch, turned the tide of his fortunes, and led to that success by which he was subsequently reinstated on the throne. This celebrated battle was fought about three quarters of a mile from the town, at a place called The Old Road, which crosses a small stream subsequently denominated Battle-well.

The town is pleasantly situated on an eminence rising from the bank of the river Avon, by which it is almost encircled, and over which is a stone bridge of seven arches, uniting it with the parish of Bengworth, which is within the borough: it consists of two principal, and some inferior streets, of which the High-street is particularly spacious. From the foundations of houses being discoverable in various parts of the environs, it appears to have been of greater magnitude than it is at present. The country adjacent is remarkable for its interesting scenery, and has consequently attracted many respectable families to the town and neighbourhood. The vale of Evesham is celebrated for the extreme richness and fertility of its soil, which, by the successful mode of cultivation, produces earlier and more abundant crops than that of any other part of the country: near the town, on both sides of the river, large portions of ground have been converted into gardens, horticulture constituting the chief occupation of the labouring class; asparagus attains an unequalled perfection in this soil, and is extensively cultivated, and vegetables of every kind are, by means of the river Avon, conveyed hence to the principal towns in the surrounding district. Though favoured by the navigable river Avon, it has never become the seat of any particular branch of trade or manufacture; there are some corn-mills, and a mill for extracting oil from linseed. The market is on Monday: fairs are held on the 2nd of February, the Monday next after Easter, Whit-Monday, and the 21st of September, the last being famous for the show of strong black horses. King Henry VIII., in the thirty-eighth year of his reign, granted and sold to Sir Philip Hobby the three fairs, tolls, customs, &c., together with the market.

The inhabitants were incorporated by a charter granted by James I., in the third year of his reign, which confirmed their prescriptive privileges, and conferred others. The government is vested in a mayor, seven aldermen, twelve capital burgesses, a recorder and chamberlain, who, with twenty-four assistants, form the common council. The mayor is chosen on the Tuesday next after St. Bartholomew's day; the mayor, the recorder, and four of the aldermen, are justices of the peace: the mayor is almoner and clerk of the market; he is also entitled to deodands, the goods of felons, and tolls of fairs and markets, with other manorial rights. A court of record, at which the mayor or recorder presides in person, or by deputy, assisted by two of the senior aldermen, is held every Tuesday, for the recovery of debts to the amount of £100, by charter of James I.: a court of session is also held on the Friday after the county quarter sessions. The assizes for the county, now holden at Worcester, were formerly held here. The corporation possess the privilege of trying and executing for all capital offences except high treason: the last infliction of this punishment occurred in 1740, when a female was burnt for petty treason. The town hall is a plain building in the market-place, in which the courts are held, and assemblies take place during the season. The borough returned members to parliament in the 23rd of Edward I., but after that king's reign it discontinued till the commencement of that of James I., since which period it has uninterruptedly returned two representatives. The right of election is vested in the burgesses, of whom there are about seven hundred: the mayor is the returning officer. The influence possessed by Lord Northwick enables him to ensure the return of one member.

The borough comprises the parishes of All Saints, St. Lawrence, and Bengworth, formerly in the peculiar jurisdiction of the abbot of Evesham, now in the archdeaconry and diocese of Worcester; the last, lying on the eastern bank of the river, was added to the borough by the charter of James I. The living of All Saints' is a discharged vicarage, rated in the king's books at £10. 16. 0½., endowed with £200 private benefaction, £400 royal bounty, and £600 parliamentary grant, and in the patronage of the Crown. The church was formerly a chapel to the abbey, and is said to have been built about 1350, but probably earlier : it is an elegant structure in the later style of English architecture, with a tower and spire ; the porch at the western entrance is of very beautiful construction, embattled, and having pinnacles at the corner : on the south side is a small chapel, built by abbot Clement Lichfield, the roof of which is finely groined, and beautifully adorned with fan tracery. The living of the parish of St. Lawrence is a perpetual curacy, united to the vicarage of All Saints, endowed with £600 royal bounty, and in the patronage of the Crown. The church, which is in ruins, exhibits a rich specimen of the later style of English architecture : attached to it is a chapel of exquisite beauty ; the tower and spire are of earlier construction. There are places of worship for Baptists, the Society of Friends, Wesleyan Methodists, and Unitarians. The free grammar school was endowed originally by abbot Lichfield. Henry VIII., after the dissolution of the abbey, refounded this school, restoring only a part of its previous revenue. The charter which James granted to the inhabitants remodelled the institution, when it was called the free school of Prince Henry. The master receives £10 annually from the crown, with a house rent-free, and some minor emoluments. In Bengworth is also a school, founded in 1709, pursuant to the will of John Deacle, Esq., alderman of London, dated three years previously, whereby he bequeathed £2000 for the endowment of a free school for the benefit of thirty poor boys, who are clothed, educated, and apprenticed. The nomination of the boys is vested in the churchwardens and overseers of the parish ; and, should there not be a sufficient number of poor boys in Bengworth, in the mayor and capital burgesses of Evesham. John Gardner, of London, gave £4. 6. 8. annually, with the addition of 18s. per annum, arising from some tenements in the town, towards the instruction, in the English language, of twenty-five poor boys belonging to the parishes of All Saints and St. Lawrence. Several benefactions to the poor, and for apprenticing children, are recorded on tablets in the churches of the respective parishes. In the parish of Bengworth was an ancient castle, which, in 1169, was attacked by the abbot William D'Andeville, who destroyed it, and erected the present church on its site ; it is built on the surface of the soil without sinking for a foundation. Ten years ago, on levelling a bank in the grounds belonging to B. Cooper, Esq., called the Moat-arches, about sixty yards from the church, the foundation of a large room, sixty feet by twenty-five, was discovered, which furnished sufficient stone to build a convenient house. Walter of Evesham, a monkish writer of great celebrity, and John Feckenham, of Feckenham, in this county, received the early part of their education in the abbey here. John Bernardi, of Italian extraction, but born here, was a daring, adventurous soldier ; he was committed to Newgate for suspected treason, where he died. Sir Charles Cocks, Bart., on his elevation to the peerage, on the 17th of May, 1784, assumed the title of Lord Somers, Baron of Evesham, which is held by the present Earl Somers.

EVINGTON, a parish in the hundred of GARTREE, county of LEICESTER, 3¾ miles (E.S.E.) from Leicester, containing 257 inhabitants. The living is a vicarage, in the jurisdiction of the peculiar court of the lord of the manor of Evington, rated in the king's books at £7 16. 8., and in the patronage of the Bishop of Lincoln. The church is dedicated to St. Denis.

EWART, a township in the parish of DODDINGTON, eastern division of GLENDALE ward, county of NORTHUMBERLAND, 5 miles (N.N.W.) from Wooler, containing 150 inhabitants. There is a small endowment for the education of children. This place is pleasantly situated between the rivers Till and Glen, where it is supposed there was formerly a church and a burial-ground. In 1814, two ancient bronze sword blades were found in the park.

EWE (ST.), a parish in the eastern division of the hundred of POWDER, county of CORNWALL, 4 miles (E.N.E.) from Tregoney, containing 1663 inhabitants. The living is a rectory, in the archdeaconry of Cornwall, and diocese of Exeter, rated in the king's books at £21, and in the patronage of Thomas Carlyon, Esq. The Wesleyan Methodists have a place of worship here. There are extensive copper and tin mines and works in this parish.

EWELL, a parish in the hundred of BEWSBOROUGH, lathe of ST. AUGUSTINE, county of KENT, 2½ miles (N.W.) from Dovor, containing 340 inhabitants. The living is a vicarage, in the archdeaconry and diocese of Canterbury, rated in the king's books at £6. 13. 4., endowed with £200 private benefaction, and £400 royal bounty, and held by sequestration under the Archbishop of Canterbury. John Angle, Esq. was patron in 1784. The church is a small edifice, dedicated to St. Mary and St. Peter. This village, situated in the beautiful valley between Barham Downs and the Land's End, at Dovor, was formerly called Temple-Ewell, from its having formed part of the possessions of the Knights Templars so early as the year 1185 : a building on a hill to the north is still called the Temple Farm ; but the remains of the ancient mansion of the Templars, which stood near this spot, are said to have been destroyed about seventy years since. In this parish rises the principal stream of the river Dour, or Idle, which falls into the sea at Dovor.

EWELL, a parish partly in the first division of the hundred of REIGATE, but chiefly in the first division of the hundred of COPTHORNE, county of SURREY, 5½ miles (N.W. by N.) from Kingston, on the road to Worthing, containing, with the liberty of Kingswood, which is in the hundred of Reigate, 1737 inhabitants. The village was anciently of more importance than it is at present, and in the parish was the splendid palace of Nonsuch, erected by Henry VIII., and taken down in the reign of Charles II. There are still some remains of that celebrated edifice, which, for costly magnificence and splendid decoration, was, as its name implied, unequalled by any building of the kind. They consist chiefly of the walls of the inner court, including a quadrangular area of half an acre, in the centre of which was the banqueting-house, twenty-five feet square, and three stories in height ; and of some of the bastions by which the palace was defended : the ascent into the court was by three double flights of stone steps, still in tolerable preservation ; and in an adjoining field, called Diana's Dyke, was a cold bath.

decorated with statues of Diana and Actæon, which was used by Queen Elizabeth, who occupied the palace during the latter part of her life, but which is at present only a small pond. The remains of this once stately pile are carefully preserved by Mr. Calverley, who has erected a mansion in the ancient style of English architecture, near the site: in the grounds, several Roman coins have been discovered, among which were one of Antoninus, and one of Constantine. The village is well paved, and partially lighted with oil, and the inhabitants are amply supplied with water. There are several gunpowder and flour-mills set in motion by the river Kingsmill, a stream which has its source in the parish, and falls into the Thames at Kingston. The market, formerly held on Thursday, has long been discontinued: the fairs are, May 12th for cattle, and October 29th, a very large mart for sheep, at which from thirty to forty thousand are frequently sold. The parish is within the jurisdiction of a court held at Kingston, for the recovery of debts to any amount: courts leet and baron are held at Michaelmas. The living is a vicarage, in the archdeaconry of Surrey, and diocese of Winchester, rated in the king's books at £8, and in the patronage of Sir Leweu Powell Glyn, Bart. The church, dedicated to St. Mary, is an ancient structure, and has received an addition of one hundred and eighty-one free sittings, towards defraying the expense of which, the Incorporated Society for the enlargement of churches and chapels granted £50. The rectory-house is an ancient edifice; in the grounds several fossils and coins have been found within the last few years; among the latter was one of Trajan. There is a place of worship for Independents. A National school, to which some bequests for the education of children have been assigned, was established in 1816: about one hundred and seventy children are taught in this school, which is chiefly supported by subscription.

EWELME, a parish in the hundred of EWELME, county of OXFORD, 3¼ miles (N.E. by E.) from Wallingford, containing 573 inhabitants. The living is a rectory annexed to the Regius Professorship of Divinity, in the University of Oxford, in the archdeaconry and diocese of Oxford, rated in the king's books at £21. 10. 5. At this place, called from the elms Ewelme (vulgarly Newelme), William de la Pole, Duke of Suffolk, erected, in 1437, a mansion, a neat hospital, and a handsome church, dedicated to St. Mary, in which his lady was buried: her tomb is remarkably elegant, having no less than fifty alabaster figures of angels about it. The hospital, called God's House, for two priests and thirteen poor men, under the control of the Regius Professor of divinity at Oxford, was valued, in the 26th of Henry VIII., at £20 per annum: it still exists, with an endowment for a reader and twelve poor men: There is also a free school. The church and hospital stand on the west side of a hill, but the mansion is in a low situation. An urn full of Roman coins was found on Ewelme common, near the Roman Iknield-street, and another on Harcourt hill, two miles from the village. The Earl of Macclesfield has the title of Viscount Parker, of Ewelme.

EWEN, a tything in the parish of KEMBLE, hundred of MALMESBURY, county of WILTS, 7 miles (N.E. by N.) from Malmesbury. The population is returned with the parish.

EWERBY, a parish in the hundred of ASWARD-HURN, parts of KESTEVEN, county of LINCOLN, 3¾ miles (E. by N.) from Sleaford, containing 315 inhabitants. The living is a discharged vicarage, in the archdeaconry and diocese of Lincoln, rated in the king's books at £6. 10. 10., and in the patronage of the Crown. The church is dedicated to St. Andrew. Here is a small endowed school, with a garden attached.

EWHURST, a parish in the hundred of KINGSCLERE, Kingsclere division of the county of SOUTHAMPTON, 6 miles (N.W.) from Basingstoke, containing 18 inhabitants. The living is a discharged rectory, in the archdeaconry and diocese of Winchester, rated in the king's books at £1. 6. 8., endowed with £200 private benefaction, and £200 royal bounty, and in the patronage of Sir Peter Pole, Bart. The church is dedicated to St. Mary. On the summit of a hill in this parish, from which an extensive and pleasing view of the adjoining counties may be obtained, are some tumuli, and yew trees of great antiquity.

EWHURST, a parish in the second division of the hundred of BLACKHEATH, county of SURREY, 9¼ miles (W. by N.) from Godalming, containing 821 inhabitants. The living is a rectory, in the archdeaconry of Surrey, and diocese of Winchester, rated in the king's books at £12. 7. 3½., and in the patronage of the Crown. The church, dedicated to St. Peter and St. Paul, is chiefly in the early English style. On a common, called the Churt, or East Churt, is a large camp called Holmbury, supposed to be of Roman construction.

EWHURST, a parish in the hundred of STAPLE, rape of HASTINGS, county of SUSSEX, 4 miles (E. by N.) from Roberts-Bridge, containing 1225 inhabitants. The living is a rectory, in the archdeaconry of Lewes, and diocese of Chichester, rated in the king's books at £12. 2. 6., and in the patronage of the Provost and Fellows of King's College, Cambridge. The church, dedicated to St. James, has portions in the early English, with insertions in the decorated style. The Rother runs on the northern side of the parish. Fairs for cattle and pedlary are held May 21st and August 5th.

EWSHOTT, a tything in the parish and hundred of CRONDALL, Basingstoke division of the county of SOUTHAMPTON, 3½ miles (E.) from Odiham, containing 489 inhabitants.

EWYAS-HARROLD, a parish in the hundred of WEBTREE, county of HEREFORD, 12½ miles (S.W.) from Hereford, containing 412 inhabitants. The living is a perpetual curacy, in the archdeaconry of Brecon, and diocese of St. David, endowed with £200 private benefaction, and £400 royal bounty, and in the patronage of the Bishop of St. David's. The church, dedicated to St. Michael, is a small edifice, with a massive tower in the early English style. Here was anciently a castle, which, according to Dugdale, was built by William Fitz-Osborne, Earl of Hereford, after the Conquest; but Leland observes that it was probably erected by King Harold, prior to his elevation to the throne, who conferred it upon an illegitimate son, also named Harold, from whom the place is supposed to have received its distinguishing appellation. A prior and a small convent of monks settled here about 1100, from the abbey of St. Peter, in Gloucester, and continued till 1358, when the revenue being insufficient for their support, they were again united to the abbey.

EXBOURNE, a parish in the hundred of BLACK TORRINGTON, county of DEVON, 4¾ miles (E. by S.) from Hatherleigh, containing 503 inhabitants. The living is a rectory, in the archdeaconry of Totness, and diocese of Exeter, rated in the king's books at £27. 11. 8. The Rev. F. Belfield was patron in 1793. The church is dedicated to St. Mary. A fair for cattle and pedlary is held annually on the third Monday in April.

EXBURY, a chapelry in the parish of FAWLEY, in that part of the hundred of BISHOP'S WALTHAM which is in the New Forest (East) division of the county of SOUTHAMPTON, 9½ miles (E. by N.) from Lymington, containing, with the tything of Leap, 311 inhabitants. This chapelry lies on the left bank, and near the mouth of the Beaulieu river, which falls into the Isle of Wight channel, at the Preventive station between Stone and Needs Bar points. There are salt-works at the village; also a ferry over the river to St. Leonard's.

EXELBY, a township in the parish of BURNESTON, wapentake of HALLIKELD, North riding of the county of YORK, 2¼ miles (S. E. by E.) from Bedale, containing, with Leeming and Newton, 562 inhabitants. The sum of about £40 per annum is applied to the instruction of the poor children of the townships of Exelby, Leeming, and Newton.

EXETER, a city and a county of itself, locally in the hundred of Wonford, county of DEVON; of which it is the chief town, 10 miles (N. N. W.) from Exmouth, 44 (N. E.) from Plymouth, and 176 (W. by S.) from London, containing 23,479 inhabitants. Geoffrey of Monmouth affirms that Exeter was a British city prior to its establishment as a Roman station, and various circumstances concur to prove the fact. It was by the Britons called *Caer-Wisc*, i. e. city of the water; also *Caer Rydh*, or the red city, from the colour of the adjacent soil. After its capture by the Romans, who made it a stipendiary town, it was denominated *Isca*, with the addition of *Danmoniorum*, to distinguish it from *Isca* (now Usk), in Monmouthshire. That it was once occupied by the Romans is evident from the numerous coins and other relics which have been dug up at different times, and more particularly in July, 1778, when small statues of Mercury, Mars, Ceres, and Apollo, the largest not exceeding four inches and a half in height, evidently the Penates, or household gods, of that people, together with fragments of urns, tiles, and tesselated pavement, were discovered. The city is said to have been honoured at one time with the name of *Augusta*, from the circumstance of its having been occupied by the second Augustan legion, commanded by Vespasian, the conqueror of Britannia Prima, which included Danmonium. It was for a considerable time the capital of the West Saxon kingdom, and was afterwards occupied by the Danes, after the violation of a solemn treaty made with Alfred, the Saxon monarch. Alfred, however, invested the city, and compelled the enemy to capitulate, with a promise of evacuating all their holds within the West Saxon territory: it was afterwards attacked by the Danish

Arms.

marauders in 894, and was again relieved by Alfred. Exeter was at a very early period distinguished for its religious establishments, and contained so many monastic foundations that the Cornish Britons and Saxon pagans are reported to have called it in derision "Monk-town." On the accession of Athelstan, however, the Britons and Saxons who had not embraced Christianity, and who till now had formed a considerable portion of its population, were expelled, and the number of its religious institutions was augmented by the foundation of a Benedictine monastery, dedicated to St. Peter, which may be regarded as the origin of the present cathedral. The town is greatly indebted for its early importance to Athelstan, who is said to have established two mints in it, and to have regularly fortified it with towers and a wall of hewn stone, from which circumstance, most probably, it was denominated *Exan-ceastre*, or *Exacestre*, i. e. the castellated city of the Exe, from which its present name is derived. In 968, King Edgar restored the monastery founded by his predecessor, Athelstan, which had been destroyed by the Danes, and appointed Sydemann to the abbacy. At this time the West Saxon see of Sherborne, of which, prior to 924, Tawton, near Barnstaple, was the head, having been sub-divided into several, Crediton became the seat of the Devonshire diocese, and Sydemann was ultimately raised to the bishoprick. In 1003, Sweyn, King of Denmark, landed on the western coast with a formidable force, to avenge the slaughter of his countrymen, and laid siege to Exeter, which, after a vigorous resistance for two months, was treacherously given up by its governor, and, with its inhabitants, devoted to merciless destruction. The monastery of St. Peter shared in the common ruin; nor did the city recover from its devastation till the accession of Canute, when it began to resume its former importance, and the monks of St. Peter their former privileges. In the reign of Edward the Confessor, Exeter had attained to such magnitude, wealth, and security, that the sees of Crediton and St. Germans (Cornwall) were united under one bishop, and Exeter was made the head of the diocese. The ceremonies attendant on this change were commensurate with its importance; and the church of the abbey of St. Peter was erected into the cathedral church, in the presence of Edward, whose chaplain, Leofric, was installed first bishop of the united see. The monks were now removed to Westminster abbey, and twenty-four secular canons were appointed by the new bishop to perform the service of the Cathedral.

The citizens, instigated by Githa, mother of Harold, refused to receive a Norman garrison, and having recourse to arms, were joined by the neighbouring inhabitants of Cornwall and Devonshire. On the approach of William to punish their revolt, sensible of the unequal contest, they submitted to his authority, and delivered hostages for their obedience. This agreement having been broken by a meeting of the populace, the Conqueror appeared before the walls of the city, and ordering the eyes of one of the hostages to be put out, the inhabitants surrendered at discretion. The principal persons in the city, consequently, went forth in procession to acknowledge the supremacy of the Norman conqueror, who qualified his severities by some acts of favour; enforcing the payment of "a grievous fine," but renewing all their privileges, and merely altering the gates in commemoration of his triumph. Githa escaped with her treasures, and took refuge in Flanders. To prevent a revolt in future, William erected a citadel in Exeter, the government of which he entrusted to Baldwin de Brioniis, who, being elevated to the great barony of Oakhampton, was, by virtue of his office, Earl of Devon, and sheriff for the county. The castle having been garrisoned in 1136 by the partizans of the Empress Matilda, held out against Stephen for three months, but was compelled to surrender from want of water. Stephen, however, acted with clemency, and Henry II. subsequently rewarded the loyalty of the citizens by a grant of additional privileges. In 1284, Hugh Courtenay, then Earl of Devon, greatly injured the trading interests of Exeter, by obstructing the navigation of the river Exe, hitherto navigable for vessels of considerable burden. The alleged occasion of this is curious: in the market-place were three pots of fish, and the earl's caterer wanted the whole; the bishop's was equally unreasonable; and the dispute being referred to the mayor, he allotted one to the earl, a second to the bishop, and the third to the use of the town generally. This, and other equally unimportant matters, so offended the earl that he erected a large dam, or wen, across the Exe at Topsham, where he built a quay, and considerably curtailed the trade of the port. In 1286 Edward I. held a parliament at Exeter, augmented the privileges of the borough, and gave it a new common seal. The Black Prince remained here several days with his royal prisoner of France, and subsequently visited the city in 1371. In 1469, the Duchess of Clarence, with others of the royal adherents, took refuge in Exeter, which was besieged by Sir William Courtenay, one of Edward's generals; the siege, however, was raised at the mediation of the clergy. In 1470, Edward IV. arrived in pursuit of the Duke of Clarence and the Earl of Warwick; and sometime after the battle of Tewkesbury, that prince, with his queen and infant son, were entertained here for several days. Richard the Third's visit to Exeter is alluded to by Shakspeare. In 1488, Edward Courtenay, Earl of Devon, was made free of the city, being the first honorary freeman on record. In 1497, Exeter sustained a violent assault from Perkin Warbeck, the pretended Richard of York, and claimant of the crown: the inhabitants, however, successfully resisted the impostor till the arrival of the Earl of Devon, when Perkin retreated to Taunton. The loyalty of the citizens was afterwards rewarded by Henry VII., who presented them with his sword. In 1501, Catherine of Arragon remained here several days, on her way from Plymouth to London. On the 2nd of July, 1549, Exeter was invested by a strong body of the popish adherents; the citizens withstood the attack till the 5th of August, when John, Lord Russell, having defeated the rebels at Clist heath, dispersed the assailants. The privations endured by the inhabitants during the siege were of the severest kind, and such was their gratitude for deliverance, that the day of Lord Russell's entry into the city (August 6th) was consecrated an annual festival.

Exeter is distinguished for numerous proofs of loyal attachment, which has been extended even to the unfortunate among foreign monarchs, as in the case of Don Antonio, the deprived King of Portugal. So sensible was Queen Elizabeth of the loyalty of the Exonians,

that, with other more substantial proofs of her favour, she presented the corporation with the honourable motto Semper Fidelis. During the parliamentary war, Exeter continued firm to the royal cause; but the lord lieutenant of the county, who was of the opposite party, disarmed the citizens, and garrisoned the castle with parliamentarian troops. It was, however, subsequently taken by Prince Maurice and Sir John Berkeley, the latter of whom was appointed governor. The city was now regarded as a place of great security, and the queen, being near the time of her confinement, took refuge within its walls. Her accouchement took place in Bedford House, where she was delivered of the Princess Henrietta Maria, afterwards baptized in the cathedral. Charles I. visited Exeter on his way to and return from Cornwall, and the infant princess remained here till the surrender of the city, after a vigorous blockade of more than two months, to General Fairfax, in April, 1646. During the stay of the parliamentary forces, the cathedral was shamefully defaced, and divided into places of worship for Presbyterians and Independents. The palace, with other buildings adjoining, was turned into barracks, and the chapter-house converted into a stable. During the Protectorate of Cromwell, two zealous royalists, who had attempted to restore Charles II., were by Cromwell's order beheaded in the city. On the restoration of Charles II., the city again testified its loyalty with much enthusiasm; and the king, on his visit, in 1671, presented the corporation with a portrait of his sister Henrietta, then Duchess of Orleans. On the appearance of the Prince of Orange, in November 1688, the inhabitants submitted to him, and that monarch established a mint here. In August, 1787, George III., with his queen and three of the princesses, visited Exeter. Pestilential diseases have formerly raged here, as in most other towns, with destructive effect: the plague is said to have been fatal to a great number in 1569. In 1586 one of the judges of assize, several of the grand jury, and others, fell victims to the gaol distemper. The plague was again prevalent in 1603 and 1625; and in 1777, no less than two hundred and eighty-five persons died of the small pox.

This city, which has been denominated "The Capital of the West," occupies the flat summit and the declivities of a hill, rising gradually from the eastern bank of the river Exe, but abruptly steep on the western side, in the midst of a fertile and undulating country, surrounded on all sides by scenes of beauty, or spots of interest. Its salubrious air, cleanliness, good market, and proximity to several delightful watering-places, tend greatly to enhance its eligibility as a place of residence. That portion of it which is within the walls is an oblong quadrangle, about two thousand six hundred and seventy yards in compass, divided by two spacious principal, and intersected by two inferior, streets: the four divisions thus produced are denominated the North, South, East, and West wards. Fore-street, occupying the acclivity, and High-street, the summit of the hill, together form a noble thoroughfare, running in a north-easterly direction from the river, which makes a curve round the lower end of the city, on the south-west. Exeter, with its suburbs, contains many handsome rows of modern houses, particularly in the eastern part of the town, in which are situated the cathedral, Bedford Circus, Southernhay Place, and Northernhay Place in front of which are enclosed pleasure grounds, and the public baths, erécted in 1821, having a handsome exterior of classical design, and internally replete with every accommodation. The town is well paved, partly lighted with gas by a company established in 1816, and supplied with water from the river, by water-works erected in 1694, at its western extremity. At the western entrance is a handsome stone bridge over the river Exe, erected, after repeated failures caused by the rapidity of the current, in 1778, at an expense of £20,000, a little above the site of an ancient bridge of twelve arches, originally erected in 1250. To the north of the city are the cavalry barracks, and at some distance to the south-west the artillery barracks, both comprising extensive ranges of buildings. The Devon and Exeter Institution, for the general promotion of science, &c., was established in 1813. On the ground floor are two spacious rooms forming the library, which at present contains ten thousand volumes, under the care of a resident librarian, with numerous natural and artificial curiosities, a model of the cathedral in wood, and miniature representations of Mont Blanc, the Simplon, &c., besides some good paintings: it is supported by two hundred and thirty proprietors, who pay a premium of £40, and £2 annually. The affairs of the institution are managed by a committee, consisting of a president, vice-president, a treasurer, and twenty-one of the proprietors. In Fore-street is a public subscription library, founded in 1807, and containing two thousand five hundred volumes. The tradesmen and mechanics' institution, formed in 1825, now consists of two hundred members, and is attended by masters in the mathematics, architecture, and the French language: it contains a good library, reading-rooms, &c., and in the winter season public lectures are delivered. The freemasons' grand provincial lodges, 53d, 98th, 178th, and the East Devon Military lodge, 272nd, are held here. In a handsome modern building near the Northern Hay walk are the public rooms, erected by subscription, in 1820: the ball-room, measuring eighty feet by forty, is superbly fitted up, and lighted by a handsome dome. The theatre is a neat modern structure, erected on the site of a former one destroyed by fire: its scenic arrangements are good, and the decorations appropriate: it is frequently visited by the London performers. The races generally take place in July or August, on Haldon, or Hall down, an excellent race-course in the vicinity.

The port of Exeter extends from the coast near Lyme-Regis, to the Ness Point at Teignmouth. A little above Topsham the tide is arrested by the "Lower Weir," there being another between this and the city. Leland alludes to the intention of the citizens to remedy the inconvenience, but we do not hear of its completion till 1580, after which, lighters of sixteen tons' burden were enabled to come from Topsham to the city quay. In 1699, a canal was cut nearly to Topsham, navigable for vessels of one hundred and fifty tons; it was completed at an expense of £20,000, communicating with the river about three miles from the city. On the 14th of September, 1827, this canal was re-opened with great pomp, its line having been extended about two miles and a half farther to the south, for the admission of vessels of larger tonnage. On the quay are the custom-house and wharfinger's office; and near

it are extensive iron-foundries, fulling-mills, timber wharfs, &c. A large basin is in progress of excavation opposite the quay, where vessels of considerable burden may float and discharge their cargoes. There are now about twenty-five vessels, of from seventy to one hundred tons' burden,- trading between this and London, three to Liverpool, five to Bristol, ten to Plymouth, and one to Falmouth and Penzance. The principal exports are woollen goods and manganese; the imports, wine, hemp, tallow, grocery, &c. The trade of Exeter, at a very early period, was chiefly in the article of wool, the market for this commodity having been removed hither from Crediton, in 1538. Fulling-mills existed here in the time of Edward I.: the weavers and fullers were united to the merchant adventurers, and incorporated by Elizabeth. It formerly exported woollen cloth to Italy, Turkey, &c.: and it is said that before the year 1700, eight out of ten of the citizens were engaged in that trade, which decreased during the American war. The cotton-works, and manufactories for kerseymere and shawls, have also declined; though there is some probability of the latter being revived. The manufacture at present consists chiefly of coarse cloth. The governors of the Bank of England have recently established a branch bank here. The West of England Fire and Life Insurance Company, which was formed in 1807, with a capital of £600,000, has agents in all the principal towns in England. The markets are held by prescription: the principal market day is Friday; there is, however, a daily sale for butcher's meat, fish, and vegetables; besides a market for pork, poultry, butter, &c., on Tuesday and Friday, on which latter day is also a market for corn, cattle, and serges. The fairs are on the third Wednesday in February, third Wednesday in May, last Wednesday in July, and the second Wednesday in December: there is a great market on the second Friday in every month.

Corporate Seal.

The city was anciently held in demesne by the crown: its earliest charter was granted by Henry I., and confirmed by Henry II. and Richard I. It is supposed to have been first governed by a mayor in the reign of John, in the year 1200, at which time the mayor's office was held for life. In 1312, the mayor and bailiffs were made justices of the peace. Edward III. granted them the cognizance of pleas: the charters of Edward IV. and Henry VII. confirmed their privileges, and Henry VIII. constituted Exeter a county of itself. Extended privileges were granted by Charles I., and in 1684, a new charter of incorporation was obtained from Charles II., but never enrolled. In 1770, George III. renewed and confirmed the charter, by which the government is vested in a mayor, recorder, eight aldermen, fourteen common council-men, assisted by a town clerk and deputy, and subordinate officers. The mayor is elected annually from two previously nominated and approved by the twenty-four, and he and the recorder and aldermen are justices of the peace, the latter holding office for life. The remaining officers are, the mayor's chaplain, chamberlain, under sheriff, surveyor, sword-bearer, coroner for the city and county of Exeter, bailiff, four serjeants at mace, constables for the four wards of the city, others for those of the county of the city, and additional constables for the whole city and county, &c. The corporation hold a court of assize for the city and county of the city twice a year at the guildhall: the assizes for the county of Devon are held in the sessions house within the castle: a court of quarter sessions is also held in both places. The Devon county court, for the recovery of debts under 40s., is held every fourth Tuesday in the castle, where there is also an insolvent debtors' court three times a year; and there is a debtors' court at the guildhall, where also the mayor's court, for the decision of petty offences, is held every Monday and Saturday. The court of requests, for the recovery of debts under 40s., by an act passed in the 13th of George III., is held every fortnight. The court of provosty of the city of Exeter, or Provost's court, is held every Saturday throughout the year, for the recovery of debts to any amount above 40s.: it is held by prescription, traced by roll to the 14th of Edward I., in the year 1286: the officers constituting the court are the receiver, and three other stewards, also called provosts, or bailiffs, two of whom form a quorum, and are assisted by the town clerk, who is the prothonotary of the court, and the processes are executed by four serjeants at mace. Attendance is given at the guildhall by the magistrates every morning at eleven o'clock, to hear complaints, &c.; and in the castle the magistrates for the hundred hold petty sessions every Friday: a general court day is held by the corporation of the poor, on the first Tuesday in every month.

Exeter has sent two members to parliament ever since the reign of Edward I.: the right of election is vested in the freeholders and freemen generally, the number of whom is about one thousand two hundred: the sheriff is the returning officer. The guildhall was formerly fronted by a chapel dedicated to St. George, which was demolished in 1592: the present façade projects into the street, and is a curious specimen of ancient English and Italian architecture: the common hall is spacious, and has an arched roof, supported by grotesque figures: it contains portraits of Charles I., his daughter the Princess Henrietta, General Monk, and others. The sessions house, within the walls of Rougemont castle, was erected in 1773: it exhibits a neat stone front, and is complete in its internal arrangement. The new city prison, erected in 1819, is a large brick building for felons and debtors; the front is a house for the governor. The county gaol, a short distance north of the city, erected in 1796, is very spacious, and judiciously planned for the classification of prisoners; in the centre is the governor's house, with a chapel attached; on each side are wings, two stories in height. The bridewell, erected in 1809, near the same spot, consists of three detached buildings diverging from the area around the keeper's house: each wing contains two distinct wards, with a spacious airing-yard to each ward. The chapel, in the keeper's house, is so divided that the different classes of prisoners do not see each other. The buildings include also spacious work-shops, a masons' yard, and a treadmill. The sheriff's debtors' ward, south-west of the city, was erected in 1818.

Arms of the Bishoprick.

Exeter was, in the reign of Edward the Confessor, erected into a see, the jurisdiction of which extends over the counties of Devon and Cornwall, with the exception of the deanery of St. Burian, in the latter county: the authority of rural dean is exercised in this diocese. The ecclesiastical establishment consists of a bishop, dean, sub-dean, precentor, chancellor, treasurer, four archdeacons, and twenty-four prebendaries, of whom nine are residentiary canons. Antiquaries are at variance concerning the character and magnitude of the cathedral, as it existed at the time of the union of the sees of Devon and Cornwall. According to an old record at Oxford, a new church was commenced by Bishop Warlewast, in 1112, and continued by his successors till completed by Bishop Marshall, who died in 1206. It is also said to have been finished according to the original plan of Warlewast; consequently the entire building must have corresponded in character with its two massive Norman towers. On the accession of Bishop Quivil, in 1280, the cathedral, with the exception of the towers, was rebuilt in the early style of English architecture, and is justly regarded as one of the most superb ecclesiastical structures in the kingdom. Among the successors of Quivil who contributed towards the completion of his design, Bishops Stapleton and Grandison were distinguished by their munificence. Under the episcopacy of the latter, the nave was lengthened and the roof vaulted: the west front was probably erected in the time of his successor, Brantingham; and in 1420, under the superintendence of Bishop Lacey, the whole as it now appears was completed. The west front is splendidly decorated with a profusion of canopied niches, statuary, and elegant tracery: the principal entrance is in the centre of an elaborately carved screen, divided, by projecting and highly enriched buttresses, into compartments, in which are two series of arches, of which the lower, surmounted by an open battlement, contains statues, in a sitting posture, of several of the kings arrayed in their robes, and of others in armour; in the upper stories and on the buttresses are several statues of monarchs in an erect posture, and in the central niche is one of a king sitting with his foot on a globe, holding in one hand a book, and in the other a sceptre; below which are the arms of the see quartered with those of the ancient Saxon monarchs, in a shield supported by kneeling angels. Above the screen is a noble window of nine lights, with elegant tracery. On the north and south sides of the cathedral are the massive Norman towers, of which the lower parts, opening into the nave, form the transepts. The interior exhibits a striking combination of majestic grandeur and graceful simplicity; the nave is separated from the aisles by massive clustered columns, but of elegant proportion, and above the finely pointed arches which support the vaulted roof, are a triforium of singular beauty, and a noble range of clerestory windows filled with rich tracery: the choir, which is separated from the nave by a screen of exquisite design, is of similar style and of equal elevation, and has a continuation of the triforium and clerestory, the windows

X 2

of which, as well as those of the cathedral in general, exhibit the finest specimens of tracery in the decorated style to be found in the kingdom. On the south side of the choir are some stalls of exquisite beauty, and the bishop's throne, reaching to the clerestory windows at an elevation of sixty feet, is a specimen of tabernacle-work of unequalled magnificence. To the north and south of the lady chapel are those of St. Mary Magdalene and St. Gabriel, and in various parts of the cathedral are others richly adorned with sculpture, in one of which, dedicated to St. Edmund, is held the consistorial court on every Friday during term. In the north aisle of the choir are the splendid monuments of Sir Richard and Bishop Stapleton; and among many others equally deserving attention, is the tomb of Bishop Stafford, of beautiful design and elaborate execution. The length of the cathedral is three hundred and ninety feet, from east to west, and one hundred and forty from the extremities of the transepts. The chapter-house is a beautiful edifice, partly in the early, and partly in the later style of English architecture; the roof is of oak, carved in panels on the slope, and the intervals above the beams are filled with tabernacle-work. The episcopal palace is an ancient structure, containing several noble apartments, and a chapel. The deanery is celebrated as having been honoured by the visits of Charles II., William III., and George III.

The city comprises the parishes of All Hallows, All Hallows on the Walls, St. Edmund, St. George, St. John, St. Kerrian, St. Lawrence, St. Martin, St. Mary Arches, St. Mary Major, St. Mary Steps, St. Olave, St. Pancras, St. Paul, St. Petrock, St. Sidwell, St. Stephen, and Holy Trinity, the parochial chapelries of St. David and St. Sidwell, and the extra-parochial precincts of the Cathedral Close, Bedford, and Bradninch, all in the archdeaconry and diocese of Exeter. The living of All Hallows' is a discharged rectory, rated in the king's books at £6. 4. 7., endowed with £800 royal bounty, and in the patronage of the Rector of St. Stephen's. The living of All Hallows' on the Walls is a discharged rectory, rated in the king's books at £5. 4. 9½., and in the patronage of the Dean and Chapter: the church having been demolished, the service was transferred to that of St. Mary Steps in 1805. The living of St. Edmund's is a discharged rectory, rated in the king's books at £10. 16. 8., endowed with £400 private benefaction, £400 royal bounty, and £400 parliamentary grant, and in the patronage of the Mayor and Corporation. The living of St. George's is a discharged rectory, rated in the king's books at £9. 13. 8., endowed with £400 royal bounty, and £1400 parliamentary grant, and in the patronage of the Crown. The living of St. John's is a rectory not in charge, endowed with £400 private benefaction, £700 royal bounty, and £1200 parliamentary grant, and in the patronage of the Crown. The living of St. Kerrian's is a discharged rectory united to that of St. Petrock's, the former rated in the king's books at £5. 18. 6½., the latter at £14. 10. 2., endowed with £200 private benefaction, and £1200 royal bounty, and in the patronage of the Dean and Chapter. The living of the parish of St. Lawrence is a discharged rectory, endowed with £400 private benefaction, and £600 royal bounty, and in the patronage of the Crown. The living of St. Martin's is a discharged rectory united with that of St. Pancras', the former rated in the king's books at £8. 14. 6.,

and the latter at £4. 13. 4., endowed with £200 private benefaction, £800 royal bounty, and £200 parliamentary grant, and in the patronage of the Dean and Chapter. The living of the parish of St. Mary Arches is a discharged rectory, rated in the king's books at £10, endowed with £600 private benefaction, £800 royal bounty, and £1000 parliamentary grant, and in the patronage of the Bishop. The living of St. Mary Major's is a discharged rectory, rated in the king's books at £15. 14. 9½., endowed with £200 private benefaction, £800 royal bounty, and £1000 parliamentary grant, and in the patronage of the Dean and Chapter. The living of the parish of St. Mary Steps is a discharged rectory, rated in the king's books at £8. 6. 8., endowed with £400 private benefaction, £1200 royal bounty, and £1600 parliamentary grant. The Rev. William Carwithen was patron in 1825. The living of St. Olave's is a discharged rectory, rated in the king's books at £7. 13. 4., endowed with £400 royal bounty, and £400 parliamentary grant, and in the patronage of the Crown. The living of St. Paul's is a discharged rectory, rated in the king's books at £8. 2. 6., endowed with £200 private benefaction, £200 royal bounty, and £400 parliamentary grant, and in the patronage of the Dean and Chapter. The living of St. Stephen's is a discharged rectory, rated in the king's books at £7. 17. 3½., endowed with £200 royal bounty, and in the patronage of the Bishop. The living of the Holy Trinity parish is a discharged rectory, rated in the king's books at £11. 16. 4., endowed with £200 private benefaction, £200 royal bounty, and £200 parliamentary grant, and in the patronage of the Dean and Chapter. The living of the parochial chapelry of St. David is a perpetual curacy, in the patronage of the Vicar of Heavitree: the chapel was rebuilt in 1816, on the site of the ancient edifice. That of St. Sidwell's is also a perpetual curacy, endowed with £1400 parliamentary grant, and in the patronage of the Vicar of Heavitree: the chapel, rebuilt in 1812, is a spacious and handsome structure in the later style of English architecture, with a lofty square tower, surmounted by an octangular spire. On an eminence to the south-west of the city is the cemetery of St. Bartholomew, which was consecrated in 1639. Owing to the increase of population, chapels of ease are about to be built in some of the above parishes. There are places of worship for Baptists, the Society of Friends, Independents, Wesleyan and other Methodists, and Unitarians, a Roman Catholic chapel, and a Synagogue.

The free grammar school was founded by the citizens, before the date of the charter of Charles I., and in 1633 the corporation instituted certain ordinances for its better government: it is open to the sons of freemen gratuitously. There are fifteen exhibitions, to either Cambridge or Oxford, belonging to this seminary : viz., six of £36 each, of which two are for boys of the county of Devon, two for boys of the county of Cornwall, and two for the sons of freemen of the city; three of £30 each, for boys of any county, educated here; and eight of £8. The school-room forms part of the building called St. John's hospital, a convent of Augustine friars, founded in 1239, the revenue of which at the dissolution was £102 12. 9.; the present income, arising from various endowments, is nearly £800 per annum. Adjoining it is the mayor's chapel; and beneath the school-room and library there is a large open hall, for the sale of cloths, &c.: there are four masters, the first of them residing rent-free upon the spot. Within St. John's hospital is the Blue-coat school, founded by Hugh Crossing and others, in the year 1661; twenty-five boys, admitted from seven to ten years of age, are maintained, clothed, and educated, till they attain the age of fourteen, when they are dismissed with £6, as an apprentice fee: they are appointed by the governors, "from the city and county of Exeter, with the exception of those for whom a specific mode of nomination is appointed by the donors." The College school, at Mount Radford, is pleasantly situated, with extensive grounds attached, and was established in 1826, for the purpose of general instruction: it is supported by a number of shareholders, and managed by a body of directors; the principal is resident, together with one director, and the several masters receive boarders. The Blue Maids' school, for the instruction, clothing, and maintenance of seven poor girls, who, on leaving school, receive an apprentice fee of £4, was founded in 1672, by Sir John Maynard and Mrs. Elizabeth Stirt, and endowed with lands producing more than £100 per annum. St. Mary Arches parochial school was founded in 1686, by W. Wootton, for the instruction, on Dr. Bell's system, of forty-four boys, of whom thirty are clothed. The episcopal charity schools, originating with Bishop Blackall, in 1709, and supported by subscriptions, are open to all children of the parishes in Exeter, and the out-parish of St. Thomas: one hundred and seventy-six boys, and one hundred and thirty girls, are clothed and educated. The Ladies' school, in which fifty poor girls are educated, was established in 1804, and is supported by subscription. The Devon and Exeter Central school, "for promoting the education of the poor in the principles of the established church," was founded in 1811, and is supported by subscription: about four hundred and thirty boys, and two hundred and seventy girls, are taught to read and write, on the Madras system. The Exeter British school was established in 1807, for the instruction of children, without regard to sect or party; there are about one hundred and thirty boys, and as many girls in it. The Devon and Exeter infant school was established in 1825: there is a second school of the same kind, called "The West of England," &c. The dissenters' charity school, in St. Sidwell's parish, was established in 1780; the house had previously been used as an academy for dissenting ministers, and had a valuable library attached to it, but failing to obtain support, it was closed in 1772: the present school is supported by benefactions, subscriptions, &c., for clothing and educating about fifty male and female children. Between seven hundred and eight hundred children attend the Exeter Episcopal Sunday schools: there are also Sunday schools attached to most of the dissenting places of worship.

The Devon and Exeter hospital was opened for patients in 1743, and the present number of beds exceeds two hundred: it is supported by subscription, and has a considerable income arising from funded property: the affairs of the hospital are under the direction of a president, vice-presidents, and eighteen members, elected from the subscribers and benefactors: four physicians, four surgeons, and an apothecary, are attached to the institution. The Exeter dispensary is similarly supported. The Lunatic asylum, founded in 1795, is supported by an income arising from benefactions and legacies, and the payments received for the board of private patients: it is managed by a president, treasurer, two physicians, a surgeon, apothecary, matron, &c. An eye infirmary, and an institution for the instruction of the deaf and dumb, have been established, the latter of which is open to the poor of the counties of Devon, Cornwall, Dorset, and Somerset. A Female penitentiary was established in 1819. Here are also a Humane society; a society for the relief of clergymen, their widows, and orphans; a society for supplying the poor with clothing, coal, baby-linen, and medicine; and a lying-in charity. The Exeter workhouse is situated on the London road, a short distance from the city, and is of great extent; it was finished under an act of parliament, in 1707, and forms a large quadrangle, with a chapel in the centre: there are a house for the governor, spacious committee-rooms, and sufficient accommodation for several hundreds of the poor; the average number of inmates is about two hundred and forty. The Devon and Exeter savings bank was established in 1815. The Magdalene hospital is said to have been founded before the Crusades, for persons afflicted with leprosy; and, in 1244, the government of it was vested in the corporation, under whose management it still remains: since the extinction of the leprosy, it has been open to six poor scrofulous persons: the income is about £65 per annum: the ancient chapel is in ruins.

St. Catherine's almshouse was founded in 1457, for thirteen aged people, by John Stevens, who gave 17s. 4d. per annum to each of the pensioners; to which other benefactions have been added, making a total income of £32. Wynard's hospital was established in 1436, for providing lodging and subsistence to twelve infirm and elderly men, who are appointed by the corporation, and by Mr. Kennaway, who has the nomination of four of the inmates: the chapel attached to this institution is a handsome structure, the officiating minister of which is appointed by Mr. Kennaway. Grendon's, or the Ten Cells' almshouses, were founded in 1406, by S. Grendon, Esq., for ten unmarried men or women: they have an income of about £50 per annum, and are inhabited by ten widows. In 1479, John Palmer founded an almshouse for four poor women; it is managed by the corporation, who also nominate the three occupants of Moore's almshouse, founded in 1514. Hurst's almshouses were founded in 1568, for twelve poor tradesmen, or their widows, and are endowed with nearly £100 per annum. There is also in the parish of St. Mary Arches, an almshouse for two married couple, and two single persons, among whom the sum of 7s. 8d. is distributed weekly. Flaye's almshouses, consisting of six tenements, for the widows of poor clergymen and decayed tradesmen, were founded in 1634, the corporation being appointed trustees of the charity: the income is about £100 per annum. Six poor parishioners of St. Mary Arches are appointed by the corporation to the almshouse founded in 1669, by Christopher Lethbridge, Esq., which Sir Thomas Lethbridge endowed with £15. 12. per annum, to be divided equally among the pensioners. In St. John's parish is an endowed almshouse for six poor persons, founded by Alice Brooking. The city almshouses, for twelve aged people, rebuilt in 1764, with funds originating in a bequest by Richard Lant, in 1675, have an income of £170 per annum. Atwill's almshouses were founded and endowed by the corporation, with the arrears of Mr.

Atwill's charity, in 1771, for fifteen aged woollen manufacturers, appointed by the corporation: the annual income of this charity amounts to about £320. In St. Sidwell's parish are the ancient chapel and eight almshouses of St. Anne; the former has been lately repaired, and is open for divine service every Wednesday; the pensioners, who are appointed by the Dean and Chapter, receive each a quarterly allowance from the almshouse, and a weekly one from the Dean and Chapter: there was formerly an hermitage annexed to the chapel. There are also an old chapel and almshouses in the adjoining parish of Heavitree; besides which in this parish is an almshouse for four poor women, founded in 1676, by Mr. John Webb, the rental of the land belonging to which is about £30. A singular benefaction was made by one Griffin Ameridith, who bequeathed in trust to the corporation the annual proceeds of his lands at Sidbury, to be laid out in the purchase of shrouds and coffins for the bodies of malefactors executed at this place. The incorporated company of weavers and fullers meet twice a year in Tucker's hall; viz., in the months of August and November, for the purpose of arranging several charitable affairs with which they are entrusted: they give away twenty suits of clothes annually; and to such of the freemen's sons as have been educated in the school attached to this foundation, £5 each towards an apprentice fee. In addition to the above, there are various lands in the possession of the different parishes, the proceeds of which are applicable to general purposes of charity, and numerous individual bequests and donations.

Exeter still retains some proud vestiges of its ancient institutions and mural fortifications. In the vicinity are several ancient encampments, among which may be particularized that at Stoke Hill; it is semi-circular, and more than two hundred and fifty paces in diameter. The north, south, and east gates were taken down for the improvement of the city; but the walls in some places exhibit the original elevation, and may be correctly traced throughout. On the highest ground in the city, the north-west angle, stand the venerable remains of the Norman castle, supposed to occupy the site of that founded by Athelstan: it was denominated Rougemont castle from having been erected on a mound of red earth. A collegiate chapel was founded within its walls, by Avenell, the grandson of Baldwin de Brioniis, to which were attached four prebends: it served for the purpose of the assize chapel after the Reformation, but was taken down in 1782: its principal gateway, a lofty and picturesque object, still remains, as does also the greater part of the outer walls, from the summit of which is a delightful prospect over the city, on the south-east. The Benedictine priory of St. Nicholas is said to have been founded by William the Conqueror, and was at first subordinate to the abbey of Battle, in Sussex; it afterwards obtained from the parent house a renunciation of superior authority, the presentation remaining with the Abbot of Battle. At the dissolution, the revenue was £154. 12., when it was conveyed to the corporation, who demolished the buildings for the sake of the materials, and subsequently sold the property in lots. The walls may be traced to a considerable extent; and in Mint-lane are the remains of the crypt, with its massive Norman arches, &c. On the site of the ancient church stands the Roman Catholic chapel, opened in 1792. Here were also Franciscan and Dominican convents: the latter was converted, after its suppression, into a mansion belonging to the Bedford family; the site is now occupied by Bedford Crescent. In the neighbourhood are some remains of Polleshoo priory, founded in the reign of Richard I., of which, at the dissolution, the revenue was £170. 2. 3. At Cowick, in the parish of St. Thomas, there was also a monastery. Among the'most distinguished natives of this city, may be enumerated Josephus Iscanus, or Joseph of Exeter, a Latin poet of the twelfth century; his contemporary, Baldwin, Archbishop of Canterbury; John Hooker, who wrote a history of Exeter, in the sixteenth century; Sir Thomas Bodley, founder of the Bodleian library at Oxford; Dr. John Barcham, an eminent writer on heraldry, born in 1572; Matthew Lock, a composer of music in the seventeenth century; Lord Chancellor King, a distinguished lawyer and theological writer; the Rev. Thomas Yalden, a poet of eminence; Simon Ockley, a learned Orientalist; Dr. James Foster, a non-conformist divine, and theological writer of celebrity; William Jackson, an ingenious musical composer; Andrew Brice, author of a topographical dictionary; and the late Chief Justices Gibbs and Gifford. Exeter gives the titles of earl and marquis to the family of Cecil.

EXFORD, a parish in the hundred of CARHAMPTON, county of SOMERSET, 8½ miles (N. W. by N.) from Dulverton, containing 373 inhabitants. The living is a rectory, in the archdeaconry of Taunton, and diocese of Bath and Wells, rated in the king's books at £18. 2. 8½., and in the patronage of the Master and Fellows of Peter House, Cambridge. The church is dedicated to St. Mary Magdalene. Exford takes its name from its situation at one of the fords on the river Exe, over which is a stone bridge of three arches. The environs, for many miles, were at one time a forest, called Exmoor. Many curious plants and flowers grow here, and several barrows are scattered over the tract, together with circular intrenchments thrown up for religious rites or feats of exercise. A mile and a half westward from the church are vestiges of some very ancient iron-works, in which tradition says the entire wood of the forest has been consumed.

EXHALL, a parish in the county of the city of Coventry, 4¾ miles (N. by E.) from Coventry, containing 775 inhabitants. The living is a perpetual curacy, in the archdeaconry of Coventry, and diocese of Lichfield and Coventry. T. W. Knightly, Esq. was patron in 1805. The church is dedicated to St. Giles. There is a small sum for the education of children.

EXHALL, a parish in the Stratford division of the hundred of BARLICHWAY, county of WARWICK, 2½ miles (S. E. by S.) from Alcester, containing 209 inhabitants. The living is a rectory with the curacy of Wixford, in the archdeaconry and diocese of Worcester, rated in the king's books at £8. 17. 3½., endowed with £200 private benefaction, £200 royal bounty, and £300 parliamentary grant, and in the patronage of the Crown. The church is dedicated to St. Giles.

EXMINSTER, a parish in the hundred of EXMINSTER, county of DEVON, 5 miles (S. E. by S.) from Exeter, containing 928 inhabitants. The living is a vicarage, in the archdeaconry and diocese of Exeter, rated in the king's books at £12, and in the patronage of the Governors of Crediton Church Corporation

Trust. The church is dedicated to St. Martin. There is a charity school partly supported by the governors, and partly by subscription. At this village, which is very pleasantly situated on the west side of the river Exe, a fair is held on the first Thursday in May. The Exeter canal runs through the parish.

EXMOOR, an extra-parochial liberty in the hundred of WILLITON and FREEMANNERS, county of SOMERSET, containing 113 inhabitants. This was formerly a forest, and it is said that most of the wood was consumed in some iron-works near Exford, where the pits from which the ore was dug are still visible : a considerable part of this wild romantic waste has lately been brought into cultivation. In the time of the Druids, the forest was one of the spots where their religious rites were celebrated, and here are several circular intrenchments, which it is supposed were thrown up for that purpose.

EXMOUTH, a fashionable bathing-place, and chapelry, partly in the parish of WITHYCOMBE-RAW-LEIGH, but chiefly in that of LITTLEHAM, eastern division of the hundred of BUDLEIGH, county of DEVON, 11 miles (S. E. by S.) from Exeter, and 169½ (W. S.W.) from London. The population is returned with the respective parishes. This place, as its name implies, is situated at the mouth of the river Exe, on the coast of the English channel. The landing of the Danes here, in 1001 and 1003, probably first made it the object of attention as a maritime station, and occasioned the erection of a castle, to defend the entrance to the haven. The port appears to have been of some consequence in the beginning of the thirteenth century ; it sent two members to a council of state held at Westminster in the 14th of Edward III., and furnished ten ships, and one hundred and ninety-three men, towards the great naval armament of that king, at the commencement of his war with France. The Earl of March, afterwards Edward IV., on the defeat of the Yorkists at Ludlow, in 1459, fled into Devonshire, with the Earls of Salisbury, Warwick, and others, and took shipping at Exmouth, whence they sailed to Calais. During the great civil war, this place was alternately held by the royalist and parliamentary forces, and was finally taken by the latter in March, 1646. Whatever may have been the importance of Exmouth in former ages, it seems to have fallen into a state of decay, and about a century ago it was described as a small hamlet, inhabited chiefly by fishermen. Since that period it has attained celebrity as a bathing-place, being one of the oldest, and at present one of the most frequented, in the county. This is partly owing to the salubrity and mildness of the air, the town being open to the south-west, and sheltered by a hill from the east winds. It stands on the eastern side of the river, where two projecting sand banks form a partial enclosure, leaving an opening of about one-third of the width of the harbour. The river is here a mile and a half across; and, though the entrance is somewhat difficult, the harbour is extremely convenient, and the bar will admit of the passage of ships of more than three hundred tons' burden. The town, which is irregularly built, occupies the base and acclivity of a promontory called the Beacon Hill, the summit of which affords a noble view, extending from Buryhead, the southern boundary of Torbay, to the city of Exeter. On the strand are some good shops and lodg-ing-houses, with a convenient market-house, recently erected at the expense of Lord Rolle ; though that part of the town on the cliff facing the sea towards the south is more pleasantly situated. On this commanding eminence are two hotels and boarding-houses, one of which includes a subscription library, and billiard and card-rooms: and on the western beach are two pleasing specimens of Grecian architecture, in imitation of the temples of Theseus and the Winds, at Athens. Among various contemplated improvements in the neighbourhood is the formation of a new line of road between this place and Sidmouth, about a mile in length, intended to be lined with cottages. Exmouth is well supplied with water. There is no trade but that occasioned by the influx of visitors ; but among the lower classes most of the women are employed in lace-making. A small weekly market is held for provisions ; and there are fairs on the 25th of April and the 28th of October. The chapel, dedicated to St. Margaret, is the chief ornament of the town, occupying a conspicuous station on the Beacon Hill, and is a chapel of ease to the vicarage of Littleham : it was erected in 1825, by Lord Rolle, at the expense of £12,000 ; and it consists of a body and aisles, with a lofty square tower of great beauty, in the English style of architecture. Here are places of worship for the Independents and Wesleyan Methodists. Nearly two hundred children are educated in a National school founded by Lord Rolle, and endowed by Lady Rolle in 1816.

EXNING, a parish in the hundred of LACKFORD, county of SUFFOLK, 2 miles (N.W.) from Newmarket, containing 695 inhabitants. The living is a vicarage, with the curacy of Landwade, in the archdeaconry of Sudbury, and diocese of Norwich, rated in the king's books at £13. 7. 6., and in the patronage of the Dean and Chapter of Canterbury. The church is dedicated to St. Martin. There is a place of worship for Wesleyan Methodists.

EXTON, a parish in the hundred of ALSTOE, county of RUTLAND, 5½ miles (N.E. by E.) from Oakham, containing 735 inhabitants. The living is a discharged vicarage, with the rectory of Horn united, in the archdeaconry of Northampton, and diocese of Peterborough, rated in the king's books at £8. 7. 8., endowed with £200 private benefaction, and £200 royal bounty. Sir Gerard Noel Noel, Bart. was patron in 1817. The church, dedicated to St. Peter and St. Paul, is principally in the later English style, with a handsome steeple. There is an endowed school, founded in 1702 by Henry Forster, Esq., of which the justices of the peace for the county are patrons.

EXTON, a parish in the hundred of WILLITON and FREEMANNERS, county of SOMERSET, 4 miles (N. by E.) from Dulverton, containing 301 inhabitants. The living is a rectory, in the archdeaconry of Taunton, and diocese of Bath and Wells, rated in the king's books at £14. 12. 11. J. Everard, and J. Jeffery, Esqrs. were patrons in 1822. The church is dedicated to St. Peter. The village stands on an eminence overlooking the river Exe, from which it derives its name.

EXTON, a parish in the hundred of FAWLEY, Fawley division of the county of SOUTHAMPTON, 4¾ miles (N.E. by E.) from Bishop's Waltham, containing 293 inhabitants. The living is a rectory, in the peculiar jurisdiction of the incumbent, rated in the king's books at £10. 6. 0½., and in the patronage of the Bishop of Winchester. The church is principally in the early

English style, with some insertions of a later date. This parish is within the jurisdiction of the Cheyney Court held at Winchester every Thursday, for the recovery of debts to any amount.

EXTWISTLE, a joint township with Brierscliffe, in that part of the parish of WHALLEY which is in the higher division of the hundred of BLACKBURN, county palatine of LANCASTER, 3¼ miles (E.N.E.) from Burnley, containing 1407 inhabitants.

EYAM, a parish in the hundred of HIGH PEAK, county of DERBY, comprising the townships of Eyam and Woodland-Eyam, and the hamlet of Foolow, and containing 1516 inhabitants, of which number, 1021 are in the township of Eyam, 1½ mile (N.W. by W.) from Stony-Middleton. The living is a rectory, in the archdeaconry of Derby, and diocese of Lichfield and Coventry, rated in the king's books at £13. 15. 5. The Duke of Devonshire was patron in 1826. The church is dedicated to St. Helen. There is a place of worship for Wesleyan Methodists. A free school is endowed with about £12 per annum, for which twenty poor children are educated: the school-house was rebuilt in 1826, by voluntary contribution. In September and October, 1665, the infection having been conveyed hither in a package from London, four-fifths of the inhabitants of the village were carried off by the plague. This parish is within the honour of Tutbury, duchy of Lancaster, and within the jurisdiction of a court of pleas held at Tutbury every third Tuesday, for the recovery of debts under 40s. Ann Seward, poetess and novelist, was a native of this place, of which her father was rector.

EYDON, a parish in the hundred of CHIPPING-WARDEN, county of NORTHAMPTON, 9½ miles (S. by W.) from Daventry, containing 548 inhabitants. The living is a rectory, in the archdeaconry of Northampton, and diocese of Peterborough, rated in the king's books at £16. 16. 3., and in the patronage of the Crown. The church, which is dedicated to St. Nicholas, has lately received an addition of ninety-seven sittings, of which seventy are free, the Incorporated Society for the enlargement of churches and chapels having granted £45 towards defraying the expense.

EYE, a parish in the hundred of WOLPHY, county of HEREFORD, 3½ miles (N.) from Leominster, comprising the townships of Ashton, Eye-Moreton, and Luston, and containing 678 inhabitants. The living is a discharged vicarage, in the archdeaconry and diocese of Hereford, rated in the king's books at £7. 19. 2., and in the patronage of the Crown. The church is dedicated to St. Peter and St. Paul. There is a charity school supported by subscription. A court leet is held occasionally.

EYE, a parish in the liberty of PETERBOROUGH, county of NORTHAMPTON, 3¼ miles (N.E.) from Peterborough, containing 747 inhabitants. The living is a perpetual curacy, in the archdeaconry of Northampton, and diocese of Peterborough, endowed with £200 private benefaction, £400 royal bounty, and £600 parliamentary grant, and in the patronage of the Bishop of Peterborough. The church is dedicated to St. Matthew. There is a place of worship for Wesleyan Methodists.

EYE, a joint liberty with Dunsden, in that part of the parish of SONNING which is in the hundred of BINFIELD, county of OXFORD, 5 miles (S. by W.) from Henley upon Thames, containing 845 inhabitants.

EYE, a borough, market town, and parish, having separate jurisdiction, though locally in the hundred of Hartismere, county of SUFFOLK, 20½ miles (N.) from Ipswich, and 89½ (N.E. by N.) from London, containing 1882 inhabitants. The name of this place, anciently *Eay*, is derived from its situation on a tract of land almost surrounded with water, and in the adjoining fields small rudders, iron rings, and other articles of shipping tackle, have been frequently turned up by the plough. Soon after the Conquest, Robert, son of Robert Malet, who had accompanied William I. to England, having obtained the honour of Eye (of which he was afterwards dispossessed for taking part with Robert, Duke of Normandy), erected a castle here, of which there are still some slight remains at the foot of the Mill Hill. The same Robert Malet also founded a Benedictine monastery, dedicated to St. Peter, to which was annexed the episcopal see at Dunwich. In this monastery was preserved St. Felix' book of the Gospels, written in large Lombardic characters, and called the Red Book, on which the people used to be sworn, and which was removed from the abbey at Dunwich when that place was destroyed by the sea. The revenue at the dissolution was £184. 9. 7.: the remains of the buildings, which are to the east of the town, have been converted into stables. The town is pleasantly situated in a valley, surrounded on all sides by streams of excellent water, and within a distance of two miles from the high road from London to Norwich. A news-room is supported by subscription. The principal branch of manufacture is that of British lace, which, since the introduction of machinery, has been declining. The market is on Tuesday for corn, and there is also a market for butter and vegetables on Saturday: the fairs are on Whit-Monday, for pigs and toys; and July 22nd, for lambs and cattle. The government, by charter of incorporation from King John, confirmed by Queen Elizabeth and William III., is vested in two bailiffs, a recorder, ten capital burgesses, and twenty-four common council-men, assisted by a town clerk and other officers. The bailiffs are chosen annually on the Saturday preceding, and sworn into office on, the 29th of September: the late bailiffs act as coroners for the following year: the town clerk is appointed by the bailiffs and ten principal burgesses, and the other officers are chosen by the common council-men. The freedom of the borough is inherited by the eldest son only of a freeman, whether born within the borough or not; acquired by servitude to a master living within the borough during the whole term of apprenticeship, or obtained by gift. The bailiffs are justices of the peace, the county magistrates having concurrent jurisdiction within the borough. The corporation have the power to hold a court of record every Saturday, under a charter of the 9th of William III., for the recovery of debts to any amount, but this court has not been held since Jan 1st., 1816. Courts leet are held annually within a month after Lady-day and Michaelmas. The town-hall is a handsome building in the centre of the town, adjoining the house of industry. A new gaol has been erected, which is a

Seal and Arms.

lofty and commodious edifice, well adapted to its purpose. The elective franchise was conferred in the thirteenth of Elizabeth, since which time the borough has regularly returned two members to parliament: the right of election is vested in the free burgesses generally, in number about two hundred, who are chiefly in the interest of Marquis Cornwallis : the bailiffs are the returning officers.

The living is a vicarage, in the archdeaconry of Sudbury, and diocese of Norwich, rated in the king's books at £11. 14. 7., and in the patronage of Major General Sir Edward Kerrison, Bart. The church, dedicated to St. Peter and St. Paul, is a spacious and handsome structure, with a fine square tower in the later style of English architecture : in the chancel is a very ancient tomb much defaced, and in the north aisle a curious piece of sculpture representing the good Samaritan. There are places of worship for Baptists and Wesleyan Methodists. A free grammar school, the founder of which is unknown, is endowed by the corporation with £10 per annum for the master, and with the rents of some land for the support of an usher ; there are twenty boys at present on the foundation of this school, which has two exhibitions to Cambridge for sons of freemen born in the borough. A National school for children of both sexes is supported by subscription. An almshouse was founded in 1636, by Mr. Nicholas Bedingfield, who endowed it with certain lands and houses in Eye, for the support of four poor widows, or aged unmarried women. Marquis Cornwallis enjoys the inferior title of Baron Cornwallis, of Eye, in the county of Suffolk.

EYFORD, an extra-parochial liberty, in the upper division of the hundred of SLAUGHTER, county of GLOUCESTER, 2½ miles (W. by S.) from Stow on the Wold, containing 67 inhabitants. The Duke of Shrewsbury had a mansion here, in which he received a visit from William III. ; and in a summer-house, now destroyed, Milton is said to have written a great part of his "Paradise Lost."

EYKE, a parish in the hundred of LOES, county of SUFFOLK, 3¾ miles (E. N. E.) from Woodbridge, containing 396 inhabitants. The living is a discharged rectory, in the archdeaconry of Suffolk, and diocese of Norwich, rated in the king's books at £15, endowed with £200 private benefaction, and £200 royal bounty. The Rev. Jacob Chilton was patron in 1776. The church is dedicated to All Saints.

EYNESBURY, a parish in the hundred of TOSELAND, county of HUNTINGDON, ½ a mile (S.) from St. Neot's, containing 903 inhabitants. The living is a rectory, in the archdeaconry of Huntingdon, and diocese of Lincoln, rated in the king's books at £32. 3. 9. William Palmer, Esq. was patron in 1808. The church, dedicated to St. Mary, was built in the reign of James II.

EYNESFORD, a parish in the hundred of AXTON, DARTFORD, and WILMINGTON, lathe of SUTTON at HONE, county of KENT, 6 miles (S. E.) from Foot's Cray, containing, with the hamlet of Crockinhill, 1077 inhabitants. The living is a vicarage, in the peculiar jurisdiction of the Archbishop of Canterbury, rated in the king's books at £12.: there is also a sinecure rectory, rated at £12. 16. 8. The Archbishop of Canterbury appoints the rector, and the rector presents to the vicarage. The church, dedicated to St. Martin, is of early Norman

construction, and, though it has been greatly altered by subsequent repairs, still exhibits a very curious ornamented door-way. The Baptists have a place of worship here. There is a school at Crockinhill, for the instruction of the children of this parish, founded by Thomas Palmer, in 1809, and endowed by himself and others : besides this, nine children are sent to the charity school at Tonbridge, on the foundation of Sir Thomas Dyke. Eynesford, through which the Darent passes, takes its name from a noted ford on that river, on the east bank of which are the ruins of a castle, supposed to have been erected in the Norman times by a family named De Eysford.

EYTHORN, a parish in the hundred of EASTRY, lathe of ST. AUGUSTINE, county of KENT, 6¼ miles (N. N. W.) from Dovor, containing 390 inhabitants. The living is a rectory, with the curacy of Sutton, in the archdeaconry and diocese of Canterbury, rated in the king's books at £15. 12. 6., and in the patronage of the Earl of Guildford and T. Papillon, Esq., alternately. The church, dedicated to St. Peter and St. Paul, has portions in the later English style. There is a place of worship for Baptists. A fair for toys and pedlary is held on Midsummer-day. At the southern extremity of this parish is a Roman intrenchment, and near Eythorn Court Wood a large barrow or tumulus.

EYTHORPE, a hamlet in the parish of WADDESDON, hundred of ASHENDON, county of BUCKINGHAM, 4 miles (W.) from Aylesbury. The population is returned with the parish. Here was formerly a chapel, now demolished.

EYTON, a parish in the hundred of WOLPHY, county of HEREFORD, 2¼ miles (N. W. by N.) from Leominster, containing 125 inhabitants. The living is a perpetual curacy, in the archdeaconry and diocese of Hereford, endowed with £400 private benefaction, and £1200 royal bounty, and in the patronage of the Governors of Lucton school. The church is dedicated to All Saints. The boys of this parish are entitled to free instruction at Lucton school. The river Lugg runs between this place and Kingsland.

EYTON, a township in that part of the parish of ABBERBURY which is in the hundred of FORD, county of SALOP, 7 miles (W.) from Shrewsbury, containing 65 inhabitants.

EYTON upon SEVERN, a chapelry in the parish of WROXETER, Wellington division of the hundred of BRADFORD (South), county of SALOP, 6¾ miles (N. W. by N.) from Much Wenlock. The population is returned with the parish. The chapel is dedicated to All Saints.

EYTON upon the WILD MOORS, a parish in the Wellington division of the hundred of BRADFORD (South), county of SALOP, 2½ miles (N.) from Wellington, containing 390 inhabitants. The living is a discharged rectory, annexed to the vicarage of Wellington, in the archdeaconry of Salop, and diocese of Lichfield and Coventry, rated in the king's books at £2. 14. 9½., and in the patronage of T. Eyton, Esq. The church is dedicated to All Saints : there is no burial-ground at this place. Edward, the celebrated Lord Herbert of Chirbury, was born here in 1581 : in 1625 he was created a baron of the kingdom of Ireland, and in 1631 was elevated to the English peerage : his lordship died in 1648.

EYWORTH, a parish in the hundred of BIGGLES-WADE, county of BEDFORD, 4½ miles (E. by N.) from Biggleswade, containing 111 inhabitants. The living is a discharged vicarage, in the archdeaconry of Bedford, and diocese of Lincoln, rated in the king's books at £6. 13. 4. Lord Yarborough was patron in 1792. The church, which is dedicated to All Saints, contains some interesting monuments.

F.

FACCOMBE, a parish in the hundred of PASTROW, Kingsclere division of the county of SOUTHAMPTON, 8½ miles (N. by E.) from Andover, containing 305 inhabitants. The living is a rectory, in the archdeaconry and diocese of Winchester, rated in the king's books at £26. 2. 3½., and in the patronage of the Rev. Edwin Lance. The church, dedicated to St. Michael, contains some ancient monuments of the Lucies. There is a chapel of ease at Tangley, in this parish. The Wesleyan Methodists have a place of worship here. The Wansdyke, or Wodensdyke, supposed to have been one of the boundaries during the Heptarchy, passes through the parish.

FACEBY, a chapelry in the parish of WHORLTON, western division of the liberty of LANGBAURGH, North riding of the county of YORK, 4½ miles (S.W. by S.) from Stokesley, containing 178 inhabitants. The living is a perpetual curacy with that of Carleton, in the archdeaconry of Cleveland, and diocese of York, endowed with £200 royal bounty, and £200 parliamentary grant.

FADDILEY, a township in the parish of ACTON, hundred of NANTWICH, county palatine of CHESTER, 4¾ miles (W. by N.) from Nantwich, containing 291 inhabitants. A domestic chapel was built at Woodhey by the relict of Sir Thomas Wilbraham, who, in 1703, endowed it with a rent-charge on the manor of Newton, in Staffordshire, of £25 per annum, of which £20 is paid to a minister appointed by the Earl of Dysart, £2 to the clerk, and £3 for repairs. There is a place of worship for Wesleyan Methodists.

FADMORE, a township in the parish of KIRKBY-MOORSIDE, wapentake of RYEDALE, North riding of the county of YORK, 6¾ miles (N. E.) from Helmsley, containing 162 inhabitants.

FAILSWORTH, a township in the parish of MAN-CHESTER, hundred of SALFORD, county palatine of LANCASTER, 4¼ miles (N.E. by E.) from Manchester, containing 3358 inhabitants.

FAIRBURN, a township in the parish of LEDSHAM, upper division of the wapentake of BARKSTONE-ASH, West riding of the county of YORK, 2¼ miles (N. N.W.) from Ferry-Bridge, containing 426 inhabitants. It is situated on the banks of the Aire, and abounds with limestone. A cut has been made from a canal in the vicinity, and a tunnel is about to be constructed under the village, for the greater convenience of the lime-works.

FAIRFIELD, a chapelry in the parish of HOPE, hundred of HIGH PEAK, county of DERBY, 1 mile (E. N.E.) from Buxton, containing 482 inhabitants. The living is a perpetual curacy, in the peculiar jurisdiction and patronage of the Dean and Chapter of Lichfield.

The chapel is dedicated to St. Peter. Anthony Swann, in 1662, bequeathed £4 a year for teaching ten children; in 1693, Rowland Swann left a trifling sum for books; and in 1771, the commissioners of enclosures allotted land of the annual value of £10, in augmentation of the master's salary.

FAIRFIELD, a parish in the hundred of ALOES-BRIDGE, lathe of SHEPWAY, county of KENT, 6¼ miles (W. by N.) from New Romney, containing 86 inhabitants. The living is a perpetual curacy, in the archdeaconry and diocese of Canterbury, and in the patronage of the Dean and Chapter of Canterbury. The church is dedicated to St. Thomas à Becket.

FAIRFIELD, a hamlet in the parish of ASHTON under LINE, hundred of SALFORD, county palatine of LANCASTER, 3¾ miles (E. by S.) from Manchester. The population is returned with the parish. The Moravians have an establishment here; the ground plot forms a spacious square area, the houses in which are neatly built of brick: there is also a chapel with a burial-ground.

FAIRFIELD, a hamlet in that part of the parish of STOGURSEY which is in the hundred of WILLITON and FREEMANNERS, county of SOMERSET, 9½ miles (N. W. by W.) from Bridg-water. The population is returned with the parish. Here was formerly a chapel.

FAIRFIELD-HEAD, a township in the parish of ALLSTONEFIELD, northern division of the hundred of TOTMONSLOW, county of STAFFORD, 7½ miles (N.E. by E.) from Leek, containing 1135 inhabitants.

FAIRFORD, a market town and parish in the hundred of BRIGHTWELLS-BARROW, county of GLOUCES-TER, 24 miles (S.E. by E.) from Gloucester, and 80 (W. by N.) from London, containing 1547 inhabitants. The name of this place is of uncertain etymology, being derived either from the Saxon word *faran*, to pass, or the words *fair* and *ford*, in allusion to the convenience it possesses for crossing the river Colne, on which it is situated, near the confluence of that river with the Thames. About the middle of the ninth century, the manor of Fairford belonged to the kings of Mercia; and at the period of the Norman survey, to Maud, the consort of William I.; and after various changes, it came into the possession of Henry VII., who sold it to John Tame, a merchant. The town is situated at the foot of the Cotswold hills, and consists principally of one long street, irregularly formed, and neither lighted nor paved : there are several good detached houses, but the buildings in general are mean : the inhabitants are supplied with water from wells and springs as well as from the Colne, across which are two neat bridges. A market is held on Thursday, by charter obtained about 1668; and there are fairs on May 14th and Nov. 12th.

The parish is divided into three tythings, viz., the borough, which is governed by its own constable, East End, and Mill-town End, each of which has a tything-man. The living is a vicarage, in the archdeaconry and diocese of Gloucester, rated in the king's books at £13. 11. 5½., and in the patronage of the Dean and Chapter of Gloucester. The church, dedicated to the Virgin Mary, presents a fine specimen of the style of English architecture which prevailed about the end of the fifteenth century, and is also an object of considerable interest for its curious windows of painted glass : it consists of a nave, aisles, and chancel, with a central tower, and is ornamented with buttresses, battlements, pinnacles, and canopied niches, formerly filled with statues : the aisles are separated from the nave and chancel by light clustered pillars, sustaining six pointed arches on each side : an elegantly carved oak screen separates the chancel from the nave and aisles; the former contains some stalls and tabernacle-work : there is also a very fine oak ceiling, and the pavement of the church is chequered with blue and white stone. The erection of this beautiful edifice is attributed to John Tame, Esq., a rich London merchant, who, in trading to Italy about 1492, captured a Flemish vessel bound for Rome, on board of which was a quantity of stained glass ; having purchased the manor of Fairford, he commenced building the church in 1493, but his death taking place in 1500, it was finished by his son, Sir Edmund Tame, Knt. The stained glass was found sufficient to fill twenty-eight windows, with four or more compartments in each ; some of the figures, however, have been displaced, and others mutilated, owing to the glass having been removed in the reign of Charles I., to preserve it from being destroyed by the puritans. The paintings are exceedingly well executed, but by an unknown artist, and consist of representations of events in Scripture history, of figures of the Fathers of the Christian church and of some of the Roman emperors. Of these windows twenty-five only remain : the best is the third in the north aisle, which represents the Salutation of the Virgin, with a fine perspective of the interior of the temple : the great east and west windows retain their original perfection ; the subject of the former is Christ's entry into Jerusalem, remarkable for the splendour of its colours ; that of the latter is the last Judgment, exhibiting a grotesque and fearful assemblage of imagery : they are protected by a lattice of wire, constructed in 1725. In the north aisle is an altar-tomb, with brasses, exhibiting effigies of the founder and his wife, with escutcheons and commemorative inscriptions ; there are also monuments to the memory of Sir Edward Tame and other persons of distinction. There are places of worship for Baptists and Independents. A bequest of £1000 was made, in 1704, by the Hon. Elizabeth Farmor, daughter of Lord Lempster, to be expended in land, for the maintenance of an afternoon lecture every Sunday in the church, and for the foundation and support of a free school, which is also endowed with a subsequent bequest of £500 by her cousin, Mrs. Mary Barker, besides other benefactions. The schoolroom was erected in 1738 : the total annual income is £136. 19.; the disbursements are, £60 to the master, £25 to the mistress, and £5 for books : sixty boys and sixty girls are instructed on the National plan, the schools being now connected with the central establishment. The nomination of the lecturer, schoolmaster, and scholars, was vested in Samuel Barker, Esq., and his heirs. Lady Mico, sister to Elizabeth, wife of Andrew Barker, Esq., gave £400, to apprentice four boys annually, which was vested in the purchase of lands in Lechlade, and yields an income of £68. 10.; and she likewise left a weekly gift of bread to the poor, who enjoy the benefit of several other benefactions. This town gives the title of viscount to the Earl of Hillsborough.

FAIRHAUGH, a township in the parish of Allen-TON, western division of Coquetdale ward, county of Northumberland, 13 miles (N.N.W.) from Rothbury, containing 8 inhabitants, and only one house.

FAIRLIGHT, a parish in the hundred of Guestling, rape of Hastings, county of Sussex, 2½ miles (E.N.E.) from Hastings, containing 477 inhabitants. The living is a vicarage, in the archdeaconry of Lewes, and diocese of Chichester, rated in the king's books at £6. 9. 2., and in the patronage of the Rev. Mr. Pierce. The church, dedicated to St. Andrew, is in the early style of English architecture. The parish is bounded on the south by the English channel, and the Royal Military canal terminates here.

FAIRSTED, a parish in the hundred of Witham, county of Essex, 4 miles (W.N.W.) from Witham, containing 263 inhabitants. The living is a rectory, in the archdeaconry of Colchester, and diocese of London, rated in the king's books at £6. 13. 4., and in the patronage of the Bishop of London. The church is dedicated to St. Mary.

FAITH (ST.), a parish within the liberty of the soke, and adjacent to the city, of Winchester, county of Southampton, containing, with the extra-parochial liberty of the Hospital of St. Cross, 372 inhabitants. The living is a rectory not in charge, with the chaplaincy of the Hospital of St. Cross annexed to it, in the peculiar jurisdiction and patronage of the Bishop of Winchester.

FAKENHAM, a market town and parish in the hundred of Gallow, county of Norfolk, 25½ miles (N.W.) from Norwich, and 109 (N.N.E.) from London, containing, with the hamlet of Alethorpe, 1635 inhabitants. Its ancient name was Fakenham-Lancaster, but the adjunct is not used. The town is pleasantly situated on a declivity north of the river Yare ; the streets are paved with flint-stone, and partially lighted with oil; the inhabitants are plentifully supplied with water from springs. Here were formerly a manufactory for crape and bombazine, and some celebrated salt pits, but they have all been discontinued. The market is on Thursday, for corn and cattle, and is well attended by dealers from a considerable distance : two fairs, on Whit-Tuesday and November 22nd, principally for cattle, are held on Hampton Green, about one mile from the town. The county magistrates hold here a session for the hundred every month ; and courts leet and baron for the manor are held annually. The quarter sessions for this district were formerly held at Fakenham and Walsingham alternately; but they have been transferred hence to Holt, and the sessions-house has been converted into a school-room : there is a court-house for transacting parochial business. The inhabitants are exempted from serving on juries, &c. The living is a rectory, in the archdeaconry of Norfolk, and diocese of Norwich, rated in the king's books at £35. 6. 8., and in the patronage of the Master and Fellows of Trinity College, Cambridge. The church, dedicated to St. Peter, is a handsome and commodious edifice, consisting of a nave, aisles, chancel, and south porch, with a stately tower of stone at the west end, where is a noble door-way surmounted by a lofty window divided into six compartments, and sub-divided by horizontal mullions and tracery mouldings ; on each side of the door is a canopied niche, the buttresses of which are adorned with panelling : the font is octangular, and richly embellished with carvings of the arms of the duchy of Lancaster. An organ has been recently presented by the rector, to whom the parishioners are likewise indebted for some emblematical designs in stained glass which decorate the chancel window. There are places of worship for Baptists, Independents, and Primitive and Wesleyan Methodists. A Lancasterian school for boys is supported by voluntary contributions, and there is a National school for girls. Lady Mary Townshend bequeathed a house and land in 1672, directing the proceeds to be applied in apprenticing poor children.

FAKENHAM (MAGNA), a parish in the hundred of BLACKBOURN, county of SUFFOLK, 5 miles (S. S. E.) from Thetford, containing 214 inhabitants. The living is a discharged rectory, in the archdeaconry of Sudbury, and diocese of Norwich, rated in the king's books at £11. 10. 5., and in the patronage of the Duke of Grafton. The church is dedicated to St. Peter.

FAKENHAM (PARVA), a hamlet (formerly a parish) in the parish of EUSTON, hundred of BLACKBOURN, county of SUFFOLK, 4½ miles (S.S.E.) from Thetford. The population is returned with Euston. The living, a rectory not in charge, is united to that of Euston, in the archdeaconry of Sudbury, and diocese of Norwich. The church, which was dedicated to St. Andrew, has been demolished.

FALDINGWORTH, a parish in the wapentake of LAWRESS, parts of LINDSEY, county of LINCOLN, 5 miles (S.W.) from Market-Raisen, containing 276 inhabitants. The living is a rectory, in the archdeaconry of Stow, and diocese of Lincoln, rated in the king's books at £15. 8. 1½., and in the patronage of Earl Brownlow. The church is dedicated to All Saints. There is a free school with an endowment of £5 per annum.

FALFIELD, a chapelry in the parish, and lower division of the hundred, of THORNBURY, county of GLOUCESTER, 4 miles (N. E. by E.) from Thornbury, containing, with Moorton, 844 inhabitants.

FALKENHAM, a parish in the hundred of COLNEIS, county of SUFFOLK, 8½ miles (E. S. E.) from Ipswich, containing 285 inhabitants. The living is a discharged vicarage, in the archdeaconry of Suffolk, and diocese of Norwich, rated in the king's books at £7. 11. 3., and in the patronage of the Crown. The church is dedicated to St. Ethelbert. The navigable river Deben runs through the parish.

FALKINGHAM, or FOLKINGHAM, a market town and parish in the wapentake of AVELAND, parts of KESTEVEN, county of LINCOLN, 26½ miles (S.S.E.) from Lincoln, and 102½ (N. by W.) from London, containing 759 inhabitants. This town is supposed to have originated from a baronial castle in the vicinity, said to have been built by Henry de Beaumont, lord of the manor in the reign of Edward I., which having been garrisoned by the royalists in the time of Charles I., was subsequently demolished by order of Cromwell: it occupies an elevation which commands an extensive view over the fens. The streets are clean and well paved, and the inhabitants well supplied with water from springs. There is a small market on Thursday; fairs are held on Ash-Wednesday, Palm-Monday, and May 19th, for horses and sheep; June 15th and 16th, for horses and cattle; July 3d, for hemp and hardware; and on the

Thursday after Old Michaelmas-day, and November 22d, for horses, cattle, &c. A court leet is held annually for the manor, on the 1st or 2d of November: the petty sessions for the parts of Kesteven, formerly held here, have been removed to Bourn. In the year 1808, a new prison, or house of correction, was erected on the site of the ancient castle, at an expense of £6600, which was defrayed by a rate on the county; in 1825, a further sum of £8000 was expended in making considerable additions: it is now capable of containing from sixty to seventy prisoners, and is intended for a district which comprises five market towns and two hundred and eleven villages: the jurisdiction and superintendence are vested in the magistrates for the parts of Kesteven, who appoint six officers belonging to the prison, viz., a chaplain, surgeon, surveyor, keeper, matron, and turnkey. There are ten day-rooms and airing-yards, used by the five classes of male and female prisoners, as directed by act of parliament in the 4th of George IV., and within the walls are a chapel and a tread-mill. The male prisoners sentenced to hard labour are employed at the tread-wheel, and the females in knitting and spinning, and they are severally allowed one-fourth of their earnings; prisoners not committed for hard labour, who work voluntarily, receive one-half, and those committed for trial three-fourths. The living is a rectory, with the vicarage of Laughton united, in the archdeaconry and diocese of Lincoln, rated in the king's books at £21. 12. 3½., and in the patronage of Sir Gilbert Heathcote, Bart. The church, which is dedicated to St. Andrew, is a spacious and handsome structure, principally in the later style of English architecture; the chancel is of earlier date, and exhibits some fine decorated windows; and the tower, which is the most remarkable part of the edifice, has a rich battlement and eight pinnacles. The free grammar school is open to all the children of the parish: the master has a salary of £30 per annum, in addition to £40 per annum which is chargeable on land near the town, and was bequeathed by J. R. Brokesby, Esq.; other benefactions have been made to provide clothing for a certain number of the scholars.

FALLOWDON, a township in the parish of EMBLETON, southern division of BAMBROUGH ward, county of NORTHUMBERLAND, 7½ miles (N. N.E.) from Alnwick, containing 112 inhabitants. Thomas Wood, Esq., in 1764, bequeathed a rent-charge of £5 a year upon an estate in this township, for teaching poor children.

FALLOWFIELD, a township in the parish of ST. JOHN, LEE, southern division of TINDALE ward, county of NORTHUMBERLAND, 3¼ miles (N.) from Hexham, containing 93 inhabitants. A rich vein of lead-ore is wrought in the neighbourhood. About half a mile south of the remains of the Roman wall is Written Crag, on which is legibly inscribed " PETRA FLAVI CARANTINI. "

FALLOWLEES, a township in the parish of ROTHBURY, western division of COQUETDALE ward, county of NORTHUMBERLAND, 5¾ miles (S.S.W.) from Rothbury, containing 3 inhabitants.

FALLYBROOM, a township in the parish of PRESTBURY, hundred of MACCLESFIELD, county palatine of CHESTER, 1¾ mile (N. W. by W.) from Macclesfield, containing 31 inhabitants.

FALMER, a parish in the hundred of YOUNSMERE,

rape of Lewes, county of Sussex, 4 miles (N.E.) from Brighton, containing 437 inhabitants. The living is a discharged vicarage, with the rectory of Stanmer united, in the archdeaconry of Lewes, and diocese of Chichester, rated in the king's books at £6.10.10., endowed with £250 private benefaction, and £200 royal bounty, and in the patronage of the Earl of Chichester.

Arms.

FALMOUTH, a parish in the hundred of Kerrier, county of Cornwall, comprising the sea-port and market town of Falmouth, which possesses exclusive jurisdiction, and containing 6374 inhabitants, exclusively of a portion of the parish of Budock, which extends into Falmouth, in which there are 4392 persons, 54 miles (S.W.) from Launceston, and 267 (W.S.W.) from London. The name of this place is derived from its situation at the mouth of the river Fal: the origin of the town may be dated subsequently to the year 1600, but the haven was well known long before that period, and resorted to by ships bound for British ports, having been considered one of the most secure and commodious in Great Britain. The earliest mention of it in history occurs in the reign of Henry IV., when the Duchess Dowager of Bretagne landed here on her arrival in England, to celebrate her nuptials with that monarch. Until 1613 there was only a single house of entertainment for sea-faring persons, and perhaps a few fishermen's cottages on the site of the present town, at which period John (afterwards Sir John) Killigrew, to whom the ground belonged, began to build several new houses, and met with much opposition from the corporations of Penryn, Truro, and Helston, who united to petition King James against the work, stating the evil consequences they anticipated to their own interests, should a town be built at Falmouth harbour. The matter was referred to the lords of the council, and by them decided in Killigrew's favour; the buildings therefore proceeded rapidly, and the town soon became a place of great trade. Soon after 1670, Sir Peter Killigrew, Bart. constructed a new quay, and procured an act of parliament to secure certain duties to be paid to himself and his heirs; and the subsequent establishment of the post-office packets to Lisbon, the West Indies, &c., contributed much to the increasing prosperity of the place. In 1664, the houses in Falmouth amounted to two hundred; before 1700, they had increased to nearly three hundred and fifty; about 1750, to between five and six hundred; and, in 1811, there were 647 inhabited houses in the town and suburbs within the parish, exclusively of seventy-two in the adjoining parish of Budock. In its infancy this town was called Smithick, under which appellation it is mentioned in a resolution of the House of Commons, in January, 1653, appointing a weekly market; the first record which mentions the name of Falmouth is the charter of incorporation, bearing date 1661. It was made a separate parish in 1664, having up to that period been a part of Budock, a portion of which still extends into this town.

The town is agreeably situated on the south-western shore of that branch of the harbour which stretches to Penryn, and consists principally of one main street, which, under different names, extends about a mile in length, paved, well lighted with gas, and amply supplied with water. The buildings in general are modern and have a neat appearance; behind are rising grounds which overlook the harbour and the town. On each side of the entrance to the harbour are the castles of St. Mawes and Pendennis; the latter, which is on the western side, being built upon a peninsular eminence, two miles in circumference at the base, and rising upwards of three hundred feet above the level of the sea, has a very majestic appearance: it is strongly fortified, and contains commodious barracks, storehouses, and magazines, with apartments for the lieutenant-governor. The castle of St. Mawes, on the opposite side, in the parish of St. Just, is inferior, both in size and situation. There are reading and billiard-rooms and a theatre: a musical society, called the Philharmonic Society, has been established.

The trade of Falmouth, from its advantageous position, soon became extensive, and it is now one of the principal ports in the West of England, being scarcely inferior to any in its advantages as a rendezvous for outward and homeward bound fleets. In many instances, vessels have made their voyage from this harbour, while those from Plymouth and Portsmouth have been forced back by contrary winds, before they could reach the mouth of the channel: outward bound ships from Liverpool, Bristol, Greenock, &c. rendezvous here to join convoy, and thus avoid a tedious navigation up and down the channel; while, for a similar reason, the masters and supercargoes of homeward bound vessels call to ascertain the state of the British and continental markets, or to receive orders from their owners or correspondents for regulating their further proceedings. This port has for many years carried on a very extensive foreign trade; it was one of the first ports in the western counties to which the privileges of the bonding act were extended, and is the only tobacco port in the counties of Cornwall and Devon: its jurisdiction extends from Helford river westward, to the Deadman point eastward. The imports are,—from America, wood, wheat, flour, staves, rice, &c.; from Spain and Portugal, fruit, wine, wool, salt, &c.; from Holland, oak-bark, grain, &c.; from Russia and the north of Europe, hemp, tallow, tar, pitch, iron, linen, sail-cloth, timber, and occasionally grain; from the Mediterranean, fruit, oil, silk, &c.; from France, grain, flour, fruit, wine and brandy; and from Ireland, salt provisions, flour, feathers, &c. It formerly exported a great quantity of pressed pilchards to the West Indies and Italy; but this fish has lately been very scarce; the exports now chiefly consist of the produce of the tin and copper mines and manufactories, and of wine, brandy, &c., which had been imported under the bonding act; there is also a considerable trade with Jersey in fruit and cider. A quantity of mining apparatus and hardware has been exported hence to the Brazilian and Mexican mines. The number of vessels that entered inwards from foreign ports in 1826 was, forty-seven British, and ten foreign; and the number that cleared outwards, twenty-eight British. Several regular trading vessels from Falmouth to London, Bristol, Ireland, &c., bring in large supplies of grocery, ship chandlery, &c., and take in return to London a quantity of tin, &c. Falmouth is supposed to have become a station for post-office packets about the year 1688; the present establishment consists of five packets on the Lisbon station, and thirty-four to other parts of the world. At Falmouth and St. Mawes there was formerly a very extensive pilchard fishery, fourteen thousand hogsheads having been exported hence in one season; but from the decrease of fish, little has been done for the last two years. Here is some employment in ship-building and rope-making. Markets are held on Tuesday, Thursday, and Saturday, for butchers' meat, fish, and other provisions: and there are two fairs, on August 7th and October 10th, for cattle. The market-house was built in 1813, at the expense of Lord Wodehouse, and has a fountain of spring water in the centre. This town was incorporated by charter of Charles II., in 1661: the municipal body consists of a mayor, seven aldermen, twelve burgesses, with a recorder and town clerk; the latter officers are appointed by the King, on the petition of the corporation; the serjeants at mace and constables are appointed by the corporation. The mayor is elected from the aldermen, and the aldermen from the burgesses, by a majority of the whole body. They hold a court of quarter session by charter; and a court of record, for sums not exceeding one hundred marks, was appointed by the charter to be held every second Thursday before the mayor, recorder, and aldermen, or their deputies, or any three of them; its jurisdiction extends only to the town itself, but this court has not been held since May, 1785. The mayor, his predecessor, and the recorder, are by charter justices of the peace, with exclusive jurisdiction. The county magistrates meet at the Green Bank hotel on the second Thursday in every month, to hold a petty session for the eastern division of the hundred of Kerrier.

The living is a rectory, in the peculiar jurisdiction of the Bishop of Exeter, rated in the king's books at £3, and in the patronage of Lord Wodehouse. The church, built soon after the Restoration, and dedicated to the memory of Charles I., " King and Martyr," was made parochial in 1664, by act of parliament. A handsome chapel of ease was erected about two years since, by private subscription, and a grant from the Incorporated Society for the enlargement of churches, &c., at the north-west end of the town, within the parish of Budock; the site was presented by Lord de Dunstanville. There are places of worship for Baptists, Bryanites, the Society of Friends, Independents, Primitive and Wesleyan Methodists, and Unitarians, likewise a synagogue, and a neat Roman Catholic chapel, the latter built in 1820. Here are classical and mathematical schools for one hundred boys, established in 1825, by the subscriptions of seventy-five shareholders, at £15 each, whose property is vested in fifteen trustees; the ground for the institution was given by Lord Wodehouse. Extensive charitable institutions for educating the children of the poor are supported by voluntary contributions: the principal are, a school on the National plan, established about the year 1801, in which thirty boys and thirty girls are clothed and instructed in reading, writing, and arithmetic, and the latter in needle-work; a Sunday school connected with the church, in which about three hundred children are taught; a Lancasterian school for sixty girls, instituted in 1811, supported by general subscription, but patronised chiefly by some ladies of the Society of Friends; one of a similar kind, for from two

hundred to two hundred and fifty boys, established also under the direction of the Society of Friends; besides some infant schools. The merchants' hospital, for the relief and support of maimed and disabled seamen belonging to the port of London, and the widows and children of such as should be killed or drowned in the merchants' service, was established here about 1750, under the powers of an act of parliament passed in the 20th of George II., authorising any out-port, desirous of establishing an hospital for seamen belonging to such port, to appoint fifteen trustees for its management, who are annually elected by the owners and commanders of vessels belonging to the port, and confirmed by the corporation in London, established under the same act: a treasurer, receiver, and secretary, are appointed by the trustees, who meet monthly at the packet office to transact business. The present income of this hospital is about £300 per annum; the regular pensioners, widows and children of deceased mariners, who receive relief, are numerous. All merchant ships and packets registered at this port claim a right for their seamen, on payment of sixpence per month each, to the benefits of the establishment. The widows' retreat, an almshouse containing ten small rooms, for the residence of as many poor widows, was erected in 1810, at the expense of Lord Wodehouse. A dispensary was established about the year 1807, and soon afterwards a benevolent society for the relief of the poor, and especially of strangers, under the management of a visiting committee; to facilitate their examination of cases, the town is divided into several districts. In 1800, a lying-in charity was established; in 1812, a humane society; and in 1817, a provident society and savings bank: in addition to these are several benefit societies and masonic lodges. The interest of £300 three per cent. consols. was bequeathed by the late Mrs. Daval, of Chiswick, to be applied alternately to the relief of poor widows, and apprenticing the son of a poor widow. Near Pendennis are the remains of an intrenchment made by Cromwell during the civil war. Falmouth confers the title of earl on the family of Boscawen of Tregothnan. Dunstanville Terrace, or Green Bank, is an appendage of this town, but situated in the parish of Budock.

FALSGRAVE, a township within the jurisdiction of the borough of SCARBOROUGH, North riding of the county of YORK, 1 mile (S. W. by W.) from Scarborough, containing 345 inhabitants.

FALSTONE, a parish in the north-western division of TINDALE ward, county of NORTHUMBERLAND, 8 miles (W. N. W.) from Bellingham, comprising the townships of Falstone, Plashets, and Wellhaugh quarter, and containing 501 inhabitants. The living is a perpetual curacy, in the archdeaconry of Northumberland, and diocese of Durham, endowed with £400 private benefaction, and £400 royal bounty, and in the patronage of the Governors of Greenwich Hospital. The church, which was rebuilt in 1825, has received an addition of one hundred and five free sittings, the Incorporated Society for the enlargement of churches and chapels having granted £100 towards defraying the expense. Falstone is one of the six parishes into which the late extensive parish of Simonburn was divided by act of parliament, in 1811; it is a large and mountainous district, abounding with coal, and affording also good pasturage for sheep. The North Tyne has its source in a morass here, and receives the Kilder and numerous rivulets as it runs through the parish. The river Liddle, or Liddel, issues also from the same morass, and pursues its course into Scotland. There are several mineral springs in the neighbourhood, one of which, near the head of the Tyne, is said to be equally powerful and efficacious with those at Gilsland Spa. At a place called the Bells are the remains of an ancient religious building, contiguous to which is a cemetery.

FAMBRIDGE (NORTH), a parish in the hundred of DENGIE, county of ESSEX, 5 miles (N. N. W.) from Rochford, containing 147 inhabitants. The living is a discharged rectory, in the archdeaconry of Essex, and diocese of London, rated in the king's books at £4. 13. 4., and in the patronage of the Crown. The church is dedicated to the Holy Trinity. North and South Fambridge are separated by the river Crouch, over which there is a ferry.

FAMBRIDGE (SOUTH), a parish in the hundred of ROCHFORD, county of ESSEX, 3½ miles (N. N. W.) from Rochford, containing 107 inhabitants. The living is a rectory, in the archdeaconry of Essex, and diocese of London, rated in the king's books at £17. E. Stephenson, Esq. was patron in 1809. The church is dedicated to All Saints.

FANGFOSS, a parish in the Wilton-Beacon division of the wapentake of HARTHILL, East riding of the county of YORK, 4 miles (N.W.) from Pocklington, containing, with Spittle, 154 inhabitants. The living is a perpetual curacy, endowed with £1000 royal bounty, and in the peculiar jurisdiction and patronage of the Dean of York.

FARCETT, a chapelry in the parish of STAND-GROUND, hundred of NORMAN-CROSS, county of HUNTINGDON, 2¾ miles (S. by E.) from Peterborough, containing 499 inhabitants. The chapel is dedicated to St. Mary.

FAREHAM, a market town and parish, in the hundred of FAREHAM, Portsdown division of the county of SOUTHAMPTON, 12 miles (E.S.E.) from Southampton, and 73 (S.W.) from London, on the road from Southampton to Portsmouth, containing 3677 inhabitants. This town, situated on the north-west branch of Portsmouth harbour, which is here crossed by a bridge, is mentioned in Domesday-book as having, from its maritime situation, been formerly much exposed to the invasions of the Danes. It is a neat and flourishing town, occupying an elevated site, neither lighted nor regularly paved, but well supplied with water. Several of the inhabitants are connected with the naval establishment at Portsmouth. There is a handsome assembly-room, erected about thirty years ago, in which, during the winter season, assemblies are held monthly. Ship-building is here carried on, though upon a small scale, being confined to sloops and small vessels : there are also a rope-walk, and a manufactory for fine red bricks and Dutch or porcelain tiles. The town has a considerable trade in corn, coal, timber, &c. ; and vessels of three hundred tons' burden can sail up to the port. The corn market is one of the largest in the county, and the market day is every alternate Monday : there is a fair for cattle and cheese, &c., on the 29th and 30th of June. The local government is vested in a bailiff, two constables, and two ale-tasters : the officers for the town and hundred of Fareham are annually chosen by a jury, at the manorial court leet held by the steward

of the Bishop of Winchester ; and petty sessions are held here weekly for the division of Portsdown. The living is a vicarage, in the peculiar jurisdiction of the incumbent, rated in the king's books at £8. 12. 6., and in the patronage of the Bishop of Winchester. The church, dedicated to St. Peter and St. Paul, is a handsome edifice, rebuilt about fifteen years ago, with the exception of the chancel, which is of early English architecture. Independents and Wesleyan Methodists have each a place of worship. Here is a National school, at which about eighty boys and fifty girls are educated ; it was established in 1813, and about two years ago a suitable school-room was erected. In 1721, William Price gave by will £200, for the erection of a charity school ; and an estate in this parish, with another in the parish of Alverstoke, from the produce of which a salary of £35 per annum is paid to a master for teaching thirty poor boys, chosen by the minister and churchwardens, who are trustees of the charity, and receive £6 per annum for their trouble ; the overplus of the rents, after paying for books and clothing the children, is distributed among poor widows. The funds have been augmented by money arising from the sale of timber, and other sources ; and the present income, including rents and dividends on funded property, amounts to £264. 10. 8. per annum.

FAREWELL, a parish in the southern division of the hundred of OFFLOW, county of STAFFORD, 2 miles (N. W.) from Lichfield, containing, with Charley, 202 inhabitants. The living is a perpetual curacy, in the peculiar jurisdiction of the Dean and Chapter of Lichfield, endowed with £600 royal bounty, and in the patronage of the Marquis of Anglesey. The church is dedicated to St. Bartholomew. Roger, Bishop of Chester, or Lichfield, founded, about 1140, a religious house, to the honour of the Blessed Virgin Mary, for canons regular, who afterwards gave place to Benedictine nuns ; it was suppressed by Wolsey.

FARFORTH, a parish in the Wold division of the hundred of LOUTH-ESKE, parts of LINDSEY, county of LINCOLN, 6¼ miles (S. by W.) from Louth, containing, with Maiden-Well, 94 inhabitants. The living is a discharged rectory, with the vicarage of Maiden-Well, united in 1753 to the rectory of Ruckland, in the archdeaconry and diocese of Lincoln, rated in the king's books at £6. 6. 8. The church is dedicated to St. Peter.

FARINGDON, a parish in the hundred of SEL-BORNE, Alton (North) division of the county of SOUTH AMPTON, 3 miles (S. by W.) from Alton, containing 479 inhabitants. The living is a rectory, in the archdeaconry and diocese of Winchester, rated in the king's books at £18. 6. 0½. Lewis Cage, Esq. was patron in 1797. The church is dedicated to All Saints. Langston harbour bounds the parish on the south and south-east.

FARLAM, a parish in ESKDALE ward, county of CUMBERLAND, comprising the townships of East Farlam, and West Farlam, and containing 663 inhabitants, of which number, 491 are in the township of East Farlam, 3 miles (E. by S.) from Brampton, and 172 in that of West Farlam. The living is a perpetual curacy, in the archdeaconry and diocese of Carlisle, endowed with £800 royal bounty, and £1000 parliamentary grant, and in the patronage of the Earl of Carlisle. The church is dedicated to St. Thomas a Becket. A considerable quantity of limestone is obtained and burnt: there are coalworks in the adjoining parish of Hayton.

FARLEIGH (EAST), a parish in the hundred of MAIDSTONE, lathe of AYLESFOLD, county of KENT, 2½ miles (S. W. by W.) from Maidstone, containing 1143 inhabitants. The living is a vicarage, in the peculiar jurisdiction of the Archbishop of Canterbury, rated in the king's books at £6. 16. 8., and in the patronage of the Crown. The church has at the west end a tower and spire. An ancient stone bridge of five arches crosses the Medway at the entrance to the village. Here are almshouses for five poor persons.

FARLEIGH (WEST), a parish in the hundred of TWYFORD, lathe of AYLESFORD, county of KENT, 3¼ miles (W. S. W.) from Maidstone, containing 364 inhabitants. The living is a vicarage, in the archdeaconry and diocese of Rochester, rated in the king's books at £6. 10. 5., and in the patronage of the Dean and Chapter of Rochester. The church, dedicated to All Saints, is principally in the early style of English architecture. This place, which rises gradually from the southern bank of the Medway, has been the residence of genteel families for centuries; the houses are prettily detached, and there are communications with the opposite side of the river by three bridges, viz., Barnjet, St. Helen's, and Teston.

FARLEIGH-HUNGERFORD, a parish in the hundred of WELLOW, county of SOMERSET, 7 miles (S. E.) from Bath, containing 174 inhabitants. The living is a discharged rectory, in the archdeaconry of Wells, and diocese of Bath and Wells, rated in the king's books at £8. 11. 8., and in the patronage of John Houlton, Esq. The church is dedicated to St. Leonard. The river Frome runs through the parish, and the neighbourhood abounds with a species of marble, good for roads, and with the best freestone rock for ornamental buildings in the kingdom. Farleigh castle was erected in 1170, by Sir Thomas Hungerford; only two of the towers are now standing, those at the north-eastern angle having been demolished in 1797: the chapel contains several ancient monuments to the Hungerfords. Margaret, Countess of Salisbury, daughter of George, Duke of Clarence, and the last of the Plantagenets, was born here; this princess was married to Sir Richard Pole, a kinsman of Henry VII., and was the mother of the celebrated Cardinal Pole; also of Lord Henry Montague, who being accused of high treason, the Countess was implicated in the charge, and sentenced to be beheaded; after a violent struggle with the executioner, she suffered death in the 23rd of Henry VIII. A Roman tesselated pavement was discovered in 1685, and more recently a bath and other vestiges of a Roman villa were found, on digging in a field about half a mile north-westward from the castle.

FARLEIGH-WALLOP, a parish in the hundred of BERMONDSPIT, Basingstoke division of the county of SOUTHAMPTON, 3¼ miles (S. S. W.) from Basingstoke, containing 84 inhabitants. The living is a rectory, united to the rectory of Cliddesden, in the archdeaconry and diocese of Winchester, rated in the king's books at £9. 12. 6., and in the patronage of the Earl of Portsmouth. The church is dedicated to St. John.

FARLETON, a township in the parish of MELLING, hundred of LONSDALE, south of the sands, county palatine of LANCASTER, 8¼ miles (N. E. by E.) from Lancaster, containing 91 inhabitants.

FARLETON, a township in the parish of BEETHAM, KENDAL ward, county of WESTMORLAND, 3 miles (N.) from Burton in Kendal, containing 102 inhabitants. The Kendal and Lancaster canal passes on the western side of the village. Farleton Knot, a lofty rock of limestone rising above the village, has on its summit several springs.

FARLEY, a township in the parish of ALVETON, southern division of the hundred of TOTMONSLOW, county of STAFFORD, 4¼ miles (E. by N.) from Cheadle, containing 398 inhabitants.

FARLEY, a parish in the second division of the hundred of TANDRIDGE, county of SURREY, 5 miles (S. E.) from Croydon, containing 84 inhabitants. The living is a discharged rectory, in the archdeaconry of Surrey, and diocese of Winchester, rated in the king's books at £4. 16. 5½., endowed with £200 private benefaction, and £200 royal bounty, and in the patronage of the Warden and Fellows of Merton College, Oxford. The church is dedicated to St. Mary.

FARLEY, a chapelry in the parish and hundred of ALDERBURY, county of WILTS, 5 miles (E.) from Salisbury, containing 229 inhabitants. This chapelry is within the peculiar jurisdiction of the Treasurer in the Cathedral Church of Salisbury. The chapel was rebuilt by Sir Stephen Fox, who was born here in 1627; he also founded, in 1678, an almshouse, and endowed it with £188 per annum, arising out of the manor of Mannington, for the support of a chaplain, or warden, six men, and six women: it is a plain brick building, forming three sides of a quadrangle, the centre of which is appropriated to the chaplain, who has, besides, the charge of a free school, established by the same benevolent individual.

FARLEY-CHAMBERLAYNE, a parish in the hundred of KING'S SOMBOURN, Andover division of the county of SOUTHAMPTON, 5¾ miles (W. by S.) from Winchester, containing, with Slackstead, 201 inhabitants. The living is a rectory, in the archdeaconry and diocese of Winchester, rated in the king's books at £10. 12. 1., and in the patronage of Paulet St. John Mildmay, Esq. The church is dedicated to St. John. On an eminence, termed Beacon hill, are vestiges of an ancient encampment.

FARLINGTON, a parish in the hundred of PORTSDOWN, Portsdown division of the county of SOUTHAMPTON, 2¼ miles (W. by S.) from Havant, containing, with the extra-parochial liberty of Mudlands, 553 inhabitants. The living is a rectory, in the archdeaconry and diocese of Winchester, rated in the king's books at £9. 13. 4., and in the patronage of Edward Tew Richards, Esq. The church, among other recent improvements, has received two hundred and forty-seven free sittings, the Incorporated Society for the enlargement of churches and chapels having granted £250 towards defraying the expense. An enclosure, called Mudlands, once covered by the sea, was afterwards subject to occasional inundations, until additional precautions were taken after a great storm in November, 1824. A fine spring rises in the adjoining marshes, and flows into cisterns, from which the water is forced by a steam-engine, about half a mile up the slope, towards Portsdown, into a larger reservoir, whence the town of Portsmouth, about six miles distant, is supplied.

FARLINGTON, a chapelry in the parish of SHEriff-Hutton, wapentake of Bulmer, North riding of the county of York, 6¼ miles (E. S. E.) from Easingwould, containing 170 inhabitants. The chapel is dedicated to St. Leonard. There are sundry small benefactions, the interest of which is applied to teaching six children.

FARLOW, a joint chapelry with Kingston-Lisle, in that part of the parish of Sparsholt which is in the hundred of Shrivenham, county of Berks, 5¼ miles (W.) from Wantage, containing 357 inhabitants. The chapel, which was dedicated to St. James, has been demolished.

FARLOW, a chapelry in that part of the parish of Stottesden which is in the hundred of Wolphy, county of Hereford, 5¼ miles (N. W. by N.) from Cleobury-Mortimer, containing 345 inhabitants. The chapel is dedicated to St. Giles.

FARLSTHORP, a parish in the Wold division of the hundred of Calceworth, parts of Lindsey, county of Lincoln, 1¾ mile (S. E.) from Alford, containing 101 inhabitants. The living is a discharged vicarage, in the archdeaconry and diocese of Lincoln, rated in the king's books at £5. 6. 8., and endowed with £200 royal bounty. Henry Kipling, Esq. was patron in 1814. The church is dedicated to St. Andrew.

FARMANBY, a township partly in the parish of Ellerburn, but chiefly in that of Thornton-Dale, Pickering lythe, North riding of the county of York, 3 miles (E. S. E.) from Pickering, containing 403 inhabitants. There is an estate in this township belonging to the Dean and Canons of Windsor, part of which is called *Monklands*.

FARMBOROUGH, a parish in the hundred of Keynsham, county of Somerset, 3¾ miles (S. E. by E.) from Pensford, containing 752 inhabitants. The living is a rectory, in the archdeaconry of Bath, and diocese of Bath and Wells, rated in the king's books at £10. 2. 11. J. F. Gunning, Esq. was patron in 1823. The church is dedicated to All Saints. There is a place of worship for Wesleyan Methodists.

FARMCOT, a chapelry in the parish of Lower Guyting, lower division of the hundred of Kiftsgate, county of Gloucester, 2¼ miles (E.) from Winchcombe. The population is returned with the parish.

FARMINGTON, a parish in the hundred of Bradley, county of Gloucester, 2 miles (E. N. E.) from North Leach, containing 245 inhabitants. The living is a rectory, in the archdeaconry and diocese of Gloucester, rated in the king's books at £16. 5. 5. E. Waller, Esq. was patron in 1824. The church is dedicated to St. Peter. The old fosse-way bounds the parish on the north.

FARNBOROUGH, a parish in the hundred of Compton, county of Berks, 5 miles (W. by N.) from East Ilsley, containing 210 inhabitants. The living is a rectory, in the archdeaconry of Berks, and diocese of Salisbury, rated in the king's books at £12. 8. 4., and in the patronage of the Rev. George Price. The church is dedicated to All Saints.

FARNBOROUGH, a chapelry in the parish of Chelsfield, hundred of Ruxley, lathe of Sutton at Hone, county of Kent, 4¼ miles (S. E. by S.) from Bromley, containing 553 inhabitants. The chapel, dedicated to St. Giles the Abbot, was rebuilt in 1639, in which year the ancient structure was destroyed by a tempest. Farnborough, a corruption of *Fearnberga*, derived its name from the quantity of fern growing here: it had anciently a market and two fairs, but the former has been long since disused, and one fair only is now held, on September 12th. Farnborough gives the title of baron to the family of Long, created July 8th, 1826.

FARNBOROUGH, a parish in the hundred of Crondall, Basingstoke division of the county of Southampton, 5½ miles (N. E. by N.) from Farnham, containing 287 inhabitants. The living is a discharged rectory, in the archdeaconry and diocese of Winchester, rated in the king's books at £7. 12. 11., and in the patronage of —— Greenwood, Esq. and others. The Basingstoke canal passes through the parish.

FARNBOROUGH, a parish in the Burton-Dassett division of the hundred of Kington, county of Warwick, 6½ miles (E. by S.) from Kington, containing 356 inhabitants. The living is a discharged vicarage, in the archdeaconry of Coventry, and diocese of Lichfield and Coventry, rated in the king's books at £5. 12., endowed with £200 private benefaction, and £200 royal bounty. W. Holbeche, Esq. was patron in 1812. The church is dedicated to St. Botolph. John Freckleton, about 1764, bequeathed property for the benefit of the poor of Aston, Cleydon, Dasset, and Farnborough; and in 1812, Viscount Andover left £100, producing together an income of about £42, which is applied to the education of seventy children of these parishes. The Oxford canal enters the county at the northern boundary of the parish.

FARNDALE, a chapelry comprising the township of Farndale High Quarter, in the parish of Lastingham, and the township of Farndale Low Quarter, in the parish of Kirkby-Moorside, wapentake of Ryedale, North riding of the county of York, 13 miles (N. W.) from Pickering, and containing 499 inhabitants.

FARNDALE-EASTSIDE, a township in the parish of Lastingham, wapentake of Ryedale, North riding of the county of York, 11 miles (N. W. by N.) from Pickering, containing 455 inhabitants.

FARNDISH, a parish in the hundred of Willey, county of Bedford, 4½ miles (S.W. by S.) from Higham-Ferrers, containing 73 inhabitants. The living is a rectory, in the archdeaconry of Bedford, and diocese of Lincoln, rated in the king's books at £10. C. Chester, Esq. was patron in 1784. The church is dedicated to St. Michael.

FARNDON, a parish in the higher division of the hundred of Broxton, county palatine of Chester, comprising the townships of Barton, Churton by Farndon, Clutton, Crewe, and Farndon, and containing 857 inhabitants, of which number, 429 are in the township of Farndon, 8¾ miles (S.) from Chester. The living is a perpetual curacy, in the archdeaconry and diocese of Chester, endowed with £600 private benefaction, £200 royal bounty, and £600 parliamentary grant, and in the patronage of Earl Grosvenor. The church, dedicated to St. Chad, was garrisoned in the civil war, and in consequence sustained great injury during the siege of Holt castle, in 1645; in 1658 it was repaired: it has a curious stained window, representing several gentlemen who commanded in Chester during the war. There is a place of worship at the township of Barton for Calvinistic Methodists. Farndon is bounded on the west by the navigable river Dee, which is crossed by an ancient bridge of eight arches, communicating with the town of Holt, in Flintshire. A charity school was erected in 1629, and endowed with land producing about £14 per annum, with a small croft and garden occupied by the master, who conducts the school on the Madras system. John Speed, the celebrated English topographer and historian, was born here in 1552.

FARNDON, a hamlet in the parish of WOODFORD, hundred of CHIPPING-WARDEN, county of NORTHAMPTON, 9½ miles (S.S.W.) from Daventry. The population is returned with the parish.

FARNDON, a parish in the southern division of the wapentake of NEWARK, county of NOTTINGHAM, 2¼ miles (S.W. by W.) from Newark, containing 499 inhabitants. The living is a discharged vicarage, with the curacies of Balderton, and Fiskerton, in the archdeaconry of Nottingham, and diocese of York, rated in the king's books at £6. 13. 4., endowed with £400 royal bounty, and in the patronage of the Prebendary of Farndon in the Cathedral Church of Lincoln. The church, dedicated to St. Peter, is a large and lofty edifice. The parish is bounded on the west by the river Trent, and is intersected by the Roman fosse-road. There is a small endowment for teaching children.

FARNDON (EAST), a parish in the hundred of ROTHWELL, county of NORTHAMPTON, 2 miles (S.S.W.) from Market-Harborough, containing 250 inhabitants. The living is a rectory, in the archdeaconry of Northampton, and diocese of Peterborough, rated in the king's books at £13. 1. 0½., and in the patronage of the President and Fellows of St. John's College, Oxford. The church is dedicated to St. John the Baptist. There is a mineral spring in the parish.

FARNHAM, a parish partly in the hundred of CHALK, county of WILTS, but chiefly in that part of the hundred of CRANBORNE which is in the Shaston (West) division of the county of DORSET, 8 miles (W. by N.) from Cranborne, containing, with the tything of Farnham-Tollard, 283 inhabitants. The living is a discharged rectory, in the archdeaconry of Dorset, and diocese of Bristol, rated in the king's books at £7. 10., and in the patronage of the Crown. The church is dedicated to St. Lawrence. There is a fair for cheese on the 21st of August.

FARNHAM, a parish in the hundred of CLAVERING, county of ESSEX, 3¼ miles (W. by N.) from Stansted-Mountfitchet, containing 470 inhabitants. The living is a rectory, in the archdeaconry of Colchester, and diocese of London, rated in the king's books at £23. 8. 9., and in the patronage of the President and Fellows of Trinity College, Oxford. The church, dedicated to St. Mary, has lately received an addition of seventy free sittings, the Incorporated Society for the enlargement of churches and chapels having granted £18 towards defraying the expense.

FARNHAM, a township in the parish of ALLENTON, western division of COQUETDALE ward, county of NORTHUMBERLAND, 6 miles (W.) from Rothbury, containing 36 inhabitants.

FARNHAM, a parish in the hundred of PLOMESGATE, county of SUFFOLK, 2¾ miles (S.W.) from Saxmundham, containing 213 inhabitants. The living is a perpetual curacy, in the archdeaconry of Suffolk, and diocese of Norwich, endowed with £15 per annum private benefaction, and £800 royal bounty. D. Long North, Esq. was patron in 1827. The church is dedicated to St. Mary.

FARNHAM, a parish in the hundred of FARNHAM, county of SURREY, comprising the market town of Farnham, the chapelry of Bagshot, and the tythings of Culverlands with Tilford, Runfold, Runwick, and Wrecklesham with Bourn, and containing 5413 inhabitants, of which number, 3132 are in the town of Farnham, 10 miles (W. by S.) from Guildford, and 38 (S.W.) from London, on the road to Southampton. This place, originally called Fernham, from the fern growing on the extensive heaths by which on all sides, except the south-west, it is for many miles surrounded, was by Ethelbald, King of the West Saxons, annexed to the see of Winchester. In 893, Alfred obtained a signal victory over the Danes, who were ravaging this part of the country; and in the reign of Stephen, Henry de Blois, brother of that monarch, and Bishop of Winchester, erected, on a hill commanding the town, a castle of great strength and of considerable extent, which is said to have been seized by the Dauphin of France, in his expedition against King John. In the following reign, this castle having become a retreat for the mal-contents, was demolished by Henry III., in the war with the barons; but was subsequently rebuilt by the bishops of Winchester, with greater magnificence, as the episcopal palace. During the parliamentary war, the castle was garrisoned for the king, but being besieged by Waller, the parliamentary general, it fell into his hands, and was afterwards dismantled and nearly destroyed. The principal remains are some portions of the walls, and the keep, which still retains vestiges of its ancient strength: the deep fosse, by which the castle was surrounded, is on the north side occupied by a plantation of forest trees. At the Restoration the inhabited part was greatly improved by Bishop Morley, who expended £8000 in repairs: it has been since modernised, and is still the principal residence of the bishops of the diocese, and contains an extensive and valuable library belonging to the see. The park, three miles in circumference, commands a fine view of the valley in which the town is situated, and of the adjoining country to the south and south-east. To the east of the palace is a noble avenue of ancient elms, forming a delightful promenade, nearly a mile in length, which the inhabitants of the town enjoy by prescriptive right.

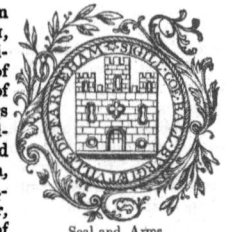

Seal and Arms.

The town is situated on the river Wey, and consists of four principal streets, diverging nearly at right angles from the market-place in the centre, and of several smaller streets, roughly paved, and lighted with oil by subscription during the winter. The houses are mostly well built, many of them are handsome, and the general appearance of the place is respectable and prepossessing: the inhabitants are supplied with spring water from pumps, and in the centre of the town is a reservoir of soft water, brought from the hills on the north by pipes, which crossing the park, first supply the castle. The view of the castle from the market-place, though partially obstructed by the market-house, is picturesque, and the environs abound with pleasing and richly varied scenery: to the south are fertile meadows bounded by hills crowned with wood, and to the north are extensive plantations of hops, for which the soil is peculiarly favourable. The manufacture of cloth, formerly carried on to a considerable extent, has been superseded by the cultivation of hops, which has prevailed here for about one hundred and fifty years, and at present constitutes the staple trade of the town. The hops, from the favourable nature of the soil, and the peculiar care bestowed on their culture, possess a decided superiority over those produced in any other part of the kingdom, and invariably obtain a higher price : they are almost exclusively sent to Weyhill fair, near Andover, where they are sold to the west country dealers. On the banks of the Wey are several flour-mills, from which considerable supplies are sent to the London market by the Basingstoke canal, which crosses the high road within four miles of the town. The market, which was formerly well supplied with corn, is on Thursday : the fairs are on Holy Thursday and Midsummer-day, for horses, cattle, sheep, and hogs, and November 13th, for horses and cattle. Farnham was anciently a borough, and returned members to parliament from the 4th of Edward II. till the 38th of Henry VI. : it had a charter of incorporation granted by the bishops, under which the government was vested in two bailiffs and twelve burgesses ; but these privileges were so little regarded that the vacancies in the number of the burgesses were not filled up, and in 1790, the bailiffs having been indicted for not repairing the bridges at Tilford, surrendered their charter to the bishop, and sent the records of the borough to the castle. The town is within the jurisdiction of the county magistrates, who hold here petty sessions for the division : the bishop holds a court leet in the spring, at which tythingmen and constables are appointed, and a court baron every third week, for the recovery of debts under 40s.

The living is a vicarage, in the archdeaconry of Surrey, and diocese of Winchester, rated in the king's books at £29. 9. 5., and in the patronage of the Archdeacon. The church, dedicated to St. Andrew, is a spacious and handsome structure in the later style of English architecture, with a low tower at the west end; it has a very fine east window of five lights, with elegant tracery. In 1825, the gallery over the north aisle was enlarged with two hundred and twenty additional free sittings, by a grant from the Incorporated Society for the enlargement of churches and chapels, and a similar increase of ninety-three free sittings for females was made in the gallery over the south aisle, by subscription. There is a place of worship for Independents, and also one at Tilford. A free grammar school had existed here prior to 1611, to which Dr. Harding, President of Magdalene College, Oxford, in that year, bequeathed a rent-charge of £10 per annum, which has been augmented by subsequent benefactions; the present income, nearly £30 per annum, is paid to the master, who receives private boarders, and pays to a schoolmaster in the town a certain sum for teaching the poor children that apply for gratuitous instruction. A National school, to which benefactions amounting to £25 per annum have been made, is principally supported by subscription. Almshouses for the residence and maintenance of eight aged persons were founded in 1619, by Andrew Windsor, who endowed them with a farm at Buscott, in the county of Berks, producing, with subsequent benefactions,

about £80 per annum. At the distance of about two miles south of the town are the remains of the abbey of Waverley, founded in 1128, by Giffard, Bishop of Winchester, for monks of the Cistercian order, then introduced into England (the abbot, according to Gale, being accounted the superior of that order in this country), the clear annual revenue of which, at the dissolution, was £174. 8. 3. : the remains consist of part of the south aisle of the church, in the windows of which, within the memory of the present generation, were many specimens of the rich stained glass with which the church was decorated ; and part of the dormitory, refectory, and the cloisters, richly mantled with ivy, and extending in detached portions over a space of three or four acres : stone coffins and numerous sepulchral remains having been frequently discovered on the spot. Peter de Rupibus, Bishop of Winchester, died at Farnham, and was buried at Winchester, but his heart was deposited at Waverley, and is said to have been dug up entire about six years since, enclosed in a leaden box, containing a saline liquid. Nicholas de Farnham, successively physician to Henry III., Bishop of Chester and Durham, and author of several works on the practice of physic and the nature of herbs ; and the Rev. Augustus Montague Toplady, A.M. an eminent controversial divine of the last century, were natives of this place.

FARNHAM, a parish in the lower division of the wapentake of Claro, West riding of the county of York, comprising the townships of Farnham, Ferensby, and Scotton, and containing 548 inhabitants, of which number, 141 are in the township of Farnham, 2¼ miles (N.) from Knaresborough. The living is a vicarage, within the peculiar jurisdiction of the court of the honour of Knaresborough, rated in the king's books at £6. 12. 1., endowed with £200 private benefaction, £800 royal bounty, and £1700 parliamentary grant, and in the patronage of the Rev. Thomas Collins, and the Rev. Timothy Shann. The church is a neat structure, situated on an eminence. The river Nidd bounds the parish on the west. A copper mine was opened in 1757, but the adventurers failed of success.

FARNHAM-ROYAL, a parish in the hundred of Burnham, county of Buckingham, 3½ miles (N.) from Eton, containing, with the hamlets of Hedgerley-Dean and Seer-Green, and a portion of Salt-hill, 1149 inhabitants. The living is a rectory, in the archdeaconry of Buckingham, and diocese of Lincoln, rated in the king's books at £12. 16. 0½., and in the patronage of the Provost and Fellows of Eton College. The church is dedicated to St. Mary. There is a place of worship for Dissenters. Mrs. Elizabeth Hetherington, in 1777, gave £140 towards the foundation of a school, the proceeds of which, with sundry contributions, have been recently appropriated to the erection of a school-house.

FARNHAM-TOLLARD, a tything in the parish of Farnham, in that part of the hundred of Cranborne which is in the Shaston (West) division of the county of Dorset, containing 208 inhabitants.

FARNHILL, a joint township with Cononley, in the parish of Kildwick, eastern division of the wapentake of Staincliffe and Ewcross, West riding of the county of York, 3¾ miles (S.S.E.) from Skipton, containing 1350 inhabitants.

FARNHURST, a parish in the hundred of Ease-

Z 2

BOURNE, rape of CHICHESTER, county of SUSSEX, 5 miles (N. by E.) from Midhurst, containing 593 inhabitants. The living is a perpetual curacy, in the archdeaconry and diocese of Chichester, endowed with £200 private benefaction, £200 royal bounty, and £1700 parliamentary grant. W. S. Poyntz, Esq. was patron in 1796. The church is in the early style of English architecture.

FARNINGHAM, a parish in the hundred of AXTON, DARTFORD, and WILMINGTON, lathe of SUTTON at HONE, county of KENT, 5½ miles (S. E. by E.) from Foot's Cray, containing 586 inhabitants. The living is a vicarage, in the peculiar jurisdiction and patronage of the Archbishop of Canterbury, rated in the king's books at £9. 5. 10. The church, dedicated to St. Peter and St. Paul, is principally in the early style of English architecture, having at the west end a handsome flint tower, and containing brasses and other remnants of antiquity, with an octagonal font curiously and elaborately carved. Farningham, anciently Fremingham, signifying the village by the brook, is situated on the high road from London to Maidstone, on the river Darent, which is crossed by a bridge of four arches, and has some paper-mills on its banks: it had formerly a market on Tuesday, and a fair for four days, commencing annually on the eve of St. Peter's day; there is still a fair for horses and cattle on the 15th of October.

FARN-ISLANDS, a cluster of small islands in the parish of HOLY ISLAND, in ISLANDSHIRE, county palatine of DURHAM, seventeen in number, extending about 7 miles (S. E.) from Holy Island. The largest of them, called House Island, which lies nearly two miles to the eastward of Bambrough castle, is remarkable as the spot where St. Cuthbert passed a few of the latter years of his life, and whereon a priory subordinate to Durham was subsequently founded for Benedictine monks, whose revenue at the dissolution was £12. 17. 8. Ethelwold, St. Bartholomew, and Thomas, prior of Durham, among other celebrated devotees, since the time of St. Cuthbert, sequestered themselves in this place. A square tower, the ruins of a church, and other buildings, are still remaining, also a stone coffin, in which it is said the body of St. Cuthbert was first laid. At the northern end is a deep chasm, through which in stormy weather the sea forces its way with such violence as to form a fine *jet d'eau* sixty feet high, called the Churn. A light-house has been erected on House island, and another upon Staples island, three miles to the eastward, the passage between which is open to large ships, and is termed Scar road from the Oxscar rocks lying about mid-channel. There are from five to eight fathoms of water both in this road and in Budle bay. These islands produce kelp, and there are a few seals.

FARNLEY, a chapelry in that part of the parish of OTLEY which is in the upper division of the wapentake of CLARO, West riding of the county of YORK, 2 miles (N. N. E.) from Otley, containing 179 inhabitants. The living is a perpetual curacy, in the archdeaconry and diocese of York, endowed with £1000 royal bounty, and £200 parliamentary grant, and in the patronage of the Vicar of Otley.

FARNLEY, a chapelry in that part of the parish of ST. PETER, LEEDS, which is within the liberty of LEEDS, though locally in the wapentake of Morley, West riding of the county of YORK, 3½ miles (W. by S.) from Leeds, containing 1332 inhabitants. The living is a perpetual curacy, in the archdeaconry and diocese of York, endowed with £1000 private benefaction, £800 royal bounty, and £600 parliamentary grant, and in the patronage of the Vicar of Leeds.

FARNLEY-TYAS, a chapelry in that part of the parish of ALMONDBURY which is in the upper division of the wapentake of AGBRIGG, West riding of the county of YORK, 4 miles (S. S. E.) from Huddersfield, containing 900 inhabitants. Here is a free school.

FARNSFIELD, a parish in the liberty of SOUTHWELL and SCROOBY, though locally in the wapentake of Thurgarton, county of NOTTINGHAM, 4 miles (N. W. by W.) from Southwell, containing 811 inhabitants. The living is a discharged vicarage, in the peculiar jurisdiction and patronage of the Chapter of the Collegiate Church of Southwell, rated in the king's books at £4. The church is dedicated to St. Michael. There is a place of worship for Wesleyan Methodists. A free school is endowed with a house and certain land of the annual value of £20.

FARNWORTH, a chapelry in the parish of DEAN, hundred of SALFORD, county palatine of LANCASTER, 2¼ miles (S. S. E.) from Great Bolton, containing 2044 inhabitants. The chapel, a handsome structure, has been recently erected by the Commissioners appointed under the act for building additional churches, at an expense of £8000. There is a place of worship for Independents. In this township are extensive coal and vitriol works, spinning and power-loom mills, and one of the best paper manufactories in the kingdom. A school-house, erected on land given by James Roscoe, in 1715, was endowed, in 1728, with £300 by Nathan Dorning. The commissioners of enclosures, in 1798, allotted certain land to the trustees of this school, and in 1825 the school-room was rebuilt; there is also a house and garden for the master. An infant school, and a school for the children of Wesleyan Methodists, are supported by subscription.

FARNWORTH, a chapelry in the parish of PRESCOT, hundred of WEST DERBY, county palatine of LANCASTER, 5¾ miles (W.) from Warrington. The population is returned with the parish. The living is a perpetual curacy, in the archdeaconry and diocese of Chester, endowed with £200 private benefaction, £200 royal bounty, and £600 parliamentary grant, and in the patronage of the Vicar of Prescot. The chapel is dedicated to St. Wilfrid. There is a commodious free grammar school, in which about twenty boys are instructed in English and the classics; the annual income, arising from various donations and bequests, is about £60.

FARRINGDON, a parish in the eastern division of the hundred of BUDLEIGH, county of DEVON, 4¾ miles (N. E.) from Topsham, containing, with a portion of the tything of Clist-Sackville, 379 inhabitants. The living is a rectory, in the archdeaconry and diocese of Exeter, rated in the king's books at £8. 8. 1½., and in the patronage of the Bishop of Exeter. John Weare, in 1691, bequeathed £3 a year for teaching four children, and to purchase books. In pursuance of the will of Walter Wotton, in 1708, a house was conveyed to trustees for the purpose of a school, with an endowment of £56: the house was burnt down many years since, but the inhabitants erected another, with apartments for the master, and a room for vestry meetings. At

Bishop's Clist was formerly a chapel, endowed for two chaplains by Bishop Bronscombe, to which was annexed an hospital for twelve blind or infirm clergymen. Clist house was garrisoned by Fairfax, during the civil war in 1645.

FARRINGDON, a chapelry in the parish of IWERNE-COURTNAY, hundred of REDLANE, Sturminster division of the county of DORSET, 5½ miles (S. S. W.) from Shaftesbury. The population is returned with the parish. The chapel is dedicated to St. Mary. Farringdon, anciently Ferendone, is mentioned in the *Inquisitio Gheldi*, as giving name to a hundred, which in after times was transferred to Redlane. There is a medicinal spring in the neighbourhood.

FARRINGDON (GREAT), a parish comprising the market town of Farringdon, the chapelry of Little Coxwell, and the tything of Hospital, in the hundred of FARRINGDON, and the tything of Wadley, or Littleworth with Thrupp, in the hundred of SHRIVENHAM, county of BERKS, and containing 2784 inhabitants, of which number, 2271 are in the town of Farringdon, 35 miles (W. N. W.) from Reading, and 68 (W. by N.) from London. Here the Saxon kings had a palace, in which Edward the Elder expired. The town acquired some celebrity during the war between the Empress Maud and Stephen, from a castle erected by Robert, Earl of Gloucester, which he defended for the empress with distinguished bravery, until want of provisions compelled him to surrender, on which Stephen levelled it with the ground. In 1203, the site was granted by King John, for the erection of an abbey for monks of the Cistercian order, which subsequently became a cell to the monastery of Beaulieu, in Hampshire; and in 1218, a charter for a market was obtained by the abbot of Beaulieu. During the civil commotions in the reign of Charles I., Farringdon house was garrisoned for the king, and a large body of the parliamentary forces sustained a repulse before it a short time prior to the reduction of Oxford. It was one of the last places which surrendered, and it is worthy of remark, that Sir Robert Pye, the proprietor of the house and manor at that period, held a commission under the commonwealth, and commanded the assailants. The property afterwards reverted to him, and was retained by his descendants till 1788, when Henry James Pye, Esq., who was poet-laureate during a great part of the reign of George III., disposed of the mansion, which he had then recently erected, and of the estate, to William Hallet, Esq., sometime member for the county. Farringdon is a small town, but neat, well built, and paved, lighted with oil, and abundantly supplied with water from a noted spring called Port-well. It is pleasantly situated in the fertile vale of White Horse, a little more than two miles from the Isis, at the junction of two great roads, the constant travelling along which is a source of great advantage to the town. There is no prevailing branch of manufacture: hops are cultivated in the vicinity to a considerable extent. The navigation of the Thames, or Isis, which flows within two miles of the town, furnishes a medium for the conveyance of coal from the mines of Gloucestershire and Somersetshire, and of other heavy articles from London. The market, which is noted for corn is on Tuesday: fairs are held February 13th, and on Whit-Tuesday, for horses and cattle; on the next Tuesdays before and after Old Michaelmas, which are statute fairs; and October 29th, for cattle and pigs, which latter are slaughtered here, and sold in large quantities. The market-house, standing in the centre of the town, is a compact building enclosed by iron rails; the upper part is used for the town-hall, in which all public business is transacted. The local affairs of the town are managed by a bailiff, who, together with the constables, is appointed at the manorial court: and the county magistrates hold petty sessions for the division every alternate Tuesday, or as occasion may require, at the town-hall. The living is a vicarage; it was formerly a prebend in Salisbury Cathedral, but is now a lay fee in the peculiar jurisdiction and patronage of the Lord of the Manor, rated in the king's books at £14. 1. 3. The church, dedicated to All Saints, is a spacious cruciform edifice in the earliest style of English architecture: a plain square tower rises from the intersection, and was formerly surmounted by a spire, which was partly thrown down during the siege of Farringdon house; the lower part only is remaining, and rises but little above the roof of the church. In the interior are some ancient monuments, especially one to the memory of Sir Henry Unton, K. G., ambassador to France in the reign of Elizabeth, and who challenged the Duke of Guise for speaking disrespectfully of that queen. At Little Coxwell, in this parish, is a chapel of ease. There is a place of worship for Baptists. The National school, which was erected in 1825, at a short distance from the town, on the road to Wantage, is a neat stone building; it was intended to accommodate two hundred boys, and is supported chiefly by voluntary contributions. There is likewise a school for female infants, conducted on the Lancasterian system; and various benefactions have been made for the purpose of apprenticing poor boys. In the immediate vicinity of the town is Farringdon hill, rising gradually from the vale, and surmounted by a small grove, which is visible as a land-mark at a great distance: it commands a fine view of the rich vale, and of parts of the counties of Oxford, Gloucester, and Wilts. Within this parish, about two miles northward, is Radcot bridge, an ancient structure, near which a battle was fought in the reign of Richard II., between the insurgent barons and Robert de Vere, Marquis of Dublin, the king's favourite, who was defeated, and compelled to swim across the Thames in order to effect his escape. Near the town are the remains of an ancient causeway, supposed by some writers to be of Roman origin, but by others, and with more probability, assigned to the Norman baron, Robert D'Oyley, who is believed to have constructed it soon after the Conquest.

FARRINGDON (LITTLE), a chapelry in that part of the parish of LANGFORD which is in the hundred of FARRINGDON, county of BERKS, though locally in the hundred of Bampton, county of Oxford, 2 miles (N. E.) from Lechlade, containing 140 inhabitants. This chapelry is within the peculiar jurisdiction of the Prebendary of Langford in the Cathedral Church of Salisbury.

FARRINGTON, a township in the parish of PEN-WORTHAM, hundred of LEYLAND, county palatine of LANCASTER, 4¾ miles (S.) from Preston, containing 513 inhabitants. A school-room was erected by subscription in 1812, towards the support of which £30 is annually paid from the funds of Penwortham free school: one hundred boys and girls are educated at a trifling charge.

FARRINGTON-GURNEY, a chapelry in the parish of CHEWTON-MENDIP, hundred of CHEWTON, county of SOMERSET, 8¼ miles (N. E. by N.) from Wells, containing 526 inhabitants. The chapel is dedicated to St. John the Baptist. There is a place of worship for Wesleyan Methodists. The adjunct to the name is derived from the Gournays, its ancient possessors, of whom Sir Thomas de Gournay was concerned in the murder of Edward II. at Berkeley castle, for which his estates were confiscated, and Farrington has since been annexed to the duchy of Cornwall. A coal mine is wrought here.

FARSLEY, a township in the parish of CALVERLEY, wapentake of MORLEY, West riding of the county of YORK, 4¼ miles (E.N.E.) from Bradford, containing, with the township of Calverley, 2605 inhabitants. There is a place of worship for Baptists.

FARTHINGHOE, a parish in the hundred of KING'S SUTTON, county of NORTHAMPTON, 3¾ miles (N.W. by W.) from Brackley, containing 476 inhabitants. The living is a rectory, in the archdeaconry of Northampton, and diocese of Peterborough, rated in the king's books at £16. The Earl of Wilton was patron in 1794. The church is dedicated to St. Michael. Captain Philip Thicknesse, a noted tourist and miscellaneous writer, was born here in 1719.

FARTHINGSTONE, a parish in the hundred of FAWSLEY, county of NORTHAMPTON, 7 miles (N.W.) from Towcester, containing 265 inhabitants. The living is a rectory, in the archdeaconry of Northampton, and diocese of Peterborough, rated in the king's books at £13. 18. 11½., and in the patronage of the Bishop of Lincoln. The church is dedicated to St. Mary. On the brow of a hill is an ancient intrenchment with a lofty keep mount, called Castle Dykes, much obscured with woods, and intersected from east to west by a large ditch : in digging among the ruins, a vaulted room was discovered, with another beneath it. On the declivity of a contiguous hill is an area of an irregular form, called the Castle Yard, with trenches on all sides except the south-west, at the bottom of which are huge heaps of cinders, earth, and pebbles.

FARWAY, a parish in the hundred of COLYTON, county of DEVON, 3 miles (S. by E.) from Honiton, containing 346 inhabitants. The living is a rectory, in the archdeaconry and diocese of Exeter, rated in the king's books at £15. 6. 8., and in the patronage of the Rev. T. Putt. The church, dedicated to St. Michael, has some piers and other portions in the Norman style. A school was endowed in 1795, by Mrs. Hannah Atkinson, with the dividends of certain stock, producing about £7. 10. per annum.

FAUGH, a joint township with Fenton, in the parish of HAYTON, ESKDALE ward, county of CUMBERLAND, 8½ miles (E. by S.) from Carlisle, containing 331 inhabitants.

FAULD, a township in the parish of HANBURY, northern division of the hundred of OFFLOW, county of STAFFORD, 7¼ miles (S.E. by E.) from Uttoxeter, containing 48 inhabitants.

FAULKBOURN, a parish in the hundred of WITHAM, county of ESSEX, 2 miles (N.W.) from Witham, containing 168 inhabitants. The living is a rectory, in the archdeaconry of Colchester, and diocese of London, rated in the king's books at £6. 13. 4., and in the patronage of J. J. C. Bullock, Esq. The church is dedicated to St. Germanus.

FAVERSHAM, or FEVERSHAM, a sea port, market town, and parish, having separate jurisdiction, locally in the hundred of Faversham, lathe of SCRAY, county of KENT, containing 4208 inhabitants, of which number, 3919 are in the town of Faversham, 9 miles (W.) from Canterbury, 18 (E.N.E.) from Maidstone, and 47 (E.) from London, on the road to Dover.

Arms.

This town is of great antiquity, having been inhabited by the Britons prior to the Roman invasion. It was held in royal demesne in 811, and is called, in a charter granted by Kenulf, King of Mercia, "The king's little town of Febresham." In 930, King Athelstan held a council here, " to enact laws, and devise methods for their future observance." It is returned in Domesday-book as being held by William the Conqueror, by the name of *Favreshant ;* and he is said to have given the advowson to the abbey of St. Augustine, in Canterbury, and the manor to one of his favourite Normans, as a reward for his services. In 1147, a celebrated abbey for twelve Cluniac monks was founded here by Stephen, who, with Matilda, his consort, and his eldest son, Eustace, Earl of Boulogne, were interred within its walls, as were also several other persons of renown. The town has obtained peculiar privileges, and numerous charters from various kings. Selden states that the endowments and privileges granted by Stephen were confirmed by successive sovereigns, and that the abbots sat in thirteen several parliaments, in the reigns of Edward I. and Edward II., but that, on account of their reduced state and poverty, they ceased to do so after the eighteenth year of the latter monarch's reign. It appears that an acrimonious feeling had existed for a considerable length of time between the monks and the people of Faversham, who endured with reluctance the imposts and exactions of the former. Among these grievances were claims, by way of composition, for allowing the inhabitants to send their swine to pannage, for exposing their wares to sale in the market, for the liberty of brewing, &c.; in which state matters continued till the time of Henry VIII., when this monastery shared the fate of the other religious houses. At that period its clear revenue was estimated at £286. 12. 6¾., but the full annual value, according to a record published by Jacob, was £355. 15. 2. In 1539, the year after its surrender, the chief parts of the monastery were destroyed, and the ground on which it stood was granted to Sir Thomas Cheney, Lord Warden of the cinque-ports, together with some adjoining lands. The two entrance gates were remaining within the last fifty years, but being in a ruinous state they were taken down, and there is nothing now but some portions of the outer walls. James II. having been seized at Shellness point, on his first attempt to quit the kingdom, after the landing of the Prince of Orange, in 1688, was detained at Faversham, and subsequently escaped from Rochester.

The town is situated on a branch of the river Swale, called East Swale, and consists of four principal streets. During the last fifty years it has undergone very material improvement, part of which consists in the opening of a spacious avenue from the London road into Preston-street, and the erection of a bridge over the stream at the bottom of West-street, which took place in 1773. In 1789, an act was passed for paving, watching, and lighting the town, which is also well supplied with spring water. Many of the houses are large and handsome, and there are an assembly-room, a theatre, and a public subscription library. Faversham has long been distinguished for its manufacture of gunpowder, which is said to have been established here prior to the reign of Elizabeth, but restricted to private individuals till 1760, when government constructed buildings with due regard to additional security. Nevertheless, in 1767, a store containing twenty-five barrels of gunpowder blew up, and considerably damaged the town a much more disastrous occurrence took place on the 17th of April, 1781, through the explosion of seven thousand pounds of gunpowder, by which the corning-mill and dusting-house were blown to atoms, the workmen killed, and the buildings in Faversham and Davington either wholly or partially unroofed, and otherwise greatly damaged; so tremendous was the report that it was heard at the distance of twenty miles. Government granted pecuniary aid for the relief of the suffering inhabitants, and an act was passed for the greater safety of gunpowder-works, one of the provisions of which was the removal of the stores into the marsh, a considerable distance below the town. During the late war, the quantity of powder annually manufactured here was twelve or thirteen thousand barrels, affording employment to nearly four hundred persons. Since the peace of 1815, the Crown has disposed of the works near the town, but retained the more distant works; the former have become the property of a private manufacturer, who conducts the business on a reduced scale. Faversham is nevertheless a place of considerable traffic, as more than forty thousand quarters of corn, besides a considerable quantity of hops, fruit, wool, and other articles of merchandise, are shipped every year for London: there is also a manufactory for Roman cement, and ship-building is carried on to a small extent.

The port in the reign of Elizabeth had eighteen vessels, from five to forty-five tons' burden. The quay mentioned by Leland, under the appellation of *Thorn*, has long been in disuse, and in its stead three new quays, or wharfs, have been constructed close to the town. The navigation of the river has been much improved of late; vessels of one hundred tons' burden can generally come up to the wharf with the tides, and the channel will now admit of ships drawing eight feet water to sail up at spring tides. About thirty coasting vessels, of from forty to one hundred and fifty tons' each, belong to the port: there are a custom-house and an excise-office. The number of vessels which entered inwards from foreign parts, in 1826, was eighty-five British, and four foreign; and the number that cleared outwards, eleven British and one foreign. The management and support of the navigation are vested in the corporation, and the expenses are defrayed by town droits of twopence per quarter on grain, and four-pence per ton, or load, on all other goods exported or imported, which have been levied from time immemorial. The oyster fishery is very considerable, and constitutes a prominent article of trade. The com-

pany of free fishermen and free dredgermen of the hundred of Faversham, as tenants under the lord of the manor, are under his jurisdiction and protection, and he appoints a steward, who holds two courts annually, called Admiralty Courts, or Water Courts, at which all regulations for the benefit of the fishery are made. To be a free dredger, it is necessary to have served a seven year's apprenticeship to a freeman, and also to be a married man. The right of this fishery was originally an appurtenance to the manor of Milton, but was detached from it by King John, who conferred it upon Faversham abbey, together with the property in the grounds. The markets are on Wednesday and Saturday, besides which there is a cattle market monthly, and an annual fair on Michaelmas-day.

Seal.

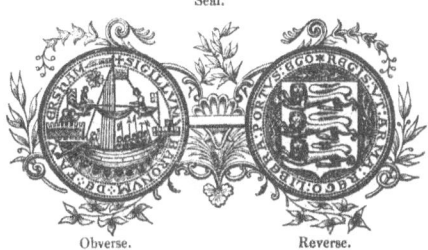

Obverse.   Reverse.

From an early period this town has been a member of the port of Dovor, as one of the cinque-ports, and this connexion may probably account for many of the privileges it has obtained. The oldest charter now extant is that of the 36th of Henry III., in which its freemen are styled "Barons;" other charters of confirmation, with extended privileges, have been given by subsequent monarchs, and that under which it is now governed was granted in the 37th of Henry VIII., by which the government is vested in twelve jurats, of whom one is annually chosen mayor, twenty-four common council-men, assisted by a town clerk, two chamberlains, two serjeants at mace, and other officers. The mayor is chosen annually on the 30th of September; the jurats are chosen by the mayor and the greater part of their own body; and one half of the common council-men are elected by the mayor and jurats, the other half by the common council; the twelve jurats are justices of the peace. A company of mercers was established by a by-law of the corporation in 1616, con sisting of a master, two wardens, and eight assistants, who have the power of admitting persons to the freedom of the company, of which the mayor is always master, and two of the jurats are chosen wardens; the town clerk is the clerk of the company. The freedom of the town is obtained by servitude and by purchase, the fee of which is £10; and every son of a freeman inherits the privilege on coming of age: the freedom of the port is obtained by servitude and marriage; it comprises the freedom of the town, but the converse does not hold. The mayor holds a court of session twice a year, at which all offenders, except for high treason, are tried, and this court has adjournments monthly. He also holds a court of record for the recovery of debts to any amount, but no process has been issued for thirty years. There is a court of requests for the recovery of debts above

2s. and under 40s., by an act passed in the 25th of George III.; and a similar one for the hundred, by the same act, the jurisdiction of which extends to Whitstable, Doddington, and Boughton. The guildhall was erected in 1574, and enlarged in 1814; the upper part is appropriated to the holding of the courts, and the lower part to the use of the market : the gaol was built in 1812.

The living is a discharged vicarage, in the archdeaconry and diocese of Canterbury, rated in the king's books at £26. 17. 6., and in the patronage of the Dean and Chapter of Canterbury. The church, dedicated to St. Mary, was founded prior to the Conquest, and given by William the Conqueror to the abbey of St. Augustine, at Canterbury. The present edifice is a spacious cruciform structure of flint, partly in the decorated, and partly in the later style of English architecture, with a light tower at the west end, crowned with pinnacles, and surmounted by an octagonal spire, seventy-three feet high. The interior of the west end was rebuilt in 1755, from a design by the late George Dance, Esq., at an expense of about £2500, raised partly by assessments on the inhabitants, and partly by a donation from the corporation ; but the tower and spire are of more recent erection. At the west end of the south aisle is a large room, now used as a school-room, and beneath this is a crypt, or chapel, divided in the centre by three round pillars sustaining pointed arches. The monuments are numerous, but not particularly interesting. There are places of worship for Baptists, Independents, and Wesleyan Methodists. The grammar school, situated on the north side of the church-yard, was founded by Dr. Cole, a native of Kent, and Warden of All Souls' College, Oxford, in the 18th of Henry VIII., who bequeathed to the abbot and convent of Faversham divers lands in the neighbourhood, for a school, in which " the novices of the abbey were to be instructed in grammar ;" but at the dissolution the lands became vested in the crown, and continued so until the 18th of Elizabeth, when a charter was obtained for re-founding it ; the mayor, jurats, and commonalty of Faversham, with their successors, being constituted governors, with a common seal. The master is appointed by the warden, or sub-warden, and six senior fellows of All Souls' College, Oxford, and in default of their nomination, the Archbishop of Canterbury appoints. The annual produce of the endowment is £200, the whole of which, after deducting the expense of repairs, with other incidental charges, averaging about £30 a year, is paid to the master. The school is open for classical instruction to all boys of the town and neighbourhood. Here are also two small charity schools, established in the year 1716, and supported principally by subscriptions, for instructing and clothing youth of both sexes. A National school was established in 1814, which is endowed with various benefactions, producing about £60 a year, and further supported by subscription, in which one hundred and seventy boys, and two hundred girls, receive instruction. Almshouses for six poor widows were founded in 1614, and endowed by Thomas Menfield with £24 per annum. Henry Wreight has erected six more, and allows the inmates a weekly sum ; he has also built six for decayed dredgers. Thomas Napleton, in 1721, founded and endowed almshouses for six poor men, who receive £25

per annum each ; and there are also some almshouses unendowed, and tenements for poor persons. Dr. John Wilson, an eminent musician and gentleman of the chapel royal in the reigns of Charles I. and Charles II., and musical professor in the University of Oxford, was born here in 1595 : this is also the birthplace of Dr. Marsh, Bishop of Peterborough. Faversham gives the title of baron to the family of Duncombe.

FAVINLEY, otherwise FARNLAWS, a township in that part of the parish of HARTBURN which is in the north-eastern division of TINDALE ward, county of NORTHUMBERLAND, 13 miles (W. by N.) from Morpeth, containing 16 inhabitants.

FAWCET-FOREST, a township partly in the parish of ORTON, EAST ward, partly in that of SHAP, WEST ward, but chiefly in that part of the parish of KENDAL which is in KENDAL ward, county of WESTMORLAND, 7 miles (N.N.E.) from Kendal, containing 54 inhabitants. This wild and extensive district was anciently called *Fauside*, and belonged to Byland abbey, Yorkshire.

FAWDINTON, a township in that part of the parish of CUNDALL which is in the wapentake of BIRDFORTH, North riding of the county of YORK, 5¾ miles (N. E. by N.) from Boroughbridge, containing 39 inhabitants.

FAWDON, a township in that part of the parish of GOSFORTH which is in the western division of CASTLE ward, county of NORTHUMBERLAND, 4 miles (N.N.W.) from Newcastle upon Tyne, containing 747 inhabitants. In 1801, there were only twenty-six inhabitants, the increase being caused by the establishment of extensive collieries.

FAWDON, a joint township with Clinch and Hareside, in the parish of INGRAM, northern division of Coquetdale ward, county of NORTHUMBERLAND, 9¾ miles (S. by E.) from Wooler, containing 80 inhabitants.

FAWKHAM, a parish in the hundred of AXTON DARTFORD, and WILMINGTON, lathe of SUTTON at HONE, county of KENT, 5¾ miles (S. E. by S.) from Dartford, containing 168 inhabitants. The living is a rectory, in the archdeaconry and diocese of Rochester, rated in the king's books at £6. 9. 4½., and in the patronage of V. D. Folk, Esq. and Miss Selby alternately. The church, dedicated to St. Mary, is principally in the early style of English architecture.

FAWLER, a hamlet in that part of the parish of CHARLBURY which is in the hundred of BANBURY, county of OXFORD, 4¾ miles (N. by E.) from Witney, containing 147 inhabitants.

FAWLEY, a parish in the hundred of KINTBURY-EAGLE, county of BERKS, 5½ miles (S.) from Wantage, containing, with the tythings of South Fawley and Whatcombe, 212 inhabitants. The living is a vicarage not in charge, in the archdeaconry of Berks, and diocese of Salisbury, and in the patronage of Mr. and Mrs. Wroughton. The church is dedicated to St. Mary.

FAWLEY, a parish in the hundred of DESBOROUGH, county of BUCKINGHAM, 3 miles (N. by W.) from Henley upon Thames, containing 276 inhabitants. The living is a rectory, in the archdeaconry of Buckingham, and diocese of Lincoln, rated in the king's books at £11. 10. 10., and in the patronage of — Freeman, Esq. The church, dedicated to St. Mary, was repaired and fitted up in 1748, at the expense of John Freeman, Esq : the altar, font, pulpit, and pews, belonged to the chapel at Canons.

the seat of the Duke of Chandos, which had been pulled down the year preceding. Fawley-court was garrisoned by the king's troops in 1642, whereby many valuable manuscripts, books, &c., the property of its celebrated owner, Sir Bulstrode Whitlock, were destroyed.

FAWLEY, a chapelry in the parish of FOWNHOPE, hundred of GREYTREE, county of HEREFORD, 8 miles (N. by W.) from Ross. The chapel is dedicated to St. John the Baptist.

FAWLEY, a parish partly in the hundred of REDBRIDGE, comprising the tythings of Brightminstone and Stone, but chiefly in that part of the hundred of BISHOP'S WALTHAM which is in the New Forest (East) division of the county of SOUTHAMPTON, 6 miles (S. S. E.) from Southampton, containing 1684 inhabitants. The living is a rectory, in the peculiar jurisdiction of the incumbent, rated in the king's books at £34. 13. 6½., and in the patronage of the Bishop of Winchester. The church is dedicated to All Saints; in the windows are some curious specimens of painted glass. At Exbury, in this parish, is a chapel of ease. There is a place of worship for Wesleyan Methodists. The parish is bounded on the east by the Southampton water.

FAWNS, a township in the parish of KIRKWHELPINGTON, north-eastern division of TINDALE ward, county of NORTHUMBERLAND, 13¼ miles (W.) from Morpeth, containing 8 inhabitants. It consists only of a single farm, anciently called Le Fawings.

FAWSLEY, a parish in the hundred of FAWSLEY, county of NORTHAMPTON, 5 miles (S. by W.) from Daventry, containing 22 inhabitants. The living is a vicarage, in the archdeaconry of Northampton, and diocese of Peterborough, rated in the king's books at £7. 9. 7. Sir C. Knightley, Bart, was patron in 1819. The church, dedicated to St. Mary, contains several fine monuments of the Knightley family, lords of this manor since the time of Henry III.; and at whose mansion, Fawsley park, the parliamentarian party came to their decisive resolutions previously to the breaking out of the great civil war. A weekly market was formerly held on Thursday. Dr. John Wilkins, a celebrated divine and mathematician, was born here in 1614.

FAXFLEET, a township in that part of the parish of SOUTH CAVE which is within the liberty of ST. PETER of YORK, though locally in the Hunsley-Beacon division of the wapentake of Harthill, East riding of the county of YORK, 7 miles (S.W.) from South Cave, containing 163 inhabitants.

FAXTON, a chapelry in the parish of LAMPORT, hundred of ORLINGBURY, county of NORTHAMPTON, 6 miles (W. S.W.) from Kettering, containing 85 inhabitants. The chapel is dedicated to St. Denis. Lady Danvers, in 1730, founded an almshouse for four poor persons, and endowed it with a rent-charge of £2 per annum; and Jane Kensey, in 1736, bequeathed £100, the interest to be applied in aid of this charity.

FAZAKERLEY, a township in the parish of WALTON on the HILL, hundred of WEST DERBY, county palatine of LANCASTER, 4¼ miles (N.E.) from Liverpool, containing 418 inhabitants. There is a small schoolhouse with a trifling endowment in land, the gift of Samuel Turner, in 1725.

FAZELY, a chapelry in that part of the parish of TAMWORTH which is in the southern division of the hundred of OFFLOW, county of STAFFORD, 1½ mile (S.)

from Tamworth, containing 1128 inhabitants. The living is a perpetual curacy, in the archdeaconry of Stafford, and diocese of Lichfield and Coventry, endowed with £3100 parliamentary grant, and in the patronage of Sir Robert Peel, Bart., whose late father, about the year 1810, erected and liberally endowed the chapel, which has since received an addition of one hundred and twenty free sittings, the Incorporated Society for the enlargement of churches and chapels having granted £60 towards defraying the expense. There is a place of worship for Wesleyan Methodists; also a National school, well supported. The Roman road Watling-street, the Birmingham and Fazely canal, and the Coventry canal, pass through the chapelry, which abounds with coal and stone. There are extensive printing and bleaching-works, and some woollen, nail, and edge-tool manufactures. A court leet is held once in three years: there are fairs for cattle, on March 21st, the second Mondays in January, February, April, September, and December; the third Mondays in July, August, and November; the last Mondays in May and June, and the first Monday after Old Michaelmas-day.

FEARBY, a township in the parish of MASHAM, eastern division of the wapentake of HANG, North riding of the county of YORK, 2 miles (E.) from Masham, containing 214 inhabitants.

FEARNHEAD, a joint township with Poulton, in the parish of WARRINGTON, hundred of WEST DERBY, county palatine of LANCASTER, 2½ miles (N.E.) from Warrington, containing 631 inhabitants.

FEATHERSTON, a township in the parish of HALTWHISTLE, western division of TINDALE ward, county of NORTHUMBERLAND, 3¾ miles (S. W.) from Haltwhistle, containing 239 inhabitants. Featherston castle, which has been recently repaired and enlarged by its present noble owner, was from an early period the seat of the Featherstonehaugh family, one of whom, Timothy, raised a troop of horse for the king during the civil war, and was knighted under the royal banner; but having been taken prisoner at the battle of Worcester, in 1651, he was beheaded, and his estate sold by parliament to the Earl of Carlisle.

FEATHERSTONE, a chapelry in that part of the parish of WOLVERHAMPTON which is in the eastern division of the hundred of CUTTLESTONE, county of STAFFORD, containing 49 inhabitants.

FEATHERSTONE, a parish comprising the townships of Ackton and Whitwood, in the lower division of the wapentake of AGBRIGG, and the townships of Featherstone and Peerston-Jaglin, in the upper division of the wapentake of OSGOLDCROSS, West riding of the county of YORK, and containing 945 inhabitants, of which number, 337 are in the township of Featherstone, 3½ miles (W.) from Pontefract. The living is a discharged vicarage, in the archdeaconry and diocese of York, rated in the king's books at £5. 8. 6½., endowed with £200 private benefaction, and £200 royal bounty, and in the patronage of the Dean and Canons of Christ Church, Oxford. The church is dedicated to All Saints.

FECKENHAM, a parish in the upper division of the hundred of HALFSHIRE, county of WORCESTER, 7 miles (E. by S.) from Droitwich, containing 2383 inhabitants. The living is a discharged vicarage, in the archdeaconry and diocese of Worcester, rated in the king's books at £9, endowed with £400 private benefaction,

£400 royal bounty, and £1500 parliamentary grant, and in the patronage of the Rev. Edward Neal. The church is dedicated to St. John the Baptist. There is a place of worship for Independents. A free grammar school was founded by Sir Thomas Cookes, Bart., and endowed with £50 per annum, arising out of lands in the neighbourhood, a regular attendance at which for two years renders young men eligible to scholarships established by the founder in Worcester College, Oxford; but preference is given to those educated at the school at Bromsgrove. This place gave name to an adjoining forest, and has long been noted for the manufacture of needles and fish hooks. There are fairs for cattle on March 26th and September 30th : a court leet is held in October, when a constable is chosen. John de Feckenham, an eminent Roman Catholic divine, and the last abbot of Westminster, was born here ; he held disputations with Cranmer, Ridley, and Latimer, but performed kind offices for many others of the persecuted protestants in the reign of Mary.

FEERING, a parish in the Witham division of the hundred of LEXDEN, county of ESSEX, 1¼ mile (N.N.E.) from Kelvedon, containing 615 inhabitants. The living is a discharged vicarage, in the archdeaconry of Colchester, and diocese of London, rated in the king's books at £11, and in the patronage of the Bishop of London. The church is dedicated to All Saints. The parish is separated from Kelvedon by the river Pont, or Blackwater, over which there is a light and elegant bridge.

FELBRIGG, a parish in the northern division of the hundred of ERPINGHAM, county of NORFOLK, 3 miles (S.W.) from Cromer, containing 165 inhabitants. The living is a discharged rectory with the rectory of Metton united, in the archdeaconry of Norfolk, and diocese of Norwich, rated in the king's books at £6. 18. 4., and in the patronage of Rear Admiral Windham. The church is dedicated to St. Margaret.

FELIX-KIRK, a parish comprising the township of Felix-Kirk, within the liberty of RIPON, West riding, and the chapelry of Boltby, and the townships of Sutton under Whitestone Cliffe, and Thirlby, in the wapentake of BIRDFORTH, North riding, of the county of YORK, containing 1008 inhabitants, of which number, 113 are in the township of Felix-Kirk, 4 miles (N.E. by E.) from Thirsk. The living is a vicarage, in the archdeaconry of Cleveland, and diocese of York, rated in the king's books at £10, and in the patronage of the Archbishop of York. The church is dedicated to St. Felix. At Mount-St. John, in this parish, the Knights of St. John of Jerusalem had formerly a preceptory.

FELIXSTOW, a parish in the hundred of COLNEIS, county of SUFFOLK, 11½ miles (S.E. by E.) from Ipswich, containing 385 inhabitants. The living is a vicarage, with the vicarage of Walton united, in the archdeaconry of Suffolk, and diocese of Norwich, rated in the king's books at £5. 9. 7., and in the patronage of Mr. Eagle and others. The church is dedicated to St. Peter and St. Paul. The river Deben falls into the North sea on the east of this parish. Roger Bigod, in the reign of William II., gave the church of St. Felix to the monks of Rochester, who established therein a cell of Benedictine monks, which was suppressed in 1528, and its possessions granted to Cardinal Wolsey, towards the endowment of his intended colleges.

FELKINGTON, a township in the parish of NOR-HAM, otherwise Norhamshire, county palatine of DUR-HAM, though locally to the northward of the county of Northumberland, 14½ miles (N. by W.) from Wooler, containing, with Grievestead, 186 inhabitants.

FELKIRK, a parish in the wapentake of STAIN-CROSS, West riding of the county of YORK, 6¼ miles (N.E. by N.) from Barnesley, comprising the townships of Brierly, Havercroft with Cold Hiendley, South Hiendley, and Shafton, and containing 1042 inhabitants. The living is a vicarage, in the archdeaconry and diocese of York, rated in the king's books at £7. 1. 10½., and in the patronage of the Archbishop of York. The church is dedicated to St. Peter. Prudence Berry, in 1637, bequeathed £6 towards the support of a schoolmaster in the parish, in augmentation of whose salary, £10.17.4. is paid by Viscount Galway, for teaching poor children of the township of Havercroft.

FELLISCLIFFE, a township in the parish of HAMPSTHWAITE, lower division of the wapentake of CLARO, West riding of the county of YORK, 8 miles (W.) from Knaresborough, containing 382 inhabitants. This township is within the peculiar ecclesiastical jurisdiction of the court of the honour of Knaresborough.

FELLSIDE, a township in the parish of WHICK-HAM, western division of CHESTER ward, county palatine of DURHAM, 5½ miles (S. W.) from Newcastle, containing 455 inhabitants. The late Earl of Strathmore, in 1812, erected a handsome chapel in the grounds of Gibside hall, one of the seats of the family.

FELLY, a hamlet in the parish of ANNESLEY, northern division of the wapentake of BROXTOW, county of NOTTINGHAM, 8 miles (S.W. by S.) from Mansfield, containing 71 inhabitants. Ralph Brito and his son, in 1156, gave a church and an old hermitage, then standing here, to the monks of Radford, or Wirksop, who built a priory for Black canons, in honour of the Blessed Virgin Mary ; at the time of its dissolution it had five or six religious whose revenue was valued at £61. 4. 8.

FELMERSHAM, a parish in the hundred of WILLEY, county of BEDFORD, 7 miles (N.W. by N.) from Bedford, containing, with the hamlet of Radwell, 390 inhabitants. The living is a discharged vicarage, with the vicarage of Pavenham united, in the archdeaconry of Bedford, and diocese of Lincoln, rated in the king's books at £13. 13. 4., and in the patronage of the Master and Fellows of Trinity College, Cambridge. The church, dedicated to St. Mary, is a handsome edifice in the early style of English architecture. The river Ouse runs through the parish, and is crossed by a bridge at Radwell.

FELMINGHAM, a parish in the hundred of TUN-STEAD, county of NORFOLK, 2½ miles (W.S.W.) from North Walsham, containing 361 inhabitants. There are two livings, one a discharged vicarage, rated in the king's books at £6, and in the patronage of the Bishop of Norwich, and the other a discharged rectory, endowed only with a fourth part of the great tithes, and £600 royal bounty, rated at £6 ; they are in the archdeaconry of Norfolk, and diocese of Norwich. John Seaman, Esq. was patron in 1804. The church is dedicated to St. Andrew.

FELPHAM, a parish in the hundred of AVISFORD, rape of ARUNDEL, county of SUSSEX, 8 miles (S.W.) from Arundel, containing 581 inhabitants. The living comprises a rectory and a discharged vicarage, the former a sinecure, in the archdeaconry and diocese of Chichester, rated together in the king's books at £29. 6. 8., and in the patronage of the Dean of Chichester. The church is dedicated to St. Mary. The parish is situated on the shore of the English channel, and the lands are occasionally subject to inundations from the sea.

FELSHAM, a parish in the hundred of THEDWESTRY, county of SUFFOLK, 6¾ miles (W. by S.) from Stow-Market, containing 389 inhabitants. The living is a rectory, in the archdeaconry of Sudbury, and diocese of Norwich, rated in the king's books at £8. 4. 7. The Rev. Joseph Gould was patron in 1822. The church is dedicated to St. Peter. There is a fair on the 16th of August, for sheep, lambs, and toys.

FELSTEAD, a parish in the hundred of HINCKFORD, county of ESSEX, 4 miles (E.S.E.) from Great Dunmow, containing 1724 inhabitants. The living is a vicarage, in the archdeaconry of Middlesex, and diocese of London, rated in the king's books at £13. 6. 8., and in the patronage of the Hon. W. T. L. P. Wellesley. The church, dedicated to the Holy Cross, has lately received an addition of seventy free sittings, the Incorporated Society for the enlargement of churches and chapels having granted £50 towards defraying the expense; in it is a superb monument to the memory of Lord Rich, who, in the reign of Elizabeth, founded a free school and an almshouse, the former of which has been long supported by some of the principal families in the county. Sydney Boteler, in 1690, gave a rent-charge of £7. 12. per annum, for clothing and teaching six children, and other purposes.

FELTHAM, a parish in the hundred of SPELTHORNE, county of MIDDLESEX, 4 miles (S.W.) from Hounslow, containing 962 inhabitants. The living is a discharged vicarage, in the archdeaconry of Middlesex, and diocese of London, rated in the king's books at £8, endowed with £200 private benefaction, and £200 royal bounty. The Rev. Joseph Morris was patron in 1818. The church is dedicated to St. Dunstan.

FELTHORPE, a parish in the hundred of TAVERHAM, county of NORFOLK, 7 miles (N.W. by N.) from Norwich, containing 370 inhabitants. The living is a discharged rectory, in the archdeaconry and diocese of Norwich, rated in the king's books at £4, endowed with £200 royal bounty, and in the patronage of the Bishop of Norwich. The church is dedicated to St. Margaret.

FELTON, a parish in the hundred of BROXASH, county of HEREFORD, 8 miles (N.E. by N.) from Hereford, containing 135 inhabitants. The living is a discharged vicarage, in the archdeaconry and diocese of Hereford, rated in the king's books at £4. 12. 2., endowed with £600 private benefaction, and £800 royal bounty, and in the patronage of Thomas Hill, and Philip Barneby, Esqrs. The church is dedicated to St. Michael.

FELTON, a parish comprising the townships of Acton with Old Felton, Elyaugh, Felton, Greens with Glantlees, and Swarland, in the eastern division of Coquetdale ward, the townships of Bockenfield, Eshott, and East and West Thriston with Shothaugh, in the eastern division, and the townships of Brinkburn South side, in the western division, of MORPETH ward, county of NORTHUMBERLAND, containing 1516 inha-

bitants, of which number, 554 are in the township of Felton, 9 miles (S.) from Alnwick. The living is a vicarage, in the archdeaconry of Northumberland, and diocese of Durham, rated in the king's books at £3. 13. 4., and in the patronage of the Crown. The church, dedicated to St. Michael, stands on an eminence on the north side of the Coquet, which winds beautifully through the parish, and is crossed by a stone bridge of three arches to the westward of the village. On the south side of the river there is a neat place of worship for Presbyterians. Fairs for cattle, sheep, &c. are held on the first Monday in May and the first in November. The barons of Northumberland did homage at Felton to Alexander, King of Scotland, which so exasperated King John, that in 1216 he caused the village to be burned.

FELTON, county of SOMERSET. ——— See WHITCHURCH.

FELTON (OLD), a joint township with Acton, in that part of the parish of FELTON which is in the eastern division of COQUETDALE ward, county of NORTHUMBERLAND, 8 miles (S.) from Alnwick, containing 91 inhabitants.

FELTON (WEST), a parish in the hundred of OSWESTRY, county of SALOP, 5 miles (S.E. by E.) from Oswestry, containing 1035 inhabitants. The living is a rectory, in the archdeaconry of Salop, and diocese of Lichfield and Coventry, rated in the king's books at £20. 12. 6., and in the patronage of the Earl of Craven. The church is dedicated to St. Michael. The Ellesmere canal passes the boundary of this parish. There is a remarkable well in the township of Woolston, dedicated to St. Winifred. John Dovaston, Esq., a man of learning, science, and ingenuity, was born here in 1740, died on the 31st of March, 1808: the limited education which he received was at the village school, and the varied and extensive abilities which he afterwards displayed were self-acquired. The estate, called the Nursery, is now in the occupation of his son, J. F. M. Dovaston, Esq., who has distinguished himself by his poetical attainments, his sportive genius, and lively imagination.

FELTWELL, a parish comprising the consolidated parishes of St. Mary and St. Nicholas, in the hundred of GRIMSHOE, county of NORFOLK, 6½ miles (S.) from Stoke-Ferry, containing 1153 inhabitants. The living is a rectory, in the archdeaconry of Norfolk, and diocese of Norwich, rated in the king's books at £23. 17. 3½., and in the patronage of the Crown and the Bishop of Ely, alternately. There is a place of worship for Wesleyan Methodists. A fair for toys, &c. is held on the 20th of November.

FENBY, a hamlet in the parish of ASHBY, wapentake of BRADLEY-HAVERSTOE, parts of LINDSEY, county of LINCOLN, 6½ miles (S. by W.) from Great Grimsby. The population is returned with the parish.

FENCOT, a hamlet in the parish of CHARLTON upon OTMORE, hundred of PLOUGHLEY, county of OXFORD, 4¼ miles (S. by W.) from Bicester, containing, with Murcot, 274 inhabitants.

FENCOTT, a township in the parish of DOCKLOW, hundred of WOLPHY, county of HEREFORD, 4½ miles (N.W.) from Bromyard. The population is returned with the parish.

FENHAM, a township in that part of the parish of ST. ANDREW, NEWCASTLE, which is in the western division of CASTLE ward, county of NORTHUMBERLAND.

$1\frac{1}{2}$ mile (W.N.W.) from Newcastle on Tyne, containing 87 inhabitants. Coal is obtained here.

FENITON, a parish in the hundred of HAYRIDGE, county of DEVON, 4 miles (W. by S.) from Honiton, containing 321 inhabitants. The living is a rectory, in the archdeaconry and diocese of Exeter, rated in the king's books at £16. 18. $6\frac{1}{2}$., and in the patronage of the Rev. J. Rogers, Mr. Wolley, and the Northcote family, alternately. The church, dedicated to St. Andrew, has a very rich wooden screen. The villages of Colestock and Corscombe are in this parish. Feniton bridge was the scene of a sanguinary contest, in which Sir J. Russell and Lord Grey defeated the Cornish insurgents, in the reign of Edward VI.

FENROTHER, a township in the parish of HEBBURN, western division of MORPETH ward, county of NORTHUMBERLAND, 5 miles (N.W. by N.) from Morpeth, containing 99 inhabitants.

FEN-STANTON, a parish in the hundred of TOSELAND, county of HUNTINGDON, $2\frac{1}{2}$ miles (S. by E.) from St. Ives, containing 776 inhabitants. The living is a discharged vicarage with the perpetual curacy of Hilton annexed, in the archdeaconry of Huntingdon, and diocese of Lincoln, rated in the king's books at £11. 11. $5\frac{1}{2}$., and in the patronage of the Master and Fellows of Trinity Hall, Cambridge. The church is dedicated to St. Peter and St. Paul. Joseph Ellis, in 1728, endowed a school with about £10 a year, for teaching four children of Fen-Stanton, and four of Fen-Drayton. The river Ouse runs through the parish.

FENTON, a joint township with Faugh, in the parish of HAYTON, ESKDALE ward, county of CUMBERLAND, 8 miles (E.) from Carlisle, containing 331 inhabitants.

FENTON, a chapelry in the parish of BECKINGHAM, wapentake of LOVEDEN, parts of KESTEVEN, county of LINCOLN, $7\frac{1}{4}$ miles (E.S.E.) from Newark, containing 99 inhabitants. The chapel is dedicated to All Saints.

FENTON, a hamlet in the parish of KETTLETHORPE, wapentake of WELL, parts of LINDSEY, county of LINCOLN, $9\frac{3}{4}$ miles (N.W. by W.) from Lincoln, containing 198 inhabitants.

FENTON, a hamlet in the parish of WOOLER, eastern division of GLENDALE ward, county of NORTHUMBERLAND, $4\frac{3}{4}$ miles (N. by W.) from Wooler. The population is returned with the parish. There is a fair for cattle, sheep, and horses, on the 27th of September.

FENTON (KIRK), a parish partly within the liberty of ST. PETER of YORK, East riding, but chiefly in the upper division of the wapentake of BARKSTONE-ASH, West riding, of the county of YORK, comprising the townships of Biggin, Little Fenton, and Kirk-Fenton, and containing 693 inhabitants, of which number, 416 are in the township of Kirk-Fenton, 5 miles (S.E. by S.) from Tadcaster. The living is a discharged vicarage, in the peculiar jurisdiction and patronage of the Prebendary of Kirk-Fenton in the Cathedral Church of York, rated in the king's books at £6. 13. 4.

FENTON (LITTLE), a township in the parish of KIRK-FENTON, partly within the liberty of ST. PETER of YORK, East riding, and partly in the upper division of the wapentake of BARKSTONE-ASH, West riding, of the county of YORK, $6\frac{1}{2}$ miles (S. E. by S.) from Tadcaster, containing 113 inhabitants.

FENTON-CALVERT, a township in the parish

of STOKE upon TRENT, northern division of the hundred of PIREHILL, county of STAFFORD, $2\frac{3}{4}$ miles (E.S.E.) from Newcastle under Line. The population is returned with the parish.

FENTON-VIVIAN, a township in the parish of STOKE upon TRENT, northern division of the hundred of PIREHILL, county of STAFFORD, $2\frac{1}{4}$ miles (E.) from Newcastle under Line. The population is returned with the parish.

FENWICK, a township in the parish of STAMFORD-HAM, north-eastern division of TINDALE ward, county of NORTHUMBERLAND, $13\frac{1}{2}$ miles (N.W. by W.) from Newcastle upon Tyne, containing 76 inhabitants. Fenwick tower, which was the seat of the ancient family of the same name, has long been in ruins; in pulling down a part of it in 1775, two hundred and twenty-six gold nobles of the reigns of Edward III., Richard II., and David II. of Scotland, were found.

FENWICK, a township in the parish of CAMPSALL, upper division of the wapentake of OSGOLDCROSS, West riding of the county of YORK, $5\frac{1}{2}$ miles (S.W.) from Snaith, containing 295 inhabitants. There is a place of worship for Wesleyan Methodists.

FEOCK, a parish in the western division of the hundred of POWDER, county of CORNWALL, 5 miles (S.) from Truro, containing 1093 inhabitants. The living is a discharged vicarage, in the archdeaconry of Cornwall, and diocese of Exeter, rated in the king's books at £11, and in the patronage of the Bishop of Exeter. The church is dedicated to St. Feock; it has a low detached tower at the distance of twenty feet from the main building. There is a place of worship for Wesleyan Methodists. The parish is bounded on the east by Truro river, on the west by a creek of Falmouth harbour, and on the south by Carrick roads.

FERENSBY, a township in the parish of FARNHAM, lower division of the wapentake of CLARO, West riding of the county of YORK, $2\frac{1}{2}$ miles (N.E. by N.) from Knaresborough, containing 110 inhabitants. This township is within the peculiar ecclesiastical jurisdiction of the court of the honour of Knaresborough.

FERNHAM, a hamlet in the parish and hundred of SHRIVENHAM, county of BERKS, $2\frac{1}{4}$ miles (S. by E.) from Great Farringdon, containing 183 inhabitants.

FERNILEE, a township in the parish of HOPE, hundred of HIGH PEAK, county of DERBY, containing 422 inhabitants. Thomas Ouff, in 1786, bequeathed an estate, from the proceeds of which £18 a year is paid for teaching eight children.

FERRIBY (NORTH), a parish in the county of the town of KINGSTON upon HULL, East riding of the county of YORK, comprising the townships of North Ferriby and Swanland, and containing 765 inhabitants, of which number, 347 are in the township of North Ferriby, $5\frac{1}{4}$ miles (S. E.) from South Cave. The living is a discharged vicarage, in the archdeaconry of the East riding, and diocese of York, rated in the king's books at £8. 13. 4., endowed with £400 private benefaction, £200 royal bounty, and £2300 parliamentary grant, and in the patronage of Sir Robert Peel, Bart. The church, dedicated to All Saints, appears to be a part only of a more spacious structure, and contains some handsome monuments. Two annuities of £10 each, one the gift of Luke Lillington, Esq., in 1773, the other that of Sir Henry Etherington, Bart., in 1781, are paid to a schoolmaster for teaching poor children. The parish is bounded on the south by the Humber. A priory of Knights Templars, founded here by Lord Eustace Vescy, was, at the suppression of that order, converted into a priory of Augustine canons, whose revenue at the dissolution was valued at £95. 11. 7.

FERRIBY (SOUTH), a parish in the northern division of the wapentake of YARBOROUGH, parts of LINDSEY, county of LINCOLN, 3¼ miles (W. by S.) from Barton upon Humber, containing 453 inhabitants. The living is a discharged rectory, in the archdeaconry and diocese of Lincoln, rated in the king's books at £12. 17. 6., and in the patronage of the Bishop of Lincoln. The church, dedicated to St. Nicholas, is remarkable as standing north and south. There is a place of worship for Wesleyan Methodists. The Humber bounds the parish on the north.

FERRING, a parish in the hundred of POLING, rape of ARUNDEL, county of SUSSEX, 3¾ miles (W.) from Worthing, containing 286 inhabitants. The living is a discharged vicarage, in the archdeaconry and diocese of Chichester, rated in the king's books at £6. 8. 4., and in the patronage of the Prebendary of Ferring in the Cathedral Church of Chichester. The church, which is in the early style of English architecture, is dedicated to St. Andrew, in honour of whom a church, or monastery, was built here so early as the time of Offa, King of Mercia, of which there were some remains in the reign of Edward III.

FERRY (EAST), a chapelry in the parish of SCOTTON, wapentake of CORRINGHAM, parts of LINDSEY, county of LINCOLN, 7¼ miles (N. by E.) from Gainsborough, containing 151 inhabitants. The chapel is dedicated to St. Mary. There is a place of worship for Wesleyan Methodists.

FERRY-BRIDGE, a hamlet in the parish of FERRY-FRYSTONE, upper division of the wapentake of OSGOLDCROSS, West riding of the county of YORK, 21½ miles (S. S. W.) from York. The population is returned with the parish. This place derives its importance from its situation on the great north road; there are some excellent inns, and the houses are in general well built: a handsome stone bridge here crosses the river Aire. The possession of this pass was warmly contested by the rival armies of York and Lancaster, since which period numerous skeletons, pieces of armour, and other military relics, have been often found in the neighbourhood. There is a place of worship for Wesleyan Methodists.

FERRY-HILL, a chapelry in the parish of MERRINGTON, south-eastern division of DARLINGTON ward, county palatine of DURHAM, 5¾ miles (E. N. E.) from Bishop-Auckland, containing 574 inhabitants. The chapel has lately received an addition of three hundred and fifty-two sittings, of which two hundred and fifty-six are free, the Incorporated Society for the enlargement of churches and chapels having granted £250 towards defraying the expense. There are collieries in the neighbourhood. At an early period the convent of Durham had a chapel here, dedicated to St. Ebbe and St. Nicholas, a court-house, swannery, and fish pool; there are still some remains of the swan-house.

FERSFIELD, a parish in the hundred of DISS, county of NORFOLK, 4¼ miles (W. N. W.) from Diss, containing 325 inhabitants. The living is a rectory, in the archdeaconry of Norfolk, and diocese of Norwich, rated

in the king's books at £6. 6. 8. Frederick Nassau, Esq. was patron in 1803. The church is dedicated to St. Andrew.

FETCHAM, a parish in the second division of the hundred of COPTHORNE, county of SURREY, 1¼ mile (W.) from Leatherhead, containing 377 inhabitants. The living is a rectory, in the archdeaconry of Surrey, and diocese of Winchester, rated in the king's books at £21. 10. 5. The Rev. J. G. Bolland was patron in 1818. The church is an ancient structure of flints, pebbles, chalk, and Roman tile, and, though now small, appears to have been formerly large and cruciform. The bones of about twenty human bodies, a small pike, and some knife blades, were found near this spot in 1758; and on the top of the hill other bones have been discovered, supposed to be the remains of those Saxons who were killed in the pursuit of the Danes, after the battle of Ockley, in 851, which seems to be countenanced by the name of Standard hill having been given to a neighbouring eminence.

FEWCOT, a hamlet in the parish of STOKE-LYNE, hundred of PLOUGHLEY, county of OXFORD, 4 miles (N. W.) from Bicester, containing 148 inhabitants.

FEWSTON, a parish in the lower division of the wapentake of CLARO, West riding of the county of YORK, comprising the townships of Blubberhouses, Clifton with Norwood, Fewston, Thurcross, and Great Timble, and containing 1989 inhabitants, of which number, 610 are in the township of Fewston, 7 miles (N. by W.) from Otley. The living is a discharged vicarage, in the peculiar jurisdiction of the court for the honour of Knaresborough, rated in the king's books at £5, endowed with £200 royal bounty, and in the patronage of the Crown. The church is dedicated to St. Mary Magdalene.

FIDDINGTON, a joint tything with Natton, in the parish of ASHCHURCH, lower division of the hundred of TEWKESBURY, county of GLOUCESTER, 3 miles (E. by S.) from Tewkesbury, containing 166 inhabitants.

FIDDINGTON, a parish in the hundred of CANNINGTON, county of SOMERSET, 7¼ miles (W. N. W.) from Bridg-water, containing 185 inhabitants. The living is a discharged rectory, in the archdeaconry of Taunton, and diocese of Bath and Wells, rated in the king's books at £6. 10. 2½., and in the patronage of the Rev. H. W. Rawlins. The church is dedicated to St. Martin.

FIELD, a township in the parish of LEIGH, southern division of the hundred of TOTMONSLOW, county of STAFFORD, 4½ miles (W.) from Uttoxeter, containing 72 inhabitants.

FIELD-DALLING, a parish in the northern division of the hundred of GREENHOE, county of NORFOLK, 5 miles (E. by N.) from Little Walsingham, containing 322 inhabitants. The living is a discharged vicarage, in the archdeaconry and diocese of Norwich, rated in the king's books at £5. 8. 1¼., and endowed with £400 royal bounty. Mrs. Smith was patroness in 1811. The church is dedicated to St. Andrew. Maud de Harscolye, in the time of Henry II., founded here a priory, as a cell to the Cistercian abbey of Savigny in Normandy, which, after the suppression of Alien houses, was granted by Richard II. to the Carthusian monastery near Coventry, and subsequently to the priory of Mountgrace.

FIFEHEAD-MAGDALEN, a parish in the hundred

of REDLANE, Sturminster division of the county of DORSET, 6 miles (W. by S.) from Shaftesbury, containing 296 inhabitants. The living is a vicarage, in the archdeaconry of Dorset, and diocese of Bristol, rated in the king's books at £7, and in the patronage of the Bishop of Bristol. The church is dedicated to All Saints.

FIFEHEAD-NEVILLE, a parish in the hundred of PIMPERNE, Blandford (North) division of the county of DORSET, 10½ miles (N.W. by W.) from Blandford-Forum, containing 95 inhabitants. The living is a discharged rectory with that of Bellchalwell, in the archdeaconry of Dorset, and diocese of Bristol, rated in the king's books at £5. 1. 5½., and in the patronage of Lord Rivers. The church is dedicated to All Saints.

FIFIELD, a parish in the hundred of CHADLINGTON, county of OXFORD, 4½ miles (N. by W.) from Burford, containing 136 inhabitants. The living is a perpetual curacy, in the peculiar jurisdiction of the Chancellor of the Cathedral Church of Salisbury, endowed with £16 per annum and £200 private benefaction, £600 royal bounty, and £300 parliamentary grant, and in the patronage of the Hon. and Rev. Hugh Percy. The church is dedicated to St. John the Baptist. The river Evenlode skirts part of the parish. Jane Bray, in 1715, gave a rent-charge of £4. 10. a year for teaching poor children.

FIFIELD, a hamlet in that part of the parish of BENSINGTON which is in the hundred of DORCHESTER, county of OXFORD, 3 miles (N. E.) from Wallingford, containing only 2 inhabitants.

FIFIELD-BAVANT, a parish in the hundred of CHALK, county of WILTS, 6¾ miles (S. W.) from Wilton, containing 42 inhabitants. The living is a discharged rectory, in the archdeaconry and diocese of Salisbury, rated in the king's books at £7. 10., and in the patronage of the Crown.

FIGHELDEAN, a parish in the hundred of AMESBURY, county of WILTS, 4¼ miles (N.) from Amesbury, containing 437 inhabitants. The living is a discharged vicarage with a sinecure rectory, in the peculiar jurisdiction and patronage of the Treasurer in the Cathedral Church of Salisbury, rated in the king's books at £37. The church is dedicated to St. Michael.

FILBY, a parish in the eastern division of the hundred of FLEGG, county of NORFOLK, 3 miles (W. by N.) from Caistor, containing 424 inhabitants. The living is a rectory, in the archdeaconry of Norfolk, and diocese of Norwich, rated in the king's books at £11. 1. 5½. Charles Lucas, Esq. was patron in 1820. The church is dedicated to All Saints. There are places of worship for Wesleyan Methodists and Unitarians.

FILEY, a parish partly in PICKERING lythe, North riding, but chiefly in the wapentake of DICKERING, East riding, of the county of YORK, 2½ miles (N. by E.) from Hunmanby, containing, with the townships of Gristhorpe and Libberston, which are in Pickering lythe, 1128 inhabitants. The living is a perpetual curacy, in the archdeaconry of the East riding, and diocese of York, endowed with £400 private benefaction, £600 royal bounty, and £1600 parliamentary grant, and in the patronage of Humphrey Osbaldeston, Esq. The church is dedicated to St. Oswald. The parish is bounded on the east by the bay of the same name. It has a considerable fishery, and is much resorted to in the bathing season. There is a mineral spring, the water of which has properties similar to that at Scarborough.

FILGROVE, a joint parish with Tyrringham, in the hundred of NEWPORT, county of BUCKINGHAM, 3¾ miles (N.) from Newport-Pagnell, containing 204 inhabitants. The living, a rectory, is united to that of Tyrringham, in the archdeaconry of Buckingham, and diocese of Lincoln, rated in the king's books at £5. 19. 7. The church, which was dedicated to St. Mary, is in ruins.

FILKINS, a hamlet in the parish of BROADWELL, hundred of BAMPTON, county of OXFORD, 5 miles (S. by W.) from Burford, containing 508 inhabitants.

FILLEIGH, a parish in the hundred of BRAUNTON, though locally in the hundred of South Molton, county of DEVON, 3¾ miles (W. N. W.) from South Molton, containing 307 inhabitants. The living is a rectory, in the archdeaconry of Barnstaple, and diocese of Exeter, rated in the king's books at £12. 5. 2½., and in the patronage of Earl Fortescue. The church, dedicated to St. Paul, was built by Earl Fortescue in 1732. There is a charity school, chiefly supported by the Earl and Countess, in which about fifty children are educated and clothed. Limestone and a hard stone of a blueish tinge, used for building, are obtained in the parish, and perfect *nautili* have been found here.

FILLINGHAM, a parish in the western division of the wapentake of ASLACOE, parts of LINDSEY, county of LINCOLN, 10 miles (N. by W.) from Lincoln, containing 279 inhabitants. The living is a rectory, in the archdeaconry of Stow, and diocese of Lincoln, rated in the king's books at £22, and in the patronage of the Master and Fellows of Balliol College, Oxford. The church is dedicated to St. Andrew. There are fairs for pigs on the Thursday in Easter week and on Nov. 22d. In the grounds of Summer castle, an embattled edifice built by Sir Cecil Wray, in 1760, are vestiges of a Roman camp, where coins, spear-heads, and fragments of armour have been discovered.

FILLONGLEY, a parish in the Atherstone division of the hundred of HEMLINGFORD, county of WARWICK, 6½ miles (N. W. by N.) from Coventry, containing 980 inhabitants. The living is a discharged vicarage, in the archdeaconry of Coventry, and diocese of Lichfield and Coventry, rated in the king's books at £8. 9. 9., and in the patronage of the Crown. The church is dedicated to St. Mary and All Saints: to the southward of it are the ruins of an ancient castle, and on the north-east, the area and mounds of another, called Castle hills, are still visible. There is a free school for all the children of the parish, founded by Richard Walker, and endowed with a farm-house and twenty-nine acres of land, the rent of which is equally divided between the master and mistress. William Avery, in 1732, left certain houses and lands, from the proceeds of which £10 a year is paid for teaching ten boys, and £10 for clothing them in blue; and Ayliffe Green bequeathed a house with thirty-one acres of land for similar purposes, the boys to be dressed in green. Several fine trout streams have their sources in the parish.

FILTON, a parish in the lower division of the hundred of BERKELEY, county of GLOUCESTER, 3½ miles (N. by E.) from Bristol, containing 210 inhabitants. The living is a discharged rectory, in the peculiar jurisdiction of the Bishop of Bristol, rated in the king's books at £7, endowed with £200 private benefaction, and £200 royal bounty. Mrs. Manley was patroness in 1824. The church, dedicated to St. Peter, is chiefly in the decorated style of English architecture.

FIMBER, a chapelry in the parish of WETWANG, partly within the liberty of ST. PETER of YORK, and partly in the wapentake of BUCKROSE, East riding of the county of YORK, 8¾ miles (W. by N.) from Great Driffield, containing 104 inhabitants. This chapelry is within the peculiar jurisdiction of the Prebendary of Wetwang in the Cathedral Church of York.

FINBOROUGH (GREAT), a parish in the hundred of STOW, county of SUFFOLK, 2¾ miles (W. by S.) from Stow-Market, containing 392 inhabitants. The living is a discharged vicarage, in the archdeaconry and diocese of Norwich, rated in the king's books at £5. 1. 3., and in the patronage of the Bishop of Ely. The church is dedicated to St. Andrew.

FINBOROUGH (LITTLE), a parish in the hundred of STOW, county of SUFFOLK, 3¾ miles (S. W. by S.) from Stow-Market, containing 70 inhabitants. The living is a discharged perpetual curacy, in the archdeaconry of Suffolk, and diocese of Norwich, rated in the king's books at £1. 13. 4., endowed with £600 royal bounty, and in the patronage of the Provost and Fellows of King's College, Cambridge. The church is dedicated to St. Mary.

FINCHAM, a parish in the hundred of CLACKCLOSE, county of NORFOLK, 5 miles (E. N. E.) from Downham-Market, containing 708 inhabitants. It formerly comprised two parishes; St. Martin's, a discharged vicarage, and St. Michael's, a discharged rectory, in the archdeaconry of Norfolk, and diocese of Norwich, now consolidated, rated jointly in the king's books at £17. 6. 8, and in the patronage of the Crown and the Rev. R. Forby, alternately. There is a place of worship for Wesleyan Methodists. A fair for horses and toys is held on March 3rd, and there is a show of horses on August 9th.

FINCHAMPSTEAD, a parish in the hundred of CHARLTON, county of BERKS, 3¾ miles (S.S.W.) from Wokingham, containing 552 inhabitants. The living is a rectory, in the archdeaconry of Berks, and diocese of Salisbury, rated in the king's books at £12. 9. 4½. Rev. Ellis St. John was patron in 1819. The church is dedicated to St. James. Henry VI. granted a charter for an annual fair on Whit-Monday and the two following days, which has fallen into disuse; but at West-court, within the parish, there is a fair for cattle on April 23rd.

FINCHINGFIELD, a parish in the hundred of HINCKFORD, county of ESSEX, 5½ miles (E. by N.) from Thaxted, containing 2007 inhabitants. The living is a vicarage, in the archdeaconry of Middlesex, and diocese of London, rated in the king's books at £18. R. Marriot, Esq. was patron in 1810. The church is dedicated to St. John the Baptist. There is a place of worship for Independents. William Bendlowes, in 1576, founded an almshouse for four widows, towards the maintenance of whom Sir Robert Kempe left £5 per annum; he also bequeathed £5 a year for a school; and Ann Cole, in 1730, gave a rent-charge of £6.3., for teaching and apprenticing children.

FINCHLEY, a parish in the Finsbury division of the hundred of OSSULSTONE, county of MIDDLESEX, 7 miles (N. W. by N.) from London, containing 2349 inhabitants. The living is a rectory, in the archdeaconry of Middlesex, and diocese of London, rated in

the king's books at £20, and in the patronage of the Bishop of London. The church, dedicated to St. Mary, is a stone edifice in the later English style, consisting of a nave, chancel, and north aisle, and containing several ancient monuments. Here are places of worship for Independents and Wesleyan Methodists. The great north road through Highgate passes to the east of the parish church, and it is joined by a new road from St. John's Wood, Paddington. A market for pigs is held here every Monday. This place is within the jurisdiction of a court of requests for the recovery of debts under 40s., held at Kingsgate-street, Holborn. In 1489, Robert Waren gave land at Finchley for charitable uses, which, together with property arising from other benefactions, was vested in certain trustees, who erected an almshouse for six poor persons: the income is about £280 per annum, part of which is applied in repairing the church and highways, relieving the poor, and other purposes, the sum of £10 per annum being paid to a National school, which is further supported by subscription. Finchley common, stated to contain one thousand and ten acres of land now enclosed, is situated partly in this parish and partly in those of Friern-Barnet and Hornsey. On this spot General Monk drew up his army in 1660; and here also a detachment of troops encamped during the summer of 1780, after the riots in London, occasioned by the meeting of the Protestant Association under Lord George Gordon.

FINDERN, a chapelry in the parish of MICKLEOVER, hundred of MORLESTON and LITCHURCH, county of DERBY, 5 miles (S. W. by S.) from Derby, containing 363 inhabitants. The chapel is dedicated to All Saints. There is a place of worship for the Unitarians. The Trent and Mersey canal passes through the chapelry. John Allsop, in 1714, bequeathed land and premises, now producing £50 a year, for the maintenance of a schoolmaster, to teach the children of Findern, Willington, and Stenson; there is also a bequest by John Erpe, of 13s. per annum, applied to the same purpose.

FINDON, a parish in the hundred of BRIGHTFORD, rape of BRAMBER, county of SUSSEX, 4 miles (W. S. W.) from Steyning, containing 477 inhabitants. The living is a discharged vicarage, in the archdeaconry and diocese of Chichester, rated in the king's books at £13. 3. 9., and in the patronage of the President and Fellows of Magdalene College, Oxford. The church, dedicated to St. John the Baptist, is mostly in the early English style, with an east window of decorated architecture. There are fairs on Holy Thursday for pedlary, and on September 14th for sheep.

FINEDON, otherwise THINGDON, a parish in the hundred of HUXLOE, county of NORTHAMPTON, 3¼ miles (N. E. by N.) from Wellingborough, containing 1159 inhabitants. The living is a vicarage, in the archdeaconry of Northampton, and diocese of Peterborough, rated in the king's books at £10. 17. 1. Sir E. Dolben, Bart. was patron in 1810. The church, dedicated to St. Mary, is a large and handsome edifice, mostly in the decorated style: the tower, battlements, and spire, are fine specimens of later English architecture: the font is a large cubical mass of stone, with the angles sloped off, so as to make the plan of the upper face octagonal. There is a place of worship for Wesleyan Methodists.

FINESHADE, a parish in the hundred of CORBY, county of NORTHAMPTON, 8 miles (N. N. W.) from Oundle, containing 76 inhabitants. The living is a donative, in the patronage of C. Kirkman, Esq. The church is dedicated to St. Mary. On the ruins of Castle-Hymel, which was demolished in the reign of King John, a priory of Black canons was founded by Richard Engain, Lord of Blatherwike, in honour of the Blessed Virgin, the revenue of which, at the dissolution, was estimated at £62. 16.

FINGALL, a parish in the western division of the wapentake of HANG, North riding of the county of YORK, comprising the townships of Akebar, Burton-Constable, Fingall, and Hang-Hutton, and containing 398 inhabitants, of which number, 126 are in the township of Fingall, 5 miles (E. N. E.) from Middleham. The living is a rectory, in the archdeaconry of Richmond, and diocese of Chester, rated in the king's books at £18. 18. 4., and in the patronage of Marmaduke Wyvill, Esq. The church is dedicated to St. Andrew.

FINGEST, a parish in the hundred of DESBOROUGH, county of BUCKINGHAM, 5½ miles (N.W. by W.) from Great Marlow, containing 295 inhabitants. The living is a discharged rectory, in the archdeaconry of Buckingham, and diocese of Lincoln, rated in the king's books at £6. 7. 11., endowed with £200 private benefaction, and £200 royal bounty, and in the patronage of the Prebendary of Dultingcot in the Cathedral Church of Wells. The church, dedicated to St. Bartholomew, exhibits some remains of Norman architecture; the font is circular and enriched with arches. There is a bequest in land, by the Rev. Francis Edmunds, for teaching and clothing twelve children.

FINGLAND, a township in the parish of BOWNESS, ward and county of CUMBERLAND, 6½ miles (N.) from Wigton, containing 128 inhabitants.

FINGRINGHOE, a parish in the hundred of WINSTREE, county of ESSEX, 4¼ miles (S.E. by S.) from Colchester, containing 472 inhabitants. The living is a discharged vicarage, in the archdeaconry of Colchester, and diocese of London, rated in the king's books at £13. 7. Peter Firmin, Esq. was patron in 1826. The church is dedicated to St. Andrew. The river Colne is navigable on the east, and Geeton creek on the south side of the parish.

FININGHAM, a parish in the hundred of HARTISMERE, county of SUFFOLK, 6¼ miles (W. S. W.) from Eye, containing 435 inhabitants. The living is a discharged rectory, in the archdeaconry of Sudbury, and diocese of Norwich, rated in the king's books at £10. 10. 5. The Right Hon. J. H. Frere was patron in 1825. The church is dedicated to St. Bartholomew. A fair for lean cattle and toys is held on the 4th of September.

FINMERE, a parish in the hundred of PLOUGHLEY, county of OXFORD, 8 miles (N. E. by N.) from Bicester, containing 395 inhabitants. The living is a rectory, in the archdeaconry and diocese of Oxford, rated in the king's books at £8. 9. 4½., and in the patronage of the Duke of Buckingham. The church is dedicated to St. Michael. The river Ouse runs through the parish.

FINNINGLEY, a parish comprising the township of Aulkey, in the Hatfield division of the wapentake of BASSETLAW, county of NOTTINGHAM, and the township of Blaxton, in the soke of DONCASTER, West riding of the county of YORK, 4 miles (N. by E.) from Bawtry, and containing 782 inhabitants. The living is a rectory, in the archdeaconry of Nottingham, and diocese of York, rated in the king's books at £13. 4. 9½. J. Harvey, Esq. was patron in 1826. The church is dedicated to St. Oswald. There is a school for educating and clothing a limited number of boys; it was established by the rector, and has been since extended by private contributions.

FINSTHWAITE, a parochial chapelry in the parish of COULTON, hundred of LONSDALE, north of the sands, county palatine of LANCASTER, 8½ miles (N. E. by N.) from Ulverstone. The population is returned with the parish. The living is a perpetual curacy, in the archdeaconry of Richmond, and diocese of Chester, endowed with £600 private benefaction, and £600 royal bounty, and in the patronage of the land-owners. The chapel, which is dedicated to St. Peter, was consecrated and made parochial in 1725. There is a small endowment for a school, the gift of James Dixon, in 1729. Finsthwaite is bounded on the north-east by the outlet of Winandermere lake.

FINSTOCK, a hamlet in that part of the parish of CHARLBURY which is in the hundred of BANBURY, county of OXFORD, 4¼ miles (N.) from Witney, containing 497 inhabitants.

FIRBANK, a chapelry in the parish of KIRKBY-LONSDALE, LONSDALE ward, county of WESTMORLAND, 10½ miles (N.) from Kirkby-Lonsdale, containing 209 inhabitants. The living is a perpetual curacy, in the archdeaconry of Richmond, and diocese of Chester, endowed with £200 private benefaction, and £600 royal bounty, and in the patronage of the Vicar of Kirkby-Lonsdale. The chapel and burying-ground are on the edge of an extensive moor. The chapelry is bounded on the west by the river Lune, which separates it from Yorkshire.

FIRBECK, a parish partly in the liberty of ST. PETER of YORK, and partly in the southern division of the wapentake of STRAFFORTH and TICKHILL, West riding of the county of YORK, 4½ miles (S. W. by S.) from Tickhill, containing 226 inhabitants. The living is a perpetual curacy, in the archdeaconry and diocese of York, endowed with £1200 royal bounty, and in the peculiar jurisdiction and patronage of the Chancellor in the Cathedral Church of York. The church, dedicated to St. Peter, has lately received an addition of one hundred and fourteen free sittings, the Incorporated Society for the enlargement of churches and chapels having granted £120 towards defraying the expense.

FIRBY, a township in the parish of WESTOW, wapentake of BUCKROSE, East riding of the county of YORK, 5 miles (S.W. by S.) from New Malton, containing 44 inhabitants.

FIRBY, a township in that part of the parish of BEDALE which is in the eastern division of the wapentake of HANG, North riding of the county of YORK, 1¼ mile (S. by E.) from Bedale, containing 76 inhabitants.

FIRLE (WEST), a parish in the hundred of TOTNORE, rape of PEVENSEY, county of SUSSEX, 4¾ miles (S. E. by E.) from Lewes, containing 644 inhabitants. The living is a vicarage, united to that of Beddingham, in the archdeaconry of Lewes, and diocese of Chichester, rated in the king's books at £13. 9. 4½. The church is dedicated to St. Peter.

FIRSBY, a parish in the Wold division of the wapentake of CANDLESHOE, parts of LINDSEY, county of LINCOLN, 5 miles (S. E. by E.) from Spilsby, containing 119 inhabitants. The living is a discharged rectory, with the vicarage of Great Steeping united, in the archdeaconry and diocese of Lincoln, rated in the king's books at £12. 0. 2., endowed with £200 royal bounty, and in the patronage of the Rev. Joseph Walls. The church is dedicated to St. Andrew. Steeping river runs through the parish, in which there are several good springs of water; one near the church is slightly chalybeate.

FIRSBY (EAST), a parish in the eastern division of the wapentake of ASLACOE, parts of LINDSEY, county of LINCOLN, 6½ miles (W. by S.) from Market-Raisen, containing 29 inhabitants. The living is a discharged rectory, held by sequestration, in the archdeaconry of Stow, and diocese of Lincoln, rated in the king's books at £6. 13. 4. The church, dedicated to St. James, has fallen into ruins ; the parishioners resort to Saxby church.

FIRSBY (WEST), a township adjoining East Firsby, in the eastern division of the wapentake of ASLACOE, parts of LINDSEY, county of LINCOLN, 8½ miles (W. by S.) from Market-Raisen, containing 34 inhabitants.

FISHBOURN (NEW), a parish in the hundred of Box and STOCKBRIDGE, rape of CHICHESTER, county of SUSSEX, 1¼ mile (W.) from Chichester, containing 288 inhabitants. The living is a rectory, in the peculiar jurisdiction of the Dean of Chichester, rated in the king's books at £5. 10., and in the patronage of the Crown. The church, dedicated to St. Peter and St. Mary, is in the early style of English architecture; it has lately received an addition of forty-six sittings, of which thirty-one are free, the Incorporated Society for the enlargement of churches and chapels having granted £50 towards defraying the expense. The parish is bounded on the west by Chichester harbour.

FISHBOURN (OLD), a hamlet in the parish of NEW FISHBOURN, hundred of Box and STOCKBRIDGE, rape of CHICHESTER, county of SUSSEX, 2 miles (W.) from Chichester. The population is returned with the parish.

FISHBURN, a township in the parish of SEDGEFIELD, north-eastern division of STOCKTON ward, county palatine of DURHAM, 9¼ miles (S. E. by S.) from Durham, containing 192 inhabitants. There is a place of worship for Wesleyan Methodists ; also a school, endowed with £5 per annum by the trustees of Lord Crewe.

FISHERTON-ANGER, a parish in the hundred of BRANCH and DOLE, county of WILTS, containing 1253 inhabitants. The living is a discharged rectory, in the archdeaconry and diocese of Salisbury, rated in the king's books at £13. W. H. F. Talbot, Esq. was patron in 1804. The church is dedicated to St. Clement. There are places of worship for Baptists and Wesleyan Methodists. This place is situated on the bank of the river Avon, which separates it from the city of Salisbury : over the river is an ancient stone bridge, at the foot of which formerly stood the county gaol ; the site has been converted into a market garden, and a new gaol erected on the road leading to Devizes. The Salisbury infirmary is situated in this village. A house of Black friars was endowed by Edward I.

FISHERTON de la MERE, a parish forming a distinct portion of the hundred of WARMINSTER, though locally in that of Dunworth, county of WILTS, 10 miles (W. by S.) from Amesbury, containing, with the

VOL. II.

tything of Bapton, 290 inhabitants. The living is a discharged vicarage, in the archdeaconry and diocese of Salisbury, rated in the king's books at £8. 17. John Davis, Esq. was patron in 1820.

FISHERWICK, a township in that part of the parish of St. MICHAEL, LICHFIELD, which is in the northern division of the hundred of OFFLOW, county of STAFFORD, 3½ miles (E.) from Lichfield, containing 91 inhabitants. The Birmingham and Fazeley canal crosses the south-west angle of the township.

FISHLAKE, a parish in the southern division of the wapentake of STRAFFORTH and TICKHILL, West riding of the county of YORK, comprising the chapelry of Sykehouse, and the township of Fishlake, and containing 1274 inhabitants, of which number, 723 are in the township of Fishlake, 4½ miles (W.) from Thorne. The living is a vicarage, in the archdeaconry and diocese of York, rated in the king's books at £13. 3. 9., endowed with £400 private benefaction, and £1600 parliamentary grant, and in the patronage of the Dean and Chapter of Durham. The church is dedicated to St. Cuthbert. The Rev. Richard Rands, in 1641, founded and endowed a school for the education of children unlimitedly : the property consists of a school-house and garden, with certain lands producing an income of £102. 13. a year : forty children are now educated.

FISHLEY, a parish in the hundred of WALSHAM, county of NORFOLK, ¾ of a mile (N.) from Acle, containing, with the parish of Upton, 465 inhabitants. The living is a discharged rectory, in the archdeaconry and diocese of Norwich, rated in the king's books at £5. Robert Dundas, Esq. and others were patrons in 1801. The church is dedicated to St. Mary.

FISHTOFT, a parish in the wapentake of SKIRBECK, parts of HOLLAND, county of LINCOLN, 3 miles (E. S. E.) from Boston, containing 456 inhabitants. The living is a rectory, in the archdeaconry and diocese of Lincoln, rated in the king's books at £19. 6. 8., and in the patronage of Francis Thirkill, Esq. The church is dedicated to St. Guthlake. The parish is bounded on the south by the river Witham. There is an endowed school.

FISHWICK, a township in the parish of PRESTON, hundred of AMOUNDERNESS, county palatine of LANCASTER, 1¾ mile (E.) from Preston, containing 284 inhabitants.

FISKERTON, a parish in the wapentake of LAWRESS, parts of LINDSEY, county of LINCOLN, 4½ miles (E.) from Lincoln, containing 294 inhabitants. The living is a rectory, in the archdeaconry of Stow, and diocese of Lincoln, rated in the king's books at £12. 1. 8., and in the patronage of the Dean and Chapter of Peterborough. The church, dedicated to St. Clement, is a handsome structure, having portions of Norman architecture, and a tower at the west end ; it was partly rebuilt early in the fifteenth century. There is a ferry over the Trent to the village of Stoke, and along the bank of the river are several coal wharfs and warehouses.

FISKERTON, a chapelry in the parish of ROLLESTON, southern division of the wapentake of THURGARTON, county of NOTTINGHAM, 3 miles (S. E.) from Southwell, containing 342 inhabitants. The chapel is dedicated to St. Mary. There is a place of worship for Wesleyan Methodists. Ralph de Ayncourt having given the manor to Thurgarton priory, of which he was the founder, there were placed in the manor-house a few

Black canons, who had a chapel, dedicated to the Blessed Virgin, and several benefactions given them.

FITLING, a township in the parish of HUMBLETON, middle division of the wapentake of HOLDERNESS, East riding of the county of YORK, 11 miles (E. N. E.) from Kingston upon Hull, containing 119 inhabitants.

FITTLETON, a parish in the hundred of ELSTUB and EVERLEY, county of WILTS, 8¼ miles (W. by S.) from Ludgershall, containing, with the tything of Hacklestone, 298 inhabitants. The living is a rectory, in the archdeaconry and diocese of Salisbury, rated in the king's books at £23, and in the patronage of the President and Fellows of Magdalene College, Oxford. The church is dedicated to All Saints.

FITTLEWORTH, a parish in the hundred of BURY, rape of ARUNDEL, county of SUSSEX, 3¼ miles (S.E. by E.) from Petworth, containing 631 inhabitants. The living is a vicarage, in the archdeaconry and diocese of Chichester, rated in the king's books at £6. 13. 4., and in the patronage of the Bishop of Chichester. The church has portions in the early English and decorated styles of architecture. The river Rother bounds the parish on the south, and is there crossed by a bridge.

FITZ, a parish in the hundred of PIMHILL, county of SALOP, 5½ miles (N.W. by N.) from Shrewsbury, containing 229 inhabitants. The living is a discharged rectory, in the archdeaconry of Salop, and diocese of Lichfield and Coventry, rated in the king's books at £5. 5. 10., and in the patronage of the Crown. The church is dedicated to St. Paul. The river Perry runs through the parish, which is bounded by the Severn.

FITZHEAD, a parish in the western division of the hundred of KINGSBURY, county of SOMERSET, 2¾ miles (E. by N.) from Wiveliscombe, containing 300 inhabitants. The living is·a perpetual curacy, in the peculiar jurisdiction of the Prebendary of Wiveliscombe in the Cathedral Church of Wells, endowed with £400 private benefaction, and £600 royal bounty. The church, dedicated to St. Mary, has a tower at the west end.

FIVEHEAD, a parish in the hundred of ABDICK and BULSTONE, county of SOMERSET, 5 miles (S.W. by W.) from Langport, containing 326 inhabitants. The living is a discharged vicarage, in the archdeaconry of Taunton, and diocese of Bath and Wells, rated in the king's books at £7. 2. 8., endowed with £200 private benefaction, and £200 royal bounty, and in the patronage of the Dean and Chapter of Bristol. The church, dedicated to St. Martin, is a neat building, with an embattled tower at the west end.

FIXBY, a township in the parish of HALIFAX, wapentake of MORLEY, West riding of the county of YORK, 3½ miles (N.N.W.) from Huddersfield, containing 345 inhabitants.

FLADBURY, a parish in the middle division of the hundred of OSWALDSLOW, county of WORCESTER, 4 miles (E.) from Pershore, comprising the chapelries of Stock with Bradley, Throckmorton, and Wyre-Piddle; the township of Hill with Moor, and the hamlet of Hob-Lench, otherwise Abbots-Lench, and containing 1387 inhabitants. The living is a rectory, in the peculiar jurisdiction of the rector, rated in the king's books at £81. 10., and in the patronage of the Bishop of Worcester. The church is dedicated to St. John the Baptist. In Ethelred's reign, a society of religious bersons was established here subordinate to the church

of Worcester. The navigable river AVON has a ferry over it at this place.

FLAGG, a township in the parish of BAKEWELL, hundred of HIGH PEAK, county of DERBY, 6 miles (W.) from Bakewell, containing 220 inhabitants.

FLAMBOROUGH, a parish in the wapentake of DICKERING, East riding of the county of YORK, 4 miles (E. N. E.) from Bridlington, containing 917 inhabitants. The living is a perpetual curacy, in the archdeaconry of the East riding, and diocese of York, endowed with £400 royal bounty, and £1400 parliamentary grant, and in the patronage of the Archbishop of York and Sir W. Strickland, Bart. alternately. The church is dedicated to St. Oswald. There are places of worship for Primitive and Wesleyan Methodists. Some writers suppose this parish to derive its name from the Saxon Fleam-burg, and assert that Ida, the Saxon, landed at the Head; others infer that its appellation originated from the "flame," or light, anciently placed on the cliffs, to direct mariners in the navigation of the German ocean. Though in ancient times the place was of some note, the Danes, in their hostile attacks upon England, frequently making it one of their principal stations, it can only at the present time be considered as a fishing village. Flamborough Head is a lofty promontory overlooking the village, forming a magnificent object, and one of the greatest natural curiosities in the kingdom. The cliffs, which are of limestone rock, white as snow, extend in a range from five to six miles, and rise in many places to an elevation of three hundred feet perpendicularly from the sea. At the base are several extensive caverns, formed by some mighty convulsion of nature, or worn by the action of the water. The scenery is very grand and imposing. On the extreme point of the promontory, at the distance eastward of nearly a mile and a half from the village, and at an elevation of about two hundred and fifty feet, a light-house, with revolving points, was erected in 1806. In the summer season, these cliffs are the resort of a vast number of aquatic birds, from various regions, to build their nests and rear their young; boys are frequently let down the rocks by means of ropes fastened to stakes, and bring away with them bushels of eggs for the use of the sugar-house at Hull. Some vestiges of Danish structures are still visible in the parish; viz., an ancient ruin at the west end, called "the Danes' Tower," and the intrenchments around it, denominated "Little Denmark."

FLAMSTEAD, a parish in the hundred of DACORUM, county of HERTFORD, 2¾ miles (N.W.) from Redbourn, containing 1392 inhabitants. The living is a perpetual curacy, in the archdeaconry of Huntingdon, and diocese of Lincoln, endowed with £800 parliamentary grant, and in the patronage of the Master and Fellows of University College, Oxford, to whom the rectory, rated in the king's books at £41. 6. 8., was devised by Robert Gunsley, in 1618, on condition that, besides paying a stipend to the curate, they should maintain four scholars at a grammar school, affording them a stipulated allowance yearly after their removal to college, the selection to be made equally from the grammar schools of Rochester and Maidstone, of scholars born in the county of Kent. The church is dedicated to St. Leonard. The village, not far from which is the Roman Watling-street, stands upon the summit of a high ridge of land which rises abruptly from the south-western side of the valley through which the river Ver runs, and was in ancient times called Verlam-stedt, in allusion to its situation near that river. There is a small sum for the education of children. An almshouse for two widowers and two widows was founded in 1669, by Thomas Saunders. Esq., who endowed them with a rent-charge of £5. A priory, dedicated to St. Giles, is stated by Leland to have been founded at Woodchurch, in this neighbourhood, by Roger de Tony, for a prioress and nuns, the demesnes of which, at the dissolution of religious houses, lapsed to the crown, and were granted by Henry VIII. to Sir Richard Page, Knt., to whose mansion Edward VI., in his infancy, being in an infirm state of health, was sent for the benefit of a salubrious air.

FLASBY, a joint township with Winterburn, in the parish of GARGRAVE, eastern division of the wapentake of STAINCLIFFE and EWCROSS, West riding of the county of YORK, 4½ miles (N.W. by N.) from Skipton, containing 134 inhabitants.

FLASHBROOK, a township in the parish of AB-DASTON, northern division of the hundred of PIREHILL, county of STAFFORD, containing, with Batchacre, formerly deemed extra-parochial, 127 inhabitants.

FLAT-HOLMES, an island in the parish of UP-HILL, hundred of WINTERSTOKE, county of SOMERSET, 7 miles (N. W. by W.) from Uphill. The population is returned with the parish. It is about a mile and a half in circumference, commanding a delightful prospect of the Bristol channel. On the highest point of land is a light-house, at an elevation of about eighty feet.

FLAUNDEN, a chapelry in the parish of HEMEL-HEMPSTEAD, hundred of DACORUM, county of HERT-FORD, 5½ miles (W.S.W.) from King's Langley, containing 277 inhabitants. The chapel, dedicated to St. Mary Magdalene, stands at the distance of about a mile from the village, in a sequestered valley watered by a stream commonly called the Chesham river.

FLAVEL (FLYFORD), county of WORCESTER.— See FLYFORD-FLAVEL.

FLAWBOROUGH, a chapelry partly in the parish of ORSTON, northern division of the wapentake of BINGHAM, and partly in the parish of STAUNTON, southern division of the wapentake of NEWARK, county of NOTTINGHAM, 8 miles (S. by W.) from Newark. That part which is in the parish of Staunton contains 85 inhabitants, and the population of the other part is included in the return for Orston.

FLAWITH, a township in the parish of ALNE, partly in the liberty of ST. PETER of York, and partly in the wapentake of BULMER, North riding of the county of YORK, 5½ miles (S.W.) from Easingwould, containing 94 inhabitants.

FLAX-BOURTON, a parish in the hundred of PORTBURY, county of SOMERSET, 5½ miles (W. S. W.) from Bristol, containing 192 inhabitants. The living is a perpetual curacy, annexed to the rectory of Nailsea, in the archdeaconry of Bath, and diocese of Bath and Wells.

FLAXBY, a township in the parish of GOLDSBO-ROUGH, upper division of the wapentake of CLARO, West riding of the county of YORK, 3¾ miles (E. by N.) from Knaresborough, containing 78 inhabitants. There is a free school endowed with about £15 a year.

FLAXLEY, a parish in the hundred of ST. BRIA-

VELLS, county of GLOUCESTER, 3 miles (N. by E.) from Newnham, containing 196 inhabitants. The living is a perpetual curacy, in the archdeaconry of Hereford, and diocese of Gloucester. Sir T. Crawley was patron in 1810. In the reign of Stephen, an abbey for Cistercian monks, dedicated to the Blessed Virgin, was built here by Roger Fitz-Milo, second earl of Hereford, the revenue of which at the dissolution amounted to £112. 13. 1.: the chief part was burnt down in 1777. There are establishments for smelting iron-ore, and works which produce weekly twenty tons of pig iron of excellent quality: the wheels which set in motion the bellows and hammers are turned by a powerful stream of water, which falls into the Severn near Newnham.

FLAXTON on the MOOR, a township partly with in the liberty of ST. PETER of York, East riding, and partly in that part of the parish of BOSSALL which is in the wapentake of BULMER, North riding of the county of YORK, 9 miles (N.E. by N.) from York. The population of the former part is returned with the liberty of St. Peter; the latter contains 299 inhabitants. There is a place of worship for Wesleyan Methodists. In 1807, a lead box, containing about three hundred small Saxon silver coins, in high preservation, some silver rings, and several pieces of spurs, were turned up by the plough in a field near this place.

FLECKNEY, a parish in the hundred of GARTREE, county of LEICESTER, 7¼ miles (N.W. by W.) from Market-Harborough, containing 450 inhabitants. The living is a perpetual curacy, in the archdeaconry of Leicester, and diocese of Lincoln, and in the patronage of Lady Byron. The church is dedicated to St. Nicholas. The Union canal runs through the eastern part of this parish.

FLEDBOROUGH, a parish in the northern division of the wapentake of THURGARTON, county of NOT-TINGHAM, 5½ miles (E. by N.) from Tuxford, containing 75 inhabitants. The living is a rectory, in the archdeaconry of Nottingham, and diocese of York, rated in the king's books at £9. 7. 6., and in the patronage of Earl Manvers. The church is dedicated to St. Gregory.

FLEET, a parish in the hundred of UGGSCOMBE, Dorchester division of the county of DORSET, 4 miles (W. by N.) from Weymouth, containing 132 inhabitants. The living is a discharged vicarage, in the archdeaconry of Dorset, and diocese of Bristol, rated in the king's books at £5. 6. 8., endowed with £200 private benefaction, and £200 royal bounty. J. Gould, Esq. was patron in 1802. The church is a small ancient edifice dedicated to the Holy Trinity. The parish is supposed to take its name from its situation near the Fleet water. A market and fair were granted in the 28th of Henry III., which have been discontinued.

FLEET, a parish in the hundred of ELLOE, parts of HOLLAND, county of LINCOLN, 2 miles (E. by S.) from Holbeach, containing 776 inhabitants. The living is a rectory, in the archdeaconry and diocese of Lincoln, rated in the king's books at £15. Joseph Dodds, Esq. was patron in 1807. The church, the steeple of which is at some distance from it, is dedicated to St. Mary Magdalene. A large quantity of Roman copper coins, chiefly of the Emperor Galienus, was found here not many years since.

FLEETHAM, a township in the parish of BAM-BROUGH, northern division of BAMBROUGH ward, county

Q B 2

of NORTHUMBERLAND, 6 miles (S. E. by S.) from Belford, containing 94 inhabitants.

FLEMPTON, a parish in the hundred of THINGOE, county of SUFFOLK, 4¾ miles (N. N.W.) from Bury-St. Edmund's, containing 129 inhabitants. The living is a rectory with the rectory of Hengrave, in the archdeaconry of Sudbury, and diocese of Norwich, rated in the king's books at £5. The Rev. R. S. Dixon was patron in 1826. The church is dedicated to St. Catherine. The navigable river Lark runs on the north of this parish.

FLETCHING, a parish in the hundred of RUSHMONDEN, rape of PEVENSEY, county of SUSSEX, 3¾ miles (N. W. by W.) from Uckfield, containing 1690 inhabitants. The living is a discharged vicarage, in the archdeaconry of Lewes, and diocese of Chichester, rated in the king's books at £3. 6. 8. The Earl of Sheffield was patron in 1786. The church is dedicated to St. Andrew and St. Mary. A National school has been established, and a neat school-house was erected in 1824. A fair for the sale of pedlary is held here on the Monday preceding Whit-Sunday. The river Ouse runs through the parish, and there are several chalybeate springs. A Roman military way was discovered some years since on St. John's common.

FLETTON, a parish in the hundred of NORMAN-CROSS, county of HUNTINGDON, 1 mile (S. by E.) from Peterborough, containing 159 inhabitants. The living is a rectory, in the archdeaconry of Huntingdon, and diocese of Lincoln, rated in the king's books at £9. 3. 9. The Earl of Carysfort was patron in 1798. The church is dedicated to St. Margaret. In digging a well in this parish, in the year 1739, fossil shells and wood were found at the depth of thirty feet.

FLIMBY, a parish in ALLERDALE ward below Darwent, county of CUMBERLAND, 2½ miles (S. by W.) from Maryport, containing, exclusively of seamen, 376 inhabitants. The living is a perpetual curacy, in the archdeaconry and diocese of Carlisle, endowed with £600 royal bounty, and £1400 parliamentary grant, and in the patronage of the Landowners. The church, which was rebuilt in 1794, is dedicated to St. Nicholas. This parish was anciently a chapelry in the parish of Cammerton, from which it was separated in 1545: it lies on the sea coast, and abounds with coal.

FLINTHAM, a parish in the northern division of the wapentake of BINGHAM, county of NOTTINGHAM, 6½ miles (S.W.) from Newark, containing 546 inhabitants. The living is a discharged vicarage, in the archdeaconry of Nottingham, and diocese of York, rated in the king's books at £6. 2. 6., endowed with £400 private benefaction, and £400 royal bounty, and in the patronage of the Master and Fellows of Trinity College, Cambridge. The church is a spacious edifice dedicated to St. Augustine. There is a place of worship for Wesleyan Methodists. In 1727, Robert Hacker bequeathed certain lands, the income of which, about £20 per annum, is applied to the instruction of children: the school-house was erected in 1779. Harleford ferry over the Trent to Bleasby is in this parish. The village, which is of a considerable size, is situated near the fosse, or Roman road; several urns and coins have been found.

FLINTON, a township in the parish of HUMBLETON, middle division of the wapentake of HOLDERNESS, East riding of the county of YORK, 9¼ miles (N. E.) from Kingston upon Hull, containing 125 inhabitants.

FLITCHAM, a parish in the Lynn division of the hundred of FREEBRIDGE, county of NORFOLK, 4¾ miles (E. by N.) from Castle-Rising, containing 346 inhabitants. The living is a perpetual curacy, in the archdeaconry and diocese of Norwich, endowed with £600 royal bounty, and £200 parliamentary grant, and in the patronage of Thomas W. Coke, Esq. In the reign of Henry III. a priory of the order of St. Augustine was founded at this place, as a cell to Walsingham abbey, by Robert d'Aiguillon, the revenue of which was valued at the dissolution at £55. 5. 6.; the walls and offices remain. Here is a hill with a square area, surrounded by a trench, where, in the reign of William Rufus, the hundred court was held.

FLITTON, a parish in the hundred of FLITT, county of BEDFORD, comprising the chapelry of Silsoe, and the township of Flitton, and containing 1069 inhabitants, of which number, 501 are in the township of Flitton, 1¼ mile (W.) from Silsoe. The living is a discharged vicarage, in the archdeaconry of Bedford, and diocese of Lincoln, rated in the king's books at £11. 7. 8., and in the patronage of the Dean and Canons of Christ Church, Oxford. The church, an ancient edifice, dedicated to St. John the Baptist, contains several monuments, amongst which is a figure in brass of Thomas Hill, who died in 1601, at the great age of one hundred and twenty-eight years. Southward from the village, which was anciently called *Flitcham*, is Pallox hill, remarkable in the beginning of the last century for a gold mine discovered in it, which was seized for the king, and leased to a refiner; the produce, however, being too inconsiderable, it was soon abandoned.

FLITWICK, a parish in the hundred of REDBORNE-STOKE, county of BEDFORD, 2¾ miles (S. by W.) from Ampthill, containing 489 inhabitants. The living is a discharged vicarage, in the archdeaconry of Bedford, and diocese of Lincoln, rated in the king's books at £7. 17., endowed with £200 private benefaction, and £200 royal bounty. The Duke of Bedford was patron in 1820. The church is dedicated to St. Peter and St. Paul. A monastery, or cell to Dunstable priory, was erected here in 1170, by Philip de Sannerville.

FLIXBOROUGH, a parish in the northern division of the wapentake of MANLEY, parts of LINDSEY, county of LINCOLN, 11 miles (N. W. by W.) from Glandford-Bridge, containing 216 inhabitants. The living is a rectory, with the vicarage of Burton upon Stather united, in the archdeaconry of Stow, and diocese of Lincoln, rated in the king's books at £13. 10. Sir Robert Sheffield, Bart. was patron in 1822. The church is dedicated to All Saints. The parish, in which are some petrifying springs, is bounded on the west by the river Trent. Sir Edward Anderson, Bart., a Chief Justice of the Common Pleas in the reign of Elizabeth, was born at this place.

FLIXTON, a parish in the hundred of SALFORD, county palatine of LANCASTER, comprising the townships of Flixton and Urmston, and containing 2249 inhabitants, of which number, 1604 are in the township of Flixton, 7 miles (W. S.W.) from Manchester. The living is a perpetual curacy, in the archdeaconry and diocese of Chester, endowed with £600 private benefaction, £200 royal bounty, and £1400 parliamentary grant, and in the peculiar jurisdiction and patronage of the Prebendary of Flixton in the Cathedral Church of Lichfield and Coventry. The church, a neat edifice, is dedicated to

St. Michael. There is a place of worship for Wesleyan Methodists. The rivers Stowell and Mersey run through the parish.

FLIXTON, a parish in the hundred of MUTFORD and LOTHINGLAND, county of SUFFOLK, 3 miles (W.N. W.) from Lowestoft, containing 34 inhabitants. The living is a discharged rectory, united to that of Blundeston, in the archdeaconry of Suffolk, and diocese of Norwich. The church is dedicated to St. Andrew.

FLIXTON, a parish in the hundred of WANGFORD, county of SUFFOLK, 3 miles (S. W.) from Bungay, containing 209 inhabitants. The living is a discharged vicarage, in the archdeaconry of Suffolk, and diocese of Norwich, rated in the king's books at £6. A. Adair, Esq. was patron in 1820. The church is dedicated to St. Mary. At this place was an Augustine nunnery, founded by Mareny, Baroness Creke, in 1258, and valued at the dissolution at £23 per annum.

FLIXTON, a township in the parish of FOLKTON, wapentake of DICKERING, East riding of the county of YORK, 6¾ miles (S.) from Scarborough, containing 267 inhabitants. An hospital was founded here in the reign of Athelstan, by one Acchorn, a knight, for an alderman and fourteen brethren and sisters, " to preserve travellers from wolves and other wild beasts:" it was restored and confirmed in the 25th of Henry VI., by the name of Carman's Spittle, but was dissolved before the 26th of Henry VIII : a farm-house occupies its site.

FLOCKTON, a chapelry comprising Nether Flockton and Over Flockton, in the parish of THORNHILL, lower division of the wapentake of AGBRIGG, West riding of the county of YORK, 6¼ miles (E. by S.) from Huddersfield, containing 988 inhabitants. The living is a perpetual curacy, in the archdeaconry and diocese of York, endowed with £200 private benefaction, and £200 royal bounty, and in the patronage of the Rector of Thornhill. The Independents have here a place of worship. There is a small sum for the education of children. The chapelry abounds with coal mines.

FLOOKBOROUGH, a chapelry in the parish of CARTMELL, hundred of LONSDALE, north of the sands, county palatine of LANCASTER, 5¼ miles (E. S. E.) from Ulverstone. The population is returned with the parish. The living is a perpetual curacy, in the archdeaconry of Richmond, and diocese of Chester, endowed with £400 private benefaction, and £400 royal bounty, and in the patronage of Lord G. Cavendish. The church is dedicated to St. John the Baptist. This place, now a small village, was formerly a market town.

FLOORE, a parish in the hundred of NOBOTTLE-GROVE, county of NORTHAMPTON, 7¼ miles (W.) from Northampton, containing 861 inhabitants. The living is a vicarage, in the archdeaconry of Northampton, and diocese of Peterborough, endowed with one-third of the great tithes of the hamlet of Glasthorpe, which is in this parish, rated in the king's books at £17, and in the patronage of the Dean and Canons of Christ Church, Oxford. The church, dedicated to All Saints, has portions in the decorated, with considerable insertions in the later, style of English architecture. The river Nen bounds the parish on the south and west.

FLORDON, a parish in the hundred of HUMBLE-YARD county of NORFOLK, 3¼ miles (N. by W.) from St. Mary Stratton, containing 159 inhabitants. The living is a discharged rectory, in the archdeaconry of Norfolk,

and diocese of Norwich, rated in the king's books at £6. 13. 4. Sir W. R. Kemp, Bart. was patron in 1816. The church is dedicated to St. Michael.

FLOTTERTON, a township in the parish of ROTHBURY, western division of COQUETDALE ward, county of NORTHUMBERLAND, 3¾ miles (W.) from Rothbury, containing 92 inhabitants.

FLOWTON, a parish in the hundred of BOSMERE and CLAYDON, county of SUFFOLK, 5¾ miles (W.N.W.) from Ipswich, containing 150 inhabitants. The living is a discharged rectory, in the archdeaconry of Suffolk, and diocese of Norwich, rated in the king's books at £3. 9. 9½., endowed with £200 royal bounty. H. S. Thornton, Esq. was patron in 1815. The church is dedicated to St. Mary.

FLYFORD-FLAVEL, a parish in the upper division of the hundred of PERSHORE, county of WORCESTER, 8¾ miles (E. by S.) from Worcester, containing 159 inhabitants. The living is a discharged rectory, in the archdeaconry and diocese of Worcester, rated in the king's books at £5. 4. 9½. Thomas Sheldon, Esq. was patron in 1823. The church is dedicated to St. John the Baptist.

FLYFORD-GRAFTON, a parish in the upper division of the hundred of PERSHORE, county of WORCESTER, 8 miles (E.) from Worcester, containing 241 inhabitants. The living is a rectory, in the archdeaconry and diocese of Worcester, rated in the king's books at £20. 0. 10. The Earl of Coventry was patron in 1797. The church is dedicated to St. John the Baptist. Here is an endowed school.

FOBBING, a parish in the hundred of BARSTABLE, county of ESSEX, 3½ miles (E.) from Horndon on the Hill, containing 407 inhabitants. The living is a rectory, in the archdeaconry of Essex, and diocese of London, rated in the king's books at £21, and in the patronage of the Crown. The church is dedicated to St. Michael. This parish has Shell-haven and the Thames on the south, and Holly and East havens on the east.

FOCKERBY, a township in the parish of ADLINGFLEET, lower division of the wapentake of OSGOLDCROSS, West riding of the county of YORK, 10 miles (S.E.) from Howden, containing 106 inhabitants. Here is a free school, formerly a grammar school, endowed with land producing £60 per annum, the gift of Mr. Skerne: the master is appointed by the Master and Fellows of Catherine Hall, Cambridge, to which hall there are eight exhibitions, founded by the same individual, whose niece, Mrs. Mary Ramsden, in 1743, founded six fellowships and ten scholarships in the same, preference being given to youths born in the county of York, and more particularly to such as had been educated in the free school at Fockerby.

FOGGATHORPE, a township in the parish of BUBWITH, Holme-Beacon division of the wapentake of HARTHILL, East riding of the county of YORK, 6½ miles (N.) from Howden, containing 137 inhabitants. There is a place of worship for Wesleyan Methodists.

FOLESHILL, a parish in the county of the city of COVENTRY, 2½ miles (N.E. by N.) from Coventry, containing 4937 inhabitants. The living is a vicarage not in charge, in the archdeaconry of Coventry, and diocese of Lichfield and Coventry, and in the patronage of the Crown. The church is dedicated to St. Lawrence. There are places of worship for Independents and Wesleyan Methodists.

FOLKE, a parish in the hundred of SHERBORNE, Sherborne division of the county of DORSET, 3¼ miles (S. E. by S.) from Sherborne, containing 269 inhabitants. The living is a rectory, in the peculiar jurisdiction of the Dean of Salisbury, rated in the king's books at £9. 12. 3½. The Rev. W. Chafin and the Dean and Chapter of Salisbury were joint patrons in 1777. The church is dedicated to St. Lawrence.

Corporate Seal.

FOLKESTONE, a parish in the hundred of FOLKE-STONE, lathe of SHEPWAY, county of KENT, comprising the sea-port and market town of Folkestone, which has a separate jurisdiction, the hamlet of Ford, and part of the hamlet of Sandgate, and containing 4541 inhabitants, of which number, 3989 are in the town of Folkestone, 37¼ miles (E. S. E.) from Maidstone, and 71 (E. S. E.) from London. This place, called by the Saxons *Fulcestane*, and in Domesday-book *Fullcheston*, is by some antiquaries supposed to have been a Roman station, though its particular name has not been ascertained. A great quantity of Roman coins has been found here, and on one of the hills in the immediate vicinity of the town are the remains of a quadrilateral fortification, of which the vallum and fosse are plainly discernible. Though supposed to have been a *Castra Stativa* of the Romans, it was probably only one of those forts which that people, in the reign of Theodosius the Younger, erected at different intervals for the defence of the southern coast, and of which, or of other similar fortifications, traces may be observed along the whole ridge of hills which terminates the plain. Eadbald, the sixth king of Kent, built a castle here, on the high cliff, close to the sea-shore, which having been reduced to a heap of ruins by the Danes, and Earl Godwin, when he ravaged this coast in 1052, it was rebuilt by William de Albrincis, or de Averenches, who became lord of this place after the Norman Conquest, and it continued to be the chief seat of the barony till it was destroyed, and also the cliff on which it stood, by the encroachments of the sea. King Eadbald, some time after he had built the castle, founded within its precincts a priory for nuns of the Benedictine order, of which his daughter Eanswithe became first one of the sisters, and afterwards abbess. This convent having been destroyed during the Danish ravages, a convent for Benedictine monks was erected on its site, by Nigel de Mundeville, lord of Folkestone, in 1095, who made it a cell to the abbey of Lonley, in Normandy. Not long after, the sea having so far wasted that part of the cliff upon which it stood as to endanger the buildings, the monks removed to a new situation, immediately to the south of the present church. This priory being afterwards made denizen, escaped the general fate of the Alien priories in the reign of Henry V., and existed until the general dissolution, when its revenue was estimated at £63. 0. 7.: the only part of the monastic buildings remaining is a Norman arched door-way; but their foundations may be traced for a considerable distance. Before the reign of Henry I. Folkestone was made a member of the town and port of Dovor, one of the cinque-ports, its freemen being styled the barons of the town of Folkestone. King Edward III. re-incorporated the inhabitants by the title of the mayor, jurats, and commonalty of the town of Folkestone. In the year 1378, the greater part of it was burned by the united forces of the Scots and French; this devastation, added to the continual encroachments made upon it by the sea, reduced it to a very low and inconsiderable state, in which it continued until the last century, when, by the establishment of a fishery, and a lucrative trade with France, it encreased in opulence and importance; and since that time, from the salubrity of the air, the pleasantness of its situation, and the excellence of its beach, it has become a fashionable and well-frequented place for sea-bathing.

The town is situated on the shore of the English channel, opposite Boulogne, and in a hollow between two cliffs rising precipitously to the height of ninety feet above the level of the sea, stretching into an extended and very fertile plain, terminated on the east by the beautiful bay of East Ware, and extending on the west for nearly three miles, through small but rich glens, to Romney Marsh, being bounded on the north by a bold ridge of picturesque hills. The houses, irregularly built of brick, stand chiefly on the acclivities of the western cliff, on the summit of which is the church; the streets are narrow and indifferently paved, and the inhabitants are supplied with water by two rivulets, one of which flows through the centre of the town. The environs are pleasant, and the high grounds command an extensive view of the French coast. There are hot and cold baths fitted up with every convenience, and a bathing-machine on the beach: the hamlet of Sandgate is also much frequented as a bathing-place by such as are fond of retirement.

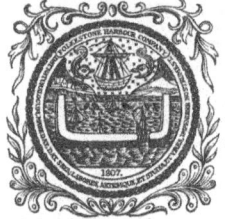

Seal of the Harbour Company.

Folkestone, as a member of the cinque-port of Dovor, enjoys special privileges: the harbour, which was small, and protected by jetties, was formerly kept in repair by voluntary contributions; but these eventually proving insufficient, an act was passed in 1766, imposing a small duty on coal brought to the port, to be applied to that purpose. It was afterwards judged necessary to construct a new and more capacious harbour, but, from the great accumulation of shingle, it is still very incomplete; and a large sum of money would be requisite for the erection of sluices, and other works necessary to render it capable of affording anchorage for a very considerable number of vessels. To this harbour belongs a great number of fishing boats, which in the mackarel season are employed in catching that fish for the London market. When the mackarel season is over, the Folkestone boats frequently go off to the coasts of Suffolk and Norfolk, to catch herrings. There is a small custom-house establishment belonging to the out-port of Dovor, under a supervisor, surveyor, and other officers. At a short distance from the church is a battery of four guns. The market, granted by King John, is on Thursday the market-house is now being rebuilt, upon a more extended scale: there is a fair on the 28th of June.

The corporation consists of a mayor, twelve jurats, and twenty-four common council-men, with a recorder, chamberlain, and town-clerk. The mayor, who is coroner by virtue of his office, is chosen yearly on the 8th of September; and, together with the jurats, who are justices of the peace within the liberty, holds a court of session generally once a year; they have also power to hold a court of record under the charter of the 20th of Charles II., for the recovery of debts to any amount exceeding 40s., and in which fines of lands are levied. A new and spacious Guildhall, is now being erected, with jury-room and council-chamber adjoining. There is a common gaol and house of correction, of which the Earl of Randor is hereditary gaoler, appointing a deputy. A court of requests is held for the recovery of debts not exceeding 40s.

The living is a perpetual curacy, in the archdeaconry and diocese of Canterbury, endowed with £200 private benefaction, and £700 parliamentary grant, and in the patronage of the Archbishop of Canterbury. The church, dedicated to St. Mary and St. Eanswith, anciently that of the priory, is a cruciform structure of sand-stone, in the early style of English architecture, with a tower in the centre supported by very large piers, from which spring pointed arches : the western division of the building has been contracted in its dimensions, part of it having been blown down in December, 1705. In the south aisle is a curious altar-tomb of variegated marble, with figures of two armed knights. There are places of worship for Baptists, the Society of Friends, and Wesleyan Methodists. Dr. William Harvey bequeathed £200 for the benefit of the poor of this town, and his nephew and executor, Sir Eliab Harvey, in 1674, in fulfilment of this bequest, founded a school for twenty poor children, and endowed it with part of the income of an estate in the parish of Lympne, from which the master receives a salary of about £36 per annum : the scholars are nominated by the mayor and jurats, who, with several other trustees, have the management of the school. About a mile and a half south of the town, on the summit of a lofty hill, are ancient earthworks, supposed to have been those of the Roman fortress. At Ford, about half a mile from the town in the same direction, is a chalybeate spring. The most celebrated natives appear to have been Dr. Harvey, born in 1578, who discovered the circulation of the blood; and John Phillepott, Somerset Herald, and one of the principal Kentish antiquaries, born about the close of the sixteenth century. Folkestone gives the title of viscount to the family of Bouverie, Earls of Radnor.

FOLKINGHAM, county of LINCOLN. —See FALKINGHAM.

FOLKINGTON, a parish in the hundred of LONGBRIDGE, rape of PEVENSEY, county of SUSSEX, 4¼ miles (S.W. by S.) from Haylsham, containing 186 inhabitants. The living is a discharged rectory, in the archdeaconry of Lewes, and diocese of Chichester, rated in the king's books at £12, and in the joint patronage of the Earl of Plymouth and Earl Delawarr. The church, dedicated to St. Peter, is in the early style of English architecture, with later insertions.

FOLKSWORTH, a parish in the hundred of NORMAN-CROSS, county of HUNTINGDON, 1½ mile (N.W. by W.) from Stilton, containing 203 inhabitants. The living is a rectory, in the archdeaconry of Huntingdon,

and diocese of Lincoln, rated in the king's books at £8. 6. 3. The Rev. W. Wilkinson was patron in 1820. The church is dedicated to St. Helen.

FOLKTON, a parish in the wapentake of DICKERING, East riding of the county of YORK, comprising the townships of Flixton and Folkton, and containing 411 inhabitants, of which number, 144 are in the township of Folkton, 6 miles (S. by E.) from Scarborough. The living is a discharged vicarage, in the archdeaconry of the East riding, and diocese of York, rated in the king's books at £8. 11. 10½., endowed with £200 private benefaction, and £200 royal bounty : there is also a sinecure rectory, rated at £15. H. Osbaldeston, Esq. was patron in 1817. The church is dedicated to St. John the Evangelist.

FOLLYFOOT, a township in the parish of SPOFFORTH, upper division of the wapentake of CLARO, West riding of the county of YORK, 5 miles (N.W. by W.) from Wetherby, containing 293 inhabitants. There is a place of worship for Wesleyan Methodists.

FONTHILL (BISHOP'S), a parish in the hundred of DOWNTON, locally in the hundred of Mere, county of WILTS, 1½ mile (E. by N.) from Hindon, containing 228 inhabitants. The living is a rectory, in the archdeaconry and diocese of Salisbury, rated in the king's books at £10, and in the patronage of the Bishop of Winchester. The church, dedicated to All Saints, is principally in the early style of English architecture.

FONTHILL (GIFFORD), a parish in the hundred of DUNWORTH, county of WILTS, 1¾ mile (S.E.) from Hindon, containing 471 inhabitants. The living is a rectory, in the archdeaconry and diocese of Salisbury, rated in the king's books at £13. 10., and in the patronage of the Executors of the late Mr. Farquhar. The church is dedicated to St. Nicholas. In this parish was the magnificent mansion belonging to William Beckford, Esq., called Fonthill Abbey.

FONTMELL (MAGNA), a parish in that part of the hundred of SIXPENNY-HANDLEY which is in the Shaston (West) division of the county of DORSET, 4¼ miles (S.) from Shaftesbury, containing, with the tything of Hartgrove, 733 inhabitants. The living is a vicarage with the curacy of West Orchard, in the archdeaconry of Dorset, and diocese of Bristol, rated in the king's books at £7. 10. : the prebend, or rectory, to which the vicarage is united, is rated at £18. Mrs. Salkeld was patroness in 1819. The church, dedicated to St. Andrew, is chiefly in the later English style. There is a place of worship for Wesleyan Methodists.

FOOLOW, a township in the parish of EYAM, hundred of HIGH PEAK, county of DERBY, 2¾ miles (E. by N.) from Tidswell, containing 298 inhabitants. There is a place of worship for Wesleyan Methodists.

FOOTHOG, a township in that part of the parish of CWMYOY which is in the hundred of EWYASLACY, county of HEREFORD, 10 miles (N.N.W.) from Abergavenny, containing 87 inhabitants.

FORCETT, a parish in the western division of the wapentake of GILLING, North riding of the county of YORK, comprising the townships of Barforth, Carkin, Forcett, and Ovington, and containing 417 inhabitants, of which number, 86 are in the township of Forcett, 7 miles (N. by E.) from Richmond. The living is a perpetual curacy, in the archdeaconry of Richmond, and diocese of Chester, endowed with £400 royal bounty, and £1400 parliamentary grant, and in the patronage of the Vicar of Gilling. The church, dedicated to St. Cuthbert, is a neat structure. There are remains of a Roman intrenchment in the parish.

FORD, a hamlet in that part or the parish of DINTON which is in the hundred of AYLESBURY, county of BUCKINGHAM, 4 miles (S. S. W.) from Aylesbury. The population is returned with the parish. Here was formerly a chapel.

FORD, a joint township with Bidstone, in the parish of BIDSTONE, lower division of the hundred of WIRRALL, county palatine of CHESTER, 8½ miles (N.) from Great Neston, containing 257 inhabitants.

FORD, a hamlet in the parish of NORTH WINGFIELD, hundred of SCARSDALE, county of DERBY. The population is returned with the parish. The celebrated non conformist divine, William Bagshaw, called the Apostle of the Peak, was a native of this place.

FORD, a chapelry in the parish of BISHOP-WEARMOUTH, northern division of EASINGTON ward, county palatine of DURHAM, 3½ miles (W.) from Sunderland, comprising the villages of High and Low Ford, and containing 791 inhabitants. The living is a perpetual curacy, in the archdeaconry and diocese of Durham, and in the patronage of the Rector of Bishop-Wearmouth. The chapel was built in 1817, by Captain Thomas James Maling, R.N., who likewise endowed it. Low Ford is situated upon the river Wear, across which there is a ferry, called Hylton Ferry, and where there are two vards for ship-building, copperas works, and an earthenware manufactory.

FORD, a chapelry in the hundred of WOLPHY, county of HEREFORD, 4 miles (S. E. by S.) from Leominster, containing 31 inhabitants. The living is a perpetual curacy, in the archdeaconry and diocese of Hereford, endowed with £200 private benefaction, and £800 royal bounty, and in the patronage of Richard Arkwright, Esq.

FORD, a joint township with Orrell, in the parish of SEPHTON, hundred of WEST DERBY, county palatine of LANCASTER, 5½ miles (N. by W.) from Liverpool, containing 217 inhabitants.

FORD, a parish in the western division of GLENDALE ward, county of NORTHUMBERLAND, 9 miles (N.N.W.) from Wooler, containing 1807 inhabitants. The living is a rectory, in the archdeaconry of Northumberland, and diocese of Durham, rated in the king's books at £24, and in the patronage of the Marquis of Waterford. The church is dedicated to St. Michael. There are places of worship for Baptists and Presbyterians. The parish contains a considerable quantity of coal, limestone, freestone, whin stone, and slate. About seventy children are educated in a charity school, of whom thirteen boys and thirteen girls are clothed at the expense of the Marquis of Waterford. There are several other schools in the parish. On the western side of the village is Ford castle, erected in 1287, by Sir William Heron, and rebuilt by the late Lord Delaval: two towers, the remains of the former castle, are retained in the present structure. This castle was demolished by the Scots in 1385, under the earls of Fife, March, and Douglas; and, prior to the battle of Flodden, it was captured by King James' troops. In 1549, it was again taken by the Scots, who demolished a great part of it. Courts leet and baron are held annually

about Easter, for the recovery of small debts, at which the steward of the manor presides. Floddon-field, in this parish, was the scene of the celebrated battle fought on the 9th of September, 1513, by the Scotch under King James IV., and the English commanded by the Earl of Surrey, in which the former were defeated, and their king slain. The top of the hill is now covered with fir trees. As some workmen were digging in a field near Floddon, in 1810, they discovered a large pit filled with human bones.

FORD, a parish in the hundred of FORD, county of SALOP, 4¾ miles (W. by N.) from Shrewsbury, containing 212 inhabitants. The living is a perpetual curacy, in the archdeaconry of Salop, and diocese of Hereford, rated in the king's books at £6. 13. 4., endowed with £400 private benefaction, and £400 royal bounty, and in the patronage of W. E. Tomline, Esq. The church is dedicated to St. Michael. The Roman Watling-street runs through the parish, which is bounded by the river Severn.

FORD, a parish in the hundred of AVISFORD, rape of ARUNDEL, county of SUSSEX, 5½ miles (S.S.W.) from Arundel, containing 83 inhabitants. The living is a discharged rectory, in the archdeaconry and diocese of Chichester, rated in the king's books at £9. 6. 8., and in the patronage of the Bishop of Chichester. The church is principally in the decorated style of English architecture. The Portsmouth and Arundel canal passes through this parish, which is bounded on the east by the river Arun.

FORD, a tything in the parish of IDMISTON, hundred of ALDERBURY, county of WILTS, containing 20 inhabitants.

FORDHALL, a hamlet in the parish of WOOTTON-WAVEN, Henley division of the hundred of BARLICHWAY, county of WARWICK, containing, with Aspley, 106 inhabitants.

FORDHAM, a parish in the hundred of STAPLOE, county of CAMBRIDGE, 5½ miles (N.) from Newmarket, containing 1042 inhabitants. The living is a discharged vicarage, in the archdeaconry of Sudbury, and diocese of Norwich, rated in the king's books at £13. 6. 8., and in the patronage of the Master and Fellows of Jesus College, Cambridge. The church is dedicated to St. Mary. The Independents have a place of worship here. There are six almshouses for poor widows, erected by Thomas Hinson, in 1626. A small Gilbertine priory was founded in the reign of Henry III., by Sir Robert de Fordham, as a cell to the great monastery of the same order at Sempringham in Lincolnshire, scarcely a vestige of which remains. James I., when coursing in this parish, took refreshment at a place still called "the King's Path," and killed a hare near the spot; this circumstance being commemorated upon a beam still preserved in the church, by a carved representation of two greyhounds pursuing a hare.

FORDHAM, a parish in the Colchester division of the hundred of LEXDEN, county of ESSEX, 6 miles (N.W. by W.) from Colchester, containing 696 inhabitants. The living is a rectory, in the archdeaconry of Colchester, and diocese of London, rated in the king's books at £14. 4. 2. The Countess de Grey was patroness in 1804. The church is dedicated to All Saints.

FORDHAM, a parish in the hundred of CLACKCLOSE, county of NORFOLK, 2½ miles (S.) from Downham-Market, containing 136 inhabitants. The living is a perpetual curacy, in the archdeaconry of Norfolk, and diocese of Norwich, endowed with £800 royal bounty. E. R. Pratt, Esq. was patron in 1823.

FORDINGBRIDGE, a market town and parish in the hundred of FORDINGBRIDGE, New Forest (West) division of the county of SOUTHAMPTON, 20 miles (W. by N.) from Southampton, through Ringwood, and 92 (SW. by W.) from London, containing, with the tything of Godshill, sometimes deemed extra-parochial, 2602 inhabitants. This town is noticed in Domesday-book under the name of Forde, in which it is further stated to have contained a church and two mills. It has suffered repeatedly by fire, and particularly at the beginning of the last century. It is pleasantly situated on the borders of the New Forest, and on the banks of the Upper Avon, which is here navigable, and crossed by a bridge of seven arches at the south-east entrance into the town which is plentifully supplied with good water. There is a sail-cloth manufactory, and there was formerly one for bed-ticks and checks to a considerable extent, but of these only a small quantity is now made. The market is on Friday; and an annual fair is held on the 9th of September, chiefly for amusement. The living is a vicarage, in the archdeaconry and diocese of Winchester, rated in the king's books at £30. 2. 3½., and in the patronage of the Provost and Fellows of King's College, Cambridge. The church, dedicated to St. Mary, consists of a nave and aisles, with a small north transept, over which rises a square tower and two chancels parallel with each other, one east of the nave, the other beyond the north aisle and transept: the tower is about seventy feet high, and of excellent workmanship: the south chancel is the most ancient part of the building, and is supposed to have been erected about the commencement of the thirteenth century. The west window, which is very large, is a beautiful specimen of the decorated English style. There is a chapel of ease at Ibsley, in this parish. Here are places of worship for the Society of Friends and Independents. In 1801, Catherine Eycott Bulkeley gave £200 three per cent. consols. in trust, to apply the dividends towards the support of the Sunday school; and in 1824, Sarah Dale bequeathed £50 for the same purpose: this charity is further supported by voluntary contributions. A rent-charge of £5, payable every fourth year, was given by John Dodington, in 1638, to apprentice poor children of this parish. There are the remains of several ancient encampments in the neighbourhood, the principal of which is at Godshill, about two miles from the town.

FORDINGTON, a parish in the liberty of FORDINGTON, Dorchester division of the county of DORSET, ¼ a mile (E. S. E.) from Dorchester, containing 1275 inhabitants. The living is a discharged vicarage, in the peculiar jurisdiction of the Dean of Salisbury, rated in the king's books at £15, and in the patronage of the Prebendary of Fordington in the Cathedral Church of Salisbury. The church, dedicated to St. George, is an ancient cruciform structure, partly of Norman and partly of English architecture. This place anciently formed part of the town of Dorchester, and derived its name from the ford over the river Frome, across which there are now several bridges in the neighbourhood.

In the 29th of Edward III., Queen Isabel procured a grant of a market on Tuesdays, and a fair on the eve, day, and morrow of St. George. In the parish are many barrows, some of them very large; and Roman coins are frequently ploughed up. In 1747, above two hundred skeletons, the supposed remains of those who fell in the Danish wars, were discovered at the depth of four or five feet, the skulls being remarkably thick, and many of the teeth very sound: they were re-interred in the church-yard, or in pits dug on the place. Many other skeletons have been found, from time to time, in this neighbourhood.

FORDLEY, formerly a distinct parish, now united to MIDDLETON, in the hundred of BLYTHING, county of SUFFOLK, 3¾ miles (N. E. by E.) from Saxmundham, containing 351 inhabitants. The living is a discharged rectory, united to the rectory of Middleton, in the archdeaconry of Suffolk, and diocese of Norwich, rated in the king's books at £5. The church, dedicated to the Holy Trinity, was situated in Middleton church-yard, but has long since been demolished.

FORDON, a chapelry in the parish of HUNMANBY wapentake of DICKERING, East riding of the county of YORK, 12½ miles (N. by E.) from Great Driffield, containing 48 inhabitants.

FORDWICH, a parish, and a member of the town and port of SANDWICH, locally in the hundred of Downhamford, lathe of ST. AUGUSTINE, county of KENT, 2 miles (E. by N.) from Canterbury, containing 242 inhabitants. The living is a discharged rectory, in the archdeaconry and diocese of Canterbury, rated in the king's books at £5. 15. 2. Earl Cowper was patron in 1802. The church is dedicated to St. Mary. Fordwich is situated upon the river Stour, which is navigable as far as the bridge that crosses it a little above the village, and upon which are extensive flour-mills. In Domesday-book it is recorded as the "small borough of Forewich," and later authorities state it to have been a borough by prescription, governed by a mayor, jurats, and commonalty, with a high steward, treasurer, and town clerk. The mayor, who by virtue of his office was also coroner, and the jurats, who were justices, had the privilege of holding a general session of the peace and gaol delivery, together with a court of record.

FOREBRIDGE, a township in the parish of CASTLE-CHURCH, eastern division of the hundred of CUTTLESTONE, county of STAFFORD, ¾ of a mile (S. E.) from Stafford. The population is returned with the parish. Here is a free school endowed with £15 per annum, in which about fifty children are taught.

FOREMARK, a parish in the hundred of REPTON and GRESLEY, county of DERBY, 6½ miles (S. S. W.) from Derby, containing, with the township of Ingleby, 203 inhabitants. The living is a perpetual curacy, in the archdeaconry of Derby, and diocese of Lichfield and Coventry, endowed with £400 royal bounty, and £200 parliamentary grant, and in the patronage of Sir Francis Burdett, Bart. The church, dedicated to our Saviour, is a plain small edifice. The old parochial church, which was an appendage to the priory at Repton, stood in the hamlet of Ingleby, on the banks of the Trent, about one mile to the east; but falling into decay, the present edifice was erected by the then possessor of Foremark, at his own expense; and consecrated in 1662. There is a small sum for the education of children. In the parish is a singular rocky bank, the centre of which presenting the appearance of an edifice in ruins, tradition asserts to have been the residence of an anchorite, whence it has derived the name of Anchor Church. Human bones have been dug up on this spot; and the faint traces of a figure somewhat sepulchral are yet left beneath the rock.

FOREST, a joint township with Frith, comprising Ettersgill, Middle-Forest, and Harwood parts, in the parish of MIDDLETON in TEESDALE, south-western division of DARLINGTON ward, county palatine of DURHAM, 4½ miles (N.W.) from Middleton, containing 723 inhabitants. This township contains several lead mines, and abounds with romantic scenery: it is bounded on the south by the Tees, where that river, rolling over a rocky bed, forms several cascades, two of which, Caldron Snout and High Force, rank amongst the most remarkable waterfalls in the kingdom.

FOREST, county palatine of CHESTER. See MACCLESFIELD-FOREST.

FOREST-HILL, a parish in the hundred of BULLINGTON, county of OXFORD, 5 miles (E. by N.) from Oxford, containing 157 inhabitants. The living is a perpetual curacy, in the archdeaconry and diocese of Oxford, endowed with £200 private benefaction, £600 royal bounty, and £500 parliamentary grant, and in the patronage of the Rector and Fellows of Lincoln College, Oxford. The church is dedicated to St. Nicholas. The children of this parish are entitled to gratuitous instruction in the school at Stanton-St. John, founded by Dame Elizabeth Holford.

FOREST-QUARTER, a township in the parish of STANHOPE, north-western division of DARLINGTON ward, county palatine of DURHAM, 7 miles (N.W.) from Stanhope, containing 3735 inhabitants. This township contains the market town called St. John's Chapel, and several hamlets. At Copt Hill is a chapel built by Dr. Barrington, late Bishop of Durham, who endowed it with land which now lets for £15 per annum. There are places of worship for the Primitive and Wesleyan Methodists within the township. The bishop also erected two school-rooms, one at Wear's Head, and the other at Lane Head, both schools being conducted on the National plan.

FORMBY, a chapelry in the parish of WALTON on the HILL, hundred of WEST DERBY, county palatine of LANCASTER, 8¾ miles (W.) from Ormskirk, containing 1257 inhabitants. The living is a perpetual curacy, in the archdeaconry and diocese of Chester, endowed with £400 private benefaction, £600 royal bounty, and £200 parliamentary grant, and in the patronage of the Rector of Walton. The chapel is dedicated to St. Peter. There are two free schools for the education of children, one situated near the Cross, called the Higher or Upper school, and the other at the north end of Formby, near Ainsdale, the income of both being about £34 per annum, the bequest of Richard Marsh, in 1703: upwards of one hundred children are instructed. The township had anciently a chartered market, which has fallen into disuse.

FORNCETT (ST. MARY), a parish in the hundred of DEPWADE, county of NORFOLK, 3 miles (W.N.W.) from St. Mary Stratton, containing 274 inhabitants. The living is a rectory, with the rectory of Forncett-St. Peter united, in the archdeaconry of Norfolk, and dio-cese of Norwich, rated jointly in the king's books at £20, and in the patronage of the Duke of Norfolk, for a fellow of St. John's College, Cambridge. There is a fair for toys on the 11th of September.

FORNCETT (ST. PETER), a parish in the hundred of DEPWADE, county of NORFOLK, 2¾ miles (W. by N.) from St. Mary Stratton, containing 638 inhabitants. The living is a rectory united to the rectory of Forncett-St. Mary, in the archdeaconry of Norfolk, and diocese of Norwich.

FORNHAM (ALL SAINTS), a parish in the hundred of THINGOE, county of SUFFOLK, 2¼ miles (N.N.W.) from Bury-St. Edmund's, containing 305 inhabitants. The living is a rectory with the rectory of Westley, in the archdeaconry of Sudbury, and diocese of Norwich, rated in the king's books at £19. 10. 5., and in the patronage of the Master and Fellows of Clare Hall, Cambridge. The navigable river Lark runs through the parish. There are the remains of an ancient priory formerly connected with the abbey of Bury, now converted into a dwelling-house.

FORNHAM (ST. GENEVEVE), a parish in the hundred of THEDWESTRY, county of SUFFOLK, 4¼ miles (N.N.W.) from Bury-St. Edmund's, containing 144 inhabitants. The living is a discharged rectory united to that of Risby, in the archdeaconry of Sudbury, and diocese of Norwich, rated in the king's books at £7. 1. 0½. The church was burnt down about twenty years since, and has not been rebuilt. The navigable river Lark runs through the parish.

FORNHAM (ST. MARTIN), a parish in the hundred of THEDWESTRY, county of SUFFOLK, 2 miles (N.) from Bury-St. Edmund's, containing 222 inhabitants. The living is a discharged rectory, in the archdeaconry of Sudbury, and diocese of Norwich, rated in the king's books at £7. 11. 3. George Hogg, Esq. was patron in 1814. The navigable river Lark runs through the parish.

FORRABURY, a parish in the hundred of LESNEWTH, county of CORNWALL, 2½ miles (N.E.) from Bossiney, containing 223 inhabitants. The living is a discharged rectory, in the archdeaconry of Cornwall, and diocese of Exeter, rated in the king's books at £4. 12. 8½., endowed with £200 royal bounty, and in the patronage of Thomas John Phillips, Esq. The church is dedicated to St. Simphorian. This was formerly a place of some importance, its decay being attributed to the destruction of Tintagel and Botreaux castles, on which it was dependent. The parish is bounded on the north-west by the Bristol channel.

FORSBROOK, a township in the parish of DILHORNE, northern division of the hundred of TOTMONSLOW, county of STAFFORD, 2¾ miles (W.S.W.) from Cheadle, containing 665 inhabitants.

FORSCOTE, a parish in the hundred of WELLOW, county of SOMERSET, 7½ miles (S. S. W.) from Bath, containing 115 inhabitants. The living is a discharged rectory, in the archdeaconry of Wells, and diocese of Bath and Wells, rated in the king's books at £4. 19. 2. Sir Hugh Smith, Bart. was patron in 1806. The church, dedicated to St. James, is a small neat edifice. There are some mills on the banks of a stream which runs through this parish.

FORSTER'S BOOTH, a hamlet partly in the parish of COLD HIGHAM, and partly in that of PATTISHALL, hundred of TOWCESTER, county of NORTHAMPTON, 3¼ miles (N.N.W.) from Towcester. The population is returned with the respective parishes.

FORTHAMPTON, a parish in the lower division of the hundred of TEWKESBURY, county of GLOUCESTER, 2½ miles (W.) from Tewkesbury, containing 474 inhabitants. The living is a perpetual curacy, endowed with £1400 private benefaction, £1000 royal bounty, and £600 parliamentary grant, and in the patronage of J. Yorke, Esq. The church is dedicated to St. Mary. The navigable river Severn runs through the parish, and frequently inundates the meadows on its banks. Forthampton court, a private mansion, was formerly the residence of the abbots of Tewkesbury.

FORTON, a township in the parish of GARSTANG, hundred of AMOUNDERNESS, county palatine of LANCASTER, 4 miles (N.) from Garstang, containing 587 inhabitants. The Independents have a place of worship here. There is an endowment of about £20 per annum, the bequests of different individuals, for the education of children.

FORTON, a joint tything with Tatworth, in the parish of CHARD, eastern division of the hundred of KINGSBURY, county of SOMERSET, 1½ mile (S.E.) from Chard, containing 437 inhabitants.

FORTON, a parish in the western division of the hundred of CUTTLESTONE, county of STAFFORD, 1½ mile (N.E. by N.) from Newport, containing, with the township of Meer, 702 inhabitants. The living is a rectory, in the archdeaconry of Stafford, and diocese of Lichfield and Coventry, rated in the king's books at £20. 19. 2., and in the patronage of Sir J. F. Boughey, Bart. The church is dedicated to All Saints.

FOSDYKE, a parish in the wapentake of KIRTON, parts of HOLLAND, county of LINCOLN, 6 miles (N.N.W.) from Holbeach, containing 424 inhabitants. The living is a perpetual curacy annexed to the rectory of Algarkirk, in the archdeaconry and diocese of Lincoln. The church is dedicated to All Saints.

FOSTON, a parish in the hundred of GUTHLAXTON, county of LEICESTER, 6¾ miles (S. by E.) from Leicester, containing 24 inhabitants. The living is a rectory, in the archdeaconry of Leicester, and diocese of Lincoln, rated in the king's books at £14. 2. 3½., and in the patronage of Sir C. Lamb. The church is dedicated to St. Bartholomew.

FOSTON, a parish in the wapentake of LOVEDEN, parts of KESTEVEN, county of LINCOLN, 5¾ miles (N.W. by N.) from Grantham, containing 426 inhabitants. The living is a perpetual curacy annexed to the vicarage of Long Bennington, in the archdeaconry and diocese of Lincoln. The church is dedicated to St. Peter. Sir Thomas Manners Sutton, Knt., a baron of the exchequer, was elevated to the peerage by the title of Baron Manners of Foston, in the county of Lincoln, on the 20th of April, 1807, on being appointed Lord Chancellor of Ireland.

FOSTON, a parish in the wapentake of BULMER, North riding of the county of YORK, comprising the townships of Foston and Thornton upon Clay, and containing 264 inhabitants, of which number, 91 are in the township of Foston, 11¼ miles (N.E. by N.) from York. The living is a rectory, in the archdeaconry of Cleveland, and diocese of York, rated in the king's books at £14, and in the patronage of the Crown. The church is dedicated to All Saints.

FOSTON upon the WOLDS, a parish in the wapentake of DICKERING, East riding of the county of YORK, comprising the townships of Brigham, Foston upon the Wolds, Gembling, and Great Kelk, and containing 648 inhabitants, of which number, 300 are in the township of Foston upon the Wolds, 6½ miles (E.S.E.) from Great Driffield. The living is a discharged vicarage, in the archdeaconry of the East riding, and diocese of York, rated in the king's books at £15. 8. 6½., endowed with £400 royal bounty, and £1200 parliamentary grant, and in the patronage of the Crown. The church is dedicated to St. Andrew. The Wesleyan Methodists and Calvinistic Dissenters have each a place of worship here.

FOTHERBY, a parish in the wapentake of LUDBOROUGH, parts of LINDSEY, county of LINCOLN, 3¼ miles (N. by W.) from Louth, containing 198 inhabitants. The living is a discharged vicarage, in the archdeaconry and diocese of Lincoln, rated in the king's books at £3, endowed with £800 royal bounty, and in the patronage of the Crown. The church is dedicated to St. Mary.

FOTHERINGHAY, a parish in the hundred of WILLYBROOK, county of NORTHAMPTON, 3½ miles (N. N. E.) from Oundle, containing 309 inhabitants. The living is a perpetual curacy, in the archdeaconry of Northampton, and diocese of Peterborough. Thomas Belsey, Esq. was patron in 1814. The church, dedicated to St. Mary and All Saints, is a handsome edifice in the later English style: it has an ancient stone pulpit, and the font is a very fine one: several distinguished members of the Plantagenet family are interred in it. It was formerly collegiate, and at one period the conventual church of a nunnery, the inmates of which were translated to De la Pré, near Northampton. Edmund of Langley, son to Edward III., procured a license to erect a college, but his death prevented the execution of the design. He left two sons, Edward and Richard, the former of whom founded and endowed the college, which was confirmed by Henry V., who also bestowed upon it certain lands that belonged to Alien priories. Edward IV. made the college of his own foundation, and enlarged the buildings. At the dissolution its revenue amounted to about £419 per annum. On the north side of the church is a free school, endowed with £20 per annum, for a master, payable out of the exchequer by the receiver for the county. The village, in which a fair for horses is held on the third Monday after July, was anciently a considerable town: the adjoining country is much esteemed for its excellent pasture and corn land. It is pleasantly situated on the river Nen, over which is a bridge of freestone, erected in 1722 by the Marquis of Halifax, in lieu of a wooden one built in 1573 by Queen Elizabeth. Fotheringhay castle was a strong and handsome structure, with double ditches, keep, &c. In the reign of Henry III., when the many strong holds encouraged the nobility to rebel, it was surprised by William, Earl of Albemarle, who laid waste the surrounding country. It was the birthplace of Richard III., the scene of the trial of Mary Queen of Scots, and the place of her execution. James I., Mary's son, on his accession to the throne, demolished the castle; its site may however still be traced: some remains of the college walls are also visible, and part of the cloisters.

FOTHERLY (HIGH), a township in the parish of BYWELL-ST. PETER, eastern division of TINDALE ward, county of NORTHUMBERLAND, 3 miles (S.S.W.) from Bywell, containing 92 inhabitants.

FOULBY, a hamlet in the parish of WRAGBY, partly in the lower division of the wapentake of AGBRIGG, and partly in the upper division of the wapentake of OSGOLDCROSS, West riding of the county of YORK, 5 miles (E. S. E.) from Wakefield.

FOULDEN, a parish in the southern division of the hundred of GREENHOE, county of NORFOLK, 5 miles (E. by S.) from Stoke-Ferry, containing 467 inhabitants. The living is a discharged vicarage, united to the rectory of Oxborough, in the archdeaconry of Norfolk, and diocese of Norwich, rated in the king's books at £10. 1. 10. The church is dedicated to All Saints.

FOULMIRE, a parish in the hundred of THRIPLOW, county of CAMBRIDGE, 5½ miles (N. E.) from Royston, containing 541 inhabitants. The living is a rectory, in the archdeaconry and diocese of Ely, rated in the king's books at £29. 14. 2., and in the patronage of the Earl of Hardwicke. The church is dedicated to St. Mary. There was anciently a market at this place.

FOULNESS, an island and a parish in the hundred of ROCHFORD, county of ESSEX, 9 miles (E. by N.) from Rochford, containing 565 inhabitants. The living is a discharged rectory, within the jurisdiction of the court of the Commissary of Essex and Herts, concurrently with the Consistorial court of the Bishop of London, rated in the king's books at £15, and in the patronage of the Earl of Winchelsea. The church, dedicated to St. Mary, is nearly in the centre of the island, the floods having frequently prevented the inhabitants from attending their respective places of worship on the main land. There is a small endowment for the education of children. The circumference of Foulness is about twenty miles, exclusively of a tract called the Saltings, which is not yet em banked from the sea. Courts leet and baron are occasionally held by the lord of the manor. There is a fair for toys on the 10th of July.

FOULNEY, an island in the parish of DALTON in FURNESS, hundred of LONSDALE, north of the sands, county palatine of LANCASTER, 7 miles (S. by E.) from Dalton.

FOULRIDGE, a township in that part of the parish of WHALLEY which is in the higher division of the hundred of BLACKBURN, county palatine of LANCASTER, 1¼ mile (N.) from Colne, containing 1307 inhabitants. This neighbourhood is remarkable for romantic scenery.

FOULSHAM, a market town and parish, in the hundred of EYNSFORD, county of NORFOLK, 18 miles (N. W.) from Norwich, and 108 (N. N. E.) from London, containing 835 inhabitants. In 1770 this town was almost totally destroyed by fire, but it has been rebuilt in a superior manner, and now contains many good dwelling-houses. There is a market for corn every Tuesday fairs are held on Easter Tuesday for petty chapmen, and on the first Tuesday in May for cattle and toys ; and there is a statute fair for hiring servants on the first Tuesday after Michaelmas-day. The living is a rectory, in the archdeaconry of Norfolk, and diocese of Norwich, rated in the king's books at £27. 14. 9½., and in the patronage of the Rev. Henry Nicholas Astley. The church, dedicated to the Holy Innocents, is a noble building of flint and stone : the tower is ninety feet high, and is ornamented with pinnacles.: part of the chancel window is of painted glass. In the church and churchyard are some curious monuments. The Baptists have a place of worship here.

FOULSTON, a township in the parish of KIRK-BURTON, upper division of the wapentake of AGBRIGG, West riding of the county of YORK, 7¾ miles (S.S.E.) from Huddersfield, containing 1264 inhabitants.

FOULTON, a hamlet in the parish of RAMSEY, hundred of TENDRING, county of ESSEX, 3½ miles (S.W. by W.) from Harwich. The population is returned with the parish. Here was formerly a chapel, long since demolished.

FOUNTAIN'S-EARTH, a township in the parish of KIRKBY-MALZEARD, lower division of the wapentake of CLARO, West riding of the county of YORK, 3¾ miles (S.W. by W.) from Ripon, containing, with the chapelry of Middlesmoor, 441 inhabitants. An abbey of the Cistercian order was founded here in 1132, for thirteen Benedictine monks of St. Mary's near York, who leaving their house with the design of observing a more strict and reformed rule, obtained from Thurstan, Archbishop of York, a grant of land sufficient for their purpose. It was dedicated to the honour of the Blessed Virgin, and was endowed with great revenues, said to be worth, at the dissolution, £1173. 0. 7. The abbey was situated in a valley environed by well-wooded hills, on the banks of a small stream called the Skell : the ruins, occupying an area of about two acres, are considered the most extensive and interesting monastic remains in the kingdom ; they are partly in the Norman, and partly in the early style of English architecture, and consist of the church, with its lofty tower, two cloisters, the chapter-house, refectory, dormitory, and kitchen, besides the appendages of the gate, the mill, and the bridge.

FOVANT, otherwise FOFFONT, a parish in the hundred of CAWDEN and CADWORTH, county of WILTS, 7 miles (W. by S.) from Wilton, containing 523 inhabitants. The living is a rectory, in the archdeaconry and diocese of Salisbury, rated in the king's books at £17, and in the patronage of the Earl of Pembroke. The church is dedicated to St. George.

FOWBERRY, a township in the parish of CHATTON, eastern division of GLENDALE ward, county of NORTHUMBERLAND, 3 miles (E.N.E.) from Wooler. The population is returned with the parish. In 1532 this place was plundered by the Scots.

FOWEY, a borough, seaport, market town, and parish, in the eastern division of the hundred of POWDER, county of CORNWALL, 29 miles (S.W. by S.) from Launceston, and 234½ (S.W. by W.) from London, containing 1455 inhabitants. This town, the name of which was formerly spelt *Fawey*, is a place of ancient origin, and rose into importance during the wars that occurred in the reigns of Edward I. and III. and Henry V. In the reign of Edward III., its ships refusing to strike when required, as they sailed by Rye and Winchelsea, were attacked by the ships of those ports, but defeated them ; in commemoration of which gallant conduct they bore their arms united with the arms of those two cinque-ports, which gave rise to the appellation of the "Gallants of Fowey." To the fleet of Edward III. before Calais, this place contributed forty-seven ships, being

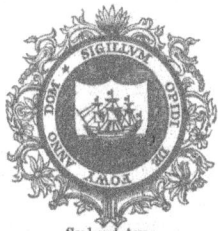

Seal and Arms.

a greater number than was supplied by any other port in England : it also furnished seven hundred and seventy mariners, which was a greater proportion than that of any other town except Yarmouth. Fowey was attacked and partly burnt by the French, in 1457 ; and being subsequently threatened by them in the reign of Edward IV., that monarch caused two towers, the ruins of which are yet visible, to be built at the public charge for its security ; but he was subsequently so much displeased with the inhabitants, for attacking the French during a truce which was proclaimed with Louis XI., that he took away all their ships and naval stores, together with a chain drawn across the river, between the two forts, which was carried to Dartmouth. In the parliamentary war, it was, at first, one of the royal garrisons : in 1644, the town and harbour were taken possession of by the Earl of Essex, with several ships and seventeen pieces of ordnance ; and here his army was mostly quartered when it surrendered to the king. The fortress and haven were held by the royalists till March, 1646, when they were delivered up, with thirteen pieces of ordnance, to Sir Thomas Fairfax. The Dutch under Admiral de Ruyter made an unsuccessful attempt on the harbour in 1667.

The town is situated at the mouth of the river Fowey, extending a mile along its eastern bank ; and the scenery around the harbour is at once beautifully grand and interesting : the cliffs on the opposite side of the river, across which there is a ferry for passengers, are of the boldest character. The streets, however, are both narrow and irregular, with numerous angles, rendering it difficult for carriages to drive through the town. There is a spacious market-house, over which is the town-hall, erected some years since, by Viscount Valletort and Philip Rashleigh, Esq., then representatives for the borough. Though at one time a place of considerable commercial importance, but little of this now remains, except what arises from its Pilchard fishery, in which most of the inhabitants are engaged, and which affords employment to a great number of vessels. It is computed that upwards of twenty-eight thousand hogsheads of fish are annually brought into this port : it has also a few vessels engaged in the timber and coal trade, two or three London traders, and some small country barges. In 1827, the coasting tonnage inwards amounted to twenty-nine thousand four hundred and ninety-nine tons, and the same outwards to fifty-six thousand four hundred and fifty-six tons. The copper-ores shipped during the same year amounted to about twenty-eight thousand tons ; the china, clay, and stone, shipped in 1827, amounted to twelve thousand tons : from all which it appears that the general trade of the place is considerably on the increase. The number of vessels that entered inwards from foreign parts during the year 1826, was eighteen British, and twenty-one foreign ; and the number that cleared outwards, four British. The market is on Saturday ; and fairs are held on Shrove-Tuesday, May 1st, and September 10th. The tolls of the market and fairs, and the harbour dues, are vested in the corporation, subject to the payment of a fee-farm rent of 40s. The harbour is esteemed the best outlet to the westward of all the ports in the west of England, being at all times safe, and affording such excellent anchorage, that vessels of a thousand tons' burden can ride in safety, and enter at the lowest tide,

drawing three fathoms of water, and go into deeper water above. The shores are bold and free from danger ; and ships in distress may run in with perfect safety, without cable or anchor. The fort of St. Catherine, constructed for the protection of the harbour in the reign of Henry VIII., still exists, and has four guns mounted upon it ; and between this and the town are two small forts of more modern erection.

Fowey was incorporated by charter of James II. Another charter was granted by William and Mary, in 1690 ; and a third in 1819, under which the corporation consisted of a mayor, recorder, eight aldermen, a town clerk, and assistants ; but a writ of ouster was brought against them for the abuse of their chartered privileges, and judgment having been recorded against them in Trinity Term, 1827, no attempt has been made to elect another mayor, hold sessions, nor do any other corporate acts ; and the county magistrates have ever since acted within and for the borough. Under the charter of 1819, the mayor and free burgesses were empowered to hold a court of record for the recovery of debts not exceeding £100 ; but no process has been issued from this court since 1823. The only courts now held are those of the lord of the manor, including a court leet, and a court baron. The borough sent members to a national council in the 14th of Edward III., but first returned representatives to parliament in the 13th of Elizabeth, since which it has continued to send two members. The elective franchise is vested in the inhabitants of the borough paying scot and lot, and in such of the tenants of the duchy manor as are capable of being portreeves of the borough, viz., those of the duke's tenants only who have been admitted on the court rolls of the manor of the borough, whose lands, being freehold, were anciently, and still continue to be, held immediately of the duchy of Cornwall, as parcel of the manor, and whose title to such lands has been presented at a court baron, by a sworn homage, or jury, of the freeholders of the manor : the portreeve is the returning officer, and the number of electors about sixty, who are in the patronage of Joseph Thomas Austen, Esq.

The living is a discharged vicarage, in the archdeaconry of Cornwall, and diocese of Exeter, rated in the king's books at £10, and in the patronage of J. T. Austen, Esq. The church, dedicated to St. Fimbarrus, is a handsome edifice, consisting of a nave, two aisles, with a lofty pinnacled tower at the west end : it was rebuilt in 1336, and again rebuilt, or much altered, and its present tower erected, about 1466 : in the north aisle is a fine altar-tomb of marble, with a recumbent statue in alabaster, and an inscription to the memory of John Rashleigh, Esq., who died in 1582 ; and there are also several other monuments belonging to the families of Rashleigh and Treffry. There are places of worship for Wesleyan Methodists and Independents. A school, for educating thirty children of voters, was founded here by a bequest from Shadrack Vincent, in 1700, and endowed with £500, to be invested in the purchase of land : it was formerly a grammar school, but is now conducted as a school for teaching English, writing, &c : the master has a salary of £30 a year, paid out of the rent of the land. There is another charity school, for educating twenty-five children of both sexes, the mistress of which has a salary of £8. 10. per annum. In the reign of Charles I., Philip Rashleigh, Esq. built an almshouse here for eight poor widows, and endowed it with the great tithes of the parish of St. Wenn: the widows receive 2s. 9d. each weekly, but are prohibited from begging, or receiving any other eleemosynary relief. The castellated mansion of Place-house, on an eminence near the church, anciently the residence of the Treffry family, but now that of the Austen family, is a curious relic of early domestic architecture; and an oriel, projecting from the south side of it, is very richly ornamented with tracery. The ruins of the block-houses, erected for the defence of the harbour in the reign, and by the command, of Edward IV., are also still to be seen.

FOWNHOPE, a parish in the hundred of GREYTREE, county of HEREFORD, 7 miles (S.E.) from Hereford, containing 866 inhabitants. The living is a vicarage, with the vicarage of Woolhope and the perpetual curacy of Fawley, in the archdeaconry and diocese of Hereford rated in the king's books at £6. 9. 9½., and in, the patronage of the Dean and Chapter of Hereford. The church is dedicated to St. Mary. The village is pleasantly situated on the east bank of the Wye. About half a mile to the north of it is an eminence crowned by an ancient camp; and not far distant is a second camp, occupying the summit of another eminence, called Capler-hill: the latter is double-trenched and called Woldbury; the former has no distinct appellation. The Capler-hill is finely wooded, and from its summit the prospects are rich and extensive.

FOXCOTE, a chapelry in the parish and hundred of ANDOVER, Andover division of the county of SOUTHAMPTON, 2 miles (N.W.) from Andover, containing 96 inhabitants.

FOXCOTT, a parish in the hundred and county of BUCKINGHAM, 2 miles (N.E.) from Buckingham, containing 119 inhabitants. The living is a rectory, in the archdeaconry of Buckingham, and diocese of Lincoln, rated in the king's books at £9. 9. 4½., and in the patronage of the Duke of Buckingham. The church is dedicated to St. Leonard.

FOXEARTH, a parish in the hundred of HINCKFORD, county of ESSEX, 3½ miles (N.W.) from Sudbury, containing 436 inhabitants. The living is a rectory, in the archdeaconry of Middlesex, and diocese of London, rated in the king's books at £10. 4. 4½. The Rev. J. Pemberton was patron in 1810.

FOXHALL, a parish in the hundred of CARLFORD, county of SUFFOLK, 4¼ miles (E. by S.) from Ipswich, containing 217 inhabitants. The living is a perpetual curacy, annexed to the rectory of Brightwell, in the archdeaconry of Suffolk, and diocese of Norwich. The church, which was dedicated to All Saints, has been demolished.

FOXHAM, a chapelry in the parish of BREMHILL, hundred of CHIPPENHAM, county of WILTS, 5 miles (N.E. by E.) from Chippenham. The population is returned with the parish. The chapel is dedicated to St. John the Baptist.

FOXHOLES, a parish in the wapentake of DICKERING, East riding of the county of YORK, comprising the chapelry of Butterwick, and the township of Foxholes with Boythorp, and containing 262 inhabitants, of which number, 169 are in the township of Foxholes with Boythorp, 10½ miles (N. by W.) from Great Driffield. The living is a rectory, in the archdeaconry of the East

riding, and diocese of York, rated in the king's books at £22. D. Sykes, Esq. was patron in 1815. There is a place of worship for Wesleyan Methodists.

FOXLEY, a parish in the hundred of EYNSFORD, county of NORFOLK, 2 miles (S. by E.) from Foulsham, containing 250 inhabitants. The living is a discharged rectory, in the archdeaconry of Norfolk, and diocese of Norwich, rated in the king's books at £6. 13. 4. E. Lombe, Esq. was patron in 1792. The church is dedicated to St. Thomas.

FOXLEY, a parish in the hundred of MALMESBURY, county of WILTS, 2½ miles (W. S. W.) from Malmesbury, containing 71 inhabitants. The living is a discharged rectory, in the archdeaconry of Wilts, and diocese of Salisbury, rated in the king's books at £3. 17. 8¼., endowed with £10 per annum private benefaction, and £200 royal bounty, and in the patronage of Lord Holland. This parish is bounded on the north by a branch of the Lower Avon. Lord Holland is Baron Holland, of Foxley.

FOXT, a joint township with Moorage, in that part of the parish of IPSTONES which is in the southern division of the hundred of TOTMONSLOW, county of STAFFORD, 4 miles (N. N. E.) from Cheadle, containing 415 inhabitants.

FOXTON, a parish in the hundred of THRIPLOW, county of CAMBRIDGE, 6 miles (S. S. W.) from Cambridge, containing 368 inhabitants. The living is a vicarage, in the archdeaconry and diocese of Ely, rated in the king's books at £11. 2. 11., and in the patronage of the Bishop of Ely. The church, erected about the year 1456, is dedicated to St. Lawrence. A market and two fairs were anciently held here; one fair is still held at Easter.

FOXTON, a joint township with Shotton, in the parish of SEDGEFIELD, north-eastern division of the hundred of STOCKTON ward, county palatine of DURHAM, 9 miles (N. W. by W.) from Stockton upon Tees, containing 63 inhabitants.

FOXTON, a parish in the hundred of GARTREE, county of LEICESTER, 3 miles (N.W. by W.) from Market-Harborough, containing 383 inhabitants. The living is a discharged vicarage, in the archdeaconry of Leicester, and diocese of Lincoln, rated in the king's books at £7. 3. 4., endowed with £200 royal bounty, and in the patronage of the Crown. The church is dedicated to St. Andrew. There is a place of worship for Particular Baptists. The Union canal runs through the village.

FOY, a parish partly in the hundred of GREYTREE, but chiefly in the upper division of the hundred of WORMELOW, county of HEREFORD, 3¾ miles (N.) from Ross, containing, with the township of Eaton-Tregoes, 293 inhabitants. The living is a vicarage, in the archdeaconry and diocese of Hereford, rated in the king's books at £13. 6. 8., and in the patronage of the Rev. John Jones. The church is dedicated to St. Mary.

FRADLEY, a hamlet in the parish of ALREWAS, northern division of the hundred of OFFLOW, county of STAFFORD, 4¼ miles (N. E.) from Lichfield, containing 426 inhabitants.

FRADSWELL, a chapeiry in the parish of COLWICH, southern division of the hundred of PIREHILL, county of STAFFORD, 7¼ miles (E. by S.) from Stone, containing 219 inhabitants. The chapelry is within the peculiar jurisdiction of the Prebendary of Colwich and Bishop's Itchington in the Cathedral Church of Lichfield.

FRAISTHORP, a parish in the wapentake of DICK-ERING, East riding of the county of YORK, 4¾ miles (S.S.W.) from Bridlington, containing, with the chapelry of Awburn, 91 inhabitants. The living is a perpetual curacy, in the archdeaconry of the East riding, and diocese of York, endowed with £600 royal bounty, and in the patronage of Sir W. Strickland, Bart.

FRAMCOTE, a chapelry in the parish of LOWER, or POWER GUYTING, lower division of the hundred of KIFTSGATE, county of GLOUCESTER, 3 miles (E.) from Winchcombe. The population is returned with the parish.

FRAMFIELD, a parish in the hundred of LOXFIELD-DORSET, rape of PEVENSEY, county of SUSSEX, 1½ mile (S.E.) from Uckfield, containing 1437 inhabitants. The living is a discharged vicarage, in the peculiar juris-diction of the Archbishop of Canterbury, rated in the king's books at £13. 6. 8., and in the patronage of the Rev. Mr. Cooper. The church, dedicated to St. Tho-mas à Becket, has portions in the early and decorated styles of English architecture. In 1719, Robert Smith bequeathed £200, the interest of one moiety of which was to be applied to the education of poor children ; and in 1764, this fund was increased with a bequest in land by the Rev. Thomas Wharton, now producing £50 a year : thirty children are instructed. There were for-merly iron-works in the parish; and on the road side, near Stone bridge, was a famous mineral spring, which entirely disappeared a few years ago, upon the owner draining a piece of boggy ground between it and a fish pond below.

FRAMINGHAM (EARL), a parish in the hundred of HENSTEAD, county of NORFOLK, 5 miles (S.E.) from Norwich, containing 56 inhabitants. The living is a dis-charged rectory united to the rectory of Bixley, in the archdeaconry of Norfolk, and diocese of Norwich, rated in the king's books at £3. 6. 8. The church, a small Norman edifice, is dedicated to St. Andrew.

FRAMINGHAM (PIGOT), a parish in the hun-dred of HENSTEAD, county of NORFOLK, 5½ miles (S.E. by S.) from Norwich, containing 304 inhabitants. The living is a discharged rectory, in the archdeaconry of Norfolk, and diocese of Norwich, rated in the king's books at £3. 6. 8., and in the patronage of the Bishop of Norwich.

FRAMLINGHAM, a market town and parish in the hundred of LOES, county of SUFFOLK, 18 miles (N.E. by N.) from Ipswich, and 87 (N.E.) from Lon-don, containing 2327 inhabitants. This place is of very remote antiquity, having been one of the chief towns of the Iceni, a British tribe in alliance with the Romans, to whom their king, Prasatagus, bequeathed a part of his dominions, in the hope of securing to his queen, Boadicea, the undisturbed possession of the re-mainder. On the death of Prasatagus, the Roman pro-curator took possession of the whole, and on Boadicea's remonstrating, ordered her to be scourged like a slave, and violated the chastity of her daughters. Boadicea, in revenge for this outrage, excited the Trinobantes and other tribes to revolt, and heading her own forces with masculine intrepidity, obtained a victory over the Romans, of whom seventy thousand were slain in battle, though she was subsequently defeated and lost her life, or, as some say, took poison. At what time the castle was originally built is uncertain, but it is a very ancient structure, and it is known that

a fortress existed here in the time of Redwald, third king of the East Angles, who occasionally retired to it from his court at Rendlesham. The castle was also the retreat of King Edmund the Martyr, who, when pursued by the Danes, fled from Dunwich, and took refuge within its walls, whence endeavouring to escape, when closely besieged, he was overtaken, and beheaded at Hoxne. In 1173, it became the temporary asylum of Prince Henry, whom Queen Eleanor, his mother, had incited to rebel against his father, Henry II. And upon the death of Edward VI., in 1553, Mary retired to this castle, where she was joined by the inhabitants of Suffolk and the neighbouring counties, who, to the number of thirteen thousand, accompanied her to London, to take posses-sion of the crown. The castle was a spacious and noble structure, the surrounding walls including an irregular quadrilateral area of nearly an acre and a half ; they were forty-four feet in height, and eight feet in thickness, de-fended by thirteen square towers of considerably greater elevation, of which, one towards the east, and one towards the west, were watch-towers : the whole was surrounded by a double moat, over the inner of which was a draw-bridge. The walls are in a tolerably perfect state, and in front of the gateway-tower are the arms of the Howards, Mowbrays, Brothertons, &c., all quar-tered in one shield, having lions for supporters, and for the crest, a lion passant. In the interior, the build-ings of which were demolished about the year 1670, an almshouse for aged men, who are supported by an en-dowment by Sir Robert Hitcham, and a workhouse for the poor, have been built with the materials of the castle. The town is pleasantly situated on a hill, near the source of the river Ore, which rises to the north of the castle, and falls into the sea at Orford ; it contains many respectable and well built houses, is lighted with oil by subscription, and amply supplied with water ; the air is salubrious, the approaches good, and the town generally improving. The trade is principally in malt : the market is on Saturday, for corn, and occasionally for cattle ; the fairs are on Whit-Monday, and October 11th, for toys.

The living is a rectory, in the archdeaconry of Suf-folk, and diocese of Norwich, rated in the king's books at £43. 6. 8., and in the patronage of the Master and Fellows of Pembroke Hall, Cambridge. The church, dedicated to St. Michael, is a stately structure, part-ly in the decorated, and partly in the later, style of English architecture, with a lofty square embattled tower, strengthened with buttresses ; over the west en-trance, a representation of St. Michael encountering the dragon is finely sculptured in relievo : the chancel, which, both in style and workmanship, is superior to the rest of the church, is supposed to have been added in the reign of Edward VI. : the roof of the nave, which is of oak curiously carved, is supported by octangular pillars, and that of the chancel by clustered columns of very graceful proportion. The church con-tains several fine monuments, and the ashes of many illustrious personages; among the former are the monu-ments of Henry Howard, Earl of Surrey ; Henry Fitz-roy, Duke of Richmond, natural son of Henry VIII. ; the two wives of Thomas, Duke of Norfolk, who was beheaded in the reign of Elizabeth ; and the wife of Sir Robert Hitcham. There is a chapel of ease at Saxtead, in this parish. Here are places of worship for Independents, Wesleyan Methodists, and Unitarians. The free school was founded in 1636, by Sir Robert Hitcham, Knt., who endowed it with lands producing an ample revenue for the instruction in writing, reading, and arithmetic, of forty boys, to each of whom he allowed an apprentice fee of £10; the number of scholars has been recently increased to fifty. There are four Sunday schools, in which five hundred children are instructed, partly supported by subscription, and partly by the charitable bequests of Sir Robert Hitcham, who also founded an almshouse for twelve aged widows, or widowers, who receive each a weekly allowance in money, and an annual supply of coal and a gown, on which they wear a badge with the arms of the founder: the alms-people are required to attend morning prayer at the parish church daily, for which purpose Sir Robert Hitcham bequeathed £20, now increased to £30 per annum, to the minister, and £5 per annum to the clerk and sexton; the school and almshouse are under the management of the Master and Fellows of Pembroke Hall, Cambridge. Thomas Mills, in 1708, bequeathed estates producing at present nearly £700 per annum, for the foundation of almshouses for eight aged persons; and also for the education of children, and the relief of the poor: there are likewise several other bequests for charitable purposes. In 1823, some remains of elephants' tusks were dug up at the depth of ten feet from the surface, in a field to the north of the town. Robert Hawes, who compiled a history of the hundred of Loes, still in manuscript, and to whom, as a zealous investigator of antiquities, the Master and Fellows of Pembroke Hall, Cambridge, presented a silver cup and cover, was buried here in 1731.

FRAMLINGTON (LONG), a parish in the eastern division of COQUETDALE ward, county of NORTHUMBERLAND, comprising the townships of Brinkburn High ward, Brinkburn Low ward, and Long Framlington, containing 815 inhabitants, of which number, 563 are in the township of Long Framlington, 11 miles (N.N.W.) from Morpeth. The living is a perpetual curacy, in the archdeaconry of Northumberland, and diocese of Durham, and in the patronage of the Vicar of Felton. There is a place of worship for Presbyterians. The interest of £500, the bequest of Mrs. Tate, in 1825, is appropriated to the maintenance of a school for educating twenty poor children. Within the last few years the village has been much improved by the erection of several neat houses and shops. It was formerly very badly supplied with water, but in 1821, a liberal subscription was raised to sink a public well, from which the inhabitants have now an abundant supply. Fairs for the sale of sheep, black cattle, &c., are held on the second Tuesday in July, and on October 25th. Limestone, freestone, and coal, are found in the parish. The Hall-hill, at this place, is supposed to have been the site of a Roman station, and the remains of a triple intrenchment are still visible. At Evergreen, near the same place, are foundations of a building supposed to have been a fort. At the north-western extremity of the parish is a long narrow tract of wild and dreary moor-land, containing about one thousand acres. Here is a great number of cairns, composed of loose stones, but their situation is remote and difficult of access. On a farm called Canada are large heaps of slag, or *scoriæ*, such as is produced by smelting iron-stone, which operation is

supposed to have been done by the Romans, as the road called the Devil's causeway passes near this place.

FRAMPTON, a parish (formerly a market town) in the liberty of FRAMPTON, Bridport division of the county of DORSET, 5¾ miles (N. W. by W.) from Dorchester, and 130 (S. W.) from London, containing 418 inhabitants. The name of this place properly belonged to the site of an ancient priory, and is derived from the river Frome which passes it: in Domesdaybook it is written *Frantone,* and, when that record was compiled, the priory was a cell to the abbey of St. Stephen, at Caen in Normandy. It was purchased, by license of Richard II., by Sir John Devereaux, Knt.; it afterwards fell to the crown, and was granted by Henry V. to his brother, the Earl of Bedford, after whose death it was given to the collegiate church of St. Stephen, in Westminster. In the 14th of Elizabeth, the manor and advowson were given to Sir Christopher Hatton, who sold them to John Brown, Esq., in whose family they now remain. A handsome residence was erected in 1704, upon the site of the priory, by Robert Brown, Esq. A market on Thursday, now disused, was granted by Edward III., and four fairs by succeeding monarchs; of the latter two only are now held, on March 9th and May 4th, for cattle, horses, &c. Courts leet and baron are held annually, at which the constable and tythingmen for the liberty are appointed. The living is a discharged vicarage, in the archdeaconry of Dorset, and diocese of Bristol, rated in the king's books at £11. 9. 7., and in the patronage of F. J. Brown, Esq. The church, which is dedicated to St. Bartholomew, was built in the reign of Edward IV., and is adorned with several devices of that monarch; it consists of a nave, aisles, and chancel, with a tower at the west end having battlements and pinnacles, erected in 1695 by Robert Browne, Esq., the old tower having fallen down: the pulpit is ornamented with three curiously carved figures in niches; one of these is much defaced, the other two represent monks, one holding the sun in his right hand and a book in his left, the other a cross and a book: the entire edifice has been recently altered and repaired, at the expense of the patron. The above-mentioned Robert Browne, by will dated in 1734, left £40 per annum for the support of the minister, likewise an annuity of £15, and a house for a schoolmaster, to be appointed by the lord of the manor, for the instruction of children of both sexes. A National school for boys and girls is supported by subscription.

FRAMPTON, a tything in the parish of SAPPERTON, hundred of BISLEY, county of GLOUCESTER, 6¼ miles (W. by N.) from Cirencester, containing 181 inhabitants.

FRAMPTON, a parish in the wapentake of KIRTON, parts of HOLLAND, county of LINCOLN, 3¼ miles (S.) from Boston, containing 688 inhabitants. The living is a discharged vicarage, in the archdeaconry and diocese of Lincoln, rated in the king's books at £18. 19. 4., endowed with £200 private benefaction, and £1100 parliamentary grant, and in the patronage of Charles Keightley Tunnard, Esq. The church is dedicated to St. Mary. There is an endowed school, in which all the children of the parish are taught gratuitously.

FRAMPTON-COTTERELL, a parish in the upper division of the hundred of LANGLEY and SWINEHEAD, county of GLOUCESTER, 4¾ miles (W. by S.) from

Chipping-Sodbury, containing 1610 inhabitants. The living is a rectory, in the archdeaconry and diocese of Gloucester, rated in the king's books at £11. 16. 0½., and in the alternate patronage of the Duke of Beaufort and the representatives of the late Mr. Hughes. The church is dedicated to St. Peter. Independents and Wesleyan Methodists have each a place of worship here. Frampton derives its name from being situated on the river Frome.

FRAMPTON upon SEVERN, a parish in the lower division of the hundred of WHITSTONE, county of GLOUCESTER, 6¼ miles (N. by W.) from Dursley, containing 996 inhabitants. The living is a discharged vicarage, in the archdeaconry and diocese of Gloucester, rated in the king's books at £7. 11., endowed with £410 private benefaction, and £400 royal bounty. J. Dunsford, Esq. was patron in 1813. The church, dedicated to St. Mary, has portions in the decorated style, and a handsome tower with pinnacles. There is a place of worship for Independents. In the year 904, the Danes were overtaken at this place, and attacked by an army of Mercians and West Angles, by whom they were totally routed, and three of their kings slain. Frampton is situated on the river Frome, near its confluence with the Severn, whence it derives its name. The Gloucester and Berkeley canal passes close to the village. A fair, called Frying-pan fair, is held on the 14th of February. At this place is particularly observable that remarkable influx of the river, at the coming in of the tide, termed "the Hygre," and "the Bore, or Boar:" the water rolls in with a head of foam three or four feet high, stretching like a moving weir across the stream. About 1750, the Earl of Berkeley constructed a bulwark near it, called Hock Crib, to prevent the river from encroaching on the land.

FRAMSDEN, a parish in the hundred of THREDLING, county of SUFFOLK, 4 miles (S. E.) from Debenham, containing 702 inhabitants. The living is a vicarage, in the archdeaconry of Suffolk, diocese of Norwich, rated in the king's books at £10. 0. 2½., and in the patronage of the Countess of Dysart. The church is dedicated to St. Mary. There was formerly a monastery at this place.

FRANKBY, a township in the parish of WEST KIRBY, lower division of the hundred of WIRRALL, county palatine of CHESTER, 7 miles (N. N. W.) from Great Neston, containing 66 inhabitants.

FRANKLEY, a chapelry in the parish of HAGLEY, lower division of the hundred of HALFSHIRE, county of WORCESTER, 3¾ miles (S.E. by S.) from Hales-Owen, containing 189 inhabitants. The chapel is dedicated to St. Leonard. Lord Lyttleton is baron of Frankley.

FRANKTON, a parish in the Rugby division of the hundred of KNIGHTLOW, county of WARWICK, 4½ miles (W. by S.) from Dunchurch, containing 253 inhabitants. The living is a rectory, in the archdeaconry of Coventry, and diocese of Lichfield and Coventry, rated in the king's books at £5. 12. 1. The Rev. John Biddulph was patron in 1805. The church is dedicated to St. Nicholas.

FRANSHAM (GREAT), a parish in the hundred of LAUNDITCH, county of NORFOLK, 6¼ miles (N.E. by E.) from Swaffham, containing 322 inhabitants. The living is a rectory, in the archdeaconry and diocese of Norwich, rated in the king's books at £7. 15. 10. VOL. II.

F. R. Reynolds, Esq. was patron in 1791. The church is dedicated to All Saints.

FRANSHAM (LITTLE), a parish in the hundred of LAUNDITCH, county of NORFOLK, 5¾ miles (E. N. E.) from Swaffham, containing 228 inhabitants. The living is a discharged rectory, in the archdeaconry and diocese of Norwich, rated in the king's books at £6. 8. 4. E. Swatman, Esq. was patron in 1803. The church is dedicated to St. Mary.

FRANT, or FANT, a parish partly in the hundred of WASHLINGSTONE, lathe of AYLESFORD, county of KENT, but chiefly in the hundred of ROTHERFIELD, rape of PEVENSEY, county of SUSSEX, 2 miles (S. by E.) from Tunbridge Wells, containing 1727 inhabitants. The living is a vicarage, in the archdeaconry of Lewes, and diocese of Chichester, rated in the king's books at £8. 5. 5., and in the patronage of the Rector of Rotherfield. The church, which is partly in the early and partly in the decorated style of English architecture, has lately received an addition of four hundred and ninety sittings, two hundred and eighty of which are free, the Incorporated Society for the enlargement of churches and chapels having granted £350 towards defraying the expense. This parish, which is within the liberty of the duchy of Lancaster, is bounded on the north and south by two branches of the river Medway: it contains some mineral springs, and vestiges of several iron-works. In that part of it which is in the county of Sussex are the ruins of Beigham, or Bayham, abbey, founded by the Premonstratensian canons of Brockley, at the instance of Robert de Turneham, or Thornham, who, about the year 1200, gave all his lands at this place for that purpose: it was dedicated to the Virgin Mary, and was originally established at Beaulieu, near Brockley; but the monks removed, with those at Otteham, to this place: the monastery was one of those which Cardinal Wolsey obtained for the endowment of his intended colleges: its revenue, in the 17th of Henry VIII., was £152. 9. 4. The ruins, consisting of portions of the walls of the nave and transepts of the abbey church, are situated in the gardens of Bayham Park, a seat belonging to Marquis Camden, to whom it gives the title of viscount.

FRATING, a parish in the hundred of TENDRING, county of ESSEX, 6 miles (E. S. E.) from Colchester, containing 263 inhabitants. The living is a discharged rectory united to the rectory of Thorrington, in the archdeaconry of Colchester, and diocese of London, rated in the king's books at £10.

FRECKENHAM, a parish in the hundred of LACKFORD, county of SUFFOLK, 3¼ miles (S.W. by W.) from Mildenhall, containing 366 inhabitants. The living comprises a discharged vicarage and a rectory, within the peculiar jurisdiction of the Bishop of Rochester, the former rated in the king's books at £3. 15. 2½., the latter at £16. 11. 5½, endowed with £220 private benefaction, and £200 royal bounty, and in the patronage of the Master and Fellows of Peter House, Cambridge. The church is dedicated to St. Andrew. The river Lark is navigable on the north of this parish, where it receives a smaller stream, which runs through the village.

FRECKLETON, a township in the parish of KIRKHAM, hundred of AMOUNDERNESS, county palatine of LANCASTER, 2 miles (S.) from Kirkham, containing 875 inhabitants. The Independents have a place of worship

2 D

here. There is a large sacking and sail-cloth manufactory in this township.

FREEBY, a chapelry in the parish of MELTON-MOWBRAY, hundred of FRAMLAND, county of LEICESTER, 3½ miles (E.N.E.) from Melton-Mowbray, containing 110 inhabitants. The chapel is dedicated to St. Mary. There is a place of worship for Independents. The Melton-Mowbray and Oakham canal runs to the south of this place.

FREEFOLK, a chapelry in the parish of WHITCHURCH, hundred of EVINGAR, Kingsclere division of the county of SOUTHAMPTON, 1½ mile (E.N.E.) from Whitchurch, containing 68 inhabitants. The living is a perpetual curacy, in the archdeaconry and diocese of Winchester, and in the patronage of the Bishop of Winchester. Here is a very large paper-mill, where the paper used for the Bank of England notes is manufactured.

FREEFORD, a hamlet in that part of the parish of ST. MICHAEL, LICHFIELD, which is in the northern division of the hundred of OFFLOW, county of STAFFORD, 2¼ miles (S.E.) from Lichfield, containing 14 inhabitants.

FREEHOLDERS' QUARTER, a township in the parish of LONGHORSLEY, western division of MORPETH ward, county of NORTHUMBERLAND, containing 109 inhabitants.

FREETHORPE, a parish in the hundred of BLOFIELD, county of NORFOLK, 4 miles (S.) from Acle, containing 304 inhabitants. The living is a discharged vicarage with the rectory of Reedham, in the archdeaconry and diocese of Norwich, endowed with £400 royal bounty. The church is dedicated to All Saints.

FREMINGTON, a parish in the hundred of FREMINGTON, county of DEVON, 3 miles (W. by S.) from Barnstaple, containing 1099 inhabitants. The living is a vicarage, in the archdeaconry of Barnstaple, and diocese of Exeter, rated in the king's books at £20. 0. 5., and in the patronage of the Rev. C. Hill. The church is dedicated to St. Peter. There is a place of worship for Independents. Fremlington is mentioned in ancient records as a borough, and it once sent members to parliament in the reign of Edward III. In the neighbourhood are beds of limestone, enclosed in a stratum of blueish building stone; pipe and potters' clay are also found. At Fremington Pill, a small æstuary of the river Tor, coal barges discharge their cargoes, and merchant vessels await the spring tides. A salvage is claimed by the lord of the manor.

FRENCH-MOOR, a tything in the parish of BROUGHTON, hundred of THORNGATE, Andover division of the county of SOUTHAMPTON, 7¼ miles (N.W.) from Romsey, containing 44 inhabitants.

FRENSHAM, a parish comprising the tything of Dockingfield, in the hundred of ALTON, Alton (North) division of the county of SOUTHAMPTON, and the tything of Chart with Pitfold, in the hundred of FARNHAM, county of SURREY, 4 miles (S.) from Farnham, and containing 1433 inhabitants. The living is a perpetual curacy, in the archdeaconry of Surrey, and diocese of Winchester, endowed with £5 per annum, and £100 private benefaction, £200 royal bounty, and £200 parliamentary grant, and in the patronage of Robert Colmer, Esq. The church, dedicated to St. Mary, has lately received an addition of two hundred and eighty one sittings, of which two hundred and thirty are free, the Incorporated Society for the enlargement of churches and chapels

having granted £150 towards defraying the expense. The river Wey runs through the parish, in which also are two extensive sheets of water, and a mineral spring.

FRENZE, otherwise THORPE (PARVA), a parish in the hundred of DISS, county of NORFOLK, 1¼ mile (E. by N.) from Diss, containing 60 inhabitants. The living is a discharged rectory, in the archdeaconry of Norfolk, and diocese of Norwich, rated in the king's books at £2. 13. 4., and endowed with £200 royal bounty. James Smith, Esq. was patron in 1824. The church is dedicated to St. Andrew.

FRESDON, a tything in the parish of HIGHWORTH, hundred of HIGHWORTH, CRICKLADE, and STAPLE, county of WILTS, containing 24 inhabitants.

FRESHFORD, a parish in the hundred of BATH-FORUM, county of SOMERSET, 4¾ miles (S.E.) from Bath, containing 587 inhabitants. The living is a discharged rectory, in the archdeaconry of Bath, and diocese of Bath and Wells, rated in the king's books at £7. 7. 8½., and in the patronage of the Rev. George Bythersea. The church, dedicated to St. Peter, is a very neat structure. There is a place of worship for Wesleyan Methodists. The Frome takes a winding course through the parish from south to north-west, and then north, when it falls into the Avon, which forms the boundary of the parish on the northern side. The Kennet and Avon canal runs parallel with the Avon, at the distance of about half a mile from the village, which is pleasantly situated on the southern declivity of a hill, finely wooded, and abounding with rich and extensive views. The hills in the neighbourhood contain ample stores of the Bath stone, limestone, and fullers' earth. There is an extensive manufactory for fine broad cloth. The ruins of an old hermitage and friary, probably connected with Hinton abbey, may still be seen, as may also the remains of a Roman encampment.

FRESHWATER, a parish in the liberty of WEST MEDINA, Isle of Wight division of the county of SOUTHAMPTON, 1¾ mile (S. S. W.) from Yarmouth, containing 876 inhabitants. The living is a rectory, in the archdeaconry and diocese of Winchester, rated in the king's books at £9. 8. 4., and in the patronage of the Master and Fellows of St. John's College, Cambridge. The church, dedicated to All Saints, has lately received an addition of seventy-four sittings, of which forty-three are free, the Incorporated Society for the enlargement of churches and chapels having granted £25 towards defraying the expense. There is a place of worship for Wesleyan Methodists. In 1714, David Urry gave a messuage and lands, now producing £27 per annum, for the education of sixteen boys. This parish has the English channel on the south and west; on the north is the Isle of Wight channel, whence the river Yar is navigable to the village. To the west of Freshwater Gate, a small creek in the centre of Freshwater-bay is the extensive natural opening to the sea, called Freshwater-cave, the depth of which is about one hundred and twenty feet, the principal entrance being about twenty feet high and thirty-five wide. The prospect from the light-house, on the highest point of the Freshwater cliffs, is exceedingly fine, and includes a full view of the Needles. That eminent mathematician and natural philosopher, Dr. Robert Hooke, Gresham professor of geometry, and author of several esteemed publications, was born in this village in the year 1635.

FRESSINGFIELD, a parish in the hundred of HOXNE, county of SUFFOLK, 7¼ miles (E. N. E.) from Eye, containing 1231 inhabitants. The living is a vicarage with the rectory of Withersdale, in the archdeaconry of Suffolk, and diocese of Norwich, rated in the king's books at £17. 17. 1., and in the patronage of the Master and Fellows of Emanuel College, Cambridge. The church is dedicated to St. Peter and St. Paul. Archbishop Sancroft was born in this parish, in which he founded and endowed a school.

FRESTON, a parish in the hundred of SAMFORD, county of SUFFOLK, 3½ miles (S.) from Ipswich, containing 189 inhabitants. The living is a discharged rectory, in the archdeaconry of Suffolk, and diocese of Norwich, rated in the king's books at £6. 7. 6., and in the patronage of the Rev. J. Bond. The church is dedicated to St. Peter. The village is situated on the banks of the river Orwell, and abounds with beautiful and picturesque scenery, the view of which is greatly enriched by the old ruin called Freston Tower.

FRETHERNE, a parish in the upper division of the hundred of WHITSTONE, county of GLOUCESTER, 9½ miles (W. N. W.) from Stroud, containing 210 inhabitants. The living is a discharged rectory, in the archdeaconry and diocese of Gloucester, rated in the king's books at £5. 6. 8. The Rev. J. H. Dunsford was patron in 1824. The church is dedicated to St. Mary. This is supposed to be the place called in the Saxon Chronicle *Fethanleag*, where Ceawlin, King of Wessex, obtained a victory over the Britons in 584. Fretherne cliff rises sixty feet above the surface of the Severn, on the bank of which it is situated. The Clifford family had anciently a castle in this parish.

FRETTENHAM, a parish in the hundred of TAVERHAM, county of NORFOLK, 2¼ miles (S. W. by W.) from Coltishall, containing 248 inhabitants. The living is a rectory with that of Stanninghall, in the archdeaconry and diocese of Norwich, rated in the king's books at £10. Lord Suffield was patron in 1807. The church is dedicated to St. Peter.

FRICKLEY, a joint parish with Clayton, in the northern division of the wapentake of STRAFFORTH and TICKHILL, West riding of the county of YORK, 10½ miles (E. by N.) from Barnesley, containing, with Clayton, 360 inhabitants. The living is a perpetual curacy with Clayton, in the archdeaconry and diocese of York, endowed with £200 parliamentary grant. S. Andrew Ward, Esq. was patron in 1821.

FRIDAYTHORPE, a parish partly within the liberty of ST. PETER of YORK, but chiefly in the wapentake of BUCKROSE, East riding of the county of YORK, 9 miles (N.E. by N.) from Pocklington, containing 275 inhabitants. The living is a discharged vicarage, rated in the king's books at £4. 13. 4., and in the peculiar jurisdiction and patronage of the Prebendary of Wetwang in the Cathedral Church of York. There is a place of worship for Wesleyan Methodists.

FRIERMERE, a chapelry in that part of the parish of ROCHDALE which is in the hundred of SALFORD, county palatine of LANCASTER, 1 mile (N.) from Delph. The population is returned with the parish. The living is a perpetual curacy, in the archdeaconry and diocese of Chester, endowed with £800 royal bounty, and £1600 parliamentary grant, and in the patronage of the Vicar of Rochdale. The chapel was consecrated in 1768.

FRIERNING, county of ESSEX. See FRYERNING.

FRIESDEN, a joint chapelry with Nettlesden, in the parish of PIGLESTHORNE, hundred of COTTESLOE, county of BUCKINGHAM, 2 miles (N.E.) from Berkhampstead, containing 108 inhabitants.

FRIESTHORPE, a parish in the wapentake of LAWRESS, parts of LINDSEY, county of LINCOLN, 5¾ miles (S.W. by S.) from Market-Raisen, containing 45 inhabitants. The living is a discharged rectory, in the peculiar jurisdiction and patronage of the Dean and Chapter of Lincoln, rated in the king's books at £4. 10., and endowed with £400 royal bounty.

FRIESTON, a parish in the wapentake of SKIRBECK, parts of HOLLAND, county of LINCOLN, 3¼ miles (E.) from Boston, containing 862 inhabitants. The living is a discharged vicarage united to the vicarage of Butterwick in 1751, in the archdeaconry and diocese of Lincoln, rated in the king's books at £16. 11. 10., endowed with £200 private benefaction, and £300 parliamentary grant. G. Scholey, Esq. was patron in 1816. There is a place of worship for Wesleyan Methodists.

FRILFORD, a chapelry in the parish of MARCHAM, hundred of OCK, county of BERKS, 4 miles (W.) from Abingdon, containing 152 inhabitants.

FRILSHAM, a parish in the hundred of FAIRCROSS, county of BERKS, 6¼ miles (S.S.E.) from East Ilsley, containing 171 inhabitants. The living is a rectory, in the archdeaconry of Berks, and diocese of Salisbury, rated in the king's books at £8, and in the patronage of Robert Floyd, Esq. The church is dedicated to St. Frideswide. Here is a school endowed with the interest of £200.

FRIMLEY, a chapelry in that part of the parish of ASH which is in the first division of the hundred of GODLEY, county of SURREY, 4 miles (S.W. by S.) from Bagshot, containing 1284 inhabitants. The living is a perpetual curacy, in the archdeaconry of Surrey, and diocese of Winchester, endowed with £200 private benefaction, £200 royal bounty, and £1500 parliamentary grant, and in the patronage of the Warden and Fellows of Winchester College. The church has recently been rebuilt, and contains four hundred and fifty free sittings, the Incorporated Society for the enlargement of churches and chapels having granted £400 towards defraying the expense.

FRINDSBURY, a parish in the hundred of SHAMWELL, lathe of AYLESFORD, county of KENT, 2 miles (N. by W.) from Rochester, containing 1562 inhabitants. The living is a vicarage, in the archdeaconry and diocese of Rochester, rated in the king's books at £10. 13. 11½., and in the patronage of the Bishop of Rochester. The church, dedicated to All Saints, stands on a commanding eminence rising from the Medway, along the course of which river, and over the town of Rochester, the view from the church-yard is extremely fine. There is a place of worship for Wesleyan Methodists. The parish is bounded on the south and east by the Thames, and the Thames and Medway canal unites in it with the Medway, on the banks of which are several wharfs. Brickmaking is carried on to some extent, and chalk is found in the parish. Upnor castle, erected by Queen Elizabeth to defend the passage of the Medway, was for some time used as a powder magazine: it is surrounded by a moat, and consists of a central building, of an oblong form, connected with a round tower at each end.

FRING, a parish in the hundred of SMITHDON, county of NORFOLK, 8 miles (S.W. by W.) from Burnham-Westgate, containing 139 inhabitants. The living is a perpetual curacy, in the archdeaconry of Norfolk, and diocese of Norwich, endowed with £200 private benefaction, £200 royal bounty, and £500 parliamentary grant, and in the patronage of the Dean and Chapter of Norwich. The church is dedicated to All Saints.

FRINGFORD, a parish in the hundred of PLOUGHLEY, county of OXFORD, 3¼ miles (N.N.E.) from Bicester, containing 289 inhabitants. The living is a rectory, in the archdeaconry and diocese of Oxford, rated in the king's books at £12. 16. 0½., and in the patronage of the Crown. The church is dedicated to St. Michael.

FRINSTED, a parish in the hundred of EYHORNE, lathe of AYLESFORD, county of KENT, 4½ miles (S. by W.) from Sittingbourne, containing 152 inhabitants. The living is a rectory, in the archdeaconry and diocese of Canterbury, rated in the king's books at £9. 11. 8. S. T. Pattenson, Esq. was patron in 1822. The church is dedicated to St. Dunstan.

FRINTON, a parish in the hundred of TENDRING, county of ESSEX, 13 miles (S.E.) from Manningtree, containing 45 inhabitants. The living is a discharged rectory, in the archdeaconry of Colchester, and diocese of London, rated in the king's books at £7. 6. 8. W. Lushington, Esq. was patron in 1818. This parish lies on the shore of the North sea, which is continually encroaching on the land.

. FRISBY, a chapelry in the parish of GAULBY, hundred of GARTREE, county of LEICESTER, 8½ miles (E. by S.) from Leicester, containing 18 inhabitants. The chapel is desecrated.

FRISBY on the WREAK, a parish in the eastern division of the hundred of GOSCOTE, county of LEICESTER, 4½ miles (W.S.W.) from Melton-Mowbray, containing 376 inhabitants. The living is a discharged vicarage, in the archdeaconry of Leicester, and diocese of Lincoln, rated in the king's books at £7. 16. 8., and in the patronage of the Crown. The church is dedicated to St. Thomas à Becket. There is a place of worship for Wesleyan Methodists. The river Wreak runs through the parish.

FRISKNEY, a parish in the Marsh division of the wapentake of CANDLESHOE, parts of LINDSEY, county of LINCOLN, 4 miles (S.W.) from Wainfleet, containing 1268 inhabitants. The living is a vicarage, in the archdeaconry and diocese of Lincoln, rated in the king's books at £15. 6. 8., and in the patronage of W. H. Booth, Esq. The church is dedicated to All Saints. There is a place of worship for Wesleyan Methodists.

FRISTON, a parish in the hundred of PLOMESGATE, county of SUFFOLK, 3 miles (S.E.) from Saxmundham, containing 452 inhabitants. The living is a vicarage united to that of Snape, in the archdeaconry of Suffolk, and diocese of Norwich, rated in the king's books at £5, and endowed with £200 royal bounty. The church is dedicated to St. Mary.

FRISTON, a parish in the hundred of WILLINGDON, rape of PEVENSEY, county of SUSSEX, 3 miles (W. by S.) from East Bourne, containing 62 inhabitants. The living is a vicarage united to that of East Dean, in the archdeaconry of Lewes, and diocese of Chichester,

rated in the king's books at £7. This parish has Cuckmere haven on the west, and the English channel on the south.

FRITH, a joint township with Wrenbury, in the parish of WRENBURY, hundred of NANTWICH, county palatine of CHESTER, 6 miles (S.W. by W.) from Nantwich, containing 526 inhabitants.

FRITHAM, a tything in that part of the parish of BRAMSHAW which is in the hundred of NEW FOREST, New Forest (East) division of the county of SOUTHAMPTON, 3½ miles (N.W.) from Lyndhurst. The population is returned with the parish.

FRITHELSTOCK, a parish in the hundred of SHEBBEAR, county of DEVON, 2 miles (W.) from Great Torrington, containing 632 inhabitants. The living is a perpetual curacy, in the archdeaconry of Barnstaple, and diocese of Exeter, endowed with £200 private benefaction, £400 royal bounty, and £1000 parliamentary grant, and in the patronage of Mrs. Prudence Johns. The church is dedicated to St. Mary and St. Gregory. There is a charity school, with a small endowment given by Mr. and Mrs. Gay. In the reign of Henry III., Sir Robert Beauchamp founded a small house of Augustine canons, dedicated to the Virgin Mary, St. Gregory, and St. Edmund, and valued at the dissolution at £127. 2. 4. per annum : a small portion of the conventual church is yet remaining.

FRITH-VILLE, an extra-parochial liberty, in the western division of the soke of BOLINGBROKE, parts of LINDSEY, county of LINCOLN, containing 272 inhabitants. This liberty, with six others, was created such by an act of parliament in 1812, on account of the drainage of about fourteen thousand acres in Wildmore Fen, and in the East and West Fens. The inhabitants attend the chapel of Carrington.

FRITTENDEN, a parish in the hundred of CRANBROOKE, lathe of SCRAY county of KENT, 4¼ miles. (N.E. by N.) from Cranbrooke, containing 799 inhabitants. The living is a rectory, in the archdeaconry and diocese of Canterbury, rated in the king's books at £15. 18. 9., and in the patronage of J. L. Hodges, Esq. The church, dedicated to St. Mary, is principally in the decorated style of English architecture.

FRITTON, a parish in the hundred of DEPWADE, county of NORFOLK, 2½ miles (E. by N.) from St. Mary Stratton, containing 275 inhabitants. The living is a discharged rectory, in the archdeaconry of Norfolk, and diocese of Norwich, rated in the king's books at £9, endowed with £200 private benefaction, and £200 royal bounty. The Rev. T. Howes was patron in 1797. The church is dedicated to St. Catherine.

FRITTON, a parish in the hundred of MUTFORD and LOTHINGLAND, county of SUFFOLK, 7½ miles (N.W.) from Lowestoft, containing 174 inhabitants. The living is a discharged rectory, in the archdeaconry of Suffolk, and diocese of Norwich, rated in the king's books at £6. 13. 4. Miss Buckle was patroness in 1788. The church is dedicated to St. Edmund.

FRITWELL, a parish in the hundred of PLOUGHLEY, county of OXFORD, 5 miles (N. W. by N.) from Bicester, containing 476 inhabitants. The living is a discharged vicarage, in the archdeaconry and diocese of Oxford, rated in the king's books at £7. 9. 4. J. F. Willes, Esq. was patron in 1799. The church is dedicated to St. Olave.

FRIZINGTON (HIGH and LOW), a township in the parish of ARLECDON, ALLERDALE ward above Darwent, county of CUMBERLAND, 3 miles (E. by S.) from White-haven. The population is returned with the parish. In this township is a chalybeate spring, the water of which is said to possess the same virtues as that at Harrogate. Iron-ore is obtained here.

FROBURY, a tything in that part of the parish of KINGSCLERE which is in the hundred of KINGSCLERE, Kingsclere division of the county of SOUTHAMPTON, $\frac{3}{4}$ of a mile (N. W.) from Kingsclere, with which the population is returned.

FROCESTER, a parish in the lower division of the hundred of WHITSTONE, county of GLOUCESTER, $5\frac{1}{2}$ miles (W. by S.) from Stroud, containing 437 inhabitants. The living is a discharged vicarage, in the archdeaconry and diocese of Gloucester, rated in the king's books at £10. 5. 10. Lord Ducie was patron in 1814. The church is dedicated to St. Peter. The village is situated at the foot of a lofty hill, from the top of which may be obtained an extensive and beautiful view of the vale, watered by the Severn. A college of prebendaries is said to have anciently existed here, which having been suppressed, its revenue was given to the abbey of St. Peter at Gloucester.

FRODESLEY, a parish in the hundred of CON-DOVER, county of SALOP, $8\frac{3}{4}$ miles (W. by N.) from Much Wenlock, containing 179 inhabitants. The living is a discharged rectory, in the archdeaconry of Salop, and diocese of Lichfield and Coventry, rated in the king's books at £4. 14., and in the patronage of the Rev. T. R. Gleadow, M.A. The church, dedicated to St. Mark, was rebuilt in 1809, in a plain but very neat style. Several years ago, coal mines were opened, but they do not present the appearance of having been much worked. The Roman Watling-street, on the line of the present turnpike-road, runs through the parish.

FRODINGHAM, a parish in the eastern division of the wapentake of MANLEY, parts of LINDSEY, county of LINCOLN, $8\frac{1}{2}$ miles (W. N. W.) from Glandford-Bridge, comprising the townships of Bromby and Scunthorpe, and containing 406 inhabitants. The living is a discharged vicarage, in the archdeaconry of Stow, and diocese of Lincoln, rated in the king's books at £12. 16. 8., and endowed with £200 royal bounty — Healey, Esq. was patron in 1827. The church is dedicated to St. Lawrence.

FRODINGHAM (NORTH), a parish in the northern division of the wapentake of HOLDERNESS, East riding of the county of YORK, $5\frac{1}{2}$ miles (S. E. by E.) from Great Driffield, containing 575 inhabitants. The living is a discharged vicarage, in the archdeaconry of the East riding, and diocese of York, rated in the king's books at £5, endowed with £20 per annum private benefaction, and £600 royal bounty. The Rev. Francis Drake was patron in 1809. The church is dedicated to St. Elgin. There are places of worship for Independents, and Primitive and Wesleyan Methodists. Frodingham had formerly the privilege of a weekly market : it is situated about half a mile eastward from the river Hull, over which there is a bridge, and is navigable thence to Hull, but the superior locality for trade enjoyed by the neighbouring town of Great Driffield, caused the ancient charter of this place to be transferred thither about seventy years ago, from which pe-

riod the market has been discontinued. There is a trifling endowment, the gift of the Rev. Samuel Hunter, in 1803, for teaching four children.

FRODINGHAM (SOUTH), a township in that part of the parish of OWTHORNE which is in the southern division of the wapentake of HOLDERNESS, East riding of the county of YORK, 4 miles (N.) from Patrington, containing 71 inhabitants.

FRODSHAM, a parish in the second division of the hundred of EDDISBURY, county palatine of CHESTER, comprising the market town of Frodsham, the chapelry of Alvanley, the lordship of Frodsham, and the townships of Helsby, Kingsley, Manley, Newton, and Norley, and containing 5451 inhabitants, of which number, 1556 are in the town of Frodsham, 10 miles (N. E. by N.) from Chester, and 192 (N. N. W.) from London. Frodsham is mentioned in Domesday-book as being the property of the Earl of Chester. The town, situated on an eminence on the banks of the river Weever, near its confluence with the Mersey, consists of a broad street, a mile in length, extending along the road from Chester to Warrington, and another branching from it and leading to the church : at the east end is a stone bridge of four arches, over the Weever, which is here navigable, and at the west end anciently stood a Norman castle. A charter was granted about 1220, by Ranulph de Blundeville, sixth earl of Chester, to the burgesses of Frodsham, which was pleaded in reply to a writ of *Quo Warranto*, issued in the 22nd of Henry VII., and confirmed in the 33d of Henry VIII. and 21st of Elizabeth ; but the manor having been separated from the earldom about the beginning of the seventeenth century, the chartered privileges of the burgesses expired. Courts leet and baron are now held twice a year, and there are two presentments, one for the borough and fee, and the other for the borough and lordship; and for each of these townships a constable is appointed and sworn in court. The lord of the manor has the tolls of a market held on Saturdays, and of two fairs, on the 15th of May and the 21st of August : the market, owing to the vicinity of Warrington, is inconsiderable. The principal branch of trade carried on is the refining of salt, besides which here are flour-mills and cotton factories. In the township of Manley is a quarry of excellent freestone. The living is a vicarage, in the archdeaconry and diocese of Chester, rated in the king's books at £23. 13. $11\frac{1}{2}$., and in the patronage of the Dean and Canons of Christ Church, Oxford. The church, dedicated to St. Lawrence, is situated on elevated ground, adjacent to the village of Overton, but within the township of Frodsham : it is built of red freestone, and appears to be of high antiquity, as the nave displays manifest traces of Norman architecture. An organ was erected in 1790, and the organist receives a salary arising from a tenement called the Organ Lot. Wesleyan Methodists have a place of worship here. There is a free school, built about 1660, near the church : the master is chosen by twenty-four feoffees, consisting of the vicar and churchwardens, with four feoffees out of the township and lordship, three out of Kingsley, and two each from Norley, Newton, Alvanley, Manley, and Hellesby : he has a good house in Overton, and a salary of more than £100 per annum from lands at Frodsham, and a rent-charge on an estate at Christleton : the usher receives £7 per annum from an estate in Overton. Mrs. Gastrell bequeathed a rent-charge of £10 per annum, upon an estate near the town, to the Warrington Society, for the relief of widows and orphans of the clergy in the archdeaconry of Chester; and there are various charitable benefactions of less importance.

FROGGATT, a township in the parish of BAKE-WELL, hundred of HIGH PEAK, county of DERBY, 2 miles (N. E. by E.) from Stony-Middleton, containing 179 inhabitants.

FROME-SELWOOD, a market town and parish in the hundred of FROME, county of SOMERSET, 25 miles (N. E.) from Ilchester, and 105 (W. by S.) from London, containing 12,411 inhabitants. This place takes its name from the river, called by the Saxons, *Frau*, now Frome, which, passing by the town, runs into the Avon, near Bristol; and its adjunct, from its situation in an ancient and extensive forest, formerly infested with hordes of banditti, whose depredations were a terror to the surrounding neighbourhood, but from which they were expelled, by cutting down large tracts of woodland, and establishing small farms. A monastery was founded here in 705, and dedicated to St. John the Baptist, by Aldhelm, afterwards Bishop of Sherborne; it was plundered in the Danish wars, and the monks were dispersed, but the church continued till the middle of the twelfth century; and the remains, together with those of a chapel belonging to a small nunnery dedicated to St. Catherine, have been converted into tenements for the poor. The town is pleasantly situated on the north-east declivity of a hill, in the ancient Forest of Selwood, and consists chiefly of a great number of streets, irregularly built, and inconveniently narrow, but from their situation tolerably clean. A new opening through the town has recently been made, forming a very handsome street, with well built houses on each side. The buildings in general are constructed of small rough stone, and roofed with stone dug in the neighbourhood; the inhabitants are well supplied with water, and the town has been recently improved by the erection of a commodious market-house and other buildings. Over the Frome, which abounds with excellent trout and eels, is a neat stone bridge of five arches: the environs are pleasant, and contain some handsome seats. Frome has long been celebrated for its woollen manufacture, of which the principal articles are broad cloths and kerseymeres, of very superior quality: the manufacture of wool-cards is also carried on to a great extent, and formerly they were supplied from this place to almost every town in England. Frome has long been in great repute for the excellent quality of its beer, which is kept to a great age. The principal market is on Wednesday, and there is a smaller one on Saturday: the fairs are on February 24th and November 25th, for cattle and cheese. The county magistrates hold here petty sessions for the division; and a bailiff, two constables, and a tythingman for the town-tything, are chosen annually at the court leet of the Earl of Cork and Orrery; a constable and a tythingman for the West Woodlands are appointed at the court leet of the Marquis of Bath; and a tythingman for the East Woodlands is chosen at the hundred court at Frome.

The living is a vicarage, in the archdeaconry of Wells, and diocese of Bath and Wells, rated in the king's books at £22, endowed with £1200 private bene-faction, and £1800 parliamentary grant, and in the patronage of the Marquis of Bath. The parochial church, dedicated to St. Peter, is a spacious structure, consisting of a nave, north and south aisles, chancel, and four sepulchral chapels, with a square tower surmounted by a spire, and a north and south porch; within it are many handsome and interesting monuments. Christ Church, erected in 1818, by subscription among the inhabitants, is a handsome edifice in the later style of English architecture, containing nine hundred sittings, four hundred of which are free, the Incorporated Society for the enlargement of churches and chapels having granted £100 towards defraying the expense: the living is a perpetual curacy, in the patronage of the Vicar of Frome. In the Woodlands, three miles south of the town, a church was erected in 1712, by Thomas, Lord Viscount Weymouth, who made the living a perpetual curacy, by endowing it with £60 per annum, arising from an estate at Pennard, in this county, to be paid to a minister appointed by his successors in the estate of Longleat; it is further endowed with £30 per annum, by the will of the Hon. Henry Frederick Thynne, and also with the clear profits of the estate of Codrington in this parish. The church is a handsome edifice, with a tower surmounted by an octagonal spire; the woodlands which surround it are the only parts of the ancient Forest of Selwood which exhibit any traces of their former character. There are places of worship for Baptists, the Society of Friends, Independents, Wesleyan Methodists, and Presbyterians. The free grammar school was founded in the reign of Edward VI., and is endowed with £6 per annum, which, from time immemorial, has been paid out of the Treasury, to which, £5 per annum has been subsequently added, but all documents relating to its foundation and further endowment are lost: there are no scholars at present on the foundation; the master takes private pupils, and the premises consist only of a large school-room and ante-room. A charity school, in which thirty-seven boys are clothed and educated for four years, at the end of which time they are apprenticed, is supported from the funds of certain lands vested in twenty trustees. Adjoining the school are almshouses for thirty-one aged women, supported out of the same funds, which produce an annual income of nearly £70, arising partly from property given by the original founder, William Leversedge, in the reign of Edward IV., and partly from subsequent benefactions. In that part of the town called Keyford is an asylum, founded in 1790, by Robert Stevens, Esq., who endowed it with £12,000 four per cent. Bank annuities, for the maintenance, clothing, and education of forty girls, to be placed out also in service, or as apprentices; and with £7000 in the same funds, for the maintenance of twenty aged men, natives of the parish: the annual income is at present nearly £800: the premises form a handsome quadrangular range of building commodiously arranged and appropriated to both these purposes. A National school, a capacious and handsome building, has been recently erected by subscription, in which two hundred boys, and one hundred and twenty-five girls, are at present instructed.

FROMEHAMPTON, a township in the parish of MARDEN, hundred of BROXASH, county of HEREFORD,

5½ miles (N. N. E.) from Hereford. The population is returned with the parish.

FROOME (BISHOP'S), a parish in the hundred of RADLOW, county of HEREFORD, comprising the townships of Bishop's Froome, Eggleton, Halmonds-Froome, Leadon, and Walton, and containing 897 inhabitants, of which number, 298 are in the township of Bishop's Froome, 4½ miles (S. by E.) from Bromyard. The living is a vicarage, in the archdeaconry and diocese of Hereford, rated in the king's books at £8. 5. 10., and in the patronage of the Rev. John Hopton. The church is dedicated to St. Mary. There is an endowed free school.

FROOME (CANON), a parish in the hundred of RADLOW, county of HEREFORD, 6 miles (N. W. by N.) from Ledbury, containing 105 inhabitants. The living is a discharged vicarage, in the archdeaconry and diocese of Hereford, rated in the king's books at £4. 13. 4., endowed with £400 private benefaction, and £400 royal bounty, and in the patronage of the Rev. John Hopton. The church is dedicated to St. James. The river Froome bounds the parish on the north.

FROOME (CASTLE), a parish in the hundred of RADLOW, county of HEREFORD, 7 miles (N. N. W.) from Ledbury, containing 180 inhabitants. The living is a rectory, in the archdeaconry and diocese of Hereford, rated in the king's books at £5. 13. 4., and in the patronage of Francis Freeman, Esq. The church is dedicated to St. Michael. The river Froome runs through the parish, in which there is a considerable quantity of limestone, also stone for building.

FROOME (HALMONDS), a township in the parish of BISHOP'S FROOME, hundred of RADLOW, county of HEREFORD, 5 miles (S. by E.) from Bromyard, containing 275 inhabitants.

FROOME (ST. QUINTIN), a parish in the hundred of TOLLERFORD, Dorchester division of the county of DORSET, 9½ miles (E. by N.) from Beaminster, containing 120 inhabitants. The living is a rectory with Evershot, in the archdeaconry of Dorset, and diocese of Bristol, rated in the king's books at £15. 7. 1., and in the patronage of the Crown. The church is dedicated to St. Mary. The parish derives its name from its situation on the river Frome, and its prefix from its ancient lords the St. Quintins. At Caldwell, within the parish, there was anciently a chapel.

FROOME-VAUCHURCH, a parish in the hundred of TOLLERFORD, Dorchester division of the county of DORSET, 7½ miles (N. W. by W.) from Dorchester, containing 105 inhabitants. The living is a rectory, united in 1772 to that of Batcombe, in the archdeaconry of Dorset, and diocese of Bristol, rated in the king's books at £7. 11. 0½., and in the joint patronage of the Dowager Countess of Sandwich and the Marquis of Cleveland. George Browne, in 1774, gave a rent-charge of £21 per annum, for teaching children.

FROSTENDEN, a parish in the hundred of BLYTHING, county of SUFFOLK, 4¼ miles (N. N. W.) from Southwold, containing 390 inhabitants. The living is a discharged rectory, in the archdeaconry of Suffolk, and diocese of Norwich, rated in the king's books at £12. Sir Thomas Gooch, Bart. was patron in 1806. The church is dedicated to All Saints.

FROSTERLEY, a hamlet in the parish of STANHOPE, north-western division of DARLINGTON ward,

county palatine of DURHAM, 3¼ miles (W.) from Walsingham. The population is returned with the parish. Here was formerly a chapel, which has long since gone to decay, but its site still retains the name of Chapel Close. There is a place of worship for Wesleyan Methodists. John Hinks, in 1735, and Mary Todd, in 1824, bequeathed property for the endowment of a school, now producing an annual income of about £40. A school-room, with a house for the master, was erected by subscription in 1747.

FROWLESWORTH, a parish in the hundred of GUTHLAXTON, county of LEICESTER, 4¾ miles (N. W. by N.) from Lutterworth, containing 301 inhabitants. The living is a rectory, in the archdeaconry of Leicester, and diocese of Lincoln, rated in the king's books at £12. 10., and in the patronage of the Trustees of the Rev. S. G. Noble. The church is dedicated to St. Nicholas. An almshouse was founded in 1725, by Chief Baron Smith, and liberally endowed with land and money for the maintenance of eighteen widows, who receive £20 per annum each.

FROXFIELD, a chapelry in the parish and hundred of EAST-MEON, Alton (South) division of the county of SOUTHAMPTON, 3¾ miles (N. W. by W.) from Petersfield, containing 548 inhabitants. The living is a perpetual curacy annexed to the vicarage of East-Meon, in the peculiar jurisdiction of the vicar thereof, and in the patronage of the Bishop of Winchester. The chapel is dedicated to St. Peter. Robert Love, in 1721, bequeathed £1000, with which a free school was founded and endowed for the education of twenty of the poorest boys of Froxfield, being, in 1767, farther endowed with £300, the bequest of Francis Beckford, Esq.: the income is about £55 per annum, for which twenty-two boys are instructed.

FROXFIELD, a parish in the hundred of KINWARDSTONE, county of WILTS, 3¼ miles (W. by S.) from Hungerford, containing 508 inhabitants. The living is a discharged vicarage, in the archdeaconry and diocese of Salisbury, rated in the king's books at £8. 16. 4., endowed with £200 private benefaction, and £200 royal bounty, and in the patronage of the Dean and Canons of Windsor. The church is dedicated to All Saints. There is a noble almshouse, founded in 1686, by Sarah, Duchess Dowager of Somerset, who bequeathed considerable landed and other property for its erection, and for the maintenance of thirty widows, the number to be increased to fifty, when the revenue should exceed £400 per annum. Twenty apartments were added to the original building in 1775, the whole forming an oblong quadrangle, with a small chapel within it, the minister of which has an annual stipend of £70. Thirty widows of clergymen, from any part of England, and twenty widows of laymen, not having an income of more than £20 per annum, are eligible to this charity, the allowance to each of whom is £21 a year. The government is vested in twelve trustees, chosen from the nobility and gentry of the county, who nominate the steward, chaplain, apothecary, and porter of the establishment.

FROYLE, a parish in the hundred of ALTON, Alton (North) division of the county of SOUTHAMPTON, 3¼ miles (N. E.) from Alton, containing 734 inhabitants. The living is a discharged vicarage, in the archdeaconry and diocese of Winchester, rated in the king's books at

£11. 12. 3½., endowed with £200 private benefaction, and £200 royal bounty, and in the patronage of the Rev. Sir Thomas Miller, Bart. The church is dedicated to St. Mary. Three children of this place are entitled to partake of the benefit of education at St. Andrew's school, Holybourn. The river Wey runs through the parish.

FRYERNING, a parish in the hundred of CHELMS-FORD, county of ESSEX, 1 mile (N. W. by W.) from Ingatestone, containing 612 inhabitants. The living is a rectory, in the archdeaconry of Essex, and diocese of London, rated in the king's books at £9, and in the patronage of the Warden and Fellows of Wadham College, Oxford. The church is dedicated to St. Mary.

FRYSTONE (FERRY), a parish in the upper division of the wapentake of OSGOLDCROSS, West riding of the county of YORK, ¾ of a mile (W.N.W.) from Ferry-Bridge, containing 777 inhabitants. The living is a discharged vicarage, in the peculiar jurisdiction of the Dean and Chapter of York, rated in the king's books at £5. 19. 2., endowed with £200 private benefaction, and £200 royal bounty, and in the patronage of the Sub-Chanter and Vicars Choral of the Cathedral Church of York. The church is dedicated to St. Andrew.

FRYSTONE (MONK), a parish in the lower division of the wapentake of BARKSTONE-ASH, West riding of the county of YORK, comprising the townships of Burton-Salmon, Hillam, and Monk-Frystone, and containing 860 inhabitants, of which number, 409 are in the township of Monk-Frystone, 4 miles (N. N. E.) from Ferry-Bridge. The living is a perpetual curacy, in the archdeaconry and diocese of York, endowed with £200 private benefaction, and £1300 parliamentary grant, and in the patronage of the Prebendary of Wistow in the Cathedral Church of York.

FRYTON, a township in that part of the parish of HOVINGHAM which is in the wapentake of RYEDALE, North riding of the county of YORK, 6¾ miles (W. N. W.) from New Malton, containing 62 inhabitants.

FUGGLESTONE (ST. PETER), a parish in the hundred of BRANCH and DOLE, county of WILTS, ¾ of a mile (E.) from Wilton, containing, with Bemerton, 528 inhabitants. The living is a rectory with that of Bemerton, in the archdeaconry of Wilts, and diocese of Salisbury, rated in the king's books at £24, and in the patronage of the Earl of Pembroke. According to Leland, Ethelred, King of the West Saxons, having been slain by the Danes in 827, was buried here. An hospital for leprous brethren and sisters, dedicated to St. Giles and St Anthony, is stated to have been founded at this place by Adelicia, second queen of Henry I.: its revenue, at the time of the general dissolution, was valued at £5. 13. 4.; the establishment was continued, and now supports a master (who must be a clergyman), and four poor people, who have a certain yearly allowance. Of the ancient building, only the ruinous chapel remains, in which it is said the royal foundress was interred.

FULBECK, a parish in the wapentake of LOVEDEN, parts of KESTEVEN, county of LINCOLN, 10¼ miles (N. by E.) from Grantham, containing 555 inhabitants. The living is a rectory, in the archdeaconry and diocese of Lincoln, rated in the king's books at £20. 15. 7½. Colonel Henry Fane was patron in 1807. The church is dedicated to St. Nicholas : its exterior is in the later style of English architecture, but the interior exhibits portions in the Norman, early English, and decorated styles, with a very fine Norman font.

FULBOURN, in the hundred of FLENDISH, county of CAMBRIDGE, 5 miles (E. N. E.) from Cambridge, comprising the parishes of All Saints and St.Vigors, and containing together 1023 inhabitants : the living of the former is a vicarage, rated in the king's books at £14. 17., and in the patronage of the Bishop of Ely ; and that of the latter a rectory, rated at £25. 15. 2½., and in the patronage of the Master and Fellows of St. John's College, Cambridge : they are in the archdeaconry and diocese of Ely. Both churches were situated in one church-yard, but one having fallen into decay, it was taken down in 1776 : the benefices still continue distinct. There is a place of worship for Independents. On the north side of the church-yard are some ancient almshouses for eleven poor persons. Elizabeth March, in 1722, bequeathed a farm, now producing about £100 a year, for the endowment of schools in the parishes of Fulbourn, Haddenham, Brinkley, Fen-Ditton, and Histon, equally.

FULBROOK, a chapelry in the parish of BURFORD, hundred of CHADLINGTON, county of OXFORD, ¾ of a mile (N. E. by N.) from Burford, containing 351 inhabitants. The chapel, dedicated to St. James, has lately received an addition of sixty-seven sittings, of which forty-one are free, the Incorporated Society for the enlargement of churches and chapels having granted £60 towards defraying the expense.

FULBROOK, a parish in the Snitterfield division of the hundred of BARLICHWAY, county of WARWICK, 4 miles (N. E. by N.) from Stratford upon Avon, containing 77 inhabitants. The living is a rectory, united in 1428 to the perpetual curacy of Sherbourne, in the archdeaconry and diocese of Worcester, rated in the king's books at £0. 14. 2. The church has been demolished.

FULFORD, a tything partly in the parishes of CHERITON-FITZPAINE and SHOBROOKE, in the western division of the hundred of BUDLEIGH, but chiefly in the parish and hundred of CREDITON, county of DEVON, 1½ mile (E. by N.) from Crediton, with which the population is returned.

FULFORD, a chapelry in the parish of STONE, southern division of the hundred of PIREHILL, county of STAFFORD, 4¾ miles (N. E.) from Stone. The population is returned with the parish. The living is a perpetual curacy, in the archdeaconry of Stafford, and diocese of Lichfield and Coventry, endowed with £200 private benefaction, £200 royal bounty, and £1200 parliamentary grant, and in the patronage of W. Allen, Esq. The chapel, dedicated to St. Nicholas, has lately received an addition of one hundred and eight free sittings, the Incorporated Society for the enlargement of churches and chapels having granted £150 towards defraying the expense. Quarries of excellent stone are wrought in the parish. A school-house was built pursuant to the will of George Hiatt, who in 1735 bequeathed £300 for the support of a master ; the income is £12. 10. a year, and the average number of scholars fifteen. Eleven other children are taught by a schoolmistress for £3. 10., the bequests of Thomas Shalcross and Thomas Porter.

FULFORD-AMBO, a parish partly within the liberty of ST. PETER of YORK, but chiefly in the wapentake of OUZE and DERWENT, East riding of the county of YORK, comprising the townships of Fulford-Gate and

Fulford-Water, and containing 847 inhabitants, of which number, 812 are in the township of Fulford-Gate, 1½ mile (S.) from York. The living is a perpetual curacy, in the archdeaconry and diocese of York, endowed with £800 private benefaction, £800 royal bounty, and £600 parliamentary grant, and in the patronage of Thomas Key, Esq. The church is dedicated to St. Oswald. There is a place of worship for Wesleyan Methodists. The York barracks, and a lunatic asylum, called the Retreat, in connexion with the Society of Friends, are situated in this parish. John Key, Esq., in 1771, assigned a messuage and rent-charge of £9. 12. a year, for the education of twenty children.

FULFORD-WATER, a township in the parish of Fulford-Ambo, partly in the liberty of St. Peter of York, and partly in the wapentake of Ouze and Derwent, East riding of the county of York, 2½ miles (S. by E.) from York, containing 35 inhabitants.

FULHAM, a parish in the Kensington division of the hundred of Ossulstone, county of Middlesex, containing, with the chapelry of Hammersmith, 15,301 inhabitants, of which number, 6492 are in the township of Fulham, 4 miles (S. W. by W.) from London. This place, situated on the north bank of the Thames, consists of several irregularly built streets, some of which are paved, and lighted with gas, and is amply supplied with water from the river and from springs. It is a place of considerable antiquity, the Danes having fixed their head-quarters here during their invasion of England in 879; from which, after wintering there, they set sail for Flanders in the spring. In 1642, the Earl of Essex, the parliamentary general, caused a bridge to be built, on barges and lighters, across the Thames, from Fulham to Putney, for the conveyance of his army and artillery into Surrey; and the parliamentary army under Sir Thomas Fairfax was quartered here in 1647. The manor, which appears to have belonged to the see of London from the end of the seventh century, was sold by order of the parliamentary commissioners in 1647, but restored in 1660; and the manor-house, or palace of Fulham, has been, from a very early period, the usual summer residence of the bishops of London. It is built of brick, the oldest part having been erected in the reign of Henry VII., by Bishop Fitz-James. The edifice consists of buildings surrounding two courts; on the north side of the inner court is the chapel, the windows of which are ornamented with stained glass, the greater part of which was removed from the chapel of London House, Aldersgate-street. Bishop Compton, distinguished as a botanist in the beginning of the last century, improved the gardens by the introduction of a number of curious plants and forest trees, particularly from North America. In the vicinity of Fulham are several extensive nursery-grounds, and much of the land is occupied by market-gardeners, who are noted for the cultivation of asparagus. A manufactory for earthenware, in imitation of porcelain, was established in 1684; but this has been long since superseded by a manufactory for brown stoneware. There is an extensive malt-kiln. About 1763, the manufacture of carpets and tapestry was introduced on a small scale, but the undertaking was soon abandoned from want of success. Near Wormholt, or Wormwood Scrubs, is a detached portion of the parish through which the Paddington canal passes: a design

has been projected to form a communication with this canal and the Thames, by a navigable line commencing near Fulham, but the undertaking has not been carried into effect further than Kensington, where there is a basin. This place is connected with Putney in Surrey by a wooden bridge over the Thames, built by Mr. Philips, carpenter to George II. Fulham is within the jurisdiction of a court of requests for the recovery of debts under 40s., held in Kingsgate-street, Holborn.

The living comprises a rectory and a vicarage, in the archdeaconry of Middlesex, and diocese of London, the former a sinecure, rated in the king's books at £26, and in the patronage of the Bishop of London; and the latter rated at £10, in the patronage of the Rector. The church, dedicated to All Saints, is an ancient stone structure, consisting of a nave, aisles, and chancel, with a handsome tower at the west end, in the decorated English style: within it is a single stone stall, with a canopy ornamented with quatrefoils; and some ancient sepulchral monuments. Among the distinguished persons interred here may be mentioned Dr. William Butts, physician to Henry VIII.; Dr. Richard Zouch, professor of Civil Law at Oxford, in the reign of Charles I.; Bishops Compton, Gibson, Sherlock, and Lowth; Dr. Richard Fiddes, author of a Life of Cardinal Wolsey; and Dr. William Cadogan, an eminent physician, who died in 1797. There is a chapel at Walham Green, dedicated to St. John, which was erected in 1829, at the expense of £9683. 17. 9., raised by subscription and a grant from the parliamentary commissioners: it contains one thousand three hundred and seventy sittings, of which five hundred and forty-four are free. In the Fulham division of the parish, on the south side of the road between Kensington and Hammersmith, is a proprietary chapel, erected in 1813 at the expense of Richard Hunt, Esq., and dedicated to St. Mary; and in the Hammersmith division are the church of St. Paul, and the chapel of St. Peter, the latter built by parliamentary grant in 1829. There is a place of worship for Independents. A library is supported by subscription. A National school for boys, and another for girls, containing about three hundred children of both sexes, eighty of whom are clothed, were established in 1811, and endowed with the produce of various benefactions, amounting to about £50 per annum; but they are principally supported by voluntary contributions. An infant school was established in 1830. Sir William Powell, Bart., in 1680, founded twelve almshouses for poor widows, and endowed them with property producing £51 per annum, to which considerable additions have been made by subsequent benefactors. Dr. Thomas Turner, in 1706, bequeathed £100, directing the produce to be applied in apprenticing poor children; and there are many other donations for charitable purposes.

FULKING, a hamlet in that part of the parish of Edburton which is in the hundred of Poynings, rape of Lewes, county of Sussex, 4½ miles (S.W.) from Hurst-Pierpoint, containing 177 inhabitants.

FULLAWAY, a tything in the parish of Allcannings, hundred of Swanborough, county of Wilts, 4 miles (E. by N.) from Devizes, containing 14 inhabitants.

FULLETBY, a parish in the hundred of Hill, parts of Lindsey, county of Lincoln, 3½ miles (N. E.) from Horncastle, containing 254 inhabitants. The living is a rectory, in the archdeaconry and diocese of Lincoln, rated in the king's books at £21. 2. 8½. Mr. Rockliffe was patron in 1784. The church is dedicated to St. Andrew.

FULMER, a parish in the hundred of STOKE, county of BUCKINGHAM, 4½ miles (S. E.) from Beaconsfield, containing 340 inhabitants. The living is a rectory not in charge, in the archdeaconry of Buckingham, and diocese of Lincoln, and in the patronage of the Dean and Canons of Windsor. The church, dedicated to St. James, was built at the expense of Sir Marmaduke Darell, in 1610. Fulmer was formerly a chapelry to the rectory of Datchet, but was separated therefrom, and made a distinct parish, in the reign of Edward VI.

FULMODESTON, a parish in the hundred of GALLOW, county of NORFOLK, 5 miles (E.) from Fakenham, containing, with Croxton, 331 inhabitants. The living is a rectory, in the archdeaconry of Norfolk, and diocese of Norwich, rated in the king's books at £10, and in the patronage of the President and Fellows of Corpus Christi College, Cambridge. The church is dedicated to St. Mary. There is a chapel of ease at Croxton, in this parish.

FULNECK, a hamlet in the parish of CALVERLEY, wapentake of MORLEY, West riding of the county of YORK, 6 miles (S.W.) from Leeds. The Moravians have one of their principal establishments here ; it was commenced about 1748, and now forms a considerable village, wherein various trades are carried on, which supply the community with most of their articles of consumption : the buildings, which occupy an extensive terrace, comprise a hall containing a chapel, the minister's dwelling, separate school-houses for boys and girls, a house for single men, another for single women, a third for widows, and several others for those who have families.

FULNETBY, a chapelry in the parish of RAND, western division of the wapentake of WRAGGOE, parts of LINDSEY, county of LINCOLN, 4 miles (W.N.W.) from Wragby, containing 52 inhabitants.

FULSHAW, a township in the parish of WILMSLOW, hundred of MACCLESFIELD, county palatine of CHESTER, 6 miles (N.W.) from Macclesfield, containing 256 inhabitants.

FULSTOW, a parish in the wapentake of BRADLEY-HAVERSTOE, parts of LINDSEY, county of LINCOLN, 7¼ miles (N.) from Louth, containing 389 inhabitants. The living is a vicarage, in the archdeaconry and diocese of Lincoln, rated in the king's books at £8. 10. 3., endowed with £800 royal bounty, and in the patronage of the Crown. The church is dedicated to St. Lawrence. There is a place of worship for Wesleyan Methodists.

FULWELL, a township in the parish of MONK-WEARMOUTH, eastern division of CHESTER ward, county palatine of DURHAM, 2 miles (N.N.W.) from Sunderland, containing 118 inhabitants. On removing a bank of earth, in 1759, a human skeleton, nine feet and a half in length, was found, with two Roman coins near its right hand ; and in working the limestone quarries several years ago, a square pit was discovered, containing a considerable quantity of stags' horns, in pieces three or four inches long, lying in a substance resembling animal matter.

FULWOOD, a township in that part of the parish of LANCASTER which is in the hundred of AMOUNDER-

NESS, county palatine of LANCASTER, 3 miles (N.) from Preston, containing 430 inhabitants. A school-house was erected about 1722, out of funds bequeathed for that purpose by John Hatch, who endowed it with £80, the income arising from which is applied towards the education of twenty-five children.

FUNDENHALL, a parish in the hundred of DEPWADE, county of NORFOLK, 5 miles (N.W. by W.) from St. Mary Stratton, containing 307 inhabitants. The living is a perpetual curacy, in the archdeaconry of Norfolk, and diocese of Norwich, and in the patronage of T. T. Berney, Esq. The church is dedicated to St Nicholas.

FUNTINGTON, a parish in the hundred of BOSHAM, rape of CHICHESTER, county of SUSSEX, 5 miles (W.N.W.) from Chichester, containing 847 inhabitants. The living is a perpetual curacy, in the archdeaconry and diocese of Chichester, endowed with £10 per annum private benefaction, £200 royal bounty, and £1000 parliamentary grant, and in the patronage of the Dean and Chapter of Chichester.

FURLAND, a tything in the parish and hundred of CREWKERNE, county of SOMERSET. The population is returned with the parish. Here was formerly a chapel.

FURNESS-ABBEY, county palatine of LANCASTER. See DALTON in FURNESS.

FURTHO, a parish in the hundred of CLELEY, county of NORTHAMPTON, 2 miles (N.N.W.) from Stony-Stratford, containing, with a small portion of the hamlet of Old Stratford, 12 inhabitants. The living is a rectory, in the archdeaconry of Northampton, and diocese of Peterborough, rated in the king's books at £7, and in the patronage of the Principal and Fellows of Jesus College, Oxford. The church is dedicated to St. Bartholomew. The Roman Watling-street passes along the south-western boundary of this parish.

FYFIELD, a parish in the hundred of OCK, county of BERKS, 4½ miles (W.N.W.) from Abingdon, containing 407 inhabitants. The living is a vicarage not in charge, in the archdeaconry of Berks, and diocese of Salisbury, endowed with £1200 private benefaction, £400 royal bounty, and £1200 parliamentary grant, and in the patronage of the President and Fellows of St. John's College, Oxford. The church is dedicated to St. Nicholas.

FYFIELD, a parish in the hundred of ONGAR, county of ESSEX, 2¾ miles (N.E. by N.) from Chipping-Ongar, containing 583 inhabitants. The living is a rectory, in the archdeaconry of Essex, and diocese of London, rated in the king's books at £25. 7. 6., and in the patronage of the Crown. The church is dedicated to St. Nicholas. A free school was endowed with lands by Dr. Walker, in 1692.

FYFIELD, a parish in the hundred of ANDOVER, Andover division of the county of SOUTHAMPTON, 4¾ miles (W. by N.) from Andover, containing, with the hamlet of Redenham, 201 inhabitants. The living is a rectory, in the archdeaconry and diocese of Winchester, rated in the king's books at £11. 12. 11., and in the patronage of the Crown. The church is dedicated to St. Nicholas.

FYFIELD, a tything in the parish of ENDFORD, hundred of ELSTUB and EVERLEY, county of WILTS, 8 miles (W.) from Ludgershall, containing 138 inhabitants.

FYFIELD, a chapelry in that part of the parish of

OVERTON which is in the hundred of SELKLEY, county of WILTS, 2¾ miles (W.) from Marlborough. The population is returned with the parish.

FYLINGDALES, a parish in the liberty of WHITBY-STRAND, North riding of the county of YORK, 4½ miles (S.E. by S.) from Whitby, containing 1702 inhabitants. The living is a perpetual curacy, in the archdeaconry of Cleveland, and diocese of York, endowed with £600 royal bounty, and £1400 parliamentary grant, and in the patronage of the Archbishop of York. The church, dedicated to St. Stephen, has lately received an addition of one hundred and forty-two sittings, of which one hundred and twelve are free, the Incorporated Society for the enlargement of churches and chapels having granted £150 toward defraying the expense.

G.

GADDESBY, a chapelry in the parish of ROTHLEY, eastern division of the hundred of GOSCOTE, county of LEICESTER, 6 miles (S.W.) from Melton-Mowbray, containing 282 inhabitants. It is within the peculiar ecclesiastical jurisdiction of the Lord of the Manor of Rothley. The chapel is dedicated to St. Luke.

GADDESDEN (GREAT), a parish in the hundred of DACORUM, county of HERTFORD, 2½ miles (N.W. by N.) from Hemel-Hempstead, containing 1096 inhabitants. The living is a discharged vicarage, in the archdeaconry of Huntingdon, and diocese of Lincoln, rated in the king's books at £10. 1. 10. Mrs. Halsey was patroness in 1820. The church is dedicated to St. John the Baptist. This village, which consists of a few scattered houses, derives its name from the river Gade, upon the south-west bank of which it is situated.

GADDESDEN (LITTLE), a parish in the hundred of DACORUM, county of HERTFORD, 5¾ miles (N. by E.) from Berkhampstead, containing 531 inhabitants. The living is a rectory, in the archdeaconry of Huntingdon, and diocese of Lincoln, rated in the king's books at £11. 12. 8½., and in the patronage of the Trustees of the late Earl of Bridgewater. The church is dedicated to St. Peter and St. Paul.

GAGINGWELL, a hamlet in the parish of CHURCH-ENSTONE, hundred of CHADLINGTON, county of OX-FORD, containing 63 inhabitants.

GAINFORD, a parish comprising the chapelry of Denton, and the township of Houghton-Lee-Side, in the south-eastern division; and the chapelries of Barnard-Castle and Whorlton, and the townships of Bolam, Gainford, Headlam, Ingleton, Langton, Marwood, Morton-Tynemouth, Pierse-Bridge, Staunton with Streatlam, Summerhouse, Westwick, and a part of Cleatlam, in the south-western division, of DARLINGTON ward, county palatine of DURHAM, and containing, including the whole population of Cleatlam, 6508 inhabitants, of which number, 500 are in the township of Gainford, 7¾ miles (W. by N.) from Darlington. The living is a vicarage, in the archdeaconry and diocese of Durham, rated in the king's books at £39. 6. 0½., and in the patronage of the Master and Fellows of Trinity College, Cambridge. The church, dedicated to St. Mary, was built by Egfrid, Bishop of Lindisfarne; it has been frequently repaired, and a gallery was erected on the north side by the late John Walton Elliot, Esq. There is a place of worship for Wesleyan Methodists. In 1691, the Rev. Henry Greswold left £100, directing the interest to be applied to the education of children. This place was anciently a seigniory, endowed with special liberties. In 1293, Agnes de Valentia had lands and free warren here, a place of execution, and various other privileges of a royal franchise. There are some mineral springs in the parish, and an abundance of coal and limestone. The village is pleasantly situated on the north bank of the Tees, and consists, of one spacious street of good buildings, extending along the high road, parallel with the river. The Marquis of Cleveland, as lord of the manor, holds courts leet and baron monthly, in the court-house at Barnard-Castle. On the road between Gainford and Pierse-Bridge is a stone deeply buried in the earth, of a form very like that of a Roman altar, called the White Cross. In digging on Gainford Green, many human skulls were discovered, the supposed remains of some Scots who suffered decapitation.

GAINSBOROUGH, a parish in the wapentake of CORRINGHAM, parts of LINDSEY, county of LINCOLN, comprising the market town of Gainsborough, and the hamlets of Morton, East Stockwith, and Walkerith, and containing 6761 inhabitants, of which number, 5893 are in the town of Gainsborough, 18¼ miles (N.W. by N.) from Lincoln, and 147 (N. by W.) from London. This town, which is situated on the eastern bank of the river Trent, appears to have been founded by a tribe of Saxons, soon after their first invasion of Britain : under the Heptarchy, it belonged first to the kingdom of Northumberland, and then to that of Mercia. In 868, Alfred the Great celebrated his nuptials at this place, with Ealswitha, the daughter of a Mercian nobleman ; and here the Danes, in 1013, landed under the command of their king Sweyn, and commenced their devastations, which terminated in the subjugation of the kingdom. Matthew of Westminster says that Sweyn was assassinated at this place whilst revelling with his followers ; but other historians consider Thetford in Norfolk to have been the scene of his death. On this event his son Canute, who was at Gainsborough, was chosen king of England by the Danes; but Ethelred II. returning from Normandy, where he had taken refuge, his troops attacked the Danes, compelled Canute to flee from England, and wreaked their fury on his adherents. In the beginning of the war between Charles I. and the parliament this town was placed by the king under the government of the Earl of Kingston, who, being taken prisoner and sent to Hull, was unfortunately shot by the royalists, by mistake, in crossing the Humber : it was taken by the parliamentarians, but shortly after retaken by the Marquis of Newcastle, who placed it under the protection of a new governor. In 1643, Cromwell, on his way to York, encountered a party of royalists near Gainsborough, when they were defeated, and their commander, General Cavendish, brother of the Marquis of Newcastle, and Colonel Markham, of Allerton, fell in the conflict. As evidence of the military contests which have taken place here, it may be mentioned, that in paving the streets many human bodies have been found, which appeared to have been promiscuously interred after battle.

The town chiefly consists of one long street running parallel with the river, with a cross street leading from its bank to the cattle market : a new street, called Spring-gardens, has been formed within a few years, and a considerable number of buildings has been raised on the south side of the town. The streets are well paved, and were first lighted with gas in 1825; the inhabitants are supplied with water from the Trent, by means of an engine. A handsome stone bridge of three arches was erected across the river in 1791, which has contributed materially to the improvement of the town. A theatre has been formed out of part of an ancient structure, called the Old Hall, said to have been built by John of Gaunt; it is open for six weeks at the October mart. A room in the present town-hall is occasionally used for assemblies; and races are held annually in the North Marsh. Here are two extensive rope-walks, four steam-mills for bruising linseed, several malt-houses, three ship-yards, and a few brass and iron-foundries. The town is favourably situated for the purposes of commerce, and enjoys a very fair proportion for an inland town. The Trent is navigable for vessels of two hundred tons' burden, and a considerable trade to the Baltic is carried on; a great quantity of corn is also shipped for the London and other markets; and the counties of Stafford, Nottingham, and Leicester, are chiefly supplied with foreign produce through this port. Before the completion of the Grand Junction canal, the whole of the Staffordshire ware was shipped here for London. The annual number of vessels which entered inwards, on an average, from 1812 to 1816, was about three hundred, and that which cleared outwards about two hundred and sixty. Besides those entered at the custom-house (which was established in 1820), many small craft are employed in the trade to Hull, and the counties of York, Leicester, Nottingham, &c., along the Trent and the various canals which intersect this part of the country. The market is on Tuesday; and there are two fairs, or marts, one commencing on Easter-Monday, and the other on the 20th of October, both lasting ten days; and a large market for wool on the Monday before July 5th, and every alternate Monday until August 5th, then on the Friday following for the last day. The highest civil officer is a burgess-constable, elected annually at a court leet : a court baron is also held twice a year, soon after Easter and Michaelmas, at which the steward of the manor presides : here is also a court for the recovery of small debts. The quarter sessions for the north parts of Lindsey were formerly held at the town-hall, but they have been removed to Kirton. The gaol is a small building, lately erected at the bottom of Church-lane, near the workhouse.

The living is a vicarage, in the archdeaconry of Stowe, and diocese of Lincoln, rated in the king's books at £22. 16. 8., and in the patronage of the Prebendary of Corringham in the Cathedral Church of Lincoln. The church, dedicated to All Saints, appears to have been founded and endowed by the Knights Templars, about the year 1209. In 1736 the nave was taken down, and the rebuilding of it completed in 1748, at an expense of £5230, which was raised by a duty on coal brought to the town, aided by a parochial rate. The tower affords a fine specimen of the later style of English architecture, and contrasts curiously with the modern portion of the building. There are places of worship for Baptists, the Society of Friends, Independents, Primitive and Wesleyan Methodists, and Presbyterians. Mrs. Sarah Mott, of Doncaster, in 1704, bequeathed £300 to be invested in lands, from the produce of which three poor boys are apprenticed annually. In 1708, Joshua Tyler bequeathed land, chargeable with the payment of £5 per annum, for the education of children. In 1731, Mr. Wharton gave, by will, land to the trustees of the free school, directing the proceeds to be applied in clothing and educating children, and providing bread for the poor. In 1736, Mrs. E. Hopkinson bequeathed £365, the interest to be applied to clothing poor women, and to the education of children. In 1781, Miss Hickman gave £200 for the education of poor girls, and the benefit of the poor generally; and she subsequently gave land for the erection of a school-room, and a house for the master. The free school was founded by letters patent granted by Elizabeth, in 1590, and endowed with a rent-charge of £30 per annum on the estates of the crown, which was never paid, so that it is, consequently, only nominally free : the master has the gratuitous use of the school-room, dwelling-house, and play-ground, and receives a quarterage for the education of children. A school on the Madras system is supported by subscription, wherein about two hundred children are instructed; and thirty girls are also educated on the same plan, at a school-room in the old Methodist chapel yard. The Old Hall is a curious structure, forming three sides of a quadrangle, and occupying nearly half an acre of ground; it is in the ancient style of domestic architecture : part of it is said to have been built by John of Gaunt, Duke of Lancaster, the western wing by a member of the Burgh family, about 1490, and the eastern one, about 1600, by a member of the family of Hickman, in whose possession it remains; it has been converted into small tenements or workshops, and the theatre. Near North-holme, on the hills eastward from the town, is a spring possessing tonic qualities, similar to those of the Buxton waters, but of a different degree of temperature. This is the birthplace of William de Gainsborough, the firm defender of the doctrine of the pope's infallibility, who was advanced by Boniface VIII. to the see of Worcester, at which place he died, in 1308. Simon Patrick, Bishop of Ely, was born here in 1626; as also was his brother, John Patrick, one of the translators of Plutarch.

GALBY, county of LEICESTER. See GAULBY.

GALHAMPTON, a hamlet in the parish of NORTH CADBURY, hundred of CATSASH, county of SOMERSET, 1¼ mile (S.) from Castle-Carey, containing 362 inhabitants.

GALLOW-HILL, a township in that part of the parish of BOLAM which is in the western division of MORPETH ward, county of NORTHUMBERLAND, 8¾ miles (W. S. W.) from Morpeth, containing 74 inhabitants. This place derives its name from the circumstance of its having once been the place of execution for the barony of Bolam.

GALTON, a tything in the parish and liberty of OWERMOIGNE, Blandford (South) division of the county of DORSET, 9 miles (S. E.) from Dorchester. The population is returned with the parish.

GAMBLESBY, a township in the parish of ADDINGHAM, LEATH ward, county of CUMBERLAND, 10 miles

(N. E.) from Penrith, containing 279 inhabitants. Independents and Wesleyan Methodists have each a place of worship here.

GAMELSBY, a joint township with Biglands, in the parish of AIKTON, ward and county of CUMBERLAND, 3¾ miles (N. by E.) from Wigton, containing 191 inhabitants. There is a place of worship for Wesleyan Methodists.

GAMLINGAY, a parish in the hundred of LONGSTOW, county of CAMBRIDGE, 2¼ miles (N. E. by N.) from Potton, containing 1256 inhabitants. The living is a vicarage, in the archdeaconry and diocese of Ely, rated in the king's books at £5, and in the patronage of the Bishop of Ely: there is also a sinecure rectory, rated at £15. 14. 2., and in the patronage of the Warden and Fellows of Merton College, Oxford. The church is a handsome edifice, dedicated to St. Mary. There is a place of worship for Baptists. In this parish is an almshouse for eight poor widows, endowed with a bequest of £2000 South Sea Annuities, by Mrs. Elizabeth Lane; and a small charity school has a trifling endowment. A market was formerly held here, but it has for many years been discontinued, having been transferred to the neighbouring town of Potton, in Bedfordshire.

GAMPSTON, a hamlet in that part of the parish of WEST BRIDGFORD which is in the southern division of the wapentake of BINGHAM, county of NOTTINGHAM, 2¼ miles (S. E.) from Nottingham, containing 102 inhabitants.

GAMSTON, a parish in the South-clay division of the wapentake of BASSETLAW, county of NOTTINGHAM, 3½ miles (S.) from East Retford, containing 385 inhabitants. The living is a rectory, in the archdeaconry of Nottingham, and diocese of York, rated in the king's books at £11. 16. 5½., and in the patronage of the Crown. The church, dedicated to St. Peter, has a tower with eight pinnacles in the later English style.

GANEREW, a parish in the lower division of the hundred of WORMELOW, county of HEREFORD, 3 miles (N. E. by N.) from Monmouth, containing 118 inhabitants. The living is a discharged rectory, in the archdeaconry and diocese of Hereford, rated in the king's books at £1. 10., and in the patronage of Joseph Pyrke, Esq. The church, dedicated to St. Swithin, is said to be that in which Vortigern, Prince of Dumnonium, was interred. There is a place of worship for Wesleyan Methodists. The river Wye bounds the parish on the south-east: a considerable quantity of limestone is obtained in the vicinity. There are two hills, called Great and Little Doward; on the slope of the former are the remains of an ancient fortification, distinguished by the name of Arthur's Hall, and on the summit of the latter are traces of another, near which broad arrow heads have been found.

GANSTEAD, a township in that part of the parish of SWINE which is in the middle division of the wapentake of HOLDERNESS, East riding of the county of YORK, 4½ miles (N. E. by N.) from Kingston upon Hull, containing 61 inhabitants.

GANTHORPE, a township in the parish of TERRINGTON, wapentake of BULMER, North riding of the county of YORK, 7 miles (W. by S.) from New Malton, containing 106 inhabitants. Here is a school, endowed by the Earl of Carlisle with about £20 per annum.

GANTON, a parish in the wapentake of DICKERING, East riding of the county of YORK, 9¼ miles (S. S. W.) from Scarborough, containing, with Brompton, 278 inhabitants. The living is a discharged vicarage, in the archdeaconry of the East riding, and diocese of York, rated in the king's books at £5. 2. 6. Sir Thomas Legard, Bart. was patron in 1828. The church is dedicated to St. Nicholas.

GARBOLDISHAM, a parish in the hundred of GUILT-CROSS, county of NORFOLK, 4¼ miles (S. S. E.) from East Harling, containing 700 inhabitants. The living is a rectory consolidated with that of All Saints, in the archdeaconry of Norfolk, and diocese of Norwich, rated in the king's books at £19. 16. 0½. C. M. Montgomery, Esq. was patron in 1815. The church is dedicated to St. John the Baptist.

GARENDON, an extra-parochial liberty, in the western division of the hundred of GOSCOTE, county of LEICESTER, 2 miles (W.) from Loughborough, containing 43 inhabitants. An abbey for Cistercian monks, dedicated to the Blessed Virgin, was founded here in 1133, by Robert Bossu, Earl of Leicester, the revenue of which, at the dissolution, amounted to £186. 15. 2.

GARFORD, a chapelry in the parish of MARCHAM, hundred of OCK, county of BERKS, 5 miles (W. by S.) from Abingdon, containing 192 inhabitants.

GARFORTH (WEST), a parish in the lower division of the wapentake of SKYRACK, West riding of the county of YORK, 7 miles (E.) from Leeds, containing 731 inhabitants. The living is a rectory, in the archdeaconry and diocese of York, rated in the king's books at £8. 17. 8½. The Rev. J. Whitaker was patron in 1797. The church is dedicated to St. Mary. Here are places of worship for Independents and Wesleyan Methodists. There is a small sum for the education of children; the school-house was erected by subscription in 1818.

GARGRAVE, a parish in the eastern division of the wapentake of STAINCLIFFE and EWCROSS, West riding of the county of YORK, comprising the townships of Bank-Newton, Cold Coniston, Eshton, Flasby with Winterburn, and Gargrave, and containing 1659 inhabitants, of which number, 972 are in the township of Gargrave, 4½ miles (W. N. W.) from Skipton. The living is a vicarage, in the archdeaconry and diocese of York, rated in the king's books at £12. 13. 11½. John Marsden, Esq. was patron in 1806. The church, dedicated to St. Andrew, is principally in the later English style. Here is a place of worship for Wesleyan Methodists. There is a small endowed school. This place is situated close to the Leeds and Liverpool canal, upon which it has extensive warehouses: the principal branch of business is the cotton manufacture. A court for the recovery of debts under 40s. is held every three weeks, of which the Duke of Devonshire is chief bailiff. The river Aire runs through the village. There are a Roman pavement and encampment in the parish.

GARMONDSWAY-MOOR, a township in the parish of BISHOP's MIDDLEHAM, north-eastern division of STOCKTON ward, county palatine of DURHAM, 6¾ miles (S. E. by S.) from Durham, containing 35 inhabitants. This place is said to have derived its name from Garmundus the Dane. The ancient *Via Garmundi*, along which King Canute travelled barefooted to the shrine of St. Cuthbert, at Durham, passed through it, and gave name to the township.

GARRETT, a hamlet in the parish of WANDSWORTH, western division of the hundred of BRIXTON, county of SURREY, 7 miles (S. W. by S.) from London. The population is returned with the parish. A mock election formerly took place here on the dissolution of every parliament; which circumstance gave rise to Foote's diverting comedy of "the Mayor of Garrett." An iron railway from Wandsworth to Croydon, and thence to Merstham near Reigate, passes through this place.

GARRIGILL, a chapelry in the parish of ALDSTONE, LEATH ward, county of CUMBERLAND, 3 miles (E. S. E.) from Aldstone Moor, containing 1288 inhabitants. The Independents and Primitive and Wesleyan Methodists have each a place of worship. Mines belonging to the London Lead Company afford employment to many of the inhabitants. Fairs for cattle and sheep are held on the third Friday in May, and the first Friday in September.

GARRISON-SIDE, an extra-parochial liberty, locally in the county of the town of Kingston upon Hull, East riding of the county of YORK, containing 173 inhabitants.

GARRISTON, a township in the parish of HAUKSWELL, western division of the wapentake of HANG, North riding of the county of YORK, 4¼ miles (N. N. E.) from Middleham, containing 52 inhabitants.

GARSDALE, a chapelry in the parish of SEDBERGH, western division of the wapentake of STAINCLIFFE and EWCROSS, West riding of the county of YORK, 6 miles (E.) from Sedbergh, containing 679 inhabitants. The living is a perpetual curacy, in the archdeaconry of Richmond, and diocese of Chester, endowed with £400 private benefaction, £400 royal bounty, and £400 parliamentary grant, and in the patronage of the Crown. The church is dedicated to St. John the Baptist. There is a small sum for the education of children.

GARSDON, a parish in the hundred of MALMESBURY, county of WILTS, 2 miles (E. by N.) from Malmesbury, containing 183 inhabitants. The living is a rectory, in the archdeaconry of Wilts, and diocese of Salisbury, rated in the king's books at £10. 9. 9½., and in the patronage of P. Methuen, Esq. The church is dedicated to All Saints.

GARSINGTON, a parish in the hundred of BULLINGTON, county of OXFORD, 5 miles (S.E. by E.) from Oxford, containing 595 inhabitants. The living is a rectory, annexed to the Headship of Trinity College, Oxford, in the archdeaconry and diocese of Oxford, rated in the king's books at £14. 19. 9½. The church, dedicated to St. Mary, is an ancient structure.

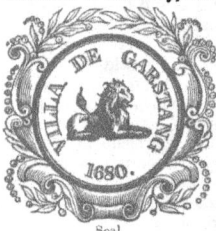
Seal.

GARSTANG, a parish in the hundred of AMOUNDERNESS, county palatine of LANCASTER, comprising the market town of Garstang, the chapelry of Pilling, the townships of Barnacre with Bonds, Billisborrow, Cabus, Catteral, Claughton, Forton, Kirkland, Nateby, Winmarleigh, Nether Wyersdale, and a part of Clevely, and the hamlet of Holleth; and containing, including the whole population of Clevely, 7403 inhabitants, of which number, 936 are in the town of Garstang, 11 miles (S. by E.) from Lancaster, and 229 (N.W. by N.)

from London. The name appears to be of Saxon origin, and the place was anciently called *Gayrstang*, probably from *Garri*, a Saxon thane, who is said to have been its first resident lord. Though not a station of the Romans, it was situated on one of their great roads leading from *Lugovallum* (now Carlisle), to *Condate*, (now Kinderton, in Cheshire). At the close of the last century, a Roman shield of brass, of curious workmanship, was found in the neighbourhood, which is now among the Towneley collection in the British Museum. An oaken box also, strong, but roughly constructed, and fastened by wooden pins, was turned up by the plough in this parish; which, on being opened, was found to contain a fine collection of celts, spear-heads, and other instruments, partly Roman and partly British. During the parliamentary war, this parish was the scene of some unimportant operations, and the castle of Greenhaugh, which is in the neighbourhood, was held for the king, by the Earl of Derby, in 1643. When the Scottish adherents to the Pretender made their incursion into England, in 1715, they halted at Garstang, before taking possession of Preston, and in the following year, some of the rebels were executed at this place.

The town is situated on the river Wyre, on the road between Preston and Lancaster: the more ancient part consists of houses indifferently built, the streets being irregularly formed; but great improvements have lately been introduced: the streets are now well paved, the town lighted, and a few houses of respectability have recently been added. The trade and manufactures are not very considerable: several looms are employed in weaving linen and cotton goods, and there are some cotton mills, and a large calico-printing establishment in the neighbourhood; but the town derives its greatest advantages from its situation as a thoroughfare. The market is on Thursday; and a market for cattle is held every alternate Thursday, between the first Thursday in Lent and Holy Thursday. Fairs are held on Holy Thursday, July 10th, and Nov. 22nd. An impulse has lately been given to the trade of the town and parish by the facilities afforded by the Lancaster canal, which crosses the river Wyre by a handsome aqueduct, near the end of the principal street, thus forming a communication with the Trent, Severn, and Mersey; and from the Wyre, which winds round the town on the eastern and southern sides, a tolerable supply of fish is obtained. The inhabitants were first incorporated by a charter granted in 1314; but this was superseded by a new one granted by Charles II., in 1680, with additional privileges, by which the government of the town was vested in a bailiff and seven capital burgesses, elected annually on the 29th of September. In case of the death or removal of a burgess, the remainder elect another from among the freemen: the bailiff is chosen from among the capital burgesses. The freedom is obtained by birth, by apprenticeship to a freeman, or by gift from the corporation. The bailiff holds a court of pie-powder at the fairs: the borough is co-extensive with the township. A court baron, held twice a year, possesses jurisdiction for the recovery of small debts, but little use is now made of it. The town-hall, which is the principal public edifice, and is situated in the market-place, was built at the expense of the corporation in 1755, on the site of a former edifice: the lower part serves for a corn exchange, and the upper for transacting public business: the petty sessions for the hundred of Amounderness are held in it.

The living is a vicarage, in the archdeaconry of Richmond, and diocese of Chester, rated in the king's books at £14. 3. 4., and in the patronage of the Rev. John Pedder. The church, dedicated to St. Helen, is a stately structure, situated about a mile and a half from the town, in that part of the parish called Garstang Church Town, in the township of Kirkland: having been injured by the overflowing of the river Wyre, near which it stands, it was repaired in 1746, and again in 1811, when the walls of the nave and chancel were raised, and the whole received a new roof, at an expense of £1200, which was defrayed jointly by the parishioners and Thomas Strickland Standish, Esq., the lay impropriator. There is a chapel within the town, the living of which is a perpetual curacy, endowed with £400 private benefaction, £600 royal bounty, and £500 parliamentary grant, and in the patronage of the Vicar of Garstang: there is another chapel at Pilling, which is in the patronage of the Lord of the Manor. The Independents, Wesleyan Methodists, and Roman Catholics, have each a place of worship here. The free school was built about the year 1756, partly from the funds of the corporation, and partly by subscription, and endowed with a bequest of £150, from John Morland, Esq., and £5 per annum, the gift of William Baylton, the proceeds of which are paid to the master for instructing four children, two others being educated at the expense of the corporation: besides which, there are between sixty and seventy scholars who pay quarterage. The Roman Catholics support also both a day and a Sunday school. Three miles west of Garstang is Pilling-moss, the scene of a phenomenon, of which the following account is given in the Philosophical Transactions, No. 475, January 26th, 1744-5:—" A part of Pilling-moss was observed to rise to a surprising height; and after a short time it sank as much below the level, and moved slowly towards the south side; and in half an hour it covered twenty acres of land, improved land adjoining to that part of the moss which moved, in a concave circle, containing about one hundred acres, was nearly filled up with moss and water. That part of the moss which sank remained like the bed of a river, running from north to south, above a mile in length, and half a mile in breadth." A considerable portion of the moss has been reclaimed of late years, and successfully converted to agricultural purposes, while the margin supplies an abundance of turf, which compensates in a measure for the scarcity of coal.

GARSTON, a chapelry in the parish of CHILDWALL, hundred of WEST DERBY, county palatine of LANCASTER, 6 miles (S. E.) from Liverpool, containing 874 inhabitants. The living is a perpetual curacy, in the archdeaconry and diocese of Chester, endowed with £730 private benefaction, £600 royal bounty, and £600 parliamentary grant. Richard Watt, Esq. was patron in 1811. There are extensive works at this place for refining salt, which afford employment to about one hundred persons: the material from which the salt is made is brought from Northwich, in Cheshire.

GARSTON (EAST), a parish situated partly in the hundred of WANTAGE, partly in the hundred of MORETON, but chiefly in the hundred of LAMBOURN, county of BERKS, 2¾ miles (E. S. E.) from Lambourn, containing 637 inhabitants. The living is a discharged vicarage, in the archdeaconry of Berks, and diocese of Salisbury, rated in the king's books at £13. 6. 8., and in the patronage of the Dean and Canons of Christ Church, Oxford. The church is dedicated to All Saints. Here is a place of worship for Wesleyan Methodists. There is a small sum for the education of children.

GARTHORP, a township in the parish of LUDDINGTON, western division of the wapentake of MANLEY, parts of LINDSEY, county of LINCOLN, 13 miles (W. by S.) from Barton upon Humber, containing 500 inhabitants.

GARTHORPE, a parish in the hundred of FRAMLAND, county of LEICESTER, 5¾ miles (E. N. E.) from Melton-Mowbray, containing 115 inhabitants. The living is a discharged vicarage, in the archdeaconry of Leicester, and diocese of Lincoln, rated in the king's books at £7. 5. 2., and in the patronage of the Lord of the Manor. The church, dedicated to St. Mary, has portions in the decorated style. The small river Eye runs through the parish.

GARTON, a parish in the middle division of the wapentake of HOLDERNESS, East riding of the county of YORK, containing, with the townships of Garton and Owstwick, part of which latter is in the parish of Rooss, 299 inhabitants, of which number, 160 are in the township of Garton, 12 miles (N. E. by E.) from Kingston upon Hull. The living is a discharged vicarage, in the archdeaconry of the East riding, and diocese of York, rated in the king's books at £6. 1. 0½., endowed with £400 royal bounty, and in the patronage of the Crown. The church is a neat structure, dedicated to St. Michael. Here is a place of worship for Wesleyan Methodists.

GARTON upon the WOLDS, a parish partly in the liberty of ST. PETER of YORK, and partly in the wapentake of DICKERING, East riding of the county of YORK, 3 miles (W. N. W.) from Great Driffield, containing 357 inhabitants. The living is a discharged vicarage, in the archdeaconry of the East riding, and diocese of York, rated in the king's books at £5. 6. 8., endowed with £600 royal bounty, and in the patronage of the Crown. The church is dedicated to St. Michael. There is a place of worship for Wesleyan Methodists. A school is partly supported by the proceeds of a share in the Driffield canal, bequeathed by the late Mrs. Jane Cook.

GARVESTONE, a parish in the hundred of MITFORD, county of NORFOLK, 5 miles (S. S. E.) from East Dereham, containing 330 inhabitants. The living is a discharged rectory, in the archdeaconry and diocese of Norwich, rated in the king's books at £7. 16. Sir W. Clayton, Bart. was patron in 1828. The church is dedicated to St. Margaret.

GARWAY, a parish in the lower division of the hundred of WORMELOW, county of HEREFORD, 7 miles (N. W.) from Monmouth, containing 522 inhabitants. The living is a perpetual curacy, in the archdeaconry and diocese of Hereford, endowed with £200 private benefaction, £800 royal bounty, and £1000 parliamentary grant, and in the patronage of W. H. Jenkins, Esq. The church is dedicated to St. Michael. Here is a place of worship for Baptists. Mrs. Frances Scudamore, in 1715, bequeathed an estate, now producing a rental of £64, in trust, to the minister and churchwardens of Garway, Kentchurch, and Llangaron, for apprenticing two or more children of one of those parishes every year alternately; and the residue for distribution, in like manner, among six poor widows.

GASPER, county of SOMERSET. See BROOK.

GASTHORPE, a parish in the hundred of GUILT-CROSS, county of NORFOLK, 4¼ miles (S.) from East Harling, containing 113 inhabitants. The living is a rectory not in charge, united to that of Riddlesworth, in the archdeaconry of Norfolk, and diocese of Norwich. The church, which was dedicated to St. Nicholas, has fallen to ruins.

GATCOMB, a parish in the liberty of WEST MEDINA, Isle of Wight division of the county of SOUTHAMPTON, 3¾ miles (S. S. W.) from Newport, containing 247 inhabitants. The living is a rectory, in the archdeaconry and diocese of Winchester, rated in the king's books at £25. 18. 9., and in the patronage of the University of Oxford, in trust for the Principal of St. Edmund's Hall. The church is dedicated to St. Olaye. There is a small endowed school.

GATCOMBE, a hamlet in the parish and hundred of COLYTON, county of DEVON, 2½ miles (S. W.) from Colyton, with which the population is returned. Here was formerly a chapel.

GATEFORTH, a township in the parish of BRAYTON, lower division of the wapentake of BARKSTONE-ASH, West riding of the county of YORK, 5 miles (S. W. by W.) from Selby, containing 192 inhabitants.

GATELEY a parish in the hundred of LAUNDITCH, county of NORFOLK, 5½ miles (S. E. by S.) from Fakenham, containing 104 inhabitants. The living is a discharged vicarage with the rectory of Brisley, in the archdeaconry and diocese of Norwich, rated in the king's books at £3. 2. 8½. The church is dedicated to St. Helen.

GATENBY, a township in the parish of BURNESTON, wapentake of HALLIKELD, North riding of the county of YORK, 4¾ miles (E.) from Bedale, containing 88 inhabitants.

GATESGILL, a joint township with Raughton, in the parish of DALSTON, ward and county of CUMBERLAND, 6¼ miles (S. by W.) from Carlisle, containing 294 inhabitants.

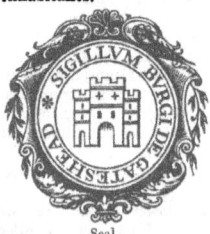

Seal.

GATESHEAD, a parish in the eastern division of CHESTER ward, county palatine of DURHAM, 1 mile (S. S. E.) from Newcastle, and 14 (N. by E.) from Durham, containing, with the seamen of registered shipping, 11,767 inhabitants. This place is situated on the southern bank of the Tyne, opposite to Newcastle, with which it has a communication by a stone bridge. It is supposed by some antiquaries to have been a Roman station, called *Gabrosentum*, which signifies Goat's Head, this having been the sign of the principal inn, and corresponding with the appellation of *Caput Capræ* referred to by Bede; but the only indication of Roman residence here arises from the discovery of Roman coins, and from the vicinity of the Watling-street. The earliest authentic notice of this place is connected with the account given by Simeon of Durham, of the insurrection of the Northumbrians, and the murder of

Bishop Walcher, who was slain whilst endeavouring to make his escape from the church of Gateshead, which had been set on fire by his assailants, in 1080. Hugh Pudsey, Bishop of Durham, in 1164, granted to the burgesses a charter of privileges nearly similar to those enjoyed by the burgesses of Newcastle. The subsequent history of Gateshead relates to the frequent contests between the bishops of Durham and the corporation of Newcastle, concerning the navigation of the Tyne, and the right of building quays on its banks, which ultimately terminated in favour of the latter. On the dissolution of the see of Durham, in 1552, an act of parliament was passed for annexing this town to the borough of Newcastle; but the rights of the bishoprick having been restored soon after by Queen Mary, Gateshead reverted to its former jurisdiction. From the earliest period of authentic record, this town was governed by a bailiff appointed by the Bishop of Durham, till 1695, since which the supreme municipal authority has been exercised by two stewards, who are annually elected by the borough holders and freemen. The borough contains one hundred and forty-four burgage tenements, but, as more than one of these may be held by the same individual, the number of borough-holders seldom exceeds one hundred, and in addition to these, are ten or eleven freemen. The town comprises a line of irregular edifices distinguished by the appellations of High-street and Bridge-street, from which diverge Hillgate, formerly St. Mary's Gate, and several streets of inferior importance. Some local improvements have been effected under the authority of an act of parliament for cleansing, lighting, and watching the streets, passed in 1814; and an act passed in 1824, empowering the trustees, under the Durham and Tyne Bridge road act, to form a road from the eastern side of the High-street to the southern gate of the church-yard. In 1818, a company was formed for the purpose of lighting the town with gas. The inhabitants are plentifully supplied with water from a reservoir at a short distance from the town, whence it is brought by means of pipes. There were anciently several incorporated trading companies, similar to those of Newcastle, but they have long since become extinct. The principal manufactories at present are those for cast and wrought iron and glass, which are very extensive; there are also collieries, chemical laboratories, and whiting manufactories. A market formerly held here, on Tuesday and Friday in each week, was discontinued about the commencement of the sixteenth century. Two fairs for the hiring of servants were established in 1822, and are held on the second Monday in April, and the first Monday in November. A halmote court is held annually before the steward of the manor; and petty sessions for the district are held here every Saturday.

The living is a rectory, in the archdeaconry and diocese of Durham, rated in the king's books at £27. 13. 4., and in the patronage of the Bishop of Durham. The church, dedicated to St. Mary, is a cruciform structure, appearing to have been founded at a remote period, but considerably altered by modern reparations. The tower and part of the western end of the nave were rebuilt in 1740, and the roof was altered in 1764; but there are some decorated pillars and arches remaining, and a Norman south door-way under a modern porch. A handsome window of painted glass, representing the Annunciation of the Blessed Virgin, and adorned with armorial bearings, was presented by Mr. Joseph Price, in 1819, and put up in the southern transept; and an organ, which cost five hundred guineas, raised by subscription, was completed in January 1824. The chapel of St. Edmund was built by subscription in 1808 : divine service is performed in it on Sundays, and it is used for a National school on the other days of the week. The hospital of St. Edmund, to which it belongs, was founded in 1248, by Bishop Farnham, who endowed it for a master and three chaplains : this establishment survived the Reformation, but its charters having been lost, and its revenue partly converted to purposes of private advantage, it was refounded by James I., in 1610, for a master and three poor brethren, the master to be the rector of Gateshead. In 1810, an act of parliament was procured, which altered the constitution of the hospital, and the brethren are now thirteen in number, three elder, and ten younger, who are all appointed by the master. The annual revenue is about £455, of which sum, the master receives one-third, the chaplain £40, each of the elder brethren £25 with a house, and each of the younger £12. The ruins of the old chapel of St. Edmund, affording a beautiful specimen of early English architecture, are still remaining, as is also a portion of the old house of the brethren. Here are two places of worship for Methodists of the New Connexion, four for Wesleyan Methodists, and one for Presbyterians. The Anchorage school, held in an apartment over the vestry-room of St. Mary's church, is stated to derive its name from the circumstance of anchorage dues of that part of the Tyne which had formerly belonged to the Bishop of Durham having been paid here. Its establishment took place previously to 1658, and its endowment arises from the interest on £300, given by Theophilus Pickering, D.D., in 1701, towards the support of a free school, for instruction in English and classical literature, and navigation: the master, besides his salary, receives one shilling a quarter from each of the fifteen boys who are upon the foundation, and is permitted to take as many other pupils as the schoolroom will accommodate : the master and free scholars are appointed by the rector. The National school was formed in 1808, and removed in 1810 to St. Edmund's chapel, whence it is called the Chapel school. An almshouse in the High-street, founded in 1731, through the bequest of Thomas Powell, is now used as the poor-house for the parish; and there is an unendowed almshouse in Hillgate for six poor women, given to the parish by John Bowman, in 1689. A subscription news-room was established in 1820 : there is a society for the prosecution of felons, the oldest institution of the kind in Great Britain.

GATESHEAD-FELL, a parish in the eastern division of Chester ward, county palatine of Durham, 3 miles (S.) from Newcastle. The population is returned with Gateshead. It formerly constituted a part of the parish of Gateshead, from which it was separated in pursuance of an act of parliament passed in 1808. The living is a rectory not in charge, in the archdeaconry and diocese of Durham, and in the patronage of the Bishop of Durham. The church, dedicated to St. John, was commenced in May 1824, and consecrated August 30th, 1825, having been erected at the expense of

VOL. II.

£2742, towards which the Society for building new churches contributed £350 : it contains one thousand sittings, five hundred of which are free. Here are places of worship for Baptists and Wesleyan Methodists. The quarries of the Fell are famous for producing excellent grind-stones; and there are numerous coal mines. Notwithstanding their division, the parishes of Gateshead and Gateshead-Fell constitute one constablewick as before, and the inhabitants of both contribute jointly towards the maintenance of the poor, the management of whom since 1821 has been entrusted to a select vestry. In 1068, William the Conqueror here gained a victory over Malcolm II., King of Scotland, who had invaded the kingdom in support of Edgar Atheling.

GATTON, a borough and parish, in the second division of the hundred of Reigate, county of Surrey, 22 miles (E. by N.) from Guildford, and 18 (S. by W.) from London, containing 135 inhabitants. This was formerly a considerable town, and had a castle; but it is now an insignificant village, only distinguished by the privilege of sending two members to parliament, which it has enjoyed since the 29th of Henry VI. The right of election is vested in the freeholders and inhabitants paying scot and lot; and the constable for the manor is the returning officer : the patronage of the borough belongs to Sir Mark Wood, Bart. The living is a rectory, in the archdeaconry of Surrey, and diocese of Winchester, rated in the king's books at £9. 2. 8½., and in the patronage of Sir M. Wood, Bart. The river Mole has its source in this parish; and here is a quarry of white stone which will bear exposure to a high degree of heat, and is therefore much used in the construction of ovens, furnaces for glass-houses, &c.

GAULBY, a parish in the hundred of Gartree, county of Leicester, 8 miles (E. S. E.) from Leicester, containing, with the chapelry of Frisby, 114 inhabitants. The living is a rectory, in the archdeaconry of Leicester, and diocese of Lincoln, rated in the king's books at £18. 2. 6., and in the patronage of G. A. Legh-Keck, Esq. The church is dedicated to St. Peter.

GAUTBY, a parish in the southern division of the wapentake of Gartree, parts of Lindsey, county of Lincoln, 6½ miles (W. N. W.) from Horncastle, containing 118 inhabitants. The living is a discharged rectory, in the archdeaconry and diocese of Lincoln, rated in the king's books at £6. 3. 4., endowed with £200 private benefaction, and £200 royal bounty, and in the patronage of the Crown. The church is dedicated to All Saints.

GAWCOTT, a chapelry in the parish and within the liberty of the borough of Buckingham, county of Buckingham, 2 miles (S. W.) from Buckingham, containing 566 inhabitants. The living is a perpetual curacy, in the archdeaconry of Buckingham, and diocese of Lincoln, endowed with £200 private benefaction, and £1100 parliamentary grant, and in the patronage of certain Trustees. The ancient chapel, dedicated to St. Catherine, was demolished, but a new one was opened in 1828.

GAWSWORTH, a parish in the hundred of Macclesfield, county palatine of Chester, 3½ miles (S.W. by S.) from Macclesfield, containing 804 inhabitants. The living is a rectory, in the archdeaconry and diocese

2 F

of Chester, rated in the king's books at £7. 4. 4½., and in the patronage of the Earl of Harrington. The church, dedicated to St. James, is a handsome structure. There is a small sum for the education of children. The New Macclesfield canal, connecting the Grand Trunk with the Peak Forest, passes through the eastern side of the parish. Courts leet and baron are held annually.

GAYDON, a chapelry in the parish of BISHOP'S ITCHINGTON, Kington division of the hundred of KINGTON, county of WARWICK, 3 miles (N. E.) from Kington, containing 187 inhabitants. It is within the peculiar ecclesiastical jurisdiction of the Prebendary of Colwich and Bishop's Itchington in the Cathedral Church of Lichfield. The chapel is dedicated to St. Giles. The inhabitants marry and bury at Chadshunt, which is a parochial chapelry within the same parish.

GAYHURST, a parish in the hundred of NEWPORT, county of BUCKINGHAM, 2¾ miles (N.W.) from Newport-Pagnell, containing, with the extra-parochial liberty of Gorefields, 90 inhabitants. The living is a rectory, united in 1736 with that of Stoke-Goldington, in the archdeaconry of Buckingham, and diocese of Lincoln, rated in the king's books at £6. 0. 2½., and in the patronage of Miss Anne Barbara Wrighte. The church, dedicated to St. Peter, was completed in 1728, by means of a sum of money bequeathed for that purpose by Mr. Wrighte, lord of the manor. The river Ouse runs through the parish, and there is a chalybeate spring in the neighbourhood.

GAYLES, a township in the parish of KIRKBY-RAVENSWORTH, western division of the wapentake of GILLING, North riding of the county of YORK, 5 miles (N. W. by N.) from Richmond, containing 218 inhabitants.

GAYTON, a township in the parish of HESWALL, lower division of the hundred of WIRRALL, county palatine of CHESTER, 3 miles (N. W. by N.) from Great Neston, containing 153 inhabitants. There is a ferry over the Dee into Flintshire, the æstuary at this place being nearly four miles broad.

GAYTON, a parish in the Lynn division of the hundred of FREEBRIDGE, county of NORFOLK, 7¼ miles (E.) from Lynn-Regis, containing 545 inhabitants. The living is a discharged vicarage, in the archdeaconry and diocese of Norwich, rated in the king's books at £8. 6. 8., and in the patronage of the Bishop of Norwich. The church is dedicated to St. Nicholas. Here is a place of worship for Wesleyan Methodists. William de Scohies founded a Benedictine priory here in the reign of William the Conqueror.

GAYTON, a parish in the hundred of TOWCESTER, county of NORTHAMPTON, 4¼ miles (N. by E.) from Towcester, containing 389 inhabitants. The living is a rectory, in the archdeaconry of Northampton, and diocese of Peterborough, rated in the king's books at £15. 5. 2½., and in the patronage of the Master and Fellows of Sidney Sussex College, Cambridge. The church is dedicated to St. Mary. The Grand Junction canal runs through this parish.

GAYTON, a parish in the southern division of the hundred of PIREHILL, county of STAFFORD, 6 miles (N. E.) from Stafford, containing 284 inhabitants. The living is a perpetual curacy, in the archdeaconry of Stafford, and diocese of Lichfield and Coventry, endowed with £600 royal bounty, and £400 parliamentary grant,

and in the patronage of Mr. Fitzgerald. The church is dedicated to St. John the Baptist. There is a trifling sum for the education of children.

GAYTON le MARSH, a parish in the Marsh division of the hundred of CALCEWORTH, parts of LINDSEY, county of LINCOLN, 5¾ miles (N. by W.) from Alford, containing 276 inhabitants. The living is a rectory, in the archdeaconry and diocese of Lincoln, rated in the king's books at £13. 10. 2½., and in the patronage of the Crown. The church is dedicated to St. George.

GAYTON-THORPE, a parish in the Lynn division of the hundred of FREEBRIDGE, county of NORFOLK, 8 miles (N. W. by N.) from Swaffham, containing 187 inhabitants. The living is a rectory, in the archdeaconry and diocese of Norwich, rated in the king's books at £6. A. Hamond, Esq. was patron in 1818. The church is dedicated to St Mary.

GAYTON le WOLD, a parish in the Wold division of the hundred of LOUTH-ESKE, parts of LINDSEY, county of LINCOLN, 6¼ miles (W. by S.) from Louth, containing 122 inhabitants. The living is a discharged rectory, in the archdeaconry and diocese of Lincoln, rated in the king's books at £8. 11. 0., and in the patronage of the Crown. The church is dedicated to St. Peter.

GAYWOOD, a parish in the Lynn division of the hundred of FREEBRIDGE, county of NORFOLK, ¾ of a mile (E. by N.) from Lynn-Regis, containing 474 inhabitants. The living is a rectory, in the archdeaconry and diocese of Norwich, rated in the king's books at £5. 13. 4., and in the patronage of W. Bagge, Esq. The church is dedicated to St. Faith. The inhabitants of the neighbouring parish of Bawsey, having no church, attend at Gaywood. The river Gaywood runs through the parish, in which there are two mineral springs.

GAZELEY, a parish in the hundred of RISBRIDGE, county of SUFFOLK, 5¼ miles (E. by N.) from Newmarket, containing, with the hamlet of Higham Green, 644 inhabitants. The living is a discharged vicarage with Kentford, in the archdeaconry of Sudbury, and diocese of Norwich. The church is dedicated to All Saints.

GEDDING, a parish in the hundred of THEDWESTRY, county of SUFFOLK, 6¾ miles (W.) from Stow-Market, containing 144 inhabitants. The living is a discharged rectory, in the archdeaconry of Sudbury, and diocese of Norwich, rated in the king's books at £4. 13. 4., and in the patronage of the Mayor and Corporation of Ipswich. This place is situated on the river Orwell.

GEDDINGTON, a parish in the hundred of CORBY, county of NORTHAMPTON, 3½ miles (N. E. by N.) from Kettering, containing 751 inhabitants. The living is a discharged vicarage, in the archdeaconry of Northampton, and diocese of Peterborough, rated in the king's books at £5 11. 0½., endowed with £400 royal bounty, and in the patronage of the Duke of Buccleuch. The church is dedicated to St. Mary Magdalene. To the north-east of it there was formerly a royal seat, called the Castle, or Hall Close, where Henry II. held a parliament in 1188, to raise money for a crusade. In the centre of the village stands one of the elegant crosses erected by Edward I. to the memory of his consort Eleanor.

GEDLING, a parish in the southern division of the

wapentake of THURGARTON, county of NOTTINGHAM, $3\frac{1}{2}$ miles (N. E. by E.) from Nottingham, containing, with the township of Stoke-Bardolph, and the hamlet of Charlton, 2017 inhabitants. The living comprises a rectory and a vicarage, in medieties, the former rated in the king's books at £14. 6. 0½., and the latter at £6. 16. 8., in the archdeaconry of Nottingham, and diocese of York, and in the patronage of the Earl of Chesterfield. The church is dedicated to All Saints.

GEDNEY, a parish in the wapentake of ELLOE, parts of HOLLAND, county of LINCOLN, 3 miles (E.) from Holbeach, containing, with the chapelry of Gedney-Hill, 1786 inhabitants. The living is a vicarage, in the archdeaconry and diocese of Lincoln, rated in the king's books at £30. 11. 10½., and in the patronage of the Crown. There is also a sinecure rectory, rated at £23. 11. 0½., and in the patronage of the Crown for two terms, and of W. Clayton, Esq. for one. The church, dedicated to St. Mary Magdalene, is a beautiful structure, supposed to have been built by the abbots of Crowland, who had a house and large possessions in the parish: it contains fifty-three windows, those of the north aisle having considerable remains of painted glass. In this parish are vestiges of intrenchments, supposed to have been the site of Roman fortifications.

GEDNEY-HILL, a chapelry in the parish of GEDNEY, wapentake of ELLOE, parts of HOLLAND, county of LINCOLN, $6\frac{3}{4}$ miles (E.) from Crowland, containing 344 inhabitants. The living is a perpetual curacy, in the archdeaconry and diocese of Lincoln, and in the patronage of certain Feoffees of land bequeathed for charitable uses. The chapel is dedicated to the Holy Trinity. Several coins of Antoninus have been found here.

GELDESTONE, a parish in the hundred of CLAVERING, county of NORFOLK, $2\frac{1}{4}$ miles (N. W. by W.) from Beccles, containing 284 inhabitants. The living is a discharged rectory, in the archdeaconry and diocese of Norwich, rated in the king's books at £6, endowed with £200 royal bounty, and in the patronage of the Crown. The church is dedicated to St. Michael.

GEMBLING, a township in the parish of FOSTON upon WOLDS, wapentake of DICKERING, East riding of the county of YORK, $7\frac{1}{4}$ miles (E. by S.) from Great Driffield, containing 87 inhabitants.

GENNYS (ST.), a parish in the hundred of LESNEWTH, county of CORNWALL, 10 miles (N. by E.) from Camelford, containing 680 inhabitants. The living is a vicarage, in the archdeaconry of Cornwall, and diocese of Exeter, rated in the king's books at £8. Sir W. Molesworth, Bart. was patron in 1783. This parish is situated on the coast of the Bristol channel.

GEORGE (ST.), a parish in the hundred of BARTON-REGIS, county of GLOUCESTER, 2 miles (E.) from Bristol, containing 5334 inhabitants. The living is a vicarage not in charge, in the archdeaconry of Dorset, and diocese of Bristol, and in the patronage of the Mayor and Corporation of Bristol. The church was consecrated in 1756. This place, which is bounded on the south by the Avon, was constituted a distinct parish by act of parliament in the 24th of George II., having been previously part of the out-parish of St. Philip and St. Jacob, Bristol; and was called Easton (East-town) from its situation, and more anciently Bertune. Many coal pits are worked in the parish, some of which are of a very unusual depth. There are several small bequests for the education of children. Anciently there was an hospital for lepers, dedicated to St. Lawrence.

GEORGEHAM, a parish in the hundred of BRAUNTON, county of DEVON, 8 miles (N. W. by W.) from Barnstaple, containing 811 inhabitants. The living is a rectory, in the archdeaconry of Barnstaple, and diocese of Exeter, rated in the king's books at £40. 17. 11. Sir A. Chichester, Bart. was patron in 1783. The church is dedicated to St. George. Here is a charity school with a small endowment, in which between twenty and thirty children are instructed.

GERMANS (ST.), a borough, market town, and parish, in the southern division of the hundred of EAST, county of CORNWALL, 19 miles (S. by E.) from Launceston, and 227 (W.S.W.) from London, containing 2404 inhabitants. The town is situated in a beautiful valley, on the borders of a creek called St. Germans, formed by the rivers Tidi and Lynher, which, uniting with the Tamar, fall into the sea: the Tidi becomes navigable two miles above St. Germans, at a place called Tiddiford. In the southern part of the parish, which is bounded by the English channel, there is a beacon. This place derived its name from St. Germanus, Bishop of Auxerre, who is supposed to have resided here during a visit which he made to Cornwall, in the fifth century. Athelstan having conquered the Cornish Britons, in the early part of the tenth century, founded here the see of a bishop, which, in the reign of Canute, was removed to Crediton, and subsequently to Exeter. The loss of ecclesiastical authority probably contributed to the decay of the town, the market, then held on Sundays, having become very inconsiderable when the Norman survey was made. Leland mentions it as a poor fishing town; but he adds, the glory of it stood by the priory, which was a convent of Augustine canons, whose revenue at the dissolution amounted to £227.4.8.: its site is occupied by Port Eliot, a modern mansion belonging to the Earl of St. Germans. The market, which was altered from Sunday to Friday, has long been discontinued; but fairs for cattle are held May 28th and August 1st. The town is governed by a portreeve, chosen annually at the court leet for the manor. It has returned two representatives to parliament ever since 1562: the right of election is vested in householders who have resided twelve months within the borough: the portreeve is the returning officer. The patronage belongs to the Earl of St. Germans.

The living is a perpetual curacy, in the peculiar jurisdiction of the Bishop of Exeter, endowed with £1200 parliamentary grant, and in the patronage of the Dean and Canons of Windsor. The church, dedicated to St. Germanus, consists of the nave and aisles of the conventual church, with a fine Norman doorway at the west end, between two low towers: within it are several monuments of the families of Eliot, Glanvill, and Scawen, among which is a magnificent tomb erected in memory of Edward Eliot, uncle of the first Lord Eliot, with a recumbent statue of the deceased, and other figures, executed by Rysbrack; and here is also the monument of Walter Moyle, an eminent writer, the friend and correspondent of Locke, who died in 1721. Nicholas Honey, in 1657, gave land in this parish for the support of a schoolmaster, and other charitable purposes; and here is a parish school, assisted by the benefactions of Lord St. Germans. St. Germans gives the title of earl to the family of Eliot.

GERMANS-WEEK, a parish in the hundred of LIFTON, county of DEVON, 11 miles (W. by S.) from Oakhampton, containing 324 inhabitants. The living is a perpetual curacy, in the archdeaconry of Totness, and diocese of Exeter, endowed with £800 royal bounty, and £200 parliamentary grant, and in the patronage of the Dean and Chapter of Bristol.

GERMOE, a parish in the hundred of KERRIER, county of CORNWALL, 5¾ miles (W. by N.) from Helston, containing 830 inhabitants. The living is a perpetual curacy united to the vicarage of Breage, in the archdeaconry of Cornwall, and diocese of Exeter. Here is a place of worship for Wesleyan Methodists. On the north side of the church-yard is a singular edifice, called St. Germoe's chairs, consisting of a stone seat divided into three parts by pillars in the Norman style, with pointed arches, and placed in a recess similarly decorated. The parish, in which are the famous Godolphin tin mines, derives its name from St. Germoe, or Germoch, said to have been an Irish king.

GERRANS, a parish in the western division of the hundred of POWDER, county of CORNWALL, 7 miles (S.W. by S.) from Tregony, containing 732 inhabitants. The living is a rectory, in the peculiar jurisdiction and patronage of the Bishop of Exeter, rated in the king's books at £15. 12. 6. The church is dedicated to St. Gurons. Here is a place of worship for Wesleyan Methodists. This parish lies at the upper end of St. Mawe's harbour, and is bounded on the east by the English channel. On an estate called Cargurrell, at this place, is the ancient fortification called *Dingerein*, supposed by Whitaker to have been the residence of King Gerennius.

GESTINGTHORPE, a parish in the hundred of HINCKFORD, county of ESSEX, 3 miles (N.E.) from Castle-Hedingham, containing 694 inhabitants. The living is a discharged vicarage, within the jurisdiction of the Commissary of Essex and Herts, concurrently with the Bishop of London, rated in the king's books at £7, endowed with £200 private benefaction, and £200 royal bounty: there is also a sinecure rectory, rated at £13. 6. 8. J. T. H. Elwes, Esq. was patron in 1804. The church is dedicated to St. Mary.

GIDDING (GREAT), a parish in the hundred of LEIGHTONSTONE, county of HUNTINGDON, 5 miles (S.W.) from Stilton, containing 496 inhabitants. The living is a discharged vicarage, in the archdeaconry of Huntingdon, and diocese of Lincoln, rated in the king's books at £8. 5. 2., and in the patronage of Lord Sondes. The church, dedicated to St. Michael, contains a curious bason for holy water, resembling a Norman capital. A salary is paid by Lord Sondes to a master for teaching reading, writing, and arithmetic, to twenty poor boys.

GIDDING (LITTLE), a parish in the hundred of LEIGHTONSTONE, county of HUNTINGDON, 5¾ miles (S.W.) from Stilton, containing 64 inhabitants. The living is a discharged rectory, in the archdeaconry of Huntingdon, and diocese of Lincoln, rated in the king's books at £7. 6. 4., endowed with £200 royal bounty, and in the patronage of the Crown. The church is dedicated to St. John.

GIDDING (STEEPLE), a parish in the hundred

of LEIGHTONSTONE, county of HUNTINGDON, 6 miles (S.W. by S.) from Stilton, containing 93 inhabitants. The living is a discharged rectory, in the archdeaconry of Huntingdon, and diocese of Lincoln, rated in the king's books at £8. 17. 8½. J. Heathcote, Esq. was patron in 1807. The church is dedicated to St. Andrew.

GIDLEY, a parish in the hundred of WONFORD, county of DEVON, 8¼ miles (S.E. by E.) from Oakhampton, containing 121 inhabitants. The living is a discharged rectory, in the archdeaconry and diocese of Exeter, rated in the king's books at £14. 19. 0½. Henry Rattray, Esq. was patron in 1791. The church is dedicated to the Holy Trinity. In the reign of Henry II. the ancient family of Prous had a castle here, of which there are still some remains.

GIGGLESWICK, a parish (formerly a market town) in the western division of the wapentake of STAINCLIFFE and EWCROSS, West riding of the county of YORK, comprising the townships of Giggleswick, Rathmill, Settle, and Stainforth, and containing 2817 inhabitants, of which number, 746 are in the township of Giggleswick, ¾ of a mile (W. by N.) from Settle. The living is a discharged vicarage, in the archdeaconry and diocese of York, rated in the king's books at £21. 3. 4., endowed with £200 private benefaction, and £200 royal bounty. J. Coulthurst and J. Hartley, Esqrs. were patrons in 1782. The church, dedicated to St. Alkald, is principally in the later English style. Here is a free grammar school, founded by Edward VI. in the 7th year of his reign, in which Archdeacon Paley was educated: the income is estimated at £1140 per annum. The founder ordained that it should consist of a master and an usher; and that eight inhabitants should be a body corporate, and have power to act as governors; that it should be free for the classical instruction of all boys, without any restriction or qualification as to residence. Between sixty and seventy boys are educated, and there is one exhibition to the University. Agnes Hargraves also bequeathed a close of land for the instruction of children. At the foot of a ledge of rocks, in this parish, called the Scar, rises a spring, noted for ebbing and flowing, though distant nearly thirty miles from the sea : the water has been known to rise and fall nineteen inches in five minutes.

GILBERDIKE, a township in the parish of EASTRINGTON, wapentake of HOWDENSHIRE, East riding of the county of YORK, 5½ miles (E. by N.) from Howden, containing 640 inhabitants.

GILCRUX, a parish in ALLERDALE ward below Darwent, county of CUMBERLAND, 5½ miles (N. by W.) from Cockermouth, containing 377 inhabitants. The living is a discharged vicarage, in the archdeaconry and diocese of Carlisle, rated in the king's books at £5. 14. 2., and in the patronage of the Bishop of Carlisle. The church, dedicated to St. Mary, stands on an artificial eminence, and is in the early style of English architecture. The parish is bounded on the west by the river Ellen. Numerous springs rise in the village, and uniting form a considerable stream. There is also a spring of saline water called Tom Tack, at a short distance to the eastward. Coal is obtained in abundance, and there are quarries of freestone in the parish. Joseph Tordiff, in 1799, gave £800 stock, in the three per cents., producing £24 per annum, for the education of twenty-four children.

GILDEN-WELLS, a township in the parish of LAUGHTON en le MORTHEN, partly within the liberty of ST. PETER of YORK, and partly in the southern division of the wapentake of STRAFFORTH and TICKHILL, West riding of the county of YORK, 5¾ miles (N.N.W.) from Worksop, containing 83 inhabitants.

GILDERSOME, a chapelry in that part of the parish of BATLEY which is in the wapentake of MORLEY, West riding of the county of YORK, 4½ miles (S.W. by W.) from Leeds, containing 1592 inhabitants. The living is a perpetual curacy, in the archdeaconry and diocese of York, endowed with £1000 royal bounty, and £1200 parliamentary grant. The chapel has lately received an addition of one hundred and forty-three free sittings, the Incorporated Society for the enlargement of churches and chapels having granted £200 towards defraying the expense. There are places of worship for Baptists and Wesleyan Methodists. Bolton Hargrave, Esq., in 1749, bequeathed £10 a year for the education of children. Here is a scribbling-mill; and the manufacture of cotton is also carried on.

GILES (ST.), a parish in the hundred of FREMINGTON, county of DEVON, 3 miles (E. by S.) from Great Torrington, containing 786 inhabitants. The living is a perpetual curacy, in the archdeaconry and diocese of Exeter, and in the patronage of the Dean and Fellows of Christ Church College, Oxford. The church, among other monuments, contains one to the memory of Tristram Risdon, the antiquary. Robert Lovett, in 1710, bequeathed £30, the produce of which is applied to apprenticing children. There are almshouses for four poor widows, founded by an ancestor of Lord Rolle, who allows each of the inmates £1. 5. per annum. Stevenston, a mansion belonging to Lord Rolle, was taken possession of in the civil war, by Sir Thomas Fairfax, February 16th, 1646.

GILES (ST.) on the HEATH, a parish in the hundred of BLACK TORRINGTON, county of DEVON, 4½ miles (N. by E.) from Launceston, containing 301 inhabitants. The living is a perpetual curacy, in the archdeaconry of Cornwall, and diocese of Exeter, and in the patronage of Lord Valletort. There is a trifling endowment, the bequest of Roger Harvey in 1767, for teaching children.

GILL, a township in the parish of GREYSTOCK, LEATH ward, county of CUMBERLAND, 6¼ miles (W. by S.) from Penrith, containing, with the township of Motherby, 112 inhabitants.

GILLIMOOR, a township in the parish of KIRBY-MOORSIDE, wapentake of RYEDALE, North riding of the county of YORK, 7 miles (N.E.) from Helmsley, containing 195 inhabitants. There is a place of worship for Wesleyan Methodists.

GILLING, a parish comprising the chapelries of South Cowton and Eryholme, and the township of North Cowton, in the eastern division, and the townships of Eppleby and Gilling in the western division, of the wapentake of GILLING, North riding of the county of YORK, and containing 1673 inhabitants, of which number, 921 are in the township of Gilling, 3 miles (N. by E.) from Richmond. The living is a vicarage, in the archdeaconry of Richmond, and diocese of Chester, rated in the king's books at £23. 11. 5½., and in the patronage of John Wharton, Esq. The church, dedicated to St. Agatha, retains some traces of Norman architecture, and was appropriated, in 1224, to the monastery of St. Mary, in York. There is a place of worship for Wesleyan Methodists. Gilling is a place of great antiquity, and remarkable as the scene of the murder of Oswyn, King of Deira, by his host, Oswin of Bernicia; in expiation of which crime, a monastery was founded on the spot, by Queen Eanfleda, but not the slightest vestige of it now remains. There are quarries of excellent freestone, with materials drawn from which most of the bridges in the North riding are built. Sir Thomas Wharton, in 1678, founded Hartforth free school, for thirty children, and endowed it with an estate now producing about £125 a year. There is also a school, endowed with £20 per annum by Matthew Hutchinson, in which eighty children are educated on the National plan.

GILLING, a parish in the wapentake of RYEDALE, North riding of the county of YORK, comprising the townships of Cawton, Gilling, and Grimston, and containing 329 inhabitants, of which number, 168 are in the township of Gilling, 5¼ miles (S.) from Helmsley. The living is a rectory, in the archdeaconry of Cleveland, and diocese of York, rated in the king's books at £13. 10., and in the patronage of the Master and Fellows of Trinity College, Cambridge. The church, dedicated to the Holy Cross, contains a vault belonging to the family of Fairfax. The castle was built by Alan, Earl of Richmond, soon after the Conquest, to repel the frequent attacks of the Saxons and Danes, for the recovery of their lost estates. The Hon. Anne Fairfax, in 1793, left £400, now producing £20 a year, for teaching thirty children.

GILLINGHAM, a parish in the liberty of GILLINGHAM, Shaston (West) division of the county of DORSET, 4 miles (N.W. by W.) from Shaftesbury, containing, with the chapelry of Bourton, 3059 inhabitants. The living, a vicarage, is a royal peculiar within the jurisdiction of the Lord of the Manor, rated in the king's books at £40. 17. 6., and in the patronage of the Bishop of Salisbury. The church, dedicated to the Blessed Virgin Mary, is a large edifice partly in the Norman style, with a chantry chapel attached to it, and a high tower. There is a place of worship for Wesleyan Methodists. A library of six hundred volumes, given by Thomas Freke, Esq., is deposited in the vicarage-house, for the use of the vicars. The river Stour runs through the parish, which lies in the northernmost part of the county, bordering on the counties of Somerset and Wilts; it is of great extent, being about forty-one miles in circumference, and includes the ancient Forest of Selwood, which was disafforested by Charles I., on condition that the lessee should maintain four hundred deer for the king's use. About half a mile eastward from the church, on the road to Shaftesbury, are traces of the ancient palace of the Saxon and Norman kings, who made it their residence when they came to hunt in the forest. The manufacture of linen has been carried on here from a very early period, but the inhabitants derive their principal profits from the rich pastures and dairy-lands abounding in the parish. There are fairs for horses, bullocks, and sheep, on Trinity-Monday and September 12th. John Grice and others, in 1526, founded and endowed a free school, which was in much repute during the parliamentary war, and in which the celebrated Hyde, afterwards Earl of Clarendon, received part of his education. Edmund Ironside, in 1016, having vanquished Canute at Pen in Somersetshire, the pursuit is said to have extended hither, which is probable from the number of pits now discernible in the neighbourhood, on the supposed field of a second battle.

GILLINGHAM, a parish in the hundred of CHATHAM and GILLINGHAM, lathe of AYLESFORD, county of KENT, 1½ mile (E. by N.) from Chatham, containing 6209 inhabitants. The living is a vicarage, in the peculiar jurisdiction of the Archbishop of Canterbury, rated in the king's books at £15. 13. 11½., and in the patronage of the Principal and Fellows of Brasenose College, Oxford. The church, dedicated to St. Mary Magdalene, was formerly remarkable for containing what was deemed a miraculous image of the Virgin, called "Our Lady of Gillingham," to which frequent pilgrimages were made; it is a spacious fabric with a chapel on each side of the chancel, which exhibits some slight portions of Norman architecture. The font is in the same style, very capacious, and surrounded by semicircular arches rising from single pillars: some fragments of the richly stained glass remain, with which most of the windows were formerly filled by the family of Beaufitz, lords of Twydiall, some of whom lie buried here. Memorials of the Romans may be discerned within its walls. On the south side of the church-yard are foundations of an extensive building, once the archiepiscopal palace, the hall of which has been converted into a barn, and where a coin of the Emperor Antoninus has been discovered. There is a place of worship for Wesleyan Methodists. This ancient village, which is recorded in Domesday-book by the name of Gelingeham, though now inconsiderable, was, previously to the rapid rise of the neighbouring town of Chatham, a place of note, and its harbour on the Medway was a principal station for the Royal navy. In the reign of Elizabeth it possessed four quays, viz., Twydall, Midflete, Dean Med End, and Beggar Hyde, together with various ships and boats. Charles I. erected a fort for the protection of the royal dock-yard and navy, which proving ineffectual to resist the Dutch in their celebrated expedition up the river, in 1667, was subsequently enlarged, and distinguished by the name of Gillingham castle, though it was never considered of great strength. At present, however, the entire neighbourhood is strongly fortified with outposts connected with Chatham lines, within which, at the western extremity of the parish, is the populous village of Brompton, situated on the brow of a hill overlooking the royal dock yard of Chatham, and chiefly inhabited by artizans and others employed therein. This parish is within the jurisdiction of a court of requests held in the city of Rochester, for the recovery of debts under £5. Elizabeth Petty, in 1723, bequeathed a rent-charge of £19. 10. a year, for teaching fifteen children of Gillingham and Chatham; and Philip Tidd, in 1733, gave a cottage, garden, orchard, &c., to be occupied by a poor widow of the parish, who, should teach six children. Gillingham was anciently much exposed to the ravages of the Danes, and it is asserted that six hundred noblemen, who landed here in the retinue of Alfred and Edward, were murdered upon the spot by Earl Godwin. William of Gillingham, the early historian, who flourished in the reign of Richard II.; and William Adams, the discoverer of Japan, to which island he began his voyage in 1598, were born here.

GILLINGHAM, comprising the united parishes of All Saints and St. Mary, in the hundred of CLAVERING, county of NORFOLK, 1¼ mile (N. by W.) from Beccles, containing 369 inhabitants. The livings united form a discharged rectory with Winston and Windale, in the archdeaconry of Norfolk, and diocese of Norwich, rated jointly in the king's books at £10. 6. 8. Wolf Lewis, Esq. was patron in 1797. The church, dedicated to St. Mary, is principally of Norman architecture; that of All Saints was demolished in 1748, but the ruined tower still remains, and, being overgrown with ivy, presents a venerable and interesting appearance.

GILLMONBY, a township in the parish of BOWES, western division of the wapentake of GILLING, North riding of the county of YORK, 5 miles (S. W. by W.) from Barnard-Castle, containing 175 inhabitants.

GILLMORTON, a parish in the hundred of GUTHLAXTON, county of LEICESTER, 3 miles (N. E. by N.) from Lutterworth, containing 718 inhabitants. The living is a rectory, in the archdeaconry of Leicester, and diocese of Lincoln, rated in the king's books at £17. 14. 9½. The Rev. D. J. Burdett was patron in 1809. The church is dedicated to All Saints.

GILSTONE, a parish in the hundred of BRAUGHIN, county of HERTFORD, 3½ miles (W. by S.) from Sawbridgeworth, containing 213 inhabitants. The living is a rectory, in the archdeaconry of Middlesex, and diocese of London, rated in the king's books at £10. 3. 4., and in the patronage of the Bishop of London. The church has a quadrangular western tower, embattled and surmounted by a spire. There are an endowed almshouse, and a trifling rent-charge towards the support of a school for girls.

GIMINGHAM, a parish in the northern division of the hundred of ERPINGHAM, county of NORFOLK, 4 miles (N.) from North Walsham, containing 300 inhabitants. The living is a rectory with that of Trunch, in the archdeaconry of Norfolk, and diocese of Norwich, rated in the king's books at £11. 11. 10½., and in the patronage of the Master and Fellows of Catherine Hall, Cambridge. The church is dedicated to All Saints.

GINGE (WEST), a tything in the parish of LOCKINGE, hundred of WANTAGE, county of BERKS. The population is returned with the parish.

GIPPING, a chapelry in the hundred of STOW, county of SUFFOLK, 4 miles (N.N.E.) from Stow-Market, containing, with the hamlet of Stow-Market, 107 inhabitants. The living is a donative, endowed with ten acres of land here, and a farm of about one hundred acres, in the parish of Earl Stonham, and in the patronage of C. Tyrrell, Esq. The chapel is said to have been built in the fifteenth century, by Sir James Tyrrell, Knight. The river Gipping runs through the chapelry, a small stream, but enlarging considerably in its course to Ipswich, gives name to that port, which was called originally Gippovicus, the town on the Gipping, and corrupted gradually into Gippwich and Ipswich.

GIRSBY, a township in that part of the parish of SOCKBURN which is in the wapentake of ALLERTONSHIRE, North riding of the county of YORK, 6½ miles (S. W. by W.) from Yarm, containing 85 inhabitants. It is separated from the rest of the parish by the river Tees, which bounds it on the north.

GIRTON, a parish in the hundred of NORTH STOW, county of CAMBRIDGE, 3 miles (N. N. W.) from Cambridge, containing 326 inhabitants. The living is a rectory, in the archdeaconry and diocese of Ely, rated in the king's books at £18. 4. 4½. Sir S. V. Cotton, Bart. was patron in 1807. The church is dedicated to St. Andrew : its tower is in the later style of English architecture.

GIRTON, a parish in the northern division of the hundred of NEWARK, county of NOTTINGHAM, 8 miles (S. E. by E.) from Tuxford, containing, with Mering, which is deemed extra-parochial, 189 inhabitants. The living is a perpetual curacy, in the archdeaconry of Nottingham, and diocese of York.

GISBURN, a parish in the western division of the wapentake of STAINCLIFFE and EWCROSS, West riding of the county of YORK, comprising the townships of Gisburn, Gisburn-Forest, Horton, Middop, Nappa, Newsholme, Paythorne, Rimmington, and Swinden, and containing 2530 inhabitants, of which number, 690 are in the township of Gisburn, 10½ miles (W. by S.) from Skipton. The town is situated in a fertile plain, near the eastern bank of the river Ribble, and at a short distance from the borders of Lancashire. A market, which was formerly held here on Mondays, has been discontinued ; but there is a market or fair for cattle every alternate Monday throughout the year, and fairs annually on Easter Monday and the 18th and 19th of September. In the township of Rimmington is a vein of lead-ore which contains a considerable portion of silver. A court leet for the manor is held annually in May, and another in November, at one of which a constable is appointed for the township. The living is a vicarage, in the archdeaconry and diocese of York, rated in the king's books at £11. 6. 8., endowed with £200 parliamentary grant, and in the patronage of the Crown. The church, dedicated to St. Mary, is a neat edifice, including a nave, aisles, and a chancel, with a square tower, in the later style of English architecture; the windows are ornamented with stained glass. Here is a school with a small endowment for the education of seven poor children. On an eminence near the Ribble is a square fort, called Castle Haugh, and near it a barrow, in which was found a coarse earthen urn, indicating a burial-place of the ancient Britons.

GISBURN-FOREST, a township in the parish of GISBURN, western division of the wapentake of STAIN-CLIFFE and EWCROSS, West riding of the county of YORK, 8 miles (S.) from Settle, containing 457 inhabitants.

GISLEHAM, a parish in the hundred of MUTFORD and LOTHINGLAND, county of SUFFOLK, 4½ miles (S. W. by S.) from Lowestoft, containing 222 inhabitants. The living is a discharged rectory, in the archdeaconry of Suffolk, and diocese of Norwich, rated in the king's books at £13. 6. 8., and in the patronage of the Crown. The church is dedicated to the Holy Trinity. The parish is bounded on the east by the North sea.

GISLINGHAM, a parish in the hundred of HARTISMERE, county of SUFFOLK, 5 miles (W. by S.) from Eye, containing 620 inhabitants. The living is a rectory, in the archdeaconry of Sudbury, and diocese of Norwich, rated in the king's books at £26. 1. 5½. Nath. Collyer, Esq. was patron in 1797. The church is dedicated to St. Mary. There is a place of worship for Wesleyan Methodists.

GISSING, a parish in the hundred of DISS, county

of NORFOLK, 4¼ miles (N. N. E.) from Diss, containing 544 inhabitants. The living is a rectory, in the archdeaconry of Norfolk, and diocese of Norwich, rated in the king's books at £14. 16. 5½. The Rev. Sir W. R. Kempe, Bart. was patron in 1816. The church, dedicated to St. Mary, has a low round tower at the west end. There is a place of worship for Wesleyan Methodists.

GITTISHAM, a parish in the eastern division of the hundred of BUDLEIGH, county of DEVON, 2¾ miles (S. W. by W.) from Honiton, containing 351 inhabitants. The living is a rectory, in the archdeaconry and diocese of Exeter, rated in the king's books at £21. 8. 11½., and in the patronage of the Rev. T. Putt. Sir Thomas Putt, in 1686, founded a charity school, and endowed it with a rent-charge of £10 a year for teaching twenty children.

GIVENDALE, a township in that part of the parish of RIPON which is within the liberty of RIPON, though locally in the wapentake of Claro, West riding of the county of YORK, 2 miles (S. E.) from Ripon, containing 31 inhabitants.

GIVENDALE, or GWENDALE (GREAT), a parish in the Wilton-Beacon division of the wapentake of HARTHILL, East riding of the county of YORK, comprising the townships of Great Givendale and Grimthorpe, and containing 89 inhabitants, of which number, 60 are in the township of Great Givendale, which is partly within the liberty of St. Peter of York, 3½ miles (N. by E.) from Pocklington. The living is a discharged vicarage, in the peculiar jurisdiction and patronage of the Dean of York, rated in the king's books at £4. 18. 4., endowed with £700 private benefaction, and £400 royal bounty.

GLAISDALE, a parish in the eastern division of the liberty of LANGBAURGH, North riding of the county of YORK, 10 miles (W. S. W.) from Whitby, containing 1043 inhabitants. The living is a perpetual curacy, in the archdeaconry of Cleveland, and diocese of York, endowed with £200 private benefaction, £400 royal bounty, and £1500 parliamentary grant, and in the patronage of the Archbishop of York. The church was built in 1793, upon the site of a more ancient edifice, consecrated in 1388. A place of worship for Wesleyan Methodists was erected by subscription in 1821. Samuel Prudom, in 1741, and John Brodrick, in 1758, gave £2 per annum each, for which eight boys are instructed.

GLANDFORD, a parish in the hundred of HOLT, county of NORFOLK, 1½ mile (S. by W.) from Clay, containing, with the parish of Bayfield, 93 inhabitants. The living is a perpetual curacy annexed to the rectories of Blakeney and Cockthorpe, in the archdeaconry and diocese of Norwich. The church is dedicated to St. Martin.

GLANDFORD-BRIGG, or BRIDGE, a market town and chapelry in the parish of WRAWBY, southern division of the wapentake of YARBOROUGH, parts of LINDSEY, county of LINCOLN, 24 miles (N. by E.) from Lincoln, and 153 (N. by W.) from London, containing 1674 inhabitants. This place was originally only a small fishing hamlet; it is now a well built town, enjoying a plentiful supply of water from the river Ancholme, a branch of which runs through it, another passing at the distance of a quarter of a mile westward. The bridge has lately been taken down, and a new one is now being erected. A considerable trade n corn, coal, and timber, is carried on; and here are several fur manufactories, besides tanneries and fellmongers' establishments; and it is asserted, that more persons are employed here in dressing rabbit-skins than in any other provincial town in the kingdom. A great improvement has been made by draining the Ancholme level, the expense attending which is defrayed by a tax on land, and a duty on the tonnage of the river. The market is on Thursday, and a fair is held on the 5th of August. The petty sessions are held here once a fortnight; and the town is within the jurisdiction of a court of requests for the recovery of debts under £5, held at Alford every month, under an act passed in the 47th of George III. The chapel, dedicated to St. Mary, was erected in 1699, at the joint expense of four gentlemen, who endowed it with certain estates vested in their respective heirs, and the trustees of the free school. The Society of Friends, Independents, and Primitive and Wesleyan Methodists, have each a place of worship; and there is a chapel for the Roman Catholics. The free grammar school was founded in 1669, pursuant to the will of Sir John Nelthorpe, Bart., who endowed it with certain lands vested in trustees for that purpose. Boys born in the town of Brigg, and in all other parishes where the founder possessed estates, are entitled to gratuitous instruction in the Latin and Greek languages; and all other boys, wheresoever born, were to be taught reading, writing, and accounts, free of expense, by a master and an usher, for each of whom the founder desired that a house should be erected: the number of scholars is limited to eighty. In the reign of John, a hospital was founded here by Adam Paynel, which was a cell to the abbey of Selby in Yorkshire; but all traces of it have disappeared.

GLANTLEES, a joint township with Greens, in that part of the parish of FELTON which is in the eastern division of COQUETDALE ward, county of NORTHUMBERLAND, 7½ miles (S. S.W.) from Alnwick, containing 76 inhabitants.

GLANTON, a township in the parish of WHITTINGHAM, northern division of COQUETDALE ward, county of NORTHUMBERLAND, 9¼ miles (W.) from Alnwick, containing 474 inhabitants. There is a place of worship for Presbyterians; and the township has recently been much improved by the erection of several handsome houses. On a lofty eminence called Glanton Pike was formerly a beacon. Several stone coffins, and urns containing pieces of charcoal and burnt bones, were discovered about 1716; also weapons which evidently belonged to the Britons. There is a petrifying well, at the bottom of which shell marl is found.

GLAPTHORN, a parish in the hundred of WILLYBROOK, county of NORTHAMPTON, 1½ mile (N. W. by N.) from Oundle, containing 354 inhabitants. The living is a discharged vicarage, united with that of Cotterstock, in the archdeaconry of Northampton, and diocese of Peterborough. The church is dedicated to St. Leonard.

GLAPWELL, a township partly in the parish of BOLSOVER, hundred of SCARSDALE, county of DERBY, 5¼ miles (N.W.) from Mansfield, containing 110 inhabitants. Here was formerly a chapel, which in 1240 belonged to Darley abbey, but of which no later account exists than in 1511.

GLASCOED, a hamlet in that part of the parish of

Usk which is in the lower division of the hundred of Usk, county of MONMOUTH, 3¾ miles (S. W. by W.) from Usk, containing 201 inhabitants. There is a place of worship for Baptists.

GLASCOTE, a joint township with Bolehall, in that part of the parish of TAMWORTH which is in the Tamworth division of the hundred of HEMLINGFORD, county of WARWICK, 1½ mile (S.E.) from Tamworth, containing 414 inhabitants.

GLASS-HOUSE-YARD, a liberty in the Finsbury division of the hundred of OSSULSTONE, county of MIDDLESEX, containing 1358 inhabitants.

GLASSONBY, a township in the parish of ADDINGHAM, LEATH ward, county of CUMBERLAND, 8 miles (N. E. by N.) from Penrith, containing 153 inhabitants.

GLASTON, a township in the parish of ALDINGHAM, hundred of LONSDALE, north of the sands, county palatine of LANCASTER, 3 miles (S.E.) from Dalton. The population is returned with the parish. Glaston may be termed the modern port of Lancaster; it is situated on the river Lune, and has a spacious dock opened in 1787, and capable of receiving twenty-five large merchant vessels, the cargoes of which are discharged here and forwarded by smaller craft to Lancaster. A canal passes from the dock and forms a junction with the Preston and Lancaster canal.

GLASTON, a parish in the hundred of WRANDIKE, county of RUTLAND, 2 miles (E.N.E.) from Uppingham, containing 188 inhabitants. The living is a rectory, in the archdeaconry of Northampton, and diocese of Peterborough, rated in the king's books at £12. 16. 10½., and annexed to the Mastership of Peter House, Cambridge. The church is dedicated to St. Andrew. William Roberts, in 1725, gave £100 for the education of ten children, the interest of which is applied to that purpose.

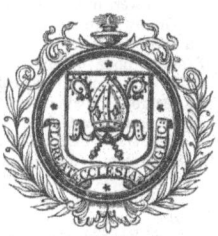

Seal.

GLASTONBURY, a market town having separate jurisdiction, locally in the hundred of Glaston-Twelve-Hides, county of SOMERSET, 7½ miles (N. by E.) from Somerton, and 124 (W. by S.) from London, containing 2630 inhabitants. This place, which is of very great antiquity, is situated in a marshy tract, called by the Britons *Avalon*, from its abounding with apples; and *Ynys-wytryn*, or the glassy island: by the Saxons it was named *Glastn-ey*, a term of similar signification, and after the erection of its monastery, which formed a small town, it was called *Glastn-a-byrig*, from which its present name is immediately deduced. That it is a place of very remote antiquity is certain, but its origin is involved in so much obscurity, that it is difficult to separate its authentic from its legendary history. It is chiefly distinguished for its celebrated abbey, said to have been originally founded by Joseph of Arimathea, whom Philip, the Apostle of Gaul, sent to preach the gospel in Britain, and who, having arrived in this island, rested with his companions on a small eminence, half a mile to the south-west of the present town, still called Weary-all hill, and established here the first society of Christian worshippers in Britain. In the most ancient charters of the monastery, Glastonbury is styled "The fountain and origin of all religion in the realm of Britain." When the church erected by Joseph had fallen into decay, Devi, Bishop of St. David's, rebuilt it on the same spot, and on its subsequent decay, it was restored by twelve persons from the northern parts of England. St. Patrick, who came from Ireland about 439, is said to have spent thirty years of his life in this convent, and to have formed the brethren, who previously lived in huts scattered round the church, into a regular community, restoring also the primitive form of Christianity, which after the death of Lucius, the first Christian king of Britain, had fallen into disuse. About the year 530, David, Archbishop of Menevia, with seven of his suffragans, retired to this place, and greatly improved the church, to the east end of which he added a chapel, dedicated to the Holy Virgin, and enriched the altar with a sapphire of inestimable value. The celebrated King Arthur, after the fatal battle with his nephew Mordred, was interred in this isle : his remains are said to have been discovered in the reign of Henry II., who ordering a search to be made, a leaden cross was found, with a Latin inscription in the rude characters of that age, to this effect, " Here lies the famous King Arthur, buried in the Isle of Avalon." Beneath was observed a coffin-like excavation in the solid rock, containing the bones of a human body, supposed to be those of Arthur, which were then deposited in the church, and covered with a sumptuous monument. St. Augustine, on his arrival in Britain, visited Glastonbury, and attempted to introduce into the abbey the rules of the order of St. Benedict, but the measure was not attended with success. The monastery, during the Heptarchy, had been much favoured by successive monarchs, and in 708, Ina, King of the West Saxons, took down the conventual buildings, which were greatly dilapidated, and rebuilt the abbey from its foundation in a style of superior splendour. In 942, Dunstan, who was appointed abbot by King Edred, and to him that monarch gave the unlimited command of his treasury for the improvement of the monastery; he enlarged the conventual buildings in a style of unrivalled magnificence, and in a short time completed an establishment, which, under his superintendence, became the " pride of England, and the glory of Christendom, " furnishing superiors to all the religious houses in the kingdom. Edgar, who had a palace within two miles of the town, in a romantic situation, at a place still called " Edgarley," now a hamlet in the parish of St. John, endowed the abbey with several estates, and invested the monks with extensive privileges. The abbots were sovereigns within the Isle of Avalon, into which neither the king nor any of the bishops could enter without their permission; they sat among the barons in parliament, and enjoyed a revenue superior to that of most monasteries in the kingdom. Of the palace of Edgar there are no other vestiges than two wolves' heads and a pelican, placed in the front of a modern house; the former conveying a direct allusion to the tax imposed by him on the Welch princes, for the extirpation of wolves within the realm. At the time of the Conquest, William, not content with curtailing the power of the abbots, and with exacting tribute from the monastery, deprived them of their privileges, and

seized on their possessions; he imposed on the monks an abbot of his own nomination, whose tyranny ultimately compelled him to retire into Normandy. Under his successor, the abbey recovered many of the estates of which it had been deprived; and during the abbacy of Henry de Blois, brother of King Stephen, whose liberality and prudence equally promoted the interest of the monks, and the cultivation of literature among them, it regained the greater part of its confiscated wealth, and retrieved its prior fame and importance. A considerable portion of the abbey having been destroyed by fire in 1184, it was restored by Henry II., who granted the abbots a charter, confirming all the privileges which had been obtained from his predecessors; but its internal tranquillity was greatly interrupted by the violent contentions between the monks and the bishop of Wells, with respect to the nomination of the abbots, which continued, with trifling intermissions, until the Reformation. In 1276, the abbey was much injured by the shock of an earthquake, which threw down the church of St. Michael on the Torr Hill. The strict discipline prevailing in the establishment for a time delayed its preconcerted fate; but, in 1539, its venerable abbot, Whytyng, refusing to surrender to the commissioners of Henry VIII., was arraigned and condemned for high treason, and, with two of his monks, being drawn on a sledge to Torr Hill, was hanged and quartered; his head was placed over the entrance to the abbey, and his members were exposed at Bath, Bridg-water, Wells, and Ilchester. At the dissolution of this celebrated monastery, which had flourished from the earliest introduction of Christianity into Britain, the revenue was £3508. 13. 4¾. The abbey and its dependencies comprehended a space of nearly sixty acres : the ruins consist chiefly of the chapel of St. Joseph, and fragments of the conventual church: the prevailing character of the chapel is Norman, but the details and enrichment, which are in good preservation, are in the early style of English architecture. The remains of the church are of a less embellished character, but exhibit much of the pure simplicity of the early English style, with some portions of a later date. The abbot's kitchen is the most entire, and is probably of more recent erection than the other buildings: it is of an octagonal form, having four fire-places; the roof is finely vaulted, and from the centre rises an octagonal pyramid, crowned with a double lantern, of curious design: the ruins are richly overspread with ivy, and present a striking memorial of departed grandeur.

The town stands on the declivity of a considerable eminence nearly in the centre of the county, and consists of a spacious street forming the principal thoroughfare, intersected nearly at right angles by another of smaller extent : the houses are in general low, but there are several of more recent erection and of more respectable appearance; and many houses in different parts of the town have been built entirely of stone taken from the ruins of the abbey. The George Inn was anciently appropriated by the abbots as a place of entertainment for pilgrims visiting the shrine of St. Dunstan, and still retains much of its original character and decoration : the old manor-house and tribunal of justice are interesting relics; and a beautiful modern building, harmonising in its style of architecture with the venerable remains by which it is surrounded, has been erected by the present proprietor of the abbey land. The town is well-paved and lighted by act of parliament, and supplied with water from a fine spring issuing from the ridge of a hill, three quarters of a mile distant, and collected in an ancient reservoir of stone, whence it is conveyed by pipes into the town. The principal branches of manufacture are those of stockings and a coarse sort of gloves, which have superseded the woollen manufacture formerly carried on here, and at present afford employment to several hundred persons in the town and neighbourhood. It is in contemplation to form a communication between this town and Bridg-water, by means of a canal from the river Parret, at Boroughbridge. The market days were formerly Tuesday and Saturday, the former has been discontinued, and the latter is now only for butchers' meat: the fairs are on the Wednesday in Easter-week, September 19th, called the Torr fair, principally for horses, October 10th, and the Monday week after St. Andrew's day. The government, by charter of Queen Anne, is vested in a mayor, recorder, seven superior, and sixteen inferior, burgesses, assisted by a town clerk, two coroners, and subordinate officers. The mayor, who is chosen annually from the superior burgesses, the recorder, who must be a barrister of three years standing, and the late mayor, are justices of the peace within the borough. The corporation hold quarterly courts of session for the trial of all offenders within the borough; and a court leet for the hundred is held in the town.

Glastonbury comprises the parishes of St. Benedict and St. John the Baptist, and gives name to a peculiar jurisdiction which extends over several parishes. The living of St. Benedict's is a donative annexed to the perpetual curacy of St. John's, jointly endowed with £800 private benefaction, £400 royal bounty, and £600 parliamentary grant, and in the peculiar jurisdiction and patronage of the Bishop of Bath and Wells. The churchwardens of St. John's are a body corporate with a common seal, and have estates producing at present about £500 per annum, of which part was granted in the year 1300. The churches are both interesting structures in the later style of English architecture, with towers of very graceful and highly enriched character, of which the former has open turrets and battlements, and more decoration than the latter, which is notwithstanding a fine composition. There are places of worship for Baptists, the Society of Friends, Wesleyan Methodists, and Independents, which last has an endowment of £80 per annum. A National school, in which thirty boys are instructed, is supported partly by subscription, and partly by an appropriation of £20 per annum, arising from property bequeathed by James Levinston, in 1666, for charitable uses. A rent-charge of £4, left by the Earl of Godolphin, is paid to a school-mistress for teaching ten children; and £5 per annum, arising from two turnpike deeds assigned by Mrs. Honora Gould, is paid for teaching twelve female children to read and sew. The Upper and Lower almshouses were founded by the abbots of the monastery, and since the dissolution have been supported by an annual grant from the crown; the former, which is in a greatly dilapidated state, is inhabited by ten aged men, and the latter, which has been lately rebuilt by a grant from the crown, is inhabited by ten aged women; attached to each is a small chapel, and in the hall of each, one additional tenant is allowed to reside in expectation of the first vacancy. On the summit of Torr Hill, at a short distance from the town, is the tower of St. Michael, the only part remaining of a splendid church and monastery, erected on the site of a former one which was destroyed by an earthquake in 1276; over the west entrance is a sculptured figure of St. Michael, holding in his hand a pair of scales, in one of which is the bible, and in the other the devil, aided by an imp in a fruitless effort to outweigh the sacred volume. Weary-all hill, the spot where Joseph of Arimathea and his disciples are stated to have rested after their pilgrimage, is connected with a legendary account of the origin of a species of thorn, called the Glastonbury thorn: on this hill, the legend relates, Joseph struck his staff into the ground, which immediately taking root, grew up into a flourishing tree, producing in succeeding ages what was called the holy thorn, there being still some trees of that species in the neighbourhood. Equally absurd with this is a variety of other legendary tales which have been interwoven into the history of this place. Some chalybeate springs were discovered here, which about the middle of the last century were numerously attended by invalids from Bath, Bristol, and other parts of the country, and such was the repute of their medicinal properties, that the water was sent in bottles to London. A great variety of organic remains consisting chiefly of *nautili, cornua ammonis*, bivalves, &c., have been found imbedded in the quarries near Torr Hill. Henry Fielding, the celebrated novelist, was a native of Sharpham park, in this parish; and among the many illustrious personages who have been interred here, are several of the Saxon kings, together with a numerous train of noblemen, bishops, abbots, and priors. Glastonbury formerly conferred the title of baron on the family of Greville, which became extinct on the death of the late lord without issue.

GLATTON, a parish in the hundred of Norman-Cross, county of Huntingdon, 2¼ miles (S. S. W.) from Stilton, containing 358 inhabitants. The living is a rectory, in the archdeaconry of Huntingdon, and diocese of Lincoln, rated in the king's books at £21. 8. 11½. The Rev. J. Hopkinson was patron in 1778. The church is dedicated to St. Nicholas.

GLAZELEY, a parish in the hundred of Stottesden, county of Salop, 3½ miles (S. by W.) from Bridgenorth, containing 46 inhabitants. The living is a discharged rectory, consolidated, together with that of Deuxhill, in 1760, with the rectory of Chetton, in the archdeaconry of Salop, and diocese of Hereford.

GLEMHAM (GREAT), a parish in the hundred of Plomesgate, county of Suffolk, 4½ miles (W. S. W.) from Saxmundham, containing 413 inhabitants. The living is a perpetual curacy, with the rectory of Little Glemham, in the archdeaconry of Suffolk, and diocese of Norwich, endowed with £200 private benefaction, and £200 royal bounty. The church is dedicated to All Saints.

GLEMHAM (LITTLE), a parish in the hundred of Plomesgate, county of Suffolk, 3 miles (N. E. by E.) from Wickham-Market, containing 349 inhabitants. The living is a rectory, with the perpetual curacy of Great Glemham, in the archdeaconry of Suffolk, and diocese of Norwich, rated in the king's books at £6.

Dudley Long North, Esq. was patron in 1826. The church is dedicated to St. Andrew.

GLEMSFORD, a parish in the hundred of BABERGH, county of SUFFOLK, 4¼ miles (E. N. E.) from Clare, containing 1275 inhabitants. The living is a rectory, in the archdeaconry of Sudbury, and diocese of Norwich, rated in the king's books at £30, and in the patronage of the Bishop of Ely. The church' is dedicated to St. Mary. In the time of Edward the Confessor a collegiate society of priests, under the government of a dean, was established here, and invested with several privileges, which were confirmed to them by Henry III.

GLEN (MAGNA), a parish in the hundred of GARTREE, county of LEICESTER, 6 miles (S. E.) from Leicester, containing, with the chapelry of Great Stretton, 714 inhabitants. The living is a vicarage, in the archdeaconry and diocese of Lincoln, rated in the king's books at £12. 14. 2. Sir G. Robinson, Bart. was patron in 1814. The church is dedicated to St. Cuthbert. The Leicester Union canal passes through the parish.

GLEN (PARVA), a chapelry in that part of the parish of AYLESTONE which is in the hundred of GUTHLAXTON, county of LEICESTER, 4¼ miles (S. by W.) from Leicester, containing 128 inhabitants.

GLENDON, a parish in the hundred of ROTHWELL, county of NORTHAMPTON, 3 miles (N. W. by N.) from Kettering, containing 37 inhabitants. The living is a rectory, in the archdeaconry of Northampton, and diocese of Peterborough, rated in the king's books at £8, endowed with £1200 royal bounty. Mrs. Booth was patroness in 1814. The church is dedicated to St. Helen.

GLENFIELD, a parish in the hundred of SPARKENHOE, county of LEICESTER, 3½ miles (W. N. W.) from Leicester, comprising the chapelries of Braunstone and Kirby-Muxloe, and the liberties of Braunstone-Frith, Glenfield-Frith, and Kirby-Frith, and containing 932 inhabitants. The living, is a rectory, is (exclusively of its chapelries) in the peculiar jurisdiction of the Lord of the Manor of Grosby, and in the patronage of the Trustees of the late Clement Winstanley, Esq., rated in the king's books at £13. 9. 9½. The church is dedicated to St. Peter. There is a place of worship for Wesleyan Methodists.

GLENFIELD-FRITH, a liberty in the parish of GLENFIELD, hundred of SPARKENHOE, county of LEICESTER, 4 miles (W. by N.) from Leicester, containing 4 inhabitants.

GLENTHAM, a parish in the eastern division of the wapentake of ASLACOE, parts of LINDSEY, county of LINCOLN, 8 miles (W. by N.) from Market-Raisen, containing 372 inhabitants. The living is a discharged vicarage, in the peculiar jurisdiction and patronage of the Dean and Chapter of Lincoln, rated in the king's books at £8. The church is dedicated to St. Peter; the tower and chancel are of more modern erection than the rest of the building, which is in the later style of English architecture. Here is a place of worship for Wesleyan Methodists; also an endowed almshouse. The river Ancholme runs through the parish.

GLENTWORTH, a parish in the western division of the wapentake of ASLACOE, parts of LINDSEY, county of LINCOLN, 11½ miles (N. by W.) from Lincoln, containing 275 inhabitants. The living is a discharged

vicarage, with the curacy of Spittal on the Street, in the archdeaconry of Stow, and diocese of Lincoln, rated in the king's books at £7. 17. 6. The Earl of Scarborough was patron in 1802. The church, dedicated to St. Michael, contains a sumptuous monument to the memory of Sir Christopher Wray, Knt., Lord Chief Justice in the reign of Elizabeth. Near the church is an almshouse for three poor women.

GLIDDEN, a tything in the parish and hundred of HAMBLEDON, Portsdown division of the county of SOUTHAMPTON, 8 miles (S. W.) from Petersfield. The population is returned with the parish. It is within the jurisdiction of the Cheyney Court held at Winchester every Thursday, for the recovery of debts to any amount.

GLINTON, a parish in the liberty of PETERBOROUGH, county of NORTHAMPTON, 3 miles (S. S. E.) from Market-Deeping, containing 372 inhabitants. The living is a perpetual curacy, with the rectory of Peakirk, in the archdeaconry of Northampton, and diocese of Peterborough. The church, dedicated to St. Benedict, has a tower and spire mostly in the later style of English architecture.

GLOOSTON, a parish in the hundred of GARTREE, county of LEICESTER, 5¾ miles (N. by E.) from Market-Harborough, containing 142 inhabitants. The living is a rectory, in the archdeaconry of Leicester, and diocese of Lincoln, rated in the king's books at £8. The Earl of Cardigan was patron in 1802. The church is dedicated to St. John.

GLORORUM, a township in the parish of BAMBROUGH, northern division of BAMBROUGH ward, county of NORTHUMBERLAND, 4¾ miles (E.) from Belford, containing 46 inhabitants.

GLOSSOP, a parish in the hundred of HIGH PEAK, county of DERBY, comprising the chapelries of Charlesworth, Chinley-Bugsworth with Brownside, and Mellor; the townships of Chunat, Dinting, Glossop, Great-Hamlet, Hadfield, Ludworth with Chisworth, Padfield, Simondsley, and Whitfield; the hamlets of Beard, Kinder, Olerset, Thornsett, and Whittle; and the liberty of Phoside, and containing 13,766 inhabitants, of which number, 1351 are in the township of Glossop, 10 miles (N.) from Chapel en le Frith. The living is a discharged vicarage, in the archdeaconry of Derby, and diocese of Lichfield, rated in the king's books at £12. 18. 9., endowed with £400 parliamentary grant, and in the patronage of the Duke of Norfolk. The church, dedicated to All Saints, has lately received an addition of two hundred and eighty sittings, of which one hundred and forty are free, the Incorporated Society for the enlargement of churches and chapels having granted £200 towards defraying the expense. There are several places of worship for Independents and Wesleyan Methodists within the limits of this extensive parish, the population of which has more than doubled during the last fifty years, owing to the great increase of its manufactures. There are about fifty cotton-mills, five extensive establishments for calico-printing, two clothing-mills, a manufactory for cloth, and another for brown paper. A fair for cattle, and wooden and tin ware, is held on the 6th of May, in the township of Glossop. A school, wherein about forty children are taught, is supported by a small endowment, the origin of which is unknown, and by an annual donation from the Duke of Norfolk. Glossop is

2 G 2

in the honour of Tutbury, duchy of Lancaster, and within the jurisdiction of a court of pleas held at Tutbury every third Tuesday, for the recovery of debts under 40s. On the south side of the Mersey, near Woolley Bridge, are vestiges of a Roman station, in dimensions one hundred and twenty-two yards by one hundred and twelve, called Melandra Castle; the moat towards the south-east, the four entrances, the ramparts, about nine feet in thickness, and the site of the prætorium, twenty-five yards square, are still discernible, as is the old Roman road from Brough to this place, and that to Buxton.

GLOSTERHILL, a township in that part of the parish of WARKWORTH which is in the eastern division of MORPETH ward, county of NORTHUMBERLAND, 8½ miles (S.E.) from Alnwick, containing 31 inhabitants. It is situated on the southern bank of the Coquet, near its confluence with the North sea.

Arms.

GLOUCESTER, a city, inland port, and county of itself, locally in the hundred of Dudstone and King's Barton, county of GLOUCESTER, 34 miles (N.N.E.) from Bristol, and 107 (W.N.W.) from London, on the road to South Wales, containing 9744 inhabitants. This was a town of considerable importance prior to the Roman invasion: its origin is generally ascribed to the Dobuni, a tribe of Britons who settled in this part of the country; and, either from its founder, Glowi, a native chief, or, with greater probability, from its eminence, obtained the appellation of *Caer Glou*, British words implying, according to the former supposition, the city of Glowi, or according to the latter, the fair city. Richard of Cirencester relates that this British fortress was taken in the year 47 by the Romans, who established here a colony, which he styles *Glebon*; and in the Itinerary of Antoninus, as well as other ancient writings, it is denominated *Glevum Colonia*. Its situation on the Ryknield Street, which was both a British and a Roman road here passing over the Severn, rendered it a station of importance. The exact site of the Roman station is supposed to have been a tract of land, now in tillage, to the north-east of the present city, called King's Holme, near which was a palace belonging to the Anglo-Saxon kings of Mercia, in old deeds named *Regia Domus*: on this spot have been found Roman coins, urns, and sacrificing utensils. Tradition relates that Lucius, the first Christian king of Britain, founded a bishop's see at Gloucester, in the second century, and that he was buried in the church of St. Mary de Lode, in this city. After the departure of the Romans, this place is said to have been governed by Eldol, a British chief, who was present at the massacre of the Britons by the Saxons at Stonehenge; and who, according to some writers, escaped from the carnage, and afterwards killed Hengist, the Saxon leader, at the battle of Maeshill, in Yorkshire, in 489. Gloucester having been captured by the Saxons in 577, was by them called *Gleau-ceasters*, from which its present name is derived; it first belonged to the kingdom of Wessex, and was afterwards annexed to that of Mercia. About 679, the city was considerably enlarged by Wulfhere,

King of Mercia, who founded here a priory dedicated to St. Oswald, and afterwards erected the abbey. Edgar, in a charter to the monks of Worcester, dated at Gloucester, in 964, styles this a "royal city." It was repeatedly plundered by the Danes; by whom, in the reign of Ethelred II., it was taken, and nearly destroyed by fire. The injury it suffered was, however, soon repaired; and Edmund Ironside having here taken up his quarters, after his defeat by Canute at Assandune, challenged that prince to decide their mutual claim to the kingdom by single combat, which took place in the Isle of Alney, on the south-western side of the city. Edward the Confessor often resided here in regal splendour, as also did William I. (who erected the castle on the bank of the Severn), William II., and others of his successors. According to Camden, a mint was established here in the reign of John, on whose death, in 1216, his son, Henry III., was crowned in the abbey church, by the Bishop of Winchester, in the presence of the pope's legate. This king, in 1263, having appointed Sir Maci de Besile, a Frenchman, sheriff for Gloucestershire, and constable of Gloucester castle, the citizens, and the nobility of the county, taking umbrage at the promotion of a foreigner, chose for their governor Sir William de Tracy, who, proceeding to hold a county court, was arrested by de Besile, and imprisoned in the castle. The discontented nobles then besieged and captured that fortress, which they held for some time; but at length surrendered it to Prince Edward, afterwards Edward I., who in 1279 held a parliament here, in which various laws were enacted, called "the Statutes of Gloucester." Another parliament was held at this place by Richard II. in 1378; others by Henry IV. in 1403 and 1407; and finally a parliament was summoned here by Henry V., in 1420, which, at the expiration of fourteen days, was adjourned to Westminster. When hostilities took place between Charles I. and the parliament, the citizens declared in favour of the latter; and having procured cannon, and repaired and strengthened their fortifications, with the assistance of a few regular troops under the government of Colonel Massie, they resolved to defend themselves against all opposition. In the middle of February, 1642, Lord Herbert, son of the Marquis of Worcester, besieged the city at the head of two thousand Welch royalists; and after remaining before it five weeks, surrendered himself and his followers, on the approach of an army under Sir William Waller to relieve the place. The governor took advantage of the opportunity afforded by this triumph of his party, to obtain fresh supplies of ammunition and provisions, and to prepare for another assault. On the 10th of August, 1643, the king, with a large and well appointed body of forces, laid siege to Gloucester; but his reiterated attacks were repulsed by the garrison with the utmost vigour and resolution; and after a siege of twenty-six days, and the loss of one thousand men, he was induced to retreat, on the advance of the Earl of Essex, who had marched from London to relieve the city. Previously to this siege, there were eleven parish churches in Gloucester, six of which were destroyed, together with the suburbs of the city, by order of the governor, to obstruct the approach of the enemy. The conduct of the citizens on this occasion was not forgotten at the restoration of Charles II., by whose order their walls were razed, and their fortifications destroyed, in 1662: that monarch also deprived them of their charter, but subsequently granted them a new one. In 1687, James II. visited Gloucester, in one of his progresses through the kingdom, and lodged at the deanery, where many resorted to him to be touched for the king's evil. George III., the queen, and the princesses, visited Gloucester on their route from Cheltenham in 1788, and in 1807 his late Majesty, George IV., then Prince of Wales, dined with the corporation, and received the freedom of the city.

Gloucester is pleasantly situated in a fertile vale, on the eastern bank of the river Severn, and consists principally of four spacious streets diverging at right angles from the centre of the town towards the cardinal points, and originally terminated by the East, North, South, and West gates, from which they respectively took their names. At the point of intersection was an elegant cross, surrounded by four churches, of which only one is now remaining. The West gate, on the western bank of the river, was standing till the recent erection of the new bridge, many years previously to which the other gates had been removed. This bridge is a handsome structure of stone, consisting of one arch eighty-seven feet in the span, with a plain parapet and cornice; the approaches on both sides are defended by iron palisades: from it a causeway, half a mile in length, extends across the Isle of Alney to Over, where is a noble bridge of one arch, in the construction of which the segments of a circle and an ellipsis have been combined. The streets are well paved, and lighted with gas, by a company incorporated in 1820; the houses are in general handsome and well built, and the inhabitants are amply supplied with water from the Severn, and with spring water from a reservoir at the distance of two miles and a half from the city, conveyed into their houses by pipes. The approaches are ornamented with ranges of modern substantial houses, and the entrance from Cheltenham displays many mansions in detached situations, suited for the residence of families of opulence and distinction. A horticultural society, and a permanent subscription library, have been established, and a society for the cultivation of natural history was formed in 1829. Triennial musical festivals of the united choirs of Gloucester, Worcester, and Hereford, are celebrated here, at which oratorios and selections of sacred music are performed in the cathedral, and miscellaneous concerts and balls are held in the spacious room at the shire-hall. The receipts arising from these performances, which embody the principal musical talent in the kingdom, are, after deducting the expenses, appropriated to the benefit of the widows and orphans of the necessitous clergy of the diocese. The theatre, a neat and conveniently arranged edifice in Westgate-street, is occasionally opened for dramatic performances; and races take place annually in a meadow on the bank of the Severn. The environs abound with pleasant walks, and the salubrity of the air, and agreeableness of its situation, render Gloucester desirable as a place of residence. To the east of the city a new mineral spring was discovered in 1814, round which an extensive tract of land has been tastefully laid out in pleasure grounds, affording pleasant promenades and drives; and an elegant pump-room has been erected, with other buildings, for the accommoda-

tion of visitors: near it have been built some handsome villas, and in 1823 a church, dedicated to the Holy Trinity, was erected, in the Grecian style of architecture, from a design by Mr. Rickman; the whole forming an elegant appendage to the city, under the designation of Gloucester Spa. The mineral water is a saline chalybeate, resembling that of Cheltenham; and, when fresh drawn, is transparent and sparkling; it emits a sulphureous odour, and has a brackish taste. It exudes through a thick stratum of blueish clay, which is diffused, at a certain depth, over a great part of the vale. In this clay are found large quantities of marine exuviæ, sulphuret of iron, and various saline compounds, which being in some degree soluble in the water percolating through the mass, communicate its peculiar properties. The principal salts contained in this water, of which there are several varieties, are sulphate and muriate of soda, and sulphate of magnesia: it is also impregnated with iron, held in solution by excess of carbonic acid; and from its resemblance to the Cheltenham waters it may in general be used in similar cases.

As an inland port, Gloucester had attained some eminence at an early period. The quay is mentioned as existing in the reign of Edward IV., and in the 22nd of Elizabeth the customs were granted by letters patent. In the following year the custom-house was erected, and also a wharf, or quay, for unloading vessels, called the King's quay. The rising prosperity of the port excited the jealousy of the inhabitants of Bristol, who addressed to the privy council an unavailing complaint against the establishment of the custom-house. The jurisdiction of the port, as fixed by a decree of the lords of the treasury, in 1820, extends from Chapel rock, or St. Teclas' point, at Beachley, on the north side of the Severn, below Gloucester, across the river to Aust Pill, including, on the south side, both banks, up to the West-gate bridge, in the city of Gloucester; but, according to practice, the limits of the port are from the source of the Severn, in Montgomeryshire, to Chapel rock, at Beachley. The number of vessels belonging to the port, in 1828, was two hundred and thirty, averaging fifty-four tons' burden. It carries on an extensive coasting trade, which is greatly facilitated by the advantages afforded by the river Severn, for keeping up a communication with Bristol and the coasts of Somersetshire, Devonshire, and South Wales, and a very considerable inland trade with Worcestershire, and other counties to the north. Many vessels are employed on this river in the coal trade, upwards of one hundred thousand tons of coal being annually shipped from the Shropshire and Staffordshire collieries, for distribution through the adjacent counties. Great quantities of lead, pig iron, grain, wool, hops, and other commodities, are also conveyed from the inland counties to Gloucester, Bristol, and other places, whence various kinds of goods are transmitted in return. The benefit of water-carriage has been further extended to this city by the Gloucester and Berkeley canal, which was commenced in 1793, and opened April 26th, 1827, at an expense of half a million of money, though the estimated expense was only £140,000: it extends sixteen miles and a quarter to its termination at Sharpness-point; is from seventy to ninety feet wide, and eighteen deep; and runs on a level, without any lock throughout its entire length. At each end is a capacious basin for the reception of shipping; and at Gloucester a second basin, with convenient wharfs for barges and small vessels drawing less than ten feet of water. By means of this canal, a more safe, speedy, and convenient passage is afforded for ships than by sailing up the Severn. Some opinion may be formed of the advantages it affords from the fact that, during the first two years after it was finished, seven thousand seven hundred and forty-one vessels traversed the line, the aggregate burden of which was three hundred and eighty-eight thousand five hundred and thirty tons. The Hereford and Gloucester canal, for facilitating the navigation between Hereford, Gloucester, and Bristol, was begun in 1792, and, after an expenditure of £105,000, has been carried no further than Ledbury, a distance of only seventeen miles, its proposed extent being about thirty. In addition to these advantages is the benefit of a junction with the Stroudwater canal, which opens a communication with London by means of the Thames: there is also a rail-road, extending from the quay to the town of Cheltenham.

Gloucester is said to have been a place of considerable trade before the time of the Conquest; and in addition to the mint, there was a merchants' guild, established in the reign of John, who granted the burgesses exemption from toll, and other privileges and immunities. Forges for the smelting of ore appear to have subsisted here so early as the twelfth century, and Long Smith-street derived its name from the number of artizans by whom it was inhabited: cap or felt-making, the refining of sugar, and the manufacture of glass, which formerly flourished, have been long discontinued. The principal branches of manufacture carried on at present are those of iron and pins; the latter, which was introduced in 1625 by Mr. John Tilsby, may be now considered as the staple trade of the place; the former, especially since the establishment of a foundry by Mr. Montague, in 1802, has greatly improved, and the castings lately produced are distinguished by a degree of excellence almost unrivalled: some of the medals and smaller productions are executed with such admirable skill as to be held in the highest estimation, and to find a place in the cabinets of the curious. A bell foundry has been carried on for nearly a century and a half, by the family of Mr. Rudhall, the original proprietor, in the course of which period not less than five thousand church-bells of various sizes have been cast: the trade of wool-stapling, which formerly afforded employment to many persons, has been in a great measure superseded by the dressing of hemp and flax: an establishment for the manufacture of shawls in imitation of those of France, has been discontinued for several years. The market days are Wednesday and Saturday, and there is a market for live stock on the first Monday in every month: the markets were formerly held in the open streets, but two large and commodious market-houses have been erected; one in Eastgate-street, for the sale of corn, meat, poultry, and vegetables; and the other in Southgate-street, for fish, butter, &c.: in front of the latter are two conduits, supplied with water from the reservoir at Robin Hood's hill. The cattle market is held in a spacious area judiciously appropriated to the purpose. The fairs are, April 5th, July 5th, September 28th and 29th (for cheese), and November 28th.

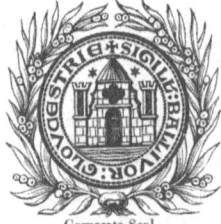

Corporate Seal.

The municipal constitution of this city has varied considerably at different periods: in 1022, the chief magistrate is said to have borne the title of præfect, and in the reign of Henry II., that of provost: under John it was constituted a borough, and governed by two bailiffs. Henry III. granted a charter of incorporation, under bailiffs or provosts, of whom there was a succession till the 1st of Richard III., who bestowed a new charter, appointing a mayor, two sheriffs, and other officers, to be annually elected by twelve aldermen, and twelve other of the most legal and discreet burgesses: he also ordained that the hundreds of Dudstone and King's Barton should be distinct from the county, and be called the county of the town of Gloucester. Henry VII. confirmed all former grants and privileges; and Henry VIII., on establishing the bishoprick of Gloucester, in 1542, directed that it should thenceforth be considered as a city. Edward VI., Elizabeth, James I., and Charles I., confirmed preceding grants; but the charter which finally extended and established the liberties and franchises of the city, and under the authority of which the corporation now act, was granted April 18th, 1672, in consideration of a payment to the king of £679. 4. 6. The government is by this charter vested in a mayor, who is also clerk of the market, and acts as marshal or steward of the royal household when His Majesty is in the city; a high steward, a recorder, twelve aldermen, any number of common council-men, which, with the mayor and aldermen, will make the corporation consist of at least thirty members, and not exceed forty, assisted by a town clerk, treasurer, chamberlain, water-bailiff, sword-bearer, four serjeants at mace, and subordinate officers. The mayor is elected annually by the aldermen from their own body, assisted by the senior common council-men, at least twenty in number, by whom also the bailiff, chamberlain, and coroner (who is generally the late mayor), are chosen at the same time: the recorder is elected by the mayor and aldermen: persons refusing to serve offices to which they are appointed are liable to fine, imprisonment, or loss of freedom. The bishop, dean, and two of the prebendaries, and the mayor, recorder, and aldermen, are justices of the peace. The freedom of the city is inherited by all the sons of freemen on attaining the age of twenty-one, and acquired by servitude to a resident freeman, by purchase, or gift of the corporation. The city is divided into four wards, to each of which constables are appointed. There were formerly twelve companies, the members of which used to accompany the mayor on public occasions with their banners; but this custom has fallen into disuse. The corporation hold quarterly courts of session, and courts of gaol delivery for the city and county of the city, with power to take cognizance of all offences except treason and misprision of treason; and a petty session every Monday and Friday, for hearing and determining affairs of police: they have the power of holding a court of record for the recovery of debts to any amount; this court, called the pie-powder court, was formerly held twice in the week, but it has not been held within the last forty years. Under charter of the 1st of William and Mary, a court of requests is held by the mayor and alderman every Monday, for the recovery of debts under 40s. The custom of Borough English prevails here. 'The assizes and quarter sessions for the county are held in this city, which is in the Oxford circuit; the average number of criminal cases at the spring assizes is from one hundred and forty to one hundred and fifty; and, at the autumn, from one hundred to one hundred and twenty. The municipal affairs of the city are transacted at a building called the Tolsey, which stands at the angle formed by Westgate and Southgate streets, on the site of a church dedicated to All Saints : it was erected in pursuance of an act of parliament passed in the 23rd of George II. : in the front is a pediment ornamented with the city arms; and in the council-chamber are portraits of the late Duke of Norfolk and of the present Duke of Gloucester. The city gaol, situated at the bottom of Southgate-street, erected in 1782, being too small, was, a few years since, enlarged and improved, with the addition of a chapel, in which divine service is regularly performed by a chaplain appointed by the corporation. Adjoining this prison a lock-uphouse has been erected, as a place of temporary confinement for vagrants and disorderly persons. The assizes were formerly held in an old edifice called the Booth-hall, situated behind the Booth-hall inn, in Westgate-street; but in 1814 a new and magnificent shire-hall, in the Grecian style of architecture, was erected, of Bath and Leckhampton stone, from a design by R. Smirke, Esq.: it stands on the south side of Westgate-street : in the front is a portico of four Ionic columns, thirty-five feet high, forming the principal entrance. The building extends three hundred feet in depth, and eighty-two in front; on one side of the portico is the entrance to the seats of the judges, and to every part except the galleries : the civil and criminal courts are nearly of the same dimensions, and of a semicircular form. From the principal entrance a stone staircase leads to an extensive room, in which the elections of members of parliament for the city and the county take place; and likewise the evening concerts at the triennial music-meetings : at the end of this room are displayed the royal arms, and over the door-way is a fine bas-relief, representing the signing of Magna Charta by King John. The county gaol stands on the bank of the Severn, and on the site of the ancient castle, the keep of which had been long used as a place of confinement previously to its entire removal to make way for the present massive and colossal edifice. It was built in consequence of an act of parliament, on the plan recommended by the celebrated Howard, and finished, in 1791, at an expense of nearly £30,000, being adapted to the classification of prisoners : there are two hundred and three separate cells, including one hundred and sixty-four sleeping-rooms, and thirty-nine work-rooms : a spacious building has been recently added for the separate confinement of debtors. The city first exercised the elective franchise in the 23d of Edward I., since which time it has returned two members to parliament: the right of election is vested in the freemen, the number of whom is about three thousand : the sheriffs are the returning officers.

Arms of the Bishoprick.

Gloucester is said to have been the see of a bishop when Britain was under the dominion of the Romans ; and Eldad is mentioned as having presided over the diocese in 490. This first bishoprick was probably suppressed when the country was conquered by the Anglo-Saxons; and the whole county of Gloucester, which formed part of the kingdom of Mercia, was, on the introduction of Christianity, included in the diocese of Lichfield. In 679 it was annexed to the newly established bishoprick of Worcester, to which it belonged till the Reformation, at which period Henry VIII., by letters patent dated September 3rd, 1541, confirmed by act of parliament, erected the city and county of the city of Gloucester, and all the county of Gloucester, into a see, to which he also annexed so much of the city and county of the city of Bristol as had formerly belonged to the diocese of Worcester. This new bishoprick was suppressed by Queen Mary, but re-established on the accession of Elizabeth. The ecclesiastical establishment consists of a bishop, dean, archdeacon, chancellor, six prebendaries, four minor canons, registrar, and other officers. On the foundation of the bishoprick the abbey church of St. Peter was constituted the cathedral church. This conventual edifice owed its origin to Wulphere, the first Christian king of Mercia, who, about 680, commenced the erection of a monastery, which was completed by his brother and successor Ethelred. It was at first a nunnery, which, being destroyed by the Danes, was refounded by Bernulf, King of Mercia, in 821, for the reception of secular priests. Canute the Dane, in 1022, ejected these priests, and introduced Benedictine monks, who, after some opposition, kept possession of the monastery, which was governed by a succession of thirty-two abbots belonging to that order, the last of whom was William Malvern, otherwise Parker, who wrote a history of the abbey, and died in retirement after the dissolution. The monastery and its possessions were surrendered to the king's commissioners in January, 1540, by the prior, Gabriel Morton, when the revenue was estimated at £1946. 5. 9. Of the monastic buildings there are no remains except the church, chapter-house, and cloisters, which escaped demolition in consequence of their being appropriated to the purposes of the episcopal establishment.

The present cathedral is one of the most magnificent ecclesiastical structures in England, combining specimens of Norman, with early and later English, architecture : it consists of a nave, choir, aisles, transepts, Lady chapel, and grand central tower, besides other parts of less importance. The oldest parts are the nave, the chantry chapels around the choir, and the crypt, or undercroft, which are supposed to have belonged to the abbey church founded by Aldred, Bishop of Worcester, a few years prior to the Norman Conquest. The roof of the nave, built by Abbot Henry Foliot, was finished in 1248. The south aisle was begun by abbot Thokey, in 1310; and the south transept was added in 1330; about which time also was commenced the erection of the north transept and the choir, which last was finished in 1457. Between 1351 and 1390, the cloisters were constructed; the west front and south porch were added in 1421; and the edifice was completed by the erection of the chapel of our Lady, and the central tower, which were begun in 1457, under the direction of Abbot Sebroke, who, dying that year, committed the execution of the work to Robert Tulley, one of the monks, who afterwards became bishop of St. David's : the chapel was finished in 1498, and the tower in 1518. Notwithstanding the variety of style in its architecture, the exterior presents a noble and impressive appearance : the tower, in particular, though of colossal dimensions, from the taste and delicacy of its ornaments has a light and airy effect, which adds greatly to the beauty of the whole . it is a square structure of three stages, rising from the intersection, and crowned with battlements and angular pinnacles. On the south side of the church are six buttresses with niches, formerly decorated with statues of tutelar saints and benefactors of the abbey, which, with other ornaments, were defaced at the Reformation, and during the usurpation of Cromwell. The west front and the south porch, in the decorated style of English architecture, display elegance of taste and symmetry of proportion. On entering the cathedral through the porch, on the left hand, is the consistory court ; and opposite the entrance, across the nave, is a gate of light open iron-work, presenting in pleasing perspective a view of the exquisite tracery of the roof of the great cloister : the western extremity is adorned with a finely painted window. The nave is separated from the aisles by massive round pillars, from which spring semicircular arches ; and its roof displays tracery which is most ornamented towards the west end. A classically correct and appropriate screen, separating the nave from the choir, was erected in 1820, displacing one of a very different character. Elegant clustered pillars rise from the base to the roof of the choir, where, by the branching of their cylinders, they contribute to form the delicately beautiful trelliswork by which it is ornamented. The sides of the choir are embellished with spiral canopies of rich tabernacle-work, carved in oak, exhibiting some of the finest specimens of English ornamental carving now extant. The high altar, which was of oak, with decorations in the Grecian style of architecture, has been very properly removed, as inconsistent with the prevailing character of the building. Before the altar is a curious pavement of painted bricks, or tiles, representing armorial bearings, the work of the monks. At the east end of the choir is a window said to be the largest in England, containing two thousand seven hundred and ninety-eight square feet of stained glass, but much decayed and mutilated. The whispering gallery is a narrow passage, twenty-five yards in extent, forming a communication between the opposite sides of the choir : its remarkable property of conveying with facility the faintest sound from one end to the other, which is mentioned by Lord Verulam in one of his philosophical works, is supposed to have been the accidental effect of the peculiar form of the gallery, not contemplated by the architect in its construction. From the aisle on the south side of the choir is an entrance, under a pointed arch, to the Lady chapel : the interior is decorated in a style corresponding with that of the choir ; and the fretted ceiling, though of inferior character, is very beautiful.

By the recent removal of an altar of stucco, the mutilated remains of the original altar-piece, which has been of the richest workmanship, and superbly decorated with curious painting and gilding, have been exposed to view. There are many tombs deserving notice ; among which may be mentioned the tomb erected by Abbot Parker, in memory of Osric, King of Northumberland, one of the founders of the monastery, who died about 729, with his effigy in freestone, in the north aisle, near the entrance to the Lady chapel ; an altar-tomb in a chapel in the same aisle, supposed to cover the remains of Robert, Duke of Normandy, son of William the Conqueror, with his statue carved in oak recumbent on it, under a wire lattice ; not far from the high altar the monument of Edward II., who was murdered at Berkeley castle, with a recumbent figure in alabaster, supposed, from the elegance of the sculpture, to be of Italian workmanship, with a more modern but beautiful canopy of tabernacle-work ; the monument of Alderman Blackleach and his wife, with their statues in white marble ; that of Mrs. Morley, with a group of statuary by Flaxman ; those of Judge Powell ; Sir George Onesiphorus Paul, Bart.; Dr. Edward Jenner, who first brought the practice of vaccination into general use ; Charles Brandon Trye, an eminent surgeon ; and Robert Raikes, Esq., who, from his unwearied exertions in promoting the increase of Sunday schools throughout the kingdom, obtained the reputation of having been the founder of these institutions, which, however, owe their origin to the Rev. Thomas Stock, rector of the parish of St. John the Baptist, in this city. The chapter-house of the monastery, situated on the north side of the cathedral, with an entrance from the cloisters, is now appropriated to the reception of the college library.

The city comprises the parishes of St. Aldate, St. John the Baptist, St. Mary de Crypt, St. Mary de Grace, St. Nicholas, St. Owen, and the Holy Trinity, and part of the parishes of St. Catherine, St. Mary de Lode, and St. Michael, all in the archdeaconry and diocese of Gloucester. The living of St. Aldate is a perpetual curacy, endowed with £200 private benefaction, and £1000 royal bounty, and in the patronage of the Crown. The living of St. Catherine is a perpetual curacy, endowed with £400 royal bounty, and in the patronage of the Dean and Chapter : the church was taken down in 1648. The living of St. John the Baptist is a discharged rectory, rated in the king's books at £14. 1. 1½., endowed with £400 private benefaction, £400 royal bounty, and £400 parliamentary grant, and in the patronage of the Crown : the church, with the exception of the ancient tower and spire, was rebuilt in 1734. The living of St. Mary de Crypt is a discharged rectory, with those of All Saints' and St. Owen's consolidated, rated in the king's books at £14. 7. 11., endowed with £400 royal bounty, and £400 parliamentary grant, and in the patronage of the Crown : the church is a spacious cruciform structure, principally in the later style of English architecture, with some remains of the Norman, early English, and decorated styles, and having a handsome tower rising from the intersection. The living of St. Mary de Grace is a perpetual curacy, consolidated with the rectory of St. Michael, and endowed with £400 royal bounty : the church was taken down by order of the corporation in 1653. The living of St. Mary de Lode is a discharged vicarage, to which that of the Holy Trinity is annexed, rated in the king's books at £10. 13. 4., endowed with £200 royal bounty, and in the patronage of the Dean and Chapter: the body of the church has been lately rebuilt in the later style of English architecture, but the chancel and tower of the old building remain; the latter formerly supported a lofty spire, which was demolished by a storm; in the north wall is an ancient tomb with a recumbent effigy, said to have been erected to the memory of Lucius, first Christian King of Britain, who is erroneously supposed to have been buried in the church. In St. Mary's square, now added to the church-yard, a monument was erected, in 1826, to the memory of Bishop Hooper, who, in the reign of Mary, suffered martyrdom on the spot. The living of St. Michael's is a discharged rectory, with the perpetual curacy of St. Mary's de Grace consolidated, rated in the king's books at £8. 16. 10., endowed with £600 royal bounty, and in the patronage of the Crown: the church, with the exception of its ancient tower, has undergone so much modern alteration as to have defaced nearly all traces of its original character. The living of St. Nicholas' is a perpetual curacy, endowed with £800 royal bounty, and £400 parliamentary grant, and in the patronage of the Mayor and Corporation: the church is an ancient structure in the early style of English architecture, with later additions and insertions; the tower, which is handsome, appears to have declined from the perpendicular by the sinking of the foundation; it is surmounted by a spire, the upper part of which has been removed for greater security. The living of St. Owen's is a perpetual curacy, consolidated with the rectory of St. Mary's de Crypt, and endowed with £200 royal bounty: the church was destroyed during the siege of the city. The living of the Holy Trinity parish is a discharged vicarage annexed to that of St. Mary's de Crypt, rated in the king's books at £9, endowed with £1000 royal bounty, and in the patronage of the Dean and Chapter: the church was taken down in 1698, since which period its beautiful tower has shared the same fate. There are places of worship for Baptists, the Society of Friends, those in the late Countess of Huntingdon's Connexion, Independents, Wesleyan Methodists, and Unitarians, a Roman Catholic chapel, and a Synagogue.

The college school, founded by Henry VIII., and originally designed for the education of youth belonging to the choir, is held in an apartment adjoining the cathedral: it is under the direction of a master and an usher, and has long enjoyed considerable reputation as a classical seminary. The school of St. Mary's de Crypt was founded and endowed in the 31st of Henry VIII., as a free grammar school, by John Cooke, or Coke, an alderman of Gloucester, and his widow: the school-room adjoins the parochial church from which it is named. It has an interest in eight scholarships, of about £50 per annum each, founded by George Townsend, Esq., in 1683, in Pembroke College, Oxford, for boys from the schools of Gloucester, Cheltenham, Chipping-Campden, and North Leach, the scholars being entitled to presentation to the livings of Colnbrook or Uxbridge. In Eastgate-street is the Blue-coat hospital, founded on a plan somewhat similar to that of Christ's Hospital, London, for the maintenance and education of twenty boys, by Sir Thomas Rich, Bart., a native of Gloucester, who, by his will dated in 1666, left

£6000, to purchase lands for the support of this charity and other beneficent purposes: the boys are taught to read and write, and six of them are apprenticed every year: the master's salary is £20 per annum. The mayor and burgesses, who are the trustees of this foundation, erected a new hospital in 1807, the former structure having become dilapidated. A National school was opened in March 1817, under the patronage of the Duke of Beaufort, which is supported by voluntary contributions: the master has a salary of £63 per annum, and the mistress one of £40: the foundation stone of the building, which stands in the London road, was laid by the Duke of Wellington, August 6th, 1815, and the structure was completed in the following year. A Lancasterian school, situated in Lower Northgate-street, has been opened for the education of two hundred boys: the master's salary is £63 per annum. The building was erected at the expense of £400; and the school, commenced in August 1813, is now supported by funds bequeathed some time previously by Mrs. Dorothy Cocks, and John Hyett, Esq., the produce of which was long applied to the reduction of the poor-rates: the government of this charity is vested in the corporation of the workhouse.

St. Bartholomew's hospital, on the north side of Westgate-street, is an almshouse for fifty-four decayed men and women, who receive weekly pensions, which, with the salaries of a chaplain, a physician, and a surgeon, are paid from the endowment, amounting to £500 per annum. Queen Elizabeth granted letters patent for the establishment of this hospital to the mayor and burgesses, through the interest of Richard Pates, Esq., recorder of the city: its revenue originally belonged to a priory founded in the reign of Henry II. The hospital was rebuilt in 1786, in the early style of English architecture. St. Mary Magdalene's, or King James's hospital, in the London road, was founded by one of the priors of Lanthony, for ten men and nine women, who have three shillings a week each, besides other allowances. Not far from this last is St. Margaret's hospital, originally a house for lepers: eight men are now supported in it, each having four shillings a week, with additional advantages. In the parish of St. Mary de Crypt is an almshouse for six poor persons, founded by Sir Thomas Bell, who died in 1566. The workhouse, or house of industry, situated in Bare Land, was founded and liberally endowed by Timothy Nourse, Esq., in 1703: it is under the management of an elective corporation: the poor are here kept employed chiefly in pin-making. Gloucester infirmary, or the county hospital for the indigent sick, is situated in Southgate-street: it was built in 1755, and is supported by funds arising from voluntary contributions: an addition has recenly been made to it, chiefly by subscription, for the reception of convalescent inmates. About half a mile from the city, on the London road, a handsome building has been erected as an asylum for lunatics. A penitentiary, called the Magdalen asylum, was established in 1821, and is supported by subscription.

Among other traces of the residence of the Romans, numerous inscribed stones, coins, &c. have at different periods been found in the city and its vicinity, chiefly at or near Kingsholm. One of the most remarkable of the relics was a *statera*, or Roman steelyard, supposed to have been the first ever discovered in Great Britain. The ancient walls of Gloucester have been entirely destroyed; and of the remains of civil monuments of the middle ages, scarcely any thing exists except the Conduit, a beautiful piece of architecture in the later English style, which formerly stood in Southgate street, but has been removed to the grounds of a private gentleman in Barton-street. Of the priory of St. Oswald, and the convents of Franciscans, Dominicans, and Carmelites, anciently subsisting here, no relics deserving of notice remain. Among the distinguished natives of Gloucester, and persons connected with the city, were, Osbern of Gloucester, a learned writer; and Benedict, author of the life of St. Dubricius, who were both monks here in the reign of Stephen; Robert of Gloucester, author of a curious chronicle in rhyme, who lived in the middle of the thirteenth century; John Rastell and John Corbett, historical writers; John Taylor, "the water poet," born in 1580; Dr. Miles Smith, Bishop of Hereford, one of the translators of the Bible; George Whitefield, founder of the Calvinistic Methodists; Dr. John Moore, Archbishop of Canterbury; and Robert Raikes, Esq.

GLOUCESTERSHIRE, a maritime county, bounded on the north and north-east by the counties of Worcester and Warwick, on the east by the county of Oxford, on the south-east by part of the counties of Berks and Wilts, on the south and south-west by the county of Somerset and the Bristol Channel, and on the west and north-west by the counties of Monmouth and Hereford: it extends from 51° 28′ to 52° 12′ (N. Lat.), and from 1° 38′ to 2° 44′ (W. Lon.), and includes one thousand two hundred and fifty-six square miles, or eight hundred and three thousand eight hundred and forty statute acres. The population, exclusively of that of Bristol, amounted in 1821 to 282,954. At the time of the second invasion of Britain by the Romans, under Claudius, in the year 66, this part of the country was inhabited by the Dobuni, who had been so much harassed and oppressed by their ambitious neighbours, the Cattieuchlani, that they submitted freely to the Romans, in order to be delivered from their former oppressors. Cogidunus, said to have been at that time prince of the Dobuni, is described by Tacitus as having persevered with great fidelity in his allegiance to the Romans, and as having therefore continued in the possession of his own territories, with some other states annexed to them. The prœtor, Ostorius Scapula, was much engaged in this county, especially in the lower part of it, where he is supposed to have formed a chain of fortifications from the Avon to the Severn, to check the inroads of the Silures from the other side of the latter river. In the first Roman division of Britain this territory was included in Britannia Prima; and in the subdivision by Constantine, it formed part of *Flavia Cæsariensis.* Under the Saxon octarchy the county was comprised within the great central kingdom of Mercia; and, bordering on the mountainous country which served as the principal retreat of the Britons, it was one of the last that were permanently annexed to that sovereignty: during the efforts made to conquer it, two important battles are recorded to have been fought within its limits; the first at Dyrham, in 578, when Ceawlin, King of Wessex, and his son Cuthwin, defeated three British kings, and gained possession of the three British cities,

Gloucester, Cirencester, and Bath; the second at Frethern, in 585, in which Cuthwin was slain, but the Britons were defeated. During the contentions of the Saxon princes among themselves, a sanguinary battle was fought near Cirencester, in 628, between Cynegils and Cwichelm, joint kings of Wessex, and Penda, King of Mercia. In 687 the Saxon kings met at Campden, to consult on the best mode of carrying on the war against the Britons. The first visit of the Danes to Gloucestershire was probably in 877, when, having plundered the kingdom of Mercia, they encamped at Gloucester, where they remained for a year; then removing to Cirencester, they wintered there, and afterwards proceeded into East Anglia, where they settled. In 894, they marched along the side of the Thames as far as Boddington, where, being reinforced by a party of the Welch, they threw up intrenchments and prepared for defence; here Alfred surrounded them with the whole force of his dominions, and destroyed a great number by famine and the sword. Tradition mentions some other places in this county as having felt the fury of these invaders, but the accounts are not confirmed by the Saxon historians. It was at Gloucester that Athelstan died, in 941; and at Pucklechurch, Edmund I. was stabbed by the robber Leof, in 946. In 1016, Edmund Ironside, after the defeat of his army at *Essandune* (Ashingdon in Essex), came to Gloucester, and having there assembled another army, was prepared again to take the field, when the Danish and English nobility, being both weary of the war, induced their kings to come to an agreement, and divide the kingdom between them by treaty; their conference on this occasion took place in the Isle of Alney, near Gloucester. In 1093, Malcolm III., King of Scotland, came to Gloucester to treat with William Rufus. In the war between Stephen and the Empress Matilda, the whole country around Gloucester espoused the cause of the empress, who at that city always found a welcome reception; and to it she is said to have escaped, by being carried in a coffin, after the siege of Winchester. Bristol, too, was one of her strongest garrisons, and in its castle Stephen was confined for nine months, until exchanged for the Earl of Gloucester, brother of the empress. In the war between Henry III. and the barons, Gloucester was captured by the latter, in 1263. In 1279, a parliament was held at Gloucester, by which those laws connected with the statute of *Quo Warranto,* known by the denomination of "the statutes of Gloucester," were enacted. In 1327, Edward II. was murdered in Berkeley castle. At Cirencester, in 1400, a conspiracy against Henry IV. was suppressed; the Duke of Surrey and the Earl of Salisbury being taken and beheaded by the inhabitants. At Tewkesbury, in 1471, was fought the great and decisive battle in which the Lancastrians were totally defeated, the Marquis of Dorset, the Earl of Devon, and three thousand men, having been slain; Margaret of Anjou, her son Prince Edward, and her general the Duke of Somerset, taken prisoners by Edward IV.; and Prince Edward assassinated, and the Duke of Somerset beheaded, after the battle. In the great contest between Charles I. and the parliament, this county was constantly the theatre of battles; and it is remarkable that the explosion of hostilities against the king took place in it, *viz.,* at Cirencester, by a personal attack upon Lord Chandos, who had been appointed to execute the royal commission of array. To gain

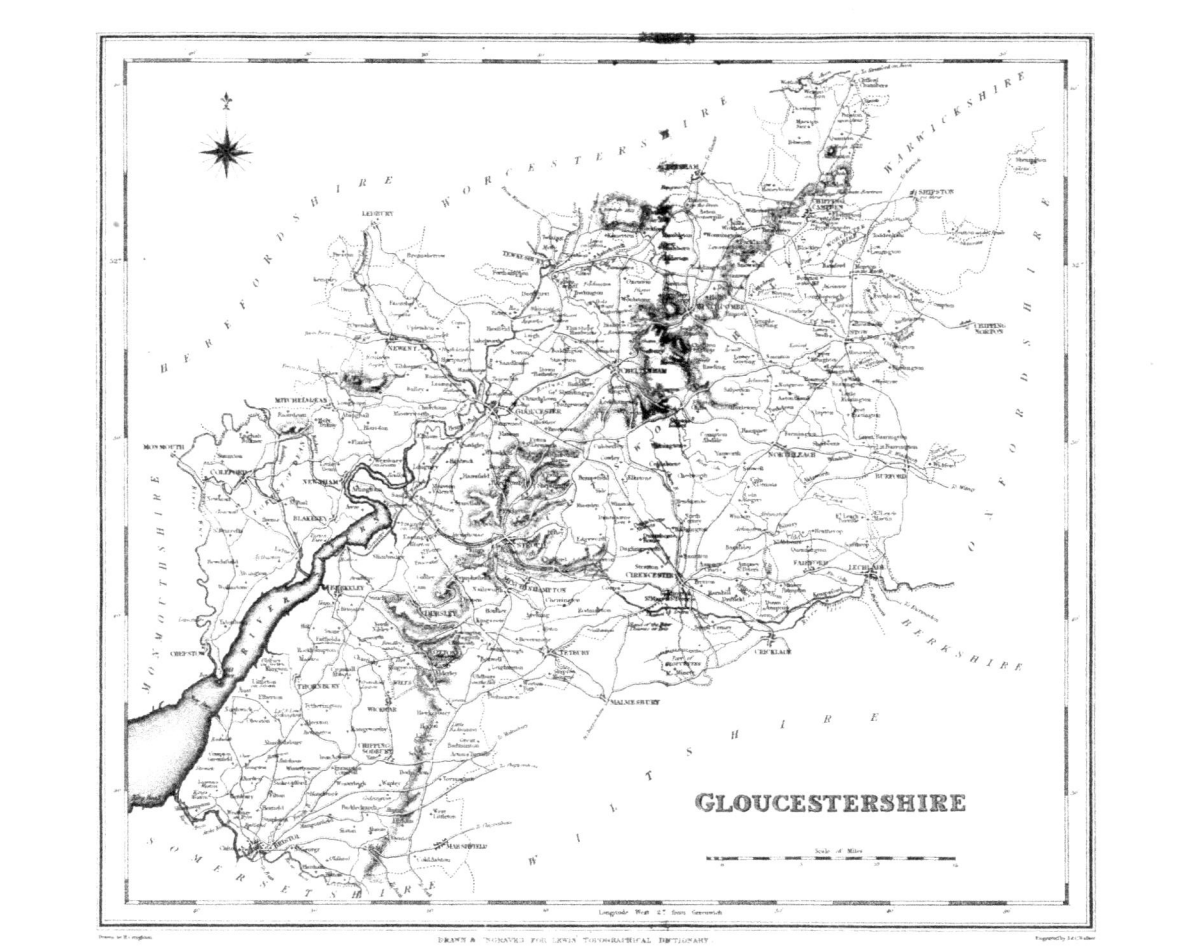

GLOUCESTERSHIRE

Scale of Miles

Longitude West 2° from Greenwich

DRAWN & ENGRAVED FOR LEWIS TOPOGRAPHICAL DICTIONARY

possession of the city of Gloucester was an object of so much importance to the success of the royal cause, that the king came in person to command the besieging army, and fixed his head-quarters for a considerable period at Matson; the city was, however, successfully defended for the parliament, by Colonel Massie, until relieved by the Earl of Essex, in September 1643. On the 2nd of February, 1642-3, Cirencester was stormed by Prince Rupert, who took one thousand two hundred prisoners; and on the 19th of March following, at Highnam, Major-General Brett, Lord John Somerset, and nearly two thousand royalists, were surprised and taken by Sir William Waller. Bristol, which had surrendered to Prince Rupert in July, 1643, was re-captured by Fairfax, in 1645. During the revolution of 1688, Lord Lovelace, on his march through Cirencester with a small party, to join the Prince of Orange, was attacked by Captain Lorange of the county militia, made prisoner, and sent to Gloucester gaol; this was the first skirmish that took place after the prince's landing.

Gloucestershire was formerly in the diocese of Lichfield, and afterwards in that of Worcester, but, by Henry VIII., in 1541, it was made a distinct bishoprick, in the province of Canterbury: it forms an archdeaconry, containing the deaneries of Campden, Cirencester, Dursley, Fairford, Forest, Gloucester, Hawkesbury, Stonehouse, Stow, and Winchcombe, and comprising three hundred and twenty-seven parishes, of which number, one hundred and thirty-nine are rectories, one hundred and one vicarages, and the remainder perpetual curacies, or united to other parishes. For civil purposes it is divided into the hundreds of Barton-Regis, Upper and Lower Berkeley, Bisley, Blidesloe, Botloe, Bradley, St. Briavells, Brightwell's Barrow, Cheltenham, Cleeve, or Bishop's Cleeve, Crowthorne and Minety, Upper and Lower Deerhurst, Lower, Middle, and Upper Dudstone and King's Barton, Upper and Lower Grumbald's Ash, Upper and Lower Henbury, Upper and Lower Kiftsgate, Duchy of Lancaster, Upper and Lower Langley and Swinehead, Longtree, Pucklechurch, Rapsgate, Upper and Lower Slaughter, Upper and Lower Tewkesbury, Upper and Lower Thornbury, Tibaldstone, Westbury, Upper and Lower Westminster, and Upper and Lower Whitstone. It contains the city of Gloucester, and locally part of that of Bristol; the borough and market towns of Cirencester and Tewkesbury, and the market towns of Berkeley, Campden, Cheltenham, Coleford, Dursley, Fairford, Minchinhampton, Lechlade, Marshfield, Mitchel-Dean, Newnham, Newent, North Leach, Painswick, Sodbury, Stow on the Wolds, Stroud, Tetbury, Thornbury, Wickwar, Winchcombe, and Wotton under Edge. Two knights are returned to parliament for the shire, two representatives for the city of Gloucester, and two for each of the boroughs: the county members are elected at Gloucester. This county is included in the Oxford circuit: the assizes and quarter sessions are held at Gloucester, where stands the common gaol, or sheriff's prison: the houses of correction are at Horsley, North Leach, Lawford's Gate, and Little Dean. There are one hundred and seventy-nine acting magistrates. The rates raised in the county for the year ending March 25th, 1827, amounted to £190,224. 1., the expenditure to £200,596. 13., of which £152,238. 2. was applied to the relief of the poor.

The natural division of the county is into the Cotswold, the Vale, and the Forest districts. The Cotswold district comprises the whole tract of hilly country from Chipping-Campden on the north, to Bath on the south, and is often divided into the Upper and Lower Cotswolds. The Vale district comprehends the whole lowlands, from Stratford upon Avon to Bristol, and is usually divided into the Vales of Evesham, Gloucester, and Berkeley; but its more natural division is into the Vales of the Severn and the Avon. These rivers are natural boundaries: the former vale includes all the low country between Tewkesbury and Bristol, and the latter the lowlands between the Upper Cotswolds and the Avon, from Tewkesbury to Stratford, wherever the river is a boundary to the county. The Forest district contains the parishes on the west side of the Severn up to Gloucester, and afterwards on the west side of the river Leden, up to where it enters the county from Herefordshire. The unsheltered state of the Cotswolds exposes them to the unmitigated effects of cold winds, and consequently throughout their whole extent a sharp climate predominates. In the denes and small vallies a milder air is felt, and in consequence of this, in former times, the villages were generally built in such sheltered situations; but since the cultivation of the higher lands, convenience has occasioned the building of houses in very exposed situations; and the hill farmer is easily distinguishable, by his more hardy complexion, from the husbandman of the vale. In the Vale district the air is comparatively mild, even in the severest weather. The climate of the Forest district is usually considered as temperate as that of the Vale; the high and otherwise exposed parts being so much sheltered by thick woods that neither northerly nor easterly winds can affect them to any considerable degree. The parts of the county which rank highest in point of picturesque beauty are the banks of the Wye and the environs of Bristol.

The general character of the soil of the Cotswolds is a shallow calcareous loam, provincially called Stonebrash, the usual depth of which is four inches, seldom exceeding seven. Under this is a stratum of rubble, or mould, and fragments of stone of the same nature as the rock on which the whole rests, which is a calcareous sand-stone, varying in some of its qualities, but known by the general name of freestone when found in large masses and deep beds. In some places, however, and more especially on the declivities, the soil inclines more to clay; and there could hardly be found a deeper or more argillaceous stratum than occurs on the banks of the rivulets running through the numerous small vallies by which this tract is intersected. There is a part of the Cotswolds lying chiefly to the south of the turnpike-road from Oxford to Bath, and extending more or less from Burford, through Cirencester and Tetbury, to Bath, which has a soil very different from that first described: the surface consists of mixed loam to the depth of from nine to twenty-four inches, under which lies a stratum of rock in thin layers, rubbly or broken, and mixed with light loam, to the depth of from four to twenty-four inches, and then a stratum of clay of various depths. This land is naturally wet, and its herbage causes the rot in sheep depastured upon it; but a considerable part has been greatly improved by draining across the natural slope of the land, so that it has become highly valuable for any purpose of husbandry, and sheep may be fed on it without danger of the rot. A great portion of the above tract is dairy land, and produces excellent cheese, similar in quality to the North Wiltshire. The soil in the Vale is various: in the northern parts of the county, as at Welford and its immediate vicinity, it is a fine black loam mixed with small pebbles and remarkably fertile; more southward it changes to a strong rich clay. These appearances continue in a greater or less degree nearly to Tewkesbury, from which place to Gloucester, on each side of the Severn, is found a red loam, formed by the long continued annual deposits of the muddy water, which, after great rains, being brought down by the river Avon, overspread the adjacent meadows. This adventitious soil is highly fertilizing, and supersedes the necessity of manure on the lands within its influence: it is also of great use for making bricks and tiles, and as a manure for light sandy lands. A soil similar to this continues, with few interruptions, for ten miles below Gloucester, when it becomes impregnated with marine salt, and mixed with sand deposited by the tide, and, though it loses much of its tenacity, it is equally if not more productive. At a distance from the Severn, on the eastern side, the soil is a strong clay, extending to the base of the hills, and in some places very stubborn. In the parish of Deerhurst, above Gloucester, and in those of Berkeley, Rockhampton, &c., below it, as also at Iron-Acton, Winterbourne, and Frampton-Cotterell, the soil is of a strong ferruginous colour: at the first mentioned places its substance is argillaceous, at the last a sandy loam; but the colour of both is probably derived from the oxyde of iron which they contain, and perhaps the great fertility of these soils is owing to the same cause. Sandy soil, with a substratum of gravel, is found in a small portion of this county. In all parts of the Vale, except where the compact limestone rocks are found, a blue clay, at different degrees of depth, forms the substratum of every soil: in some places, and more especially in the parish of Hardwick, this becomes the surface soil, and is unproductive of any but the coarsest herbage: in the higher parts of the Vale is some peaty earth, but not in abundance. Throughout a considerable part of the Forest district the soil inclines to sand; being in the northern parts little more than a decomposition of the red sand-stone, which is imbedded in large masses to a great depth, and often rises to the surface: this is the general character of the Ryelands, within the parish of Bromsberrow, and a great part of those of Dymock, Pauntley, Oxenhall, and Newent, on the high grounds; but on the lower, and nearer the level of the river Leden, the soil is of a closer and stronger texture, though retaining the same colour. It is nearly the same between Newent and Gloucester, till within a mile and a half of the city, when it changes to a black earth with silicious pebbles. The southern parts of this district have a light soil, or sandy loam, frequently of a ferruginous colour like that in the lower part of the Vale. In that portion strictly called the Forest, a kind of peaty soil prevails, interspersed with bogs and yellowish or ochreous clay.

About three hundred thousand acres of land in this county are under tillage. On the Cotswolds it is the practice to sow the crops after one ploughing, experience having proved that more frequent ploughing weakens the staple of these light soils. The average produce of wheat on the Cotswolds is fifteen bushels per acre, but in the southern parts of them somewhat more: on the loamy soils, as in the higher parts of the Vale of Evesham, and in the Lower Vale of Gloucester, it averages more than forty bushels an acre. The crops of oats are from forty to sixty bushels per acre; though not so much on the hills. Beans are the chief produce of the clay soils of the Vale, and a crop on which the farmer much depends: their average produce is from twenty to forty bushels per acre; that of peas the same. Rye is cultivated in that part of the Forest district which includes Newent, Pauntley, Oxenhall, Dymock, and Bromsberrow, here called the Ryelands. Tares or vetches are raised in every part of the county. Potatoes are more especially an object of attention in the southern parts of the county, and cultivated in a better manner than elsewhere: a hundred and fifty sacks, of three bushels each, are frequently raised on one acre of old broken up ley; but from eighty to a hundred are reckoned an average crop. The richest natural meadows and pastures are on the banks of the Severn and other rivers which run through the Vale: they are liable to be overflowed once or twice every year, and their whole manure consists of the muddy particles deposited during such inundations. Further down the Severn the quality of the herbage is changed, in consequence of the marine salt thrown over the land by the tide: these marshy meadows are generally grazing land. The meadows on each side of the Severn, in its whole course to about six miles below Gloucester, are mown every year, and most of the hay is disposed of to the range owners, for the supply of the Shropshire coal and other works, in which a great number of horses is employed: the produce of this land is nearly two tons per acre. The natural grass lands of the other parts of the Vale not within reach of these floods, are generally fertile, though not equally so with the former. The dairy being the chief object of the Vale farmers, the cattle kept are those best adapted for that purpose: notwithstanding the introduction of several varieties, in some old dairies the Gloucestershire breed of cows is still much valued. In the Higher Vale and also in the Cotswolds the long-horned cows are in most esteem. The cattle fed in the stalls are chiefly of the Herefordshire breed, and having been first worked by the breeders, at six or seven years old, are bought by the graziers at Gloucester, Hereford, Ross, &c.: calves are fattened on stages erected for the purpose. It is also customary among the Vale farmers, about the middle of summer, to buy in small Welch heifers, provincially termed *burries*, to turn into the lattermaths, which generally yield a good profit the ensuing spring. Sheep are fed in every part of the county: the principal breed is that of the Cotswolds, which is large and coarse in the wool, and at four years old will weigh from thirty to forty pounds per quarter: when crossed with the new Leicester, a practice now general, the average weight is only from twenty-two to thirty pounds per quarter, but the wool is made shorter and finer, and the carcase altogether improved. The Cotswold sheep have also been crossed with the South Down breed, the principal advantage of which consists in the improved fineness of the wool. The Vale has no peculiar breed of sheep, for the farmers are discouraged from breeding for a permanent stock by the danger of the rot. The Ryeland, or Herefordshire sheep, take their name from the district where they are found in the greatest purity : they are smaller than any other, except perhaps a few peculiar to the Forest of Dean, seldom, being three years old, exceeding twelve or fourteen pounds per quarter ; they are also beautiful in form, and superior in flesh, having remarkably fine wool. The Ryeland sheep, by crossing with the new Leicester and black-faced Shropshire, have been increased in carcase, but the quality of their wool has been deteriorated. In the Upper Vale, the improved Cotswold sheep are fattened on grass for the London market, or the markets in the neighbourhood ; and in the Vale of Berkeley, and below it, great numbers of sheep are fed on the lattermaths, for the markets of Bristol, Bath, &c. : for this latter purpose Somersetshire wethers, Mendip ewes, Wilt-shire wethers, and ewes with lambs, are chiefly pur-chased. On the lowlands, four or five miles on each side of Gloucester, the sheep chiefly fed are the Ryeland, which have here the range of extensive commons, where they quickly fatten. In the Forest district, the same sheep, with a few of the Forest breed, are fattened on grass, in summer, and on turnips, with hay or barley-meal, in winter. Hogs are fattened in every farm-yard on beans, peas, or barley meal : all sorts and mixtures of breeds are found, the greater part of them purchased in other counties, and sold at Gloucester market ; but the most frequent is a mixture of the Berkshire and the slouch-eared, or tonkey. The old Gloucestershire breed, standing high, long in the body, and white, are seldom met with in an unmixed state, and then not much esteemed. The great consumption of poultry, occasioned by the visitors of Cheltenham and Bath, increases the demand in this county, and conse-quently the price. No particular attention is paid to the breed of horses : the fairs receive their chief supply from the counties of Warwick, Stafford, Derby, and Lin-coln. The operations of tillage are more generally per-formed by horses than oxen in the Vale, where the soil is heavy, and will not bear much treading ; but on the Cotswolds, on the sandy lands of the Forest district, and in the southern parts of the Vale, oxen are chiefly used, the Herefordshire breed being preferred. The orchards of the Vale and the Forest districts form a very important part of the farmers' produce ; but on the Cotswolds, ex-cept partially on the slopes, fruit plantations are not made. About ten thousand acres in this county still remain waste, a small portion of which is in sheep downs on the Cots-wolds. On the Cotswolds, the beech and the ash are the principal trees : the former of these seems to be native ; and it is probable that at a remote period it covered most of this portion of the county. In the Vale, few tracts of woodland remain. The elm grows in almost every district ; the oak grows vigorously in different parts of the Vale, particularly in the hundred of Berkeley. In the Forest of Dean there still remains a large quantity of valuable timber. Besides the oak timber growing on the royal demesne lands, there is a considerable quantity on the estates of individuals adjacent to the Forest, and within what is agriculturally considered the Forest dis-trict. The birch trees of the Forest are remarkable for their size and beauty; the coppice woods, of which there is no great quantity, are chiefly within the Cotswold and the Forest districts.

In the Forest of Dean iron-ore exists in abundance, yet a small quantity only is raised, the greater part of that used in the furnaces being brought from Lancashire - and, notwithstanding the expense of carriage, it is more profitable for working, on account of its superior richness. Charcoal is chiefly employed in making the best wrought; iron ; while coke, made from the forest coal, is used for cast and sheet-iron. In the lower part of the Vale, veins of lead-ore are found in almost all the limestone rocks : attempts have been made to work them, but the produce has been too trifling to repay for the expense. Coal abounds in almost every part of the forest and its vicinity : the pits in the forest are numerous : much sulphur is contained in all the coal raised from them. The lower part of the Vale, including the parishes of Cromhall, Yate, Iron-Acton, Westerleigh, Pucklechurch, Stapleton, Mangotsfield, Bitton, Siston, and St. George's (within the Forest of Kingswood), equally abounds in coal, but of a less sulphureous quality. The pits in this district are very numerous, and supply the vast consumption of the Bristol manufactories, and in some degree that of Bath. Here the steam-engine is in use, and the pits are sunk to the depth of fifty fathoms, or more. Gloucester and its neighbourhood are supplied with coal from Shropshire and Staffordshire ; the coal from either of those counties being much superior to any produced in Gloucestershire. The Forest of Dean, Longhope, and adjoining places, furnish limestone for building and agriculture ; but it is inferior to that found in vast beds at the southern extremity of the county, which begin at Cromhall and diverge elliptically till they meet again in Somersetshire. The lime made of this stone is of a peculiar whiteness and great strength ; that which is burned at St.Vincent's rocks near Bristol being the best. The lime, when slaked, is closely com-pressed in casks, and becomes a considerable article of foreign and internal commerce : it is highly valued also for the purposes of agriculture, for which it is superior to any made from the calcareous grit of the Cotswolds, or the blue clay-stone of the Vale. The latter is found at various depths in beds of clay of the same colour, and, being disposed in layers of from four to ten inches thick, is useful for building. Freestone, of excellent quality for building, is raised from the Cotswold quarries ; and paving-stones, varying in quality and colour, are dug in the quarries at Frampton-Cotterell, Winterbourne, Iron-Acton, Mangotsfield, and Stapleton ; the latter are likewise found in the Forest of Dean ; as are also grits for grind-stones of various degrees of fineness, and one species of uncommon hardness and durability, esteemed the best in England for cider-mills : stone tiles are chiefly obtained in different parts of the Cotswolds. In Aust-Cliff, in the parish of Henbury, there is a fine bed of gypsum, or alabaster, which furnishes a plentiful supply for stuccoing, &c., to the masons of Bristol, Bath, and other places, but is inferior to that of Derbyshire.

The principal manufactures are those of woollen broad cloths, chiefly superfine and made of Spanish wool ; and fine narrow goods, of the stripe and fancy kind, both to a very great extent. These are carried on in the district commonly called the Bottoms, which includes parts of the several parishes of Avening, Painswick, Pitchcomb, Randwick, Minchinhampton, Stroud, Bisley, Rodbo-rough, Stonehouse, King's Stanley, Stanley-St. Leo-nard's, Woodchester, Horsley, and Eastington. There are also extensive works at Dursley, Cam, Uley, Alderley, Wickwar, and Wotton under Edge. At Cirencester are manufactured thin stuffs, composed of worsted yarn, called chinas. At Tewkesbury, frame-work knitting is the principal source of employment. Rugs and blankets are made at Nailsworth, Dursley, and North Nibley. The pin manufacture is carried on to an important extent at Gloucester. There are several mills for making fine writing-paper, as well as for paper of the coarser kinds. The manufacture of felt hats for the Bristol trade is chiefly at Frampton-Cotterell, Iron-Acton, Pucklechurch, Rangeworthy, and other villages in that neighbourhood. Flax-spinning forms a considerable part of the winter employment of the women in the upper part of the Vale of Evesham. In the Forest district are very ancient and extensive works both for the smelting of iron-ore and the manufacture of wrought-iron. The chief articles of export, besides those from the woollen cloth and pin manufactories, of the latter of which a great quantity is sent to America, are cheese, bacon, cider, perry, and all kinds of grain. Fat oxen, sheep, and pigs, are sent to the London market, as is also a considerable quantity of salmon.

The principal rivers are the Severn, the Wye, the Upper Avon, the Lower Avon, and the Isis, or Thames. The Severn, which is remarkable for the rapidity of its stream, and is navigable the whole of its course through this county, enters it near Tewkesbury, and at Maismore it divides into two channels, the city of Gloucester being situated upon the eastern; at a short distance below which they re-unite, and the width of the river increases rapidly as it passes Framilode, Newnham, and Thornbury, below which latter place it soon takes the name of the Bristol channel, and forms a grand æstuary not less than ten miles wide, which continues expanding until it mingles with the Atlantic ocean. The tide ni the Severn, well known for its boisterous and impetuous roar, comes up to Gloucester with great rapidity and violence, and the stream is turned by it as high as Tewkesbury. The greatest elevation occasioned by the tide in the river at Gloucester is nine feet, but the most usual is seven feet and a half. Its violence has often occasioned great damage to the adjoining county by sudden inundations, particularly in the years 1606, 1687, 1703, and 1737. To guard against these, much care has been taken, and great expense incurred, in making sea-walls and keeping them in repair; for the better management of which the parishes bordering on the east side of the river, from Arlingham, where the Upper Level commences, to King's Weston, where the Lower Level ends, are rated, according to the number of acres in each exposed to inundation. In each of the Levels are ten or twelve *pills*, or inlets into the country, by which the water on the surface is carried off, the works being repaired by the proprietors of the adjoining lands. The management is in the hands of commissioners of sewers, who hold meetings occasionally: the bailiwick of the Severn has often been let to farm by the crown. The fish found in the Severn are roach, dace, bleak, flounders, eels, elvers, chub, carp, trout, and perch: salmon, lampreys, lamperns, shad, soles, shrimps, cod, plaice, conger-eels, porpoises, sturgeons, and some other sea-fish, are taken within the limits of the county. The salmon, which has ever been reckoned the pride of the Severn, and in former times was caught in great abundance, is now comparatively a scarce fish. The Wye bounds this county on the west,

from the highest part of Ruer-Dean to its confluence with the Severn, separating it from Herefordshire and Monmouthshire, excepting a short interval near Monmouth, being navigable in all that part of its course: the western boundaries of the Forest of Dean form part of the celebrated scenery on the banks of this river. The Upper Avon, having passed through Warwickshire, bounds the northern extremity of Gloucestershire for two or three miles, then winding through part of Worcestershire, it enters this county about three miles above Tewkesbury, at which place it unites with the Severn, being navigable up to Stratford in Warwickshire: the fish of this river are roach, dace, bleak, carp, bream, and eels. The Lower Avon rises among the hills of North Wiltshire, and enters this county near Bath, where it becomes navigable: at Bristol it receives the waters of the Lower Frome, and, at about five miles below that city, falls into the Severn at Kingsroad: it forms the southern boundary of the county, separating it from Somersetshire, from a little above Bitton, about half way between Bath and Bristol, to its mouth. The Isis, or Thames, is generally reputed to rise at a spring called Thames-Head, in the parish of Cotes, in this county, which it shortly leaves for Wiltshire, but at Kempsford, having become navigable, it forms the boundary between that county and Gloucestershire, and so continues as far as Lechlade, where it enters Oxfordshire. The Chelt rises at Dowdeswell, and running by Cheltenham, falls into the Severn at Wainlode hill. The Leden, which rises in Herefordshire, enters this county at Preston, in the Forest district, and falls into the western channel of the Severn below Over's bridge. The Upper Frome, which rises at Brimpsfield, in Rapsgate Hundred, passes Stroud, where it is called the Stroud river, and joins the Severn at Framilode passage. The Ewelme rises at Owlpen, and flowing by Dursley, takes the name of Cam at the village of the same name, and falls into the Severn at Frampton Pill. The Middle Avon, formed by the junction of two small streams, crosses the road to Bristol at Stone, and having flowed under the walls of Berkeley castle, falls into the Severn about a mile below that town. The Winrush, remarkable for its fine trout and cray-fish, rises at Upper Guiting, passes through Bourton on the Water, and quits the county at Barrington. The Stroudwater canal, constructed about the year 1775, commences at Walbridge, in the parish of Stroud, and after a course of upwards of seven miles, opens into the Severn at Framilode. The advantages of this canal to the interests of the cloth manufacture were increased by the junction of the Thames and Severn, effected by a continuation of the above line of canal from Walbridge to Lechlade, a distance of upwards of twenty-eight miles. This part of the line, called the Thames and Severn canal, was opened in the year 1789: it has a tunnel through Sapperton-hill, two miles and three furlongs in length, fifteen feet high and fifteen feet wide, including six feet of water; while its depth from the surface is two hundred and forty feet. The Gloucester and Berkeley canal was designed to form a shorter and safer passage for vessels of large burden between Gloucester and the wider parts of the Severn; the distance being seventeen miles and a half: the basin at Gloucester was begun in 1794: from this place a rail-road extends to Cheltenham. The Hereford and Gloucester canal, intended to open a communication by water between the former city and Ledbury, Gloucester, Bristol, London, &c., was begun in 1792 : from Herefordshire it enters this county at its north-western extremity ; a tunnel, two thousand one hundred and seventy yards long, commences at Dymock and ends at Oxenhall, whence the canal descends the valley of the Leden, crosses that river by an aqueduct, and joins the western channel of the Severn at Gloucester. The road from London to Gloucester and Hereford enters the county at Lechlade, and passes through Fairford and Cirencester. The road from London to Cheltenham enters it about two miles beyond Burford, in Oxfordshire, and passes through North Leach. The road from London to Bristol enters through this county about a mile eastward from Marshfield, and, passing through that town, runs within the southern border of the county to Bristol.

Many tumuli, or barrows, are scattered over the county, but it cannot be ascertained whether any or which of them are British. The circumstance of the Romans having experienced little opposition from the Dobuni, is a probable reason why so few Roman stations and fortresses are to be found in the country which that British tribe inhabited. Ancient encampments are conspicuous on almost every eminence, but their origin is very uncertain : the principal are at Little Sodbury, Minchinhampton, Painswick, Twining, Haresfield, Tytherington, Elberton, Uley, Hatherop, North Leach, Oldbury, Cromhall, Beachley, Willersey, Staunton, and from the last place, at different intervals, along the edge of the whole Cotswold range to Bath, Henbury, and Clifton. Remains of Roman buildings, such as tesselated pavements, &c., have been discovered at Gloucester, Cirencester, Woodchester, Rodmarton, Colesborne, and Chedworth, particularly at the two first places. Roman coins have been found in various places, especially at Sapperton ; but the greater part of them are of the lower empire. Of the four great public or military roads of the Romans in Britain, three pass through Gloucestershire : the Fosse-way enters the county from the north at Lemington, and passing by North Leach and Cirencester, quits it about five miles beyond the latter town. The Iknield way enters from Oxfordshire at East Leach, and falls into the Fosse-way near Cirencester. The Ermin-street is supposed to have led from Caerleon in Monmouthshire, through Gloucester, to Cirencester and Cricklade, in its course to Southampton. Of ancient castles, only that of Berkeley, erected in the early part of the twelfth century, is entire ; there are inconsiderable remains of the castle of Beverstone, built prior to the Norman Conquest ; and more extensive relics of that of St. Briavells, built not long after the Conquest : but the most magnificent ruins of this class are those of Sudley castle, which was rebuilt about the year 1450 ; and of Thornbury castle, erected about 1511. The most remarkable ancient manor-houses remaining, wholly or in part, are, of the fifteenth century, Southam house, the manor-house of Frampton-Cotterell, Acton house, Wanswell house, and Olveston court ; of the Elizabethan age, Shipton-Cliffe house, Toddington house, Stanway house, Shurdington house, and Syston manor-house ; and of the seventeenth century, the mansion-houses of Higham, Highmeadow, Dyrham, and Hardwick ; of this last period also is the splendid mansion of the Duke of Beaufort, at Badminton. Before the Reformation

there were, according to Tanner, forty-seven monasteries, hospitals, and colleges in the county : the most considerable monastic remains are those of St. Peter's abbey at Gloucester, and of the abbeys of Tewkesbury, Cirencester, Hailes, and Kingswood. The churches are in general handsome structures ; the cathedral of Gloucester, and the churches of Tewkesbury, Cirencester, and Berkeley, exhibit the most interesting specimens of ancient ecclesiastical architecture ; the square-headed window is particularly observable in the churches in those parts of the county adjoining Somersetshire, where it is said that Henry VII. built many in reward for the attachment of that county to his cause. Fairford church is particularly distinguished for its ancient painted glass. Stone fonts of large dimensions, for immersion, are very common.

Fossils are found in great variety and abundance in almost every quarry that is opened on the Cotswolds. In the Vale, the beds of blue clay-stone are stored with the *cornua ammonis*, *conchæ rugosæ*, &c. Frethern cliff, the western shore of the Severn, near Awre, Pyrton passage, and Westbury cliff, afford similar fields of investigation for the naturalist ; as do various other parts of the county, though to a less extent. The springs which rise through beds of blue clay are often strongly saline, as at Prestbury, Cleeve, Cheltenham, Sandhurst, Hardwick, Eastington, Gloucester, &c. Of these waters, it is hardly necessary to observe that those of Cheltenham are the most celebrated.

GLOVERSTONE, a township in that part of the parish of St. Mary, Chester, which is in the lower division of the hundred of Broxton, county palatine of Chester. The population is returned with the parish.

GLUSBURN, a township in the parish of Kildwick, eastern division of the wapentake of Staincliffe and Ewcross, West riding of the county of York, 4½ miles (S.) from Skipton, containing 787 inhabitants. The manufacture of cotton is carried on here.

GLUVIAS, a parish in the hundred of Kerrier, county of Cornwall, ½ a mile (E.) from Penryn, containing, with the borough of Penryn, 3678 inhabitants. The living is a vicarage, with the perpetual curacy of Budock united, in the peculiar jurisdiction and patronage of the Bishop of Exeter, rated in the king's books at £21. 6. 10½. The church is dedicated to St. Mary Magdalene. On a moor called Glasenith, Walter Bronescomb, Bishop of Exeter, about 1270, built a collegiate church, in honour of the Blessed Virgin Mary and St. Thomas of Canterbury, for a provost, a sacrist, eleven prebendaries, seven vicars, and six choristers, whose annual revenue at the dissolution was valued at £205. 10. 6. Bohelland, in this parish, is said to have been the scene of the murder of a son by his father, which furnished the plot of Lillo's tragedy of " Fatal Curiosity :" this unnatural event happened about 1618, and the site of the house of the murderer is still pointed out, but the name of the family has been consigned to oblivion.

GLYMPTON, a parish in the hundred of Wootton, county of Oxford, 4 miles (N. by W.) from Woodstock, containing 141 inhabitants. The living is a rectory, in the archdeaconry and diocese of Oxford, rated in the king's books at £6. 16. 0½. The Rev. T. Nucella was patron in 1818. The church is dedicated to St. Mary.

GLYND, a parish in the hundred of Ringmer, rape of Pevensey, county of Sussex, 3¼ miles (E.S.E.) from Lewes, containing 250 inhabitants. The living is a discharged vicarage, in the peculiar jurisdiction of the Archbishop of Canterbury, rated in the king's books at £5. 1. 3., endowed with £200 private benefaction, and £200 royal bounty, and in the patronage of the Dean and Canons of Windsor. About sixteen children are educated by a schoolmistress, for the interest of £100 bequeathed by Mary Trevor.

GNOSALL, a parish in the western division of the hundred of Cuttlestone, county of Stafford, comprising the townships of Cowley, Gnosall, Knightley, and a part of Apeton, Alstone, Brough, and Rule, and the hamlet of Moreton, and containing 2671 inhabitants, of which number, 1038 are in the township of Gnosall, 6½ miles (W. S.W.) from Stafford. The living is a perpetual curacy, in the peculiar jurisdiction of the Lord of the Manor of Gnosall, endowed with £400 parliamentary grant, and in the patronage of the Bishop of Lichfield and Coventry. The church, dedicated to St. Lawrence, has lately received an addition of three hundred free sittings, the Incorporated Society for the enlargement of churches and chapels having granted £150 towards defraying the expense. It was given by King Stephen to the church of Lichfield, but afterwards became a royal free chapel, and had an establishment of secular canons; in the reign of Henry VIII., the Bishop of Lichfield and Coventry was titular dean, to which office no profits were attached, and there were four prebendaries, viz., of Chiltenhall, Baverley-hall, Mordhall, and Suckerhall; the first valued at £14. 6. 8., and the others at £11 each per annum. Edward Cartwright, in 1653, enfeoffed to trustees a cottage and ground for the education of fourteen children; the income is £21. 4. 6. per annum. Five others are instructed by a schoolmistress for £2 per annum, the gift of Alice Hudson in 1660.

GOADBY, a chapelry in the parish of Billesdon, hundred of Gartree, county of Leicester, 8 miles (N. by E.) from Market-Harborough, containing 96 inhabitants.

GOADBY-MARWOOD, a parish in the hundred of Framland, county of Leicester, 5½ miles (N.N.E.) from Melton-Mowbray, containing 171 inhabitants. The living is a rectory, in the archdeaconry of Leicester, and diocese of Lincoln, rated in the king's books at £16, and in the patronage of Mrs. Ann Stafford. The church, dedicated to St. Denis, has portions in the decorated style of architecture. Many Roman coins and urns, with the head of an arrow, and human bones in abundance, have been discovered at different times; and a skull of extraordinary size, the teeth perfectly white, complete in number, and the whole double, was found, about 1813, at the depth of seven feet below the surface.

GOADLAND, otherwise GOATHLAND, a chapelry in the parish and lythe of Pickering, North riding of the county of York, 13¼ miles (N. by E.) from Pickering, containing 335 inhabitants. The living is a perpetual curacy, in the peculiar jurisdiction of the Dean of York, endowed with £1200 royal bounty. The chapel, a neat edifice, was erected in 1821. In the dale of Goadland, within the ancient honour of Pickering Forest the tenants were bound to promote the breed of a large species of hawk that resorted to a cliff called Killing Nab Scar, and to secure them for the king: these birds

continue to haunt the same place, but it is remarkable that there is seldom more than one brood produced in a year.

GOAT, a joint township with Papcastle, in the parish of Bridekirk, Allerdale ward below Darwent, county of Cumberland, containing 384 inhabitants. The village is connected with the town of Cockermouth by a stone bridge across the Darwent: the knights of the shire are elected on a plot of ground within its limits; and here are some corn-mills.

GOATHILL, a parish in the hundred of Horethorne, county of Somerset, 2¼ miles (E.) from Sherborne, containing 20 inhabitants. The living is a discharged rectory, in the archdeaconry of Wells, and diocese of Bath and Wells, rated in the king's books at £3. 11. 10½. The Earl of Digby was patron in 1797. The church is dedicated to St. Peter.

GOATHURST, a parish in the hundred of Andersfield, county of Somerset, 3½ miles (S. W. by W.) from Bridg-water, containing 342 inhabitants. The living is a rectory, in the archdeaconry of Taunton, and diocese of Bath and Wells, rated in the king's books at £9. 10. 7½., and in the patronage of C. H. K. Tynte, Esq. The church, dedicated to St. Edward, contains a handsome monument to the memory of Sir C. Tynte, who sat as knight of the shire in five successive parliaments: a neat chapel serves as the mausoleum of this ancient family. The memory of a religious house is still preserved in the names Chantry and Sanctuary which distinguish parts of the aprish.

GODALMING, a market town and parish in the first division of the hundred of Godalming, county of Surrey, 4 miles (S.S.W.) from Guildford, and 34 (S. W.) from London, containing 4098 inhabitants. This place is supposed by Aubrey to have been called Goda's Alming, from Goda, Countess of Mercia, to whom it belonged, and from the circumstance of her having be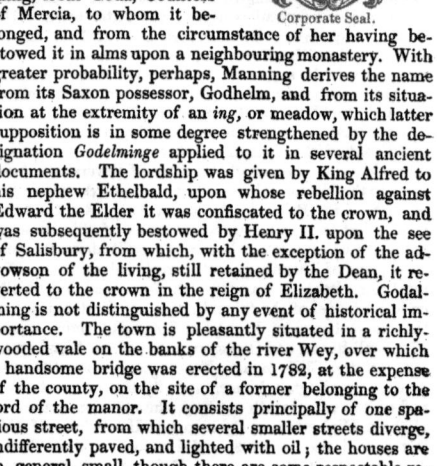

Corporate Seal.

stowed it in alms upon a neighbouring monastery. With greater probability, perhaps, Manning derives the name from its Saxon possessor, Godhelm, and from its situation at the extremity of an ing, or meadow, which latter supposition is in some degree strengthened by the designation Godelminge applied to it in several ancient documents. The lordship was given by King Alfred to his nephew Ethelbald, upon whose rebellion against Edward the Elder it was confiscated to the crown, and was subsequently bestowed by Henry II. upon the see of Salisbury, from which, with the exception of the advowson of the living, still retained by the Dean, it reverted to the crown in the reign of Elizabeth. Godalming is not distinguished by any event of historical importance. The town is pleasantly situated in a richly-wooded vale on the banks of the river Wey, over which a handsome bridge was erected in 1782, at the expense of the county, on the site of a former belonging to the lord of the manor. It consists principally of one spacious street, from which several smaller streets diverge, indifferently paved, and lighted with oil; the houses are in general small, though there are some respectable residences of modern erection, and the inhabitants are amply supplied with excellent water. The principal articles of manufacture are stockings, worsted and cotton shirts, and drawers, silk, paper, parchment, with tanned and oiled leather, and a considerable trade is carried on in timber, bark, and hoops, of which great quantities are shipped for London. The river Wey, at an expense of £8000, subscribed in shares, was in 1780 made navigable to the town, where a convenient wharf has been constructed; and the Wey and Arun canal passes through the parish. The market is on Wednesday, for corn, and on Saturday also for poultry and vegetables; the fairs are on February 13th and July 10th, at the former a great quantity of hoops is sold. The inhabitants received a charter of incorporation, in 1575, from Queen Elizabeth, by which the government is vested in a warden, bailiff, and eight assistants. The warden is annually elected on Michaelmas-day, from three assistants, nominated for that purpose by the inhabitants; the bailiff is elected at the same time by the warden, and, both having filled the office, they are exempt from serving again for three years; the assistants hold their office for life. The corporation do not exercise magisterial authority, the town being within the jurisdiction of the county magistrates. Courts leet and baron are held annually, at the former of which, constables, tythingmen, and other officers, are appointed. The town-hall is a neat edifice, erected in 1814, by public subscription, and is commodiously arranged for the transaction of public business.

The living is a vicarage, in the archdeaconry of Surrey, and diocese of Winchester, rated in the king's books at £23. 17. 11., and in the patronage of the Dean of Salisbury. The church, dedicated to St. Peter and St. Paul, is an ancient cruciform structure in the early style of English architecture, with later insertions, and having a tower surmounted by a spire. There are places of worship for General Baptists, the Society of Friends, Independents, and Wesleyan Methodists. Almshouses for ten aged persons were founded in 1618, by Mr. Richard Wyatt, who bequeathed £500 for their erection, and lands producing, with subsequent benefactions, more than £150 per annum, for their endowment; they are under the control of the Master and Wardens of the Carpenters' Company, who nominate the brethren: the premises comprise ten tenements under one roof, each containing a lower and an upper room; in the centre is a commodious chapel, and behind are two acres and a half of garden ground in allotments. There are a National and a Lancasterian school supported by subscription, in which four hundred children of both sexes are instructed, and part of an estate, producing nearly £300 per annum, left by Mr. Henry Smith, for the relief of the poor, is appropriated to the clothing and apprenticing of poor children. Near Busbridge is Old Minster field, the site of an ancient chapel mentioned in Domesday-book. The Rev. Owen Manning, F. R. S. and F. S. A., author of the History and Antiquities of the county of Surrey, and thirty-seven years vicar of this parish, was buried here in 1801.

GODDINGTON, a parish in the hundred of PLOUGHLEY, county of OXFORD, 5½ miles (N. E.) from Bicester, containing 110 inhabitants. The living is a rectory, in the archdeaconry and diocese of Oxford, rated in the

king s books at £7. 18. 9., and in the patronage of the President and Fellows of Corpus Christi College, Oxford. The church is dedicated to the Holy Trinity.

GODLEY, a township in the parish of MOTTRAM in LONGDEN DALE, hundred of MACCLESFIELD, county palatine of CHESTER, 6 miles (N. E. by E.) from Stockport, containing 514 inhabitants. Godley is a corruption of Godleigh, the name of its possessors in the reign of John. The manufacture of cotton here is principally carried on by hand-loom weaving, and there is some business in the making of hats.

GODMANCHESTER, a corporate town and parish in the hundred of TOSELAND, county of HUNTINGDON, ¾ of a mile (S. E. by S.) from Huntingdon, containing 1953 inhabitants. The town, situated on the banks of the Ouse, over which there is a bridge, is supposed to occupy the site of the Roman station *Durolipons*, and Roman coins have frequently been dug up in the neighbourhood.

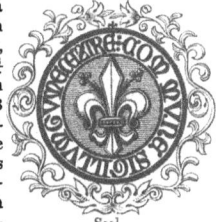

Seal.

Under the dominion of the Danes, the name was changed to Gormanchester, from Gormund, or Guthrum, a Danish chief, who is said to have founded a castle here in the reign of Alfred the Great. A fair is held annually on Easter Tuesday, chiefly for horses. In 1605, a charter of incorporation was granted, incorporating the inhabitants under the government of two bailiffs, twelve assistants, with a recorder, high steward, and town clerk: the bailiffs are chosen annually; and the bailiffs for the preceding years act as coroners. A commission of the peace was granted to the borough in 1637, under which the bailiffs acted as justices till September 8th, 1702, since which they have not exercised any magisterial authority. A court of pleas, for the recovery of debts under 40s., is held every three weeks. The living is a vicarage, in the archdeaconry of Huntingdon, and diocese of Lincoln, rated in the king's books at £17. 0. 5., and in the patronage of the Dean and Chapter of Westminster. The church, dedicated to St. Mary, has some portions in the later English style, particularly some windows and an entrance porch, which are tolerably well executed. A free grammar school was founded by charter of Elizabeth, in 1561, and endowed with landed property at Godmanchester, by Richard Robins, in 1576, but the only funds at present belonging to it are £20 per annum, from Emanuel College, Cambridge. There are several charitable benefactions for apprenticing poor children.

GODMANSTONE, a parish in the hundred of CERNE, TOTCOMBE, and MODBURY, Cerne sub-division of the county of DORSET, 5 miles (N. N. W.) from Dorchester, containing 128 inhabitants. The living is a rectory, in the archdeaconry of Dorset, and diocese of Bristol, rated in the king's books at £13. 6. 8. J. Goodenough, Esq. was patron in 1824. The church is dedicated to the Holy Trinity.

GODMERSHAM, a parish in the hundred of FELBOROUGH, lathe of SCRAY, county of KENT, 6¼ miles (N. E. by N.) from Ashford, containing 414 inhabitants. The living is a vicarage with the perpetual curacy of Challock annexed, in the peculiar jurisdiction and patronage of the Archbishop of Canterbury, rated in the king's books at £9. 3. 9. The church, dedicated to St. Lawrence, has in it eight stalls; it was formerly appropriated to the prior and monks of Canterbury, and had a chantry. The priors resided in a house near the church, which is still called the priory, and retains much of its ancient appearance: they had liberty of free warren, and obtained the privilege of a weekly market, which has been long disused. The river Stour runs through the parish. There are eight almshouses, also a charity school which is supported by voluntary contributions.

GODNEY, a chapelry in the parish of MEARE, hundred of GLASTON-TWELVE-HIDES, county of SOMERSET, 2½ miles (N. N. W.) from Glastonbury. The population is returned with the parish. The living is a perpetual curacy, within the jurisdiction of the peculiar court of Glastonbury, endowed with £1000 royal bounty. The chapel, dedicated to the Holy Trinity, stands upon the site of a more ancient edifice; at the west end is an inscription stating that it was restored, in 1737, by Peter Davis, Esq., Recorder of Wells.

GODOLPHIN, a hamlet in the parish of BREAGE, hundred of KERRIER, county of CORNWALL, 5¾ miles (N. W. by W.) from Helston. It was anciently called Godolcan, and has been long celebrated for its tin mines: it gave name to the family of Godolphin, who were its lords in the time of William the Conqueror. Sir Francis Godolphin, by his perseverance and success in mining, increased the customs more than £10,000 per annum in the reign of Elizabeth. Sidney, son of Sir William Godolphin, Bart., a distinguished statesman, was created Baron Godolphin of Rialton, in 1689, which title is now extinct.

GODSFIELD, an extra-parochial liberty, in the hundred of BOUNTISBOROUGH, Fawley division of the county of SOUTHAMPTON, 3 miles (N. N. E.) from New Alresford, containing 8 inhabitants.

GODSHILL, a tything in the parish and hundred of FORDINGBRIDGE, New Forest (West) division of the county of SOUTHAMPTON, 2 miles (E. by N.) from Fordingbridge, containing 158 inhabitants.

GODSHILL, a parish in the liberty of EAST MEDINA, Isle of Wight division of the county of SOUTHAMPTON, 5½ miles (S. S. E.) from Newport, containing 1214 inhabitants. The living is a discharged vicarage, with the rectory of Neighton and the curacy of Whitwell, in the archdeaconry and diocese of Winchester, rated in the king's books at £37. 17. 6., and in the patronage of the Provost and Fellows of Queen's College, Oxford. The church, dedicated to All Saints, has lately received an addition of one hundred and sixty free sittings, the Incorporated Society for the enlargement of churches and chapels having granted £50 towards defraying the expense. Here is a place of worship for Wesleyan Methodists. A free school was founded in 1593, by Philip Andrews and others, who endowed it with an annuity of £5, in aid of which, Lady Ann Worsley, in 1615, gave twenty marks a year, and Sir Richard Worsley bequeathed a rent-charge of £11. 6. 8., also a messuage called the Chantry-house, wherein the school was then kept. Richard Gard, in 1617, gave £5 per annum towards the support of an usher, whose salary is £10, and the master's £11. 6. 8.: the children are taught in a school-house erected in 1804, by Lord Yarborough.

GODSTONE, a parish in the first division of the hundred of TANDRIDGE, county of SURREY, 19 miles (S. by E.) from London, containing 1210 inhabitants. The living is a rectory, with the vicarage of Walkinstead, in the archdeaconry of Surrey, and diocese of Winchester, and in the patronage of the Rev. Charles James Hoare. The church, dedicated to St. Nicholas, has lately received an addition of one hundred and nineteen sittings, of which seventy-eight are free, the Incorporated Society for the enlargement of churches and chapels having granted £80 towards defraying the expense. There is also a chapel endowed with about £30 per annum, to which is annexed some provision for the education of children. David Maynard, in 1709, gave £200, producing £10 per annum, for which seventeen children are instructed. The petty sessions for the division are held here monthly. Some good stone quarries are worked in the parish, whence it is said to derive its name. There is a mineral spring containing sulphate of magnesia, and of similar properties to the Cheltenham water.

GODWICK, a parish in the hundred of LAUNDITCH, county of NORFOLK, 5¾ miles (S. S. W.) from Fakenham. The population is returned with the parish of Tittleshall. The living is a discharged rectory, united to that of Tittleshall, in the archdeaconry and diocese of Norwich, rated in the king's books at £1. 10. 10. The church has been demolished.

GOLBORN-BELLOW, a township in the parish of TATTENHALL, lower division of the hundred of BROXTON, county palatine of CHESTER, 7 miles (S. E.) from Chester, containing 86 inhabitants.

GOLBORN-DAVID, a township in that part of the parish of HANDLEY which is in the lower division of the hundred of BROXTON, county palatine of CHESTER, 6½ miles (S. E. by S.) from Chester, containing 76 inhabitants.

GOLBORNE, a township in the parish of WINWICK, hundred of WEST DERBY, county palatine of LANCASTER, 2 miles (N. N. E.) from Newton in Makerfield, containing 1310 inhabitants. William Street, in 1791, conveyed to certain trustees a dwelling-house, schoolroom, and garden, which, with the proceeds of £120 raised at the same time by subscription, are enjoyed by a schoolmaster, for teaching six children.

GOLCAR, a chapelry in the parish of HUDDERSFIELD, upper division of the wapentake of AGBRIGG, West riding of the county of YORK, 3¼ miles (W. by S.) from Huddersfield, containing 2606 inhabitants. There is a chapel now building by the Commissioners appointed under the act passed in the 58th of George III., for promoting the erection of additional churches.

GOLDCLIFF, a parish in the lower division of the hundred of CALDICOTT, county of MONMOUTH, 4½ miles (S. E.) from Newport, containing 268 inhabitants. The living is a discharged vicarage, with that of Nash, in the archdeaconry and diocese of Llandaff, rated in the king's books at £13. 2. 6., endowed with £200 private benefaction, and £200 royal bounty, and in the patronage of the Provost and Fellows of Eton College. The church, dedicated to St. Mary Magdalene, was founded and liberally endowed in 1113, by Robert de Chandos, who, by the desire of Henry I., gave it to the abbey of Bec, in Normandy, upon which a prior and twelve Black monks were placed here. In 1442, after the suppression of Alien priories, it was made a cell to the abbey of Tewkesbury, and at the dissolution possessed a revenue of £ 144. 18. 1. The parish is bounded by the Bristol channel on the south, at which point the cliff, whence its name is derived, rises abruptly from the extremity of a marshy flat, to a height of about one hundred feet above the level of the sea; it is a single rock consisting of horizontal strata of limestone, under which is a body of hard brown grit, full of yellow *micæ*.

GOLDHANGER, a parish in the hundred of THURS-TABLE, county of ESSEX, 4¼ miles (E.N.E.) from Maldon, containing 459 inhabitants. The living is a rectory, in the archdeaconry of Colchester, and diocese of London, rated in the king's books at £25. 19. 4½. N. Westcombe, Esq. was patron in 1798. The church is dedicated to St. Peter. The parish is bounded on the south by the Blackwater river and Osey island. There are very extensive salterns, at which the manufacture of salt from sea-water is carried on with considerable success by the agency of steam: they are recorded in Domesday-book as existing at the time of the Norman survey.

GOLDINGTON, a parish in the hundred of BARFORD, county of BEDFORD, 1¾ mile (N. E. by E.) from Bedford, containing 426 inhabitants. The living is a vicarage, in the archdeaconry and diocese of Lincoln, rated in the king's books at £8. 9. 4½., and in the patronage of the Duke of Bedford. The church is dedicated to St. Mary. The navigable river Ouse bounds the parish on the south. There is a lofty conical mound, the remains of an ancient fortification, called Castle hill. In the reign of Henry II., Simon Beauchamp founded a monastery in honour of St. Paul, and removed hither the Black canons of the priory of St. Paul's, Bedford; at the dissolution its revenue was estimated at £343. 15. 5.

GOLDSBOROUGH, a parish in the upper division of the wapentake of CLARO, West riding of the county of YORK, comprising the townships of Coneythorp, Flaxby, and Goldsborough, and containing 385 inhabitants, of which number, 195 are in the township of Goldsborough, 2¾ miles (E.S.E.) from Knaresborough. The living is a rectory, in the archdeaconry of Richmond, and diocese of Chester, rated in the king's books at £10. 1. 0½. The Earl of Harewood was patron in 1803. The church is dedicated to St. Mary.

GOLDSHAW-BOOTH, a chapelry in that part of the parish of WHALLEY which is in the higher division of the hundred of BLACKBURN, county palatine of LANCASTER, 3 miles (N.E. by N.) from Haslingden, containing 819 inhabitants. The living is a perpetual curacy, in the archdeaconry and diocese of Chester, endowed with £1000 royal bounty, and £1400 parliamentary grant, and in the patronage of the Vicar of Whalley. The chapel has received an addition of three hundred and eighty sittings, of which, three hundred are free, the Incorporated Society for the enlargement of churches and chapels having granted £300 towards defraying the expense. Heald yarn is manufactured here.

GOLTHO, a parish in the western division of the wapentake of WRAGGOE, parts of LINDSEY, county of LINCOLN, 1½ mile (W. by S.) from Wragby, containing 95 inhabitants. The living is a perpetual curacy with Bullington, in the peculiar jurisdiction of the Bishop of Lincoln, and in the patronage of T. Mainwaring, Esq.

GOMELDON, a tything in the parish of IDMISTON,

hundred of ALDERBURY, county of WILTS, containing 50 inhabitants.

GOMERSALL, a township comprising Great Gomersall and Little Gomersall, in the parish of BIRSTALL, wapentake of MORLEY, West riding of the county of YORK, containing 5952 inhabitants. Great Gomersall is 5¾ miles (S.E.), and Little Gomersall 6¼ (S.E. by S.), from Bradford. The Independents, Moravians, and Wesleyan Methodists, have each a place of worship here. Blankets and woollen cloths are manufactured to a considerable extent, and there are coal works in the immediate neighbourhood. Though the village of Birstall is within the limits of this township, it gives name to the parish of which Gomersall forms a part.

GOMERSHAY, a tything in the parish of STALBRIDGE, hundred of BROWNSHALL, Sturminster division of the county of DORSET, 1 mile (W.) from Stalbridge, containing 88 inhabitants.

GONALDSTON, a parish in the southern division of the wapentake of THURGARTON, county of NOTTINGHAM, 4¾ miles (S.S.W.) from Southwell, containing 96 inhabitants. The living is a rectory, in the archdeaconry of Nottingham, and diocese of York, rated in the king's books at £7. 19. 2. W. Leland, Esq. was patron in 1811. The church is dedicated to St. Lawrence. There is an endowed school for six boys, also an ancient hospital, called the Spittle, founded by William Heriz in the reign of Henry III.

GONERBY (GREAT), a parish in the soke of GRANTHAM, parts of KESTEVEN, county of LINCOLN, 1½ mile (N.N.W.) from Grantham, containing 743 inhabitants. The living is a vicarage not in charge, united to that of North Grantham, in the archdeaconry and diocese of Lincoln. The church, dedicated to St. Sebastian, has an embattled tower surmounted by a spire.

GONERBY (LITTLE), a joint township with Manthorp, in the soke and borough of GRANTHAM, parts of KESTEVEN, county of LINCOLN, ½ a mile (N.W.) from Grantham, containing, with Manthorp, 1175 inhabitants.

GOODERSTONE, a parish in the southern division of the hundred of GREENHOE, county of NORFOLK, 4¼ miles (E.N.E.) from Stoke-Ferry, containing 439 inhabitants. The living is a discharged vicarage, in the archdeaconry of Norfolk, and diocese of Norwich, rated in the king's books at £6. 12., endowed with £200 royal bounty. E. Horrex, Esq. was patron in 1816. The church, dedicated to St. George, is built of boulder-stones, having at the west end a large square tower of flint, with quoins and battlements of freestone: the south aisle was formerly the chantry of St. George's guild, be sides which several others were held in the church: in the chancel are six stalls used by the chantry priests.

GOODLEIGH, a parish in the hundred of BRAUNTON, county of DEVON, 2¾ miles (E. by N.) from Barnstaple, containing 351 inhabitants. The living is a rectory, in the archdeaconry of Barnstaple, and diocese of Exeter, rated in the king's books at £14. 19. 4½. The Rev. W. Churchward was patron in 1791. The church is dedicated to St. Gregory. Here is a place of worship for Independents. The river Yeo runs through the parish, which is noted for the production of cherries.

GOODMANHAM, a parish partly in the liberty of ST. PETER of YORK, but chiefly in the Holme-Beacon division of the wapentake of HARTHILL, East riding of the county of York, 1¼ mile (N.E. by N.) from Market-Weighton, containing 240 inhabitants. The living is a rectory, in the archdeaconry of the East riding, and diocese of York, rated in the king's books at £12.11.8. The Rev. W. Blow was patron in 1819. The church, dedicated to All Saints, is principally in the Norman style of architecture, with later additions. Stukeley says " the Apostle Paulinus built the parish church of God-mundham, where is the font in which he baptized the heathen high priest Colfi : " there is reason to suppose, from the appearance of the structure, that the materials for its erection were taken from the ruins of the chief pagan temple in Northumbria, which stood in the neighbourhood, at or near the *Delgovitia* of the Romans, the site being still plainly traceable by numerous artificial mounds, now called the Howe hills.

GOODNESTON, a parish in the hundred of Favers-HAM, lathe of Scray, county of Kent, 2 miles (E.) from Faversham, containing 66 inhabitants. The living is a discharged rectory, united to the vicarage of Graveney, in the archdeaconry and diocese of Canterbury, rated in the king's books at £5. 2. 6. The church is dedicated to St. Bartholomew.

GOODNESTONE, a parish in the hundred of Wing-HAM, lathe of St. Augustine, county of Kent, 2½ miles (S.E.) from Wingham, containing 432 inhabitants. The living is a perpetual curacy, in the archdeaconry and diocese of Canterbury, and in the patronage of Sir B. C. Bridges, Bart. The church, dedicated to the Holy Cross, is principally in the early style of English architecture, and was partly erected by the ancestors of Sir John Boys, the gallant defender of Donnington castle, who died in 1664, and was buried here.

GOODRICH, or GODERICH, a parish in the lower division of the hundred of Wormelow, county of Here-FORD, 5¼ miles (S.W. by S.) from Ross, comprising the townships of Glewston, Goodrich, and Huntisham, and containing 711 inhabitants. The living is a vicarage, in the archdeaconry and diocese of Hereford, rated in the king's books at £8, and in the patronage of the Bishop of Hereford. The church is dedicated to St. Giles; for the repairing and beautifying of it there is a bequest by Mr. Gardner, producing £23 per annum. A bridge has been lately built across the Wye, at an expense of £8000, by which there is a free communication with the Forest of Dean. Richard Talbot, lord of Goderich castle, founded and endowed, in 1347, a small priory of Black canons, in honour of St. John the Baptist, the revenue of which, at the dissolution, was valued at £15. 8. 9. On a lofty and beautifully wooded hill are the majestic remains of the old castle of the Talbots, and near it there is another recently erected by Dr. Meyrick, in the ancient baronial style, forming prominent and interesting objects in the general beauty of the scene. Some years ago, two human skeletons were discovered in the vicinity, lying across each other. The Right Hon. Frederick John Robinson was elevated to the peerage by the title of Viscount Goderich, on the 25th of April, 1827.

GOOLE, a township in that part of the parish of Snaith which is in the lower division of the wapentake of Osgoldcross, West riding of the county of York, 5 miles (S.) from Howden, containing 450 inhabitants. This township is within the peculiar jurisdiction of the ecclesiastical court of Snaith. Goole, which is gradually rising in wealth and importance, is situated at the conflux of the Dutch river with the Ouse, across which there is a new bridge, and in the vicinity are spacious docks ; several additional buildings have been erected since the recent extension of the Ouse navigation. There is a place of worship for Independents. A free school for twelve children is endowed with lands producing an income of £21 per annum.

GOOSEY, a joint chapelry with Circourt, in that part of the parish of Stamford in the Vale which is in the hundred of Ock, county of Berks, 3¾ miles (N.W.) from Wantage, containing 159 inhabitants. The chapel is dedicated to All Saints.

GOOSNARGH, a chapelry in the parish of Kirk-HAM, hundred of Amounderness, county palatine of Lancaster, 6¼ miles (N.N.E.) from Preston, containing, with the township of Newsham, 1852 inhabitants. The living is a perpetual curacy, in the archdeaconry of Richmond, and diocese of Chester, endowed with £400 private benefaction, £400 royal bounty, and £200 parliamentary grant, and in the patronage of the Vicar of Kirkham. A free grammar school is endowed with various bequests producing £40 per annum, which is paid to the master, and with £30 a year, the bequest of Henry Colborne, for the maintenance of an usher. An hospital for decayed persons was founded and richly endowed by the Rev. William Bushell, D.D., in 1735.

GOOSTREY, a joint chapelry with Barnshaw, in that part of the parish of Sandbach which is in the hundred of Northwich, county palatine of Chester, 5½ miles (N.E. by E.) from Middlewich, containing 298 inhabitants. The living is a perpetual curacy, in the archdeaconry and diocese of Chester, endowed with £600 private benefaction, and £600 royal bounty, and in the patronage of the Vicar of Sandbach. The interest of £200 was bequeathed to the minister in 1684, by Elizabeth Staplehurst, for teaching the children in the parish.

GOPSALL, an extra-parochial liberty, in the hundred of Sparkenhoe, county of Leicester, 4¼ miles (N.W. by W.) from Market-Bosworth, containing 7 inhabitants. Here was formerly a cell to the abbey of Merevale, in the county of Warwick. Gopsall is in the honour of Tutbury, duchy of Lancaster, and within the jurisdiction of a court of pleas held at Tutbury every third Tuesday, for the recovery of debts under 40s.

GORE-END, a member of the town and port of Dovor, in the parish of Birchington, locally in the hundred of Ringslow, or Isle of Thanet, lathe of St. Augustine, county of Kent, 4½ miles (W.) from Margate. The population is returned with the parish.

GOREFIELDS, an extra-parochial liberty, in the hundred of Newport, county of Buckingham, 3 miles (N.W.) from Newport-Pagnell. There was formerly a monastery at this place, but from its early destruction nothing particular is now known of it.

GORING, a parish in the hundred of Langtree, county of Oxford, 6¼ miles (S. by W.) from Walling-ford, containing 867 inhabitants. The living is a perpetual curacy, in the archdeaconry and diocese of Oxford, endowed with £600 private benefaction, £200 royal bounty, and £1200 parliamentary grant. S. Gardener, Esq. was patron in 1822. The church is dedicated to St. Thomas à Becket. There is a place of worship for Independents. Henry Alnutt, Esq., in 1724, bequeathed an estate in trust, among other purposes, for apprenticing children of the parishes of Goring, Cassington, Checkendon, Ipstone, and Southstoke : the income is about £450 a year, for which they are educated, partly clothed, and apprenticed. The Iknield street here crosses the Thames into Berkshire. A priory of nuns of the order of St. Augustine was founded in the reign of Henry II., and dedicated to the Blessed Virgin Mary, the revenue of which at the dissolution was valued at £60. 5. 6.

GORING, a parish in the hundred of POLING, rape of ARUNDEL, county of SUSSEX, 2½ miles (W.) from Worthing, containing 476 inhabitants. The living is a discharged vicarage, in the archdeaconry and diocese of Chichester, rated in the king's books at £7. 10. W.W. Richardson, Esq. was patron in 1812. The church, dedicated to St. Mary, is in the early style of English architecture.

GORLESTON, a parish in the hundred of MUTFORD and LOTHINGLAND, county of SUFFOLK, containing 1928 inhabitants. The living is a discharged vicarage, with which the rectory of South Town was consolidated in 1520, in the archdeaconry of Suffolk, and diocese of Norwich, rated in the king's books at £11. Mrs. Astley was patroness in 1814. The church is dedicated to St. Andrew. There are places of worship for Independents and Wesleyan Methodists. The parish is bounded on the east by the North sea, and on the north by Bredonwater, where a bridge connects the village of Gorleston, or Little Yarmouth as it is sometimes called, with the town of Great Yarmouth. A house of Augustine friars was founded in the reign of Edward I.; and an hospital for lepers existed here in 1372.

GORRAN, a parish in the eastern division of the hundred of POWDER, county of CORNWALL, 5¾ miles (E. S. E.) from Tregoney, containing 1203 inhabitants. The living is a vicarage, in the archdeaconry of Cornwall, and diocese of Exeter, rated in the king's books at £20, and in the patronage of the Bishop of Exeter. There is a place of worship for Wesleyan Methodists. The vicarage-house, called Polgarran, was the residence of Mr. Anthony Wills, who, with his six sons, joined the Prince of Orange (afterwards William III.), on his landing in England : one of the sons became a distinguished general in the reign of George I. At Port East, on the coast of the English channel, a great quantity of pilchards is cured for exportation.

GORTON, a chapelry in the parish of MANCHESTER, hundred of SALFORD, county palatine of LANCASTER, 4 miles (E.S.E.) from Manchester, containing 1604 inhabitants. The living is a perpetual curacy, in the archdeaconry of Richmond, and diocese of Chester, endowed with £400 private benefaction, and £400 royal bounty, and in the patronage of the Warden and Fellows of the Collegiate Church of Manchester. The chapel is dedicated to St. James. A school-room, with a dwelling-house for the master, has been erected by subscription : the pupils pay quarterage. In Gorton Vale there is a reservoir comprising seventy-one acres, formed by the Manchester water-works company, for the partial supply of that town. The several branches of spinning, manufacturing, and printing cotton, are carried on here.

GOSBECK, a parish in the hundred of BOSMERE and CLAYDON, county of SUFFOLK, 4¾ miles (E. by N.) from Needham, containing 308 inhabitants. The living is a discharged rectory, in the archdeaconry of Suffolk,

and diocese of Norwich, rated in the king's books at £8. 5. 5. John Vernon, Esq. was patron in 1813. The church, dedicated to St. Mary, stands half a mile eastward from the village.

GOSBERTON, a parish in the wapentake of KIRTON, parts of HOLLAND, county of LINCOLN, 6 miles (N. by W.) from Spalding, containing 1618 inhabitants. The living is a discharged vicarage, in the archdeaconry and diocese of Lincoln, endowed with £200 private benefaction, £200 royal bounty, and £400 parliamentary grant, and in the patronage of the Dean and Chapter of Lincoln. The church is dedicated to St. Peter and St. Paul.

GOSEBRADON, a parish in the hundred of ABDICK and BULSTONE, county of SOMERSET, 5 miles (N.) from Ilminster. The living is a sinecure rectory, in the archdeaconry of Taunton, and diocese of Bath and Wells, rated in the king's books at £1. 2. 6. The church has been demolished, and there is neither house nor inhabitant in the parish.

GOSFIELD, a parish in the hundred of HINCKFORD, county of ESSEX, 2¾ miles (W.S.W.) from Halstead, containing 598 inhabitants. The living is a discharged vicarage, in the archdeaconry of Middlesex, and diocese of London, rated in the king's books at £8, endowed with £400 private benefaction, and £200 royal bounty. The Duke of Buckingham was patron in 1782. The church is dedicated to St. Catherine. A portion of Gosfield-hall exhibits a good specimen of the domestic style of architecture prevalent in the reign of Henry VIII.

GOSFORD, a township in the parish of KIDLINGTON, hundred of WOOTTON, county of OXFORD, 4¾ miles (N.) from Oxford, containing 47 inhabitants. According to Tanner, here was a house of sisters of the order of St. John of Jerusalem, who removed about 1180 to Buckland, in Somersetshire : the estate, which was given to them by Robert D'Oily and his son, continued in the possession of the hospitallers, who built an oratory or chapel here about the year 1234, until the period of the dissolution.

GOSFORTH, a parish in ALLERDALE ward above Darwent, county of CUMBERLAND, 6¾ miles (S.E.) from Egremont, comprising the townships of High Bolton, Low Bolton, and Bornwood, and containing 888 inhabitants. The living is a discharged rectory, in the archdeaconry of Richmond, and diocese of Chester, rated in the king's books at £17. 14. 7., and endowed with £400 parliamentary grant. Mrs. W. Senhouse was patroness in 1827. The church is dedicated to St. Mary. In the church-yard is an ancient stone pillar, which was formerly surmounted by a cross. Several rivulets run through the parish, and fall, with the Bleng, into the Irt. An abundance of freestone is obtained here. On Bornwood common are fairs for cattle and horses, on April 25th and October 18th. A copper battle-axe has been recently dug up at Bolton wood, and at Sea-scales there are the remains of a druidical temple.

GOSFORTH, a parish comprising the townships of North Gosforth and South Gosforth, in the eastern division, and the townships of East Brunton, West Brunton, Coxlodge, Fawdon, East Kenton, and West Kenton, in the western division, of CASTLE ward, county of NORTHUMBERLAND, and containing 3295 inhabitants, of which number, 141 are in the township of North Gosforth, 4¼ miles (N.) from Newcastle, and 174 in that of South Gosforth, 2¾ miles (N. by E.) from

Newcastle. The living is a perpetual curacy annexed to the vicarage of St. Nicholas in Newcastle, in the archdeaconry of Northumberland, and diocese of Durham. The church, dedicated to St. Nicholas, and situated at South Gosforth, was rebuilt in 1798, and enlarged in 1819 : it is a neat edifice, with a square tower surmounted by an octagonal spire. A chapel, formerly at North Gosforth, has been demolished : the tomb-stones in the cemetery all bear dates within the seventeenth century. There are extensive coal mines in the parish.

GOSPORT, a sea port, market town, and chapelry, in the parish of ALVERSTOKE, within the liberties of ALVERSTOKE and GOSPORT, Portsdown division of the county of SOUTHAMPTON, $17\frac{1}{4}$ miles (S. E. by E.) from Southampton, and 78 (S. W.) from London, containing 6184 inhabitants. This place is mentioned by Leland, in the reign of Henry VIII., as a poor village inhabited by fishermen ; but it has risen to importance during the last century, in consequence of its vicinity to the great naval station of Portsmouth, opposite to which it is situated, on a projecting point of land on the western side of the harbour. About thirty years since a line of regular fortifications for the protection of the town was constructed, extending from Weovil to Alverstoke lake : within the works are the king's brewery and cooperage, with store-houses on a very large scale for wine, malt, hops, &c., for the navy. This place has a communication with the sea by means of a large basin and canal, with extensive quays, where vessels of considerable burden can take in their stores. There are many small sloops belonging to Weovil, which are employed in the conveyance of various articles for the use of the vessels in the harbour. The approach to Gosport from the sea presents a noble prospect, including the forts, storehouses, and other extensive buildings. There are several streets, the principal of which extends from the harbour to the fortifications, but it is somewhat interrupted by the market-house ; and along the shore are various ranges of buildings, consisting chiefly of neat and well-built houses. There is a small theatre : assemblies are held once a month, and concerts frequently take place. Stokes bay, to the south-west of Gosport, is justly celebrated for the excellence of its anchorage, affording security to an unlimited number of vessels. Near Forton lake, a creek of Portsmouth harbour, about one mile north of Gosport, is the new military hospital connected with the establishment at Portsmouth : it consists of four ranges of building connected by an arcade, with offices, &c. In each range are six large wards, with proper accommodations for attendants. On the north side of the lake, near its entrance, is the magazine, in which and in a smaller building dependent upon it, on an island above, all the powder for the service of this port is stored. The magazine, which is bomb-proof and strongly arched, communicates with the harbour by a small cut. Near it are the ruins of an ancient castle, called Borough castle. Near Forton, on the road to Gosport, is an extensive range of buildings, formerly used for the custody of prisoners of war, with an hospital and proper offices, the whole secured by a strong enclosure.

The Royal hospital at Haslar, for the reception of sick and wounded seamen of the Royal navy, was built in 1762, through the influence of the Earl of Sandwich.

It is situated near the extremity of the point of land which bounds the west side of the entrance to Portsmouth harbour, and consists of an extensive front and two wings : the airing-ground, which is almost a mile in circumference, is surrounded by a wall twelve feet high. Opposite the grand entrance is a neat guard-house. The wards are all uniform, sixty feet long, and twenty-four broad ; each containing accommodations for twenty patients, with apartments for nurses, &c. In 1818, one of the principal wings of the building was appropriated to the reception of seamen and marines labouring under lunacy, who had been previously placed in an asylum at Hoxton. Within the area there are several other buildings for the use of the governor, lieutenants, and other officers and servants belonging to the institution, which consists of-more than two hundred and sixty persons : the chapel is a neat edifice, seventy-two feet in length, and thirty-six broad. The hospital is capable of receiving upwards of two thousand sick or wounded men ; and the annual expenses of the establishment, during the time of war, amount to upwards of £5000. About three quarters of a mile south-westward from Haslar hospital is Fort Monkton, a modern and regular fortification, exceedingly strong, on which are mounted thirty-two pieces of heavy ordnance : to the westward ranges a strong redoubt, which, together with the fort, secures this part of the coast. On the shore to the eastward, a high and massive stone wall has been erected, to preserve the land from the encroachments of the sea. Still further to the east, and near the extremity of the neck of land which bounds the entrance to the harbour on this side, is the Block-house, a very strong fort with a powerful battery. Numerous ferry-boats ply between Gosport and Portsmouth, the width of the harbour being here about three-quarters of a mile.

There are several breweries, and a very extensive iron foundry for the manufacture of various articles for the use of the shipping, especially anchors. The markets are on Wednesday, Friday, and Saturday; and there are fairs on May 4th and October 10th. The living is a perpetual curacy, in the peculiar jurisdiction of the Bishop of Winchester, endowed with £200 private benefaction, and £200 royal bounty, and in the patronage of the Rector of Alverstoke. The church, dedicated to the Holy Trinity, is a spacious building on the south side of the town : the organ was formerly in the chapel of the magnificent mansion of Canons, belonging to the Duke of Chandos. There are places of worship for Independents and Wesleyan Methodists, and a Roman Catholic chapel ; and the Independents have also an academy for the education of missionaries and other candidates for the ministry. An almshouse for seven poor widows was founded and endowed by Edward Piachy, in 1693; and several charity schools have been established here by subscription.

GOSWICK, a hamlet in the parish of HOLY ISLAND, ISLANDSHIRE, county palatine of DURHAM, situated northward of the county of Northumberland, adjoining Berwick upon Tweed. The population is returned with the parish. This place, lying contiguous to a small bay of the North sea, occupies the entrance to the fordable sands between the main land and Holy Island.

GOTHAM, a parish in the southern division of the wapentake of RUSHCLIFFE, county of NOTTINGHAM, $7\frac{1}{2}$ miles (S. S. W.) from Nottingham, containing 625 inhabitants. The living is a rectory, in the archdeaconry of Nottingham, and diocese of York, rated in the king's books at £19. 8. 6½., and in the patronage of Lord St. John, the Duke of Portland, Earl Howe, and George Savile Foljambe, Esq., in rotation. The church is dedicated to St. Lawrence. There is a place of worship for Wesleyan Methodists. A school is supported by the voluntary contributions of Earl Howe and the rector. Limestone and gypsum are obtained in the parish; the latter, when burnt and pulverised, makes an excellent plaister for floors.

GOTHERINGTON, a hamlet in the parish of Bishop's Cleeve, hundred of Cleeve, or Bishop's Cleeve, county of Gloucester, 4 miles (W. by N.) from Winchcombe, containing 348 inhabitants.

GOUDHURST, a parish partly in the hundred of Cranbrooke, but chiefly in the hundred of Marden, lathe of Scray, county of Kent, 13 miles (S. by W.) from Maidstone, containing 2579 inhabitants. The living is a vicarage, in the archdeaconry and diocese of Rochester, rated in the king's books at £26. 19. 2., and in the patronage of the Dean and Chapter of Rochester. The church, dedicated to St. Mary, is a handsome structure, situated on the declivity of a lofty hill, which commands a fine view over the counties of Kent, Surrey, and Sussex. There is a place of worship for Wesleyan Methodists. Goudhurst consists mostly of large well-built houses, erected on five different roads, uniting near a large pond in the centre of the village: it had formerly a market on Wednesday, and a considerable business in the manufacture of cloth, both which have decayed, but wool-stapling is still carried on to a small extent. There is a fair for cattle on the 26th and 27th of August.' John Horsemonden, in 1670, bequeathed a rent-charge of £40; and Thomas Bathurst, in 1718, gave another of £6, which sums are applied to the instruction of children.

GOULSBY, a parish in the northern division of the wapentake of Lindsey, parts of Lindsey, county of Lincoln, 6¾ miles (S.W.) from Louth, containing 244 inhabitants. The living is a discharged vicarage, in the archdeaconry and diocese of Lincoln, rated in the king's books at £6. 0. 2., and endowed with £600 royal bounty. M. B. Lister, Esq. was patron in 1824. The church is dedicated to All Saints. There is a place of worship for Wesleyan Methodists.

GOURNAL, a chapelry comprising Lower Gournal and Over Gournal, in the parish of Sedgley, northern division of the hundred of Seisdon, county of Stafford: Lower Gournal is 1¾ mile (W.N.W.), and Over Gournal 2 miles (N.W.), from Dudley. The population is returned with the parish. The living is a perpetual curacy, in the archdeaconry of Stafford, and diocese of Lichfield and Coventry, endowed with £400 private benefaction, and £800 parliamentary grant. The chapel is dedicated to St. James.

GOWDALL, a township in that part of the parish of Snaith which is in the lower division of the wapentake of Osgoldcross, West riding of the county of York, 1½ mile (W.) from Snaith, containing 243 inhabitants. This township is within the peculiar jurisdiction of the ecclesiastical court of Snaith.

GOWTHORPE, a chapelry in the parish of Swardeston, hundred of Humbleyard, county of Norfolk. The population is returned with the parish. The curacy

is consolidated with the rectory of Intwood, in the archdeaconry of Norfolk, and diocese of Norwich. The chapel is dedicated to St. James the Apostle.

GOWTHORPE, a joint township with Youlthorpe, in the parish of Bishop-Wilton, partly within the liberty of St. Peter of York, and partly in the Wilton-Beacon division of the wapentake of Harthill, East riding of the county of York, 4½ miles (N.W. by N.) from Pocklington, containing 111 inhabitants.

GOXHILL, a parish in the northern division of the wapentake of Yarborough, parts of Lindsey, county of Lincoln, 5½ miles (E. by S.) from Barton upon Humber, containing 736 inhabitants. The living is a discharged vicarage, in the archdeaconry and diocese of Lincoln, rated in the king's books at £14. 18. 4., endowed with £200 royal bounty, and in the patronage of the Crown. The church is dedicated to All Saints. There is a place of worship for Wesleyan Methodists.

GOXHILL, a parish in the northern division of the wapentake of Holderness, East riding of the county of York, 11½ miles (E.N.E.) from Beverley, containing 70 inhabitants. The living is a discharged rectory, in the archdeaconry of the East riding, and diocese of York, rated in the king's books at £8. The Rev. C. Constable was patron in 1818. The church, dedicated to St. Giles, and standing upon an eminence amidst lofty trees, is of considerable antiquity; it has lately undergone a thorough repair. To the southward of the village are the remains of an ancient edifice, the upper story of which was probably a chapel, lighted by large pointed windows, and the lower, consisting of several vaulted apartments, the offices of a mansion.

GOYTREY, a parish in the upper division of the hundred of Abergavenny, county of Monmouth, 5 miles (N.N.W.) from Usk, containing 513 inhabitants. The living is a discharged rectory, in the archdeaconry and diocese of Llandaff, rated in the king's books at £4. 7. 6., and in the patronage of the Earl of Abergavenny. The church is dedicated to St. Peter. The parish is bounded on the north-east by the river Usk, and the Brecon and Abergavenny canal passes through it.

GRABY, a hamlet in the parish of Aslackby, wapentake of Aveland, parts of Kesteven, county of Lincoln, 4 miles (S.E. by S.) from Falkingham, containing 21 inhabitants.

GRACE-DIEU, an extra-parochial liberty, in the western division of the hundred of Goscote, county of Leicester, 5 miles (E. by N.) from Ashby de la Zouch. The population is returned with the parish of Belton. A priory for nuns of the order of St. Augustine was founded in the reign of Henry III., by Roesia de Verdon, in honour of St. Mary and the Holy Trinity, which at the dissolution had a revenue valued at £101. 8. 2.

GRACE-DIEU PARK, an extra-parochial liberty, in the lower division of the hundred of Ragland, county of Monmouth, 4½ miles (W. by S.) from Monmouth. The population is returned with the parish of Dingestow. An abbey of the Cistercian order was founded here in 1226, by John of Monmouth, Knt., in honour of the Blessed Virgin, which at the dissolution contained only two monks, whose revenue was valued at £26. 1. 4.

GRADE, a parish in the hundred of Kerrier, county of Cornwall, 9½ miles (S.S.E.) from Helston, containing 355 inhabitants. The living is a rectory, in the archdeaconry of Cornwall, and diocese of Exeter, rated in the king's books at £11. 1. 5½., and in the patronage of John Rogers, Esq. The church is dedicated to the Holy Cross. The parish is bounded on the east by Cadgwith cove.

GRAFFHAM, a parish in the hundred of LEIGHTONSTONE, county of HUNTINGDON, 4¾ miles (E. by N.) from Kimbolton, containing, with the hamlet of East Perry, 267 inhabitants. The living is a rectory, in the archdeaconry of Huntingdon, and diocese of Lincoln, rated in the king's books at £16. 14. 4½. Lady O. Sparrow was patroness in 1825. The church is dedicated to All Saints.

GRAFFHAM, a parish in the hundred of EASEBOURNE, rape of CHICHESTER, county of SUSSEX, 4¾ miles (S.E.) from Midhurst, containing 343 inhabitants. The living is a rectory, in the archdeaconry and diocese of Chichester, rated in the king's books at £9. 10. 5. John Sargent, Esq. was patron in 1805. The church, dedicated to St. Giles, is partly in the early, and partly in the decorated, style of English architecture.

GRAFTON, a township in the parish of TILSTON, higher division of the hundred of BROXTON, county palatine of CHESTER, 4½ miles (N.W. by N.) from Malpas, containing 21 inhabitants.

GRAFTON, a township in the parish of BECKFORD, hundred of TIBALDSTONE, county of GLOUCESTER, 7 miles (N.E. by E.) from Tewkesbury. The population is returned with the parish. In 1764, in consequence, it is supposed, of some incessant rains, a tract of six-teen acres of land fell from the side of Breedon hill, and covered the fields at the bottom.

GRAFTON, a township in that part of the parish of ALL SAINTS, HEREFORD, which is in the hundred of WEBTREE, county of HEREFORD, containing 45 inhabitants.

GRAFTON, a township in that part of the parish of LANGFORD which is in the hundred of BAMPTON, county of OXFORD, 4½ miles (E.N.E.) from Lechlade, containing 81 inhabitants. This township is in the peculiar ecclesiastical jurisdiction of the Prebendary of Langford-Ecclesia in the Cathedral Church of Lincoln.

GRAFTON (EAST), a hamlet in the parish of GREAT BEDWIN, hundred of KINWARDSTONE, county of WILTS, 7¾ miles (N.) from Ludgershall. The population is returned with the parish. Here was anciently a chapel, dedicated to St. Nicholas, which has been demolished.

GRAFTON (FLYFORD), county of WORCESTER. See FLYFORD-GRAFTON.

GRAFTON (TEMPLE), a parish in the Stratford division of the hundred of BARLICHWAY, county of WARWICK, 3¼ miles (S.E. by E.) from Alcester, containing, with the township of Grafton-Arden, 336 inhabitants. The living is a perpetual curacy, in the archdeaconry and diocese of Worcester, endowed with £200 private benefaction, and £800 royal bounty. F. F. Bullock, Esq. was patron in 1825. The church is dedicated to St. Andrew.

GRAFTON-ARDEN, a township in the parish of TEMPLE-GRAFTON, Stratford division of the hundred of BARLICHWAY, county of WARWICK, 3 miles (S.E.) from Alcester. The population is returned with the parish.

GRAFTON-MANOR, an extra-parochial liberty, in the upper division of the hundred of HALFSHIRE,

county of WORCESTER, 1¾ mile (W.S.W.) from Bromsgrove, containing 45 inhabitants. The ancient mansion of the Earls of Shrewsbury at this place was nearly destroyed by fire in 1710, and the only part now remaining is the hall, but this is sufficient to show its former splendour. There is a Roman Catholic chapel, which has been recently repaired and ornamented by the present earl.

GRAFTON-REGIS, a parish in the hundred of CLELEY, county of NORTHAMPTON, 4¾ miles (E.S.E.) from Towcester, containing 214 inhabitants. The living is a discharged rectory, with that of Alderton, in the archdeaconry of Northampton, and diocese of Peterborough, rated in the king's books at £9. 9. 4½., and in the patronage of the Crown. The church is dedicated to St. Mary. Grafton was erected into an honour in the 33rd of Henry VIII., with jurisdiction, confirmed by act of parliament, over an extensive tract partly in this county and partly in Buckinghamshire. Edward IV. was here privately married to Elizabeth, relict of Sir John Gray, of Groby; this lady was the daughter of Sir Richard Woodeville, of whose family mansion at this place there are still some remains: Lady Crane resided in it during the parliamentary war, when it was garrisoned for the king. The making of lace has been introduced of late years, and is carried on to some extent. The Grand Junction canal passes through the parish. Grafton gives the title of duke to the Fitzroy family.

GRAFTON-UNDERWOOD, a parish in the hundred of HUXLOE, county of NORTHAMPTON, 4¾ miles (E.N.E.) from Kettering, containing 285 inhabitants. The living is a rectory, in the archdeaconry of Northampton, and diocese of Peterborough, rated in the king's books at £12. 16. 3. The Earl of Upper Ossory was patron in 1794. The church is dedicated to St. James.

GRAIN (ISLE of), a parish in the hundred of Hoo, lathe of AYLESFORD, county of KENT, 1¾ mile (N.W. by W.) from Sheerness, containing 254 inhabitants. The living is a vicarage, in the peculiar jurisdiction of the Archbishop of Canterbury, rated in the king's books at £9. 11. 8., and in the patronage of the Rev. George Davies. The church is dedicated to St. James. There is a place of worship for Independents. The island, which is about three miles and a half long, and two and a half broad, is formed by the Thames on the north, the Medway on the south, the junction of those two rivers on the east, and Yantlet creek on the west. There are salt pans on that side bordering upon the Medway. In the reign of Edward III., Yantlet creek, though now almost choked up, was the usual passage for vessels trading to and from London, which thus avoided a more circuitous and dangerous route; at present it is navigable, at spring tides only, for barges.

GRAINSBY, a parish in the wapentake of BRADLEY-HAVERSTOE, parts of LINDSEY, county of LINCOLN, 7 miles (S.) from Great Grimsby, containing 114 inhabitants. The living is a discharged rectory, in the archdeaconry and diocese of Lincoln, rated in the king's books at £9. 18. 4. T. Sands, Esq. was patron in 1800. The church is dedicated to St. Nicholas.

GRAINTHORPE, a parish in the Marsh division of the hundred of LOUTH-ESKE, parts of LINDSEY, county of LINCOLN, 8¼ miles (N.E. by N.) from Louth, containing, with the hamlets of Ludney and Wragholme,

503 inhabitants. The living is a perpetual curacy, in the archdeaconry and diocese of Lincoln, endowed with £200 private benefaction, £400 royal bounty, and £1000 parliamentary grant, and in the patronage of the President and Fellows of Magdalene College, Cambridge. The church is dedicated to St. Clement.

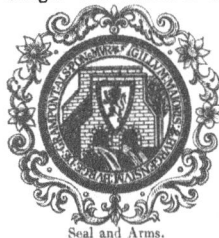

GRAMPOUND, a corporate and market town and chapelry, partly in the parish of PROBUS, but chiefly in that of CREED, western division of the hundred of POWDER, county of CORNWALL, 40 miles (S. W) from Launceston, and 247 (W.S.W.) from London, containing 668 inhabitants. This place is situated on the great road from

Seal and Arms.

London, through Plymouth, to the Land's end, and on the declivity of a hill, at the foot of which runs the river Fal. John of Eltham, Earl of Cornwall, brother of Edward III., granted a guild-merchant to the burgesses of Grampound, in 1332, which included, besides other privileges, the right of holding a market and two fairs. The market, which is inconsiderable, is on Saturday: fairs are held January 18th and June 11th; and there are two new free fairs, on the Tuesdays next after Lady-day and Michaelmas. The corporation, which exists by prescription, consists of a mayor, eight aldermen, a recorder, and town clerk. The mayor is elected on the Sunday before Michaelmas, and he nominates two aldermen, styled *Eligers*, who have the power to choose eleven freemen, forming a jury, who make presentments, appoint persons to municipal offices, and possess the right of making new freemen, whose number is indefinite. The manor is held by the corporation, under the duchy of Cornwall, at a fee farm rent of £12. 11. 4. per annum. Grampound was formerly a borough, having sent two members to parliament from the reign of Edward VI. till 1824, when, in consequence of the discovery of corrupt practices among the electors, an act of parliament was passed for disfranchising the borough, and returning two additional members for the county of York. The chapel, dedicated to St. Nunn, or St. Naunter, was a chapel of ease to the rectory of Creed, but is now falling to ruins. In 1705, John Buller gave a sum of money, directing the interest to be applied in teaching and clothing eight poor boys.

GRAMPOUND, or GRAND-PONT, a tything in that part of the parish of ST. ALDATE's, OXFORD, which is in the hundred of HORMER, county of BERKS. The population is returned with the parish. In the time of Edward I., the Crouched friars had a house here, given them by Richard Cary, sometime mayor of Oxford, which, about 1348, they left, for a house and chapel near the church of St. Peter's in the East.

GRANBY, a parish in the northern division of the wapentake of BINGHAM, county of NOTTINGHAM, 4 miles (S.E. by E.) from Bingham, containing, with Sutton, 389 inhabitants. The living is a discharged vicarage, in the archdeaconry of Nottingham, and diocese of York, rated in the king's books at £6. 3. 6½., and in the patronage of the Duke of Rutland. The church is dedicated to All Saints. There is a place of worship for Wesleyan Methodists. The river Snipe, and the Not-

VOL. II.

tingham and Grantham canal, pass through the parish. There are quarries that supply gypsum, of which plaister for flooring is made and used in this and the adjoining parishes. Granby gives the title of marquis to the family of Manners, Dukes of Rutland.

GRANDBOROUGH, a parish in the hundred of ASHENDON, county of BUCKINGHAM, 1¾ mile (S.) from Winslow, containing 286 inhabitants. The living is a discharged vicarage, in the archdeaconry of St. Alban's, and diocese of London, rated in the king's books at £8, and in the patronage of the Crown. The church, dedicated to St. John the Baptist, was formerly a chapel of ease to the vicarage of Winslow, and was pulled down in the civil war, by Cornelius Holland, the regicide, but was rebuilt after the Restoration.

GRANDBOROUGH, a parish in the Southam division of the hundred of KNIGHTLOW, county of WARWICK, 3¼ miles (S.) from Dunchurch, containing 483 inhabitants. The living is a discharged vicarage, in the archdeaconry of Coventry, and diocese of Lichfield and Coventry, rated in the king's books at £5, endowed with £600 private benefaction, and £600 royal bounty. The Bishop of Lichfield and Coventry presented by lapse in 1804. The church is dedicated to St. Paul.

GRANGE, a joint township with Claughton, in the parish of BIDSTONE, lower division of the hundred of WIRRALL, county palatine of CHESTER, 9 miles (N. by E.) from Great Neston, containing 119 inhabitants.

GRANGE, a township in the parish of WEST KIRBY, lower division of the hundred of WIRRALL, county palatine of CHESTER, 8½ miles (N.W. by N.) from Great Neston, containing 125 inhabitants. A school is supported by annual subscriptions amounting to about £30.

GRANGE, a township in the parish of LEINTWARDINE, hundred of WIGMORE, county of HEREFORD, 8 miles (W.S.W.) from Ludlow, containing, with the townships of Adforton and Payton, 212 inhabitants.

GRANGE, otherwise GRENCH, a hamlet and a member of the town and port of HASTINGS, in the parish of GILLINGHAM, locally in the hundred of Chatham and Gillingham, lathe of AYLESFORD, county of KENT, 2 miles (E. by N.) from Chatham, containing 112 inhabitants. Here was anciently a chapel, which has been demolished.

GRANGE (CHAPEL), a hamlet in the parish of OSWALD-KIRK, wapentake of RYEDALE, North riding of the county of YORK, 2¼ miles (S. by E.) from Helmsley. The population is returned with the parish.

GRANSDEN (GREAT), a parish in the hundred of TOSELAND, county of HUNTINGDON, 7¼ miles (S.E. by E.) from St. Neot's, containing 545 inhabitants. The living is a discharged vicarage, in the archdeaconry of Huntingdon, and diocese of Lincoln, rated in the king's books at £5. 7. 3½., endowed with £200 private benefaction, and £200 royal bounty, and in the patronage of the Master and Fellows of Clare Hall, Cambridge. The church is dedicated to St. Bartholomew. There is a place of worship for Baptists. A school-house was built by subscription in 1664, and endowed under the will of the Rev. B. Oley, then vicar; and in 1819 a house was erected for the master. Throughout this parish are scattered many diluvial remains, consisting of primitive and secondary rocks, and fossils

2 K

of almost every description, mineralized wood and vegetables, the vertebræ of the Ichthyosaurus, &c.

GRANSDEN (LITTLE), a parish in the hundred of LONGSTOW, county of CAMBRIDGE, 3 miles (S. W.) from Caxton, containing 261 inhabitants. The living is a rectory, in the peculiar jurisdiction and patronage of the Bishop of Ely, rated in the king's books at £18. 15. 2½. The church is dedicated to St. Peter and St. Paul. There is a small school supported by annual donations.

GRANSMOOR, a township in the parish of BURTON-AGNES, wapentake of DICKERING, East riding of the county of YORK, 7½ miles (E. by N.) from Great Driffield, containing 85 inhabitants.

GRANTCHESTER, a parish in the hundred of WETHERLEY, county of CAMBRIDGE, 2¼ miles (S. S. W.) from Cambridge, containing 344 inhabitants. The living is a discharged vicarage, in the archdeaconry and diocese of Ely, rated in the king's books at £7. 14. 4½., and in the patronage of the President and Fellows of Corpus Christi College, Cambridge. The church, dedicated to St. Mary and St. Andrew, was erected early in the fifteenth century; a portion of the interior is remarkably light and elegant. This is said to have been the *Camboritum* of Antonine, situated on the banks of the Granta, now the river Cam, the present Saxon name confirming the opinion of its having been the site of a Roman station. About the year 700, according to Bede, "Grantchester was a desolate little city, near the walls of which was found a beautiful coffin of white marble." Dr. Cay supposes the station to have extended not only as far as Cambridge, but northward, beyond the castle: foundations of buildings have been frequently discovered between the village of Grantchester and the town of Cambridge, the latter being supposed to have risen out of the ruins of the Roman station.

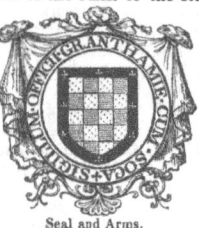

Seal and Arms.

GRANTHAM, a parish comprising the borough and market town of Grantham, and the township of Manthorp with Little Gonerby, in the soke of GRANTHAM, and the townships of Harrowby and Spittlegate, in the wapentake of WINNIBRIGGS and THREO, parts of KESTEVEN, county of LINCOLN, and containing 6077 inhabitants, of which number, 4148 are in the town of Grantham, 24 miles (S. by W.) from Lincoln, and 111 (N. by W.) from London, on the great road to York. This place being situated on the Ermin-street, which now forms part of the turnpike-road, is supposed to have been a Roman station, but there is no evidence of its having been occupied by that people; and of the origin of a castle to the east of the church, near the river Witham, of which the foundations are said to have been dug up, nothing satisfactory is recorded. The manor was held by Editha, Queen of Edward the Confessor, and continued in the crown till the reign of Henry III. A house of Franciscan, or Grey friars, was established here in 1290, the remains of which have been converted into a place of public entertainment, and the relics of a preceptory of the Knights Hospitallers, formerly existing here, now form part of the Angel Inn. During

the parliamentary war Grantham was an object of interest with the contending parties, and the scene of the first advantage gained by Cromwell over the royalists. The town is pleasantly situated on the river Witham, near the vale of Belvoir, and consists principally of four spacious streets, paved, and lighted with oil; the houses are in general of respectable appearance, and in the several approaches to the town many substantial and handsome houses have been recently erected: the inhabitants are well supplied with water. The theatre, a neat brick building, is occasionally opened, and assemblies are held at the guildhall. The environs are pleasant, being adorned with several seats and villas. There is no manufacture of importance: the trade is principally in malt, corn, and coal, of which large supplies are sent to the chief towns in the adjoining counties. By act of parliament in 1793, a navigable canal, commencing within a quarter of a mile of the town, has been constructed, which joins the Trent at Nottingham. The market is on Saturday, and is extensively supplied with corn; and in every alternate week there is a large mart for live stock: the fairs are on the first Monday in Lent, Holy Thursday, July 10th, October 26th, and December 17th, for horses and cattle.

The government, by charter of incorporation granted by Edward IV., is vested in an alderman, recorder, twelve burgesses, and twelve common council-men, assisted by a town clerk, coroner, escheator, and subordinate officers: the alderman and burgesses are justices of the peace within the borough and liberties, which constitute the soke of Grantham, comprising the parish of Grantham (with the exception of the townships of Harrowby and Spittlegate), and the parishes of Barkston, Belton, Braceby, Colsterworth, Denton, Great Gonerby, Hartaxton, Londonthorpe, Great Ponton, Sapperton, and South Stoke, which are exempt from the jurisdiction of the sheriff for the county, and subject to the bailiff of the liberties appointed by the corporation, who acts as sheriff. The freedom of the borough is inherited by birth, and acquired by servitude, gift of the corporation, or by purchase; in the last mode a non-resident pays twice as much as an inhabitant. The corporation hold quarterly courts of session for offences arising within the soke; and a court of record every Monday, under the charter of James I., for the recovery of debts not exceeding £40, at which the alderman and the recorder preside. The guildhall, a neat and commodious edifice, was rebuilt in 1787, and, in addition to the courts, contains a spacious assembly-room. The common gaol and house of correction is adapted to the classification of prisoners, and comprises six wards, six day-rooms, and six airing-yards, with a tread-wheel: it has fourteen separate cells, and is capable of receiving forty prisoners. The borough first received the elective franchise in the 7th of Edward IV., since which time it has returned two members to parliament: the right of election is vested in the freemen not receiving alms, whether resident or not, the number of whom is upwards of eight hundred: the alderman is the returning officer.

The living comprises the united vicarages of North and South Grantham, in the archdeaconry and diocese of Lincoln; the former, with the vicarages of Great Gonerby and Londonthorpe, is rated in the king's books at £19. 4. 7., and the latter, with the vicarages of Braceby and Little Gonerby, at £17. 15. 7½. : they are in the alternate patronage of the Prebendaries of North and South Grantham in the Cathedral Church of Salisbury. The church, dedicated to St. Wulfran, is a magnificent structure, partly in the early, and partly in the decorated, style of English architecture, with a very lofty tower, surmounted by an elegant spire richly crocketed : the tower communicates with the nave and aisles by three finely pointed arches, and the interior displays much variety in the piers and arches which support the roof; the chancel has a range of small clerestory windows, and a stone screen of exquisite design: under the eastern part of the church is a crypt. Among the numerous monuments, those of the greatest beauty are to the memory of Sir Thomas Bury, Chief Baron of the Exchequer in the reign of George I.; Sir Dudley Ryder, Chief Justice of the Court of King's Bench; and Captain Cust, R. N., who fell in the action at Port Louis, in 1747. The vestry-room contains a valuable library, presented to the parish by Dr. Newcome. There are places of worship for Huntingtonians, Independents, and Wesleyan Methodists. The free grammar school was founded in 1528, by Richard Fox, Bishop of Winchester, who endowed it with the revenue of two chantries, which, prior to the dissolution, belonged to the church of St. Peter, the endowment having been subsequently augmented by Edward VI.: the annual income exceeds £700, the surplus of which, after payment of the salaries to the masters, is appropriated to the establishment of exhibitions to Oxford and Cambridge, to which all scholars who have been two years in the school are eligible. Sir Isaac Newton, who was born at Coltersworth, about eight miles from Grantham, received the rudiments of his education in this school. A charity school for girls was founded by Mr. Hirst; and a Lancasterian school for boys, and another for girls, are supported by subscription. There are some almshouses, and various charitable bequests for the relief of the poor. Near the town is a chalybeate spring, but the water is not much used. This town was the native place of Bishop Fox, founder of the grammar school; and of Dr. John Still, who held the see of Bath and Wells in the reign of Elizabeth, and who is supposed to have been the author of "Gammer Gurton's Needle," the earliest comedy extant in the English language. Grantham gives the title of baron to the family of Robinson.

GRANTLEY, a joint chapelry with Winksley, in that part of the parish of RIPON which is within the liberty of RIPON, West riding of the county of YORK, 5½ miles (W. by S.) from Ripon, containing, with the township of Skeldin, 233 inhabitants. It is within the ecclesiastical jurisdiction of the peculiar court of Ripon, under the Archbishop of York. There is a school endowed by Mr. John Richmond with £6 per annum.

GRAPPENHALL, a parish in the hundred of BUCKLOW, county palatine of CHESTER, comprising the chapelry of Latchford, and the township of Grappenhall, and containing 1652 inhabitants, of which number, 400 are in the township of Grappenhall, 2¾ miles (S.E.) from Warrington. The living is a rectory, in the archdeaconry and diocese of Chester, rated in the king's books at £6. 11. 10½. The Rev. J. B. Stewart was patron in 1808. The church, dedicated to St. Wilfrid, was erected in 1539. The Duke of Bridgewater's canal passes through the parish, which is bounded on the north by the river Mersey. There is a cotton manufactory at Latchford. Courts leet and baron are annually held here. A school-house, built at the expense of the parishioners in 1712, is endowed with lands given by Mr. Thomas Johnson.

GRASMERE, a parish in KENDAL ward, county of WESTMORLAND, comprising the chapelries of Ambleside and Langdales, and the townships of Grasmere and Rydal with Loughbrigg, and containing 1778 inhabitants, of which number, 324 are in the township of Grasmere, 4 miles (N.W. by W.) from Ambleside. The living is a rectory, in the archdeaconry of Richmond, and diocese of Chester, rated in the king's books at £28. 11. 5½., and in the patronage of Lady Le Fleming. The church is dedicated to St. Oswald. Grasmere anciently formed part of the extensive parish of Kendal, in which it was a chapelry. A fair for sheep, on the first Tuesday in September, is held at the village, which is pleasantly situated upon the Rotha, a river connecting the lakes Grasmere, Rydal, and Winandermere. A school-house was built by subscription in 1685, and endowed by the then rector with £50, which, with various subsequent bequests, produces about £11 per annum, and is applied to the education of children. At the back of the village is Helm Crag, composed of huge and lofty masses of rock.

GRASSBY, a parish in the southern division of the wapentake of YARBOROUGH, parts of LINDSEY, county of LINCOLN, 3¼ miles (N.W. by N.) from Caistor, containing 299 inhabitants. The living is a discharged vicarage, in the archdeaconry and diocese of Lincoln, rated in the king's books at £5. 17. 8½. Mrs. Wilkin son was patroness in 1812. The church is dedicated to All Saints.

GRASSGARTH, a hamlet in that part of the parish of KENDAL which is in KENDAL ward, county of WESTMORLAND, 6½ miles (N.W.) from Kendal. The population is returned with the parish. A chapel, dedicated to St. Anne, was formerly situated about a quarter of a mile north-westward from that of Ings.

GRASSINGTON, a township in the parish of LINTON, eastern division of the wapentake of STAINCLIFFE and EWCROSS, West riding of the county of YORK, 9½ miles (N. by E.) from Skipton, containing 983 inhabitants. There are fairs for cattle on March 4th and September 26th, and for sheep on April 24th and June 29th. There is a place of worship for Wesleyan Methodists.

GRASSTHORPE, a township in the parish of MARNHAM, northern division of the wapentake of THURGARTON, county of NOTTINGHAM, 4½ miles (S.E. by E.) from Tuxford, containing 97 inhabitants. An ancient chapel, dedicated to St. James, has been converted into a dwelling-house.

GRATELY, a parish in the hundred of ANDOVER, Andover division of the county of SOUTHAMPTON, 6½ miles (W.S.W.) from Andover, containing 142 inhabitants. The living is a rectory, in the archdeaconry and diocese of Winchester, rated in the king's books at £15. 9. 2. The Rev. J. Constable was patron in 1819. The church is dedicated to St. Leonard. King Athelstan held his court at Grately, at which period it had five churches.

GRATTON, a hamlet in that part of the parish of YOULGRAVE which is in the hundred of HIGH PEAK, county of DERBY, 5½ miles (S. by W.) from Bakewell, containing 51 inhabitants.

GRATWICH, a parish in the southern division of the hundred of TOTMONSLOW, county of STAFFORD, 4¾ miles (W. S. W) from Uttoxeter, containing 115 inhabitants. The living is a discharged rectory, in the archdeaconry of Stafford, and diocese of Lichfield and Coventry, rated in the king's books at £4. 7. 6., endowed with £400 royal bounty, and in the patronage of Earl Talbot. The church is dedicated to St. Mary.

GRAVELEY, a parish in the hundred of PAPWORTH, county of CAMBRIDGE, 6½ miles (N.W.) from Caxton, containing 242 inhabitants. The living is a rectory, in the archdeaconry and diocese of Ely, rated in the king's books at £13. 3. 4., and in the patronage of the Master and Fellows of Jesus College, Cambridge. The church is dedicated to St. Botolph. A charity school for twelve children was founded in 1763, by the Rev. Henry Trot-man.

GRAVELEY, a parish in the hundred of BROAD-WATER, county of HERTFORD, 2 miles (N.) from Stevenage, containing 316 inhabitants. The living is a rectory, with which that of Chivesfield is consolidated, in the archdeaconry of Huntingdon, and diocese of Lincoln, rated in the king's books at £12. 0. 10., and in the patronage of the Rev. Thomas Fordham Green. The church, dedicated to St. Mary, has a square embattled tower at the west end, surmounted by a spire covered with lead. There are ruins of Chivesfield church still remaining. The old Roman road from Verulam to Chesterfield passes through the parish.

GRAVELTHORPE county of YORK.—See GREW-ELTHORPE.

GRAVENEY, a parish in the hundred of BOUGHTON under BLEAN, lathe of SCRAY, county of KENT, 3 miles (N.E. by E.) from Faversham, containing 194 inhabitants. The living is a discharged vicarage, with which the rectory of Goodneston is united, in the archdeaconry and diocese of Canterbury, rated in the king's books at £12, and in the alternate patronage of the Archbishop of Canterbury and J. H. Lade, Esq. The church, dedicated to All Saints, is principally in the early style of English architecture.

GRAVENHANGER, a township in that part of the parish of MUCKLESTON which is in the Drayton division of the hundred of BRADFORD (North), county of SALOP, 6½ miles (N.E.) from Drayton, containing 200 inhabitants.

GRAVENHURST (LOWER), a parish in the hundred of FLITT, county of BEDFORD, 3 miles (E.) from Silsoe, containing 63 inhabitants. The living is a rectory, in the archdeaconry of Bedford, and diocese of Lincoln, rated in the king's books at £7. 12. 11., and in the patronage of the Crown. The church, dedicated to St. Mary, was built by Robert de Bilhemore, whose armorial bearings are displayed on the porch, and to whose memory there is a tomb without date.

GRAVENHURST (UPPER), a parish in the hundred of FLITT, county of BEDFORD, 3 miles (E. by N.) from Silsoe, containing 291 inhabitants. The living is a perpetual curacy, in the archdeaconry of Bedford, and diocese of Lincoln, endowed with £200 royal bounty, and in the patronage of certain Trustees. The church is dedicated to St. Giles.

GRAVESEND, a market town and parish having separate jurisdiction, locally in the hundred of Tolting-trough, lathe of AYLESFORD, county of KENT, 15½ miles (N.W. by W.) from Maidstone, and 22½ (E. by S.) from London, containing, according to the census of 1821, 3814 inhabitants, which number has increased nearly two-fold since that period. This place, called in Domesday-book Graves-ham, and in the Textus Roffensis Græves-ænde, appears to have derived those names from the Saxon gerefa, a greve or reeve, implying either the habitation of the portreeve, or the limit of his jurisdiction : by some antiquaries the name is derived from græf, a coppice, denoting its situation at the extremity of a wood towards the sea. In the reign of Richard II., the French having made a descent upon this part of the coast, laid waste many of the adjacent villages, plundered and burnt the town, and carried off several of the inhabitants prisoners. It was soon afterwards rebuilt, and to indemnify the inhabitants for the loss they sustained upon that occasion, Richard II. granted them the exclusive privilege of conveying passengers to and from London, which right is still exercised under regulations adapted to the present times. In the reign of Henry VIII. two platforms were raised for the protection of the town, and a block-house was erected at Tilbury, for the defence of the river. In 1727 the greater part of the town was destroyed by a fire that broke out near the church, which edifice, with more than a hundred houses, was burnt down. George I. landed here on his first arrival from Germany, and Gravesend has been frequently distinguished by crowned heads landing and embarking at the pier.

Seal and Arms.

The town is pleasantly situated on an acclivity rising from the south bank of the river Thames, and consists of several narrow streets, paved and lighted by acts of parliament passed in the 13th and 56th of George III., and is partly in the parish of Milton, which adjoins that of Gravesend. Considerable improvements have lately taken place; among which is the recent construction of a stone pier, or quay, for the landing and embarkation of passengers in the steam-packets, which leave London in the morning, and return the same evening. Under the authority of an act passed in the 9th of George IV., every person landing or embarking at Gravesend to or from the passage boats, pays to the corporation one penny, as pier dues. The salubrity of the air, the beauty of the surrounding scenery, and the short distance from the metropolis, have, within the last few years, made Gravesend a favourite place of resort, one hundred and twenty-two thousand persons having visited it during the summer of 1829; and in proportion to the increase of visitors, preparations have been made for their accommodation. A convenient bathing-house has been fitted up with warm, cold, vapour, and shower baths; and bathing-machines are in constant attendance, and may be used with safety at any time of the tide, which here rises to the height of twenty feet above low water mark every twenty-four hours. Adjoining the bathing-house is a garden, well laid out in walks, and furnished with seats, commanding an extensive view of the river and the numerous ships which are constantly passing and repassing. There are a public subscription library, concert-rooms, and a bowling-green: the theatre is occasionally opened, and assemblies are held at the town-hall. The terrace, which is in the adjoining parish of Milton, forms an agreeable promenade, commanding a view of Tilbury Fort on the opposite shore: between it and the river are a battery mounting sixteen pieces of cannon, the custom-house and the excise office, with a commodious wharf, or quay, near which is the landing-place for troops and military stores, and at the eastern extremity is the fort, mounting sixteen pieces of ordnance, with accommodations for a commandant and some veterans of the artillery.

Gravesend being within the jurisdiction of the port of London, all outward bound ships, until recently, were here obliged to undergo a second clearing; but this practice has long been disused. Outward bound vessels take in their pilots here, and all vessels entering the port of London take in pilots from this place for the navigation of the river. A surgeon in the East India Company's service is always resident, who examines the soldiers entering that service, ascertaining also whether they have entered of their own accord, or have been trepanned into it; he also examines and registers the natives of India brought to England by the Company's ships. The outward bound Indiamen take in their supplies of fresh provisions, vegetables, liquors, ammunition, and stores at this place. A considerable number of vessels is employed in the cod and turbot fisheries; fine shrimps are also caught here in great abundance. Between Gravesend and Tilbury Fort is a ferry, called Cross Ferry, by means of which carriages, horses, and cattle are conveyed over the river; and to persons travelling from Norfolk, Suffolk, and the northern counties, into Kent or Sussex, a distance of fifty miles is thus saved. There are extensive lime and brick works, and a large manufactory for ropes and twine: ship-building and slops also been carried on to a considerable extent in a yard to the north-west of the town, in which several men of war and frigates, exclusively of smaller vessels, have been built; among the former were L'Achille of eighty guns, the Colossus of seventy-four, and the Director of sixty-four. The principal branch of trade arises from the supply of the numerous ships which on their passage outward stop to take in stores, &c., and from the number of seamen who furnish themselves with slops, for the sale of which there are numerous shops in the town. A considerable quantity of ground in the neighbourhood is appropriated to the cultivation of vegetables for the use of the shipping, and of asparagus of superior quality for the London market, for the conveyance of which, and for the promotion of the general trade, great advantages are afforded by the river Thames, and by the Thames and Medway canal, which passes to the east of the town, and just without the limits of the port of London, thereby affording the inhabitants the advantage of obtaining coal free from the orphan and other duties: on the basin of this canal a floating-bath has recently been introduced. The market days are Wednesday and Saturday, the former for corn: the fairs are, May 4th and October 24th, for horses, cloth, and various sorts of merchandise.

The inhabitants, with those of the adjoining parish of Milton, were first incorporated by charter of Queen Elizabeth, by the title of the "Portreeve, Jurats, and Inhabitants of Gravesend and Milton;" the charter was ratified and extended by Charles I., by whom the government is vested in a mayor, high steward, twelve jurats, and twenty-four common council-men, assisted by a recorder, town clerk, chamberlain, serjeant at mace, and subordinate officers. Under this charter the mayor and jurats are obliged formally to attend all foreign ambassadors, and other illustrious visitors who land at this place, and conduct them in their barges to London; or, if they prefer proceeding by land, to escort them to Blackheath. The corporation hold a court of record, under the charter of Charles I., every third Tuesday, for the recovery of debts to any amount, at which the mayor and three of the jurats preside; and a court of requests, for the recovery of debts not exceeding £5, is held on the first Friday in every month, under commissioners appointed by an act passed in the 47th of George III., the jurisdiction of which extends over the hundreds of Toltingtrough, and Axton, Dartford, and Wilmington, in the county of Kent. The corporation of London, as conservators of the rivers Thames and Medway, hold courts of conservancy for the county of Kent twice in the year. The town-hall, erected by the corporation in 1764, is a neat and commodious edifice, supported on six columns in the front, and having underneath it a convenient area for the poultry market. The arms of the corporation were those of James, Duke of Lennox, whose descendants are hereditary high stewards of Gravesend, that office being now filled by the Earl of Darnley.

The living is a rectory, in the archdeaconry and diocese of Rochester, rated in the king's books at £15, and in the alternate patronage of the Crown and the Bishop of Rochester. The church, dedicated to St. George, was erected on the site of a former edifice which was destroyed by fire, under an act passed in the 4th of George II., by which the sum of £5000 was granted to defray the expense: it is a neat and spacious edifice of brick, with quoins and cornices of stone. There are places of worship for Independents and Wesleyan Methodists. The free school was anciently founded by the corporation, and in 1703 Mr. David Varchell, then one of its members, endowed it with tenements producing at present about £70 per annum, for the clothing and instruction in reading, writing, arithmetic, and Latin, of twenty boys of the parishes of Gravesend and Milton: the endowment, in 1710, was augmented by Mr. James Fry, with a rent-charge of £14. 10., for the instruction of ten additional scholars, of which number, four are to be of the parish of Gravesend, four from Milton, and two from Chalk: there are thirty-six boys at present on the foundation of this school, which is under the management of the corporation, who, on the enlargement of the market-place, have made provision for the erection of a larger and more commodious school-house. There are various charitable bequests for the relief of the poor.

GRAVESHIP (NETHER), a township in that part of the parish of KENDAL which is in KENDAL ward, county of WESTMORLAND, 1 mile (S.) from Kendal, containing 76 inhabitants. Collinfield House, in this township, exhibits some beautiful geometrical windows, fine specimens of the style prevailing in the reign of Elizabeth. At a place called Stone-Cross barn, an ancient cross has been standing from time immemorial.

GRAYINGHAM, a parish in the wapentake of COR-RINGHAM, parts of LINDSEY, county of LINCOLN, 1½ mile (S.) from Kirton, containing 141 inhabitants. The living is a rectory, in the archdeaconry of Stow, and diocese of Lincoln, rated in the king's books at £25. 17. 6. Sir J. H. Thorold, Bart. was patron in 1820. The church is dedicated to St. Radegund.

GRAYRIGG, a chapelry in that part of the parish of KENDAL which is in KENDAL ward, county of WEST-MORLAND, 5½ miles (N. E. by E.) from Kendal, containing 229 inhabitants. The living is a perpetual curacy, in the archdeaconry of Richmond, and diocese of Chester, endowed with £400 private benefaction, and £400 royal bounty, and in the patronage of the landowners, subject to the approval of the Vicar of Kendal. The chapel was rebuilt at the expense of the inhabitants, in 1708. There is a meeting-house and burial-ground belonging to the Society of Friends, who have also an ancient cemetery at Sunny-bank, now disused. A free school was established in 1723, and a school-house erected by subscription in 1818; it is supported by the produce of sundry bequests, amounting to £27 a year.

GRAYSOUTHEN, a township in the parish of BRIGHAM, ALLERDALE ward above Darwent, county of CUMBERLAND, 3½ miles (W. by S.) from Cocker-mouth, containing 416 inhabitants. There are two collieries, a sickle manufactory, and a flax-mill in which linen thread is spun. An allotment of land, the annual rental of which is £25, was appropriated, at the time of enclosing the common, to the education of children.

GREASBROUGH, a chapelry in that part of the parish of ROTHERHAM which is in the northern division of the wapentake of STRAFFORTH and TICKHILL, West riding of the county of YORK, 2 miles (N. by W.) from Rotherham, containing 1252 inhabitants. The living is a perpetual curacy, in the archdeaconry and diocese of York, endowed with £400 private benefaction, £600 royal bounty, and £400 parliamentary grant, and in the patronage of Earl Fitzwilliam. The chapel is dedicated to the Holy Trinity. An additional chapel is now being erected by the Commissioners appointed under the late act for promoting the erection of churches and chapels. Here is a place of worship for Wesleyan Methodists.

GREASBY, a township in the parish of WEST KIRBY, lower division of the hundred of WIRRALL, county palatine of CHESTER, 7½ miles (N. N.W.) from Great Neston, containing 235 inhabitants.

GREASLY, a parish in the southern division of the wapentake of BROXTOW, county of NOTTINGHAM, 7 miles (N. W.) from Nottingham, containing 4241 inhabitants. The living is a discharged vicarage, in the archdeaconry of Nottingham, and diocese of York, rated in the king's books at £8. 5., endowed with £10 per annum and £300 private benefaction, £400 royal bounty, and £1400 parliamentary grant. Viscount Melbourne was patron in 1819. The church is a hand-some edifice, with a lofty embattled tower. Lancelot Rolleston, in 1748, founded and endowed a free school, in which twenty-two boys are taught; the annual income is about £27, with a house and garden for the master. Five pounds a year, the bequest of the Rev. John Man-sell, is paid to a schoolmistress for teaching eight children to read. The Nottingham canal passes through the south-west part of the parish, on the line of which there

are several coal wharfs, and in the neighbourhood is a railway. There are some remains of an ancient em-battled mansion called Greysley castle, to the north-ward of which are slight fragments of the Carthusian priory of Beauvale, founded in the reign of Edward III. by Nicholas de Cantilupe, and dedicated to the Holy Trinity, for a prior and twelve monks, which number was subsequently increased to nineteen, whose revenue at the dissolution was estimated at £227. 8. At the village of Kimberley, within the parish, are the ruins of an ancient chapel.

GREATFORD, a parish in the wapentake of NESS, parts of KESTEVEN, county of LINCOLN, 4¾ miles (N.W. by W.) from Market-Deeping, containing, with the cha-pelry of Wilsthorpe, 360 inhabitants. The living is a rectory, in the archdeaconry and diocese of Lincoln, rated in the king's books at £18. 10., and in the pa-tronage of the Crown. The church is dedicated to St. Thomas à Becket.

GREATHAM, a parish in the north-eastern divi-sion of STOCKTON ward, county palatine of DURHAM, comprising the townships of Claxton and Greatham, and containing 484 inhabitants, of which number, 446 are in the township of Greatham, 7 miles (N. E. by N.) from Stockton upon Tees. The living is a discharged vicar-age, in the archdeaconry and diocese of Durham, rated in the king's books at £7. 1. 8., endowed with £200 private benefaction, and £200 royal bounty, and in the patronage of the Governors of Greatham Hospital. The church occupies the site of a more ancient structure, which was pulled down in 1792, excepting some pillars and arches on each side of the nave. The " Hospital of God in Greatham" was founded and endowed with the manor of Greatham, by Robert de Stichell, Bishop of Durham, in 1272, for a master, five priests, two clerks, and forty poor brethren, selected from the episcopal manors : Bishop Anthony Bek increased the original endowment, and added one chaplain and one clerk to the establishment : Edward IV. granted a license to the master to hold a weekly market, and fairs twice a year. By the charter of James, in 1610, the number was re-duced to a master and thirteen brethren, who were con-stituted a body corporate, with a common seal, and privilege to purchase lands; at present there are a master, a chaplain, six brethren, maintained wholly in the hospital, six out-pensioners and a bailiff, upon the foundation, of which the Bishop of Durham is patron, with power to repeal ancient statutes and to make new ones. There are but slight traces of the old building remaining, the whole having been rebuilt in 1804, by the benevolent exertions of the Earl of Bridgewater, who in 1785, before succeeding to the earldom, was collated to the mastership, which he continued to hold in order to appropriate its revenue to this purpose : it has four fronts, that towards the south having an arcade of three arches in the centre, surmounted by a tower and a dome, and the apartments for the brethren fill the square : the master's house is a handsome edifice, in the garden attached to which is the chapel, rebuilt in 1788. Parkhurst's hospital was founded in 1761, and endowed by Dormer Parkhurst, Esq., then master of God's hospital, for six poor women, who have each a separate dwelling-house and garden. The revenue, arising from certain lands in the township of Stockton, is about £100 per annum, and the master of the preceding institution is the patron. On the marshes near the mouth of the Tees were formerly considerable salt works, traces of which are still to be seen.

GREATHAM, a parish in the hundred of ALTON, Alton (North) division of the county of SOUTHAMPTON, 5 miles (N. by E.) from Petersfield, containing 177 inhabitants. The living is a rectory, in the archdeaconry and diocese of Winchester, rated in the king's books at £6. 5. 10. The Rev. Edmund White was patron in 1814. The church is dedicated to St. John the Baptist.

GREATHAM, a parish in the hundred of WEST EASWRITH, rape of ARUNDEL, county of SUSSEX, 7¼ miles (N. by E.) from Arundel, containing 71 inhabitants. The living is a rectory with that of Wiggonholt consolidated, in the archdeaconry and diocese of Chichester, and in the patronage of the Devisees of the late Rev. Richard Turner. The church is in the early style of English architecture. The river Arun runs through, and the Wey and Arun canal passes by, the parish.

GREAT-HAMLET, a township in the parish of GLOSSOP, hundred of HIGH PEAK, county of DERBY, 3½ miles (N. by W.) from Chapel en le Frith, containing 705 inhabitants.

GREATWORTH, a parish in the hundred of CHIPPING-WARDEN, county of NORTHAMPTON, 6 miles (N. W. by N.) from Brackley, containing 231 inhabitants. The living is a rectory, in the archdeaconry of Northampton, and diocese of Peterborough, rated in the king's books at £9. 0. 5., and in the patronage of the Rev. H. Bradridge. The church is dedicated to St. Peter.

GREAT YATE, a township in the parish of CROXDEN, southern division of the hundred of TOTMONSLOW, county of STAFFORD, 5¾ miles (N. W. by N.) from Uttoxeter. The population is returned with the parish.

GREENCROFT, a township in that part of the parish of LANCHESTER which is in the western division of CHESTER ward, county palatine of DURHAM, 9 miles (N.W. by W.) from Durham, containing 229 inhabitants.

GREENFIELD, a hamlet in the parish of ABY, Marsh division of the hundred of CALCEWORTH, parts of LINDSEY, county of LINCOLN, 3 miles (N. W.) from Alford. The population is returned with the parish. A priory was founded, before 1153, by Eudo de Greines and Ralph his son, for nuns of the Cistercian order, in honour of St. Mary, the revenue of which at the dissolution was valued at £79. 15. 1.

GREENFIELD, a liberty in the parish of WATLINGTON, hundred of PIRTON, county of OXFORD, 7½ miles (N. N. W.) from Henley upon Thames. The population is returned with the parish.

GREENFORD, a parish in the hundred of ELTHORNE, county of MIDDLESEX, 4½ miles (N. by E.) from Hounslow, containing 415 inhabitants. The living is a rectory, within the jurisdiction of the Commissary of London, concurrently with the Bishop, rated in the king's books at £20, and in the patronage of the Provost and Fellows of King's College, Cambridge. The church, dedicated to the Holy Cross, is built of flints, with a low wooden spire at the west end; some of the windows are ornamented with stained glass. The Rev. Edward Terry, chaplain to Sir Thomas Roe, in his embassy to the Great Mogul, of which he published an account, was rector of this parish; he died here in 1660, and was buried in the church. There is a place of worship for Baptists.

GREENHALGH, a joint township with Thistleton, in the parish of KIRKHAM, hundred of AMOUNDERNESS, county palatine of LANCASTER, 3¼ miles (N. W. by N.) from Kirkham, containing 419 inhabitants. There is a school endowed with sundry bequests producing £17 per annum, for which six children are taught. The first earl of Derby erected a castle near the village, of which some slight remains are still visible.

GREENHAM, a chapelry in that part of the parish of THATCHAM which is in the hundred of FAIRCROSS, county of BERKS, 1½ mile (S. E.) from Newbury, containing 947 inhabitants. The chapel was given with Thatcham to Reading abbey by Henry I., from which period it has been considered a chapel of ease to the former, and has lately received an addition of one hundred and twenty sittings, of which seventy are free, the Incorporated Society for the enlargement of churches and chapels having granted £30 towards defraying the expense. The Knights Hospitallers had a preceptory here before the time of Henry VI.

GREEN-HAMMERTON, county of YORK.—See HAMMERTON (GREEN).

GREENHILL, an extra-parochial liberty, in the wapentake of CORRINGHAM, parts of LINDSEY, county of LINCOLN, containing 11 inhabitants.

GREENHILL-LANE, a township in the parish of ALFRETON, hundred of SCARSDALE, county of DERBY, 2¾ miles (S. S. E.) from Alfreton, with which the population is returned. An urn, containing about eight hundred Roman coins, was discovered here in 1749, by a labourer.

GREENHOW, a township in the parish of INGLEBY-GREENHOW, western division of the liberty of LANGBAURGH, North riding of the county of YORK, 5½ miles (S.E. by E.) from Stokesley, containing 102 inhabitants.

GREENHYTHE, a hamlet in the parish of SWANSCOMBE, hundred of AXTON, DARTFORD, and WILMINGTON, lathe of SUTTON at HONE, county of KENT, 3 miles (E. N. E.) from Dartford. The population is returned with the parish. Though a retired place, it is pleasantly situated on the southern bank of the Thames, across which there is a horse-ferry to West Thurrock. Great quantities of lime and flints obtained in the neighbourhood are conveyed in barges hence to London and other places. In time of peace there are usually several frigates lying here in ordinary.

GREENLEIGHTON, a township in that part of the parish of HARTBURN which is in the north-eastern division of TINDALE ward, county of NORTHUMBERLAND, 7¾ miles (S. S. W.) from Rothbury, containing 37 inhabitants. Quarries of excellent limestone are wrought here.

GREENS, a joint township with Glantlees, in that part of the parish of FELTON which is in the eastern division of COQUETDALE ward, county of NORTHUMBERLAND, containing 76 inhabitants.

GREENSIDE-HILL, a joint township with Ingram and Linop, in the parish of INGRAM, northern division of COQUETDALE ward, county of NORTHUMBERLAND, 99 miles (S. S. W.) from Wooler, containing, with Ingram and Linop, 74 inhabitants.

GREENS-NORTON, a parish in the hundred of GREENS-NORTON, county of NORTHAMPTON, 1¾ mile (N. W. by W.) from Towcester, containing 740 inhabitants. The living is a rectory, with the perpetual curacies of

Silverstone and Whittlebury consolidated, in the archdeaconry of Northampton, and diocese of Peterborough, rated in the king's books at £38, and in the patronage of the Crown. The church is dedicated to St. Bartholomew. Here was formerly a chantry, of which a barn and yard are the only remains. The parish is bounded on the south by the river Tow, and on the east by the Watling-street. Near Kingston wood is a mineral spring. A small endowed school has been incorporated with the National school lately established here. This is the birthplace of Catherine Parr, the sixth queen of Henry VIII.

GREENSTEAD, a parish within the liberty of the borough of COLCHESTER, though locally in the Colchester division of the hundred of Lexden, county of ESSEX, 1 mile (E.) from Colchester, containing 510 inhabitants. The living is a rectory, in the archdeaconry of Essex, and diocese of London, rated in the king's books at £5, and in the patronage of the Crown. The church is dedicated to St. Andrew. The navigable river Colne bounds the parish on the west.

GREENSTEAD, a parish in the hundred of ONGAR, county of ESSEX, 1¼ mile (W. by S.) from Chipping-Ongar, containing 131 inhabitants. The living is a rectory, in the archdeaconry of Colchester, and diocese of London, rated in the king's books at £6. 13. 4., and in the patronage of the Bishop of London. The church, dedicated to St. Andrew, is a small edifice, the chancel of which is of brick, and the nave very remarkable, being walled with upright trunks of trees supported by brick buttresses, with its roof rising to a point in the centre, and a wooden steeple at the west end : it is supposed to have been erected about 1013, as a shrine for the reception of the corpse of St. Edmund, on being conveyed back from London to *Beodrics worthe*, or Bury, whence it had been carried away in 1010, by Bishop Ailwin, in consequence of the invasion of the Danes under Turkil.

GREENWICH, a market town and parish in the hundred of BLACKHEATH, lathe of SUTTON at HONE, county of KENT, 6 miles (E. S. E.) from London, containing 20,712 inhabitants. This place, which derives its name from the Saxon *Grena-wic*, green creek, or bay, is first noticed in the reign of Ethelred, as having been for three years the station of the Danish fleet, when in 1011 those northern invaders made an irruption into this part of Kent, and encamping on Blackheath, made predatory incursions into the surrounding parts of the country. Having devastated the city of Canterbury, and brought away Alphege, Archbishop of the province, they detained him prisoner in their camp for more than seven months, and at length put him to death for refusing to exact from his diocese an exorbitant sum of money, as the price of his ransom : after his martyrdom, he was canonized ; and the church of Greenwich, which had been the scene of his sufferings, was dedicated to St. Alphege, in honour of his memory. The establishment of a royal residence here may be traced as far back as the reign of Edward I.; and Henry IV. dates his will, in 1408, from his manor of Greenwich, which Henry V. granted for life to Thomas Beaufort, Duke of Exeter, who died here in 1417 : it passed afterwards to Humphrey, Duke of Gloucester, and uncle of the king, who in 1433 obtained the royal license to fortify and embattle his manor-house, and to empark two hundred acres of land adjoining it : he rebuilt the

palace and enclosed the park, within which he erected a tower, on the spot where the royal observatory now stands. On its reverting to the crown, after the death of the duke in 1447, Edward IV. expended considerable sums in enlarging and beautifying the palace, which in 1466 he granted with the manor to his queen, Elizabeth. The marriage of Richard, Duke of York, with Anne Mowbray, was solemnized here with great pomp during this reign. Henry VII. resided frequently at Greenwich, where he founded a convent adjoining the palace, for a prior and twelve brethren of the order of St. Francis, which, after its dissolution in the reign of his successor, was refounded by Mary, and finally suppressed by Elizabeth, in 1559. This was also the birthplace of Henry VIII., who was baptized in the parish church, and during whose reign it was one of the principal scenes of that splendour and festivity which distinguished his court. Here his marriages with Catherine of Arragon, in 1510, and with Anne of Cleves, in 1540, were celebrated with great pomp. The princesses Mary and Elizabeth were born here, and Edward VI. kept the festival of Christmas 1502-3 in this palace, where he died in the month of July following. The assizes for the county were held here in the first, fourth, and fifth years of the reign of Elizabeth, and in 1577 the town sent two burgesses to parliament. Elizabeth made Greenwich her favourite summer residence, and Mary, daughter of James I., was baptized here with great solemnity, in 1605.

Previously to the breaking out of the parliamentary war, Charles I. occasionally resided here ; and, in 1642, the tower in the park, then called Greenwich castle, and which had been used sometimes as a place of residence for the younger branches of the royal family, frequently as a place of confinement, and occasionally as a castle, was thought to be of so much importance, that the parliament issued immediate orders to secure it for their use. When the ordinance for the sale of lands belonging to the crown was passed, in 1649, Greenwich house and park were reserved and subsequently assigned as a residence for the Lord Protector ; but the exigencies of the government induced the House of Commons to pass an act for its sale. Several of the offices and premises adjoining it were sold to different purchasers, but the palace and the park remaining unsold, in 1654, they were again, by an ordinance of the house, settled upon the Protector and his heirs. After the Restoration, Greenwich again came into the possession of the crown, and the palace having become greatly decayed, Charles II. ordered it to be taken down, and commenced the erection of a magnificent palace of freestone, one wing of which was completed at an expense of £36,000. Here that monarch occasionally resided, but no further progress was made in the work, either by himself, or his successor. Greenwich has been the place of debarkation of many illustrious visitors, and of several royal personages; among the latter may be noticed the Princess Augusta of Saxe Gotha, afterwards married to Frederick, Prince of Wales, and mother of George III., and the Princess Caroline of Brunswick, late consort of George IV. The remains of Admiral Lord Nelson were landed here, after the memorable battle of Trafalgar, in 1806, and lay in state in the hall of the hospital for three days prior to their removal for interment in the Cathedral Church of St. Paul.

Between the park and the river is that magnificent structure appropriated as an asylum for the decayed veterans and disabled seamen of the British navy, and for the maintenance and support of the widows and children of such as have fallen in the service of their country. This noble institution was established in the early part of the reign of William and Mary, and, upon the suggestion of Sir Christopher Wren, the unfinished palace of Charles II., afterwards enlarged under his gratuitous superintendence with additional buildings, was, by royal grant, appropriated to this patriotic purpose, in 1695. The king appointed nearly two hundred commissioners, including the principal officers of the state, the archbishops, bishops, judges, the lord mayor and aldermen of the city of London, the master, warden, assistants, and elder brethren of the Trinity House, to frame statutes and ordinances for the right management of the royal hospital, and, by letters patent, granted the annual sum of £2000 for completing the works, and carrying the plan into effect. By a commission issued in the reign of Queen Anne, seven of these commissioners were constituted a general court, of which the Lord High Admiral, the Lord Treasurer, or any two members of the privy council, should form a quorum. The governor and treasurer were appointed by the crown, all the other officers of the establishment by the Lord High Admiral, on the recommendation of the general court; twenty-five of the commissioners were appointed to form a standing committee, and the internal regulation of the hospital was vested in the governor and a council of officers, appointed by the Lord High Admiral. Similar commissions were issued by succeeding sovereigns, on their accession to the throne, and his late Majesty, George III., by charter, incorporated the commissioners, in whom also were vested, by act of parliament, all the estates held in trust for the benefit of the institution. By an act passed in the 10th of his present majesty, George IV., "to provide for the better management of the affairs of Greenwich Hospital," it is now placed under the authority, control, and direction, of the Lord High Admiral, or the commissioners to whom that office is usually entrusted.

The present establishment consists of a governor, lieutenant-governor, five captains, eight lieutenants, two chaplains, physician, assistant physician, surgeon, and three assistant surgeons, dispenser, and two assistants, secretary, cashier, steward, clerk of the cheque, clerk of the works, and other officers. On the opening of the hospital, in 1705, fifty-two pensioners were admitted : in the three following years the number increased to three hundred, and progressively increasing with the augmentation of the funds, it had in 1738 amounted to one thousand. Since that period the buildings have been considerably enlarged, and there are at present two thousand seven hundred and ten pensioners, who, in addition to their lodging, clothing, and maintenance, receive a weekly allowance of pocket money. Exclusively of the pensioners, there are three matrons, and one hundred and sixty-two nurses, widows of seamen, who, besides their maintenance and clothing, receive a salary of £11 per annum, for attending the pensioners when sick, and keeping their apartments and linen in order : the number of persons resident within the walls of this splendid establishment, including inferior officers and servants, is not less than three thousand five hundred.

The hospital originally was open only to seamen in the king's service, but, in 1710, the privileges were, by an act passed in the reign of Queen Anne, extended to disabled mariners in the merchants' service : mariners, as seamen, are entitled to the benefits of the hospital, and foreigners, having served two years in the British navy, are entitled to the same advantages as natives. By act of parliament in 1763, fourteen hundred out-pensioners, each of whom receive £7 per annum, were admitted on the foundation, but they have lately been transferred to the navy board. The ample funds by which this noble institution is supported have arisen from numerous sources, among which were a grant of £2000 per annum by King William ; a subscription of £8000 raised at the commencement of the work, by the original commissioners ; a grant of £19,000, the amount of various fines paid by merchants for smuggling ; the forfeited effects of Kid, a pirate, amounting to £6472. 1., granted by Queen Anne, in 1705 ; the moiety of an estate bequeathed by Robert Osbaldeston, Esq., in 1707, amounting to £20,000, with the profits of his unexpired grant of the North and South Foreland light-houses, since renewed to the hospital ; an estate devised by Mr. William Clapham, of Eltham ; the forfeited estates of the Earl of Derwentwater; a benefaction in malt-tickets of £1000. 9. 8., by some person unknown ; a legacy of £3381. 15. by John de la Fontaine, Esq.; a bequest of £2000 by Mr. Evelyn, and fines for fishing with unlawful nets and for other offences on the river Thames. With these several sums and others not detailed, an investment has been made, producing £70,000 per annum, to which may be added £30,000 per annum arising from the above mentioned forfeited estates, which are situated in the counties of Cumberland and Durham, and contain valuable mines of lead and other ores; £20,000 per annum from a contribution of six-pence per month from every seaman in the merchants' service, the profits of the market of Greenwich, given by Henry, Earl Romney, in 1700 ; a per centage on freights, and other sums, forming in the aggregate an income of nearly £130,000 per annum. The hospital is situated on a terrace fronting the Thames, eight hundred and seventy-five feet in length, and terminated at each extremity by an alcove : in the centre is a landing-place from the river, from which the view of this sumptuous pile is strikingly beautiful and magnificent, extending through a lengthened perspective of elegant building enriched by the stately domes of the hall and chapel, from each of which is continued a noble colonnade of the Doric order, three hundred and forty-seven feet in length, and terminating with the palace of Henrietta Maria, consort of Charles II., now the naval asylum, above which is seen the royal observatory on an eminence in the park. On the west side of the principal quadrangle, which is two hundred and seventy-three feet wide, and in the centre of which is a statue of George II. by Rysbrack, sculptured out of a single block of marble taken from the French by Admiral Sir George Rook, is that part of the hospital called King Charles's building. In the centre of the front towards the river is a handsome portal, leading into an inner quadrangle, separating the wing of that monarch's unfinished palace from a range of building formerly of brick, but which, having fallen into decay, was rebuilt of Portland stone in 1814, in a style of more appropriate grandeur. On each side of the portal, which is ornamented with pilasters of the Corinthian order, surmounted by an entablature of festoons and flowers, are four lofty Corinthian columns supporting an entablature and pediment; in the tympanum of that on the eastern side of the portal are the figures of Mars and Fame, finely sculptured. The east front of this range, facing the principal quadrangle, has in the centre a tetrastyle portico of the Corinthian order, with an entablature and pediment, leading also into the inner quadrangle, and at each extremity, four pilasters of the same order, with an entablature surmounted by an attic and handsome balustrade. The west front is decorated with six lofty Corinthian columns in the centre, and on each side enriched with pilasters of the same order : this range contains the apartments of the governor and lieutenant-governor, the governor's hall, council-chamber, and other offices, with wards for four hundred and seventy-six pensioners. On the east side of the principal quadrangle is that part of the hospital called Queen Anne's building, corresponding, in every respect, with the exception of some of its minuter details, with that of King Charles, and with it forming the entire front towards the river : this range, in addition to apartments for officers of the establishment, contains wards for four hundred and forty-two pensioners. To the south of these buildings are those of King William on the west, and Queen Mary on the east, erected by Sir Christopher Wren, to which there is an ascent from the principal quadrangle by a double flight of six steps, forming a terrace on the southern side, from which is a fine view of the river. In the former of these ranges is the painted hall, and in the latter the chapel of the hospital, of which the finely proportioned domes, by a projection of these ranges contracting the area of the quadrangle, are brought into a prominent point of view, in which they display with full effect the symmetry of their form and the gracefulness of their elevation. The tambour of these domes is surrounded by duplicated columns of the composite order, with projecting groups at the quoins, and the cupola is terminated by a turret surmounted by gilt vanes. The entrance to the hall is through a vestibule, in which are various emblematical paintings and portraits of several of the British admirals and benefactors to the hospital : the internal view of the dome, which is finely embellished with paintings, and from which hang many of the colours taken from the enemy, is strikingly beautiful. A large flight of steps leads from the vestibule, through a lofty and magnificent portal, into the grand saloon, one hundred and six feet in length, fifty-six in width, and fifty feet high, lighted on one side by a double range of windows, of which the jambs are empanelled and decorated with roses, and corresponding with these, on the opposite side, are recesses in which are emblematical figures painted in chiaro-oscuro. A range of lofty Corinthian pilasters, supporting a rich entablature, surrounds the saloon, the ceiling of which is exquisitely painted by Sir James Thornhill, in compartments ; in the centre are the figures of King William and Queen Mary seated on a throne, attended by the cardinal virtues, and surrounded with emblematical representations of the seasons, the signs of the zodiac, and numerous allegorical devices from mythology and history.

A series of portraits of the most distinguished admirals, and paintings of their principal naval engagements, decorate the wals, and over the great arch at the upper end of the hall are the British arms, supported by Mars and Minerva. From the saloon a flight of steps leads into the upper hall, in which the funeral car of Lord Nelson is deposited : the ceiling is decorated with paintings of Queen Anne and Prince George of Denmark, with various emblematical figures ; in the angles are the arms of England, Scotland, France, and Ireland, between which are represented the four quarters of the world, with their several emblems and productions. On the left of the entrance is a painting of the landing of the Prince of Orange, afterwards William III., and over the mantle-piece, the landing at Greenwich of George I., of whom and of his family are portraits at the upper end of the hall. To the south of the painted hall is a continuation of King William's buildings, of which the east front is of Portland stone, decorated in the centre with a pediment, in the tympanum of which is an emblematical representation of the death of Admiral Lord Nelson in alto relievo, and having a colonnade of the Doric order, three hundred and forty-seven feet in length, consisting of double columns, twenty feet high, with a return of seventy feet in length at the extremity of the range. In the centre of the east front is a handsome Doric portico leading into the quadrangle which separates the western side, erected by Sir John Vanbrugh ; this part, which is of brick, is ornamented in the centre with four massive Doric columns, nearly six feet in diameter, with an entablature and triglyphs of Portland stone : this range of building, in addition to apartments for officers, contains wards for the accommodation of five hundred and fifty-nine pensioners. Opposite to the entrance into the painted hall is the chapel of the hospital, of which the interior and roof were destroyed by fire in 1779, and restored in the most elegant style of Grecian architecture, from a design by the late Mr. James Stuart, publisher of the Antiquities of Athens. In the vestibule are statues of Faith, Hope, Meekness, and Charity, after designs by West : a flight of fourteen steps leads through folding doors of mahogany exquisitely carved, with an architrave, frieze, and cornice, of statuary marble, beautifully enriched, into the chapel, which is one hundred and eleven feet in length and fifty-two in breadth, with a lofty arched ceiling divided into compartments, and elegantly ornamented with foliage and other designs. The chapel is lighted by two ranges of windows, between which are galleries for the governor, lieutenant-governor, and principal officers, and in the lower part are seats for one thousand pensioners, exclusively of the nurses, inferior officers, and attendants. Within the entrance is a portico of four fluted columns of the Ionic order, each formed of one entire block of veined marble, fifteen feet high, which support the organ gallery; on each side of the portal are Corinthian pillars of scagliola, with bases and capitals of statuary marble, of which the shafts are twenty-eight feet high, and on each side of the altar are corresponding columns which support the roof. The altar-piece is embellished with a painting of the shipwreck of St. Paul, by West, in a richly gilt frame, twenty-five feet high and fourteen feet wide, above which are angels in statuary marble, sculptured by Bacon, and in the segment, between the cornice and the ceiling, is a painting in chiaro-oscuro of the Ascension, designed by West, and executed by Rebecca, terminating a series of subjects from the life of our Saviour, which is carried round the upper part of the chapel. To the south of the chapel is a continuation of Queen Mary's building, of Portland stone, similar in design, and, though less elaborately ornamented, corresponding in style with that of King William, and having in the front a Doric colonnade of equal length, with a return of seventy feet in length at the southern extremity. This range of building, which, like all the rest, forms a detached quadrangle, contains wards for the accommodation of one thousand one hundred and seventy pensioners. The extremities of these two last ranges form the grand south front of the hospital, between which is a singularly grand and beautiful perspective view of the river and of the country on the opposite bank. The west entrance to the hospital is formed by massive rusticated stone piers, supporting a terrestrial and celestial globe, each six feet in diameter, on which are traced the great circles of the sphere, rectified for the latitude of Greenwich. Without the walls, on the west, is the infirmary, a handsome modern quadrangular building of brick, one hundred and ninety-three feet in length and one hundred and seventy-five in breadth, containing apartments for a physician, surgeon, and apothecary, with their assistants, a surgery, dispensary, and a small chapel, and wards divided into well ventilated rooms, holding four each, for the reception of two hundred and fifty-six patients. Adjoining the infirmary is a building for the accommodation of one hundred and seventeen helpless pensioners and their nurses, with hot and cold baths, and a room containing a good medical library. The east entrance is through iron gates handsomely decorated, opposite to which is a range of brick building comprising the commissioners' board-room and the requisite offices for the secretary, cashier, steward, clerk of the cheque, and other civil officers of the establishment.

To the south of the hospital is the Naval asylum, or school, for the clothing, maintenance, and education of the children of seamen. This extensive and truly liberal institution had its origin in the establishment of the royal hospital, in which a small number of the pensioners' sons was educated, and the original school was, in 1821, incorporated with the Royal Naval asylum, which had been removed from Paddington to Greenwich in 1801. The establishment comprises an upper and a lower school: the former consists of one hundred sons of commissioned and ward-room warrant officers of the Royal Navy, and marines, presented by the Board of Admiralty collectively, and of three hundred sons of officers of the same or inferior rank, nominated in rotation by the lords and the first secretary of the admiralty, and by the commissioners, governor, and lieutenant-governor of the hospital, individually. The scholars are admitted between the ages of eleven and twelve, and are instructed in writing, arithmetic, the mathematics, navigation, and the drawing of charts on geometrical principles, by masters appointed for the purpose, the chaplain is officially head master of all the schools, and especially charged with the religious instruction of the children, and the general superintendence of the other branches of their education. Each boy has a bible and prayer-book given to him on admission, and during his continuance is supplied with all necessary books and instruments, which he is allowed to take away with him on leaving school, when he is bound apprentice to the sea service for seven years. The lower

school consists of four hundred boys and two hundred girls, children of inferior warrant and non-commissioned officers and seamen; they are admitted, from nine till twelve years of age, on petition to the governor of the hospital, according to their father's claim for service, which claims are examined monthly, and decided upon by a committee of selection: the boys are instructed in reading, writing, and arithmetic, till they are fourteen years of age, and are then apprenticed to the sea service; the girls, till of the same age, are taught reading, writing, and needle-work, and on their leaving school are placed out to trades or as household servants. The schools are supported from the general funds of the hospital, towards which are added the various sums received by the guides appointed to show the hospital to strangers, which, from its external magnificence and internal decoration, attracts numerous visitors. The present school-rooms were erected from a design by Mr. Alexander, and consist of two spacious wings, each one hundred and forty-six feet in length and forty-two in breadth, connected with the central building by a colonnade of the Tuscan order, one hundred and eighty feet long and twenty wide, affording a sheltered area for recreation in wet weather. The central building, formerly the palace of Henrietta Maria, consort of Charles II., erected in 1635, and considerably enlarged for its present purpose, contains apartments for the superintending captain, the chaplain and head master, the assistant masters, the schoolmistresses, matron, nurses, and others connected with the schools, and the school-rooms, refectory, and dormitory for the girls. In the western wing are the chapel and the upper school-room, one hundred feet long and thirty-nine wide, with a lateral recess twenty-two feet square, over which are two spacious dormitories, containing each two hundred hammocks, suspended in two tiers on each side. To the west of this wing is the gymnasium, with complete apparatus for the practice of those athletic exercises so essential in a nautical education, as tending to impart strength and agility to the body, and courage and intrepidity to the mind: in part of the ground appropriated to this purpose is a circle of lofty masts and slighter poles alternately inserted at the top into a circular beam, and in the centre a high pole with a horizontal windlas, affording a complete course of gymnastics peculiarly adapted to naval purposes. The east wing comprises the lower school-room, of equal dimensions with the upper, two similar dormitories, each containing two hundred hammocks, and a refectory one hundred and forty-three feet long and thirty-nine wide, in which eight hundred scholars dine together at four tables, and a room for washing, in which are arranged in a circle one hundred separate cisterns, and other apparatus for one hundred boys to wash at once from a running stream: connected with this part of the buildings are wash-houses, laundries, kitchen, brewhouse, bakehouse, and other requisite offices. The grounds surrounding the buildings are pleasantly laid out; and on the lawn in front of the central building is a piece of heavy ordnance mounted. To the west of the naval asylum, in a detached situation, is the infirmary belonging to the institution, a neat building of brick, arranged with due regard to the accommodation of patients, who are visited during their illness by the matron of the school, and attended by the nurses. Near the water side is an extensive iron wharf, where several smiths are employed in preparing a supply of such articles as may be wanted for immediate use.

The town is pleasantly situated at the base, and on the western declivity, of the commencement of a range of heights which forms the southern boundary of the vale of the Thames. The streets in the lower part, towards the river, are narrow and the houses mean and irregularly built ; but in the higher situations, especially on the west side of the park, towards Blackheath, many respectable houses have been erected; a spacious and handsome street, leading directly from the church towards the hospital, and forming the principal thoroughfare to Woolwich, has been already formed, and further improvements are likely to result from the erection of a new market-house, which is at present in contemplation. The town is partially paved, lighted with gas, and supplied with water from the Kent water works at Deptford : a small theatre is opened occasionally during the winter, and a literary and scientific institution has been recently established. The park, comprising nearly two hundred acres, was walled round by James I., and planted and laid out in the reign of Charles II. : the scenery is diversified with extensive lawns and stately avenues of fine old elms and chesnut trees ; the views from many of the higher grounds are extensive and magnificent, especially from the observatory, and an abrupt eminence called One Tree Hill, embracing the hospital, the winding Thames crowded with shipping, a distant view of the metropolis, and a rich variety of splendid and interesting objects. The royal observatory was erected, in 1675, on the site, and partly with the materials, of the ancient tower, built by Humphrey, Duke of Gloucester, which, with every requisite aid, was granted for that purpose by Charles II.: it was completed under the superintendence of Mr. Flamsteed, who, on the recommendation of Sir Jonas Moor, was appointed Astronomer Royal, and took possession of it in the following year. Since the time of Flamsteed, from whom it obtained the appellation of Flamsteed House, the institution has continued to improve, and is at present replete with astronomical instruments of every description, and of the most accurate construction; among these are, the instrument used by Dr. Bradley to detect the aberration of the fixed stars; a revolving circle by Troughton, of-exquisite mechanism ; and the original chronometer, by Harrison, for which parliament awarded him a considerable premium. The observatory, which is under the superintendence of an astronomer royal, appointed by the King, and six assistants, is annually visited by a deputation from the Royal Society, under whose inspection the observations made by the Astronomer Royal are annually published, pursuant to an order of his late Majesty : the longitudinal distances in England are invariably calculated from the meridian of Greenwich. The market days are Wednesday and Saturday : fairs are held annually, commencing on the Mondays at Easter and Whitsuntide, which are numerously attended. The town is within the jurisdiction of the county magistrates, who hold a petty session every Tuesday, and of whom one or two are in daily attendance. A court of requests is held every Tuesday, under an act passed in the 47th of George III., for the recovery of debts under £5, the jurisdiction of which extends over the parishes of Greenwich, Dept-

ford, Lewisham, Woolwich, Eltham, Chiselhurst, Charlton, Lea, Bromley, Beckenham, Bexley, Foot's Cray, St. Mary Cray, Orpington, Erith, and Plumstead, in the county of Kent ; and the parishes of Croydon, Carshalton, Mitcham, Beddington, Morden, Sutton, and Cheam, in the county of Surrey.

The living is a vicarage, in the archdeaconry and diocese of Rochester, rated in the king's books at £21, and in the patronage of the Crown. The ancient church, dedicated to St. Alphege, having become dilapidated, the present structure was built by act of parliament passed in the 9th of Queen Anne, for the erection of fifty churches within the city of London and its suburbs : it is a handsome edifice in the Grecian style of architecture, with a square tower, above which is a cupola supported on pillars of the Corinthian order, and surmounted by a small spire. The interior is ornamented with a painting on panel, representing a monumental effigy of Queen Elizabeth, a painting of Charles I. at his devotions, and with portraits of Queen Anne and George I. A church, dedicated to St. Mary, was erected by means of a grant from the parliamentary commissioners, in 1824, at an expense of £11,000, and contains one thousand seven hundred and thirteen sittings, of which six hundred and forty-five are free : it is a neat edifice of Suffolk white brick, in the Grecian style of architecture, with a square tower of stone, and a portico of the Ionic order. There are places of worship for Baptists, Independents, and Wesleyan Methodists, also a Roman Catholic chapel. The Grey-coat school was founded in 1643, by John Roan, Esq., who endowed it with lands and houses in the parish, producing about £700 per annum, for clothing and educating poor children ; one hundred boys are clothed and instructed in reading, writing, and arithmetic, and twenty supernumerary boys are instructed but not clothed : the management is vested in the vicar, churchwardens, and overseers of the parish. The Green-coat school was founded in 1672, by Sir William Boreman, who endowed it with lands, tenements, and fee farm rents, producing about £700 per annum, for the maintenance, clothing, and instruction of twenty poor boys of the parish : the management is vested in the Master and Wardens of the Drapers' Company, who have appropriated to it the sum of £300 given to that company for charitable uses : the endowment has been subsequently augmented with a bequest of £5000 by William Clovell, Esq., who was educated in the school : a new school-house was erected in 1788. The Blue-coat charity school, for the maintenance, clothing, and education of girls, was established in 1770, and is supported by the interest on various legacies, by an estate producing £212 per annum, bequeathed by Mrs. Elizabeth Day, and by subscription : there are twenty girls in the school : the average expenditure is £550 per annum. Queen Elizabeth's college was founded in 1576, by William Lambarde, Esq., author of the "Perambulations of Kent," who endowed it for twenty aged persons, of whom, one each is to be appointed by the Master of the Rolls and the Master and Wardens of the Drapers' Company, in whom the management is jointly vested ; six from the parish of Greenwich, appointed by the vicar and parish officers ; one from Deptford ; three from Lewisham ; one from Lee ; three from Eltham ; one from Charlton and Kedbrook ; and one from Woolwich : the original endowment has been augmented by subsequent benefactions; the inmates receive a weekly allowance of money, and an annual supply of coal. The founder, with the consent of the Bishop of Rochester, composed a form of morning and evening prayers to be used in the college, and made void his endowment should its use be prohibited by the laws of the realm. Norfolk college was founded in 1613, and dedicated to the Holy Trinity, by Henry, Earl of Northampton, who endowed it with lands and estates producing about £1500 per annum, for the support of a warden and twenty pensioners, of whom twelve are to be of this parish, and eight of the parish of Shottesham in the county of Norfolk; the management was vested by the founder in the Master and Wardens of the Mercers' Company: the building forms a neat quadrangle of brick at the east end of the town, near the river, and comprises a chapel, in which are a fine window of painted glass, and a handsome monument to the memory of the founder, removed with his remains from the chapel at Dovor castle, where he was interred. Eight almshouses were built in 1809, by subscriptions amounting to £1153, and called the Jubilee almshouses, in commemoration of the fiftieth anniversary of the accession of George III. to the throne: to these were added four more, by subscription among the Greenwich volunteer corps of infantry, in commemoration of the centenary anniversary of the accession of the house of Hanover. In 1784, several barrows were opened in the park, and various military weapons were discovered. Among the eminent men who have been interred in this parish are, William Lambarde, the Kentish antiquary, who died at West Combe, in 1601; Thomas Philpot, who published a survey of Kent from papers collected by his father, and died in 1628; Major General James Wolfe, who fell gloriously in the arms of victory at Quebec, and was buried in the old church of St.Alphege, in 1759; and Lavinia, Duchess of Bolton, who died in 1760. The learned Dr. Squire, Bishop of St. David's, was instituted to the vicarage of this parish in 1751. Of the eminent astronomers who have succeeded Flamsteed at the Royal Observatory, may be noticed Dr. Halley, who died in 1742; Dr. Bradley, who died in 1762; and the late Dr. Maskelyne, who died in 1811.

GREET, a chapelry in the parish of WINCHCOMBE, lower division of the hundred of KIFTSGATE, county of GLOUCESTER, 1 mile (N.) from Winchcombe, with which the population is returned.

GREET, a parish in the hundred of OVERS, county of SALOP, 2½ miles (W. N. W.) from Tenbury, containing 79 inhabitants. The living is a discharged rectory, in the archdeaconry of Salop, and diocese of Hereford, rated in the king's books at £5. Sir H. Edwards, Bart. was patron in 1823.

GREETHAM, a parish in the hundred of HILL, parts of LINDSEY, county of LINCOLN, 3¼ miles (E. N. E.) from Horncastle, containing 148 inhabitants. The living is a discharged rectory, in the archdeaconry and diocese of Lincoln, rated in the king's books at £10. 19. 4., and in the patronage of the Bishop of Lincoln. The church is dedicated to All Saints.

GREETHAM, a parish in the hundred of ALSTOE, county of RUTLAND, 6 miles (N. E.) from Oakham, containing 541 inhabitants. The living is a vicarage, in the archdeaconry of Northampton, and diocese of

Peterborough, rated in the king's books at £5. 3. 9., and endowed with £500 three per cent. annuities, private benefaction. The Earl of Winchelsea was patron in 1822. The church is dedicated to St. Mary.

GREETLAND, a joint chapelry with Elland, in the parish of HALIFAX, wapentake of MORLEY, West riding of the county of YORK, 3 miles (S.) from Halifax, containing 5088 inhabitants, many of whom are employed in the manufacture of coarse cloth and fancy goods. There is a place of worship for Wesleyan Methodists. An altar was found on the summit of a hill some years ago, inscribed, as dedicated by Titus Aurelius Aurelianus, to the god of the city of the Brigantes, and to the deities of the emperors.

GREETWELL, a parish in the wapentake of LAWRESS, parts of LINDSEY, county of LINCOLN, 2¼ miles (E.) from Lincoln, containing 45 inhabitants. The living is a perpetual curacy, in the archdeaconry of Stow, and diocese of Lincoln, endowed with £600 royal bounty, and in the patronage of the Dean and Chapter of Lincoln. The church is dedicated to All Saints. The river Witham bounds the parish on the south.

GREGORY (ST.), an extra-parochial liberty, contiguous to the eastern part of the city of Canterbury, in the hundred of WESTGATE, lathe of ST.AUGUSTINE, county of KENT, containing 372 inhabitants.

GREINTON, a parish in the hundred of WHITLEY, county of SOMERSET, 6½ miles (W. S. W.) from Glastonbury, containing 237 inhabitants. The living is a discharged rectory, in the archdeaconry of Wells, and diocese of Bath and Wells, rated in the king's books at £13. 0. 10. S. Kekewich, Esq. was patron in 1800. The church is dedicated to St. Michael.

GRENDON, a parish in the hundred of WYMERSLEY, county of NORTHAMPTON, 5½ miles (S. by W.) from Wellingborough, containing 597 inhabitants. The living is a discharged vicarage, in the archdeaconry of Northampton, and diocese of Peterborough, rated in the king's books at £8, endowed with £400 private benefaction, £400 royal bounty, and £400 parliamentary grant, and in the patronage of the Master and Fellows of Trinity College, Cambridge. The church is dedicated to St. Mary.

GRENDON, a parish in the Tamworth division of the hundred of HEMLINGFORD, county of WARWICK, 3¼ miles (N. W.) from Atherstone, containing, with the hamlet of Whittington, 554 inhabitants. The living is a rectory, in the archdeaconry of Coventry, and diocese of Lichfield and Coventry, rated in the king's books at £20. 3. 4., and in the patronage of Sir G. Chetwynd, Bart. The church is dedicated to All Saints. The Coventry canal passes through the parish, and coal mines are wrought in the neighbourhood.

GRENDON (BISHOP'S), a parish in the hundred of BROXASH, county of HEREFORD, 4¼ miles (W. N. W.) from Bromyard, containing 212 inhabitants. The living is a perpetual curacy, in the archdeaconry and diocese of Hereford, endowed with £800 royal bounty, and £200 parliamentary grant, and in the patronage of the Vicar of Bromyard. The church, dedicated to St. John the Baptist, was rebuilt in 1788, at the expense of six individuals of the parish, the old edifice having fallen down in 1786. There are vestiges of an ancient intrenchment in the vicinity, said to be Danish.

GRENDON-UNDERWOOD, a parish in the hundred of ASHENDON, county of BUCKINGHAM, 6¾ miles (E. by S.) from Bicester, containing 312 inhabitants. The living is a rectory, in the archdeaconry of Buckingham, and diocese of Lincoln, rated in the king's books at £15. 6. 8. W. Pigott, Esq. was patron in 1808. The church is dedicated to St. Leonard. There is a small endowment, the gift of Lady Pigott in 1678, for teaching six children.

GRENDON-WARREN, a chapelry in the parish of PENCOMBE, hundred of BROXASH, county of HEREFORD, 4¾ miles (W.) from Bromyard. The population is returned with the parish.

GRESHAM, a parish in the northern division of the hundred of ERPINGHAM, county of NORFOLK, 4¼ miles (S.W. by W.) from Cromer, containing 351 inhabitants. The living is a discharged rectory, in the archdeaconry of Norfolk, and diocese of Norwich, rated in the king's books at £6. 18. 9., and in the patronage of the Rev. John Spurgin. The church, dedicated to All Saints, has portions in the decorated style of English architecture. There are foundations of a large castellated building, which, it is said, Sir Edmund Bacon obtained license from Edward II. to embattle: it is of a quadrilateral form, with a semicircular projection at each angle, probably the remains of towers or turrets, and is surrounded by a deep fosse. Gresham gave name to the family of which Sir Thomas, the founder of the Royal Exchange and of Gresham college, was a descendant.

GRESLEY (CASTLE), a hamlet in the parish of CHURCH-GRESLEY, hundred of REPTON and GRESLEY, county of DERBY, 4 miles (S.E. by S.) from Burton upon Trent, containing 129 inhabitants. There are slight vestiges of an ancient castle built by the Gresley family, who have been resident in the parish since the period of the Norman invasion; a member of another branch of this family was one of the Conqueror's ancestors.

GRESLEY (CHURCH), a parish in the hundred of REPTON and GRESLEY, county of DERBY, 5 miles (S.E.) from Burton upon Trent, comprising the townships of Drakelow and Linton, the hamlets of Castle-Gresley and Swadlincote, and the greater portion of the hamlets of Oakthorpe and Donisthorpe, and containing, with the whole of Oakthorpe and Donisthorpe, 1951 inhabitants. The living is a perpetual curacy, in the archdeaconry of Derby, and diocese of Lichfield and Coventry, endowed with £200 private benefaction, £800 royal bounty, and £1300 parliamentary grant, and in the patronage of Sir Roger Gresley, Bart., whose remote ancestor, William, founded a priory of canons of the order of St. Augustine, in the reign of Henry I., and dedicated it to St. Mary and St. George; its revenue at the dissolution, was valued at £39. 13. 8. There are considerable potteries in the parish, which afford employment to more than six hundred persons; the clay is found in great abundance, and of good quality. Extensive collieries are also wrought, and excellent iron-stone is obtained in the neighbourhood.

GRESSENHALL, a parish in the hundred of LAUNDITCH, county of NORFOLK, 2¾ miles (N.W.) from East Dereham, containing 861 inhabitants. The living is a rectory, in the archdeaconry and diocese of Norwich, rated in the king's books at £15. 13. 4. John Hill, Esq. was patron in 1807. The church, dedicated to St. Mary, is a large cruciform pile, having a tower rising from the intersection, which was formerly surmounted by a spire, but taken down in 1698. There was also a collegiate chapel, founded by William de Stuteville in the reign of Henry III., and dedicated to St. Nicholas, the remains of which have been converted into an infirmary to the house of industry, erected here in 1776, for the hundreds of Mitford and Launditch: the college possessed a common seal, representing St. Nicholas in his pontificals; the last incumbent, who was living in 1503, had a pension of £4. 16. granted by the crown.

GRESSINGHAM, a chapelry in that part of the parish of LANCASTER which is in the hundred of LONSDALE, south of the sands, county palatine of LANCASTER, 7¼ miles (N.E.) from Lancaster, containing 201 inhabitants. The living is a perpetual curacy, in the archdeaconry of Richmond, and diocese of Chester, endowed with £800 royal bounty, and in the patronage of the Vicar of Lancaster.

GRESTY, a joint township with Shavington, in the parish of WYBUNBURY, hundred of NANTWICH, county palatine of CHESTER, 4¼ miles (E.) from Nantwich, containing 274 inhabitants.

GRETA-BRIDGE, a hamlet in the parish of BRIGNALL, western division of the wapentake of GILLING, North riding of the county of YORK, 54 miles (N.W. by N.) from York, and 242½ (N.N.W.) from London. The population is returned with the parish. It takes its name from a lofty bridge of one arch, erected in the line of the Watling-street, upon the site of a more ancient structure, over the river Greta, a little above its junction with the Tees, at each extremity of which there is a commodious inn much frequented by travellers on the great north road from London to Glasgow. There are vestiges of a Roman camp in the neighbourhood, where an altar and several coins have been discovered. Here Mr. Ward places the *Maglove* of the Notitia.

GRETTON, a chapelry in the parish of WINCHCOMBE, lower division of the hundred of KIFTSGATE, county of GLOUCESTER, 2¼ miles (N.W.) from Winchcombe, with which the population is returned. There is a place of worship for Wesleyan Methodists.

GRETTON, a parish in the hundred of CORBY, county of NORTHAMPTON, 2¾ miles (N.E.) from Rockingham, containing 687 inhabitants. The living is a discharged vicarage with the perpetual curacy of Duddington, in the peculiar jurisdiction and patronage of the Prebendary of Gretton in the Cathedral Church of Lincoln, rated in the king's books at £19. 6. 8. The church is dedicated to St. James. Here is a place of worship for Baptists. Kirby-hall, a spacious rectangular mansion erected by Sir Christopher Hatton in the reign of Elizabeth, is in this parish.

GREWELL, a chapelry in the parish and hundred of ODIHAM, Basingstoke division of the county of SOUTHAMPTON, 1¾ mile (W.) from Odiham, containing 230 inhabitants. The living is a perpetual curacy annexed to the vicarage of Odiham, in the archdeaconry and diocese of Winchester. The chapel is dedicated to St. Mary.

GREWELTHORPE, or GRAVELTHORPE, a township in the parish of KIRKBY-MALZEARD, lower division of the wapentake of CLARO, West riding of the county of YORK, 6¼ miles (N.W. by W.) from Ripon, containing 527 inhabitants.

GREY'S FOREST, a township in the parish of KIRKNEWTON, western division of GLENDALE ward, county of NORTHUMBERLAND, 7 miles (W.N.W.) from Wooler, containing 54 inhabitants.

GREYSTEAD, or GAYSTEAD, a parish in the north-western division of TINDALE ward, county of NORTHUMBERLAND, 5 miles (W. by N.) from Bellingham, comprising the townships of Chirdon and Smalesmouth, and containing 246 inhabitants. The living is a rectory not in charge, in the archdeaconry of Northumberland, and diocese of Durham, and in the patronage of the Governors of Greenwich Hospital. This parish formed part of the late extensive parish of Simonburn, which was divided in 1811, by act of parliament, into six distinct parishes. The church was consecrated in 1818. The North Tyne river runs through the parish.

GREYSTOCK, a parish in LEATH ward, county of CUMBERLAND, comprising the chapelries of Matterdale, Mungris-dale, Threlkeld, and Water-Millock, and the townships of Berrier with Murrah, Little Blencow, Greystock, Hutton-John, Hutton-Roof, Hutton-Soil, Johnby, and Motherby with Gill, and containing 2419 inhabitants, of which number, 255 are in the township of Greystock, 5 miles (W. by N.) from Penrith. The living is a rectory, in the archdeaconry and diocese of Carlisle, rated in the king's books at £40. 7. 8½., and in the patronage of Adam Askew, Esq. The church, dedicated to St. Andrew, is a spacious edifice in the decorated style of English architecture: it was made collegiate by Neville, Archbishop of York, in 1382, for a master and six canons, whose stalls still remain, but their six chantries have been demolished. Thomas de Graystoke obtained a license from Henry III. for a weekly market and an annual fair to be held here, but they have been long discontinued. There are some collieries and quarries of slate, and limestone is obtained in various parts of the parish. The ancient castle, of which only a few broken towers remain, was garrisoned for the king in 1648, but surrendered shortly afterwards to a detachment of the army under General Lambert, and was burned down by order of the parliamentary leader : the present castle was built about one hundred and sixty years ago. A copyhold court for the barony of Greystock is held at Easter and Michaelmas. There are vestiges of a Roman intrenchment, called Redstone Camp, near which have been found urns, stone coffins, and human bones ; leading from it, in a direction towards Ambleside, are traces of an ancient road, and in the same tract lie three large cairns. In the vicinity of Motherby is a circle or stones, seventeen yards in diameter, within the area of which heaps of bones have been discovered.

GRIBTHORPE, a joint township with Willitoft, in the parish of BUBWITH, Holme-Beacon division of the wapentake of HARTHILL, East riding of the county of YORK, 5¾ miles (N. by E.) from Howden, containing 145 inhabitants.

GRIMLEY, a parish in the lower division of the hundred of OSWALDSLOW, county of WORCESTER, 4½ miles (N. by W.) from Worcester, containing 666 inhabitants. The living is a discharged vicarage, in the archdeaconry and diocese of Worcester, rated in the king's books at £14. 0. 10., endowed with £10 per annum private benefaction, and £200 royal bounty, and in the patronage of the Bishop of Worcester. The church is dedicated to St. Bartholomew. There is a chapel of ease at Hallow, in this parish : on the east

flows the river Severn, over which there is a ferry. There are several plantations of hops ; and in Hallow park is a mineral spring of similar properties to the Cheltenham water.

GRIMOLDBY, a parish in the Marsh division of the hundred of LOUTH-ESKE, parts of LINDSEY, county of LINCOLN, 5 miles (E.) from Louth, containing 298 inhabitants. The living is a discharged rectory, in the archdeaconry and diocese of Lincoln, rated in the king's books at £9. 10., and in the patronage of Lord Middleton. The church is dedicated to St. Edith.

GRIMSARGH, a joint chapelry with Brockholes, in the parish of PRESTON, hundred of AMOUNDERNESS, county palatine of LANCASTER, 5 miles (N.E.) from Preston, containing, with Brockholes, 343 inhabitants. The living is a perpetual curacy, in the archdeaconry of Richmond, and diocese of Chester, endowed with £200 private benefaction, and £500 parliamentary grant, and in the patronage of the Vicar of Preston. The chapel, consecrated in 1726, is dedicated to St. Michael. There is a school-house, in which a master resides, with a school-room lately attached to it by subscription among the inhabitants, in which are taught about forty children, who pay a certain quarterage.

GRIMSBY (GREAT), a borough, sea-port, market-town, and parish, having separate jurisdiction, locally in the wapentake of Bradley-Haverstoe, parts of LINDSEY, county of LINCOLN, 35 miles (N. E. by N.) from Lincoln, and 161 (N.) from London, containing 3064 inhabitants. This place, anciently called *Grimsbye*, is

Arms.

situated on the little river Freshney, near the mouth of the Humber, and is supposed to have been the spot where the Danes landed when they first invaded Britain, towards the end of the eighth century. Camden treats as fabulous a tradition that the town was founded by a merchant named *Gryme*, who obtained great riches in consequence of having brought up an exposed child, called *Haveloc*, who proved to be of the Danish blood royal, and, after having been scullion in the king's kitchen, obtained the king's daughter in marriage: to this romantic story, whatever may be its foundation, there is a reference in the device of the seal of the corporation. A Benedictine nunnery was founded here before 1185, and subsequently convents of the Augustine and Grey friars, but of these establishments there are no remains. In the reign of Edward III. Grimsby was a considerable sea-port ; and at the siege of Calais, in 1346, it supplied the king with eleven ships and one hundred and seventy mariners, towards his naval armament. The harbour was formerly defended by two blockhouses, and the commerce of the port was very extensive till the haven became obstructed by the accumulation of sand and mud deposited by the Humber, so as to prevent the access of any vessels but sloops, in which state it continued till the beginning of the present century. The town now consists of several good streets, the houses in which are well built ; and much improvement of late years has been made in its general appearance. It has also recovered its commercial importance, chiefly through the spirited exertions of some of the principal landed proprietors in the neighbourhood, who raised a subscription for improving the harbour, and obtained an act of parliament incorporating [them under the title of " The Grimsby Haven Company." A wet and a dry dock have been constructed, at the expense of about £70,000, the works having been opened in December 1800; since which, many new buildings have been erected, especially in the vicinity of the haven. Grimsby is a port subordinate to that of Hull, and has a deputy-collector and comptroller of customs, with a coast surveyor. Coal, salt, and the produce of the countries bordering on the Baltic, constitute the principal articles of its commerce. The number of vessels that entered inwards during the year ending January 5th, 1827, was twenty-nine British and seventy-five foreign; and the number which cleared outwards, twelve British and fifty-five foreign. Ships are annually sent to the Greenland fishery, and here are a few yards for building them. There are in the town some extensive breweries; and bone-crushing, and the trade in bones for manure and other purposes, are largely carried on. The market is on Friday, and a fair is held on the 6th of June; one on the 15th of September has been discontinued.

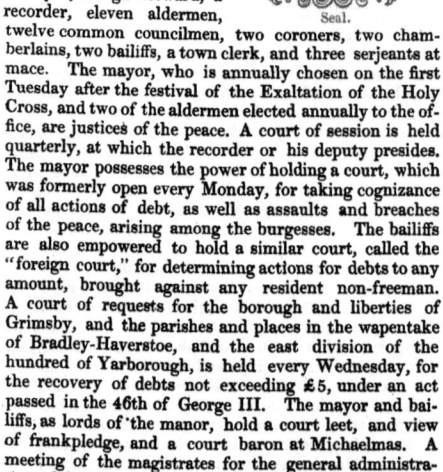

Seal.

Grimsby is one of the most ancient boroughs in England: it received its first charter from John, being either the first or second which that monarch granted. The charter whereby the town is now governed was bestowed by James II.: it ordains that the corporation consist of a mayor, a high steward, a recorder, eleven aldermen, twelve common councilmen, two coroners, two chamberlains, two bailiffs, a town clerk, and three serjeants at mace. The mayor, who is annually chosen on the first Tuesday after the festival of the Exaltation of the Holy Cross, and two of the aldermen elected annually to the office, are justices of the peace. A court of session is held quarterly, at which the recorder or his deputy presides. The mayor possesses the power of holding a court, which was formerly open every Monday, for taking cognizance of all actions of debt, as well as assaults and breaches of the peace, arising among the burgesses. The bailiffs are also empowered to hold a similar court, called the "foreign court," for determining actions for debts to any amount, brought against any resident non-freeman. A court of requests for the borough and liberties of Grimsby, and the parishes and places in the wapentake of Bradley-Haverstoe, and the east division of the hundred of Yarborough, is held every Wednesday, for the recovery of debts not exceeding £5, under an act passed in the 46th of George III. The mayor and bailiffs, as lords of the manor, hold a court leet, and view of frankpledge, and a court baron at Michaelmas. A meeting of the magistrates for the general administration of justice is held weekly, at the town clerk's office. There is a common gaol for the custody of offenders, under the jurisdiction of the mayor and justices, who appoint the gaoler. The corporation possess the exclusive right of fishing and fowling in the manors of Grimsby and Clee, and a claim on all wrecks thrown

upon their coast; and they likewise collect groundage from all ships driven on shore in gales of wind. This borough has sent two members to parliament from the 23rd of Edward I. to the present time: the mayor is the returning officer. The right of election, according to the last decision of the house of commons, is in the "freemen admitted at a full court by the mayor, aldermen, common council-men, and burgesses, such freemen being resident, and paying scot and lot, in all cases, except where no rate has taken place subsequent to their admission." All the sons of freemen born in the town are entitled to the elective franchise on coming of age, by observing the prescribed conditions, as well as every person marrying a freeman's daughter or widow, or who has obtained his freedom by servitude or redemption: the number of free burgesses at present is about three hundred. The political influence of the borough is possessed by Lord Yarborough.

The town formerly contained two parochial churches, but the parishes were united in 1586, and the church of St. Mary, then dilapidated, was suffered to fall into ruins. The living is a discharged vicarage, in the archdeaconry and diocese of Lincoln, rated in the king's books at £14. 18. 4., for the two parishes. George Robert Heneage, Esq. was patron in 1815. The remaining church, dedicated to St. James, is a spacious, handsome, cruciform structure, with a tower in the centre. Originally it was larger than it is at present; a part of the choir having fallen down about 1500, it became necessary to take the adjoining chantry down also. A considerable portion of it is in the early style of English architecture, with a western entrance of Norman character: the font is large and in the early English style, as is also a mutilated stone cross in the church-yard. The Baptists, Independents, and Primitive and Wesleyan Methodists, have each a place of worship. The free grammar school was founded in 1547, by letters patent of Edward VI., and endowed with the revenue of a suppressed chantry, which previously belonged to the church of St. James, for the support of a master to instruct the boys of parishioners gratuitously. The corporation lands are charged with the payment of £4. 5. 6. per annum to the master of this school, which is further endowed with £7 per annum given by Catherine Mason, widow. A few religious houses existed in the neighbourhood previously to the dissolution, but every vestige of them has been obliterated. Spittal-hill is supposed to have been the site of an establishment of the Knights Hospitallers of St. John of Jerusalem. In the vicinity are several deep circular pits, called *Blow Wells*, the water of which rises even with the surface of the ground, but never overflows. Dr. John Whitgift, Archbishop of Canterbury, a prelate distinguished for his piety and learning, was born here in the year 1530; and Dr. Martin Fotherby, Bishop of Salisbury in the reign of James I., was also a native of this place.

GRIMSBY (LITTLE), a parish in the wapentake of LUDBOROUGH, parts of LINDSEY, county of LINCOLN, 3¼ miles (N.) from Louth, containing 67 inhabitants. The living is a discharged vicarage, in the archdeaconry and diocese of Lincoln, rated in the king's books at £3. 6. 8., endowed with £200 private benefaction, and £400 royal bounty, and in the patronage of the Duke of St. Albans. The church is dedicated to St. Edith.

GRIMSTEAD (EAST), a chapelry in the parish of

West Dean, hundred of Alderbury, county of Wilts, 5¼ miles (E. S.E.) from Salisbury, containing 107 inhabitants.

GRIMSTEAD (WEST), a parish in the hundred of Alderbury, county of Wilts, 5 miles (S. E. by E.) from Salisbury, containing 161 inhabitants. The living is a rectory, with which the rectory of Plaitford is consolidated, in the archdeaconry and diocese of Salisbury, rated in the king's books at £7. 10. 2½., and in the patronage of the Earl of Ilchester. The line of a canal now in progress between Christchurch and Salisbury passes through the parish.

GRIMSTON, a parish in the eastern division of the hundred of Goscote, county of Leicester, 5 miles (W.N.W.) from Melton-Mowbray, containing 200 inhabitants. The living is a perpetual curacy with the vicarage of Rothley, in the peculiar jurisdiction of the Lord of the Manor of Rothley, endowed with £400 royal bounty. The church is dedicated to St. John.

GRIMSTON, a township in that part of the parish of Dunnington which is in the wapentake of Ouze and Derwent, East riding of the county of York, 3 miles (E. by S.) from York, containing 72 inhabitants.

GRIMSTON, a township in that part of the parish of Gilling which is in the wapentake of Ryedale, North riding of the county of York, 6 miles (S.) from Helmsley, containing 56 inhabitants.

GRIMSTON, a township in that part of the parish of Kirkby-Wharf which is in the upper division of the wapentake of Barkstone-Ash, West riding of the county of York, 1¾ mile (S.) from Tadcaster, containing 62 inhabitants. A school has been established and endowed by Lady Howden, for children of both sexes, who are also clothed once a year.

GRIMSTON (NORTH), a parish partly within the liberty of St. Peter of York, but chiefly in the wapentake of Buckrose, East riding of the county of York, 4½ miles (S.E. by E.) from New Malton, containing 139 inhabitants. The living is a discharged vicarage, in the peculiar jurisdiction and patronage of the Prebendary of Langtoft in the Cathedral Church of York, rated in the king's books at £6. 6. 8. The church is dedicated to St. Nicholas.

GRIMSTONE, a parish in the Lynn division of the hundred of Freebridge, county of Norfolk, 4¼ miles (S. E. by E.) from Castle-Rising, containing 918 inhabitants. The living is a rectory, in the archdeaconry and diocese of Norwich, rated in the king's books at £26. 13. 4., and in the patronage of the President and Fellows of Queen's College, Cambridge. The church is dedicated to St. Botolph.

GRIMTHORPE, a township in the parish of Givendale, or Gwendale, partly in the liberty of St. Peter of York, and partly in the Wilton-Beacon division of the wapentake of Harthill, East riding of the county of York, 3¼ miles (N.) from Pocklington, containing 29 inhabitants.

GRINDALL, a chapelry in the parish of Bridlington, wapentake of Dickering, East riding of the county of York, 4¼ miles (N.W.) from Bridlington, containing 107 inhabitants. The living is a perpetual curacy, in the archdeaconry of the East riding, and diocese of York, endowed with £1000 royal bounty. John Greame, Esq. was patron in 1816.

GRINDLETON, a chapelry in that part of the parish of Mitton which is in the western division of the wapentake of Staincliffe and Ewcross, West riding of the county of York, 3 miles (N.N.E.) from Clitheroe, containing 1125 inhabitants. The living is a perpetual curacy, in the archdeaconry and diocese of York, endowed with £800 royal bounty, and £400 parliamentary grant, and in the patronage of the Vicar of Mitton.

GRINDLEY, a joint township with Tushingham, in the parish of Malpas, higher division of the hundred of Broxton, county palatine of Chester, 4½ miles (S.E. by E.) from Malpas, containing 283 inhabitants.

GRINDLOW, a township in the parish of Hope, hundred of High Peak, county of Derby, 2¼ miles (E. N.E.) from Tidswell, containing 119 inhabitants.

GRINDON, a township in the parish of Norham, otherwise Norhamshire, county palatine of Durham, though locally to the northward of the county of Northumberland, westward of Islandshire, 7 miles (S. W.) from Berwick, containing 173 inhabitants. There are four upright stones in memory of the chieftains slain in a battle fought at this place in 1558, between the English and the Scots, when the latter were defeated.

GRINDON, a parish in the north-eastern division of Stockton ward, county palatine of Durham, comprising the townships of Grindon and Whitton, and containing 314 inhabitants, of which number, 255 are in the township of Grindon, 5½ miles (N. N.W.) from Stockton upon Tees. The living is a discharged vicarage, in the archdeaconry and diocese of Durham, rated in the king's books at £4. 11. 5½., endowed with £200 private benefaction, and £200 royal bounty, and in the patronage of the Master and Brethren of Sherbourn Hospital. The church, dedicated to St. Thomas à Becket, stands alone, about one mile and a half to the eastward of the Durham and Stockton road: there is a stone coffin in the churchyard, inscribed "Roger de Foulthorp."

GRINDON, a parish in the northern division of the hundred of Totmonslow, county of Stafford, containing 455 inhabitants, of which number, 219 are in the township of Grindon, 7¼ miles (E. by S.) from Leek. The living is a rectory, in the archdeaconry of Stafford, and diocese of Lichfield and Coventry, rated in the king's books at £15. 14. 2., and in the patronage of the Marquis of Stafford. The church is dedicated to All Saints Humphrey Hall and Samuel Nalton, in 1724, subscribed £100 towards the endowment of a school; this sum, with subsequent minor donations, now produces £8. 5. a year, for which ten children receive instruction.

GRINGLEY on the HILL, a parish in the North-clay division of the wapentake of Bassetlaw, county of Nottingham, 6 miles (E. S. E.) from Bawtry, containing 647 inhabitants. The living is a discharged vicarage, in the peculiar jurisdiction of the Lord of the Manor, rated in the king's books at £7. 18. 4., and endowed with £400 royal bounty. The Duke of Rutland was patron in 1804. The church is dedicated to St. Peter and St. Paul. The Chesterfield canal passes through the parish. There is a fair on the 12th of December for cattle and merchandise, particularly boots and shoes.

GRINSDALE, a parish in the ward and county of Cumberland, 2¾ miles (N. W. by W.) from Carlisle, containing 138 inhabitants. The living is a perpetual curacy, in the archdeaconry and diocese of Carlisle, endowed with £1000 royal bounty. Mrs. Dacre was patroness in 1804. The church, dedicated to St. Kentigern, lay for many years totally in ruins, till it was rebuilt with freestone in 1739, at the expense of Joseph Dacre, Esq.; a strong wall also has been raised to protect the cemetery from the inundations of the Eden, to which it had been previously exposed. The great Roman wall intersects the parish, and there are two large square intrenchments within its limits. Upon a rock near the river are impressions of human footsteps.

GRINSHILL, a parish within the liberty of the borough of SHREWSBURY, county of SALOP, $7\frac{1}{2}$ miles (N.N.E.) from Shrewsbury, containing 214 inhabitants. The living is a rectory, in the archdeaconry of Salop, and diocese of Lichfield and Coventry, endowed with £200 royal bounty, and £200 parliamentary grant. John Wood, Esq. was patron in 1814. The church is dedicated to All Saints. Here are noted quarries of white freestone, of which considerable quantities have been supplied for the erection of churches, bridges, and other edifices in the neighbourhood.

GRINSTEAD (EAST), a borough, market town, and parish, in the hundred of EAST GRINSTEAD, rape of PEVENSEY, county of SUSSEX, $19\frac{3}{4}$ miles (N.) from Lewes, and $29\frac{1}{2}$ (S. by E.) from London, containing 3153 inhabitants. The town is pleasantly situated on an eminence near the northern border of the county, on the road from London

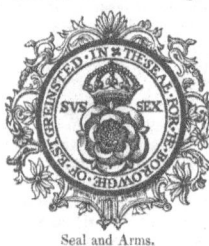

Seal and Arms.

to Brighton : it was formerly a place of considerable importance, having given name to the hundred. It is irregularly built, but contains several neat modern houses; it is paved, but not lighted, and is supplied with water from wells. The market is on Thursday; and there is a market for cattle and live stock on the last Thursday in every month : fairs are held, April 21st, July 13th, and December 11th, the first and last of which are large cattle fairs; and at Forest Row, about three miles from the town, there are fairs annually on June 25th and November 8th. East Grinstead is a borough by prescription, under a bailiff, who is chosen yearly by a jury of burgage holders, at the court leet for the manor. It has returned two members to parliament ever since the first of Edward II., the right of election being vested in the holders of thirty-six burgage tenements, twenty-nine of which belong to the Duke of Dorset, who is thus the proprietor of the borough : the bailiff is the returning officer. The Lent assizes for the county were formerly held here, but have been discontinued since 1799. This place is within the liberty of the duchy of Lancaster. The living is a vicarage, in the archdeaconry of Lewes, and diocese of Chichester, rated in the king's books at £20, and in the patronage of the Duke of Dorset. The church, dedicated to St. Swithin, is a handsome edifice in the later style of English architecture, consisting of a nave, aisles, chancel, and chantry chapels, and containing several interesting monuments. The tower, which was rebuilt after having fallen down in 1785, is a

well proportioned structure, ornamented with angular pinnacles, and surmounted by a lofty spire. There is a place of worship for a congregation in the late Countess of Huntingdon's connexion. A free school was founded in 1708, by Robert Payne, and endowed with land producing about £40 per annum, now paid to the master of a National school recently established, and principally supported by voluntary contributions, in which seventy-five children are educated. At the east end of the town is Sackville college, a charitable institution, founded in the reign of James I., by the Earl of Dorset, for the support of twenty-four aged men and women, who receive £8 per annum each, and are under the government of a warden and two gentlemen assistants : there is a neat chapel belonging to the institution, and a suite of rooms is appropriated to the use of the Duke of Dorset.

GRINSTEAD (WEST), a parish in the hundred of WEST GRINSTEAD, rape of BRAMBER, county of SUSSEX, $7\frac{1}{2}$ miles (S.) from Horsham, containing 1229 inhabitants. The living is a rectory, in the archdeaconry and diocese of Chichester, rated in the king's books at £25. 17. 6. T. Woodward, Esq. was patron in 1807. The church, dedicated to St. George, has portions in the early, decorated, and later English styles of architecture. This place was anciently of considerable note, and gave name to the hundred. A trifling sum, the gift of Mr. Dowlin in 1644, is appropriated for the education of children.

GRINSTHORPE, a hamlet in the parish of EDENHAM, wapentake of BELTISLOE, parts of KESTEVEN, county of LINCOLN, 4 miles (E. by S.) from Corby, containing 90 inhabitants.

GRINTON, a parish partly in the western division of the wapentake of HANG, and partly in the western division of the wapentake of GILLING, North riding of the county of YORK, $9\frac{1}{2}$ miles (W. by S.) from Richmond, containing, with the chapelry of Muker, and the townships of Melbecks and Reeth, which are in the wapentake of Gilling, 6300 inhabitants. The living is a discharged vicarage, in the archdeaconry of Richmond, and diocese of Chester, rated in the king's books at £12. 5. 7., and in the patronage of the Crown. The church, dedicated to St. Andrew, has been lately repaired; its windows exhibit some beautiful specimens of ancient stained glass. James Hutchinson, in 1643, gave a school-house and dwelling-house, with other premises, and £20 a year, for the maintenance of a master : the annual income is £73, which is paid to the vicar for the education of about eighty children on the National system. There are in this extensive parish considerable mines of iron, lead, and copper. On an eminence near Helagh is an ancient British encampment, approached from the east by an avenue about one hundred and twenty yards long, formed of stones, at the commencement of which is a large barrow, composed of stones and gravel, and about three hundred yards south-westward from the camp is another barrow, six yards high : there are vestiges of other intrenchments, and several cairns in the neighbourhood.

GRISTHORPE, a township in that part of the parish of FILEY which is in PICKERING lythe, North riding of the county of YORK, $5\frac{3}{4}$ miles (S.E.) from Scarborough, containing 212 inhabitants.

GRISTON, a parish in the hundred of WAYLAND, county of NORFOLK, 2 miles (S.E.) from Watton, containing 198 inhabitants. The living is a discharged vicarage, in the archdeaconry and diocese of Norwich, rated in the king's books at £7. 8. 9., and in the patronage of the Bishop of Ely. The church was anciently dedicated to St. Margaret, and had four guilds, but, in 1477, it was partly rebuilt, and dedicated anew to St. Peter and St. Paul, whose emblems, viz., cross keys and swords, still adorn its handsome tower.

GRITTENHAM, a tything in the parish of BRINK-WORTH, hundred of MALMESBURY, county of WILTS, 2½ miles (W.) from Wootton-Bassett, containing 154 inhabitants.

GRITTLETON, a parish in the northern division of the hundred of DAMERHAM, county of WILTS, 7 miles (N.W. by N.) from Chippenham, containing 354 inhabitants. The living is a rectory, in the archdeaconry of Wilts, and diocese of Salisbury, rated in the king's books at £13. 10., and in the patronage of the Rev. W. W. Burne. The church is dedicated to St. Mary. Here is a place of worship for Baptists.

GROOBY, a hamlet in the parish of RATBY, hundred of SPARKENHOE, county of LEICESTER, 4 miles (N.W. by W.) from Leicester, containing 324 inhabitants. It is in the peculiar ecclesiastical jurisdiction of the Lord of the Manor.

GROOMBRIDGE, a chapelry in that part of the parish of SPELDHURST which is in the hundred of So-MERDEN, lathe of SUTTON at HONE, county of KENT, 4 miles (W. by S.) from Tunbridge-Wells. The population is returned with the parish. The chapel has lately received an addition of one hundred free sittings, the Incorporated Society for the enlargement of churches and chapels having granted £100 towards defraying the expense.

GROSMONT, a market town and parish in the upper division of the hundred of SKENFRETH, county of MONMOUTH, 12 miles (N.) from Monmouth, and 139 (W.) from London, containing 701 inhabitants. This place, though at present consisting only of scattered cottages interspersed with a few respectable houses in the immediate vicinity of the church, and some handsome mansions in distant and detached situations, was formerly a town of considerable importance, and of great extent. Numerous remains of stone causeways, by which the adjoining meadows are intersected, are, with a high degree of probability, supposed to indicate the site of former streets, and the size and architecture of its church, unconnected with any monastic establishment of importance, tend to confirm that opinion. The castle, which, together with those of Llandeilo and Skenfreth, was erected for the defence of this part of the country, was, in the reign of Henry III., attacked by the Welch under Prince Llewellyn, but the king coming to its assistance with a powerful army, obliged them to raise the siege. In a subsequent expedition of that monarch against the Earl of Pembroke, who had placed himself under the protection of Llewellyn, the Welch having cut off the supplies of the royal army, the king retreated to Grosmont castle, and his forces encamped in the neighbourhood. While waiting here for supplies, his troops were surprised by a party of Llewellyn's cavalry, who carried off a considerable booty. The remains of the castle, which was afterwards the baronial residence of the earls of Lancaster, form an interesting and picturesque object, romantically situated on the summit of an eminence overlooking a beautiful

vale watered by the river Monnow, and bounded by the lofty mountains of Craig, Saverney, and the Garway: the walls include an area one hundred and ten feet in length, and seventy in breadth, surrounded by a moat: the principal entrance is through an arched gateway; on the right of which are the remains of the baronial hall, eighty feet in length, and twenty-seven feet wide, lighted by three fine windows on one side, and two at each end; some vestiges of the barbican may still be traced, and there are slight remains of the intrenchments to the south: the walls, richly overspread with ivy, and impending over the stream of the Monnow, the retired situation of the buildings, and the scenery of the surrounding country, combine to impart a powerful interest to this beautiful ruin. The market is on Tuesday; and fairs are held April 4th, August 10th, and October 9th, for the sale of cattle: the old market-house has been recently taken down, and a new one is at present being erected on its site, at the expense of the Duke of Beaufort. The town, which is governed by a mayor and burgesses, forms part of the duchy of Lancaster, and is included within the jurisdiction of a court baron held occasionally for the three castles of Llandeilo, or White castle, Skenfreth, and Grosmont: the petty sessions for the hundred of Ewyaslacy, in the county of Hereford, are also held here. The living is a discharged rectory, in the archdeaconry and diocese of Llandaff, rated in the king's books at £6. 5. 2½., and in the patronage of the Crown. The church, dedicated to St. Nicholas, is a spacious cruciform structure in the decorated style of English architecture, with an octagonal tower surmounted by a spire: an old tombstone in the churchyard, near the east wall of the chancel, without any inscription, is said to point out the grave of John à Kent, of whom many notable exploits are traditionally recorded. A free school was founded in 1803, by the Rev. Tudor Price, rector, who bequeathed £400 for that purpose: in 1812, Miss George added £400, the interest of which is paid to a master, for instructing the children of the poor of this parish, and those of farmers not renting land to the amount of more than £30 per annum, and six children from each of the parishes of Rolstone and Skenfreth. A Sunday school, in which from forty to fifty children are instructed, is supported by subscription. Grosmont gives the title of viscount to the Duke of Beaufort.

GROTON, a parish in the hundred of BABERGH, county of SUFFOLK, 1 mile (N. by W.) from Boxford, containing 597 inhabitants. The living is a rectory, in the archdeaconry of Sudbury, and diocese of Norwich, rated in the king's books at £8. 1. 8. J. W. Willett, Esq. and others were patrons in 1806. The church is dedicated to St. Bartholomew. There is an almshouse, with gardens attached, for four persons, purchased in 1702, and kept in repair by the parish.

GROVE, a hamlet in the parish and hundred of WANTAGE, county of BERKS, 1½ mile (N. by E.) from Wantage, containing 481 inhabitants.

GROVE, a parish in the hundred of COTTESLOE, county of BUCKINGHAM, 2½ miles (S.) from Leighton-Buzzard, containing 18 inhabitants. The living is a discharged rectory, in the archdeaconry of Buckingham, and diocese of Lincoln, rated in the king's books at £4. 13. 4., endowed with £8 per annum private benefaction, and £200 royal bounty. The Earl of Chesterfield was

2 M 2

patron in 1799. The Grand Junction canal passes through the parish.

GROVE, a parish in the South-clay division of the wapentake of BASSETLAW, county of NOTTINGHAM, 2¾ miles (E. S. E.) from East Retford, containing 106 inhabitants. The living is a rectory, in the archdeaconry of Nottingham, and diocese of York, rated in the king's books at £11. 14. 2. A. H. Eyre, Esq. was patron in 1798. The church is dedicated to St. Helen.

GRUNDISBURGH, a parish in the hundred of CARLFORD, county of SUFFOLK, 3 miles (N. W. by W.) from Woodbridge, containing 815 inhabitants. The living is a rectory, in the archdeaconry of Suffolk, and diocese of Norwich, rated in the king's books at £17. 11. 3., and in the patronage of the Master and Fellows of Trinity College, Cambridge. The church is dedicated to St. Mary. Here is a place of worship for Baptists. There is a Sunday school, towards the support of which John Lucock devised £5 a year out of certain stock invested for this and other charitable purposes.

GRUNTY-FEN-HOUSE, an extra-parochial liberty, in the southern division of the hundred of WITCHFORD, Isle of ELY, county of CAMBRIDGE. No separate return of the population has been made.

GUELDABLE, a township in that part of the parish of LEAK which is in the wapentake of BIRDFORTH, North riding of the county of YORK, containing 128 inhabitants.

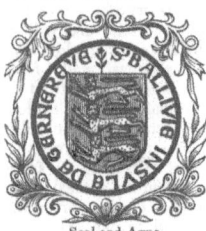

Seal and Arms.

GUERNSEY, a bailiwick, and one of the islands under the dominion of Great Britain, lying in a part of the English channel called Mount St. Michael's Bay, on the coasts of Normandy and Brittany, the port being situated in 49° 28′ (N. Lat.), and 2° 33′ (W. Lon.), 13⅓ English miles (N.W.) from Jersey, 7 (W.) from Sark, and 15 (S.W. by S.) from Alderney. It is the most westward of these islands, and the most distant from the coast of Normandy, being 26 English miles (S.W.) from Cape La Hogue, and 36 (W. by S.) from Cherbourg. The extreme length, from north-east to south-west, is about eight miles; the breadth, from north-west to south-east, nearly six; and the circumference about thirty. It contains 20,302 inhabitants, of which number, 11,173 are in the town and parish of St. Peter's Port, 838 in the parish of St. Sampson, 1215 in the Vale parish, 375 in Torteval parish, 1022 in St. Saviour's, 611 in the Forest parish, 1093 in St. Peter's du Bois, 1429 in St. Martin's, 1747 in that of the Catel, and 799 in St. Andrew's.

Respecting the early history of the island but few authentic particulars can be collected. Its surface was, in a state of nature, covered with woods and overrun with briars, when it was visited by the Romans, about seventeen years before the birth of Christ, and Octavius Augustus, then emperor, appointed a governor over it. It is the generally received opinion, that this is the island mentioned in Antoninus's Itinerary by the name of *Sarnia*; and that Alderney is called in the same Itinerary, *Riduna*; Sark, *Sarnica*; the little islands of

Herm and Jethou, *Armia* and *Sarnia*, respectively. The next mention of Guernsey is about the year 520, when it was visited by Sampson, Bishop of Dol in Brittany, who is said to have landed at what is now called St. Sampson's harbour, where he built a chapel. His successor in the bishoprick, Maglorius, prosecuted the work of converting the inhabitants to Christianity, and built a chapel in the present parish of the Vale, on a spot still called *St. Magloire*, and by the peasantry, by corruption, *St. Maliere*. At this period the inhabitants subsisted entirely by fishing; and Guernsey was reckoned, though the most distant from France, the most considerable of these islands, on account of the safety and convenience of its harbours, and the quantity of fish on its coast; and in course of time, when the fishery was well established, most of the religious houses, and many of the great families in Normandy and Brittany, were constantly supplied with fish from it. As Christianity advanced, and the population increased, chapels were built in different parts of the island, near the sea-shore, and the priests that officiated in them were allowed for their subsistence the tithe of all the fish that was caught, which custom has continued ever since.

This island, which had anciently formed part of the province of Neustria, and, with the rest of that province, was included in the kingdom of France, established by Pharamond, in 420, became, in like manner, on the cession of Neustria to the Norman invaders of France, a part of the duchy of Normandy, created about the year 892. On the diminution of the ecclesiastical revenues in Normandy, by Duke Richard, the number of monks in the abbey of Mount St. Michael, on the Norman coast, being reduced in proportion to the reduction of its income, those that were driven out retiring to Guernsey, founded, in the year 962, an abbey in that part of the island now called the Close of the Vale, dedicating it to the same patron saint. Fishing having hitherto been the only occupation of the inhabitants, their dwellings were all built close to the sea-shore; but the monks soon prevailed on them to commence clearing the land and raising corn, so that, in a few years, the greater part of the Vale was brought into cultivation. The religious soon became celebrated for their great piety, not only on the continent, but in England; they were visited by devout persons from Normandy, France, and Britain; insomuch that Guernsey acquired the name of the Holy Island, which it long retained, and by which it was designated not only in the papal bulls, but also in the charters and other acts of the Norman and English sovereigns. The Danes, in the course of their devastations towards the close of the tenth century, ravaged the monastery, and subsequently plundered the defenceless inhabitants of their corn and cattle. It was to afford means of protection from these ravages that a spacious castle was erected on an eminence in the Vale, originally called St. Michael's castle, or the castle of the Archangel, and now the Vale castle, which is still well calculated to defend the mouth of St. Sampson's harbour, where vessels of heavy burden find secure shelter. About the year 1030, when the fleet of Robert, Duke of Normandy, conveying the forces designed to support the claim of his cousins, Alfred and Edward, to the English crown, against Canute, was dispersed by a tempest, the vessel which

GUERNSEY,

AND ITS DEPENDENT ISLES.

ISLAND OF ALDERNEY

Passage of the Singes

LITTLE RUSSEL

GREAT RUSSEL

ST PETER PORT

Bargnaint Bay

Island of SARK

Scale of English Miles

West Longitude 2°.30' from Greenwich

DRAWN AND ENGRAVED FOR LEWIS' TOPOGRAPHICAL DICTIONARY.

contained the duke himself was, together with about twenty others, carried down the channel as far as Guernsey, where they would have been dashed upon the rocks, but for the fishermen, who hastened to their assistance, and piloted them into a bay on the north side of the Vale, where they moored in safety. The duke having landed, he was conducted to the abbey of St. Michael, and the stormy weather preventing his departure for some time, afforded him an opportunity of surveying the island. To reward the abbot for his hospitality, he gave to him and his successors, in fee, all the lands within the Close of the Vale for ever, by the name of the fief of St. Michael, with leave to extend the same without the Close of the Vale, towards the north-western part of the island, whenever settlers could be found to clear and cultivate the land. And to recompense the islanders for the succour they had rendered him, he left engineers and workmen to finish the castle of St. Michael, and to erect such other fortresses as might be necessary for protecting them and their property from the piratical invaders. The duke departed about a fortnight after his landing, and, in commemoration of that event, the place where his fleet lay has ever since been called *L'Ancresse*, or the Anchoring-place. In the course of a few years, the officers and artisans whom the duke had left, erected two other very strong castles : a part of one of these, called, from its marshy situation, *Le Château des Marais*, still remains in the Town parish, and, from its walls being mantled with ivy, has acquired the name of Ivy Castle : the site of the other, called the castle of Jerbourg, is on a point of land on the southern coast, now called St. Martin's point, but there are no remains of the buildings. At the same time mounds were thrown up on the most elevated parts of the island, to enable the inhabitants to observe when ships came in sight : one of these ancient alarm posts, called *La Hougue Hatenas*, remains in St. Martin's parish ; and another, called *La Hougue Fonque*, in St. Saviour's.

Robert, Duke of Normandy, when about to depart for the crusade, among the other bountiful presents which he made to the clergy of his duchy, gave tracts of land in Guernsey to the Bishop of Coutances, the Abbess of Caën, the Bishop of Avranches, the Abbot of Mount St. Michael, and the Abbot of Blanchelande, by virtue of which grants, the priory of Lihou, or Lihoumel, and the abbeys of Normoustier, Blanchelande, La Rue Frèrie, La Croix St. Geffroy, and Caën, were founded in the island. All these, except the priory of Lihou, were erected into *franc-fiefs*, the abbots holding immediately of the Duke of Normandy ; but the priory of Lihou was an *arrière-fief*, or appendage to the abbey of St. Michael. About the middle of the eleventh century, Guernsey was infested by a new race of pirates from the south coast of the bay of Biscay, who built a castle in the centre of it, called *Le Château des Sarrasins*, near the spot where the Catel church now stands. Duke William sent a force to their relief, under the command of his esquire, Sampson D'Anneville, who landed near the castle of the Vale, when a great number of the pirates was put to the sword, the remainder, with great difficulty, escaping to their ships : in reward for this service, Sampson received a considerable tract of land in the island, by the title of the fief and seigneurie D'Anneville. Other tracts being bestowed by the same sovereign upon other Norman gen-

tlemen, the greater part of Guernsey was soon brought into tillage ; and about this period it was divided into ten parishes. Each free fief had a manorial court for litigating disputes among the tenants ; and the Abbot of St. Michael, and the Seigneur D'Anneville, had *droit de haute justice*, or the privilege of judging, condemning, and executing criminals, so that the civil polity of the island was completely settled before the Norman Conquest of England.

When the French, in the reign of Edward III., made themselves masters of these islands, Guernsey remained in their possession for some time, until it was re-captured by an English fleet under Reynold de Cobham and Jeffrey de Harcourt. In the same reign it appears to have been invaded by one Ivans, a descendant of the ancient Welch princes, who was sent by the king of France, with a numerous fleet and an army of four thousand men, to reduce these islands ; and who succeeded in capturing Guernsey, after a spirited resistance : it is said to have been rescued by the arrival of eighty ships from England, when a conflict took place, in which five hundred men were killed on each side. A spot of ground in the New Town, called *La Bataille*, is supposed to derive its name from one of these sanguinary combats ; and a very ancient legend states the invaders to have been Saragozans ; to which assertion a degree of probability attaches, from the circumstance that Ivans, or Ivan of Wales, an inveterate enemy of Edward III., had been in the Spanish service, and that at that time, Henry, King of Castile, was an enemy to England, in alliance with France. In the reign of Edward IV., when Sir Richard Harliston, Vice-admiral of England, having arrived with a squadron at Guernsey, proceeded thence to re-capture Mont-Orgueil castle in Jersey, at that time in the power of the French, the men of Guernsey shared largely in the victory that followed ; and on this occasion the laurel branch is said to have been first assumed as a crest to the arms of Guernsey : these services are also recorded in the preamble of the charter granted to these islands by Henry VII., in the first year of his reign. In 1549, Leo Strozzi, admiral of the French galleys, previously to his attack upon Jersey, made an attempt upon some English ships at anchor in the road here, but was driven off by the sailors, assisted by the inhabitants.

After the decapitation of Charles I., a force was sent by Cromwell and the parliament to reduce these islands, when Guernsey was first subdued, after a vigorous defence ; but Castle Cornet held out for the king a considerable time longer : it appears, however, that the inhabitants of Guernsey were thought to have displayed on the whole less zeal for the royal cause than those of Jersey, since they deemed it expedient, upon the Restoration, to petition for the royal clemency ; in answer to which petition a general pardon was issued, wherein several individuals were specified as having given ample proofs of their loyalty. In the reign of James II., some Roman Catholic soldiers were quartered in Guernsey, and a chapel was fitted up for them in the town ; a popish priest was sent over to say mass ; and a papist was made governor ; but no sooner was the arrival of the Prince and Princess of Orange in England known here, than a plan was concerted to secure Castle Cornet, disarm the papists, and confine the lieutenant-governor. A day was accordingly fixed on, when, by rotation, the command of the castle would devolve upon a Protestant officer privy to the design, who had no sooner entered upon duty than the chief captain, accompanied by a body of the militia, seized upon and disarmed all the Popish officers and men in the town. This being done, a signal was immediately given to the commandant of the castle, who instantly summoned the garrison to arms. Being assembled on the parade, the Protestant soldiers having their muskets loaded with ball, as previously arranged, stepped out of the ranks, and, facing about, presented their pieces at the Roman Catholic soldiers, and so compelled them to lay down their arms, by which means the fortress was secured for the new king and queen.

During the late war with France this island was often under serious alarm from threatened invasion ; but the well-regulated militia force, the number of regular troops generally in barracks, the augmentation and improvement of the ancient fortifications, which took place during that period, and the erection of the new fortress of Fort George, added to the natural precipitousness of the coast, have rendered it, in case of future hostilities, almost impregnable. The force maintained by the island of Guernsey consists of one troop of cavalry, two battalions of artillery, the second being composed chiefly of invalids ; four regiments of militia, three of which are light infantry, and the royal marine corps. These regiments are clothed, equipped, and disciplined, in the same manner as the regular forces, but, since the termination of the war, they are only manœuvred six times in the course of a year. The natives are excellent marksmen, and fire not only with more precision, but with greater effect than the troops of the line, which is easily accounted for, as they are accustomed to the use of the fowling-piece from a very early age, even the peasantry being greatly addicted to the sports of the field. The superiority of the Guernsey artillery has long since been acknowledged, and although the tangent is not in use among them, the eye being the sole guide in pointing the piece, the islanders seldom miss their mark. The regular troops amount to upwards of five thousand, and the native troops to nearly three thousand ; and there are mounted on the batteries and barracks, in various parts of the island, two hundred and fifty-five pieces of ordnance, forty-seven cannonades, and four mortars.

The situation of Guernsey, in the Channel stream, produces a variety of currents on its coasts, the intricacy and rapidity of which render the navigation extremely difficult, except along the southern coast, where there is good and safe anchorage, in a sandy bottom, at the distance of a mile and a half from the shore. The dangerous rocks called the *Douore*, lie in an exact south-west direction from this island, at six leagues distance, in Lat. from 49° 10′ to 49° 16′. The form of the island is nearly triangular, and almost its whole circuit is indented by small bays and harbours. The southern coast, from the Hanois to St. Martin's point, and part of the eastern, from St. Martin's point to the town, is a continued high rock, or cliff, rising almost perpendicularly from the sea, to the height of about two hundred and seventy feet ; and, excepting a few very narrow valleys, the parishes of St. Martin, the Forest, Torteval, St. Peter of the Wood, a great part of St. Saviour's, St. Andrew's, the Catel parish, and St.

Peter's Port, are level ground, at nearly that average height from high water mark. The whole of the Vale and St. Sampson's parishes, except a few gentle elevations, are low lands, nearly on the level of high water mark ; but there is not much marshy ground, nor are they subject to inundation, even in the winter season. The low part of the island is particularly fertile ; the elevated portion, excepting nearly half of the parishes of Torteval and the Forest, is exceedingly good arable land ; and even the steep rocky elevations on the eastern and southern sides of the island, produce fine pasturage for sheep down to the water's edge. The whole island is abundantly watered by rivulets. Its general formation, geologically considered, will admit of a very natural division into two parts ; the more elevated part, to the south, consisting almost entirely of gneiss, and the low ground, or northern portion, of syenite and hornblend rock. The gneiss preserves nearly an equal elevation from the eastern shore, near the town, to the western coast, but its continuity is frequently interrupted by short and deep ravines running to the south, and by irregular vallies sloping to the west and north. The character of the gneiss is much varied by the intrusion of the strata which usually accompany that rock, but its general aspect is porphyritic, and, when newly washed by the gurge, it exhibits most beautiful specimens of that species of marble.

Vegetables are produced in great variety and of excellent quality ; those grown in the parishes of St. Sampson and the Vale are preferred. The trees, excepting the elm, are neither tall nor luxuriant. The fences in the upper, or southern, part of the island, are sometimes composed of quickset, and exactly resemble an English hedge, sometimes of high banks thickly studded with trees and underwood, and frequently of walls of hard brown stone, about four or five feet in height, the workmanship of which is usually very excellent. In the lower, or northern, division of the island, the fields are mostly enclosed by dwarf walls of stone and granite : the materials are rarely embedded in cement, but generally piled up to the height of about three feet, or even less, without regard to order or durability ; occasionally, however, the fences even in the lower parishes are of regular and solid masonry. The timber grown in the island is chiefly elm, which in quality is, probably, not excelled by any in Europe : the female elm is much used for boat-building, being, when cut into thin planks, very tough, and yet so extremely pliable, that it can be formed into almost any shape. The oak grown here is equal in quality to English oak, but there is little of it, and it is seldom allowed to attain a large size : the ash is generally inferior and but partially grown : there are chesnut and sycamore trees, but they are not numerous. Most kinds of European fruit grow in profusion ; and so genial is the climate, that myrtles and geraniums flourish in the open air, and the more hardy species of orange-tree, the Seville, will bear fruit in winter with very little shelter. The orchards, chiefly composed of apple trees, are very productive, and a great quantity of cider is made and drunk in the island. The fig-tree attains great luxuriance, and sometimes a remarkable size. The aloe frequently blossoms here. Thousands of that beautiful flower, the Guernsey lily, are exported yearly to England and France, but will not blow a second

:ime out of the island ; not even in Jersey, although in
ι more southern latitude, and better shaded. As snow
ieldom lies longer than for one or two days, and the
rummer's heat is always tempered by breezes from the
iea, the climate is peculiarly favourable to vegetation,
ιnd its salubrity is attested by the longevity of the
nhabitants. There is neither a wood nor a coppice in
ιny part of the island. There is no species of common
:ame ; but woodcocks and snipes are tolerably plenti-
ul. Most of the British song birds are occasionally
een, but the nightingale is very rarely heard. Fish are
aught in great abundance and variety : among the
ιost common are mackarel, the sea-pike or garpike,
'hitings, pollacks, bream, and rock-fish : there are
lso turbots, mullets, soles, plaice, and conger-eels,
ιe last sometimes weighing thirty or forty pounds.
hell-fish are no less plentiful : among them is the
rmer, or sea-ear (*Haliotis Tuberculata*), commonly eaten
y the poorer inhabitants, vast numbers of them being
rought to market in the early part of the year, at
'hich period they are found in the greatest abundance :
ιey adhere to rocks and moveable stones so firmly, that
; is very difficult to detach them during the ebb-tide,
ιnd in the attempt the hands are sometimes severely
ιacerated, but when the tide begins to flow they may be
:asily removed. Crabs and lobsters, of an enormous
iize, are caught off the coast ; some of the former
measure, across the body, three feet in circumference :
the spider crab, which is much smaller, is almost peculiar to this coast ; in shape it resembles the reptile after
which it is named, and is much esteemed by epicures,
as being more delicious than the common crab. Li-
chens, in great variety and beauty, are found attached
to the rocks around the island, among which the
Lichen Roccella is somewhat abundant. The mole,
snake, and toad, are not found in this island, which
is the more remarkable, as they abound in Jersey.

The agriculture of Guernsey is still in a rude state :
the same kind of plough, harrow, and almost every
other implement of husbandry, is in use now that was
employed some centuries ago ; yet the lands are clean,
being sedulously cultivated, and, from the great fertility
of the soil, yield most abundant crops. The English
plough is sometimes used, but is not generally found to
suit ; the soil, in some places, being so deep, that nothing
but the old Guernsey plough, which penetrates to the
depth of eighteen inches, will turn it up effectually.
The land, however, is subdivided into such small allotments, that few of the cultivators are able to raise
more than sufficient for their own subsistence, and
the payment of their rents. The want of manure
is chiefly supplied by a species of fucus, which is used
both as fuel and manure. The course of crops practised, with few exceptions, is of five years. First year,
wheat ; second (after sea-weed or ashes have been laid
on the stubble, usually before Christmas, and the land
has received three spring ploughings), barley sown in
April, with clover-seed ; third, clover ; fourth, after
once ploughing, wheat again ; fifth, after the ground
has been ploughed and harrowed in the autumn, the
couch burnt, and again ploughed and harrowed in January, parsnips. In this course, the ground is only
nourished by manure the second year ; the parsnips,
with the deep ploughing, being expected to answer the
purpose of a fallow for the following wheat, which, as

it is here asserted, is in general a more abundant crop
than that after potatoes or turnips with manure. Beans
and peas sometimes accompany parsnips, neither of
them being a separate article of culture. A small quantity of turnip-seed is occasionally sown after the clover-
seed in the second year, and the turnips are not supposed to do any injury, if they are removed before
the clover germinates in the following spring : three
good crops of clover are obtained in the course of the
year, the first of which usually grows above three feet
in height.

Weeding is here performed three several times,
always with the *sarcloir*, which is formed of iron, and
is from four to five inches wide at its edge, being inserted, by means of a straight spike four inches long,
into a short wooden handle, which is curved near the
centre, where it is grasped by the workman, who, when
employed in weeding, places one knee on the ground :
the *sarcloir* he thrusts under the roots of the weeds,
turns them over, and with the flat side occasionally
strikes the roots, in order to disengage from them the
adhering mould. A strong spade, peculiar to the island,
is also in use, of which the iron part is fourteen inches
long, and eleven inches across, in the widest part ; the
edge is semicircular ; the sides are narrow towards the
middle, and continue to decrease in width to within
three inches of the upper part, where it again widens,
and is inserted into a wooden bar joining the handle.
The barley is pulled up by the roots, women and
boys, as well as men, being engaged in the operation ;
usually striking it against their shoes, to free the roots
from the mould before it is laid down in rows for the
binder : it is supposed that, by this practice, a greater
bulk of straw is obtained, and that the clover crop derives considerable benefit from loosening the earth. The
barley is usually consumed in bread, but, in consequence
of the manner in which it is got in, it is found impossible to effect a complete separation of the gritty substances carried to the mill with the grain. The culture
of oats is not so general as that of barley. In bringing
new and poor land into cultivation, oats sometimes
form the first crop, and occasionally are substituted for
barley in the ordinary routine of cropping. In the sandy
district, on the south-west of the island, rye is sometimes raised ; it is of good quality, and also made into
bread. Parsnips are not in general use in this island
as human food, but principally consumed in feeding
milch cows, or fattening oxen and hogs : this plant
thrives best in a deep light loam ; with clays it does
not agree, but each soil in its turn is destined to receive it. Spade labour was formerly universal, but of
lafe years the *grande querne*, or large plough, has been
introduced, which is usually drawn by four oxen and
six horses ; it is preceded by a common plough to open
the furrow : digging would still be preferred if labourers
sufficient could be procured.

As few farmers keep more than one or two horses and
an ox, which would render deep ploughing for parsnips
and potatoes here impracticable, the custom of giving
mutual assistance during the season for that operation
has long prevailed : each farmer fixes a day for what is
termed his " grand plough," inviting his neighbours and
friends, who assemble early in the morning with their
horses and oxen, and, cheerfully contributing their own
manual labour, generally accomplish in the course of the

day the ploughing of as much land as is wanted for the growth of those vegetables ; good fare and the like kindness in return being the only recompense expected. The grass lands are very fertile, sometimes producing a ton of hay per vergee. Five vergees of grass are computed to be enough for the support of a cow ; and the custom of tethering cattle is general. This practice, as it exists in Guernsey, is certainly highly advantageous, since the fields are regularly eaten through, and, by the time the cattle have finished a meadow, the grass on which they commenced is usually forward enough to afford a second pasture. Few sheep are either bred or fattened in this island, fat sheep and oxen being generally brought from England, or France. The cows are highly celebrated, and the milk which they yield is so peculiarly rich, that it is not necessary to let it stand to produce cream, the whole being at once fit for the process of churning. The island breed of horses is a poor breed, the animals being ill shaped and usually ill fed. The hogs attain a great size, and are remarkable for the small proportions of their limbs and feet. Poultry are scarce and dear in time of continental war, but during peace the importation from Normandy and Brittany is considerable. The standard land-measure of the island is in feet, yards, perches, vergees, bouves, and carvees ; twenty-one square feet are a perch, and forty perches a vergee ; so that two vergees and a half are rather more than an English statute acre. Four vergees make a Guernsey and an Irish acre. The Guernsey vergee is equal to one thousand nine hundred and sixty square yards, which, multiplied by four, makes seven thousand eight hundred and forty square yards, being equal to an Irish acre. The denominations of the measures for corn, as established by law in the island, are quints, denerels, cabotels, bushels, and quarters. Five quints make a denerel ; three denerels a cabotel ; two cabotels a bushel ; and four bushels a quarter. The English quarter, of eight Winchester bushels, is equal to ten Guernsey bushels of wheat ; barley and other grain are measured by the same bushel, but heaped up, whereas wheat is struck. The lawful weight is the Rouen pound, being ten ounces one hundred and sixty sevenths five hundred and thirty-three-thirds more than the English avoirdupois, the English hundred weight being equal to one hundred and three, seven-ninths, Guernsey. The currency is by law said to be the money current in Normandy, and thus we see that accounts are in a great measure still kept in livres, tournois, sols, and deniers ; these livres, however, do not express the same value in both islands. In Guernsey fourteen livres, in Jersey twenty-four livres, represent a pound sterling, but both in the one and the other the relative value of a pound, in the island currency, compared with a pound in that of England, is regulated by the exchange, which rises occasionally, in the same manner as the exchange between England and other countries. In all the islands the English and French coins are current, the latter pass for ten pence to every franc of their nominal value. To the nominal value of the English coins is added that of the difference acquired by the exchange in favour of England : thus, a sovereign will sometimes pass for one pound one shilling, and sometimes for more, even for one pound one shilling and sixpence.

From time immemorial until the Revolution of 1688, the privilege of free trade in time of war, as well as of peace, between England and France, was enjoyed by these islanders, having been granted and confirmed by successive kings of England and dukes of Normandy, and even sanctioned by a bull of Pope Sixtus IV., dated in 1483, which was ordered to be published and observed in all his dominions by Charles VIII., King of France, by an ordinance dated in 1486. King William abolished this neutrality by an order in council, dated August 8th, 1689 ; upon which, this island actively engaged in privateering, and was very successful in the wars of that and the following reign ; fifteen hundred prizes having been captured by the privateers of Jersey and Guernsey in those two reigns. During the whole of the last century, the trade of the island progressively increased ; and the excise duties in England increasing also, a considerable portion of the commerce carried on was with persons engaged in the smuggling trade, until the years 1805 and 1807, when the acts of parliament for the better prevention of smuggling were passed. Before the commencement of the bonding system, this island may also be said to have served as a depôt for storing foreign goods, particularly wines and spirits, in the same manner as they are now kept in the warehouses of the London docks and the bonding ports. Guernsey unites to a central situation in Europe, a temperate climate well adapted for the keeping of wines in store ; a good harbour, the entrance to which is never obstructed by ice ; the best vaults in Europe ; and a great number of spacious and substantial warehouses : the wharfage and dues on goods in transition are very moderate. The carts employed for the carriage of wine and liquors are of peculiar construction ; the body is very low and strong ; at the end is a tail ladder : a solid iron axle passes under the body of the cart, which, rising on each side, receives the nave of a common sized wheel : in front is a capstan turned by a winch ; to the cylinder are fastened two ropes that, in loading, pass round the barrel, and draw it up the ladder, which, being then raised and rendered steady by the same ropes, serves as a back rail to the cart. These machines will carry two pipes, and can be unloaded by the carman without any other assistance.

The trading vessels belonging to the merchants of Guernsey amount to seventy-four sail, and their burden, by admeasurement, to seven thousand seven hundred and forty-three tons. The quarries afford employment to a great number of the inhabitants, a considerable quantity of granite and stone being exported. From November 30th, 1828, to November 30th, 1829, there were shipped five thousand five hundred and eighty-three tons of paving stones, six thousand and seventy feet of the same, and twelve thousand five hundred and forty-seven tons of stone chippings. During the same period, there were exported one hundred and twenty-nine cows, one hundred and eighty-one heifers, and ninety-three calves. From the port of Southampton, all the British wool allowed by parliament for the manufactures in Guernsey, Jersey, Alderney, and Sark, must be shipped ; and when the general exportation of corn is prohibited in England, a certain quantity, sufficient, with the produce of the islands, for the maintenance of the inhabitants, is allowed to be sent thither. And as the country around Southampton produces many articles which the islanders are in need of, a constant trade is carried on, and passengers find very good accommodation in the trading vessels, which are large and well-built cutters, neatly fitted up for the purpose: they generally perform the voyage in about twenty hours, and as there are several employed in this trade from Guernsey, they are continually sailing to and from the island. The regular government steam-packets, conveying the mails, sail from Weymouth to Jersey every Wednesday and Saturday, taking Guernsey in their way; but as the distance from London to Southampton is much shorter, and as steam-vessels regularly sail from that port during the summer months, the latter route is generally preferred: a constant communication is also kept up with the opposite coast of France, so that, in time of peace, this port and Jersey may be considered regular thoroughfares for passengers between England and Normandy and Brittany. During the late war, a few small smuggling vessels and privateers were built here, but the first brig launched was in October, 1815, and named by Sir John Doyle, then lieutenant-governor, *La Belle Alliance*, in memory of the decisive battle of Waterloo; since that period forty-three vessels have been built (of the aggregate burden of seven thousand two hundred and sixty tons), and twenty-four oyster smacks.

The common law of Guernsey is in substance derived from the ancient customs of Normandy, upon which the descent of property is in some measure founded. Real estates cannot be disposed of by will, but must descend to the heirs at law, and in default of such, escheat to the king, or the lord of the manor. The eldest son is here, as in Jersey, entitled to the principal dwelling, if not situate within the ancient bounds of the town of St. Peter's Port. He has also a certain portion of land, from fourteen to twenty-one perches, according to the value of the succession attached to the dwelling, as ascertained by the *douzainiers* of the parish, at whose valuation he is also entitled to purchase all the enclosures of land attached to it, the entrance to which is open to him from the house without crossing a public road. As no law exists to prevent the partition of estates below a prescribed number of vergees, land in Guernsey is infinitely divisible, but the elder frequently purchases the shares of the younger partitioners, either for rent or immediate value. Male descendants have a peculiar right to what is termed the vingtieme, which they may either claim or waive at their discretion. If claimed, the estate is measured, and one-twentieth set apart, of which the eldest son first takes his privileged portion, and the remainder is equally divided among the males. The residue of the succession is then shared by the co-heirs, two-thirds being divided among the males, and one-third among females. If the vingtieme is claimed, the whole succession, after deducting the *precipat*, as it is termed, to the eldest, is equally shared by children of both sexes. Among the most remarkable peculiarities of established usage are the two following: the children of parents who have lived for years in open adultery, but afterwards marry, are considered legitimate, and are entitled to inheritance; an insolvent person is exonerated from the payment of his debts, on surrendering upon oath the whole of his property, except his clothes, bed, and arms, and promising to make good the deficiency, if he should at any future time have it in his power so to do. Formerly, the insolvent claiming the

benefit of this law was compelled to wear a green cap, and to lay aside his girdle; but these badges of humiliation have been for some time discontinued. The contracts in Guernsey are described in a very simple style, being free from the repetitions that abound in documents of the same kind in England. The parties appear before the bailiff, and two of the magistrates of the royal court, by whom the contract is signed. When a conveyance of property is made by a married man, it is necessary that the wife should appear, and make an affidavit that she was not acting under undue influence when she consented to the transfer. All mortgages on estates are required to be registered by the *greffier*; and when a mortgage is paid off, the party has credit given him for the payment, so that an account current being kept, to which free access may always be had, the exact condition of every estate in the island may be known, and its incumbrances ascertained without difficulty. On the sale of an estate, the purchaser is only liable to such obligations and claims as are duly registered. With respect to the power of the British parliament to make enactments binding upon the inhabitants, which power has on various occasions been disputed by the magistrates of these islands, on the ground that the legislative authority over them was vested in the King alone, as Duke of Normandy, it may be observed that, in an order of council, bearing date May 7th, 1806, it is declared, that the registering of an act of parliament is not essential to its operation, and that His Majesty's subjects in these islands are bound by law to take notice of an act wherein it is especially named, although it should not be registered in the royal court there.

The assembly or convention of the states of this island, which is held only on occasions of great importance, when the general interest of the island is concerned, consists of the bailiff, twelve jurats, and *procureur* of the royal court, the beneficed clergy, and the constables and *douzainiers* of each parish, the total number being one hundred and seventy-four. The governor, or lieutenant-governor, whose consent is necessary to the holding of the states, has a deliberative voice in the assembly, but no vote; and the bailiff presides as speaker. The principal business of what are termed the states of election is, the nomination of jurats, and the appointment of the provost, in which every member has a distinct vote; but the raising of money to defray the public expenses is voted by the states of deliberation, consisting of the members above specified, but in which the constables and officers of each parish have collectively but one vote, so that the total number of votes in the latter assembly is thus reduced to thirty-two. Whenever the king's service, or the exigency of the island, requires the assembly of the states of deliberation, the bailiff, with the consent of the governor, or, in his absence, of the lieutenant-governor, or commander-in-chief for the time being, has a right to fix a day for the convention of the states, and to insert in the writs to be issued for such convention, the matters to be deliberated upon, without the concurrence of any of the jurats; but by usage long observed, the bailiff, prior to issuing such writs, communicates to the jurats in the royal court his intention of convening the states, naming the day that he proposes for the meeting, and the subjects for their consideration. These writs are prepared by the *greffier*, signed by the bailiff, and directed to the constables only, who are to communicate them to the rector, take the sense of the *touzaine* of their parish on the subject, and come prepared to give their vote accordingly. The taxes imposed by this assembly, except when they immediately regard the protection of the island, must receive the sanction of the king in council. The revenue consists of the general taxes, the harbour dues, the duties levied yearly upon licensed victuallers, or retailers of liquors in general, and the produce of lotteries. No writ from any of the British courts can extend to this island, except from the Admiralty court, which was decreed by an order in council, issued in the course of the late continental war. It is worthy of remark that although, agreeably to the numerous charters granted to these islands, the inhabitants are treated throughout the king's dominions not as aliens, but as British-born subjects, an Englishman is here considered an alien, being liable to arrest for the most trivial sum, even less than sixpence, and his bail liable to be rejected, though of known sufficiency: admission to the privileges of the island can only be granted at the pleasure of the royal court, which, after long residence, is sometimes, though rarely, conceded.

The civil and military powers appear to have been first disunited in the reign of Edward I., but in Guernsey the governor continued to appoint the bailiff until the latter part of the reign of Charles II. This island and its dependencies were under the same governor as that of Jersey until the reign of Henry VII., when the two islands were first divided into distinct governments. Although the governor has now no civil jurisdiction, his presence is sometimes required in the royal court, for enacting certain ordinances which concern the king's service, the security of the island, and the maintenance of the public peace: the court is under his immediate protection, and his authority is to be exerted, if necessary, in the execution of its decrees. This power likewise extends to the arrest and imprisonment, with the concurrence of two jurats, of any inhabitant suspected of treasonable practices; and every captain and commandant of a vessel landing passengers on the island, is obliged, under severe penalties, to make a return of them to the proper officer, and to see that such persons, as soon as it may be convenient after their arrival, attend personally to give an account of themselves. Before the governor's admission to his office he must produce his patent or commission before the royal court, and solemnly swear to maintain the liberties and immunities of the island. For a long period the governors have possessed the privilege, granted them by their patents, of executing the office by means of a deputy, whom they were formerly accustomed to appoint; but since the latter part of the reign of Charles II., the lieutenant-governor has been nominated by patent from the crown, or the king's sign manual; and when that functionary has occasion to leave the island, he delegates his authority, during absence, to the next senior military officer in command. The governors performing the office by a deputy, which has now for many years been invariably the case, take the oath before the privy council in England; the patents are transmitted with an order of council certifying such oath to have been taken, and the commissions are then registered in the royal court. The governor, whose patronage was anciently much more extensive, has still the presentation to all livings

and schools in the island, and to the offices of *greffier*, serjeant, and king's receiver. The whole of the king's rental, or dues, has for many years been granted to the governor, without his being accountable to the Exchequer for the receipt thereof, but obliging him to pay certain small allowances to some of the civil officers, &c. The governor's first duty is the care and custody of the fortifications, which have of late years been much enlarged and improved. The principal of these is Fort George, built on an eminence to the south of the town, and garrisoned by regular troops: there are barracks for upwards of five thousand men. It was begun in 1775, being named after King George III., and it is of a square figure, quite regular in its construction, defending the town and harbour of Guernsey: the barracks contain fourteen or fifteen officers, and from three to four hundred men. It is constructed for forty-five pieces of ordnance; under the ramparts are bomb-proof casemates for men and guns. The fort cannot be enfiladed from any part; there are extensive outworks in connexion with it which include the house of the chief engineer, the quarters of the officers of artillery, the store-keeper's house, and other public buildings. Of late years the militia has been re-organized, on an improved plan: every male resident without distinction, between the ages of sixteen and sixty, able to bear arms, is enrolled, trained, clothed, and accoutred, and called out occasionally for exercise and review; in time of war, all of them, in rotation, are obliged to mount guard nightly at the different batteries round the island.

The forms of the feudal system have been preserved to a greater degree in these islands than in any other part of the British dominions, although few of the ancient feudal services are exacted, and little remains of the once extensive power of the feudal courts. Anciently a court was instituted in each of the fiefs, for deciding petty broils arising on it; besides which there was a superior court, composed of a bailiff and four *chevaliers*, or knights, who held annual assizes, at which the military tenants, or lords of fiefs, attended, and appeals from the inferior courts were heard. This kind of judicature continued until the reign of King John, who, by charter, established twelve jurats instead of the *chevaliers*, who immediately checked, and in course of time effectually abolished, the feudal system. The sixteen free tenants and the thirteen *bordiers* still attend the chief pleas, or opening of the court, on the first day of the three terms, when by-laws are made for the internal government of the island. The names of the free tenants are called over immediately after those of the bailiff and jurats, but they are not now, as anciently, consulted with respect to the by-laws and ordinances, nor are they obliged to attend in person according to original custom; any one may answer for them by power of attorney, but if they do not answer at all, they are subject to a small fine. An entertainment is on those days provided for the whole court, including the military tenants and *bordiers*, at the governor's expense. The original feudal rents in kind, *viz.*, in corn, fowls, loaves of bread, eggs, and other articles, are still payable to the crown, besides some trifling sums of money in coin current in the island at the time of the original grant. When King John had lost the duchy of Normandy, he rewarded the loyalty of the islanders, who bravely resisted two attacks made by the French king, after that monarch had taken possession of the remainder of the duchy, by granting them a charter, called the Constitutions of King John, which formed the basis of the present constitution of the island, and established the royal court. This court consists of a bailiff appointed by the king, and twelve jurats chosen by the members of the states, all serving for life, unless discharged by the king and council: the officers of the court are the king's *procureur*, or attorney-general for the island; the comptroller, whose office is similar to that of solicitor-general, (these are termed the king's officers); a *provost*, or king's sheriff; the *greffier*, or registrar; and the king's serjeant. Since the establishment of the royal court, instead of the assizes being held annually, as had been previously the custom, the bailiff and jurats have administered justice three times a week in term time, and once a week during vacations, and even more frequently when necessary.

There are three terms in the year, commencing on the first Monday after January 15th, the first Monday after Easter, and the first Monday after September 29th, and each continuing for six weeks. On the first day, or opening of each term, called the *chief plaids*, or capital pleas, by-laws or ordinances are made, which have immediately the effect of law; but such of them as do not receive the royal approbation have only the same force as by-laws made by corporations in England. For the ordinary course of business, four jurats in rotation attend in each term, during which there are eight or ten court days for hearing causes in the first instance, when two jurats, with the bailiff or his deputy, who must always be present to compose a court, are sufficient: this court is called *Cour Ordinaire*, from which an appeal lies to a court of more jurats, termed *Cour d' Appeaux*, and from that again to what is termed the Court of Judgments, where at least seven jurats must be present. This latter court is held there times in each term; and if even the bailiff and all the twelve jurats are in court at the second hearing, an appeal still lies to the Court of Judgments, where only a part of them may happen to preside; and from this court alone appeals, under certain restrictions, are made to His Majesty in council. But if at the first hearing of a cause five jurats be present, appeal can then only be made directly to the Court of Judgments. The *Mobilaire* courts are held on Mondays, in which pleas for moveables or chattels are determined: the parishes are divided into two districts, called the High and the Low parishes, and the business of each is transacted on alternate Mondays, that for the Low parishes commencing first. On the Tuesday following the Monday's court for the Low parishes, judgments or final decrees are given; and on the Tuesday next after the court for the High parishes, courts of heritage are held, termed *Plaids d' Heritage*, for determining all suits relative to inheritance. The Saturdays' courts are for the passing of contracts, admiralty causes, and criminal informations; the intermediate days, either in or out of term, being devoted to the hearing of causes in general. But the Saturdays' courts for criminal causes continue from the chief pleas of Easter to the middle of July; from Michaelmas to Christmas; and from the 15th of January to the Saturday before Holy Week. When a prisoner

is charged with a capital offence, the first step taken is to make out the accusation or indictment, and to take down his answer in what is called *l'Interrogatoire*, which is a most essential document to prove the innocence of the accused when his account is corroborated by the evidence, but tending on the other hand to the proof of guilt when that account is controverted and contradicted by that evidence. The prisoner on the next Saturday, if in term time, is brought before the court, where, the accusation being read to him, he pleads guilty or not guilty, and makes choice of his counsel; he is then remanded in order that witnesses may be examined, and a day is appointed for their examination in support of the prosecution. This examination takes place before the court, which need not be composed of more than two jurats, besides the bailiff or chief magistrate: neither the prisoner, nor his counsel, is present. The witnesses are introduced one by one, and sworn, when the *greffier*, or king's officer, proceeds to set down their name, age, and deposition. When all the witnesses of the crown officers have been thus examined, another day is appointed by the court for what is called the *recollement et confrontation*, that is to say, the verification of the evidence and the confronting of the witnesses and the prisoner. At the close of this sitting the prisoner is to state what witnesses he wishes to call forward in his behalf, and what particular facts he means to prove by their evidence. A note of this is taken, and another day appointed for examining them. When all the examinations have taken place, authenticated copies of the prisoner's interrogatories, and of the depositions of the witnesses, are furnished to the prisoner's counsel, in order that he may prepare his defence. On the day of trial, the court must be composed of seven or more jurats, besides the bailiff. The prisoner's interrogatories, and the depositions of the witnesses in support of the prosecution and in behalf of the prisoner, are read; after which the prisoner's counsel (who must be one of the six advocates licensed by the court, and who is obliged to give his services *gratuitously*, if the prisoner have not the means of feeing him) is allowed to address the court at as great a length as he may think proper. The king's *procureur* then offers his opinion upon the case, and states what sentence, in his judgment, ought to be given: this is technically termed "*Les conclusions du procureur du roi.*" The king's comptroller follows much in the same way, and also gives his conclusions: the bailiff then sums up the evidence in a charge which he delivers to the jurats; after which each jurat present, from the eldest to the youngest, states his individual opinion, and the sentence is decided by a majority. Should there be an equality of opinions, the bailiff has a casting vote, and it is he who communicates the sentence of the court to the prisoner. It is not neccessary to report the proceedings to the king before a condemned criminal can suffer death: the sentence is final and irreversible, except where it may appear to the court that the criminal, though found guilty, is a fit subject for royal clemency, in which case his execution is deferred until His Majesty's pleasure can be known: all trials are conducted in the Norman French language.

The royal court-house, as the date on the tympanum of the pediment of its principal front indicates, was erected in 1799, but it was altered and embellished in 1821, by John Wilson, Esq., at an expense of £4100. The building consists of an upper and a lower court-room : the former is fifty-one feet long, by twenty-six broad, with an elevation of nineteen feet; the latter twenty-six feet by twenty, and eleven feet high. There is a spacious *greffier's* office, in which are deposited copies of all the deeds and contracts relative to every transaction in heritage property belonging to the island. There are excellent apartments for the private deliberations of the jurats, committees, &c., communicating with the upper court-room. Nearly adjoining the court-house is the new prison for felons and debtors. A debtor who cannot support himself receives ninepence per day from the creditors at whose suit he is detained, and if the gaoler fails to pay him before nine o'clock in the morning, he can claim his discharge.

The ecclesiastical jurisdiction of Guernsey was, with that of Jersey and the neighbouring islands, subjected to the Bishop of Coutances by Rollo, the first Duke of Normandy, and continued so till King John was dispossessed of that duchy in 1204, when they were united to the see of Exeter, but were soon restored to that of Coutances, to which they remained attached until, in the reign of Henry VII., they were, by a bull of Pope Alexander, annexed to the diocese of Salisbury : they were afterwards re-attached to Coutances, and formed part of that bishoprick, till Elizabeth, in 1568, transferred them to the see of Winchester. At a synod held in Guernsey June 20th, 1576, it was agreed that the ecclesiastical discipline should be strictly presbyterian, which was rigidly adhered to till the act of uniformity passed in England, in the reign of Charles II., the provisions of which extended to these islands. The Dean presented by the governor to the Bishop of Winchester, and approved by the king, entered upon his functions accordingly, and, in 1664 obtained a commission of official from the bishop, investing him with the full power of ecclesiastical jurisdiction in the island and its dependencies. The introduction of the litany and discipline of the church of England met with considerable opposition from the clergy and the people ; and even so lately as the year 1755, the dean found it necessary to apply for the aid of the magistracy to enforce it : the use of the surplice is still discontinued ; and although the sacrament of baptism is generally performed in the church, yet there is not a single font in the island. The dean holds the ecclesiastical court, whenever occasion requires it : this court consists of the dean and beneficed clergy, with a registrar and apparitor ; most of the advocates of the royal court being proctors. Before the dean, as surrogate to the bishop, the wills of persons dying in the island are proved and registered, and from him administrations are obtained for the proper distribution of the property of persons dying intestate, copies of which are regularly transmitted to the consistorial episcopal court at Winchester : the dean has also the power of granting special licenses for the solemnization of private marriages. The ceremony of confirmation, which, according to the church of England, should precede admission to the Sacrament of the Lord's Supper, is necessarily omitted in these islands, the bishop never visiting them to perform it : private instruction, competent age, and the answering of certain interrogatories at the church in the presence of the congregation, are considered as ratifying the baptismal vow. The livings are of small value, from the loss of the great tithes originally belonging to them, which were first by the papal authority appropriated to the Norman monasteries, and at the Reformation seized by the crown. The small tithes, or share of the greater, allowed by those religious houses to the incumbents, are still retained, and have been increased by what are termed *novals*, or *deserts*, namely, the tithe of land since brought into tillage. Surplice fees were formerly paid, but having been given up by the Presbyterian ministers, from aversion to the name, they have not been revived ; and the church dues for baptism, marriage, sacrament, and burial, are so very trifling that, except in the Town parish, which is populous, their amount is very small. The tithe of all grain and flax growing in the island is due to the king, and that of all apples, pears, cider, honey, calves, colts, pigs, lambs, geese, and fish, to the rector, but no tithe whatever is due to either for hay, clover, lucerne, potatoes, parsnips, or other vegetables. The *champart*, or portion of the field reserved by the chief lord, in lieu of rent, is the twelfth sheaf of the whole crop. The *presbyteries*, or parsonage-houses, are kept in repair at the expense of the respective parishes. The church service is invariably performed in the French language, excepting for the garrison, and at the new church of St. James.

The inhabitants are distinguished by several peculiarities from those of the rest of the British dominions. The Old Norman language, now gradually approximating towards the French, is generally spoken by all ranks of people ; scarcely any of the country people speak English, but many among the higher classes have acquired a tolerably correct pronunciation of it : their dress and style of living, particularly among the higher ranks, are receiving great modifications from an increasing intercourse with England. Mediocrity of fortune seems to prevail throughout the island, and a rigid economy is practised.

The island appears to have been divided into parishes soon after the Norman Conquest of England. For many years before the militia was organized, each parish had a captain, or *centenier*, who trained the men to the use of arms, and had the care of two pieces of ordnance ; but the office was discontinued when this military force was formed into regiments and better regulated. The *douzainiers* of each parish are twelve of the most respectable and intelligent inhabitants (the Town and Vale parishes excepted, the former having twenty and the latter sixteen), chosen for life by the parishioners, as their representatives in the assembly of the states on all public matters, voting individually in the choice of the jurats, or magistrates, and the sheriff, and giving their votes collectively, by the constables of their respective parishes, on other subjects requiring deliberation : they have also the regulation of all parochial matters. There are two constables in each parish, chosen annually, who preside and make part of the corps of the *Douzaine:* they may confine offenders both night and day, but must, in all cases, make their report to the bailiff and to the king's officers within twenty-four hours : they may also search for stolen property individually, but are in general accompanied by one or more of the assistant constables, particularly in town, in order to render their search more effectual. They receive the money raised for the public service from their collectors, for whom they are responsible, and apply it to the purposes intended. It is also their duty to visit, in the presence of two respectable persons, all taverns and cellars where liquors are sold, to see that such articles are wholesome, and upon finding any that are not so, to destroy them. The *curateurs*, of whom there are two in each parish, are officers exercising all the functions of churchwardens; and the office of *procureur des pauvres*, or manager of the poor, in each parish, is similar to that of an overseer : the poor-rates are collected by distinct officers, of whom there are two or more, according to the extent of the parish.

St. Peter-Port, or the Town parish, lies about the middle of the eastern coast. The town has of late years been much extended in several directions. It seems to have been formerly confined to the range of houses running parallel with the sea, from what is called Glatney to the upper part of Cornet-street. The extent of St. Peter-Port, along the coast, from the upper part of Cornet-street to the end of Long-store, is little short of a mile and a half ; and, including the New town and the Hauteville, it is about three miles in circumference. In the High-street most of the old houses have been removed, and the width greatly increased. The town, generally speaking, is well paved, and some of the streets, though narrow, have foot-ways. The streets in the Upper or New town, and the Hauteville, are straight, and the houses large and well-built, especially Saumarez-street. Owing to the improvements that have been effected in the roads, a great many English carriages are kept. Among the improvements the widening of Fountain-street, which is advancing rapidly towards completion, may be styled the most important. This street, although the principal road of communication between the harbour, town, and country, was originally only ten feet wide, which has been increased to thirty feet, and the buildings, consisting of dwelling-houses with shops, and little inferior in appearance to any in the most modern streets of London, while they surpass them in point of solidity. Pipes are now being laid down for the introduction of gas into the town. The assembly-rooms, built by subscription, in 1780, are situated in the market-place, and are supported on stone arches; the ball-room is very extensive : the public meetings are generally held here. A library was established in 1819, under the patronage of the Governor, and the Bishop of Winchester; in the reading-room are periodical publications, but no newspapers. The theatre, situated in New-street, is neatly fitted up : a company of comedians from Exeter visit the island, generally in October, and remain till Christmas. At the top of Smith-street stands Government House, a neat building, the residence of the lieutenant-governor. The church of St. James, the new college, and Castle Carey, which stand in the highest parts of the town, form very striking objects from the roads and harbour. Castle Carey was erected in 1829, at a cost of £4000; the style of its architecture is castellated English; it is two stories in height, exclusively of the basement and centre tower, or turret, and is one of the greatest ornaments to the island; it is situated near a small public park, called the New Ground, but has very little land attached to it, whence it has been denominated Castle-Lackland. There are upwards of thirty handsome villas in the immediate vicinity of the town, substantially built of native granite since 1815; and within the last ten years upwards of four hundred

houses have been erected in the town, at an expense of £200,000. Doyle's column, erected in honour of Sir John Doyle, stands on the heights between the bays of Fermain and Moulin-street : it is about one hundred feet high from the base to the top, and two hundred and fifty feet from the level of the sea, and is ascended by a winding staircase; the gallery is surrounded by an iron balustrade.

The new town stands so high that, from the level of the market-place, the side of the ravine is ascended by a flight of a hundred and forty-five steps, to the top of what is called Mount Gibel, the Moorish name *Gebal* being supposed to have been given to it by the Sarragozans, who invaded the island in the time of Edward III., and since corrupted into Gibel, with the addition of the French word *Mont*. About a quarter of a mile from this spot are the public walks, or New Ground. This plot of land, containing about eight English acres, was purchased by the parish more than half a century ago, and one-half of it laid out in groves ; the other, which is a smooth lawn, is set apart as a military parade. The vegetable market is held under the assembly-rooms, and in the open square adjoining. The principal market day is Saturday. There is a space assigned in the market-place for pork and veal, from each of the ten parishes, which is sold to the public by the farmers, on Friday and Saturday : all the weights are of brass, and marked to prevent imposition. Fish, fruit, and vegetables of excellent quality, are exposed for sale every day in the week. The butchers' market-place was constructed in 1822 : adjoining it a new fish market has recently been erected, which is not excelled by any in the United Kingdom, with the exception of that of Liverpool : it is one hundred and ninety-eight feet in length, twenty-two feet wide, and twenty-eight feet in elevation, entirely covered over, and lighted in a very tasteful manner by seven octagonal skylights, beneath which there are Venetian blinds for the purpose of ventilating the building. The fish tables, forty in number, are all of polished marble, each being supplied with fine spring water. The total cost of Fountain-street and the fish market will amount to £57,216. An extensive slaughter-house has been erected near the beach, in which all the cattle are killed : this edifice, which is of blue granite, is so judiciously constructed, as to prevent any annoyance arising from it to the town, the filth being conveyed to the beach through a pipe, and washed away by the tide at high water.

The living is a rectory, rated in the king's books at £12, and in the patronage of the Governor. The church, dedicated to St. Peter in 1312, is of more elaborate architecture than any other in the island : it consists of a nave, two aisles, and a chancel, with a tower in the centre, surmounted by a low spire. The porch on the northern side is very handsome : the pillars which support the arched roof are of granite, and on the walls are several beautiful marble monuments of modern date : it has lately undergone a thorough repair, under the direction of Mr. John Wilson ; the pews are all new, and made of Dutch wainscot. The garrison service, and the evening service, are performed in the English language. There are two chapels of ease, one called Trinity chapel, situated in County Mansell, built in 1768, and in which the service is performed in French ; the other, situated in Manor-street, is called Bethell chapel : it was built in 1791, and purchased, by an order from His Majesty's Council, in 1796, as a chapel to St. Peter-Port. St. James' church was built by subscription, expressly for the performance of the church service in English. The government is vested in elders, and the minister is paid by the congregation: it is nevertheless subject to the jurisdiction of the Bishop of Winchester, and contains one thousand three hundred and thirty-four sittings, four hundred of which are free. There are places of worship for Baptists, the Society of Friends, two for English Independents, three for French Independents, and one each for French Methodists, Primitive and Wesleyan Methodists, and Unitarians; and there is a Roman Catholic chapel, the congregation of which consists exclusively of Irish and French. The free grammar school, founded by Queen Elizabeth, has lately been rebuilt, at an expense of £12,000. It is called "The Royal College of Elizabeth," and is a fine and imposing pile of building, in the later style of English architecture, one hundred and seventy-seven feet in length from north to south, and sixty-six feet wide from east to west. It consists of a public hall, fifty-four feet by twenty-seven, and twenty-two feet and a half in elevation; seven school-rooms of lofty dimensions, each thirty-four feet by twenty-two and a half; a library, and spacious accommodation for the principal and his boarders. The centre tower, which contains the library, is one hundred feet high, with four side towers of sixty feet each. The corner stone was laid the 19th of October, 1826, and the edifice was finished in 1830, after a design by Mr. John Wilson, architect to the States. From the centre tower there is a very extensive view of the sea, of the adjacent islands, and the coast of France, as well as of the surrounding country. The institution is endowed with certain lands and rents, which, with the school-house, gardens, and meadow, adjoining, are estimated to produce to the master upwards of £300 per annum: the mastership is in the presentation of the Governor; every boy born in the island is entitled to admission, and, including the boarders, most of whom are English boys, there are upwards of one hundred and fifty scholars. In 1636, Charles I., at the request of Archbishop Laud, endowed, with an estate comprising houses in London and lands in Buckinghamshire, which had escheated to the crown, a fellowship in each of the colleges of Jesus, Exeter, and Pembroke, in the University of Oxford, for natives of Jersey or Guernsey, who have also the benefit of five scholarships, founded by Dr. Morley, Bishop of Winchester, in 1654, in Pembroke College, three for Jersey, and two for Guernsey. The town hospital was erected in 1741 and 1742, in consequence of a general meeting of the parishioners to take into consideration the state of the poor. Until then, the poor of the parish had been periodically relieved by pecuniary donations, arising from certain rents appropriated or bequeathed for that purpose, and from sundry collections at the church doors, aided, as they had been of late years, by the proceeds of a general rate. The rents above-mentioned were transferred to the new institution, and the whole placed under the management of a treasurer and other gentlemen annually chosen by the parishioners. This institution combines the objects of an hospital and a workhouse, or house of industry; and, though originally designed for parishioners only, has generally amongst its inmates a number of strangers,

who, owing to bodily infirmity, or some other substantial reason, cannot be removed to their own parish or country: it serves also as a temporary asylum for such sick strangers as are under the care of the constables, and due attention is rendered them until they are thought in a proper state to quit the island. The arrangements throughout are excellent, the inmates receiving every attention and comfort their situation requires; spinning, weaving, and various other branches of industry are carried on. There is a Magdalene ward, in which females of loose morals are kept, and who are not allowed to have any communication with the other inmates; persons afflicted with mental derangement have also separate apartments. The female children, whose number exceeds fifty, are educated, until the age of fourteen, under the personal inspection and daily attendance of some of the principal ladies of the island, after which they are received as servants in respectable families: the boys are educated until of the same age, when they are apprenticed. The building, which was considerably improved and enlarged in the years 1809 and 1810, is very commodious, with an open space of ground in front, a court-yard behind, and two gardens nearly adjoining. A National school for boys and girls has also been established in the town, in which about one hundred and forty boys and eighty girls are educated.

In 1274, the inhabitants represented to the justices of assize sent from England to the island, that a stone pier projecting into the sea, between the town and Castle Cornet, would be very useful to commerce; in consequence of which, in the following year, an order was obtained from Edward I., whereby the governor and the principal inhabitants were authorised to build a pier, and to levy, for the term of three years only, a small duty on ships coming to the island, towards defraying the expense. In violation of this order, however, the duty was not only raised by the governor for the term of three years, but was continued by him after that term, and by his successors, without their commencing the work for which it was levied, until the reign of Queen Elizabeth, when the commissioners sent to the island, placed the power of collecting the petty custom in the hands of the bailiff and jurats, and ordered them to lay it out under the inspection of the governor, by which means the south pier was begun about 1570. Sir Thomas Leighton, who governed the island in 1580 and for forty years after, was a great benefactor to the work, as was also Amice de Carteret, who was lieutenant-governor and bailiff of the island in 1608. The northern end of the pier was begun in the reign of Queen Anne, when the islanders suffering considerably by the storms, for want of a pier to the east and north of the harbour, made voluntary contributions for the erection of the north pier; and the whole work has been improved from time to time: it extends to the eastward about four hundred and sixty feet, curving inwards at the extremities, which leave an opening about eighty feet wide. The length of the south pier is seven hundred and fifty-seven feet; and they form a spacious basin, into which vessels of considerable burden can enter at high water. Castle Cornet, a fortress by which the harbour is defended, stands on a rock a little to the south-east of the pier: it is of very remote antiquity, and is supposed to have been originally constructed by the Romans. When the island was invaded by the

French, in the reign of Edward I., this castle fell into their hands, and they kept possession of it for some time. It is so well defended by batteries on all sides, that, though accessible from the town at the ebbing of every spring tide, when the intervening sands are left quite dry, it has often been successfully defended. In the reign of Charles I. it withstood a long and vigorous siege, being held for the king by Sir Peter Osborne, the lieutenant-governor, in opposition to the town, then under the influence of the parliament, who had vested the government of the island in the twelve jurats: the castle being closely blockaded, and their provisions exhausted, the garrison at length surrendered on honourable terms. A dreadful accident happened here on the 29th of December, 1672, from lightning communicating with the magazine, which blew up with a tremendous explosion, destroying a great part of the castle, and in particular some handsome new buildings, then recently erected at considerable expense by the governor, Viscount Hatton, who, together with his family and some other persons, was residing at the time in a part of the castle thrown down by the shock: several persons were killed, among whom were Lady Hatton, wife of the governor, and the Dowager Lady Hatton, his mother. Formerly the governors made this castle their place of residence, but it has ceased to be so for many years, and is placed in the care of a guard of soldiers and certain officers; it is an isolated castle, very ancient, and of a triangular form: in spring tides, at low water, it may be reached on foot. There are embrazures pierced for seventy-six pieces of ordnance; it commands the several channels of entrance to the town, and looks into St. Peter's Port.

St. Sampson's parish lies at the north-eastern extremity of the island. All the land in it was in the possession of the Duke of Normandy, until William the Conqueror rewarded Sampson d'Anneville with about one-fourth of the island, including a part of this parish, then erected into a fief, or royalty, still called the fief d'Anneville: this fief, which appears to have been the first grant to a layman in the island, is the noblest tenure in it; the lord of the seigniory ranking next after the clergy, and being so cited in the king's courts, which he is obliged by his tenure to attend three times a year, viz. at the chief pleas, or opening of the terms; he is also bound, when the king comes to the island, to attend him as his esquire during his stay. The lord holds a court yearly at Michaelmas, composed of a seneschal, three *vavasors*, or judges, a clerk, or *greffier*, and a provost: the tenants thus assembled annually choose a provost from among themselves, to collect the lord's chief rents. The living is a rectory, annexed to the vicarage of the Vale parish, rated in the king's books at £5. The church, a low edifice without either tower or spire, is chiefly remarkable for its antiquity, having been consecrated in the year 1111, and is the oldest church in the island. There is a place of worship for French Methodists. In order to facilitate the exportation of the granite from the north of the island, the harbour of St. Sampson has been rendered secure and convenient by a new breakwater and quay.

The Vale parish, lying at the northern extremity of the island, was formerly divided into two parts, at what is called the Braye du Val, by an irruption of the sea, which is supposed to have taken place about the year

1204; in consequence of which a bridge was erected to afford a communication with the part thus separated from the main land: but the sea flowing from the other extremity at the Vale church, and preventing all intercourse with the north-west, a causeway of large stones, called the Devil's bridge, or Pont du Val, was raised, for the purpose of crossing the Braye at low water, and the sea continued to flow over a large tract of land every tide, until, by the exertions of the lieutenant-governor, Sir John Doyle, this land was recovered by shutting out the sea by another bridge near the Vale church, by which eight hundred and fourteen vergees have been brought into tillage. That portion of the land which fell to the share of the crown was sold for £5000, which sum was appropriated towards defraying the expense of the new military roads across the island. In the Close of the Vale, not far from the spot where the church now stands, the fugitive monks from the Benedictine abbey of Mount St. Michael, in Normandy, about the year 962, erected a monastery, which was likewise dedicated to St. Michael, thus forming the first regular settlement in the island, and soon brought the whole Close of the Vale into cultivation. The abbot, it appears, had no regular grant of the lands from the Duke of Normandy, but assumed a property in them for the maintenance of the monastery, until the year 1032, when Robert, Duke of Normandy, father of the Conqueror, granted them to the monks by the name of the fief St. Michael, which grant the Conqueror confirmed in 1061, the fief at that time including one-fourth of the cultivated part of the island. This fief has belonged to the crown ever since the dissolution of religious houses; and the court, which consists of a seneschal, eleven *vavasors*, three provosts, a *greffier*, and a serjeant, is held thrice a year, *viz.*, on the day following each of the chief pleas of the royal court. A ceremony anciently observed at this court, of perambulating the king's highways in the island, has of late years been revived. The *chevauchée*, or cavalcade, consisting of the lieutenant-governor and the officers of his staff, with the officers and members of the court, together with the officers of the royal court, all mounted on horseback, (the bailiff also has a right to demand a horse and servant, although he has never enforced his privilege,) the horses being decorated with ribands, and led by footmen termed *peons*, dressed in white jackets and trousers, bound and ornamented with rose-coloured ribands, wearing black velvet caps, and carrying gilt-headed spears, proceed from the court-room at the Vale along the high road through the Town, St. Martin's, the Forest, St. Peter's in the Wood, and Torteval, to Plein Mont; whence, after partaking of some refreshment in a marquée provided for the purpose, they pursue their route through St. Saviour's, the King's mills, more commonly known as the Grand Moulin, and the lower part of the Catel parish, to the place from which they set out; an officer termed *porte-lance* carrying a spear erect, measuring eleven feet eight inches, elevated from the stirrup on which it rested to the height of about fourteen feet from the ground to the point: if the spear come in contact with the boughs of trees, or other projections overhanging the road, or such road is considered not in good repair and of the width of the spear's length, the owners of the adjoining lands, who are by custom bound to keep the roads in repair, are subject to fines; the lands on one side being bound to maintain a good foot-path, and those on the other a good horse or carriage road. The *peons*, who are generally the best looking young men of the island, dressed in white and decorated with ribband, &c., volunteering their services, have the privilege of saluting every woman they meet, without distinction. The Castle of St. Michael, now called Vale Castle, standing on an eminence on the eastern side of the parish, was commenced towards the close of the tenth century, to shelter the inhabitants from the ravages of the pirates that continually infested the island, and carried off the corn and cattle. It was many years in building, and three centuries after was large enough to contain both the people and their cattle, when, in case of alarm, they shut themselves up for protection. Little more of the structure remains than the outer walls, in which are some flanking towers and the old portal. Buildings have been erected within, them as barracks for a few soldiers, and upon its mouldering ramparts, the most ancient pieces of masonry now on the island, are a few pieces of ordnance. The quantity of land in this parish is four thousand three hundred vergees. The living is a vicarage, with the rectory of St. Sampson's annexed, rated in the king's books at £6. 13. 4., and in the patronage of the Governor. The church, dedicated to St. Michael the Archangel, was consecrated in 1117: it consists of a nave and aisle, with a low tower at one end, surmounted by a spire. There is a place of worship for French Methodists.

The parish of TORTEVAL lies at the western extremity of the island, and contains about one thousand three hundred and seventy vergees. The living is a rectory, with that of Forest parish united to it, rated in the king's books at £5, and in the patronage of the Governor. The church, dedicated to St. Philip, was erected by the States, at an expense of £3000, in 1817; it contains three hundred and fifty sittings. The body of the building is sixty feet long by thirty broad, being vaulted with a pointed arch, which covers the entire area. The building is of the most permanent description, its walls being of granite, roofed with brick-work and coated externally with a thick covering of Roman cement. The tower and spire, as well as the buttresses of the side walls, are circular: the spire is one hundred and twenty feet high. There is an agreeable simplicity, combined with a permanency in the appearance of this structure, seldom surpassed in a country church; the pews and doors constitute the only wood-work employed in its construction. It was consecrated by Dr. Fisher, Bishop of Salisbury, on the 5th of August, 1818. A little to the west of the signal post at Prevoté point, at the foot of a rocky steep, is a natural cavern, called *La Cave Mahie:* it is very singularly formed, about two hundred feet long, and forty or fifty wide; the vaulted roof rises from six or eight to fifty or sixty feet in height; the bottom is rough and uneven, the whole being formed by granitic points in a vertical direction, like most of the rocky cliffs throughout the island.

ST. SAVIOUR's parish lies on the western side of the island, but the exact quantity of land within its limits has not been ascertained. The living is a rectory, rated in the king's books at £10, and in the patronage of the Governor. The church, consecrated in 1154, is a commodious building, standing in a lofty

and picturesque situation, and consisting of a nave and side aisle, with a handsome tower at one end, surmounted by a very low spire. The ancient chapel of St. Apoline still remains entire, and is now used as a barn; the interior of the roof is circular, and formed of stone. There is a place of worship for French Methodists. The priory of Lihou, or Lihoumel, which stood on a small island to the south-west, communicating with the main land at low-water, is said to have been built in 1114; part of one of the walls is remaining: in the rock are two natural baths, hollowed out by the continued friction of stones washed round by the eddy of the sea: the islet is uninhabited, but contains a great number of rabbits.

The FOREST parish lies near the middle of the southern coast. The living is a rectory, united to that of Torteval parish, rated in the king's books at £7. The church, dedicated to St. Margaret, was consecrated in 1163: it is a mean building with a tiled roof, consisting of a nave and aisles, with a low tower and spire in the centre. There is a place of worship for French Methodists.

ST. PETER of the WOOD lies on the south-west side of the island, and contains two thousand seven hundred vergees. The living is a rectory, rated in the king's books at £11, and in the patronage of the Governor. The church, consecrated June 29th, 1167, is one of the best in the island in point of architecture; it stands in a picturesque situation on the declivity of Deeper valley, and consists of a nave and aisles, with a well-proportioned tower at one end. There is a place of worship for French Methodists.

ST. MARTIN's parish lies at the south-eastern extremity of the island, and contains about three thousand six hundred and fourteen vergees. Besides the king's fief, which extends into this parish, that of Sausmarez is the most considerable, and has been in the possession of the family of that name from time immemorial. Amongst other services to which the tenants of this fief are liable, they are bound to bring the seignior all his fuel and provisions, and, when required, to provide a proper vessel to convey him to and from Jersey. The court, which was formerly held thrice a year, at the chief pleas of the royal court, is now, at the will of the seignior, held but once, at Michaelmas. It appears that the command of the castle of Jerbourg was, by Edward III., vested in Matthew de Sausmarez, at that time lord of this fief, and his heirs male, who continued to be castellans as long as the fortifications existed. Of this ancient castle no vestige remains, a signal post has been erected near the spot where it stood, and a small barrack has of late years been built in this commanding and naturally strong position, which, from the deep parallel ditches on the north and south sides of the promontory, is thought to have been fortified by the Romans. The living is a rectory, rated in the king's books at £11. 13. 4., and in the patronage of the Governor. The church, consecrated in 1199, consists of a nave and aisle, with a low central tower surmounted by a spire. There is a place of worship for French Methodists.

The parish of ST. MARY DE CASTRO, generally called by corruption the Catel parish, lies near the centre of the island, and contains about five thousand four hundred and thirty vergees. The poor house, for all the country parishes, stands within it, and is conducted on a plan similar to that of the Town parish. The Vason bay, which bounds part of the parish to the westward, is conjectured, from the remains which have been dug up under the sands, to have been anciently forest or woodland. The principal feudal court in this parish is that of the fief Le Compte, a great part of which and its dependencies is included within its limits : this court, consisting of a seneschal, eight vavasors, a procureur fiscal, three provosts, a greffier, serjeant, and receiver, is held thrice a year, viz., on the second day following the chief pleas of the royal court : the escheats of persons dying without heirs, forfeitures upon condemnation to death, or upon banishment for seven years, called in French une mort civille, vareck or shipwreck found upon the fief, and other rights, appertain to the lord, which, with the change of property by death or alienation, now form the chief business of this and the other fief courts in the island. The living is a rectory, rated in the king's books at £10, and in the patronage of the Governor. The church, built on the site of the old castle erected by the piratical invaders about the middle of the eleventh century, and called the Château du Sarrazin, or Grand Geoffrey, was consecrated in 1203 : it consists of a nave and aisle, with a low central tower surmounted by a spire. A small remnant of the ancient chapel of St. George stands near the house which is called by that name.

St. Andrew's parish lies towards the southern extremity of the island, and is the only one which is not at any point contiguous to the sea : it contains about two thousand five hundred vergees of land. The minister of this parish holds a field by the service of saying the Lord's Prayer when the seignior of the fief of St. Helena holds his court. The living is a rectory, rated in the king's books at £6. 13. 4., and in the patronage of the Governor. The church, consecrated in 1204, consists of a nave and aisle, with a neat tower at one end. There are places of worship for French Independents and Wesleyan Methodists.

The remains of five Druidical temples can be distinctly traced in Guernsey : one of them is situated on a rocky ridge between the points of land formerly occupied by Le Rée, and Richmond barracks, at the western extremity of the island ; another near Norman point, on the north-east, consists of one large slab of granite, sixteen feet long, eight feet broad, and three feet thick, forming an inclined plane, and supported on rude masses of stone ; and three others on L'Ancresse common. The island of Lihou, which, like Castle Cornet in St. Peter's Port, is connected with Guernsey at low water, is situated to the north of Rocquaine bay, and is the property of Eleazar le Marchant, Esq., lieutenant-bailiff of Guernsey. Guernsey gives the inferior title of baron to the family of Finch, Earls of Aylesford.

The island of ALDERNEY, which is dependent on, and under the jurisdiction of, the states of Guernsey, is situated 6 leagues (N. E.) from that island, and 7 miles (W.) from Cape La Hogue in Normandy, from which it is separated by a strait, called by the French " Raz Blanchard," and by the English the Race of Alderney, and contains 1151 inhabitants. This island, named in old English records Aurney, Aureney, and Aurigny, by which last name it is still designated by the French geographers, is supposed to have been the Riduna of Antoninus ;
Vol. II.

but little of its history is known prior to the time of Henry III., in the fourth year of whose reign an act of parliament was passed, by which it appears that one moiety of the island belonged to that monarch, and the other moiety to the Bishop of Coutances. From an extent of the crown, made in the fourth year of the reign of James I., the whole of the island was the property of the king, who was entitled to the amends, or fines, and the perquisites of the court ; to the treiziémes, or thirteenths, upon the sale of lands; and to the wrecks, and other princely rights and royalties ; but it was subsequently granted in fee-farm to successive tenants. George III., by letters patent under the great seal, bearing date December 14th, 1763, in consideration of the surrender of the former lease, or patent, which had then become vested in John le Mesurier, Esq., and for other considerations therein specified, granted the island to the said John le Mesurier, his executors, administrators, and assigns, for ninety-nine years, with a proviso for resuming the lease at any time, upon payment to the lessee of such amount of money as should have been disbursed in improving the mansion-house, called the Governor's house, and the other premises, to be ascertained by six or more of the privy council. In this grant were included the advowson of the church and chapel, with power to levy duties upon all vessels coming into the port or harbour of the island, in the same proportion as they are levied in the harbour of St. Peter's Port in Guernsey. The rights and property of the island were purchased by government from J. le Mesurier, Esq., of Pool, who was the last governor.

The approach to the island, particularly in stormy weather, is dangerous, from the rapidity and diversity of the currents, which at spring tides rush in contrary directions, with a velocity of six miles an hour, and from the numerous rocks by which it is surrounded ; these rocks were fatal to Prince Henry, son of Henry I., who was wrecked here on his return from Normandy, in 1119 ; and, in 1744, to the Victory man of war, which was lost with the whole crew, consisting of one thousand one hundred men : the French fleet, notwithstanding, escaped through this passage after its defeat at La Hogue, in 1692. Between the north-west side of Alderney and the small island of Burhou is the passage of " Le Singe," which, though narrow, and, like the other, subject to violent agitation, has depth of water sufficient for the largest ships of war. About a mile and a half to the west is the precipitous rock Ortac, rising abruptly to the height of one hundred feet, apparently of porphyry, and forming one of the highest in a chain which stretches in this direction from Burhou. At the distance of seven miles, in the same direction, are the Caskets, a cluster of rocks rising to a height from the water of from twenty-five to thirty fathoms, and, including a few detached to the westward, about one mile in circumference : on the south-west side is a naturally-formed harbour, in which a frigate may shelter as in a dock; steps are cut in the rock, and conveniences are provided for hauling up boats : there is also a smaller and less compact harbour on the northeast side. On these rocks three lighthouses have been recently erected, and furnished with revolving reflectors : they are in a triangular position, the two southernmost, fifty feet asunder, in a direction east and west, and the third, one hundred and fifty feet to the north of the former, is on the most elevated part of the rock, twenty feet above the others, and sixty feet above the level of high water mark; the lights in clear weather may be seen at the distance of four leagues. The island, which is four miles in length, one mile and a half in breadth, and nearly ten miles in circumference, shelves considerably to the north-east, and is intersected by deep vallies: the whole of the southern and eastern parts, from La Pendante to La Clanque, is bounded by cliffs varying in elevation from one hundred to two hundred feet, and presenting picturesque and striking scenery; the northern and eastern sides are terminated with lower cliffs, alternating with small bays and flat shores. The bay of Bray is remarkably fine, affording good anchorage to vessels, and at low water the sands are very extensive: Longy bay is also commodious; and Craby harbour, in which at spring tides the water rises to the height of twenty-five feet, affords every facility for a wet dock. The east side of the island consists chiefly of reddish sand-stone, and the west side principally of porphyry, neither of which rocks are found in large masses in any of the other islands of the group. About one half of the land is in cultivation; the remainder consists of common and furze land, affording good pasturage for sheep, but insufficient for cattle. The soil, though light and sandy, is in general good, and the system of agriculture similar to that at Guernsey. The general appearance of the land is bare; few trees and no thorn hedges are to be seen, the enclosures being formed by walls of loose stones, and furze banks. Of the Alderney breed of cows, which has taken its name from this island, Jersey and Guernsey furnish by far the greater number for exportation, this island but very few. The town is situated nearly in the centre of the island, and, with the exception of the Governor's house, contains few buildings worthy of notice; it is partially paved, and well supplied with water: there is a good road to Bray harbour, and another to Longy bay, where was an ancient nunnery, subsequently used as barracks during the war, and since the peace, converted into an hospital, and depôt for military stores. The pier, near which are several houses, is of rude construction, with only one projecting arm, affording shelter to vessels only from the north-east.

The civil jurisdiction is exercised by a judge and six jurats, the former of whom is nominated by the governor, and the latter elected by the commonalty: they hold their several appointments for life, unless removed for misbehaviour, or malversation in office; and, with the king's officers, *viz.*, the king's *procureur*, or attorney-general; the king's *comptroller*, or solicitor-general; and the *greffier*, or registrar, who is also nominated by the governor, compose the court, the decision of which, however, is not necessarily definitive, being subject to an appeal to the royal court at Guernsey, and from that to the king in council. In all criminal cases the court of Alderney has only the power of receiving evidence, which is transmitted to the superior court of Guernsey, where judgment is pronounced, and the sentence of the law executed. The entire jurisprudence of the island is similar to that of Guernsey, as appears by the order of the royal commissioners sent to the island by Queen Elizabeth, in 1585. The judge and six jurats, together with the *douzainiers*,

being twelve men chosen by the commonalty for their representatives, compose the assembly of the states of the island, wherein all ordinances for its government are proposed. But the *douzainiers* have only a deliberative voice, and no vote, the judge and jurats alone deciding upon the expediency of any proposed measure. The governor, or his lieutenant, must be present at each assembly, but has no vote in it. The public acts were first registered at Alderney in 1617, and the first contract was enrolled in the year 1666. The privileges of the charter are inherited by birth, or obtained by servitude. It is not known at what time the church was built: it is an ancient edifice, not entitled to architectural notice; the tower was added to it in 1767, and a chapel near it was erected in 1763. From the year 1591 to 1607, Alderney was without an officiating minister; during that period, baptisms and marriages were solemnized at Guernsey, and registered in the parish of St. Saviour. There is a place of worship for Wesleyan Methodists. A school for boys, and another for girls, were founded by J. Le Mesurier, Esq., the last governor: the building was erected in 1790, and the institution has funded property to the amount of £400 three per cent. consols. The general hospital was erected in 1789, for the reception of patients, and is supported by subscription. The remains of the ancient nunnery have been converted into an hospital, substantially built of sand-stone, and surrounded by a strong wall; and there still exists part of a castle begun by the Earl of Essex, in the reign of Queen Elizabeth, but never finished, the ruinous foundations of which yet bear that favourite's name. The islet of Burhou, lying to the westward, is not inhabited, but is used by the governor as a rabbit-warren.

The little island of SARK, or SERK, which lies about six miles eastward of Guernsey, is also one of its dependencies, and under its immediate jurisdiction: the population, according to the census of 1821, was 488. At one part, called the *Coupée*, it is nearly divided into two portions, connected only by a high and narrow ridge not many yards wide. It was early noted for the ancient convent of St. Maglorius, a British Christian, who, fleeing with many others from the persecutions of the Pagan Saxons into Armorica, was made Bishop of Dol, and first planted Christianity in these islands, about the year 565. Queen Elizabeth granted it in fee-farm, by letters patent under the great seal, dated in 1565, to Hilary de Carteret, Esq., by the twentieth part of a knight's fee. The surface of Sark is a table land, rising a little towards the west, but having no declivity to the sea at any part, except a trifling descent at the northern extremity. The surrounding cliffs, from two to three hundred feet in height, are so very abrupt on the western side, that the largest ship may approach very near them without danger; but the eastern shore is beset with rocks running far out into the sea. The rocky scenery is very grand and picturesque; that of the *Port du Moulin* in particular, the descent to which is through a narrow pass, uncommonly wild and romantic. Such is the natural strength of the island, that although there are five landing-places, yet, except at what is called the *Creux*, where a tunnel was cut through the rock in 1588, by one of the De Carterets, scarcely any entrance is to be found without the difficulty of climbing. The landing-place nearest to Guernsey is that of *Havre Gossetin,* which is formed between the land and the little *Isle des Marchands* on the western side. The high ridge, or isthmus, which joins the main island to the smaller portion of it, called Petit Sark, is about one hundred yards long, with a precipice immediately overhanging the sea on the eastern side ; the passage on the western being in some places only three or four feet wide, and over broken rocks of terrific appearance. To the south of Petit Sark is an isolated rock, called *Etat,* much resembling in shape the Mew-stone at Plymouth ; and on the coast is a funnel, two hundred feet deep, and one hundred feet in diameter at the surface, called *Creux Terrible,* similar in appearance to the Buller of Buchan, or Tol Pedn, Penwith, near which is a spring of water, of which the specific gravity is one-eighth less than that of any other water found in the island. There are also numerous picturesque caverns excavated in the cliffs along the sea-shore. The sky is usually serene, and the air remarkably salubrious ; and the soil, which is extremely fertile, affords every necessary article of produce for the inhabitants, particularly apples, from which excellent cider is made, also turnips, parsnips, potatoes, and other vegetables, together with most kinds of grain. The grass is very sweet, and the mutton fine. Milk and butter are produced in sufficient quantities for the consumption of the inhabitants. Rabbits are also very abundant, and sea fish in great variety. The only branch of manufacture is the knitting of stockings, gloves, and waistcoats, called Guernsey jackets, which affords employment to many of the inhabitants : these are exported to Bristol and some other western ports of England, and various articles of domestic consumption brought back in return. The island, with the exception of the land held by the seignior, is divided into forty copyhold tenements, which are held under him on payment of a moderate rent. The inhabitants are principally employed in agriculture and in fishing, and dredging for oysters for the London market. A feudal court is held three times in the year, for the purpose of enacting by-laws for regulating the affairs of the island, which are in force when carried by a majority of the forty tenants, and confirmed by the consent of the seignior. The executive power is vested in a seneschal, who has cognizance of civil cases, and from whose decision an appeal lies to the Royal court at Guernsey. The church, dedicated to St. Peter, was erected in 1820, and consecrated by the Bishop of Winchester in 1829. The monastery, founded by St. Maglorius, was existing in the reign of Edward III., but it has long since gone to decay. In 1719, an earthen pot, bound with an iron hoop, was discovered, containing eighteen Gallic coins of silver gilt, which were engraved by Vertue in 1725.

The island of HERM, 3 miles (N. E.) from Guernsey, in the jurisdiction of which it is included, is about six miles in circumference, and, in 1821, contained 28 inhabitants. Since that time the population has been materially augmented by the erection of numerous houses for the accommodation of workmen employed in the quarries of granite with which the island abounds. Its appearance is diversified with hills and dales, and though upon a smaller scale than other islands of the group, it is little inferior to them in the picturesque beauty of its scenery. The northern beach, from which it rises

to a considerable elevation, is extensive, and equal in the smoothness and firmness of its sands to Worthing or Weymouth. The bay of Belvoir, on the eastern side of the island, is seated at the base of a winding and sequestered vale embosomed in hills of gradual ascent and pleasing undulation, and is the favourite retreat, during the summer, of the ladies of Guernsey, who resort to this romantic spot to collect the curious and beautiful shells which are peculiar to it. The air is mild and salubrious, and the soil is fertile, and of an average depth of three feet in that part of the island which is devoted to agriculture. The artificial grasses so much esteemed in England are indigenous to the soil, which yields in abundance wheat, barley, oats, lucerne, turnips, and every variety of agricultural produce. There are not less than thirty-three springs of pure water, which afford abundant facilities of irrigating the land in dry seasons. The principal feature in the island are its inexhaustible quarries of granite, the qualities of which have been found by experiment to be superior to any hitherto discovered. Twelve cubic feet of Herm granite are equal in weight to thirteen cubic feet of that of Aberdeen, a proof of its greater solidity; but its chief excellence consists in its wearing down rough and uniform in surface, when laid down in carriage roads, and thus affording a safer footing for horses: it can be raised from the quarries in blocks of any size and form, of which some have been raised exceeding one hundred tons in weight. The road leading to the East and West India docks in London was laid with this granite, under the direction of Mr. James Walker, civil engineer ; and on this great thoroughfare, which is traversed by the heaviest laden wagons in the kingdom, its excellent qualities of durability and resistance to friction have been fully demonstrated: it has been also laid down in Cheapside : this source of wealth was entirely neglected till the property of the island passed into the possession of the late Hon. John Lindsey, brother of the late Earl of Balcarras, who, having died before he had carried into operation his plans for working these quarries, Jonathan Duncan, Esq., son of the late governor of Bombay, who became proprietor of the island, by marriage with the daughter of Mr. Lindsey, carried that gentleman's plans into full operation on a more extended scale. Mr. Duncan, at a vast expense, constructed a harbour, in which vessels of two hundred and fifty tons' burden might, under the protection of an excellent pier, load during the most boisterous weather, in perfect safety; also an iron rail-way from the quarries to the pier, from which six hundred tons per day may be shipped with the greatest ease. He built houses for four hundred workmen, an inn, a brewery, a bakehouse, and several forges for making the various implements used in the quarries. There are some masses of stone at the northern extremity of the island, which are supposed, but upon no real authority, to be Druidical remains ; and there are portions of an ancient building, thought to have been a chapel belonging to a hermitage existing here in the sixth century. In forming the gardens of the mansion-house, some coffins and skeletons were discovered, which were, probably, the remains of some refugees, who, during the religious persecutions in the reign of Charles IX. of France, are imagined to have found an asylum in the island.

The island of JETHOU, separated from Herm by a narrow strait, and, like the former, a mass of granite, with little or no appearance of cultivation, is about a mile in circumference, and contains only nine inhabitants. The distances and bearings of the following points have carefully been ascertained by authorities on the spot. The Caskets are six leagues from Castle Cornet, bearing N. by E. ¼ E. from the most northern point of the island. Alderney is six and a half leagues from Castle Cornet, bearing N. E. by N. ½ E. from the same point. Cape la Hogue is nine leagues from the same point, and its bearing N. E. by E. ¼ E. Gros-nez point, Jersey, is six leagues from Castle Cornet, bearing S. E. by E. ¾ S.

GUESTLING, a parish in the hundred of GUESTLING, rape of HASTINGS, county of SUSSEX, 3¾ miles (W. S. W.) from Winchelsea, containing 697 inhabitants. The living is a rectory, in the archdeaconry of Lewes, and diocese of Chichester, rated in the king's books at £12. 0. 7½., and in the patronage of Sir W. Ashburnham, Bart. The church, dedicated to St. Andrew, is mostly in the later style of English architecture. Robert Bradshaw, in 1734, bequeathed £500 for the education of twenty children, which sum having been suffered to accumulate, now produces an annual income of £30 to the schoolmaster. The parish is bounded on the south by Brede channel.

GUESTWICK, a parish in the hundred of EYNSFORD, county of NORFOLK, 2½ miles (N. E. by E.) from Foulsham, containing 171 inhabitants. The living is a discharged vicarage, in the archdeaconry of Norfolk, and diocese of Norwich, rated in the king's books at £5. 0. 10., and endowed with £200 royal bounty. W. E. Bulwer, Esq. was patron in 1797. The church is dedicated to St. Peter. Here is a place of worship for Independents.

GUILDEN-MORDEN, county of CAMBRIDGE.—See MORDEN (GUILDEN).

GUILDEN-SUTTON, county palatine of CHESTER. —See SUTTON (GUILDEN).

Arms.

GUILDFORD, a borough and market town, having separate jurisdiction, locally in the first division of the hundred of Woking, county of SURREY, 30 miles (S. W.) from London, containing, exclusively of that part of the parish of St. Nicholas which is in the hundred of Godalming, 3161 inhabitants. This place, of which there is no mention either in the British or the Roman annals, is supposed to be of Saxon origin, and to have derived its name from *Guild*, a fraternity, and *Ford*, the passage over a stream. It was held in royal demesne, and, by Speed, is said to have been the residence of some of the Saxon kings. About the year 900, Alfred the Great bequeathed it to his nephew Ethelwald; and in 1036 it became memorable for the perfidious cruelty of Godwin, Earl of Kent, who, when Alfred, the son of Ethelred II., had reached Guildford, on his arrival from Normandy, by invitation of Harold Harefoot, then King of England, inhumanly massacred his retinue of six hundred Normans, and delivered him up to Harold, by whose order his eyes were put out, and he was

detained prisoner at the monastery of Ely, where he died. The castle is supposed to have been erected subsequently to the Conquest, but by whom, or at what precise time, has not been ascertained : the remains consist chiefly of the keep, which occupies the summit of a mound now forming part of a private pleasure ground, and some traces of the outer walls in the High-street and other parts of the town, which serve to mark out its former extent. Henry II. built a palace here, in which he frequently held his court, and emparked a considerable tract of land on the north side of Guildford down. It was also the occasional residence of several of his successors. Eleanor, queen of Henry III., founded here a house of Friars Preachers, which Edward II. ineffectually attempted to convert into a nunnery of the order of St. Dominic; and, according to Speed, there was also a house of Crouched friars, but of this there are not any remains.

The town is romantically situated on the declivities of two chalk hills sloping to the river Wey, which flows in a narrow channel between them, and consists principally of one spacious street, containing several handsome well-built houses. It is well paved, lighted with gas, and well supplied with water by a company. Near the site of the friary are very extensive barracks. The theatre, a neat and well-arranged edifice, is opened occasionally ; and not far from the town is a good course, where races take place annually in Whitsun-week, when a king's plate of one hundred guineas, and several subscription stakes, are run for. The trade is principally in timber, corn, malt, and beer, which are sent to the metropolis by the Wey, that river having been made navigable to the town in 1650, principally by the exertions of Sir Richard Weston, Bart. There is also an iron-foundry; and on the banks of the river are several corn-mills. The Wey and Arun canal passes through the town. The market days are Wednesday and Saturday, the latter for corn, of which there is an ample supply : the fairs, during which all persons attending them are free from arrest, are on May 4th and November 22d, for horses and cattle. A large quantity of poultry is sent to London on the market days ; and a fair for lambs is held on the Tuesday preceding Easter, and on every succeeding Tuesday till after Whitsuntide. The corn market is held in a building erected, in 1818, by subscription among the inhabitants and farmers residing in the neighbourhood : the portico is a fine specimen of the Tuscan order. The market for vegetables is kept in a noble lofty room, built in 1798, by Lords Onslow and Grantley, originally for the transaction of public business, and the holding of convivial meetings.

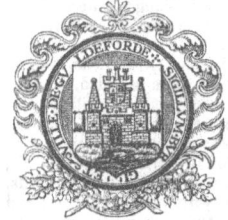

Corporate Seal.

Though Guildford was doubtless a corporate town in the time of Alfred, the first regular charter of incorporation on record is that of Henry III., subsequently confirmed by Henry VI. and Henry VIII., the latter monarch having changed the designation of the chief magistrate from seneschal to that of mayor ; and by James II., under whose charter the government is vested in a mayor, high steward, recorder, seven aldermen, and an indefinite number of bailiffs, "or approved men," seldom exceeding twenty-four, assisted by a town clerk and other officers. The mayor is elected annually on the Saturday after Michaelmas-day, from among the seven aldermen, unless there be a vacancy in that body, in which case one of the approved men is chosen, who, after having served the office of mayor, becomes alderman. The mayor, recorder, and three of the aldermen, are justices of the peace; and the late mayor and town clerk are generally chosen as coroners for the borough, though the office is elective. The freedom of the borough is obtained by servitude of seven years to a freeman; and among the privileges which it conveys is that of exemption from serving on juries at the assizes or sessions for the county, on the payment of one penny by each person, called "Head pence." The corporation hold quarterly courts of session for determining on all offences within the borough; and have power to hold a court of record every third Monday, for the recovery of debts to any amount; but this latter court has fallen into disuse. The town-hall, erected in 1683, is a neat edifice surmounted by a turret, in which is a clock, having an illuminated dial for shewing the hour at night : the interior is decorated with portraits of some of the sovereigns, and with other paintings. The elective franchise was conferred in the 23d of Edward I., since which time the borough has returned two members to parliament. The right of election is vested in the resident freemen and freeholders paying scot and lot, the number of whom is about one hundred and fifty : the mayor is the returning officer. The election of the members for the county takes place in this town. The summer assizes for the county are held alternately here and at Croydon, and the quarter sessions for the same once in the year. The petty sessions for the division are also held at Guildford. The house of correction for the county is a commodious building of red brick, completed in 1823, and adapted to the classification of prisoners : it has seven wards, seven airing-yards, seven day-rooms, and four rooms for tread-wheels.

The borough comprises the parishes of the Holy Trinity, St. Mary the Virgin, and part of that of St. Nicholas, all in the archdeaconry of Surrey, and diocese of Winchester. The living of the Holy Trinity parish is a rectory, with that of St. Mary united, rated in the king's books, the former at £11. 11. 0½., and the latter at £12.'5. 5., with an endowment of £300 private benefaction, and £300 parliamentary grant, and in the patronage of the Crown. The church is a handsome brick edifice, rebuilt in 1763, after the damage it sustained from the fall of the tower in 1740. St. Mary's is an ancient structure of flint and chalk, intermixed with pebbles, situated on the slope of a hill, and supposed to have been erected in the time of the Saxons : it consists of a nave, aisles, and chancel, with a chapel on each side, circular at the eastern extremity, having a small embattled tower : it has been recently repaired under the superintendence of the Rev. Mr. Bulse, many of its most interesting features having been judiciously restored. The living of St. Nicholas' is a rectory, rated in the king's books at £21. 0. 10., and in the patronage of the Dean of Salisbury. The church is a very ancient structure, of similar materials with those of St. Mary's, situated on the western bank of the river : it has a nave and aisles, and at the west end a tower of modern erection, and contains several interest-

ing monuments, of which the most ancient is that of a priest, whose effigy, in a recumbent posture under a niche, is clothed in a white surplice and a scarlet robe, with an embroidered gold border, fastened on the breast by a black velvet belt with a gold knot, with the inscription "Arnold Brocas, Rector, died 1395." There are places of worship for Baptists, the Society of Friends, Independents, and Wesleyan Methodists. The free grammar school was originally founded in 1509, by Mr. Robert Beckingham, of London, who endowed it with lands and tenements at Bromley, in Kent, and at Newington, in Surrey, producing £20 per annum; and by letters patent of Edward VI. it was further endowed with property belonging to suppressed chantries, which was augmented by the corporation, who purchased some land, and, with the assistance of various benefactions, erected a school-house in Trinity parish, in which are apartments for the masters, and a good library. In 1671, Joseph Nettle, Esq. devised land, producing £57. 15. per ann. for an exhibition from this school to the University of Oxford, or Cambridge. A school for clothing and educating thirty boys was founded in the reign of Elizabeth, by Mr. Thomas Baker, clothier, and endowed with the rent of a market-house, which being taken down, the school has, since 1762, been supported by voluntary contributions. There are a National and a Lancasterian school, supported by subscription, and a Sunday school, entirely supported by William Haydon, Esq. The hospital, for twelve aged men and eight unmarried women, was founded by Abbot, Archbishop of Canterbury, and incorporated by letters patent of James I., in 1622, under the title of "The Master and Brethren of the Hospital of the Blessed Trinity." Any person having served the office of mayor is eligible to the mastership; and the rector of Trinity parish may, at his option, take that office on a vacancy occurring. This institution is under the inspection of the Archbishop of Canterbury. The buildings occupy a quadrangular area, on the north side of which is a small chapel, containing some good specimens of painted glass, with the portraits of the founder and other benefactors. Four almshouses have been erected and endowed for the aged poor of the parish of St. Nicholas, and provision made for a master to teach poor children, by Caleb Lovejoy, Esq. The Poyle charity, from a bequest by Henry Smith, Esq., amounting to £600 per annum, is distributed by the mayor and aldermen, and there are several other charitable benefactions for the relief of the poor. On St. Catherine's hill are the ruins of St. Catherine's chapel. Archbishop Abbot was a native of this parish; and the Hon. Arthur Onslow, Speaker of the House of Commons, and Bishop Parkhurst, were buried in the church of the Holy Trinity. Guildford gives the title of earl to the family of North.

GUILDFORD, or GULDEFORD (EAST), a parish in the hundred of GOLDSPUR, rape of HASTINGS, county of SUSSEX, 1¾ mile (N. E. by E.) from Rye, containing 124 inhabitants. The living is a discharged rectory with that of Playden, in the archdeaconry of Lewes, and diocese of Chichester, rated in the king's books at £8. 4. 7. Thomas P. Lambe, Esq. was patron in 1807. The church is dedicated to St. Mary. A peculiar method of tything the marsh land prevails in this parish : the tenants pay three-pence per acre only while in pasture, but five shillings if ploughed. The

Kent ditch bounds the parish on the east, and the river Rother is navigable on the west.

GUILSBOROUGH, a parish in the hundred of GUILSBOROUGH, county of NORTHAMPTON, 9¼ miles (N.W. by N.) from Northampton, containing, with the hamlet of Hollowell, 950 inhabitants. The living is a vicarage, in the archdeaconry of Northampton, and diocese of Peterborough, rated in the king's books at £17. 3. 4. The Rev. Thomas Sikes was patron in 1792. The church is dedicated to St. Etheldred. Here is a place of worship for Baptists. In 1609, William Gilbert gave £100 towards the erection and support of a free school for teaching English, writing, &c., which bequest, with subsequent donations, was laid out in the purchase of the school-house, and of certain lands now producing £60 per annum, for which income about forty children receive instruction. The free grammar school was erected, in 1668, by Sir John Langham, and endowed by him with £80 a year, for the education of fifty boys. In this parish the rivers Avon and Nen have their sources, and between them are vestiges of a Roman encampment, called Borough Hill, including an area of nearly eight acres.

GUISBOROUGH, or GUILSBROUGH, a parish in the eastern division of the liberty of LANGBAURGH, North riding of the county of YORK, comprising the market town of Guisborough, and the townships of Dale-Common, Hutton-Locras, Pinchingthorpe, and Tocketts, and containing 2180 inhabitants, of which number, 1912 are in the town of Guisborough, 49 miles (N.) from York, and 244 (N. by W.) from London. This place is situated in a narrow but fertile vale, extending about four miles from the mouth of the river Tees : it consists chiefly of a spacious street of well-built houses, having a neat and pleasant appearance. A handsome town-hall was erected in 1821, in the market-place, on the site of the old toll-booth, supported on pillars and arches, the lower part serving for shambles, &c., for the market people. The market, which is well attended, is held on Tuesday ; and there are fairs on the last Tuesdays in June and July. Markets for wool take place on the last Tuesday in April, Tuesday before Whit-Sunday, the third Tuesdays in August and September, the second Tuesday in November, and the last Tuesday in March. In 1822 a mineral spring was discovered, about a mile south-east from Guisborough, which has been found to possess diuretic properties, and contains carbonic acid, with a small quantity of muriate and carbonate of soda, and other neutral salts : it is much frequented for the relief of rheumatic, scorbutic, and bilious complaints. Alum works were established at Guisborough in the reign of Queen Elizabeth, by Sir Thomas Chaloner, who brought workmen from Italy, and first introduced the manufacture of alum into England; but they have long been discontinued, and the trade transferred to Whitby. The petty sessions for the eastern division of the liberty of Langbaurgh are held in the town-hall every alternate Tuesday. The living is a perpetual curacy, in the archdeaconry of Cleveland, and diocese of York, endowed with £400 private benefaction, and £600 royal bounty, and in the patronage of the Archbishop of York. The church, dedicated to St. Nicholas, is a neat edifice, partly rebuilt in 1791. Here are places of worship for the Society of Friends, Independents, and Wesleyan Methodists. A free grammar school,

called Jesus school, was founded under letters patent of Elizabeth, in 1561, by the Rev. Robert Pursglove ; who also founded almshouses for six men and six women, and gave estates for the support of these charities, which, with other benefactions, produce an annual income of £329. 4. 4., from which the schoolmaster receives a stipend of £50 per annum, but there are no scholars on the foundation, there being little or no demand for classical instruction among the parishioners. In 1790, a school for eighty poor children, called Providence school, was established here by subscription, promoted by Mr. George Venables, who bequeathed property for its support ; and, in 1821, two new school-rooms were built, in which one hundred boys, and one hundred girls, are instructed on the National system. A priory of Augustine canons was founded here by Robert de Brus, in 1129, the revenue of which, at the dissolution, was £712. 6. 6. Walter Hemingford, a monkish historian of the thirteenth century, was a native of this place.

GUISLEY, a parish in the upper division of the wapentake of SKYRACK, West riding of the county of YORK, comprising the chapelries of Horsforth and Rawden, and the townships of Carlton, Guisley, and Yeaden, and containing 8409 inhabitants, of which number, 1213 are in the township of Guisley, 3 miles (S. by W.) from Otley. The living is a rectory, in the archdeaconry and diocese of York, rated in the king's books at £26, and in the patronage of J. L. Fox, Esq., for two turns, and of the Master and Fellows of Trinity College, Cambridge, for one. The church is dedicated to St. Oswald. Here is a place of worship for Wesleyan Methodists. In this parish are several bleaching-mills, and the manufacture of woollen cloth for the Leeds market is considerable. A free school was erected by the Rev. Robert Moore, who, in 1622, endowed it with a house and land, and in addition thereto, the Rev. Dr. Hitch, in 1676, bequeathed a portion of his estate for the support of a master, who receives the income, amounting to £50 a year, for teaching about thirty children.

GUIST, a parish in the hundred of EYNSFORD, county of NORFOLK, 2 miles (N.N.W.) from Foulsham, containing 308 inhabitants. The living is a discharged vicarage, in the archdeaconry of Norfolk, and diocese of Norwich, rated in the king's books at £5. 15. 5., endowed with £800 royal bounty. The Rev. W. Norris was patron in 1789. The church is dedicated to St. Andrew.

GULVAL, a parish in the hundred of PENWITH, county of CORNWALL, 1½ mile (N.E.) from Penzance, containing 1353 inhabitants. The living is a vicarage, in the archdeaconry of Cornwall, and diocese of Exeter, rated in the king's books at £6. 11. 0½., and in the patronage of the Crown. The church is dedicated to St. Gulwal. There is a place of worship for Wesleyan Methodists. A stream, called Dane river, from its passing under a bridge of that name, runs through the parish, in its course to Mount's bay. Several tin mines have been worked in the northern part of the parish, but being in an exhausted state, they are now almost relinquished. At Rosemorren are the remains of a cromlech, near which several sculptured stones, earthen urns containing ashes, burnt bones, an ancient belt, &c., have been found. There is a spring called Gulfwell, or the Hebrew brook, which is held in great veneration by the superstitious.

GUMLEY, a parish in the hundred of GARTREE, county of LEICESTER, 4½ miles (N. W. by W.) from Market-Harborough, containing 289 inhabitants. The living is a rectory, in the archdeaconry of Leicester, and diocese of Lincoln, rated in the king's books at £16. 2. 6., and in the patronage of the Dean and Chapter of Lincoln. The church is dedicated to St. Helen. There is a chalybeate spring in the parish.

GUNBY, a parish in the wapentake of BELTISLOE, parts of KESTEVEN, county of LINCOLN, 2¾ miles (S.W. by S.) from Colsterworth, containing 149 inhabitants. The living is a rectory, united in 1773 to that of Stainby, in the archdeaconry and diocese of Lincoln, rated in the king's books at £4. 4. 2. The church is dedicated to St. Nicholas.

GUNBY, a parish in the Wold division of the wapentake of CANDLESHOE, parts of LINDSEY, county of LINCOLN, 5¼ miles (E.) from Spilsby, containing 69 inhabitants. The living is a discharged rectory, in the archdeaconry and diocese of Lincoln, rated in the king's books at £3. 10. 2½., and in the patronage of the Duke of Rutland. The church is dedicated to St. Peter.

GUNNERSBURY, a hamlet in the parish of ACTON, Kensington division of the hundred of OSSULSTONE, county of MIDDLESEX, 5½ miles (W.) from London. The population is returned with the parish. Her Royal Highness the late Princess Amelia, youngest daughter of George III., resided in an elegant mansion at this place.

GUNNERTON, a joint chapelry with Chipchase, in the parish of CHOLLERTON, north-eastern division of TINDALE ward, county of NORTHUMBERLAND, 8½ miles (N. by W.) from Hexham, containing 409 inhabitants. Here was anciently a chapel, but not the slightest vestige of it is now visible. There are traces of a Roman encampment, and a large barrow called Money-hill, where coins have frequently been found.

GUNTHORPE, a parish in the hundred of HOLT, county of NORFOLK, 5¼ miles (W.S.W.) frm Holt, containing 317 inhabitants. The living is a discharged rectory, with that of Bale annexed, in the archdeaconry and diocese of Norwich, rated in the king's books at £13. The Rev. Charles Collyer was patron in 1798. The church is dedicated to St. Mary.

GUNTHORPE, a township in the parish of LOWDHAM, southern division of the wapentake of THURGARTON, county of NOTTINGHAM, 7¼ miles (E.N.E.) from Nottingham, containing 370 inhabitants. There is a place of worship for Wesleyan Methodists. The river Trent is here crossed by a ferry.

GUNTHORPE, anciently a hamlet in the parish of BELTON, soke of OAKHAM, county of RUTLAND, 2¼ miles (S. by E.) from Oakham, containing 7 inhabitants. Here was formerly a village, but it has been reduced to a single cottage, inhabited by a poor shepherd and his family.

GUNTHWAITE, a township in the parish of PENISTONE, wapentake of STAINCROSS, West riding of the county of YORK, 7½ miles (W.) from Barnesley, containing 86 inhabitants.

GUNTON, a parish in the northern division of the hundred of ERPINGHAM, county of NORFOLK, 4¼ miles (N.W.) from North Walsham, containing 59 inhabitants. The living is a discharged rectory, with which the vicarage of Hanworth is consolidated, in the archdeaconry of Norfolk, and diocese of Norwich, rated in the king's books at £8, and in the patronage of Lord Suffield. The church, dedicated to St. Andrew, was rebuilt, with a portico of the Doric order, by Sir William Harbord an ancestor of Lord Suffield.

GUNTON, a parish in the hundred of MUTFORD and LOTHINGLAND, county of SUFFOLK, 1½ mile (N. by W.) from Lowestoft, containing 87 inhabitants. The living is a discharged rectory, in the archdeaconry of Suffolk, and diocese of Norwich, rated in the king's books at £5. 6. 8., endowed with £200 private benefaction, and £200 royal bounty. R. Dundas, Esq. and others were patrons in 1801. The church is dedicated to St. Peter. The parish lies on the coast of the North sea.

GUNVILLE-TARRANT, county of DORSET.—See TARRANT (GUNVILLE).

GUNWALLOE, a parish in the hundred of KERRIER, county of CORNWALL, 5 miles (S.) from Helston, containing 252 inhabitants. The living is a perpetual curacy, united, with those of Cury and Germoe, to the rectory of Breage, in the archdeaconry of Cornwall, and diocese of Exeter. The church is dedicated to St. Wynwallow. Here is a place of worship for Wesleyan Methodists. A small school is supported by annual donations.

GUSSAGE (ALL SAINTS), a parish in the hundred of KNOWLTON, Shaston (East) division of the county of DORSET, 5 miles (W.S.W.) from Cranborne, containing 348 inhabitants. The living is a discharged vicarage, in the archdeaconry of Dorset, and diocese of Bristol, rated in the king's books at £6. 3. 9., and in the patronage of the Archdeacon of Dorset.

GUSSAGE (ST. ANDREW'S), a chapelry in the parish of HANDLEY, in that part of the hundred of SIX-PENNY-HANDLEY which is in the Shaston (East) division of the county of DORSET, 6¼ miles (W. by N.) from Cranborne. The population is returned with the parish.

GUSSAGE (ST. MICHAEL), a parish in the hundred of BADBURY, though locally in the hundred of Knowlton, Shaston (East) division of the county of DORSET, 6 miles (W. by S.) from Cranborne, containing 246 inhabitants. The living is a rectory, in the archdeaconry of Dorset, and diocese of Bristol, rated in the king's books at £20. 0. 2½., and in the patronage of J. and R. Randell, Esqrs. The church is a handsome edifice, with a lofty embattled tower. On the line of the London road, near Cashmore Inn, is the easternmost of seven earth-works, supposed to have been thrown up by the Belgæ across the road between this and Tarrant-Hinton, which afford reason for the opinion that the neighbourhood was the scene of some remarkable action in the time of the ancient Britons.

GUSTON, a parish in the hundred of BEWSBOROUGH, lathe of St. AUGUSTINE, county of KENT, 2 miles (N. by E.) from Dovor, containing 206 inhabitants. The living is a perpetual curacy, in the peculiar jurisdiction and patronage of the Archbishop of Canterbury, endowed with £200 private benefaction, and £400 royal bounty. The church is dedicated to St. Martin.

GUTON, a hamlet in the parish of BRANDISTONE, hundred of EYNSFORD, county of NORFOLK, 3 miles (S. E. by E.) from Reepham. The name is written *Gutheketuna* in Domesday-book, and at the period of the survey this was a considerable town, though now entirely destitute of note.

GUY'S CLIFF, a hamlet in the parish of LEEK-WOOT-TON, Kenilworth division of the hundred of KNIGHTLOW, county of WARWICK, 1¾ mile (N.N.E.) from Warwick, on the south side of the Avon. It is so called from its connexion with the legend of Guy of Warwick, of whom it is said that he retired to an ancient hermitage which existed here long before the Conquest, and to whose memory, in the reign of Henry VI., a chapel was founded, and dedicated to St. Mary Magdalene, by his descendant, Richard Beauchamp, Earl of Warwick, who placed therein two chaplains; subsequently the celebrated antiquary, John Rous, resided in it as a chantry priest. The founder caused also a gigantic statue of the famous Earl Guy to be carved out of the solid rock, which still exists, though in a mutilated state. This spot, to which is now attached an elegant modern residence, possesses great picturesque beauty.

GUYSON, a township in the parish of SHILBOTTLE, eastern division of COQUETDALE ward, county of NORTH-UMBERLAND, 8½ miles (S. by E.) from Alnwick, containing 173 inhabitants. A priory was founded here some time in the twelfth century, by Richard Tyson, and afterwards annexed to the abbey of Alnwick, by Eustace Fitz-John; its revenue, in the Lincoln taxation of temporalties, was valued at £3. 15. 4. per annum.

GUYTING (LOWER), or GUYTING-POWER, a parish in the lower division of the hundred of KIFTS-GATE, county of GLOUCESTER, 6 miles (S.E. by E.) from Winchcombe, containing, with the chapelry of Framcote, 629 inhabitants. The living is a discharged vicarage, in the archdeaconry and diocese of Gloucester, rated in the king's books at £14. 19. 5. Francis Lawson, Esq. was patron in 1797. The church, dedicated to St. Michael, is in the Norman style of architecture. In Domesday-book five salt pits are recorded to have existed here at the period of the Conquest, but there are no traces of them at present.

GUYTING (TEMPLE), a parish in the lower division of the hundred of KIFTSGATE, county of GLOUCESTER, 4¾ miles (E. by S.) from Winchcombe, containing 510 inhabitants. The living is a perpetual curacy, in the archdeaconry and diocese of Gloucester, endowed with £400 private benefaction, £600 royal bounty, and £600 parliamentary grant, and in the patronage of the Dean and Canons of Christ Church, Oxford. The church, dedicated to St. Mary, is a small but handsome edifice, with an embattled tower at the west end; it was probably built by the Knights Templars, who possessed the manor in the thirteenth century.

GWENNAP, a parish in the hundred of KERRIER, county of CORNWALL, 3½ miles (E. by S.) from Redruth, containing 6294 inhabitants. The living is a discharged vicarage, in the archdeaconry of Cornwall, and diocese of Exeter, rated in the king's books at £16. 18. 11½., and in the patronage of the Dean and Chapter of Exeter. The church, dedicated to St. Wenap, has lately received an addition of two hundred sittings, the Incorporated Society for the enlargement of churches and chapels having granted £50 towards defraying the expense. In the parish are several rich mines of tin and copper; of the latter the most productive are Weal Unity, United Mine, Weal Damsel, and Treskerby. At the village of St. Day, a weekly market on Saturday has been established for the convenience of the miners, and a small fair on the Tuesday next after the 29th of July. Here

was a chapel dedicated to the Holy Trinity, but it has been totally demolished, the tower having been pulled down in 1778. In 1827 a handsome church, or chapel, was erected. There are places of worship for Baptists and Wesleyan Methodists.

GWERNESNEY, a parish in the upper division of the hundred of USK, county of MONMOUTH, 2½ miles (E. N. E.) from Usk, containing 69 inhabitants. The living is a discharged rectory, in the archdeaconry and diocese of Llandaff, rated in the king's books at £2. 18. 6½., endowed with £200 parliamentary grant, and in the patronage of the Earl of Abergavenny. The church is dedicated to St. Michael.

GWINEAR, a parish in the hundred of PENWITH, county of CORNWALL, 7½ miles (S. W. by W.) from Redruth, containing 2383 inhabitants. The living is a vicarage, in the archdeaconry of Cornwall, and diocese of Exeter, rated in the king's books at £12, and in the patronage of the Bishop of Exeter. The church is dedicated to St. Winnear. There are several copper mines in the parish, of which the principal are Herland, Weal Alfred, and Weal Hope; the first produces also native silver.

GWITHIAN, a parish in the hundred of PENWITH, county of CORNWALL, 7½ miles (W.) from Redruth, containing 412 inhabitants. The living is a rectory united to the rectory of Phillack, in the archdeaconry of Cornwall, and diocese of Exeter. The church, dedicated to St. Gothian, has been long since demolished, and the ruins, with a considerable portion of the parish, are overwhelmed with sand, blown hither from the sea-shore by violent gales of wind. The sea-rush, the roots of which prevent the further dispersion of the sand, has been planted in sufficient quantity to protect the village from a similar fate. The river Gwithian runs through the parish, in which it is crossed by a bridge, and falls into St. Ives' bay. Several mines have been wrought at shallow levels, the lodes being very large, but relinquished from want of capital. A singular kind of sand-stone, considered by geologists a great curiosity, is obtained here, and used in building chimnies instead of brick. A remarkable spring formerly rose amongst the sands, called, from its perpetual bubbling, the Boiling well, which had never been frozen, but an adit lately driven near it has caused its disappearance. There are two moats remaining of extensive earth-works, called Trevarnon Rounds, within which cannon balls have been discovered.

GYHIRN, a chapelry in the parish of ST. MARY, WISBEACH, hundred of WISBEACH, Isle of Ely, county of CAMBRIDGE, 5½ miles (N. N. W.) from March. The living is a perpetual curacy, in the archdeaconry and diocese of Ely, endowed with £200 private benefaction, £600 royal bounty, and £500 parliamentary grant. The chapel is dedicated to St. Mary Magdalene.

H

HABBERLEY, a parish in the hundred of FORD, county of SALOP, 9 miles (S. W.) from Shrewsbury, containing 151 inhabitants. The living is a discharged rectory, in the archdeaconry of Salop, and diocese of Hereford, rated in the king's books at £4. 0. 2½., and in the patronage of John Mitton, Esq. The church is dedicated to St. Mary.

HABERGHAM-EAVES, a township in that part of the parish of WHALLEY which is in the higher division of the hundred of BLACKBURN, county palatine of LAN-CASTER, 2 miles (S.W.) from Burnley, containing 4612 inhabitants. The cotton manufacture is extensively carried on here.

HABROUGH, a parish in the eastern division of the wapentake of YARBOROUGH, parts of LINDSEY, county of LINCOLN, 10 miles (W.N.W.) from Great Grimsby, containing 286 inhabitants. The living is a discharged vicarage, united in 1740 to that of Killing-holme, in the archdeaconry and diocese of Lincoln, rated in the king's books at £8, endowed with £400 royal bounty, and in the patronage of — Pelham, Esq. The church is dedicated to St. Margaret. There is a place of worship for Wesleyan Methodists.

HABTON (GREAT), a township in the parish of KIRKBY-MISPERTON, PICKERING lythe, North riding of the county of YORK, 5¼ miles (N.W. by N.) from New Malton, containing 136 inhabitants.

HABTON (LITTLE), a township in the parish of KIRKBY-MISPERTON, PICKERING lythe, North riding of the county of YORK, 5 miles (N.W. by N.) from New Malton, containing 50 inhabitants.

HACCOMBE, an extra-parochial liberty, forming, with the parishes of Combintinhead and Stokeintinhead, and Shalden Green, a distinct portion of the hundred of WONFORD, county of DEVON, 3 miles (E.S.E.) from Newton-Abbot's, containing 27 inhabitants. The living is a rectory, in the peculiar jurisdiction of the Bishop of Exeter, rated in the king's books at £25, and in the patronage of Sir H. Carew, Bart. The church, dedicated to St. Blaize, is partly in the decorated style, and contains some very curious monuments : it was formerly collegiate, having been endowed with the great tithes of Haccombe and Quithcock, in Cornwall, for the support of an arch-priest and five inferior ones.

HACCONBY, a parish in the wapentake of AVE-LAND, parts of KESTEVEN, county of LINCOLN, 3½ miles (N. by E.) from Bourne, containing, with the hamlet of Stainfield, 321 inhabitants. The living is a discharged vicarage, united in 1732 to the vicarage of Morton, in the archdeaconry and diocese of Lincoln, rated in the king's books at £5. 17. 6. The church, dedicated to St. Andrew, has portions in the early, with insertions in the decorated and later styles of English architecture.

HACEBY, a parish in the wapentake of AVELAND, parts of KESTEVEN, county of LINCOLN, 8¼ miles (E.) from Grantham, containing 65 inhabitants. The living is a rectory, in the archdeaconry and diocese of Lincoln, rated in the king's books at £5. 2. 11. W. S. Welby, Esq. was patron in 1813.

HACHESTON, a parish in the hundred of LOES, county of SUFFOLK, 2 miles (N. by E.) from Wickham-Market, containing 534 inhabitants. The living is a discharged vicarage with that of Parham, in the arch-deaconry of Suffolk, and diocese of Norwich, rated in the king's books at £6. 1. 10. The church is dedicated to All Saints. A new school-house was erected in this parish in 1826 the school is supported partly by volun-tary subscriptions, and partly by a bequest from Richard Porter, in 1701, for the instruction of twelve poor boys.

HACKERSALL, a joint township with Preesall, in that part of the parish of LANCASTER which is in the hundred of AMOUNDERNESS, county palatine of LAN-CASTER, 8½ miles (W. by N.) from Garstang, containing 700 inhabitants.

HACKFORD, a parish in the hundred of EYNS-FORD, county of NORFOLK, 1¾ mile (W. by S.) from Reepham, containing 643 inhabitants. The living is a discharged rectory with the vicarage of Whitwell united, in the archdeaconry of Norfolk, and diocese of Norwich, rated in the king's books at £14. 10. 5. George Hunt Holley, Esq. was patron in 1812. The church is dedi-cated to All Saints.

HACKFORD, a parish in the hundred of FOREHOE, county of NORFOLK, 4 miles (W. by N.) from Wymond-ham, containing 222 inhabitants. The living is a dis-charged rectory, in the archdeaconry of Norfolk, and dio-cese of Norwich, rated in the king's books at £4. 15. 10. George Hunt Holley, Esq. was patron in 1801. The church is dedicated to St. Mary.

HACKFORTH, a township in the parish of HORN-BY, partly within the liberty of ST. PETER of YORK, but chiefly in the eastern division of the wapentake of HANG, North riding of the county of YORK, 3¾ miles (S.) from Catterick, containing 134 inhabitants.

HACKINGTON, otherwise ST. STEPHEN'S, a pa-rish in the hundred of WESTGATE, lathe of ST. AUGUS-TINE, county of KENT, 1¼ mile (N.) from Canterbury, containing 349 inhabitants. The living is a vicarage, in the archdeaconry and diocese of Canterbury, rated in the king's books at £5. 2. 3½., and in the patronage of the Archdeacon of Canterbury. The church is dedi-cated to St. Stephen. In the church-yard, in 1187, Baldwin, Archbishop of Canterbury, began a chapel in honour of St. Stephen and St. Thomas of Canter-bury, wherein he proposed to found a noble college for forty secular priests, the king and all his suffragan bishops to have a prebend, each worth forty marks a year; but the year after he had settled some secular canons at the place, the pope, at the instance of the monks at Christ Church, ordered the chapel to be levelled with the ground. The bishop erected a chapel in honour of St. Thomas à Becket at the foot of St. Thomas' hill.

HACKLESTON, a hamlet in the parish of PIDDING-TON, hundred of WYMERSLEY, county of NORTHAMP-TON, 5½ miles (S. E.) from Northampton. containing 402 inhabitants. The Particular Baptists have a place of worship here.

HACKLESTONE, a tything in the parish of FIT-TLETON, hundred of ELSTUB and EVERLEY, county of WILTS, 8¼ miles (W. by S.) from Ludgershall. The population is returned with the parish. The General and Particular Baptists have each a place of worship here.

HACKNESS, a parish in the liberty of WHITBY-STRAND, North riding of the county of YORK, compri-sing the chapelry of Harwood-Dale with Silpho, and the townships of Broxa, Hackness, and Suffield with Everley, and containing 632 inhabitants, of which num-ber, 143 are in the township of Hackness, 6½ miles (W. by N.) from Scarborough. The living is a perpetual curacy, in the archdeaconry of the East riding, and dio-cese of York, endowed with £1000 royal bounty, and in the patronage of Sir J. V. B. Johnstone, Bart. The church, dedicated to St. Peter, is a very ancient structure. The village is romantically situated in a delightful vale, from which several others run in various directions across the country: the hills which surround the vale are from one hundred to one hundred and twenty yards in perpendicular height, and their steep declivities are profusely adorned with lofty trees of the richest foliage. Springs of water, rushing in natural cascades from the sides of the hills, or falling with gentle murmurs, contribute to the beauty of the scenery; and the Derwent, which has its source in the mountainous country to the north, glides in a gentle stream past the village: the whole scene is of a most sublime character. Here was formerly a cell belonging to Whitby abbey, which, at the dissolution, contained four monks of the Benedictine order.

HACKNEY, a parish in the Tower division of the hundred of Ossulstone, county of Middlesex, 2 miles (N. E.) from London, comprising three districts, viz., Hackney St. John, South Hackney, and West Hackney, and containing 22,494 inhabitants. It is almost united to the metropolis by successive ranges of building, of which some are of handsome and respectable appearance, and was among the earliest of the adjacent villages inhabited by the more opulent merchants of London; and from its having been the first of those retreats provided with regular conveyances to that city, it is supposed to have given name to the numerous coaches which ply in the streets of the metropolis, and in the principal towns of the kingdom. Among the various mansions of distinguished persons who anciently resided here, are Brook house, at Clapton, the residence of Lord Brook (now converted into an asylum for lunatics), and the palace of the prior of the Knights of St. John of Jerusalem, in Well-street, at present let out in tenements to poor families. To the south of Lea bridge are mills, formerly belonging to the Knights Templars, and subsequently to the Knights Hospitallers of St. John of Jerusalem, having been since employed for preparing sheet-lead; they are now unoccupied. The parish is lighted with gas, and amply supplied with water: the houses are irregularly built; many of them in detached situations are handsome, and in various parts of the parish there are ranges of modern houses of neat and respectable appearance. On the site of an ancient building in the old church-yard, formerly used as a school-house, a spacious edifice has been erected, and gradually enlarged, containing sundry commodious apartments for the meetings of members of different local trusts, and for other purposes of parochial business. The environs are in many parts pleasant, and there are several nursery grounds, of which those belonging to Messrs. Loddige and Sons are noted for a great variety of scarce and curious exotic plants. A considerable quantity of land in the neighbourhood is cultivated by market-gardeners for the supply of the London market, and a much larger portion is appropriated to the pasturage of cattle. The old bridge over the river Lea was taken down in 1820, and a handsome iron bridge of one arch was erected, at an expense of £4500. The silk-manufactory at Hackney Wick, in which from six to seven hundred persons were formerly employed, has within the last two years been discontinued, and the adjoining dwelling-house, which is a handsome building, has since been commodiously fitted up in a superior style for the reception of insane persons. The principal branches of manufacture at present carried on are the making of optical glasses of every description,

the preparation of colours, dyeing, calico-printing, and calendering: there is an extensive flour-mill, and a water-mill of very great antiquity is now used for supplying the inhabitants of Clapton with water: a great number of bricks and tiles is made in the neighbourhood, and several of the fields in which the clay has been exhausted have been since advantageously cultivated or built upon. The Regent's canal passes through the western part of the parish, and the Lea river navigation through the eastern. The parish is within the jurisdiction of a court of requests held at Whitechapel, for the recovery of debts under 40s., and has been recently included within the limits of the new police act.

Until recently Hackney constituted one parish, under the designation of St. John's, consisting of a vicarage and a sinecure rectory, rated in the king's books at £20, and for all civil purposes it still continues so; but by an order of the King in council, dated March 1825, it has been divided into three districts, each of which now constitutes a distinct rectory, called respectively Hackney, South Hackney, and West Hackney, and with the consents required by the acts passed in the 58th of George III., and 3rd of George IV., and by means of the liberal sacrifices of income made both by the patron, as lessee of the rectorial tithes, and by the incumbent, the rectorial and vicarial tithes of the whole parish have been consolidated, and apportioned, with every other source of ecclesiastical emolument, among the incumbents of the three newly constituted rectories, each rector having an exclusive right to such tithes and dues as shall arise within the limits of his benefice: they are in the jurisdiction of the Commissary of London, concurrently with the Consistorial Court of the Bishop. The patronage is in W. G. D. Tyssen, Esq., as Lord of the Manor, which is co-extensive with the boundaries of the whole parish. The church of St. John the Baptist, which now constitutes the church of the central district, or Hackney (proper), was erected under an act of parliament obtained in 1791, at a short distance northward of a more ancient one, the tower of which is still standing, the new building not being considered of sufficient strength to receive the bells. It is handsomely built of brick, with a cupola and dome of stone subsequently added to it; it was consecrated in 1797, and contains sittings for upwards of three thousand persons: the roof is a singularly fine piece of mechanism, and the arches are of a bolder and wider span than those in almost any other building of similar design: the fine windows in the chancel, and one at the font, are handsomely enriched with painted glass. Among the ancient monuments removed from the old church into the vestibules of the present edifice is that of Christopher Urswick, almoner of Henry VII., and incumbent of this parish, who died in 1521. Dr. Richard Sampson, Bishop of Chichester, and afterwards of Lichfield and Coventry; David Daulben, Bishop of Bangor; and Gilbert Sheldon, Bishop of London, and afterwards Archbishop of Canterbury and Chancellor of the University of Oxford, where he built the theatre, were rectors of this parish. The church-yard is spacious and well planted. The parsonage-house has been recently rebuilt by the present incumbent, on a considerably enlarged scale.—The church of West Hackney, containing one thousand eight hundred and twenty-eight sittings, of which one thousand one hundred and ninety-two are free, is situated in Kingsland-road, and was erected by a grant from the parliamentary commissioners in 1823, at an expense of £15,302. 14.: it is a handsome edifice in the Grecian style of architecture, with a cupola and a portico of the Doric order, designed by Mr. Smirke. The site of the church, and an ample allotment of ground for a cemetery, together with an adjoining piece of land for the site of a parsonage-house, and for the purpose of a garden and slip of glebe, were given by the patron: the house was built by subscription, at an expense of about £2000.——The church of South Hackney (formerly a chapel of ease), situated in Well-street, was built in 1810, on a site given by John Dekewer, Esq.; the erection and subsequent alterations cost nearly £8000, which was defrayed by subscription: a considerable part of the church is appropriated as free sittings. In addition to the three rectories a sub-district has been apportioned from the central district, or Hackney (proper), to the chapel at Upper Clapton, called Stamford Hill chapel, and formerly proprietary, but purchased by subscription among the inhabitants, and subsequently enlarged, in aid of which the rector of the parish, and the Incorporated Society for the enlargement of churches, each contributed £200, for extending the number of free sittings. An endowment of £150 per annum has been assigned to the minister, in addition to which a transfer has been made by the rector of all dues for whatever occasional services should be performed within the chapel. There is also a small ancient chapel at Kingsland, situated partly in West Hackney parish, and partly in the parish of Islington: it was formerly attached to a lazar-house belonging to St. Bartholomew's hospital, and in the patronage of the Governors of that institution: the endowment is very insignificant, and the only other source of emolument to the minister is the pew-rents, which, from the small size of the chapel, are very inconsiderable. At Homerton, within the district attached to Stamford Hill chapel, is Ram's chapel, a private proprietary chapel, at present in disuse. There are places of worship for Baptists at Homerton and in Mare street; for Independents at Homerton, Clapton, Kingsland, Well-street, and St. Thomas' square; for Wesleyan Methodists, in Pleasant-place; and for Unitarians, in Paradise fields. Among the ministers of the Independent congregation in St. Thomas' square were Dr. William Bates, an eminent theological writer, and the Rev. Matthew Henry, author of a commentary on the Holy Scriptures; and among those of the Unitarian congregation were Dr. Price, Dr. Priestley, and the Rev. Thomas Belsham.

Mrs. Margaret Audley, in 1616, left by will £20 per annum, for the maintenance of a schoolmaster in the parish, which now forms a portion of the salary paid to the master of the parochial charity school. The parochial charity schools were established in 1714, for educating and clothing thirty boys and twenty girls, being the children of such poor inhabitants as had certified settlements in the parish: the number in each school continued to vary, until by the adoption of the Madras system of instruction, and the erection, in 1811, of a new and capacious school-house, at an expense of £4500, containing separate and sufficient accommoda-

tions in the centre of the building for a master and a mistress, and in the wings, two very large and convenient school-rooms, the guardians of the charity were enabled greatly to extend the benefit of this institution, which now affords instruction to as many children of the resident poor properly recommended, as the school-rooms will admit, one hundred of each sex being clothed also. The charity is supported by annual subscriptions, occasional benefactions, and two half yearly collections in the parish church. The schools are under the superintendence of their respective committees of visitors, and the general concerns of the institution are regulated and controlled by a committee of managers annually elected by the subscribers. The other schools in connexion with the church in the central parish, are, a school of industry in Dalston-lane, built by subscription on a piece of waste ground granted by the lord of the manor for that purpose, in which forty girls are instructed and clothed, principally by the produce of their own industry. An infant school has also been established in Homerton within the last three years, which is supported by voluntary subscriptions; it contains about one hundred children. In the district of Stamford Hill chapel, a school for boys and another for girls have been recently erected by subscription, containing at present ninety-five of the former, and seventy of the latter. There is also a school for younger children, under the superintendence of a mistress, originally established by the present rector, for the numerous population at the tile-kilns and brick-fields adjoining, but it has been recently connected with the above schools as preparatory to them. The members of the Cumberland Benevolent Institution, have also a small establishment in Church-street, for the maintenance, clothing, and instruction of seven boys and two girls, who are admitted from the age of nine to twelve, and continue till they are fourteen. The only school in connexion with the church of South Hackney is one belonging to the Rev. H. H. Norris, which was erected by him in the year 1810, on land in Grove-street, belonging to himself, and continues to be his own property: the building contains suitable accommodations for a master and a mistress, and separate school-rooms for about sixty boys and thirty girls. In West Hackney a boys' school has been recently erected by subscription, in which there are at present ninety children. There is also a considerable girls' school, the children being allowed the temporary use of a school-house in the central district, until they are enabled by the liberality of the inhabitants of West Hackney to erect one in their own. The boys' school at Homerton, in connexion with Ram's chapel, was established by subscription in 1801, and has, from legacies and benefactions a fund of £2000; and a school for girls in the same connexion, in which twenty-five are educated and clothed, is supported partly by the dividends on £950 three per cent. consols., arising from various benefactions, and by subscription. In addition to the church schools in the three newly constituted districts, there are various others in connexion with, and supported by, the several denominations of dissenters, in their respective neighbourhoods. The dissenting school in Well-street is supported partly by an income of £46 per annum, arising from benefactions and subscriptions; there are seventy boys instructed in this school. Spurstowe's almshouses, founded in 1666 by Dr. William Spurstowe, vicar of Hackney, who endowed them for six aged widows, were rebuilt in 1819, at an expense of £1352. 11. 4., which sum had accumulated from the savings of the original endowment, augmented by subsequent benefactions: the inmates are appointed at a vestry meeting, and receive a quarterly sum of money, and an annual allowance of coal. Six almshouses were built in Wells-street, for six aged men, by Henry Monger, Esq., who endowed them with an annuity of £12, to which subsequent benefactions have been added. The almshouses at Clapton were founded by Thomas Wood, Bishop of Lichfield and Coventry, who endowed them for ten aged widows, with a rent-charge of £50, and £5 per annum to a chaplain to read prayers. There are also various charitable bequests for distribution among the poor, which, in consequence of the partitioning of the parish, have been divided into three distinct portions, by the direction of the commissioners. The Retreat, for eight widows of Independent and four widows of Baptist ministers, near Paradise fields, is a handsome range of buildings, comprising six dwelling-houses, and a chapel in the centre, in the ancient style of English architecture, erected at the sole expense of Samuel Robinson, Esq., who allows each of the inmates £10 per annum, and on his decease £3 per ann. will be added to each allowance. Near St. Thomas' square are twelve almshouses, erected in 1828 by the Bakers' Company, for decayed members and their wives, adjoining which are eight additional tenements, recently erected by — Thorne, Esq., and appropriated to the same use.

The London Orphan Asylum at Clapton, founded in 1813, a spacious and handsome brick building, ornamented with columns and cornices of stone, was erected by subscription, at an expense of nearly £30,000, and comprises, in addition to a commodious chapel detached from the main building (for the exclusive benefit of the children and officers connected with the establishment, and in which the service of the church is regularly performed by the master of the school, who must be a clergyman of the established church), a centre in which are all the domestic offices, under the superintendence of a matron; and two wings, in one of which are the school-room and dormitories for the boys, under the inspection of the master, and in the other similar arrangements for the girls, under the care of the mistress: there are upwards of three hundred children in this institution, chiefly descended from respectable parents, who are maintained, clothed, and educated in virtuous and religious principles, and on their leaving the asylum, if not settled by the board of management in some permanent situation, are stimulated to good conduct by annual rewards progressively increased according to the number of annual meetings at which they have attended with certificates of character. The Metropolitan Female Asylum in Grove-street was established in 1829: it is intended to restrain poor females from deviating from the path of virtue, by affording them a temporary abode, until suitable situations can be provided for them, and to reclaim the imprudent, with a view to their emigration to the colonies. The affairs of the establishment are under the superintendence of a committee of gentlemen, and the household concerns are managed by a committee of ladies. A physician, three surgeons, and a chaplain, afford their services gratuitously. There are at present

sixty inmates; but it is contemplated to extend the benefits of the institution as soon as the patronage of the public shall enable the managers to carry into effect an object so desirable. The Hackney Church of England school is in union with the corporation of King's College, London, for the purpose of providing a course of education for youth, comprising religious instruction in conformity with the principles of the established church, classical learning, the modern languages, mathematics, and such other branches of knowledge as may be advantageously introduced. The head and second master are always to be clergymen of the established church, and graduates of one of the Universities of Oxford and Cambridge, or of Trinity College, Dublin. The second master may take boarders, with the consent of the committee of management, being pupils belonging to the school. The institution is formed by a proprietary of shareholders limited to one hundred and fifty shares of £15 each, with a discretional power in the committee to call for an additional £5. Each proprietor has the right to nominate one pupil for each share he may hold, and shall pay for each pupil, if under twelve years of age, £10. 10. per annum, and if twelve years of age, or upwards, £12. 12. per annum, the same to be in full of every charge for tuition, books, and stationery: no child is to be admitted under seven years of age. The building, situated in the Back-lane, Clapton, is wholly of brick-work, in the Grecian style of architecture, with a portico of four fluted Doric columns, which, together with the entablatures and principal front, are finished in Roman cement, to imitate stone: it contains on the basement story a school-room and hat-rooms for the students, committee and class-room, head master's room, janitor's room, and apartments for the same on the upper story. The site, about an acre in extent, including a play-ground and fives-court at the rear of the building, is enclosed on three sides by a boundary wall, and in front by an ornamental iron railing and two pair of gates, through which the principal entrance is approached by a carriage sweep of ample dimensions: the school-room is warmed by a hot-water apparatus, upon a new and improved principle: the expense of the whole was about £1750. There is another institution, designated by the name of the Hackney Grammar school, founded and supported by a proprietary of shareholders, which admits pupils of every religious denomination. The head master is a clergyman of the church of England: he is not allowed to take boarders: the number of shares are one hundred and twenty, at £15 per share: the building, situated near the old church-yard, is in the English style, and cost upwards of £1300. The Society for educating young men for the ministry, instituted in 1730, and entertaining the doctrines expressed in the catechisms of the Westminster Assembly, have a college at Homerton, for the instruction of twenty pious young men, who are not admissible under seventeen nor above twenty-two years of age: the course of studies includes the Latin, Greek, and Hebrew languages, with their application to classical and biblical literature, English composition, the mathematics, natural philosophy, the principles of, chemistry, natural history, logic, and the philosophy of the mind, general history, ecclesiastical antiquities, and scriptural divinity; besides which a professor of elocution delivers a course of lectures on that subject every session. The period of time allotted is six years : the first two are occupied solely in classical pursuits; the remainder in classical, theological, and philosophical studies. The present building of brick, which is plain and neat, and very commodious, was completed in 1823, on the site of a former one, at an expense of nearly £10,000, defrayed by subscription : it contains a good library of classical and theological works, and of others in the general branches of literature. Among the distinguished individuals interred at Hackney may be mentioned Henry, Lord Percy, Earl of Northumberland, who died at his house in this parish, June 29th, 1537, being the same earl, who, according to the assertion of Henry VIII., was contracted to Anna Boleyn, and under which pretext the sentence of divorce was pronounced between that monarch and her; Edward Vere, Earl of Oxford, a statesman, poet, and dramatist, who flourished in the reign of Elizabeth, and died in 1604 ; Dr. John Worthington, an eminent divine ; and Sir Francis D'Oliveyra, a Portuguese emigrant, who wrote against the inquisition, and died in 1783. Sir Ralph Sadleir, a distinguished statesman in the reigns of Henry VIII., Edward VI., and Elizabeth, was born here; and Howard, the great philanthropist, is supposed to have been born at Clapton, in this parish.

HACKTHORN, a parish in the eastern division of the wapentake of ASLACOE, parts of LINDSEY, county of LINCOLN, 8 miles (N. by E.) from Lincoln, containing 256 inhabitants. The living is a discharged vicarage, in the archdeaconry of Stow, and diocese of Lincoln, rated in the king's books at £4, endowed with £400 royal bounty. R. Cracroft, Esq. was patron in 1827. The church is dedicated to St. Michael.

HADDENHAM, a parish in the hundred of AYLESBURY, county of BUCKINGHAM, 3 miles (N. E. by E.) from Thame, containing 1294 inhabitants. The living is a vicarage, with the perpetual curacy of Cuddington annexed, in the archdeaconry of Buckingham, and diocese of Lincoln, rated in the king's books at £15. 17. 1., and in the patronage of the Dean and Chapter of Rochester. The church is dedicated to St. Mary. There is a place of worship for Baptists. In 1294, the monks of the convent of St. Andrew, at Rochester, obtained a charter for a weekly market to be held here on Thursday, which was discontinued in 1301 : a fair was also granted for three days, at the festival of the Assumption of the Virgin Mary. There are two mineral springs in the parish.

HADDENHAM, a parish in the southern division of the hundred of WITCHFORD, Isle of ELY, county of CAMBRIDGE, 6½ miles (S. W. by W.) from Ely, containing 1725 inhabitants. The living is a perpetual curacy, in the peculiar jurisdiction of the Bishop of Ely, and in the patronage of the Archdeacon of Ely. The church, dedicated to the Holy Trinity, is principally in the Norman style. Baptists and Wesleyan Methodists have each a place of worship. There are two sums of £10 and £17 per annum for the education of children; the former the gift of Mrs. March, the latter of Mr. Arkenstall.

HADDINGTON, a township partly in the parish of AUBORN, and partly in that of SOUTH HYCKHAM, lower division of the wapentake of BOOTHBY-GRAFFO, parts of KESTEVEN, county of LINCOLN, 7½ miles (S. W. by S.) from Lincoln, containing 108 inhabitants.

HADDISCOE, a parish in the hundred of CLAVERING, county of NORFOLK, 4¾ miles (N. N. E.) from Beccles, containing 316 inhabitants. The living is a discharged rectory united to that of Monks-Toft, in the archdeaconry of Norfolk, and diocese of Norwich, rated in the king's books at £12. The church, dedicated to St. Mary, has a Norman archway and a round tower. Here was a preceptory of Knights Templars, to which Henry III. was a considerable benefactor.

HADDLESEY (CHAPEL), a chapelry in the parish of BIRKIN, lower division of the wapentake of BARKSTONE-ASH, West riding of the county of YORK, 4½ miles (S. S. W.) from Selby, containing 199 inhabitants. The chapel is dedicated to St. John the Baptist.

HADDLESEY (WEST), a township in the parish of BIRKIN, lower division of the wapentake of BARKSTONE-ASH, West riding of the county of YORK, 5 miles (S. W.) from Selby, containing 293 inhabitants.

HADDON, a parish in the hundred of NORMANCROSS, county of HUNTINGDON, 3 miles (N. W. by N.) from Stilton, containing 112 inhabitants. The living is a rectory, in the archdeaconry of Huntingdon, and diocese of Lincoln, rated in the king's books at £11. 5. The Earl of Aboyne was patron in 1819. The church is dedicated to St. Mary.

HADDON (EAST), a parish in the hundred of NOBOTTLE-GROVE, county of NORTHAMPTON, 7½ miles (N. W.) from Northampton, containing 617 inhabitants. The living is a discharged vicarage, in the archdeaconry of Northampton, and diocese of Peterborough, rated in the king's books at £5. W. Sawbridge, Esq. was patron in 1814. The church, dedicated to St. Mary, is an ancient structure, having portions in the decorated style of architecture. There is a small provision for the education of children.

HADDON (OVER), a township in the parish of BAKEWELL, hundred of HIGH PEAK, county of DERBY, 2 miles (S. W. by S.) from Bakewell, containing 266 inhabitants. At this place is Haddon Hall, one of the ancient baronial mansions, delightfully situated on a gentle eminence overlooking the river Wye : the venerable castellated towers rising above the woods produce a magnificent effect, and as the whole building is still in nearly a perfect state, it is an object of general interest and curiosity.

HADDON (WEST), a parish in the hundred of GUILSBOROUGH, county of NORTHAMPTON, 7¼ miles (N. N. E.) from Daventry, containing 893 inhabitants. The living is a discharged vicarage, in the archdeaconry of Northampton, and diocese of Peterborough, rated in the king's books at £13. 6. 8. S. Spence, Esq. was patron in 1826. The church is dedicated to All Saints. Baptists and Wesleyan Methodists have each a place of worship. Ostor hill, a high tumulus, supposed to be that of P. Ostorius, the propraetor in Britain, is situated in this parish.

HADFIELD, a township in the parish of GLOSSOP, hundred of HIGH PEAK, county of DERBY, 11 miles (N. by W.) from Chapel en le Frith, containing 659 inhabitants. There is a neat Wesleyan Methodist chapel, with a school attached, in which upwards of four hundred children are educated. About thirty years since this district was almost entirely an agricultural one, and but thinly inhabited; but now there are many flourishing cotton factories (some of them on a large scale), which afford employment to nearly the whole of the population: there are also several good stone quarries. The river Mersey bounds the township on the north. Cattle fairs are held on the 9th of May and the 15th of October.

HADHAM (LITTLE), a parish in the hundred of Edwinstree, county of Hertford, 3 miles (W. N. W.) from Bishop's Stortford, containing 787 inhabitants. The living, with that of Much-Hadham, forms a rectory, within the jurisdiction of the Commissary of Essex and Herts, concurrently with the consistorial court of the Bishop of London.

HADHAM (MUCH), a parish in the hundred of Edwinstree, county of Hertford, 4¼ miles (W. S. W.) from Bishop's Stortford, containing 1208 inhabitants. The living is a rectory with Little Hadham, within the peculiar jurisdiction of the Commissary of Essex and Herts, concurrently with the Consistorial Court of the Bishop of London, rated in the king's books at £66. 13. 4., and in the patronage of the Bishop of London. The church is dedicated to St. Andrew. The Independents have a place of worship here. There is a small endowment for the education of six boys and six girls. Here are the remains of a palace belonging to the Bishops of London, now a private residence. Dr. John Owen, an eminent non-conformist divine, was born at this place in 1616.

HADLEIGH, a parish in the hundred of Rochford, county of Essex, 2¼ miles (W. by N.) from Leigh, containing 329 inhabitants. The living is a discharged rectory, in the archdeaconry of Essex, and diocese of London, rated in the king's books at £11. 14. 7., and in the patronage of the Rector and Fellows of Lincoln College, Oxford. The church, dedicated to St. James, is an ancient structure; the eastern end is semicircular, and in the Norman style. In the reign of Henry II., a castle was built here by Hubert de Burgh, Earl of Kent: the remains, which are picturesquely situated on the brow of a steep hill, consist chiefly of two dilapidated circular towers.

HADLEIGH, a market town and parish in the hundred of Cosford, county of Suffolk, 10½ miles (W. by S.) from Ipswich, and 64 (N. E.) from London, containing 2929 inhabitants. This town was probably founded during the Heptarchy, and it was called by the Anglo-Saxons, *Headlege*, whence it derived its modern name. Some of the kings of East Anglia were interred here; as also was Guthrum, or Gormo, a Danish chief, who submitted to Alfred the Great, and renounced paganism after the great defeat of the Danes at the battle of Ethandune: a tomb is still shown in the church as the monument of Guthrum, who died in 889; but it is obviously of much later date than the ninth century. The town is situated in a valley, the air of which is remarkably salubrious: the streets are neither lighted nor paved: the inhabitants are plentifully supplied with water from springs. The woollen manufacture formerly flourished here, but there is now only a small silk-manufactory, lately established. There is a large market, principally for corn, on Monday; another, formerly held on Saturday, has been discontinued: fairs are held on Whit-Tuesday and the 10th of October, for toys, &c. The Corn Exchange, erected by subscription in 1813, is a handsome building. This was formerly a corporate town, governed by a mayor, aldermen, and common council-men, but surrendering its charter upon a *quo*

warranto to James II., these privileges were lost, and have never been restored: it is now within the jurisdiction of the county magistrates, who hold petty sessions here. Courts baron are held for the manor, at which the steward presides. The living is a rectory, rated in the king's books at £45. 2. 1., and within the exempt deanery of Bocking, in the peculiar jurisdiction and patronage of the Archbishop of Canterbury. The church, dedicated to St. Mary, is a handsome spacious structure, surmounted by a lofty spire of wood covered with lead: it is chiefly of the later English character, and has two south porches: the aisles and clerestory are co-extensive with the nave and the chancel. In the chancel is a beautiful altar-piece, erected in 1744, by Dr. Wilkins, the incumbent, constructed of wainscot with neat cane-work, and exhibiting paintings of Moses and Aaron. The font is of great antiquity, and bears an ancient inscription in Greek characters, which being translated is, "Wash and be clean." In front of the parsonage-house is a venerable gateway with two hexagonal towers, built of brick in the year 1490, by Dr. Pykenham, Dean of Suffolk, and rector of this parish. There are places of worship for Baptists, Independents, and Wesleyan Methodists. A house in Hadleigh and some land were given by John Alabaster, in 1667, the produce to be applied for the instruction of four children in reading and writing; and, in 1701, Mrs. Anne Beaumont bequeathed an estate for the same purpose; from which benefactions united a salary of about £34 per annum is paid to a master for the instruction of twenty-four boys. A National school for an unlimited number of scholars of both sexes is supported by voluntary contributions. Twelve almshouses for decayed tradespeople, with a chapel attached, were founded by Dr. Pykenham, in the reign of Henry VII., and are under the management of the rector and the churchwardens: they are now appropriated to the accommodation of twenty-four aged persons of both sexes, and are endowed by the founder with valuable estates in Whatfield, Hadleigh, Aldham, Newton, Elmset, and Semer, and a farm at Foxearth in Essex, the bequest of Mrs. Mary Clark. Four other almshouses were founded in the reign of Edward VI., by John Raven, of Hadleigh, and endowed by him with the profits of two farms in Roydon and Holton, for the support of eight poor aged inhabitants of the parish. There are several other bequests for the benefit of the poor. Dr. William Alabaster, a learned divine of the seventeenth century, was a native of Hadleigh.

HADLEIGH (HAMLET), a chapelry in that part of the parish of Boxford which is in the hundred of Cosford, county of Suffolk, containing 201 inhabitants.

HADLEY, a joint tything with Blagrave, in the parish and hundred of Lambourn, county of Berks. The population is returned with Blagrave.

HADLEY (MONKEN), a parish in the hundred of Edmonton, county of Middlesex, ¾ of a mile (N. N. E.) from Chipping-Barnet, containing 926 inhabitants. The living is a perpetual curacy, in the jurisdiction of the Commissary of London, concurrently with the Consistorial Court of the Bishop of London, and in the patronage of John Penney, Esq. The church, dedicated to St. Mary, consists of a nave, aisles, chancel, and transept; the aisles are separated from the nave by depressed arches and clustered pillars. At the west end is a square tower of flint, on the top of which is an iron beacon. Amongst eminent persons buried here were Sir William Stamford, a learned judge and writer on the law; Dr. John Monro, a physician, author of a treatise on insanity; and Mrs. Chapone, who wrote "Letters on the Improvement of the Mind." This place was formerly a hamlet in the parish of Edmonton.

HADLOW, a parish in the lowey of TONBRIDGE, lathe of AYLESFORD, county of KENT, 3½ miles (N. E.) from Tonbridge, containing 1757 inhabitants. The living is a vicarage, in the archdeaconry and diocese of Rochester, rated in the king's books at £13, and in the patronage of the Rev. P. Monypenny. The church is a low structure dedicated to St. Mary. There are places of worship for Baptists and Wesleyan Methodists. This is an extensive parish, in which there are several hop plantations and good pasture lands. It is crossed by the river Sheet, which joins the navigable river Medway a little above Brandt bridge. At Hurlake Bolt is a flowing bolt by which, in dry seasons, the meadows can be irrigated, this plan being found highly advantageous. There is a fair on Whit-Monday.

HADNALL-EASE, a chapelry in that part of the parish of MIDDLE which is within the liberty of the borough of SHREWSBURY, county of SALOP, 5¼ miles (N. N. E.) from Shrewsbury, containing 363 inhabitants. The living is a perpetual curacy, with the rectory of Grinshill, in the archdeaconry of Salop, and diocese of Lichfield and Coventry, endowed with £400 private benefaction, and £1000 royal bounty. The chapel is dedicated to St. Mary Magdalene.

HADSOR, a parish in the upper division of the hundred of HALFSHIRE, county of WORCESTER, 1¼ mile (S. E.) from Droitwich, containing 135 inhabitants. The living is a discharged rectory, in the archdeaconry and diocese of Worcester, rated in the king's books at £6. 7. 3½. —Amphlett, Esq. was patron in 1808. The church is dedicated to St. John the Baptist. The Birmingham and Worcester canal runs through the parish.

HADSPEN, a tything in the parish of PITCOMB, hundred of BRUTON, county of SOMERSET, 1¼ mile (E.) from Castle-Cary, containing 246 inhabitants.

HADSTOCK, in the hundred of FRESHWELL, county of ESSEX, 1½ mile (S.) from Linton, containing 392 inhabitants. The living is a rectory, in the jurisdiction of the Commissary of Essex and Herts, concurrently with the Consistorial Court of the Bishop of London, rated in the king's books at £19, and in the patronage of the Bishop of Ely. The church, dedicated to St. Botolph, is an ancient structure having a curious Norman door-way. A school of industry is attended by about fifty children, and principally supported by their earnings.

HADSTON, a township in that part of the parish of WARKWORTH which is in the eastern division of MORPETH ward, county of NORTHUMBERLAND, 11 miles (N. N. E.) from Morpeth, containing 88 inhabitants.

HAGBORNE, a parish in the hundred of MORETON, county of BERKS, comprising the liberties of East Hagborne and West Hagborne, and containing 708 inhabitants, of which number, 524 are in the liberty of East Hagborne, 5½ miles (W. by S.) from Wallingford. The living is a discharged vicarage, in the archdeaconry of Berks, and diocese of Salisbury, rated in the king's books at £15. 10. 7½., endowed with £200 private benefaction,

and £300 parliamentary grant, and in the patronage of the Rev. Richard Meredith. The church, dedicated to St. Andrew, is a handsome structure in the early style of English architecture, with a square tower; the north aisle was built by John York, who died in 1413. In the village is a stone cross, surmounted by a sundial. There is a small sum for the education of children. A fair is held on the Thursday preceding the 11th of October. On the 24th of May, 1644, the parliamentary army, under the command of the Earl of Essex, quartered at this place, on their route from Reading to Abingdon.

HAGBORNE (WEST), a liberty in the parish of HAGBORNE, hundred of MORETON, county of BERKS, 6¼ miles (W. by S.) from Wallingford, containing 184 inhabitants. Here was anciently a chapel.

HAGGERSTON, a parish in the Tower division of the hundred of OSSULSTONE, county of MIDDLESEX, 1½ mile (N.E. by N.) from London. The population is returned with the parish of St. Leonard, Shoreditch. This place, formerly an inconsiderable hamlet in the parish of St. Leonard, Shoreditch, has, within the last few years, become an extensive and populous district. Many new streets have been formed, consisting of neat ranges of houses of a moderate size : the parish is partially paved, lighted with gas, and amply supplied with water. Among the larger of the various works which have been erected on the banks of the Regent's canal, which passes through the parish, are those of the Imperial and Independent Gas-light and Coke Companies, the former of which was established in 1822, for lighting the eastern district of the metropolis, and the latter incorporated in 1829. The facility afforded by the canal has contributed greatly to increase the trade of the place : there are several chemical works on an extensive scale, manufactures for japanned leather, floorcloth, and hearth-rugs; a manufactory for bone ashes, several lime-works, tile-kilns, dye-houses, and coalwharfs, affording employment to a considerable portion of the inhabitants. The parish is within the jurisdiction of a court of requests held at Whitechapel, for the recovery of debts under 40s.

Haggerston was constituted a distinct parish in 1830. The living is a vicarage, in the archdeaconry and diocese of London, and in the patronage of the Archdeacon of London. The church, dedicated to St. Mary, and erected in 1827, at an expense of £15,000, by a grant from the parliamentary commissioners, is a spacious structure, blending the early and decorated styles of English architecture, with a lofty square embattled tower of singular design, destitute of relief in the lower part, and profusely ornamented in the upper with crocketed pinnacles, with which a smaller tower rising from the centre is connected by flying buttresses ; at the western extremities of the aisles are octagonal turrets, with domed roofs surrounded by crocketed pinnacles rising from the angles : the interior, which is neatly arranged, contains one thousand nine hundred and sixty sittings, of which one thousand are free. There are places of worship for Independents and Wesleyan Methodists. Sunday schools in connexion with the established church and the dissenting congregations are supported by subscription, and an infant school is about to be established. Six almshouses, for six poor members of the Company of Goldsmiths, were founded in

1705, in Goldsmith-place, in this parish, by Mr. Richard Morrell, who endowed them with an estate for their perpetual maintenance. Fourteen almshouses, with a chapel in the centre, were erected in Kingsland-road, in 1713, by Sir Robert Geffery, Knt., for poor members of the Company of Ironmongers. On the south side of the Ironmongers' almshouses are twelve others founded by Mr. S. Harwar, citizen and draper of London, of which six are for poor freemen of the Drapers' Company, and six for poor persons of the parish. To the north of the Ironmongers' almshouses are twelve for poor freemen of the Company of Frame-work knitters and their widows, founded by Thomas Bourne, Esq., who gave £1000 for their erection, and £2000 for their endowment, to which additions have been made by subsequent benefactions.

HAGHMON (or HAUGHMOND) ABBEY, an extra-parochial liberty, in the Wellington division of the hundred of BRADFORD (South), county of SALOP, 4¼ miles (N.E.) from Shrewsbury. In 1110, William Fitz-Alan, of Clun, founded an abbey here for canons regular of the order of St. Augustine, and dedicated it to St. John the Apostle and Evangelist, the revenue of which, at the dissolution, amounted to £294. 12. 9. It forms part of the demesne of Sundorn : the remains consist of the chapter-house, which is entire, the south door-way of the nave of the church, and a range of building supposed to have been the abbot's lodging and hall, partly in the Norman, but chiefly in the early, style of English architecture. The Rev. William Clarke, Chancellor in the Cathedral Church of Chichester, and an antiquary of no mean repute, was born at this place in 1696.

HAGLEY, a parish in the lower division of the hundred of HALFSHIRE, county of WORCESTER, 2 miles (S.) from Stourbridge, containing 595 inhabitants. The living is a rectory, in the archdeaconry and diocese of Worcester, rated in the king's books at £10. 6. 5½., and in the patronage of Lord Lyttelton. The church, dedicated to St. John the Baptist, has been lately enlarged by the addition of one hundred and ninety-four sittings, one hundred and thirty-four of which are free, the Incorporated Society for the building and enlargement of churches and chapels having granted £100 towards defraying the expense : it is beautifully situated in the park of the Lyttelton estate. In 1754, the chancel was rebuilt of freestone by the first Lord Lyttelton, and decorated with an east window of rich painted glass. Among the monuments to different members of the Lyttelton family, it contains a particularly chaste one to the memory of Lucy, wife of George, the first Lord Lyttelton : his lordship, an elegant historian, poet, and miscellaneous writer, was born at this place. Hagley hall and park, the delightful residence and property of this noble family, have been celebrated by the muse of Pope, and have elicited deserved eulogy from the pens of numerous tourists and historical writers. The village contains some genteel dwelling-houses, and several highly respectable families reside in the vicinity. There is a Sunday school for boys and girls, supported by Lord Lyttelton. On Witchbury hill is a large Roman encampment.

HAGLOE, a tything in the parish of AWRE, hundred of BLIDESLOE, county of GLOUCESTER, ¾ of a mile (E.S.E.) from Blakeney. The population is returned with the parish.

HAGNABY, a parish in the western division of the soke of BOLINGBROKE, parts of LINDSEY, county of LINCOLN, 5 miles (S.W. by W.) from Spilsby, containing 91 inhabitants. The living is a discharged vicarage, in the archdeaconry and diocese of Lincoln, rated in the king's books at £8, and in the patronage of George Coltman, Esq. The church is dedicated to St. Andrew. A navigable cut, called the Catch water, passes along the southern extremity of the parish.

HAGNABY, a hamlet in the parish of HANNAY, Wold division of the hundred of CALCEWORTH, parts of LINDSEY, county of LINCOLN, 3½ miles (N.E. by N.) from Alford, containing 106 inhabitants. A Premonstratensian monastery, dedicated to St. Thomas of Canterbury, was founded here in 1175, by Herbert de Oppeby, the revenue of which, at the dissolution, amounted to £98. 7. 4.

HAGWORTHINGHAM, a parish in the hundred of HILL, parts of LINDSEY, county of LINCOLN, 4½ miles (N.W. by W.) from Spilsby, containing 533 inhabitants. The living is a rectory, in the archdeaconry and diocese of Lincoln, rated in the king's books at £14. 10. 5., and in the patronage of the Bishop of Ely. The church is dedicated to the Holy Trinity.

HAIGH, a township in that part of the parish of WIGAN which is in the hundred of WEST DERBY, county palatine of LANCASTER, 2¾ miles (N. by E.) from Wigan, containing 1300 inhabitants. A free school is supported by the rental of a house and ten acres of land, the bequest of Miles Turner, in 1634, producing about £50 per annum ; and by the interest of £100, the gift of Dame Dorothy Bradshaigh, in 1792. The "Receptacle," an almshouse for ten poor men and ten poor women of this township and those of Wigan, Blackrod, and Aspull, was erected by the same lady, and endowed with a sum now invested in the three per cent. consols., and producing £136. 13. 2. per annum : to each tenement a small plot of ground is attached. A considerable quantity of cannel coal is obtained in this district.

HAIGHTON, a township in the parish of PRESTON, hundred of AMOUNDERNESS, county palatine of LANCASTER, 3½ miles (N.N.E.) from Preston, containing 184 inhabitants.

HAILES, a chapelry in the parish of DIDBROOK, lower division of the hundred of KIFTSGATE, county of GLOUCESTER, 2 miles (N.E. by E.) from Winchcombe, containing 136 inhabitants. The living is a perpetual curacy, in the archdeaconry and diocese of Gloucester, endowed with £200 royal bounty, and in the patronage of Charles Hanbury Tracey, Esq. In 1246, Richard, Earl of Cornwall, afterwards King of the Romans and Emperor of Germany, erected here, at an expense of ten thousand marks, a noble abbey, dedicated to the Virgin Mary and All Saints, for monks of the Cistercian order, the revenue of which, at the dissolution, was estimated at £357. 7. 8.: here are still some slight remains of it.

HAILEY, a chapelry in the parish of WITNEY, hundred of BAMPTON, county of OXFORD, 1½ mile (N.) from Witney, containing 1098 inhabitants. The living is a perpetual curacy, in the archdeaconry and diocese of Oxford, endowed with £200 private benefaction, £600 royal bounty, and £1400 parliamentary grant. The chapel is dedicated to St. John the Evangelist. There is a small sum for the education of children.

HAILSHAM, a market town and parish, partly within the liberty of the borough of PEVENSEY, but chiefly in the hundred of DILL, rape of PEVENSEY, county of SUSSEX, 52 miles (E.) from Chichester, and 56¾ (S. S. E.) from London, containing 1278 inhabitants. This is a small town situated in a pleasant and fertile country, about eight miles from the sea. A market is held every alternate Wednesday; and there are fairs on April 6th and June 3rd. Hailsham is within the duchy of Lancaster. The magistrates hold a meeting here once a fortnight, on Wednesday. The living is a vicarage, in the archdeaconry of Lewes, and diocese of Chichester, rated in the king's books at £16. 6. 8., and in the patronage of E. W. Michell, Esq. The church, dedicated to St. Mary, is principally in the later style of English architecture. There is a place of worship for Baptists. A National school for boys and girls, recently erected on a common adjoining the town, is supported by subscription. In the reign of Henry II., a monastery of Premonstratensian canons was founded here, which was afterwards removed to Bayham.

HAIL-WESTON, a parish in the hundred of TOSELAND, county of HUNTINGDON, 2¼ miles (N. W.) from St. Neot's, containing 297 inhabitants. The living is a perpetual curacy, annexed to the vicarage of Southoe, in the archdeaconry of Huntingdon, and diocese of Lincoln. The church is dedicated to St. Nicholas. The Particular Baptists have a place of worship here.

HAINFORD, a parish in the hundred of TAVERHAM, county of NORFOLK, 2½ miles (W.) from Coltishall, containing 484 inhabitants. The living is a rectory, in the archdeaconry and diocese of Norwich, rated in the king's books at £6. 2. 1. Robert Marsham, Esq. was patron in 1817. The church is dedicated to All Saints.

HAINTON, a parish in the eastern division of the wapentake of WRAGGOE, parts of LINDSEY, county of LINCOLN, 6¼ miles (N. E.) from Wragby, containing 228 inhabitants. The living is a discharged vicarage, in the peculiar jurisdiction and patronage of the Dean and Chapter of Lincoln, rated in the king's books at £7. 10. 10. The church is dedicated to St. Mary.

HAISTHORP, a township in the parish of AGNES-BURTON, wapentake of DICKERING, East riding of the county of YORK, 4 miles (S. W. by W.) from Bridlington, containing 109 inhabitants.

HALAM, a parish in that part of the liberty of SOUTHWELL and SCROOBY which separates the northern from the southern division of the wapentake of THURGARTON, county of NOTTINGHAM, 1½ mile (W. by N.) from Southwell, containing 310 inhabitants. The living is a perpetual curacy, in the peculiar jurisdiction and patronage of the Chapter of the Collegiate Church of Southwell, endowed with £200 private benefaction, and £800 royal bounty. The church is dedicated to St. Michael.

HALBERTON, a parish in the hundred of HALBERTON, county of DEVON, 3½ miles (E.) from Tiverton, containing 1598 inhabitants. The living is a discharged vicarage, in the archdeaconry and diocese of Exeter, rated in the king's books at £31, endowed with £200 private benefaction, and £200 royal bounty, and in the patronage of the Dean and Chapter of Bristol. This church, dedicated to St. Andrew, once appertained to the abbey of St. Augustine in Bristol, and in the churchyard was anciently a chantry chapel. A fraternity of St. John was also attached to the church. A branch of the Grand Western canal passes through the parish.

HALDEN (HIGH), a parish in the hundred of BLACKBOURNE, lathe of SCRAY, county of KENT, 3½ miles (N. E. by N.) from Tenterden, containing 724 inhabitants. The living is a rectory, in the archdeaconry and diocese of Canterbury, rated in the king's books at £19. 4. 7., and in the patronage of the Archbishop of Canterbury. The church, dedicated to St. Mary, is a large edifice, remarkable for a singular steeple built in the reign of Henry VI. There is an endowed school, under the direction of ten trustees, possessing an estate of the value of £26 per annum, founded in 1725, by Mr. James Tylden; about twenty children are educated in it. The rivers Tarn and "the River" (so called for the sake of distinction, having no proper name,) run through the parish in their course to the Medway. The clay being of an excellent quality for common earthenware, there are many manufactories for articles of that kind. A mineral, called by the inhabitants "Crownstone," consisting of the oxyde of iron, clay, and manganese, is found here in great quantities; also hones of a particular quality, resembling those of Turkey; and strata of marble of about three quarters of an inch thick.

HALDENBY, a joint township with Eastoft, in the parish of ADLINGFLEET, lower division of the wapentake of OSGOLDCROSS, West riding of the county of YORK, 9½ miles (S. E. by S.) from Howden, containing 69 inhabitants.

HALE, a township in the parish of BOWDON, hundred of BUCKLOW, county palatine of CHESTER, 2½ miles (S. E.) from Altrincham, containing 958 inhabitants.

HALE, a parish in ALLERDALE ward above Darwent, county of CUMBERLAND, 2½ miles (S. E.) from Egremont, containing, with the hamlet of Wilton, 249 inhabitants. The living is a perpetual curacy, in the archdeaconry of Richmond, and diocese of Chester, endowed with £800 royal bounty, and in the patronage of the Earl of Lonsdale. The church, which has a small tower and spire, stands at a short distance from the village. Freestone and limestone abound in the parish.

HALE, a township in the parish and hundred of WROTHAM, lathe of AYLESFORD, county of KENT, 3¼ miles (S. S. W.) from Wrotham, with which the population is returned.

HALE, a chapelry in the parish of CHILDWALL, hundred of WEST DERBY, county palatine of LANCASTER, 7¼ miles (S.) from Prescot, containing 630 inhabitants. The living is a perpetual curacy, in the archdeaconry and diocese of Chester, endowed with £600 private benefaction, £400 royal bounty, and £300 parliamentary grant. J. Blackburn, Esq. was patron in 1818. The chapel is dedicated to St. Mary. A school was erected in 1737, by William Past, and endowed by him and Ellen Bushell, jointly, with £10 a year, for the instruction of ten children: there is also a trifling sum, the gift of Ellen Halsall, to purchase books.

HALE, a parish in the hundred of FORDINGBRIDGE, New Forest (West) division of the county of SOUTHAMPTON, 4 miles (N. E.) from Fordingbridge, containing 181 inhabitants. The living is a donative with that of Breamore, in the archdeaconry and diocese of Winchester. The church is dedicated to St. Mary. The navigable river Avon runs through the parish.

HALE (GREAT), a parish in the wapentake of As-WARDHURN, parts of KESTEVEN, county of LINCOLN, 5¾ miles (E.S.E.) from Sleaford, containing, with the township of Little Hale, 863 inhabitants. The living is a discharged vicarage, in the archdeaconry and diocese of Lincoln, rated in the king's books at £8.6., and in the patronage of the Crown. The church, dedicated to St. John the Baptist, is principally in the decorated style of English architecture.

HALE (LITTLE), a township in the parish of GREAT HALE, wapentake of ASWARDHURN, parts of KESTEVEN, county of LINCOLN, 6½ miles (E.S.E.) from Sleaford, containing 286 inhabitants.

HALE-WESTON, county of HUNTINGDON. — See HAIL-WESTON.

HALES, a parish in the hundred of CLAVERING, county of NORFOLK, 4½ miles (N.W. by N.) from Beccles, containing 252 inhabitants. The living is a perpetual curacy, in the archdeaconry of Norfolk, and diocese of Norwich. Sir Thomas Smyth, Bart. was patron in 1816. The church is dedicated to St. Margaret.

HALES-OWEN, a parish comprising the market town of Hales-Owen, in the Hales-Owen division of the hundred of BRIMSTREE, a detached portion of the county of SALOP, and the chapelry of Cradley, and the hamlets of Luttley and Warley-Wigorn, in the lower division of the hundred of HALFSHIRE, county of WORCESTER, and containing 10,946 inhabitants, of which number, 8817 are in that part of the parish which is in the county of Salop, and 1759 in the town of Hales-Owen, 35 miles (S.E.) from Shrewsbury, and 120 (N.W.) from London. This place is said to have been formerly a borough, though it does not appear to have ever returned members to parliament. King John, in the sixteenth year of his reign, gave the manor and the advowson of the church, which is stated to have been built prior to the Norman Conquest, to Peter de Rupibus, Bishop of Winchester, who founded here a priory of Premonstratensian canons, which, from parts of the walls yet remaining, though concealed by brambles and weeds, appears to have been an extensive edifice, and from the gable end of the chapter-house, in which are some fine lancet windows, to have been in the early style of English architecture. At the dissolution, its revenue was estimated at £337. 15. 6.: some vestiges of the abbot's kitchen are still visible in a farm-house near the town. Hales-Owen is more celebrated for having been the birthplace and residence of the poet Shenstone, than for any events of historical interest. The town is situated in a fertile vale watered by the river Stour, which has its source in the neighbouring hills, and surrounded with scenery of a varied and pleasing character. It consists principally of one street, in which are some respectable houses, and of some smaller streets containing humbler dwellings irregularly built. In the vicinity are several detached mansions, of which the Leasowes, the patrimonial estate and residence of Shenstone, has been deservedly eulogized for the classic taste and elegant chasteness of style with which, during his lifetime, the natural beauty of the grounds had been artificially heightened and improved. The principal branches of manufacture in the town are, nails, and some few articles of iron. The manufacture of steel is extensively carried on at Corngreaves, and some coal mines have been recently opened in the parish. The small river Stour

runs through the town, and the Netherton canal passes within half a mile of it. The market is on Monday, but is indifferently attended : the fairs are on the Mondays in Easter and Whitsun weeks. The town is within the jurisdiction of the county magistrates; and a high and low bailiff, constable, and headborough, are annually appointed at the court leet of the lord of the manor. A court of requests is held every third week, under an act passed in the 47th of George III., for the recovery of debts under £5, the jurisdiction of which extends over the parishes of Hales-Owen, Rowley-Regis, Tipton, West Bromwich, Harborne, and the manor of Bradley, in the parish of Wolverhampton, in the counties of Worcester, Salop, and Stafford.

The living is a discharged vicarage, in the archdeaconry and diocese of Worcester, rated in the king's books at £15. 8. 11½., and in the patronage of Lord Lyttelton. The church, dedicated to St. Mary and St. John the Evangelist, is a spacious structure in the Norman style of architecture, with later insertions, having a tower surmounted by a lofty spire : the interior contains a handsome monument to the memory of Major Halliday, and an urn to that of the poet Shenstone, who was buried in the church-yard in 1763. There are places of worship for Independents and Wesleyan Methodists. The free grammar school was founded under a commission for charitable uses, in 1652, and endowed with lands and tenements bequeathed by various benefactors to the parish, now producing more than £100 per ann., of which, £30 is paid to the usher, and the remainder to the master, who has also the school-house, with a good garden and six acres of land ; there are about forty boys, who are now instructed in English grammar, writing, and arithmetic. Shenstone received the rudiments of his education in this school. At Honington, in this parish, a free school was founded, in 1684, by William Smith, and endowed with lands producing about £15 per annum, for the education of twenty poor children. Dr. Adam Littleton, author of a Latin Dictionary and other works, who died in 1694; and William Caslon, the celebrated type-founder, who died in 1766; were born in this parish.

HALESWORTH, a market town and parish in the hundred of BLYTHING, county of SUFFOLK, 30½ miles (N. E. by N.) from Ipswich, and 101 (N. E.) from London, containing 2166 inhabitants. The town, which is situated in a valley on the banks of the river Blyth, is ancient and indifferently built, nearly in the form of the letter S, but contains a few good houses ; the streets are spacious and well lighted with oil, but not paved, and the inhabitants plentifully supplied with water. There is a small theatre, which is open once in two years. The river is navigable hence to Southwold, for small craft of about twenty-five tons, which are usually laden with malt and grain. There are some very large malt-houses, the trade in malting being extensive. The market is on Tuesday, for corn and provisions; and there is a fair on the 29th of October, chiefly for Scotch cattle. The magistrates of the hundred hold quarterly meetings here; and courts leet and baron for the manor are held occasionally. The living is a discharged rectory with the vicarage of Chediston, in the archdeaconry of Suffolk, and diocese of Norwich, rated in the king's books at £20, and in the patronage of J. Ward, Esq. The church, dedicated to St. Mary, is a fine edifice of flint, and has lately received an addition of two hundred and twenty-five free sittings, towards defraying the expense of which the Incorporated Society for the enlargement of churches and chapels granted £100: the tower, though low, is handsome, and is ornamented with a very splendid clock, recently put up. There are places of worship for Baptists, Independents, and Unitarians. A National school, in which two hundred children are educated, is endowed, according to the return of the Commissioners for inquiring into charities, with £30 per annum, the rent of a pew in the church, bequeathed by John Hutcher in 1816. In a school adjoining the church-yard, six poor children are instructed, by means of a benefaction of £60 left by Thomas Neale; and there is a school for twenty boys and twenty girls, endowed with a rent-charge of £17. 6. 8. bequeathed by Richard Porter, Esq. There are eight almshouses belonging to the parish, in which are fourteen poor widows, who have a small weekly allowance; and a few other benefactions have been made for different purposes.

HALEWOOD, a township in the parish of CHILDWALL, hundred of WEST DERBY, county palatine of LANCASTER, 6 miles (S.) from Prescot, containing 934 inhabitants.

HALFORD, a chapelry in the parish of BROMFIELD, hundred of MUNSLOW, county of SALOP, 8¼ miles (N.W. by N.) from Ludlow, containing 51 inhabitants.

HALFORD, or HALFORD-BRIDGE, a parish in the Kington division of the hundred of KINGTON, county of WARWICK, 4 miles (N.) from Shipston upon Stour, containing 313 inhabitants. The living is a rectory, in the archdeaconry and diocese of Worcester, rated in the king's books at £10. 9. 9½, and in the patronage of the Bishop of Worcester. The church is dedicated to St. Mary.

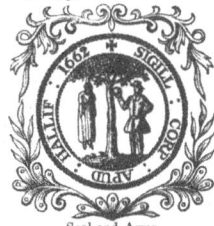

Seal and Arms.

HALIFAX, a parish in the wapentake of MORLEY, West riding of the county of YORK, comprising the market town of Halifax, the chapelries of Elland with Greetland, Heptonstall, Rastrick, and Sowerby, and the townships of Barkisland, Erringden, Fixby, Hipperholme with Brighouse, Langfield, Midgley, Norland, Ovenden, North Ouram, South Ouram, Rishworth, Shelf, Skircoat, Soyland, Stainland, Stansfield, Wadsworth, and Warley, and containing 93,850 inhabitants, of which number, 12,628 are in the town of Halifax, 42 miles (S.W.) from York, and 197 (N.N.W.) from London, on the road between those two cities. This town, though now of great magnitude and importance, is not of great antiquity; its name is not found in Domesday-book, nor is it mentioned in any ancient record before the early part of the twelfth century, when its church was granted by William, Earl of Warren, then lord of the manor, to the priory of Lewes, in Sussex. The name is supposed to have been derived from *Hali fax*, according to some signifying the holy face, in allusion to a relic called the face of St. John, preserved in a hermitage, which anciently occupied the site of the present church; or, as others think, implying the holy ways, in reference to the roads leading to the hermitage; for *fax*, in Nor-

man French, is an old plural noun denoting highways. The woollen manufacture, for which the town and neighbourhood have been distinguished for ages, prevailed so early as the year 1414, though on a very limited scale, and continued to increase from that period to 1540, during which the number of houses was gradually augmented from fifteen to five hundred and twenty. The manufacturers in the Spanish Netherlands seeking refuge from the persecutions with which they were assailed under the government of the Duke of Alva, repaired in great numbers to England, and many of them are supposed to have settled at Halifax; a conjecture which derives strength from the similarity of dialect existing between the labouring classes here and in the Low Countries, particularly Friesland. In 1642, during the great civil war, the town was garrisoned by the forces of the parliament, and the inhabitants seem to have been strongly attached to their cause. At that period an obstinate engagement took place on Halifax bank, adjoining the road to Wakefield, from which the place still retains the name of Blood Field: there are also, in different parts of the parish, vestiges of intrenchments; and tradition states it to have been the scene of various skirmishes.

For many ages a mode of trial and execution, styled the Gibbet Law, existed in the Forest of Hardwick, which was co-extensive with the parish of Halifax. The inhabitants within this forest had a custom, observed from time immemorial, that if a felon were taken within their liberty, with goods stolen either out of or within the liberty of the said forest, of the value of thirteen-pence halfpenny, he should, after three markets, or meeting-days, within the town of Halifax, next after such apprehension, be tried, and if condemned, be taken to the gibbet and have his head cut off. The following is the process of the gibbet-law: when the felon was apprehended he was immediately brought before the lord's bailiff, at Halifax, who kept the common gaol in the town, had the custody of the axe, and was the legal executioner. The bailiff then issued his summons to the constables of four several townships within the liberty, to require four frith-burgesses within each to appear before him on a certain day, to examine into the truth of the charge. At the trial the accuser and the accused were confronted before this unsworn jury, and the goods stolen were produced. If the accused party was acquitted, he was instantly liberated; if condemned, he was either executed immediately, if that was the principal market day, or placed in the stocks on the less meeting-days, with the stolen goods on his back, if portable, otherwise they were placed before him. The last executions took place in 1650, forty-nine delinquents having suffered during the preceding century; and after that period the custom was disused. The gibbet, of which some remains may still be seen at the gaol, appears to have been an engine very similar to the guillotine used in France after the Revolution.

The town is nearly three quarters of a mile in length, from east to west, but narrow and very irregular; in general it is well built, partly of brick, but principally of stone, which is very abundant in the neighbourhood. It is situated on the south-eastern declivity of a gentle eminence, but being enclosed by a chain of hills, which stretches from east to south, it seems, on being approached in that direction, to lie in a deep valley. From the boundary of Lancashire to the valley which separates the townships of Halifax and Ovenden from North Ouram, the whole substratum of the parish is grit-stone. Immediately to the east of this valley, argillaceous strata, with their general concomitants, stone and iron, appear; and to this cause, added to the abundant supply of fuel, and the rapid descent of its numerous brooks, so important in manufactures before the introduction of the steam-engine, the vicinity of Halifax is greatly indebted for its wealth and population. The parish is the largest in England, including an area of one hundred and twenty-four square miles, or seventy-nine thousand two hundred acres. The town is abundantly supplied with pure water, lighted with gas, and paved throughout. The theatre, built by subscription, is neat and commodious; and the dramatic performances take place in the months of January, February, and March. The new assembly-rooms, recently erected by subscription, are handsome, and the interior is finished with considerable taste, and with due regard to comfort: subscription assemblies are held at stated periods during the winter season: attached to the rooms are a public library, news-room, &c. There are also public baths, in a delightful valley a short distance from the road to Huddersfield, affording every accommodation for warm and cold bathing, and for swimming.

The principal articles of manufacture in the town and neighbourhood are shalloons, tammies, duroys, calimancoes, everlastings, moreens, shags, kerseys, baizes, woollen cloth (narrow and broad), coatings, and carpets. Several mills have also been erected in connexion with the cotton manufacture, which is rapidly increasing; and wool cards of superior quality are made in the neighbourhood, which abounds with coal mines and freestone quarries, the produce of the latter being shipped in considerable quantities to the metropolis. The Rochdale canal affords a medium of communication with Liverpool, Manchester, and the western district; and the Calder navigation with Hull and the eastern district. The market, which is one of the best in the north of England, is on Saturday; and there are two annual fairs for live stock, viz., on the 24th of June, and the first Saturday in November. The piece-hall, erected a few years ago by the manufacturers, is a large quadrangular building of freestone, occupying an area of ten thousand square yards, with a rustic basement story, and two upper stories, fronted with two interior colonnades, which are spacious walks leading to arched rooms, where goods in an unfinished state are deposited, and exhibited for sale to the merchants every Saturday, from ten to twelve o'clock: this structure, which was completed at an expense of £12,000, and opened on the 1st of January, 1779, unites elegance, convenience, and security; it contains three hundred and fifteen separate rooms, and is proof against fire.

This town was represented in two parliaments during the Commonwealth, but the privilege was withdrawn at the Restoration: it is governed by two constables, nominated by the inhabitants, and sworn in at the court leet of the lord of the manor of Wakefield, within which fee the town is situated. A court of requests is held under an act passed in the 33d of George III., for the recovery of debts under 40s., by the title of the "Court of Requests for the parishes of Halifax, Bradford, Keighley, Bingley, Guiseley, Calverley, Batley, Birstall, Mirfield, Hartshead cum Clifton, Almondbury, Kirkheaton,

Kirkburton, and Huddersfield, and the lordship or liberty of Tong, in the West riding of the county of York," with a reservation of the rights of the courts baron. The petty sessions for the wapentake of Morley are held here; and the magistrates attend at their office at Ward's End every Saturday, for the transaction of business relating to the district.

The living is a vicarage, in the archdeaconry and diocese of York, rated in the king's books at £84. 13. 6½., and in the patronage of the Crown. The present parish church, with the exception of part of the north wall, which appears to have been built in the time of Edward I., was erected between the years 1450 and 1470: it is a fine building in the later English style, having a nave, chancel, aisles, and two chapels, one founded by Archbishop Rokeby, who was sometime vicar of the parish, and the other by another vicar named Holdsworth: it has an embattled tower surmounted by eight pinnacles, and underneath the church, towards the east, is a crypt: the ceiling is adorned with the armorial bearings of all the incumbents, from the ordination of the vicarage, in 1274, to the present time, with those of the early benefactors to the church: several large handsome modern monuments adorn the interior. There are twelve chapels of ease in the parish, to which the vicar appoints the curates. A handsome new church of Grecian architecture was erected in 1798, by Dr. Coulthurst, then vicar, and dedicated to the Holy Trinity: the living is a perpetual curacy. Here are places of worship for Baptists, the Society of Friends, Independents, Wesleyan Methodists, and Unitarians.

The free grammar school, situated in Skircoat, was founded by letters patent of Queen Elizabeth, in 1585, under the superintendence of twelve governors selected from among the most respectable of the parishioners; they have the appointment of the head master and usher, the former of whom must have been a student for a period of five years at one of the Universities. The present school-house, with six acres of land contiguous to it, was given by Gilbert, Earl of Shrewsbury, Edward Savile, Esq., and Sir George Savile, Knt., in 1598; and several benefactions have since been added to the original endowment, among which is one by the Rev. Thomas Milner, who, by will in 1722, assigned to the Master and Fellows of St. Mary Magdalene's College, Cambridge, a reversionary grant of £1000, for founding three scholarships, for the benefit of the schools at Haversham, Leeds, and Halifax; and, in 1736, his sister added £200 for the same purpose. The master receives £80 per annum, out of which he pays an usher of his own appointment. A Blue-coat hospital was founded pursuant to the will of Nathaniel Waterhouse, in 1642, for twenty poor children, who are maintained, educated, and trained up to some useful employment, by an overseer, or master: the same benefactor founded an almshouse for twelve poor and infirm widows, to be chosen out of the town and parish of Halifax. The property left for the support of this charity produces £1181. 3. 4. per annum, out of which the schoolmaster receives about £80, the almswomen £2 each, and about £50 is expended annually in clothing the women and children; £40 per annum is applied to the augmentation of the stipends of the ministers of the chapels within the parish, and the surplus, after some deductions for other specific purposes, is paid to the master and governors of the workhouse, for the benefit of the poor. A school-house was erected in 1726, by John Smyth, Esq., of Heath, who settled an annual stipend on the school-master for teaching six poor children ; and subsequent benefactions having raised the income to £18. 16. per annum, the number of scholars has been aug-mented. There are also schools on the National and Lancasterian plans. Almshouses were founded in 1610, by Ellen Hopkinson and Jane Crowther (sisters), for eighteen poor widows of the town of Halifax, and one master to teach a certain number of poor children : these have been rebuilt, with the addition of six more rooms. Jane Crowther also, by will dated January 18th, 1613, gave a rent-charge of £8, for teaching poor children, but this design has been frustrated. There are also several institutions for the relief of the sick and destitute, among which are the dispensary, afford-ing medical and surgical aid; and the Benevolent Society, for the distribution of food and clothing to the poor. The workhouse was originally established by Nathaniel Waterhouse, in 1635, and thirteen of the most respectable inhabitants of the town were incorpo-rated by charter of Charles I., to superintend its concerns: this house being found inconvenient for the purpose of putting children to spin worsted, and make bone-lace, a new one was purchased in the year 1700, and from 1707 to 1720 the old house was used as a sessions-house by the magistrates for the West riding ; after which it was thoroughly repaired and restored to its original purpose. Several remains of British and Danish an-tiquities have, at different times, been discovered in the parish. About half a century ago, a countryman dig-ging peat on Mixenden-moor, near Halifax, struck his spade through a black polished stone, near which lay a most beautiful brass celt, in excellent preservation, four arrow-heads of black flint, a light battle-axe of a beau-tiful green pebble, and a hollow gouge, or scoop, of hard grey stone, evidently intended for the excavation of wooden vessels: the last is unique, and the whole seems to have formed part of the armour of a British soldier, who perished, perhaps two thousand years ago, among these wastes, where all remains of the body, together with the handles of the weapons, had long been entirely de-stroyed. Among the renowned characters who were born in this parish may be enumerated Henry Briggs, an emi-nent mathematician, whose discoveries relative to logarithms, born at Warley about 1556 ; Archbishop Tillotson, born in 1630, at Haughend, in the township of Sowerby, where his father was a considerable clo-thier ; Sir Henry Savile, one of the most accomplished scholars of the seventeenth century, born at Bradley, in the township of Stainland ; and Dr. David Hartley, a celebrated metaphysical writer, born in 1705, at Illing-worth, in the township of Ovenden. Daniel Defoe, the author of Robinson Crusoe ; and Sir William Herschel, the celebrated astronomer, were residents at Halifax, the latter having been organist in the church.

HALLAM (KIRK), a parish partly in the hundred of APPLETREE, and partly in the hundred of MOR-LESTON and LITCHURCH, county of DERBY, 8¾ miles (E. N. E.) from Derby, containing, with the township of Mapperley, which is in the hundred of Appletree, 433 inhabitants. The living is a discharged vicarage, in the archdeaconry of Derby, and diocese of Lichfield and Coventry, rated in the king's books at £4. 9. 7., endowed

with £600 royal bounty, and in the patronage of the Duke of Rutland. The church, which is dedicated to All Saints, is in the hundred of Morleston and Litchurch.

HALLAM (NETHER), a township in that part of the parish of SHEFFIELD which is in the southern division of the wapentake of STRAFFORTH and TICK-HILL, West riding of the county of YORK, 2 miles (W.) from Sheffield, containing 3200 inhabitants. A school-room was erected many years ago at Upper Keely, by sub-scription among the inhabitants, who also purchased land towards its support ; the annual income, including the proceeds of £150 bequeathed by Thomas, Chapman in 1801, is about £18, for which sum eighteen children are instructed. Another school-room was erected by subscription in 1791, with a dwelling-house for the master ; it is partly supported by means of a bequest of £100 from William Roncksley, in 1723, and partly from land allotted under the enclosure act in 1794 ; thirty children are taught to read in the school.

HALLAM (UPPER), a township in that part of the parish of SHEFFIELD which is in the southern divi-sion of the wapentake of STRAFFORTH and TICKHILL, West riding of the county of YORK, 3¾ miles (W.S.W.) from Sheffield, containing 1018 inhabitants.

HALLAM (WEST), a parish in the hundred of MORLESTON and LITCHURCH, county of DERBY, 8 miles (N. E. by E.) from Derby, containing 706 inhabitants. The living is a discharged rectory, in the archdeaconry of Derby, and diocese of Lichfield and Coventry, rated in the king's books at £8, and in the patronage of Francis Newdigate, Esq. The church is dedicated to St. Wilfrid. The Rev. John Scargill, in 1662, bequeath-ed £540 for the erection and endowment of a free school: the annual income is about £174, of which the master receives £60 for teaching fifty-eight children, who are each paid ninepence per week out of the same fund, according to the directions of the testator. There is a mineral spring, the water of which is similar in its qualities to the Harrogate water. A canal has been recently cut along part of the boundary of the parish, where there is a coal wharf in connexion with a neigh-bouring colliery.

HALLATON, a parish (formerly a market town) in the hundred of GARTREE, county of LEICESTER, 7 miles (N. E. by N.) from Market-Harborough, and 90 (N.N.W.) from London, containing 664 inhabitants. The name is supposed by some to be a corruption of Hollow-town, in allusion to its being situated in a valley, or hollow spot ; by others it is derived from Holy town. The market-cross is still standing, but the market has not been held within the memory of the present inhabitants. An attempt was made to revive it in 1767, which proved abortive, owing in a great measure to the badness of the roads, which were then nearly impassable in winter. Fairs are held for cattle on Holy Thursday, and on the third Thursday after it. The living is a rectory, in the archdeaconry of Lei-cester, and diocese of Lincoln, formerly in medieties, which were united in 1728 : the north mediety is rated in the king's books at £18. 13. 4., and the south mediety at £17. 6. 8. : it is held with the annexed donative of Blaston St. Michael, and is in the alternate patronage of the Rev. Calverley John Bewicke, and the Rev. George Ouseley Fenwicke. The church, dedicated to St. Michael, is a large and handsome edifice, consisting of a nave, aisles, chancel, and a western tower, with a spire: the aisles are of the same height with the nave, and lighted by fine large windows, decorated with mullions and elaborate tracery: it contains an ancient square font, supported by columns ornamented with grotesque heads. There is a place of worship for Baptists. A charity school has an endowment of £20 per annum, arising from different benefactions; and there are several charitable bequests for annual distribution among the poor.

On the western side of the town, at the distance of a mile, is the site of an ancient fortress, called Hallaton Castle hill: the most conspicuous part of the remains is a conical eminence, one hundred and eighteen feet high, and six hundred and thirty feet in circumference, on which stood the keep, occupying, with the outworks, about two acres of ground. About a quarter of a mile south-west of this spot are traces of another fortress of nearly the same extent. A battle is said to have been fought near this town, and these vestiges lend countenance to the tradition, as also does the name of Blood-wood, affixed to a neighbouring spot. Hallaton is distinguished by a singular annual custom which is thus described: on every Easter Monday the inhabitants meet on a piece of ground which was bequeathed to the use and benefit of the rector, who then provides two hare pies, a quantity of ale, and two dozen of penny loaves, to be scrambled for. Attempts have been made to put down this custom, and appropriate the bequest to charitable purposes; but so attached are the inhabitants to it, that these efforts have always failed, and on one occasion a riot was the result.

HALL-GARTH, a township in the parish of PITTINGTON, southern division of EASINGTON ward, county palatine of DURHAM, containing 304 inhabitants.

HALLING, a parish in the hundred of SHAMWELL, lathe of AYLESFORD, county of KENT, 4¾ miles (S.W.) from Rochester, containing 346 inhabitants. The living is a vicarage, in the archdeaconry and diocese of Rochester, rated in the king's books at £7. 13. 4., and in the patronage of the Dean and Chapter of Rochester. The church, dedicated to St. John the Baptist, is principally in the early style of English architecture, with a low western tower and spire. The river Medway runs through, and a ridge of hills extends quite across, the parish. The bishops of Rochester had a palace here before the Conquest: it was rebuilt some time in the twelfth century, and additions made to it about the year 1320; the remains are considerable, and the walls of the chapel nearly entire.

HALLINGBURY (GREAT), a parish in the hundred of HARLOW, county of ESSEX, 2 miles (S.E. by E.) from Bishop's Stortford, containing 678 inhabitants. The living is a rectory, in the archdeaconry of Middlesex, and diocese of London, rated in the king's books at £22. J. A. Houblon, Esq. was patron in 1812. A school is supported by annual donations of about £8.

HALLINGBURY (LITTLE), a parish in the hundred of HARLOW, county of ESSEX, 4¼ miles (N.N.E.) from Harlow, containing 470 inhabitants. The living is a rectory, in the jurisdiction of the Commissary of Essex and Herts, concurrently with the Consistory Court of the Bishop of London, rated in the king's books at £15, and in the patronage of the Governors of the Charterhouse, London. The church is dedicated to St. Mary.

HALLINGTON, a parish in the Wold division of the hundred of LOUTH-ESKE, parts of LINDSEY, county of LINCOLN, 2 miles (S.W. by W.) from Louth, containing 75 inhabitants. The living is a vicarage with Raithby, in the archdeaconry and diocese of Louth-Eske, rated in the king's books at £17. 1. 8. The church is dedicated to St. Lawrence.

HALLINGTON, a township in the parish of ST. JOHN LEE, southern division of TINDALE ward, county of NORTHUMBERLAND, 11 miles (N.N.E.) from Hexham, containing 129 inhabitants. On an eminence called the Mote-Law is a square intrenchment, with a hearth-stone in the centre, on which beacon fires were formerly kindled.

HALLIWELL, a township in the parish of DEAN, hundred of SALFORD, county palatine of LANCASTER, 1¾ mile (N.W.) from Great Bolton, containing 2288 inhabitants. Here are extensive bleaching-works.

HALLOUGHTON, a parish in that part of the liberty of SOUTHWELL and SCROOBY which separates the northern from the southern division of the wapentake of THURGARTON, county of NOTTINGHAM, 1¼ mile (S.S.W) from Southwell, containing 101 inhabitants. The living is a perpetual curacy, endowed with £1000 royal bounty, and in the peculiar jurisdiction and patronage of the Prebendary of Halloughton in the Collegiate Church of Southwell. The chapel is dedicated to St. James.

HALLOW, a chapelry in the parish of GRIMLEY, lower division of the hundred of OSWALDSLOW, county of WORCESTER, 3 miles (N.N.W.) from Worcester, containing 1081 inhabitants. The chapel is partly of Norman architecture, and partly in the early English style, with a belfry of wood and plaister, the tower having been demolished: it has lately received an addition of two hundred free sittings, the Incorporated Society for the enlargement of churches and chapels having granted £200 towards defraying the expense. The navigable river Severn runs along the eastern boundary of the chapelry. Here is a chalybeate spring.

HALLOWICKS, a hamlet in the parish of MEDMENHAM, hundred of DESBOROUGH, county of BUCKINGHAM. The population is returned with the parish. Here was formerly a chapel, which has been demolished.

HALLYSTONE, a parish in the western division of COQUETDALE ward, county of NORTHUMBERLAND, comprising the townships of Barrow, Dueshill, Hallystone, Harbottle, and Linsheeles, and containing 468 inhabitants, of which number, 132 are in the township of Hallystone, 7 miles (W. by N.) from Rothbury. The living is a perpetual curacy, annexed to that of Allenton in 1311, in the archdeaconry of Northumberland, and diocese of Durham. The church is dedicated to St. Mary. Near it are the foundations of an ancient priory, built by one of the Umfravilles, of Harbottle castle, for Benedictine nuns: the revenue, at the dissolution, was estimated at £15. 10. 8. There are also the remains of an old castle, which, for its singular strength, was used as a place of security before the union of the two kingdoms, and in which it is said a princess was born, from whom sprang the present royal family. On the southern bank of the Coquet, which runs through the parish, are vestiges of an old edifice called Barrow-Peel; and a little to the westward is Ridlee cairn hill, both supposed to have been cemeteries of the ancient Britons. Poised on the summit of a lofty hill, near which is a lake called Harbottle loch, is a large stone, called the Drake stone. There is a fine basin of water, called Lady's Well, beautifully variegated at the bottom with green and white sand, and encircled by a wall of hewn stone. On the introduction of Christianity into Northumbria, it appears that about three thousand persons were baptized at this place by Paulinus.

HALMER-END, a liberty in the parish of AUDLEY, northern division of the hundred of PIREHILL, county of STAFFORD, containing 553 inhabitants.

HALSALL, a parish in the hundred of WEST DERBY, county palatine of LANCASTER, comprising the chapelries of Lydiate, Maghull, and Melling, and the townships of Down-Holland and Halsall, and containing 3538 inhabitants, of which number, 970 are in the township of Halsall, 3 miles (W.N.W.) from Ormskirk. The living is a rectory, in the archdeaconry and diocese of Chester, rated in the king's books at £24. 11. 5½. The Misses Blundel were patronesses in 1816. The church, dedicated to St. Cuthbert, has portions in the decorated and later styles of English architecture, and a lofty spire. In the church-yard is a school-house, erected in 1595, by Edward Halsall, who bequeathed a rent-charge of £13. 6. 8. for its maintenance as a free grammar school for twelve boys. The Leeds and Liverpool canal passes through the parish. A bituminous turf, called Litturf, is found in Halsall moss, which burns like a candle.

HALSE, a hamlet in the parish of ST. PETER, borough of BRACKLEY, hundred of KING'S SUTTON, county of NORTHAMPTON, 2¾ miles (N.W. by N.) from Brackley. The population is returned with the parish. Here was formerly a chapel dedicated to St. Andrew, which has been demolished.

HALSE, a parish in the hundred of WILLITON and FREEMANNERS, though locally in the western division of the hundred of Kingsbury, county of SOMERSET, 4 miles (E.) from Wiveliscombe, containing 447 inhabitants. The living is a discharged vicarage, in the archdeaconry of Taunton, and diocese of Bath and Wells, rated in the king's books at £5. 19. 7., endowed with £600 private benefaction, £400 royal bounty, and £300 parliamentary grant. Sir J. Langham, Bart. was patron in 1793. The church is dedicated to St. James.

HALSHAM, a parish in the southern division of the wapentake of HOLDERNESS, East riding of the county of YORK, 6 miles (E. by S.) from Hedon, containing 315 inhabitants. The living is a rectory, in the archdeaconry of the East riding, and diocese of York, rated in the king's books at £13. 6. 8., and in the patronage of Sir T. Constable, Bart. The church is dedicated to All Saints: on an eminence near it is a neat mausoleum, built of white freestone faced with polished marble, having in the centre a beautiful monument to the memory of the late Sir William Constable, whose remains lie here, surrounded by those of his ancestors. Sir John Constable, in 1579, bequeathed a rent-charge of £80, for one thousand years, which was confirmed and vested in certain trustees by patent of Elizabeth, in 1584, for the purposes of a free school for eight poor children, and an hospital for eight men and two women of the parish; and to which Dame Catherine Constable added £6. 13. 4. a year, for putting out apprentices, and £10 annually for the maintenance at Trinity College, Oxford, for a term of seven years, and so on in succession, of one scholar educated here.

HALSTEAD, a market town and parish in the hundred of HINCKFORD, county of ESSEX, 17¼ miles (N.N.E.) from Chelmsford, and 47 (N. E.) from London, containing 3858 inhabitants. This town is situated on the river Colne, and on the high road from London to Norwich, through Bury-St. Edmund's : it is neither lighted nor paved, and is supplied with water from springs. In the reign of Elizabeth, the French Protestants being violently persecuted in their own country, many of them fled to England, and settling at Halstead and Colchester, introduced the manufacture of baize and says, now discontinued. A large silk-mill was erected a few years since on the site of a flour-mill, at which a considerable number of children is employed, and the trade is in a flourishing state. A market for corn is held on Friday; and there are cattle fairs on May 6th and October 29th. Courts leet and baron are held about once a year, by the lord of the manor; and the petty sessions for the division of South Hinckford are held here every Friday. There is a house of correction, in which a tread-mill has been erected. The living is a vicarage, in the peculiar jurisdiction of the Commissary of Essex and Herts, concurrently with the Consistorial Court of the Bishop of London, rated in the king's books at £17, and in the patronage of the Bishop of London. The church, dedicated to St. George, is a spacious edifice, chiefly in the later English style, except the chancel, which is decorated; and the spire is constructed of wood, in place of one destroyed by lightning about eighty years ago. It probably belonged to a college of priests, founded here in the 14th of Edward IV., the revenue of which, at the dissolution, was £26. 5. 8. Here are places of worship for Baptists, the Society of Friends, and Independents. A free grammar school was founded by Lady Ramsey, in 1594, for the education of forty children belonging to the parishes of Halstead and Colne-Engaine, and endowed with a rent-charge of £20 and a house for the master, under the patronage of the Governors of Christ's Hospital, London. Mr. Martin, in 1573, left lands producing £130 per annum; and Mrs. Holmes, in 1783, left £4000 three per cents., for the benefit of the poor of this parish. Thomas Bourchier, Archbishop of Canterbury in the reign of Edward IV., a distinguished patron of literature, was a native of Halstead.

Arms.

HALSTEAD, a parish in the hundred of CODSHEATH, lathe of SUTTON at HONE, county of KENT, 5¼ miles (N.W. by N.) from Seven Oaks, containing 243 inhabitants. The living is a rectory, in the peculiar jurisdiction and patronage of the Archbishop of Canterbury, rated in the king's books at £5. 17. 11. The church, dedicated to St. Margaret, was rebuilt, and a handsome chapel added to the north side, by the lord of the manor, in 1609; the windows of the latter were richly ornamented with stained glass, but most of it has been destroyed. There are places of worship for Baptists and Independents.

HALSTEAD, a township in that part of the parish of TILTON which is in the eastern division of the hundred of GOSCOTE, county of LEICESTER, 7¾ miles (W. S.W.) from Oakham, containing 187 inhabitants. There is a place of worship for Wesleyan Methodists.

HALSTOCK, a parish and liberty in the Sherborne division of the county of DORSET, 6½ miles (N.E. by N.) from Beaminster, containing 447 inhabitants. The living is a perpetual curacy, annexed to the vicarage of Lyme-Regis, in the peculiar jurisdiction of the Prebendary of Lyme and Halstock in the Cathedral Church of Salisbury, endowed with £400 royal bounty, and £200 parliamentary grant. The church is dedicated to St. Mary.

HALSTON, an extra-parochial liberty, in the hundred of OSWESTRY, county of SALOP, 3½ miles (E.N.E.) from Oswestry, containing 39 inhabitants. There is a domestic chapel belonging to John Mytton, Esq., who appoints the minister. The Ellesmere canal touches on the boundary of the liberty, which is crossed by a small stream called the Perry; this, by a diversion of its channel, has been made to resemble a large river, called Halston Pool, covering about forty acres. The Knights Templars had a preceptory here, dedicated to the Blessed Virgin Mary, which subsequently belonged to the hospitallers, and was valued, in the 26th of Henry VIII., at £160. 14. 10. per annum : in the reign of Mary it was re-granted to the order of St. John of Jerusalem, and in that of her successor Elizabeth it was possessed by William Horne.

HALSTOW (HIGH), a parish in the hundred of Hoo, lathe of AYLESFORD, county of KENT, 5¾ miles (N. N. E.) from Rochester, containing 350 inhabitants. The living is a rectory, in the archdeaconry and diocese of Rochester, rated in the king's books at £14. 5. 7½., and in the patronage of the Rev. B. Burt. The church is dedicated to St. Margaret.

HALSTOW (LOWER), a parish in the hundred of MILTON, lathe of SCRAY, county of KENT, 4 miles (W. N. W.) from Milton, containing 220 inhabitants. The living is a discharged vicarage, in the archdeaconry and diocese of Canterbury, rated in the king's books at £8. 2., and in the patronage of the Dean and Chapter of Canterbury. The church is dedicated to St. Margaret. Halstow is situated at the upper end of Stangate creek, by which it has a communication with the Medway a little above Sheerness. Here vessels from foreign countries, that cannot produce clean bills of health, are compelled to perform quarantine, and to remove their cargoes into two large vessels, called Lazarettos, constantly stationed for the purpose of receiving them. The road from Chatham to Sheerness, by King's ferry, crosses the creek at a ford called the Stray, south of the church. It is stated that several ships and boats belonged to this place in the reign of Elizabeth.

HALTHAM upon BAIN, a parish in the soke of HORNCASTLE, parts of LINDSEY, county of LINCOLN, 5¼ miles (S. by W.) from Horncastle, containing 196 inhabitants. The living is a discharged rectory, with which the rectory of Roughton was united in 1741, in the archdeaconry and diocese of Lincoln, rated in the king's books at £8. 11. 3., and in the patronage of the Hon. J. Dymoke. The church is dedicated to St. Benedict. The Horncastle canal, upon which two steam-vessels ply daily between Lincoln and Boston, passes through the parish.

HALTON, a parish in the hundred of AYLESBURY,

county of BUCKINGHAM, 2 miles (N. by E.) from Wendover, containing 195 inhabitants. The living is a rectory, in the peculiar jurisdiction of the Archbishop of Canterbury, rated in the king's books at £13. 6. 8. Sir. J. D. King, Bart. was patron in 1826. The church is dedicated to St. Michael.

HALTON, a chapelry (formerly a market town) in the parish of RUNCORN, hundred of BUCKLOW, county palatine of CHESTER, 3½ miles (N. N. E.) from Frodsham, containing 1066 inhabitants. The living is a perpetual curacy, in the archdeaconry and diocese of Chester, endowed with £600 private benefaction, and £600 royal bounty, and in the patronage of Sir. R. Brooke, Bart. The church is dedicated to St. Mary. The Mersey and Irwell canal, and the Duke of Bridgewater's canal, pass through the parish. Halton was given by Hugh Lupus, Earl of Chester, to his cousin Nigel, with the constablery of Chester, the earl at the same time making him his marshal : these great offices of constable of Chester and earl marshal were attached to the barony, and enjoyed by his successors the barons of Halton, who, amongst other privileges granted them by the earls, were authorised to have a castle and a prison at Halton, to hold a weekly market and two annual fairs, a court for the cognizance of various offences, and for all pleas and actions within the barony, except such as belonged to the earl's sword, and to have a master-serjeant and eight under serjeants within their fee. The castle was built soon after the Norman Conquest, on the brow of a hill commanding a very extensive prospect over a great part of Cheshire, and across the Mersey into Lancashire. Among its various distinguished possessors may be mentioned John of Gaunt, Duke of Lancaster, with whom it was a favourite residence. It was garrisoned for the king in the early part of 1643, and for the parliament in 1644. There are few remains of its ancient buildings : the habitable part of it, which appears to have been chiefly rebuilt since the civil war, has been fitted up as an inn : there is a room in which the courts for the honour are held. A charity school is endowed with about £20 per annum, arising from various benefactions. An almshouse for six poor persons was founded, in 1767, by Pusey Brooke, Esq., and endowed with £54. 12. per annum.

HALTON, a parish in the hundred of LONSDALE, south of the sands, county palatine of LANCASTER, 2½ miles (N.E. by N.) from Lancaster, containing, with the chapelry of Aughton, 1027 inhabitants. The living is a rectory, rated in the king's books at £20. 0. 7½., and in the peculiar jurisdiction and patronage of Robert Fletcher Bradshaw, Esq., as lord of the manor. Thomas Withers, in 1747, gave certain property, now producing about £14. 10. a year, for the instruction of eight children.

HALTON, a chapelry in the parish of CORBRIDGE, eastern division of TINDALE ward, county of NORTHUMBERLAND, 5 miles (N. E. by E.) from Hexham, containing 60 inhabitants. The chapel was rebuilt in 1706, principally by the subscriptions of John Douglas, Esq. and the freeholders of Whittingham : near it is Halton Tower, an ancient building crowned with four turrets, on the north side of which the remains of a much larger building may be traced.

HALTON (EAST), a parish in the eastern division of the wapentake of YARBOROUGH, parts of LINDSEY, county of LINCOLN, 7½ miles (E. by S.) from Barton upon Humber, containing 468 inhabitants. The living is a discharged vicarage, in the archdeaconry and diocese of Lincoln, rated in the king's books at £7. 18. 4., endowed with £600 royal bounty. Lord Yarborough was patron in 1792. The church is dedicated to St. Peter. There is a place of worship for Wesleyan Methodists.

HALTON (EAST), a township in that part of the parish of SKIPTON which is in the eastern division of the wapentake of STAINCLIFFE and EWCROSS, West riding of the county of YORK, 4 miles (N. E. by E.) from Skipton, containing, with Bolton, 141 inhabitants.

HALTON (WEST), a parish in the northern division of the wapentake of MANLEY, parts of LINDSEY, county of LINCOLN, 8½ miles (W.) from Barton upon Humber, containing, with the hamlet of Gunhouse, 374 inhabitants. The living is a rectory, in the archdeaconry of Stow, and diocese of Lincoln, rated in the king's books at £16, and in the patronage of the Bishop of Norwich. The church is dedicated to St. Ethelreda.

HALTON (WEST), a township in that part of the parish of ARNCLIFFE which is in the western division of the wapentake of STAINCLIFFE and EWCROSS, West riding of the county of YORK, 7 miles (S. by E.) from Settle, containing 190 inhabitants.

HALTON-GILL, a chapelry in that part of the parish of ARNCLIFFE which is in the western division of the wapentake of STAINCLIFFE and EWCROSS, West riding of the county of YORK, 11½ miles (N. E. by N.) from Settle, containing 114 inhabitants. The living is a perpetual curacy, in the archdeaconry and diocese of York, endowed with £400 royal bounty, and £200 parliamentary grant, and in the patronage of the Vicar of Arncliffe. A school was erected in 1630, by William Fawcett, and endowed by him with an annuity of £13. 6. 8., for the instruction of poor children.

HALTON-HOLEGATE, a parish in the eastern division of the soke of BOLINGBROKE, parts of LINDSEY, county of LINCOLN, 1½ mile (E. S. E.) from Spilsby, containing 460 inhabitants. The living is a rectory, in the archdeaconry and diocese of Lincoln, rated in the king's books at £16. 17. 11. Mr. and Mrs. Burrell were patrons in 1779. The church is dedicated to St. Andrew.

HALTON-SHIELDS, a township in the parish of CORBRIDGE, eastern division of TINDALE ward, county of NORTHUMBERLAND, 7 miles (N. E. by E.) from Hexham, containing 57 inhabitants. It is situated on the line of the great Roman wall, to the eastward of the station called *Hunnum*, or Halton-Chesters, and anciently garrisoned by the *Ala Saviniana*, the walls, ditches, and interior offices of which now appear in confused heaps of ruins : within its area several inscriptions have been found, together with copper coins, stags' horns, and a quantity of muscle shells ; and in 1803 a ring of pure gold, weighing somewhat less than half an ounce, was discovered in the neighbourhood.

HALTWHISTLE, a parish in the western division of TINDALE ward, county of NORTHUMBERLAND, comprising the market town of Haltwhistle, and the townships of Bellester, Blenkinsop, East Coanwood, Featherston, Hartley-Burn, Henshaw, Melkridge, Plainmellor, Ridley, Thirlwall, Thorngrafton, and Wall-Town, and containing 3583 inhabitants, of which number, 707 are in the town of Haltwhistle, 36 miles (W.) from Newcastle, and 315 (N. N. W.) from London. This town, formerly called Haltwesel, is pleasantly situated on the high road from Carlisle to Newcastle, on an eminence which commands a rich and extensive prospect of the surrounding country, and of the windings of the river Tyne through its fertile vale. The buildings are irregular, and there are but few good houses ; the streets are neither paved nor lighted, but the inhabitants are plentifully supplied with water from wells, and from brooks which are situated northward from the town. The only branch of manufacture is one of coarse baize, recently introduced. A market, in which grain is sold, is occasionally held on Thursday ; and the fairs are on the 14th of May and the 22nd of November, chiefly for cattle; those on the 12th of May and the 11th of November are statute fairs. The living is a vicarage, in the archdeaconry of Northumberland, and diocese of Durham, rated in the king's books at £12. 3. 1½., and in the patronage of the Bishop of Durham. The church, which is dedicated to the Holy Cross, stands on an eminence southward from the town ; from the church-yard there is a beautiful and extensive prospect. Here are places of worship for Primitive Methodists and Presbyterians. A charity school was founded and endowed with £35 per annum, arising from lands at Faversham, in Kent, in the year 1719, by Dorothy Capel, Baroness Dowager of Tewkesbury : the number of boys at present is about eighty : the master receives a salary of £30 per annum, with a small quarterly payment from the scholars. The vicar of this parish allows £10 per annum to a schoolmaster at Greenhead, for instructing the children of labourers. On an eminence eastward of the church are the vestiges of a fort, environed on all sides but the south by an embankment of turf ; in the centre of the enclosure is a large spring, which from neglect has converted the place into a bog. In the township of Thirlwall are the remains of a castle, formerly one of the boundary forts between England and Scotland.

HALVERGATE, a parish in the hundred of WALSHAM, county of NORFOLK, 3¾ miles (S. S. E.) from Acle, containing 449 inhabitants. The living is a discharged vicarage, in the archdeaconry and diocese of Norwich, rated in the king's books at £5, and in the patronage of the Bishop of Ely. The church is dedicated to St. Peter and St. Paul.

HALWELL, a parish in the hundred of BLACK TORRINGTON, county of DEVON, 6½ miles (S. E. by E.) from Holsworthy, containing 216 inhabitants. The living is a rectory, in the archdeaconry of Totness, and diocese of Exeter, rated in the king's books at £12. 3. 9., and in the patronage of the Crown. Good freestone is obtained in the parish.

HALWELL, a parish in the hundred of COLERIDGE, county of DEVON, 5¼ miles (S. by W.) from Totness, containing 468 inhabitants. The living is a perpetual curacy, annexed to the vicarage of Harberton, in the archdeaconry of Totness, and diocese of Devon, and in the patronage of the Dean and Chapter of Exeter. The church is dedicated to St. Leonard.

HAM, a tything in the parish and upper division of the hundred of BERKELEY, county of GLOUCESTER, ¾ of a mile (S.) from Berkeley, containing, with the chapelry of Stone, 963 inhabitants.

HAM, a parish in the hundred of EASTRY, lathe of ST. AUGUSTINE, county of KENT, 2¾ miles (S.) from Sandwich, containing 26 inhabitants. The living is a rectory, in the archdeaconry and diocese of Canterbury, rated in the king's books at £5. 6. 5½., and in the patronage of the Crown. The church is dedicated to St. George. Ham is within the jurisdiction of a court of requests held at Deal, for the recovery of debts under 40s.

HAM, a tything in that part of the parish of BAUGHURST which is in the hundred of BARTON-STACEY, Andover division of the county of SOUTHAMPTON, 7¾ miles (N. W. by N.) from Basingstoke. The population is returned with the parish.

HAM, a hamlet in the parish of KINGSTON upon THAMES, first division of the hundred of KINGSTON, county of SURREY, 9½ miles (S. W. by W.) from London, containing, with Hatch, 961 inhabitants. This place, which is pleasantly situated between Kingston and Richmond, contains several handsome mansions and detached villas. There is a pleasure fair on the 29th of May and the two following days, which is much frequented. It is in contemplation to erect a chapel of ease in this hamlet. Here is a place of worship for Independents. Ham house, a noble mansion now belonging to the Countess of Dysart, is said to have been the place where the cabinet council of Charles II., called "the Cabal," held their meetings; and James II. was ordered by the Prince of Orange to retire to Ham house just before his flight to France in 1688.

HAM, a parish in the hundred of ELSTUB and EVERLEY, though locally in the hundred of Kinwardstone, county of WILTS, 3¾ miles (S.) from Hungerford, containing 171 inhabitants. The living is a rectory, in the archdeaconry of Wilts, and diocese of Salisbury, rated in the king's books at £12. 6. 8., and in the patronage of the Bishop of Winchester. The church is dedicated to All Saints.

HAM (EAST), a parish in the hundred of BECONTREE, county of ESSEX, 6 miles (E.) from London, containing 1424 inhabitants. The living is a vicarage, in the archdeaconry of Essex, and diocese of London, rated in the king's books at £14. 3. 9., and in the patronage of the Bishop of London. The church, dedicated to St. Mary Magdalene, is partly of Norman architecture. There is a place of worship for Wesleyan Methodists. The river Thames bounds the parish on the south-east, and Bow creek separates the counties of Essex and Middlesex on the west. An almshouse for three poor men was erected and endowed with £40 per annum, by Giles Breme, in 1621; besides which considerable benefactions have been made, for various charitable purposes, by the Latimer family and others. There is an old brick tower, fifty feet high, in the garden of Greensted house, said to have been built by Henry VIII., for Anna Boleyn. Dr. Stukeley, the celebrated antiquary, who died in 1765, is buried in the church-yard.

HAM (HIGH), a parish in the hundred of WHITLEY, county of SOMERSET, 3 miles (N.) from Langport, containing, with the chapelry of Low Ham, 953 inhabitants. The living is a rectory, in the archdeaconry of Wells, and diocese of Bath and Wells, rated in the king's books at £38. 19. 2., and in the patronage of the Provost and Fellows of Worcester College, Oxford. The church, dedicated to St. Andrew, is a large structure with an em-

battled tower at the west end: the body was erected in 1476, and the chancel in 1499. There is a place of worship for Wesleyan Methodists. The Rev. Adrian Schael, in 1578, gave £120, and in 1700 the Rev. Francis Osmenton gave £30, together producing £10 a year, for the instruction of twenty children. There is also a sum of money given by Lady Dionis Hext and Lord Stawell for apprenticing poor children.

HAM (LOW), a chapelry in the parish of HIGH HAM, hundred of WHITLEY, county of SOMERSET, 2 miles (N. by E.) from Langport. The population is returned with the parish.

HAM (WEST), a parish in the hundred of BECONTREE, county of ESSEX, 4 miles (E. by N.) from London, comprising the wards of All Saints, Church-street, Plaistow, and Stratford-Langthorne, and containing 9753 inhabitants. The living is a vicarage, in the archdeaconry of Essex, and diocese of London, rated in the king's books at £39. 8. 4., and in the patronage of the Crown. The church, dedicated to All Saints, is a spacious structure with a lofty tower at the west end, and contains some handsome monuments. A charity school was founded in 1723, for ten boys: the endowment having been afterwards greatly increased by various bequests, forty boys and twenty girls are now clothed, educated, and apprenticed. A school for clothing and educating forty poor girls has also been established, in pursuance of the will, dated in 1761, of Mrs. Sarah Bonnel, who left £3000 in the funds for that purpose. The West Ham water-works, on the river Lea, supply Stratford-Langthorne, Bromley, Bow, Stepney, Bethnal-Green, and the lower part of Whitechapel. At Stratford-Langthorne an abbey was founded by William de Montfichet, in 1135, for Cistercian monks, and dedicated to the Virgin Mary and All Saints. In the year 1307, the abbot was summoned to parliament, and, at the time of the dissolution of the greater religious houses, the revenue of the abbey was estimated at upwards of £650. Margaret, the unfortunate Countess of Salisbury, beheaded on a charge of high treason in the reign of Henry VIII., resided within the precincts of the abbey about the period of its dissolution. The principal remains are a brick gateway and an ornamented arch, about three furlongs south-west of the church. George Edwards, the natural historian, who died in 1773, was born at Stratford-Langthorne.

HAMBLE en le RICE, a parish in the hundred of MANSBRIDGE, Fawley division of the county of SOUTHAMPTON, 4¾ miles (S.E.) from Southampton, containing 421 inhabitants. The living is a perpetual curacy with the vicarage of Hound, in the archdeaconry and diocese of Winchester, endowed with £1000 royal bounty. The church is dedicated to St. Andrew. The parish is bounded on the south by Southampton water. An alien priory of Cistercian monks, a cell to the abbey of Tirone, in France, dedicated to St. Andrew, was founded here in the time of Henry Blois, Bishop of Winchester; at the suppression, it was granted to New College, Oxford.

HAMBLEDON, a parish in the hundred of DESBOROUGH, county of BUCKINGHAM, 4 miles (W.) from Great Marlow, containing 1281 inhabitants. The living is a rectory, in the archdeaconry of Buckingham, and diocese of Lincoln, rated in the king's books at £35, and in the patronage of Sir Matthew White Ridley, Bart.

The church, dedicated to St. Mary, is a handsome edifice, containing three stone stalls and a circular font richly ornamented, together with some interesting monuments. There is a place of worship for Independents. A small school is supported by trifling bequests from Augustine Varnell, in 1734, and the Rev. William Fairfax, in 1763. Here was formerly a market on Monday, granted in 1315, and a fair on the festival of St. Bartholomew, in 1321. Greenland-house, in this parish, was garrisoned for the king in May 1664, and, after sustaining a long and severe siege from the parliamentary army under Major General Brown, surrendered, having been reduced to a heap of ruins.

HAMBLEDON, a parish partly in the hundred of MEON-STOKE, but chiefly in the hundred of HAMBLE-DON, Portsdown division of the county of SOUTHAMP-TON, 6 miles (E.S.E.) from Bishop's Waltham, comprising the tythings of Hambledon, Chidden, Denmead, Earvils, and Glidden, and containing 1886 inhabitants. The living is a vicarage, rated in the king's books at £26. 19. 2., in the peculiar jurisdiction of the vicar, and in the patronage of the Bishop of Winchester. The church, dedicated to St. Peter, is partly in the early, and partly in the later, style of English architecture. Fairs for horses are held on February 18th, the first Tuesday in May, and October 22nd. Windmill-down, in this parish, is noted as being frequented by the cricket-players of Hampshire and the neighbouring counties.

HAMBLEDON, a parish in the first division of the hundred of GODALMING, county of SURREY, 3½ miles (S. by W.) from Godalming, containing 381 inhabitants. The living is a rectory, in the archdeaconry of Surrey, and diocese of Winchester, rated in the king's books at £6. 7. 11. The Earl of Radnor was patron in 1810. The church is dedicated to St. Peter.

HAMBLETON, a chapelry in the parish of KIRKHAM, hundred of AMOUNDERNESS, county palatine of LAN-CASTER, 2¾ miles (N.E.) from Poulton, containing 338 inhabitants. The living is a perpetual curacy, in the archdeaconry of Richmond, and diocese of Chester, endowed with £200 private benefaction, and £400 royal bounty, and in the patronage of the Vicar of Kirkham. Eight children are educated for a trifling sum, the bequest of Matthew Lewtas, in 1791.

HAMBLETON, a parish in the hundred of MARTINS-LEY, county of RUTLAND, 3 miles (E.S.E.) from Oakham, containing 308 inhabitants. The living is a vicarage, in the archdeaconry of Northampton, and diocese of Peterborough, rated in the king's books at £10.17.1., and in the patronage of the Dean and Chapter of Lincoln. The church is dedicated to St. Andrew. Nine children are instructed for a small annuity, the gift of Mark Clayton, in 1760.

HAMBLETON, a township in the parish of BRAY-TON, lower division of the wapentake of BARKSTONE-ASH, West riding of the county of YORK, 4 miles (W.S.W.) from Selby, containing 488 inhabitants. A school-room, with a house for the master, was erected by subscription in 1796, when an allotment of land, under the enclosure act, was assigned for its support.

HAMBROOK, a chapelry in the parish of WINTER-BOURNE, upper division of the hundred of LANGLEY and SWINEHEAD, county of GLOUCESTER, 5¾ miles (N.E. by N.) from Bristol, containing 968 inhabitants.

HAMERINGHAM, a parish in the hundred of HILL, parts of LINDSEY, county of LINCOLN, 3¾ miles (E.S.E.) from Horncastle, containing 149 inhabitants. The living is a discharged rectory, with that of Scrayfield united, in the archdeaconry and diocese of Lincoln, rated in the king's books at £8. 14. 2. Mrs. Coltman was patroness in 1814. The church is dedicated to All Saints.

HAMERTON, a parish in the hundred of LEIGH-TONSTONE, county of HUNTINGDON, 7 miles (S. S. W.) from Stilton, containing 141 inhabitants. The living is a rectory, in the archdeaconry of Huntingdon, and diocese of Lincoln, rated in the king's books at £13. 15. 5., and in the patronage of James H. S. Barry, Esq. The church is dedicated to All Saints.

HAMFOLLOW, a hamlet in the parish and upper division of the hundred of BERKELEY, county of GLOUCESTER, containing 437 inhabitants.

HAMMERSMITH, a chapelry in the parish of FULHAM, Kensington division of the hundred of OSSUL-STONE, county of MIDDLESEX, 3½ miles (W. by S.) from London, on the great western road, containing 8809 inhabitants. This village, which by a continuity of buildings is almost united with Kensington, forms one of the most populous appendages to the western part of the metropolis, and is pleasantly situated on the northern bank of the river Thames. The principal street extends along the line of the turnpike-road, and a wide street, called the Broad-way, diverges from it towards the river: the houses are in general of respectable appearance, and there are some handsome ranges of modern erection: in the environs are numerous seats and elegant villas, especially towards the river, on the bank of which was Brandenburgh house, a noble mansion erected by Sir Nicholas Crispe in the reign of Charles I., which General Fairfax occupied in 1647, while the parliamentary forces were quartered in the neighbourhood, pending the proposition between Charles I. and the parliament; it was afterwards the residence of the Margrave of Anspach; and subsequently of the late Queen Caroline, since whose decease in it the building has been taken down. The streets are well paved, and lighted with gas, and the inhabitants are supplied with water by the West Middlesex Company, established at Hammersmith by act of parliament in 1806. A suspension-bridge over the Thames was commenced in 1825, and completed in 1827, from a design by Mr. Tierney Clarke, at an expense of £45,000. The distance between the suspension towers, which are forty-eight feet high, and form handsome arched entrances of the Tuscan order, is four hundred feet; from these towers are suspended eight chains, consisting of bars of wrought iron, having a dip of twenty-nine feet in the centre, from which pass perpendicular rods of iron, supporting a platform of wood overlaid with granite, six hundred and eighty-eight feet in length, with a parapet on each side: the carriage road is twenty feet broad, and the foot-path five feet wide: at the approaches are neat octagonal lodges, and on the Surrey side, the road leads directly to Barnes common, whence roads branch off to the south and south-western parts of the kingdom. A road from the bridge to join the new Brompton road is now in progress, and it is in contemplation to construct a road from Shepherd's Bush to Turnham Green. There are two large breweries, extensive nursery-grounds, and grounds for bleaching wax; and a large quantity of bricks is made in the neighbourhood : a creek which extends from the Thames to the village is navigable for barges. The petty sessions for the Kensington division are held here every Monday, and courts leet and baron in November and at Easter : the village is within the jurisdiction of the court of requests held in Kingsgate-street, Holborn, for the recovery of debts under 40s., and within the limits of the new police establishment.

Hammersmith is about to be separated from the parish of Fulham, and to be divided into two distinct parishes. The living is a perpetual curacy, in the archdeaconry of Middlesex, and diocese of London, and in the patronage of the Bishop of London. The church, erected in 1631, and dedicated to St. Paul, is a spacious and neat edifice of brick, with a square tower : against the north wall of the nave is a handsome bronze bust of Charles I., erected in grateful remembrance of his royal master, by Sir Nicholas Crispe, whose heart, in pursuance of his directions, was enclosed in an urn and placed underneath it. A church dedicated to St. Peter, and containing one thousand six hundred and one sittings, of which six hundred are free, was erected in 1829, by a grant from the parliamentary commissioners, at an expense of £12,223. 8. 4.: it is a handsome edifice of Suffolk brick, in the Grecian style of architecture, and of the Doric order, with a neat stone tower : the living is a perpetual curacy, in the patronage of the Bishop of London. St. Mary's chapel, a neat brick building, was erected in 1813, at the sole expense of the late Richard Hunt, Esq.: the living is a donative, in the gift of Charles, Edward, and Richard Hunt, Esqrs. There are places of worship for Baptists, the Society of Friends, Independents, and Wesleyan Methodists, besides a Roman Catholic chapel. A school for clothing and educating boys was founded in 1624, by Edward Latymer, Esq., who gave thirty-five acres of land, producing a rental of upwards of £540, of which a part was appropriated to the clothing of aged men; there are eighty boys in the school, and thirty men are annually clothed. A charity school, in which fifty girls are educated and clothed, is supported partly by the twelfth part of the rents of a farm now let for £450 per annum, bequeathed by the Dowager Lady Capell, and partly by subscription : there is also a Roman Catholic school at Brook-Green, supported by voluntary contributions. Sunday schools are supported by subscription. There are almshouses for four old women at Brook-Green, founded and endowed by Thomas Isles, D.D., in 1629 ; and various charitable bequests have been made for the relief of the poor. A mechanics' institution and a savings-bank have been established. In King-street is a convent of Benedictine nuns, said to have subsisted since the reign of Charles II.: at the east end of the building is the chapel, which was rebuilt in 1810, at an expense of £1600, defrayed by subscription. Near the church is an ancient mansion, supposed to have been erected at the same time as the palace at Hampton-Court; the apartments in the north part of the building are much admired for the beauty of their architecture. In a house adjoining the Dove Coffee-house, now a smoking-box belonging to the Duke of Sussex, Thomson the poet is said to have written his Seasons.

Catherine, Queen Dowager of Charles II., resided for some years in a house in the Upper Mall, in which Dr. Radcliffe subsequently lived. Sir Samuel Morland, the inventor of the speaking-trumpet; Dr. William Sheridan, author of some sermons; Thomas Worlidge, a painter and etcher of great eminence; Sir Elijah Impey, Knt., who was first appointed on the high court of judicature for the British possessions in India; George Doddington, Lord Melcombe, a distinguished courtier and statesman in the reign of George II.; and Arthur Murphy, a barrister, and a dramatic writer of celebrity, are among the eminent persons who have been interred here : Philip James De Loutherbourgh, the celebrated landscape painter, resided at this place.

HAMMERTON (GREEN), a township in that part of the parish of WHIXLEY which is in the upper division of the wapentake of CLARO, West riding of the county of YORK, 7¼ miles (S.E. by S.) from Aldborough, containing 329 inhabitants. There is a place of worship for Wesleyan Methodists.

HAMMERTON (KIRK), a parish partly in the upper division of the wapentake of CLARO, West riding, and comprising the township of Wilstrop, within the ainsty of the city of YORK, East riding, of the county of YORK, 8 miles (S.E. by S.) from Aldborough, containing 504 inhabitants. The living is a perpetual curacy, in the archdeaconry of Richmond, and diocese of Chester, endowed with £400 private benefaction, £200 royal bounty, and £300 parliamentary grant, and in the patronage of the Rev. W. Metcalfe. The church is dedicated to St. John the Baptist. There is a place of worship for Wesleyan Methodists. The manufacture of linen is carried on here.

HAMMERWICK, a parish in the southern division of the hundred of OFFLOW, county of STAFFORD, 3¾ miles (S.W. by W.) from Lichfield, containing 218 inhabitants. The living is a perpetual curacy annexed to the vicarage of St. Mary, Lichfield, in the peculiar jurisdiction of the Dean of Lichfield, endowed with £600 royal bounty, and £200 parliamentary grant, and in the patronage of certain Trustees. The Wyrley and Essington canal passes through the parish, in which the manufacture of nails is carried on.

HAMMOON, a parish in the hundred of PIMPERNE, Blandford (North) division of the county of DORSET, 7 miles (S.W. by S.) from Shaftesbury, containing 71 inhabitants. The living is a rectory, in the archdeaconry of Dorset, and diocese of Bristol, rated in the king's books at £7. 4. 2., and in the patronage of the Rev. Mr. Meech. The river Stour separates this parish from that of Manston.

HAMPDEN (GREAT), a parish in the hundred of AYLESBURY, county of BUCKINGHAM, 3¼ miles (W.N.W.) from Great Missenden, containing 281 inhabitants. The living is a rectory, consolidated in 1799 with the vicarage of Great Kimble, in the archdeaconry of Buckingham, and diocese of Lincoln, rated in the king's books at £9. 9. 7., and in the patronage of the Earl of Buckinghamshire. The church, dedicated to St. Mary Magdalene, has lately received an addition of one hundred free sittings, the Incorporated Society for the enlargement of churches and chapels having granted £30 toward defraying the expense. Among other monuments, it contains one to the memory of John Hampden, Esq., ornamented with a medallion, on which is represented a tree bearing the arms of the family and of their alliances; and at the foot of it, in bas relief, the battle of Chalgrave, in which that renowned patriot received his death wound, of which he died about three weeks afterwards, on June 24th, 1643. Queen Elizabeth was entertained here by Griffith Hampden, Esq., who, to render Her Majesty greater honour, cut an avenue, still called the Queen's gap, through his wood, for a more convenient approach to the house.

HAMPDEN (LITTLE), a parish in the hundred of AYLESBURY, county of BUCKINGHAM, 3¼ miles (N. W. by W.) from Great Missenden, containing 88 inhabitants. The living is a perpetual curacy, annexed to the rectory of Hartwell, in the archdeaconry of Buckingham, and diocese of Lincoln.

HAMPHALL, a joint township with Stubbs, in the parish of ADWICK le STREET, northern division of the wapentake of STRAFFORTH and TICKHILL, West riding of the county of YORK, 6 miles (N.W.) from Doncaster, containing 140 inhabitants. A priory of Cistercian nuns, in honour of the Blessed Virgin Mary, was founded here about 1170, by William de Clairfai and Avicia de Tarry, his wife, the revenue of which, at the dissolution, was £85. 6. 11.

HAMPNETT, a parish in the hundred of BRADLEY, county of GLOUCESTER, 1½ mile (N.W. by N.) from North Leach, containing 121 inhabitants. The living is a rectory, with which that of Stowell was united in 1660, in the archdeaconry and diocese of Gloucester, rated in the king's books at £10, and in the patronage of Lord Stowell. The church, dedicated to St. George, is principally in the early style of English architecture. A brook rises in this parish, which gives name to the adjoining town of North Leach. The old Fosse-way passes along the south-eastern boundary.

HAMPNETT (WEST), a parish in the hundred of Box and STOCKBRIDGE, rape of CHICHESTER, county of SUSSEX, 1½ mile (N. E.) from Chichester, containing 401 inhabitants. The living is a discharged vicarage, in the archdeaconry and diocese of Chichester, rated in the king's books at £7.4.4., endowed with £1000 royal bounty, and in the patronage of the Crown. The church is dedicated to St. Peter.

HAMPRESTON, a parish comprising the hamlet of Long Ham, within the liberty of WESTOVER, New Forest (West) division of the county of SOUTHAMPTON, but chiefly in that part of the hundred of CRANBORNE which is in the Shaston (East) division of the county of DORSET, 3½ miles (E.S.E.) from Wimborne-Minster, and containing 892 inhabitants. The living is a rectory, in the archdeaconry of Dorset, and diocese of Bristol, rated in the king's books at £13.10. C. and H. Warland, Esqrs. were patrons in 1806. The church, dedicated to All Saints, is partly in the early, and partly in the decorated, style of English architecture, and has lately received an addition of one hundred and ten free sittings, the Incorporated Society for the enlargement of churches and chapels having granted £20 towards defraying the expense. Hampreston was formerly a chapelry within the parish of Wimborne-Minster, but was separated from it about 1440, when license was granted to bury here. The navigable river Stour runs along the southern boundary.

HAMPSHIRE.—See SOUTHAMPTON (County of).

HAMPSTEAD, a parish in the Holborn division of VOL. II.

the hundred of OSSULSTONE, county of MIDDLESEX, 4 miles (N. by W.) from London, containing 7263 inhabitants. This place was granted by King Ethelred to the monks of St. Peter at Westminster, and the grant having been confirmed by William the Conqueror, it continued in their possession till the dissolution of the convent in the reign of Henry VIII. The ancient Grange house, of which scarcely a memorial remains, was the residence of the monastic superintendent of the manor, and the prior resided at Belsize house, which was subsequently converted into a place of public entertainment. Hampstead was anciently an inconsiderable hamlet in the parish of Hendon, from which it was separated, and made a distinct parish, in the year 1598, when its churchwardens for the first time attended the bishop's annual visitation. The election for the county members took place on the heath in 1681, and continued to be held till 1701, when it was removed to Brentford. Its pleasant situation, the salubrity of the air, and its proximity to the metropolis, had made it the residence of some of the more wealthy citizens, and from the discovery of its chalybeate springs and mineral waters, in the early part of the eighteenth century, it became the resort of numerous invalids, for whose accommodation and amusement a pump-room, tavern, and coffee and assembly-rooms, were successively erected. The water of the chalybeate spring contains oxyde of iron, muriates of soda and magnesia, sulphate of lime, and a small portion of silex, and its mean temperature at the wells is from 46 to 47° of Fahrenheit. Other saline springs were afterwards discovered at the southeastern extremity of the heath, near Pond-street, in their properties generally resembling the Cheltenham and Harrogate waters: the water continued for some time to be sent in flasks from the wells by accredited agents of the principal houses, called the Upper and Lower Flask Houses.

Hampstead is at present more regarded as a healthy and pleasant place of residence than on account of its waters, which have within the last few years fallen almost into disuse. The village is situated on the southern acclivity of a hill, on the summit of which is an extensive heath, commanding, at different elevations, varied and beautiful views of the metropolis and the adjacent country, abounding in picturesque scenery, and agreeably diversified with richly-wooded hills, extensive meadows, and sequestered vales, interspersed with elegant villas, splendid mansions, and rural cottages. The heath is divided into the Upper and Lower Heath, the Vale of Health, and other subdivisions, possessing a temperature of climate proportioned to their several elevations, or to their different degrees of shelter from the colder winds, and consequently adapted to the various constitutions of the permanent residents, or of the invalids who occasionally reside there for the recovery of their health. Numerous respectable lodging-houses have been erected for the accommodation of the latter; and to afford them opportunities of exercise and excursion through the pleasing environs of this beautiful spot, pony carriages and donkeys are in constant attendance. A telegraph has been erected on the Upper Heath, forming the first in the line of communication between Chelsea Hospital and Yarmouth. The approach from the metropolis is by an excellent road, from many points of which the view of Hampstead and Highgate is strikingly beautiful; and on ascending the hill which leads into the village, handsome ranges of modern buildings, detached mansions, and elegant villas, rise in continued succession. The village is lighted with oil, and supplied with water from a large reservoir in Shepherd's fields, and from pumps attached to the houses; the Hampstead Water Company have a reservoir on the heath, which supplies the inhabitants of Kentish Town, Camden Town, and Tottenham-Court road. Petty sessions are held here occasionally, and courts leet and baron on the Monday before Whitsuntide; a general court baron and customary court are also held annually within a month or six weeks after Christmas: the parish is within the jurisdiction of a court of requests held at Kingsgate-street, Holborn, for the recovery of debts under 40s., and is also within the limits of the new police establishment.

The living is a perpetual curacy, in the archdeaconry of Middlesex, and diocese of London, and in the patronage of Sir Thomas Maryon Wilson, Bart. The church, dedicated to St. John, a neat brick edifice, was erected in 1747, on the site of the ancient church, which was taken down: the steeple is at the east end, and among the monuments is one to the memory of Lady Erskine, beautifully executed by Bacon the younger. In 1771, William Pierce bequeathed £1700 three per cent. consols., directing the dividends to be applied in paying stipends of £24 per annum to the curate of Hampstead, and £5 per annum to the clerk, for performing divine service every Friday, £10 per annum to the Independent minister, and for other purposes. Hampstead chapel, in Well Walk, originally the pump-room of the Wells tavern, and St. John's chapel on Downshire Hill, erected in 1823, a plain neat building, are proprietary episcopal chapels. There are places of worship for Baptists, Wesleyan Methodists, and Unitarians, and a Roman Catholic chapel. National schools for children of both sexes are supported by subscription, and for apprenticing them there is a fund of £2100 three per cent. consols., arising from a bequest of £1000 by John Stock, Esq., in 1780, and subsequent benefactions. Dowager Viscountess Campden, in 1643, bequeathed £200 to be invested in land, a moiety of which was appropriated to the poor, and the remainder for apprenticing one poor child, with which sum, together with £40 given by an unknown benefactress, lands in the parish of Hendon were purchased, producing at present £83. 11. per annum. The Hon. Susannah Noel, in 1698, gave six acres of the heath land, directing the produce to be applied to placing out poor children of this parish, and other charitable uses: on this land the chapel and several houses in Well Walk have been built: the present revenue arising from the estate, which is under the management of fourteen trustees, is £95, and on the expiration of the leases the rents will probably be greatly increased. There are also several other charitable bequests for the relief of the poor. In that part of Kilburn which is in this parish was a convent of Benedictine nuns, the revenue of which, at the dissolution, was £121. 16.: near the site of this convent is a place of public entertainment, called Kilburn Wells, where is an aperient saline spring, still resorted to. In 1774 sepulchral urns, vases, earthen lamps, and other Roman antiquities were dug up in Well Walk. On the left hand of the entrance into Hampstead from London is the mansion of Sir Henry Vane,

one of the judges of Charles I., where, after the Restoration of Charles II., he was arrested, and shortly after tried and executed. Here also resided Dr. Joseph Butler, Bishop of Durham, author of the "Analogy of Religion, natural and revealed, to the constitution and course of Nature." On Haverstock Hill, a mile nearer London, is the cottage in which Sir Charles Sedley resided, afterwards occupied by Sir Richard Steele. At a house, formerly a place of public entertainment, called the Upper Flask, noticed by Richardson in his Clarissa, George Stevens, the celebrated commentator on Shakspeare, lived and died; prior to which it was the place of meeting of the Kit Cat Club. Among many distinguished persons who were interred at Hampstead were Dr. Anthony Askew, a learned critic and physician; James Mc Ardell, an engraver in mezzotinto; John Harrison, who obtained a premium from parliament for his improvements on the chronometer; Archdecon Travis; James Pettit Andrews, author of a history of Great Britain; and John Carter, an eminent antiquary.

HAMPSTEAD (EAST), a parish comprising the hamlet of Bracknell, in the hundred of COOKHAM, but chiefly in the hundred of RIPPLESMERE, county of BERKS, 4 miles (E. S. E.) from Wokingham, containing 615 inhabitants. The living is a rectory, in the archdeaconry of Berks, and diocese of Salisbury, rated in the king's books at £9. 1. 3., and in the patronage of the Dean and Canons of Christ Church, Oxford. The church is dedicated to St. Mary Magdalene. There are several chalybeate springs in the parish, and a Roman military work, called Cæsar's camp.

HAMPSTEAD-MARSHALL, a parish in the hundred of KINTBURY-EAGLE, county of BERKS, 4 miles (W. by S.) from Newbury, containing 304 inhabitants. The living is a rectory, in the archdeaconry of Berks, and diocese of Salisbury, rated in the king's books at £12. 14. 4½., and in the patronage of Earl Craven. The church is dedicated to St. Mary. The Kennet and Avon canal passes through the parish.

HAMPSTEAD-NORRIS, a parish in the hundred of FAIRCROSS, county of BERKS, 3¾ miles (S. E. by S.) from East Ilsley, containing 1111 inhabitants. The living is a discharged vicarage, in the archdeaconry of Berks, and diocese of Salisbury, rated in the king's books at £9. 18. 11½., and in the patronage of the Marquis of Downshire. The church is dedicated to St. Mary. There are two places of worship belonging to the Independents, and one for Wesleyan Methodists. In Park coppice is a large tumulus, also the remains of an intrenchment. The foundations of an ancient building, some tesselated pavement, a few coins, and a number of Roman bricks, were discovered, on excavating a field near Well house, in 1827.

HAMPSTHWAITE, a parish in the lower division of the wapentake of CLARO, West riding of the county of YORK, comprising the chapelry of Thornthwaite with Padside, and the townships of Birstwith, Felliscliffe, Hampsthwaite, and Menwith with Darley, and containing 2750 inhabitants, of which number, 490 are in the township of Hampsthwaite, 1½ mile (S. W. by W.) from Ripley. The living is a vicarage, rated in the king's books at £13. 6. 8., in the peculiar jurisdiction of the court for the honour of Knaresborough, and in the patronage of the Rev. T. M. Sham. The church is dedicated to St. Thomas à Becket. William Ridsdale, in

1711, gave a house and two guineas a year for teaching six boys of the township of Hampsthwaite; and in the same year John Richmond founded a free school at West Syke Green, in this parish, and endowed it with £14 per annum, for educating thirty boys.

HAMPTON, a township in the parish of MALPAS, higher division of the hundred of BROXTON, county palatine of CHESTER, 2¾ miles (N. E.) from Malpas, containing 207 inhabitants.

HAMPTON, a parish in the hundred of SPELTHORNE, county of MIDDLESEX, 13½ miles (W. S. W.) from London, containing, with the chapelry of Hampton-Wick, 3549 inhabitants. In the reign of Edward the Confessor, Hampton belonged to Earl Algar, a powerful Saxon nobleman, and after the Norman Conquest it was held by Walter de St. Valeri, who probably gave the advowson of the living to the priory of Takeley, in Essex, which was a cell to the abbey of St. Valeri, in Picardy; but the manor subsequently became the property of Sir Robert Gray, whose widow, in 1211, left it to the Knights Hospitallers, and they at one period had an establishment here for the sisters of that order. Cardinal Wolsey, when in the height of his power, having determined on building a palace for his principal residence in the vicinity of the metropolis, fixed on Hampton for the site of it, as being one of the healthiest and most pleasant spots in the south of England. He therefore obtained from the prior of St. John a lease of the manor and manor-house, and in 1516 commenced the erection of a magnificent mansion, which he furnished in a style of corresponding splendour; and before the structure was completed, in 1526, he presented it to the king, together with his interest in the manorial estate. In 1538, an act of parliament passed for making a royal chase, called Hampton Court chase, extending over several adjoining parishes in Middlesex and Surrey. It was enclosed and stocked with deer, but on the petition of the inhabitants, after the death of Henry VIII., the enclosure was removed, though the tract which it comprehended is still considered as a royal chase, under the superintendence of an officer called the lieutenant, or keeper of his majesty's chase of Hampton Court. The order of the Knights Hospitallers having been suppressed in England in 1540, this manor became vested in the crown, and in the same year a new act was passed creating the manor of Hampton Court an honour, the office of chief steward and feodary of which, together with that of lieutenant and keeper of the chase, has always been conferred on a personage of high rank.

Hampton Court was completed by Henry VIII., according to the design of the architect employed by Cardinal Wolsey, and being made one of the royal palaces, was a frequent and favourite residence of his majesty and the court. Edward VI. was born in it, October 12th, 1537; and at this palace, in 1543, Henry VIII. was married to his last wife, Catherine Parr. It was the occasional residence of several of the sovereigns antecedent to William III., who rebuilt a considerable part of the palace, and laid out the gardens and park in their present form. Queen Anne resided here before her accession to the throne, and her son William, Duke of Gloucester, was born in it, July 24th, 1689. George II. was the last sovereign who made Hampton Court the place of his abode, as his successors have only been casual visitors. The whole of the buildings, except

the state apartments and a suite of rooms under them called the Duke of York's apartments, are now occupied by private families, who have grants during pleasure from the Lord Chamberlain; the number of the residents, including servants, is about seven hundred. The palace, situated on the north bank of the Thames, comprises three large quadrangles, with some detached buildings; but the first quadrangle at the western entrance alone remains as originally erected by Cardinal Wolsey: it extends one hundred and sixty-nine feet from north to south, and one hundred and forty-one from east to west. The second quadrangle, called the Clock-court, from a curious astronomical clock over the gateway, has been partially remodelled from a design by Sir Christopher Wren, who erected an Ionic colonnade leading to the grand staircase and the state apartments. On the north side of this quadrangle is the great hall, built by Henry VIII., the noble roof of which was restored in 1820: it was used as a theatre in the reigns of Elizabeth and George I. and II.; and in 1830 it was fitted up for divine service while the parish church was being rebuilt. The Fountain court, or third quadrangle, was rebuilt by Sir Christopher Wren, in 1690; it is one hundred and ten feet from east to west, and one hundred and seventeen from north to south. On the south side is the king's staircase, leading to the state apartments, the walls of which are ornamented with mythological paintings by Verrio; and on the north side is the queen's staircase, with paintings on the walls by Laguerre. The principal state apartments are the guardhall, decorated with arms and armour; the presencechambers; the audience chamber; the king's drawingroom and writing closet; Queen Mary's closet; the queen's gallery, ornamented with Gobelin tapestry; the royal bed-rooms and dressing-rooms; and the long gallery, in which are the Cartoons of Raphael. The royal chapel, in which is some beautiful carved work by Grimling Gibbons, is opened for divine service every Sunday. The gardens, including the site of the palace, comprise a space of about three miles in circumference. In a hot house in the private gardens is a vine of the Black Hamburgh kind, noted for its extraordinary fertility, often bearing two thousand five hundred bunches of grapes in a season. There is a fine canal three quarters of a mile in length; and the gardens are ornamented with four beautifully sculptured marble vases. The village of Hampton stands about one mile and a half from the palace, on the north side of the Thames, over which there is a wooden bridge at Hampton Court, and there is also a ferry over the river for carriages and foot-passengers at Hampton. It contains several handsome villas, particularly one which belonged to the celebrated Garrick, on the lawn in front of which is a small temple dedicated to Shakspeare, with a statue of the great dramatist, the work of G. Garrard, A. R. A. There are eight assemblies in the course of the year at the Royal Hotel at Hampton Court; and Hampton races are held in June annually, at Moulsey Hurst, on the opposite side of the Thames. Courts leet and baron for the manor are held once a year. Hampton is within the jurisdiction of a court of requests for the recovery of debts under 40s., held at Brentford, during the summer half year, and at Uxbridge in winter.

The living is a vicarage, in the archdeaconry of Middlesex, and diocese of London, rated in the king's books at £10, and in the patronage of the Crown. The church, dedicated to the Blessed Virgin, having long been in a dilapidated state, was taken down at the commencement of 1830, and on the 13th of April, in that year, the first stone of a new edifice was laid, intended to contain one thousand four hundred persons, with four hundred and eighty free sittings : the estimated expense of the building is about £8000. Here is a place of worship for Independents. A free grammar school was founded in consequence of the bequest of lands and tenements at Hampton, by Robert Hamonde, in 1556, and the subsequent benefactions of Edmund Pigeon, in 1657, and John Jones, Esq., in 1691 : the entire annual income is £327. 10. from which the master receives £287. 13. 6., and pays £60 per annum to an usher, and about £10 per annum for books, &c. The school is open to the children of all the parishioners, and the scholars are instructed on the National system. There is a National school for girls, twelve of whom are clothed at the expense of Her Royal Highness the Duchess of Clarence, and the remainder, seventy-two in number, by subscription : there is also a Sunday school for boys, on the National plan. The school-house for the Sunday school and the school of industry was erected in 1805, on a piece of ground given by the Duke of Clarence, at the expense of £429. 6. 4., raised by voluntary contribution. Queen Anne gave £50 per annum to the poor of this parish; and there are many other considerable benefactions, for apprenticing poor children and other charitable purposes. Among the more distinguished inhabitants of this place who have been interred here, may be mentioned John Beard, patentee of Covent Garden theatre, celebrated as a public singer, who died in 1791 ; and Richard Tickell, Esq., author of a popular pamphlet entitled "Anticipation," containing satirical sketches of parliamentary debates.

HAMPTON in ARDEN, a parish in the Solihull division of the hundred of HEMLINGFORD, county of WARWICK, 4 miles (E. by N.) from Solihull, comprising the chapelries of Balsall and Knowle, and the hamlets of Kinwalsey, and Nuthurst, and containing 2772 inhabitants. The living is a vicarage, in the archdeaconry of Coventry, and diocese of Lichfield and Coventry, rated in the king's books at £15. 6. 8., and in the patronage of the Master and Brethren of the Earl of Leicester's Hospital, in Warwick. The church, dedicated to St. Mary and St. Bartholomew, had formerly a lofty spire, which was destroyed by lightning in 1643. A charter for a market and a fair was granted by Henry III. The river Blythe and the Birmingham and Warwick canal pass through the parish. George Fentham, in 1690, bequeathed certain property for the instruction of youth of both sexes : the annual proceeds are about £60, of which sum the schoolmaster receives £42, the schoolmistress £12. 12., and £5 is laid out in apprenticing children: the school-house for the boys was erected by the trustees in 1782. At Nuthurst, in this parish, was an ancient chapel, but there are not any remains of it.

HAMPTON (BISHOP'S), a parish in the hundred of GRIMSWORTH, county of HEREFORD, 4 miles (S. E. by E.) from Hereford, containing, with the township of Tupsley, 544 inhabitants. The living is a rectory, in the peculiar jurisdiction of the Dean of Hereford, rated in the king's books at £13. 13. 9., and in the patronage of the Bishop of Hereford. The church is dedicated to St. Andrew. The parish is bounded on the south by the river Wye, on the north by the Lug, both navigable for vessels of thirty tons' burden, and on the east by the river Froomy.

HAMPTON (GREAT), a parish in the lower division of the hundred of BLACKENHURST, county of WORCESTER, 1 mile (W. by S.) from Evesham, containing, with the township of Little Hampton, 324 inhabitants. The living is a discharged perpetual curacy, in the archdeaconry and diocese of Worcester, rated in the king's books at £7. 12. 3½., and in the patronage of the Dean and Canons of Christ Church, Oxford. The church, dedicated to St. Andrew, is in the later style of English architecture. The navigable river Avon is crossed by a ferry here.

HAMPTON (HIGH), a parish in the hundred of BLACK TORRINGTON, county of DEVON, 3½ miles (W.) from Hatherleigh, containing 282 inhabitants. The living is a discharged rectory, in the archdeaconry of Totness, and diocese of Exeter, rated in the king's books at £8. 19. 4½., J. M. Woolcombe, Esq. was patron in 1810. The church, dedicated to the Holy Cross, has a plain Norman door : it is situated on a very high hill, and serves as a land-mark for the surrounding country. Here is a small charity school.

HAMPTON (HILL), a hamlet in the parish of MARTLEY, upper division of the hundred of DODDINGTREE, county of WORCESTER, containing 138 inhabitants.

HAMPTON (LITTLE), a sea-port, market-town, and parish, in the hundred of POLING, rape of ARUNDEL, county of SUSSEX, 4 miles (S.) from Arundel, and 61 (S. S. W.) from London, containing 1166 inhabitants. This place, which is situated on the east bank of the river Arun, was, a few years ago, an insignificant village, but is now a considerable port, and is much frequented for sea-bathing. Some fine buildings have been erected on the beach, which commands an uninterrupted view of the coast, from Brighton to the Isle of Wight, and on the land side many beautiful and varied prospects. There are several inns distinguished for the excellence of their accommodation, and the shops are fitted up with great taste. The fineness of the sands, and the salubrity of the air, have long rendered Hampton famous as a place for bathing ; and new baths have been recently established on the beach, which comprise hot, cold, and shower baths, and apartments for shampooing, besides a reading-room furnished with the principal London and provincial news-papers. The harbour, which is regarded as superior to any other on this coast, will conveniently admit vessels drawing thirteen feet of water. The chief trade carried on is in coal and timber. There is a market for corn on Thursday, which is well attended.

The living is a vicarage, in the archdeaconry and diocese of Chichester, endowed with £200 royal bounty, and in the patronage of the Bishop of Chichester. The church, dedicated to St. Mary, is in the early English style, with some later insertions. Here is a school for eighteen boys, founded in pursuance of a bequest by John Coney, Esq., in 1805, and endowed with £600 three per cent. consols. ; and Mrs. Jane Downer, in 1763, left a small sum for the instruction of two poor girls. An institution was established in 1815, called the Little Hampton Beneficial Society, to provide relief for distressed members, and to protect them from removal by the parochial authorities when not actually chargeable upon the parish.

HAMPTON (LITTLE), a township in the parish of GREAT HAMPTON, lower division of the hundred of BLACKENHURST, county of WORCESTER, ¾ of a mile (W. by S.) from Evesham. The population is returned with the parish. The river Arun here falls into the English channel; and on its eastern bank there is a fort to defend the entrance to Arundel haven.

HAMPTON (MAISEY), a parish in the hundred of CROWTHORNE and MINETY, county of GLOUCESTER, 2¼ miles (W.S.W.) from Fairford, containing 362 inhabitants. The living is a rectory, with the perpetual curacy of Marston-Maisey, in the archdeaconry and diocese of Gloucester, rated in the king's books at £26.17.3½., and in the patronage of the President and Fellows of Corpus Christi College, Oxford. The church is dedicated to St. Mary. There are several small bequests for the support of a Sunday school.

HAMPTON (MINCHIN), a parish in the hundred of LONGTREE, county of GLOUCESTER, comprising the chapelry of Rodborough, part of the chapelry of Nailsworth, and the market town of Minchin-Hampton, 14 miles (S.) from Gloucester, and 100 (W.) from London, and containing, with Rodborough and Nailsworth, 7843 inhabitants. Shortly after the Conquest, the manor of Hampton was given to the nunnery of Caen, in Normandy, and a church was founded here, and the grant of a market procured for the town, by the abbess of Caen, in the reign of Henry III.; hence it derived its prefix of Minchin from Monachina, a diminutive of Monacha, a nun. The town is pleasantly situated on the summit and southern declivity of an eminence bordering on the vale of the Severn to the east: it consists of a long irregular street, intersected by another, partially paved, and is abundantly supplied with water from springs. There are several streams near the town, and in other parts of the parish, on which stand clothing-mills, the principal employment of the inhabitants consisting in the manufacture of woollen cloth, which has long been extensively carried on in the vicinity. A small market for provisions is held on Tuesday; and there are fairs on Trinity-Monday and October 29th.

The living is a rectory, in the archdeaconry and diocese of Gloucester, rated in the king's books at £41.13.4., and in the patronage of Richard Harris, Esq. The church, dedicated to the Holy Trinity, is a large cruciform edifice, chiefly in the decorated style of English architecture, with an octagonal tower at the intersection; and at the south end of the transept is a very large window, with a rich wheel in the tracery. In the interior are some ancient monuments and statues, and an inscription to the memory of Dr. Bradley, Astronomer Royal, who was interred in the church-yard. Here are places of worship for Baptists and Wesleyan Methodists. At Seintlieu, or Sinckley, in this parish, is a free school for the instruction of boys in writing and arithmetic, founded in 1699, in pursuance of a benefaction of £1000 by Nathaniel Cambridge, a Hamburgh merchant, which, with some additional endowment, was invested in land, producing about £110 per annum, that sum, after deductions for taxes and repairs,

being paid to the master, who has also the benefit of a house and garden, for which he is bound to receive all the boys belonging to this and the adjoining parish of Woodchester, but the average number of scholars is not more than thirty. There is a charity school for fourteen poor boys, endowed with £8 per annum, from a bequest by Ursula Tooke, in 1698, and about £25 from a bequest by Henry King, in 1699. Several benefactions have been made for apprenticing poor children, and for other purposes. An ancient unendowed almshouse here having become greatly dilapidated, the late David Ricardo, Esq., of Gatcombe park, in the vicinity, built other almshouses for eight poor persons, who receive a voluntary allowance from Mrs. Ricardo. A dispensary is supported by subscription. Amberley, or Hampton common, a large tract of unenclosed land to the westward of the town, was given to the inhabitants by Alice de Hampton, in the reign of Henry VIII.: on this common is a very extensive intrenchment, supposed to have been a Danish camp; and near it a valley, called "Woeful Danes' Bottom," where Alfred the Great is said to have obtained a victory over the Danes.

HAMPTON (NETHER), a chapelry in the parish of WILTON, hundred of CAWDEN and CADWORTH, county of WILTS, 1¾ mile (S.E. by S.) from Wilton, containing 147 inhabitants. The chapel, dedicated to St. Catherine, is principally in the later style of English architecture, but the chancel is early English.

HAMPTON (WELCH), a parish in the hundred of PIMHILL, county of SALOP, 2¾ miles (E. by N.) from Ellesmere, containing 478 inhabitants. The living is a perpetual curacy, endowed with £400 private benefaction, and £400 royal bounty, and in the peculiar jurisdiction and patronage of the Lord of the Manor, the Rev. Sir Edward Kynaston, Bart. The church is dedicated to St. Michael.

HAMPTON-CHARLES, a hamlet in that part of the parish of BOCKLETON which is in the hundred of BROXASH, county of HEREFORD, 5½ miles (N.W. by W.) from Bromyard, containing 91 inhabitants.

HAMPTON-COURT, an extra-parochial liberty, locally in the parish of Hope under Dinmore, hundred of WOLPHY, county of HEREFORD, 5½ miles (S.S.E.) from Leominster. Here is a noble and spacious mansion, on the eastern bank of the river Lug, erected by Sir Rowland Lenthall, yeoman of the robes to Henry IV., who distinguished himself at the battle of Agincourt. The buildings, which form a quadrangle, display a mixture of monastic and castellated architecture: on the north side are a gate-house and angular towers, one of which joins a chapel, with a fine timber roof ornamented with carved work; and in the windows are some armorial bearings in painted glass. The mansion is situated in the midst of a spacious lawn, surrounded by a park and pleasure grounds about eight miles in circumference.

HAMPTON-GAY, a parish in the hundred of PLOUGHLEY, county of OXFORD, 2¾ miles (E. by S.) from Woodstock, containing 86 inhabitants. The living is a perpetual curacy, in the archdeaconry and diocese of Oxford. The church is dedicated to St. Giles.

HAMPTON-LOVETT, a parish in the upper division of the hundred of HALFSHIRE, county of WORCESTER, 1½ mile (N.N.W.) from Droitwich, containing 176 inhabitants. The living is a rectory, in the archdeaconry and diocese of Worcester, rated in the king's books at £9. 16. 0½., and in the patronage of Sir John Pakington, Bart. The church is dedicated to St. Mary.

HAMPTON-LUCY, otherwise BISHOP'S HAMPTON, a parish in the Snitterfield division of the hundred of BARLICHWAY, county of WARWICK, 4¼ miles (E.N.E.) from Stratford upon Avon, containing 554 inhabitants. The living is a rectory, rated in the king's books at £51. 6. 8., in the peculiar jurisdiction of the Rector, but wills are always proved in the presence of the Bishop's registrar at Worcester, and are deposited in the registry there. George Lucy, Esq. was patron in 1815. The church is dedicated to St. Peter. A free grammar school was founded in 1635, by the Rev. Richard Hill, who endowed it with estates now producing about £143 per annum, for which about sixty boys from the parishes of Bishop's Hampton, Charlecote, Alveston, and Wasperton, receive an English education only, classical instruction not having been given for many years past. In 1723, the Rev. William Lucy, D.D., gave £2000, in support of four scholars from this establishment at St. Mary Magdalene's Hall, Oxford, but, being ineligible from the want of classical instruction, selections are now made from other foundations.

HAMPTON-POYLE, a parish in the hundred of PLOUGHLEY, county of OXFORD, 3¼ miles (E. by S.) from Woodstock, containing 153 inhabitants. The living is a rectory, in the archdeaconry and diocese of Oxford, rated in the king's books at £6. 2. 8¼., and in the patronage of the Warden and Fellows of Queen's College, Oxford. The church is dedicated to St. Mary.

HAMPTON-WICK, a chapelry in the parish of HAMPTON, hundred of SPELTHORNE, county of MIDDLESEX, 1½ mile (E. by N.) from Hampton Court, containing 1261 inhabitants. The living is a perpetual curacy, in the archdeaconry of Middlesex, and diocese of London, and in the patronage of the Vicar of Hampton. The erection of a chapel was completed in 1830, at an expense of about £4000, granted by the parliamentary commissioners; it contains eight hundred sittings, one-half of which are free. The inhabitants of Hampton-Wick are entitled to one-third part of the charitable benefactions belonging to the parish, by virtue of an agreement entered into in 1698, between the minister and officers of Hampton, and the churchwarden of Hampton-Wick; and the free school is open to the children of the chapelry. The trade is principally in malt, a considerable quantity of which is made here. This place is within the jurisdiction of a court of requests for the recovery of debts under 40s., held during the summer half year at Brentford, and during the winter at Uxbridge. A new stone bridge over the Thames to Kingston has recently been erected, instead of a former bridge of wood, said to have been one of the oldest on the river. In making an excavation for the foundation of the abutment of the new bridge, on the north side of the river, in 1826, several military weapons of beautiful workmanship, in good preservation, were found, imbedded in blue clay, at the depth of thirty feet below the surface of the soil.

HAMSEY, a parish in the hundred of BARCOMB, rape of LEWES, county of SUSSEX, 2 miles (N.) from Lewes, containing 537 inhabitants. The living is a rectory, in the archdeaconry of Lewes, and diocese of Chichester, rated in the king's books at £16. 12. 8½., and in the patronage of Sir B. W. Bridges, Bart. The church, dedicated to St. Peter, is partly of early English architecture, with portions in the later style.

HAMSTALL-RIDWARE, a parish in the northern division of the hundred of OFFLOW, county of STAFFORD, 5½ miles (E.N.E.) from Rudgeley, containing 455 inhabitants. The living is a rectory, in the archdeaconry of Stafford, and diocese of Lichfield and Coventry, rated in the king's books at £6. 1. 0½., and in the patronage of Chandos Leigh, Esq. The church is dedicated to St. Michael. The parish is bounded on the south by the river Trent. A free school, erected in 1809, by the late Rev. Thomas Leigh, is supported by Chandos Leigh, Esq., and conducted upon the National system.

HAMSTEELS, a joint township with Burnop, in that part of the parish of LANCHESTER which is in the western division of CHESTER ward, county palatine of DURHAM, 6½ miles (W.N.W.) from Durham. The population is returned with Burnop.

HAMSTERLEY, a chapelry in that part of the parish of ST. ANDREW AUCKLAND which is in the north-western division of DARLINGTON ward, county palatine of DURHAM, 6¼ miles (W.) from Bishop-Auckland, containing 552 inhabitants. The living is a perpetual curacy, in the archdeaconry and diocese of Durham, endowed with £200 private benefaction, £200 royal bounty, and £1000 parliamentary grant. W. Chator, Esq. was patron in 1825. The church is dedicated to St. James. The Baptists have a place of worship, erected in 1774, with a burial-ground, a house and garden for the minister, and a school-room. There is also a place of worship for Wesleyan Methodists. At Bidburn are extensive iron-works: coal is obtained in the neighbourhood. A school-house has been built by public subscription, and there is a mechanics' institution in the parish.

HAMWORTHY, a chapelry in the parish of STURMINSTER-MARSHALL, hundred of COGDEAN, Shaston (East) division of the county of DORSET, 1½ mile (W.) from Poole, containing 313 inhabitants. It is within the jurisdiction of the peculiar court of Sturminster-Marshall. The chapel, which was destroyed during the parliamentary war, has been recently rebuilt, and contains four hundred and fifty free sittings, the Incorporated Society for the enlargement of churches and chapels having granted £550 towards defraying the expense. The chapelry is divided into Higher and Lower Ham, the latter of which is the more considerable; it adjoins Poole harbour, which affords great facility for carrying on trade.

HANBURY, a parish in the northern division of the hundred of OFFLOW, county of STAFFORD, comprising the chapelries of Marchington and Newborough, the townships of Coton, Fauld, Hanbury, Hanbury-Woodend, Marchington-Woodlands, and the hamlet of Stubby-Lane, and containing 2516 inhabitants, of which number, 147 are in the township of Hanbury, 6¾ miles (N.W. by W.) from Burton upon Trent. The living is a vicarage, not in charge, in the archdeaconry of Stafford, and diocese of Lichfield and Coventry; and in the patronage of the Bishop of Lichfield and Coventry. The church, dedicated to St. James, is principally in the later style of English architecture, with a Norman font, and has lately received an addition of one hundred and forty-three free sittings, the Incorporated Society for the enlargement of churches and chapels having granted £261 towards defraying the expense. A school-house was built by subscription in 1815, in which from sixty to seventy children are taught; it is endowed with about £24 per annum, arising from bequests by Jane Browne and — Hawkins, Esq.

HANBURY, a parish in the Middle division of the hundred of Oswaldslow, county of Worcester, 4 miles (E. by N.) from Droitwich, containing 1042 inhabitants. The living is a rectory, rated in the king's books at £29. 16. 8., in the peculiar jurisdiction of the Rector, but wills are always proved in the presence of the Bishop's registrar at Worcester, and are deposited in the registry there: it is in the patronage of T. T. Vernon, Esq. The church, dedicated to St. John the Baptist, stands upon a very lofty eminence: it is in the early, decorated, and later, English styles of architecture, and contains some elegant monuments to the Vernons. The Birmingham and Worcester canal passes through the parish, and in the neighbourhood is a salt spring. The Rev. Thomas Vernon, in 1627, founded a charity school in this parish, and Thomas Vernon, Esq., in 1711, gave certain lands towards its support, besides £200 for apprenticing poor children.

HANBURY-WOODEND, a township in the parish of Hanbury, northern division of the hundred of Offlow, county of Stafford, containing 256 inhabitants.

HANBY, a hamlet in the parish of Lavington, otherwise Linton, wapentake of Beltisloe, parts of Kesteven, county of Lincoln, 4½ miles (W. S. W.) from Falkingham, containing 32 inhabitants.

HANDBOROUGH, a parish in the hundred of Wootton, county of Oxford, 5¼ miles (E. N. E.) from Witney, containing 885 inhabitants. The living is a rectory, in the archdeaconry and diocese of Oxford, rated in the king's books at £11. 6. 0½., and in the patronage of the President and Fellows of St. John's College, Oxford. The church, dedicated to St. Peter and St. Paul, has a fine Norman door.

HANDCHURCH, a township in the parish of Trentham, northern division of the hundred of Pirehill, county of Stafford, 3 miles (S.) from Newcastle under Line, containing 224 inhabitants.

HANDFORD, a township in the parish of Trentham, northern division of the hundred of Pirehill, county of Stafford, containing 490 inhabitants.

HANDFORTH, a joint township with Boxden, in the parish of Cheadle, hundred of Macclesfield, county palatine of Chester, 6½ miles (S. W. by S.) from Stockport, containing 1745 inhabitants.

HANDLEY, a parish comprising the township of Handley, in the higher division, and the township of Golborn-David, in the lower division, of the hundred of Broxton, county palatine of Chester, and containing 332 inhabitants, of which number, 256 are in the township of Handley, 7¾ miles (S. E. by S.) from Chester. The living is a discharged rectory, in the archdeaconry and diocese of Chester, rated in the king's books at £6. 0. 5., and in the patronage of the Dean and Chapter of Chester. The church is dedicated to All Saints.

HANDLEY, a parish in that part of the hundred of Sixpenny-Handley which is in the Shaston (East) division of the county of Dorset, 5½ miles (N. W. by W.) from Cranborne, containing, with the chapelry of Gussage-St. Andrew, and the tythings of Minchinton and Woodcots, 831 inhabitants. The living is a perpetual curacy annexed to the vicarage of Iwerne-Minster, in the archdeaconry of Dorset, and diocese of Bristol. The church is dedicated to St. Mary. A market was granted for this place at an early period, and the market-day was changed in the reign of Henry III. but it has been disused from time immemorial.

HANDSACRE, a joint parish with Armitage, in the southern division of the hundred of Offlow, county of Stafford, 3½ miles (E. S. E.) from Rudgeley, containing, with Armitage, 793 inhabitants. The living is a perpetual curacy, within the peculiar jurisdiction and patronage of the Prebendary of Handsacre in the Cathedral Church of Lichfield.

HANDSWORTH, a parish in the southern division of the hundred of Offlow, county of Stafford, 2¼ miles (N. W. by N.) from Birmingham, containing, with the hamlets of Perry-Barr and Soho, 3859 inhabitants. The living is a rectory, in the archdeaconry of Stafford, and diocese of Lichfield and Coventry, rated in the king's books at £13. 9. 2., and in the patronage of Wyrley Birch, Esq. The church, dedicated to St. Mary the Virgin, has lately received an addition of four hundred and fifty sittings, of which two hundred and fifty are free, the Incorporated Society for the enlargement of churches and chapels having granted £500 towards defraying the expense: it contains two elegant marble monuments to the memory of Messrs. Boulton and Watt, the late celebrated proprietors of the extensive manufactory called Soho, at this place, who lived, died, and were buried here; that to the memory of Mr. Watt is placed in a handsome oratory erected purposely for its reception. The river Tame runs through the parish. A school was established in 1812, on the National system, at an expense of nearly £800, defrayed out of the fund of the Bridge trust; and is supported by voluntary contributions.

HANDSWORTH, a parish partly within the liberty of St. Peter of York, and partly in the southern division of the wapentake of Strafforth and Tickhill, West riding of the county of York, 4½ miles (E. by S.) from Sheffield, containing 2173 inhabitants. The living is a rectory, rated in the king's books at £12. 4. 7., in the peculiar jurisdiction of the Chancellor in the Cathedral Church of York. The Duke of Norfolk was patron in 1801. The church is dedicated to St. Mary. A school was erected by subscription about 1778, in which ten children are taught free; there is also a dwelling-house for the master, who receives £20 a year arising from a bequest of £200 by the Rev. Francis Lockier, D.D., in 1734, and a similar sum, the gift of Mrs. Howard, widow of the late rector.

HANFORD, an extra-parochial liberty, in the hundred of Redlane, Sturminster division of the county of Dorset, 5¼ miles (N. W. by N.) from Blandford-Forum, containing 13 inhabitants. This was anciently a distinct parish: here is a chapel in which divine service is performed once every Sunday; it is the burial-place of the family of Seymour, whose mansion is situated on the south side, and northward are the foundations of an ancient village.

HANGLETON, a parish in the hundred of Fisher-gate, rape of Lewes, county of Sussex, 4½ miles (N.W.)

from Brighton, containing 52 inhabitants. The living is a discharged rectory, in the archdeaconry of Lewes, and diocese of Chichester, rated in the king's books at £11. 14. 2. Lord Whitworth, and others were patrons in 1815. The church, dedicated to St. Helen, is in the early style of English architecture.

HANHAM, a chapelry in the parish of BITTON, upper division of the hundred of LANGLEY and SWINE-HEAD, county of GLOUCESTER, 5 miles (E. S. E.) from Bristol, containing 1086 inhabitants. It is bounded on the south-west by the river Avon.

HANKELOW, a township in the parish of AUD-LEM, hundred of NANTWICH, county palatine of CHES-TER, 1½ mile (N. N. E.) from Audlem, containing 258 inhabitants.

HANKERTON, a parish in the hundred of MALMES-BURY, county of WILTS, 3½ miles (N. E.) from Malmesbury, containing, with the tything of Cloatly, 356 inhabitants. The living is a vicarage, in the archdeaconry of Wilts, and diocese of Salisbury, rated in the king's books at £8. 10. The Rev. J. Wiggett was patron in 1785. The church is dedicated to the Holy Cross.

HANLEY, a market town and chapelry in the parish of STOKE upon TRENT, northern division of the hundred of PIREHILL, county of STAFFORD, 2½ miles (N.E. by E.) from Newcastle, and 152 (N. W. by N.) from London, containing 5622 inhabitants. This place, which is situated within the populous district of the potteries, is of comparatively recent origin, and is chiefly inhabited by persons employed in those works, the proprietors of which have several handsome mansions in the neighbourhood. The streets are paved with brick, and lighted with gas under the superintendence of commissioners appointed by act of parliament in 1825, and amended in 1828, the provisions of which extend also to the adjoining hamlet of Shelton; and the inhabitants are supplied with water conveyed into their houses by pipes. The principal articles of manufacture are china and earthenware, for which there are numerous manufactories, affording employment to a considerable part of the population, including women and children. The trade is greatly facilitated by the Trent and Mersey canal, which passes through the adjoining hamlet of Shelton, forming a channel of conveyance for the various articles manufactured, and an abundant supply of coal and other things requisite for their production. The market days are Wednesday and Saturday, and a large cattle market is held four times in the year. The police of the town is also under the control of the commissioners, and a chief bailiff is annually elected from among the most respectable inhabitants, whose chief business it is to convene and preside at all public meetings of the inhabitants. The living is a perpetual curacy, in the archdeaconry of Stafford, and diocese of Lichfield and Coventry, endowed with £1100 private benefaction, £1000 royal bounty, and £200 parliamentary grant, and in the patronage of the Trustees of the chapel. By an act of parliament passed in 1827, for the endowment of new churches at Shelton and Longton, provision is made for the further endowment of the living of Hanley, and for its subsequent conversion into a distinct rectory, and the chapelry into a separate parish; and with a view to carry this measure into effect, a treaty is now in negociation for transferring the patronage to the bishop

of the diocese. The chapel, an indifferent edifice not entitled to any architectural description, is about to be rebuilt as a church for the intended rectory, by means of a grant from the parliamentary commissioners. There are places of worship for Baptists, Independents, Wesleyan and other Methodists, Unitarians, and a Roman Catholic chapel. A National school, in which five hundred children are educated, is supported by subscription; and there are Sunday schools in connexion with the established church and the several dissenting congregations, in which a great number of children is instructed.

HANLEY-CASTLE, a parish in the lower division of the hundred of PERSHORE, county of WORCESTER, 1¼ mile (N. N. W.) from Upton upon Severn, containing 1424 inhabitants. The living is a discharged vicarage, in the archdeaconry and diocese of Worcester, rated in the king's books at £12. 15., and in the patronage of Sir Anthony Lechmere, Bart. The church is dedicated to St. Mary. There is a chapel for the Roman Catholics. Courts leet and baron are held annually. A school, founded by an ancestor of the family of Lechmere, is open to children of both sexes, who are supplied with books, and taught upon Dr. Bell's system: the endowment consists of land producing an income of £160 per annum, with a school-house and garden: the classics were originally taught, and the school had formerly two small exhibitions to Balliol College, Oxford. The river Severn runs through the parish, on the margin of which there was a castle successively possessed by the Nevilles, Earls of Warwick, the De Spensers, and the Lechmeres: its remains have been converted into a farm-house.

HANLEY-CHILD, a chapelry in the parish of EASTHAM, upper division of the hundred of DODDING-TREE, county of WORCESTER, 5 miles (S. E. by E.) from Tenbury, containing 195 inhabitants.

HANLEY-WILLIAM, a parish in the upper division of the hundred of DODDINGTREE, county of WOR-CESTER, 6 miles (E. S. E.) from Tenbury, containing 124 inhabitants. The living is a rectory, in the archdeaconry of Salop, and diocese of Hereford, rated in the king's books at £5. 7. 11., and in the patronage of the Rev. R. Whitehead. The church is dedicated to All Saints.

HANLITH, a township in that part of the parish of KIRKBY in MALLAM DALE which is in the western division of the wapentake of STAINCLIFFE and EWCROSS, West riding of the county of YORK, 6 miles (E. S. E.) from Settle, containing 46 inhabitants.

HANNAY, a parish in the Wold division of the hundred of CALCEWORTH, parts of LINDSEY, county of LINCOLN, 3¾ miles (N. E. by E.) from Alford, containing with Hagnaby, 106 inhabitants. The living is a donative, endowed with £1400 royal bounty, and in the patronage of J. Grant, Esq.

HANNEY (EAST), a township in the parish of WEST HANNEY, partly in the hundred of OCK, but chiefly in the hundred of WANTAGE, county of BERKS, 3½ miles (N. N. E.) from Wantage, containing 587 inhabitants. There is a trifling endowment for teaching poor children.

HANNEY (WEST), a parish comprising the chapelry of Lyford, in the hundred of OCK, and the township of East Hanney, chiefly in the hundred of WANTAGE, county of BERKS, 3¾ miles (N. by E.) from Wantage, containing 1107 inhabitants. The living is a discharged vicarage, in the archdeaconry of Berks, and diocese of Salisbury, rated in the king's books at £22. 12. 6., and in the patronage of the Dean and Chapter of Salisbury. The church, dedicated to St. James, is principally of Norman architecture. The river Ock, on which a silk-throwing mill has been erected, runs through the parish. Richard Belcher, in 1713, bequeathed a trifling sum for teaching children, and providing bread for the poor. At Lyford there is a chapel of ease; also an almshouse, founded in 1611 by Oliver Aschcombe Esq., for ten aged persons, elected from amongst the parishioners.

HANNINGFIELD (EAST), a parish in the hundred of CHELMSFORD, county of ESSEX, 4¼ miles (S. by W.) from Danbury, containing 398 inhabitants. The living is a rectory, in the archdeaconry of Essex, and diocese of London, rated in the king's books at £13. 15. 7½., and in the patronage of the Rev. John Nottidge. The church is dedicated to All Saints.

HANNINGFIELD (SOUTH), a parish in the hundred of CHELMSFORD, county of ESSEX, 6 miles (S. S. W.) from Danbury, containing 176 inhabitants. The living is a rectory, consolidated, in 1785, with that of West Hanningfield, in the archdeaconry of Essex, and diocese of London, rated in the king's books at £10. The church is dedicated to St. Peter.

HANNINGFIELD (WEST), a parish in the hundred of CHELMSFORD, county of ESSEX, 6 miles (S. W.) from Danbury, containing 468 inhabitants. The living is a rectory, with which the rectory of South Hanningfield was consolidated in 1785, in the archdeaconry of Essex, and diocese of London, rated in the king's books at £16. 13. 4., and in the patronage of Thomas Lowden, Esq. The church is dedicated to St. Mary and St. Edward. The inhabitants are supplied with water from a public well four hundred and sixty-two feet deep.

HANNINGTON, a parish in the hundred of ORLING-BURY, county of NORTHAMPTON, 6¾ miles (N. N. W.) from Wellingborough, containing 177 inhabitants. The living is a rectory consolidated with that of Walgrave, in the archdeaconry of Northampton, and diocese of Peterborough, rated in the king's books at £10. 11. 3., and in the patronage of the Bishop of Lincoln. The church is dedicated to St. Peter and St. Paul. Dr. Francis Godwin, successively Bishop of Llandaff and Hereford, a distinguished antiquary and biographer, was born, in 1561, in this parish, of which his father was rector, and afterwards Bishop of Bath and Wells: he died in 1633.

HANNINGTON, a parish in the hundred of CHUTE-LY, Kingsclere division of the county of SOUTHAMPTON, 7½ miles (N. W. by W.) from Basingstoke, containing 245 inhabitants. The living is a rectory, rated in the king's books at £6. 7. 3½., in the peculiar jurisdiction of the Rector, and in the patronage of the Bishop of Winchester. The church is dedicated to All Saints. Han-nington is within the jurisdiction of the Cheyney Court held at Winchester every Thursday, for the recovery of debts to any amount.

HANNINGTON, a parish in the hundred of HIGH-WORTH, CRICKLADE, and STAPLE, county of WILTS, 1¾ mile (W. N. W.) from Highworth, containing 412 inhabitants. The living is a vicarage, in the archdeaconry of Wilts, and diocese of Salisbury, rated in the king's

books at £7. 0. 10., and in the patronage of Roger Montgomery, Esq. The church is dedicated to St. John the Baptist.

HANSLOPE, a parish in the hundred of NEWPORT, county of BUCKINGHAM, 4½ miles (N. N. E.) from Stony-Stratford, containing 1479 inhabitants. The living is a vicarage not in charge, with the perpetual curacy of Castle-Thorpe, in the archdeaconry of Buckingham, and diocese of Lincoln, endowed with £600 royal bounty, and £400 parliamentary grant, and in the patronage of the Mayor and Corporation of Lincoln, as impropriators of the rectory, which is rated in the king's books at £48. The church, dedicated to St. James, had formerly an octagonal fluted spire, which, with the tower, rose to the height of more than two hundred feet: it was erected in 1409, by Thomas Knight, then rector, and was destroyed by lightning in 1804. There is a place of worship for Baptists. Hanslope had the privilege of a market on Thursday, which has long been disused; it was granted to William Beauchamp, Earl of Warwick, in 1293, with a fair commencing on St. James's day and continuing fifteen days; this also has been discontinued, but a fair for cattle is held on Holy Thursday. Several of the inhabitants are employed in the manufacture of lace. Children of both sexes are put to the lace schools at the early age of five years, and when arrived at that of eleven or twelve are able to support themselves. A school was founded and endowed in 1721, by Lucy, Lady Pierrepoint, for teaching four children; besides which there are various charitable gifts to the poor, vested in the hands of feoffees, and annually distributed on St. Thomas's day.

HANTHORPE, or HARMTHORPE, a chapelry in the parish of MORTON, wapentake of AVELAND, parts of KES-TEVEN, county of LINCOLN, containing 254 inhabitants.

HANWELL, a parish in the hundred of ELTHORNE, county of MIDDLESEX, 8 miles (W.) from London, containing 977 inhabitants. The living is a rectory, in the archdeaconry of Middlesex, and diocese of London, rated in the king's books at £20, and in the patronage of the Bishop of London. The church, dedicated to St. Mary, is a small brick edifice, rebuilt in 1781, at an expense of about £1675, principally raised by subscription. There is a place of worship for Independents. The river Brent runs through the parish, and the Grand Junction canal bounds it on the west. William Hobbayne, in 1484, gave for charitable uses lands then valued at £6 a year, now producing upwards of £105, of which sum £35 per annum is applied to the support of a charity school. A lunatic asylum for the county of Middlesex is now being erected here. Dr. George Henry Glasse, rector of Hanwell, who died in 1809, was an eminent classical scholar, and distinguished himself by writing Greek poetry, and by his Greek translation of Milton's Sampson Agonistes. James Hanway, a noted traveller and philanthropist, who died in 1786, was buried at Hanwell.

HANWELL, a parish in the hundred of BLOXHAM, county of OXFORD, 3 miles (N. N. W.) from Banbury, containing 286 inhabitants. The living is a rectory, in the archdeaconry and diocese of Oxford, rated in the king's books at £17. 16. 0½., and in the patronage of the Lord of the Manor. The church is dedicated to St. Peter. There are some remains of a castle belonging to the family of Cope.

HANWOOD (GREAT), a parish within the liberty of the borough of SHREWSBURY, county of SALOP, 3¾ miles (S. W. by W.) from Shrewsbury, containing, exclusively of the township of Little Hanwood, 157 inhabitants. The living is a discharged rectory, in the archdeaconry of Salop, and diocese of Hereford, rated in the king's books at £3, endowed with £400 private benefaction, and £400 royal bounty. H. D. Warters, Esq. was patron in 1810.

HANWOOD (LITTLE), a township in the parish of PONTESBURY, hundred of FORD, though locally in the parish of Great Hanwood, within the liberty of the borough of Shrewsbury, county of SALOP. The population is returned with the parish.

HANWORTH, a parish in the hundred of SPELTHORNE, county of MIDDLESEX, 3¼ miles (S. W. by S.) from Hounslow, containing 552 inhabitants. The living is a rectory, in the jurisdiction of the Commissary of London, concurrently with the Bishop, rated in the king's books at £11. 13. 4. John Bastard, Esq., was patron in 1819. The church is dedicated to St. George. The manor-house was the occasional residence of Henry VIII., and of Elizabeth, before she ascended the throne. Thomas Killegrew, a wit, dramatist, and courtier in the reign of Charles II., is said to have been a native of this place.

HANWORTH, a parish in the northern division of the hundred of ERPINGHAM, county of NORFOLK, 5½ miles (N. by E.) from Aylsham, containing 250 inhabitants. The living is a discharged vicarage, with the rectory of Gunton, in the archdeaconry of Norfolk, and diocese of Norwich, rated in the king's books at £5. 1. 8. The church is dedicated to St. Bartholomew.

HANWORTH (COLD), a parish in the eastern division of the wapentake of ASLACOE, parts of LINDSEY, county of LINCOLN, 8¾ miles (N. N. E.) from Lincoln, containing 57 inhabitants. The living is a discharged rectory, in the archdeaconry of Stow, and diocese of Lincoln, rated in the king's books at £5. 10., and in the patronage of Robert Cracroft, Esq. The church, dedicated to All Saints, was formerly surrounded by buildings, as is evident from the number of foundations remaining.

HAPPISBURGH, a parish in the hundred of HAPPING, county of NORFOLK, 6¼ miles (E.) from North Walsham, containing 523 inhabitants. The living is a discharged vicarage, in the archdeaconry of Norfolk, and diocese of Norwich, rated in the king's books at £6. 6. 8., and in the patronage of the Bishop of Norwich. The church is dedicated to St. Mary. This parish lies on the coast of the North sea. The skeleton of a very large fish was discovered in 1659, by the fall of a cliff into the sea, which from appearances had lain buried near the summit.

HAPSFORD, a township in the parish of THORNTON, second division of the hundred of EDDISBURY, county palatine of CHESTER, 4¼ miles (S. W. by W.) from Frodsham, containing 89 inhabitants.

HAPTON, a township in that part of the parish of WHALLEY which is in the higher division of the hundred of BLACKBURN, county palatine of LANCASTER, 3½ miles (W. S. W.) from Burnley, containing 568 inhabitants.

HAPTON, a parish in the hundred of DEPWADE, county of NORFOLK, 3½ miles (N. W. by N.) from St.

Mary Stratton, containing 186 inhabitants. The living is a perpetual curacy, in the archdeaconry of Norfolk, and diocese of Norwich, and in the patronage of the Master and Fellows of Christ's College, Cambridge. The church is dedicated to St. Margaret. There is a place of worship for Unitarians.

HARAM, a township in the parish of HELMSLEY, wapentake of RYEDALE, North riding of the county of YORK, 2¼ miles (S. E. by E.) from Helmsley, containing 461 inhabitants.

HARBERTON, a parish in the hundred of COLERIDGE, county of DEVON, 2 miles (S. W. by W.) from Totness, containing 1425 inhabitants. The living is a vicarage, with the perpetual curacy of Halwell annexed, in the archdeaconry of Totness, and diocese of Exeter, rated in the king's books at £49. 2. 1., and in the patronage of the Dean and Chapter of Exeter. The church, dedicated to St. Andrew, contains a very rich stone pulpit and three stone stalls, and has lately received an addition of two hundred and seventy sittings, of which two hundred and thirty-three are free, the Incorporated Society for the enlargement of churches and chapels having granted £100 towards defraying the expense. There is a place of worship for Baptists. Henry Wyse, in 1733, erected almshouses for ten poor persons. There was formerly an endowed chapel at Washbourn in this parish.

HARBLEDOWN (ST. MICHAEL), a parish in the hundred of WESTGATE, lathe of ST. AUGUSTINE, county of KENT, 1¼ mile (W. S. W.) from Canterbury, containing 678 inhabitants. The living is a rectory, in the archdeaconry and diocese of Canterbury, rated in the king's books at £9. 2. 6., and in the patronage of the Archbishop of Canterbury. The church, dedicated to St. Michael, has lately received an addition of two hundred and eighty-four free sittings, the Incorporated Society for the enlargement of churches and chapels having granted £250 towards defraying the expense. In this parish is a very ancient hospital, called originally the hospital of the Forest of Bleane, and subsequently of St. Nicholas of Harbledown, which latter name it still retains. It was founded by Archbishop Lanfranc, in 1084, for the reception of lepers of both sexes, for whom there were separate establishments, and so remained till the dissolution, when its revenue was valued at £109. 7. 2.; but being continued, it became, in the reign of Edward VI., as it now is, a college, or asylum for decayed persons, under the patronage of the Archbishop of Canterbury, with a revenue increased by various donations to about £250. The establishment is for a master, fifteen in-brothers, who enjoy the privileges of freeholders, and as many in-sisters; they have each about six guineas a year, and elect a prior and prioress from amongst their own body; there is the same number of out-brothers and sisters, with an allowance £1. 4. a year each, also a reader, who is a clerk in orders. At the time they lived in a conventual state the inmates were accustomed to carry out into the road the upper part of a shoe set in copper and chrystal, said to have belonged to Thomas à Becket, for passing travellers to kiss. The hospital was rebuilt in the reign of James II., and is chiefly of brick: the chapel, dedicated to St. Nicholas, which was formerly parochial, is a curious ancient edifice in the Norman style, with a square tower at the south-west angle.

HARBONE, or HARBORNE, a parish in the southern division of the hundred of OFFLOW, county of STAFFORD, 3¾ miles (S. W. by W.) from Birmingham, containing, with the hamlet of Smethwick, 3350 inhabitants. The living is a vicarage, rated in the king's books at £4, endowed with £200 private benefaction, and £200 royal bounty, and in the peculiar jurisdiction and patronage of the Dean and Chapter of Lichfield. The church, dedicated to St. Peter, has a tower in the later style of English architecture, and has lately received an addition of three hundred and sixty sittings, of which two hundred and sixty are free, the Incorporated Society for the enlargement of churches and chapels having granted £250 towards defraying the expense. A schoolroom, built by subscription, has been endowed by Mr. Henry Hinckley with three tenements producing an income of £24. 15. a year, for which sum forty children receive free instruction.

HARBOROUGH (MAGNA), a parish in the Kirby division of the hundred of KNIGHTLOW, county of WARWICK, 3¾ miles (N. N. W.) from Rugby, containing 319 inhabitants. The living is a rectory, in the archdeaconry of Coventry, and diocese of Lichfield and Coventry, rated in the king's books at £14. 13. 4., and in the patronage of Lady Leigh. The church is dedicated to All Saints. The Oxford canal bounds the parish on the west.

HARBOROUGH (MARKET), a market town in the parish of BOWDEN-MAGNA, hundred of GARTREE, county of LEICESTER, 17 miles (N.) from Northampton, 15 (S. E. by S.) from Leicester, and 83 (N. W. by N.) from London, containing 1873 inhabitants. This town, in the ancient record called Testa de Nevil, is called Haverberg, from haver, a term still used in the northern counties to signify oats, and berg, a hill; which was afterwards converted into Haverbrowe, and Harborough. It is supposed to have been occupied the Romans; a square intrenchment, probably the site of a camp, having formerly existed in a field called King's Head close, at a short distance from which Roman urns and other fragments of pottery have been discovered; and in one of the streets, a sewer, or drain, was found a few years ago, in which were traces of Roman masonry. During the civil war, this town was attached to the royal cause, and was the headquarters of the king's army prior to the memorable battle of Naseby, in Northamptonshire, in 1645. The royalists formed on the morning of battle on a hill north of the town; and Cromwell's letter to the Parliament, giving an account of the battle, is dated at Harborough. The town is situated on the southern border of the county, and on the northern bank of the river Welland, and consists of one principal street and several smaller. The buildings have been much improved of late years, and it is now well paved and lighted. In the principal street is a large town-hall, built in 1788, by the Earl of Harborough, for the use of the tammy dealers, but that branch of manufacture, as well as that of shalloons, &c., having become extinct, the under part has been converted into shops, and the upper is occupied by the magistrates for official purposes. The only remaining branch of manufacture is that of carpets. The market is on Thursday: fairs are held on January 6th, February 16th, April 29th, on the Tuesday after May 2nd, Tuesday after Mid-Lent Sunday, and July 31st, for cattle; on October 19th and eight

following days, for cattle, cheese, leather, &c., on the Tuesday before November 22nd, and December 8th. The canal from Leicester passes by the town, near which it joins the Welland. The London road enters the town over a handsome stone bridge erected in 1814, at the joint expense of the counties of Leicester and Northampton. The petty sessions for the hundred of Gartree are held here occasionally; and a court leet and baron for the manor is also held, but at uncertain periods. The living is a perpetual curacy, in the archdeaconry of Leicester, and diocese of Lincoln, and in the patronage of the Dean and Canons of Christ Church, Oxford. The church, which is dedicated to St. Dionysius, is a large, handsome, and uniform edifice, and ranks among the finest in the county: it consists of a nave, aisles, and a chancel, with two tiers of windows, two porches, and a tower, having an octangular crocketed spire: it is said to have been built by John of Gaunt, about the year 1370. There are places of worship for Independents and Wesleyan Methodists. Here is a free grammar school, founded about 1614 by Robert Smith, a native of this place, and Chamberlain of London, who purchased of the lord mayor and commonalty an annuity of £10 per annum, to be paid to the master for teaching fifteen poor boys; and there is some additional endowment from subsequent benefactions, but the whole being insufficient for the support of a classical teacher, it has lately been converted into a National school, in which about one hundred boys are taught gratuitously. Harborough gives the titles of baron and earl to the family of Sherard.

HARBOTTLE, a township in the parish of HALLYSTONE, western division of COQUETDALE ward, county of NORTHUMBERLAND, 2 miles (N.W.) from Hallystone, containing 181 inhabitants. A place of worship for Presbyterians was erected in 1756. There are two fairs for sheep, on the 8th of July and the 9th of September. A free school was founded by the late William Dixon, and endowed with certain property producing £14. 10. a year, for which sixteen children are educated, besides thirteen others instructed at the expense of Thomas Clennell, Esq. The castle, now in ruins, was, in the reign of Edward I., a very strong fortress, and sustained the reiterated attacks of the whole Scottish army in 1296. Hither Margaret, Queen Dowager of Scotland, retired in 1515, after her marriage with the Earl of Angus, and here she was delivered of a daughter in 1518. The extensive remains of the building are situated on a commanding eminence overlooking the river Coquet; the walls of the great tower, being rent asunder and overhanging their bases, have a singular and striking effect.

HARBRIDGE, a chapelry in the parish and hundred of RINGWOOD, New Forest (West) division of the county of SOUTHAMPTON, 3¼ miles (N.) from Ringwood, containing 352 inhabitants. This chapelry is within the peculiar jurisdiction of the vicar of Ringwood. The river Avon is navigable through the parish.

HARBURY, otherwise HARBERBURY, a parish in the Kenilworth division of the hundred of KNIGHTLOW, county of WARWICK, 3¾ miles (W. S. W.) from Southam, containing 1045 inhabitants. The living is a discharged vicarage, in the archdeaconry of Coventry, and diocese of Lichfield and Coventry, rated in the king's books at £5. Miss Newsham was patroness in 1806. The church is dedicated to All Saints. There is a place of worship for Wesleyan Methodists. Thomas

Wagstaffe, in 1611, founded a school for teaching all the children of the parish, and endowed it with £20 a year, which is paid to the master, who resides in a house appropriated to his use.

HARBY, a parish in the hundred of FRAMLAND, county of LEICESTER, 8¾ miles (N.) from Melton-Mowbray, containing 457 inhabitants. The living is a rectory, in the archdeaconry of Leicester, and diocese of Lincoln, rated in the king's books at £20, and in the patronage of the Duke of Rutland. The church is dedicated to St. Mary. The Nottingham and Grantham canal passes through the parish. Here are several chalybeate springs, and in the village is an ancient stone cross.

HARBY, a chapelry in the parish of NORTH CLIFTON, northern division of the wapentake of NEWARK, county of NOTTINGHAM, 8½ miles (W.) from Lincoln, containing 267 inhabitants. The chapel has lately received an addition of one hundred and ten sittings, of which eighty are free, the Incorporated Society for the enlargement of churches and chapels having granted £60 towards defraying the expense. There is a place of worship for Wesleyan Methodists.

HARCOURT, a township in the parish of STANTON upon HINE HEATH, Whitchurch division of the hundred of BRADFORD (North), county of SALOP, containing 34 inhabitants.

HARDENHUISH, a parish in the hundred of CHIPPENHAM, county of WILTS, 1¼ mile (N. W.) from Chippenham, containing 70 inhabitants. The living is a rectory not in charge, in the archdeaconry of Wilts, and diocese of Salisbury, and in the patronage of T. Clutterbuck, Esq. The church is dedicated to St. Christopher Anstey, Esq., author of the New Bath Guide, and of several miscellaneous poems, died here in 1805.

HARDHAM, a parish in the hundred of BURY, rape of ARUNDEL, county of SUSSEX, 6 miles (S. E. by E.) from Petworth, containing 114 inhabitants. The living is a discharged rectory, in the archdeaconry and diocese of Chichester, rated in the king's books at £5. 5. 10., and endowed with £1600 royal bounty. Sir C. F. Goring, Bart. was patron in 1788. The church, dedicated to St. Botolph, is in the early style of English architecture. The parish is bounded on the east, north, and south by the river Arun, and partly on the west by a branch of the Rother, which there falls into the Arun. A priory of Black canons, in honour of the Holy Cross, or of St. George, was founded here, but by whom is uncertain.

HARDHORN, a joint township with Newton, in the parish of POULTON, hundred of AMOUNDERNESS, county palatine of LANCASTER, 1½ mile (S.) from Poulton, containing 392 inhabitants.

HARDINGHAM, a parish in the hundred of MITFORD, county of NORFOLK, 5¾ miles (N. W. by W.) from Wymondham, containing 461 inhabitants. The living is a rectory, in the archdeaconry of Norfolk, and diocese of Norwich, rated in the king's books at £15. 3. 4., and in the patronage of the Master and Fellows of Clare Hall, Cambridge. The church is dedicated to St. George.

HARDINGSTONE, a parish in the hundred of WYMERSLEY, county of NORTHAMPTON, 2 miles (S. S. E.) from Northampton, containing, with the hamlets of Cotton-End, Far-Cotton with Paper-Mills, and De-

lapree-Abbey, 1012 inhabitants. The living is a vicarage, in the archdeaconry of Northampton, and diocese of Peterborough, rated in the king's books at £13. 5., and in the patronage of the Crown. The church, dedicated to St. Edmund, has portions in the early style of English architecture. The river Nen, and a branch from the Grand Junction canal to Northampton, pass through the parish, and join at Cotton-End, where are commodious wharfs and warehouses. There are many fine springs of water, and some which are strongly impregnated with iron. Near the side of the London road is one of the beautiful monumental crosses erected by Edward I. to the memory of his consort Eleanor, called Queen's Cross, to the south-west of which is a commanding eminence crowned by the remains of Danes' camp, a circular fortification enclosing an area of more than four acres, and supposed to have been constructed by Sweyn, the father of Canute. In an adjoining field the skeletons of soldiers have been found, buried with their arms, consisting of swords, spears, &c., also some earthen vessels of a peculiar shape. A battle, called the battle of Northampton, was fought here, in which the Duke of Buckingham and other nobles were killed, and Henry VI. was made prisoner, in the 38th year of his reign. James Hervey, author of the Meditations, was born at this village in 1714.

HARDINGTON, a parish in the hundred of KILMERSDON, county of SOMERSET, 4½ miles (N.W. by N.) from Frome, containing 31 inhabitants. The living is a discharged rectory with that of Hemington, in the archdeaconry of Wells, and diocese of Bath and Wells, rated in the king's books at £6, and in the patronage of Sir G. Bamfylde, Bart. The church is dedicated to St. Mary.

HARDINGTON-MANDEVILLE, a parish in the hundred of HOUNDSBOROUGH, BERWICK, and COKER, county of SOMERSET, 4½ miles (S. W.) from Yeovil, containing 537 inhabitants. The living is a rectory, in the archdeaconry of Wells, and diocese of Bath and Wells, rated in the king's books at £9. 15. 7½. William Helyar, Esq. was patron in 1823. The church, dedicated to St. Mary, has lately received an addition of one hundred and ten free sittings, the Incorporated Society for the enlargement of churches and chapels having granted £80 towards defraying the expense.

HARDLEY, a parish in the hundred of LODDON, county of NORFOLK, 7 miles (S. by W.) from Acle, containing 222 inhabitants. The living is a perpetual curacy, in the archdeaconry of Norfolk, and diocese of Norwich, and in the patronage of the Mayor and Corporation of Norwich. The church is dedicated to St. Margaret. A considerable quantity of corn is sent in small craft from Hardley-staith to Yarmouth.

HARDMEAD, a parish in the hundred of NEWPORT, county of BUCKINGHAM, 5 miles (N. E. by E.) from Newport-Pagnell, containing 75 inhabitants. The living is a rectory, in the archdeaconry of Buckingham, and diocese of Lincoln, rated in the king's books at £13. 6. 10½. Robert Shedden, Esq. was patron in 1817. The church is dedicated to St. Mary.

HARDRES (LOWER), a parish in the hundred of BRIDGE and PETHAM, lathe of ST. AUGUSTINE, county of KENT, 3 miles (S.) from Canterbury, containing 213 inhabitants. The living is a rectory, in the archdeaconry and diocese of Canterbury, rated in the king's books at

£7. 19. 9½., and in the patronage of the Crown. The church is dedicated to St. Mary.

HARDRES (UPPER), a parish in the hundred of Bridge and Petham, lathe of St. Augustine, county of Kent, 4¾ miles (S.) from Canterbury, containing 243 inhabitants. The living is a rectory, with the perpetual curacy of Stelling, in the archdeaconry and diocese of Canterbury, rated in the king's books at £19. 13. 1½., and in the patronage of the Heirs of Lady Hardres. The church, dedicated to St. Peter and St. Paul, is principally in the early style of English architecture. The ancient Stane street passes through the parish. Elizabeth Denward, in 1785, gave a dwelling house and two school-rooms, with lands and certain stock in the Navy five per cents., towards the support of a master and a mistress, who teach twenty boys and twelve girls upon the National system.

HARDROW, a chapelry in the parish of Aysgarth, western division of the wapentake of Hang, North riding of the county of York, 18½ miles (W. by N.) from Middleham. The population is returned with the township of High Abbot-side. The living is a perpetual curacy, in the archdeaconry of Richmond, and diocese of Chester, endowed with £400 private benefaction, £800 royal bounty, and £400 parliamentary grant, and in the patronage of Lord Wharncliffe, who has recently endowed a school with £10. 10. per annum. Within the parish is a tremendous waterfall, called Hardrow Scarr, with immense masses of rock overhanging it on each side : during the severe frost in 1740, this cascade was entirely congealed into a stupendous cone of ice.

HARDWICK, a hamlet in the parish of Monk-Hesleton, southern division of Easington ward, county palatine of Durham, 11 miles (E. by S.) from Durham. The population is returned with the parish. Here was formerly a chapel, which has been demolished. A serpentine canal runs into Hardwick park, and passing under a handsome bridge, empties itself into a lake covering about thirty-six acres. Artificial cascades and mock ruins of a monastery, the latter formed principally of carved stones brought from the ancient priory of Guisborough, also adorn the grounds.

HARDWICK, a chapelry in the parish of Standish, upper division of the hundred of Whitstone, county of Gloucester, 5 miles (S. W. by S.) from Gloucester, containing 446 inhabitants. The chapel has a low embattled tower at the west end of the south aisle. The Gloucester and Berkeley canal passes through the chapelry. Hardwick gives the titles of baron and earl to the family of Yorke.

HARDWICK, a parish in the hundred of Depwade, county of Norfolk, 3 miles (S. S. E.) from St. Mary Stratton, containing 237 inhabitants. The living is a discharged rectory with that of Shelton, in the archdeaconry of Norfolk, and diocese of Norwich, rated in the king's books at £5. The church, dedicated to St. Margaret, has a tower circular at the base, and octagonal above. There is a place of worship for Wesleyan Methodists.

HARDWICK, a hamlet (formerly a parish) in the Lynn division of the hundred of Freebridge, county of Norfolk, 1½ mile (S. S. E.) from Lynn-Regis. The population is returned with North Runcton, with the living of which parish that of Hardwick has been con-

solidated. There was anciently an hospital for lepers, dedicated to St. Lawrence.

HARDWICK, a parish in the hundred of Orlingbury, county of Northampton, 3¼ miles (N. W. by W.) from Wellingborough, containing 87 inhabitants. The living is a rectory, in the archdeaconry of Northampton, and diocese of Peterborough, rated in the king's books at £6. 17. 6. The Rev. H. Hughes was patron in 1805. The church is dedicated to St. Leonard.

HARDWICK, an extra-parochial liberty, though locally in the parish of Hawstead, hundred of Thingoe, county of Suffolk, 1½ mile (S. by W.) from Bury-St. Edmund's. The population is returned with Hawstead. At Hardwick-house, in this liberty, lived and died Sir John Cullum, a learned antiquary, and author of the History of Hawstead.

HARDWICK (EAST), a township in the parish of Pontefract, upper division of the wapentake of Osgoldcross, West riding of the county of York, 1½ mile (N. by W.) from Pontefract, containing 96 inhabitants. Stephen Cawood, in 1653, conveyed to trustees certain estates for the purpose of erecting and maintaining a chapel and a free school, and for other charitable uses : the annual income is £132, and thirty children are educated free.

HARDWICK (PRIORS), a parish in the Burton-Dassett division of the hundred of Kington, county of Warwick, 5¾ miles (S. E.) from Southam, containing 263 inhabitants. The living is a vicarage, with the perpetual curacy of Priors-Marston, in the archdeaconry of Coventry, and diocese of Lichfield and Coventry, rated in the king's books at £23. 16. 0½. The Duke of Marlborough was patron in 1796. The church is dedicated to St. Mary. The Oxford canal passes through the parish.

HARDWICK (WEST), a township in that part of the parish of Wragby which is in the upper division of the wapentake of Osgoldcross, West riding of the county of York, 4 miles (S. W.) from Pontefract, containing 93 inhabitants.

HARDWICKE, a parish in the hundred of Cottesloe, county of Buckingham, 3½ miles (N. by W.) from Aylesbury, containing, with the hamlet of Weedon, 627 inhabitants. The living is a rectory, in the archdeaconry of Buckingham, and diocese of Lincoln, rated in the king's books at £39. 9. 7., and in the patronage of the Warden and Fellows of New College, Oxford. The church is dedicated to St. Mary. John Bridle, D. D., in 1781, founded a charity school and endowed it with lands, the proceeds of which are applied to the instruction of eighteen boys and twelve girls.

HARDWICKE, a parish in the hundred of Longstow, county of Cambridge, 5½ miles (E. by N.) from Caxton, containing 134 inhabitants. The living is a rectory, in the peculiar jurisdiction and patronage of the Bishop of Ely, rated in the king's books at £8. 14. 2. The church is dedicated to St. Mary.

HARDWICKE, a hamlet in that part of the parish of Abergavenny which is in the upper division of the hundred of Abergavenny, county of Monmouth, 2 miles (S. S. E.) from Abergavenny, containing 83 inhabitants.

HARDWICKE, a hamlet in the parish of Ducklington, hundred of Bampton, county of Oxford, 3¼ miles (S.S.E.) from Witney, containing 124 inhabitants.

HARDWICKE, a parish in the hundred of PLOUGH-LEY, county of OXFORD, 5 miles (N.) from Bicester, containing, with the parish of Tusmore, 98 inhabitants. The living is a discharged rectory, in the archdeaconry and diocese of Oxford, rated in the king's books at £5, endowed with £200 royal bounty, and in the patronage of Sir H. W. Dashwood, Bart. The church is dedicated to St. Mary.

HARDY, a joint chapelry with Chorlton, in the parish of MANCHESTER, hundred of SALFORD, county palatine of LANCASTER, 4¼ miles (S.S.W.) from Manchester. The population is returned with Chorlton, under which the account of the living is given.

HAREBY, a parish in the western division of the soke of BOLINGBROKE, parts of LINDSEY, county of LINCOLN, 4¼ miles (W.) from Spilsby, containing 71 inhabitants. The living is a discharged rectory, united in 1739 to the rectory of Bolingbroke, in the archdeaconry and diocese of Lincoln, rated in the king's books at £6. 4. 7. Earl Brownlow was patron in 1816. The church is dedicated to St. Peter and St. Paul.

HAREFIELD, a parish in the hundred of EL-THORNE, county of MIDDLESEX, 4¼ miles (N.) from Uxbridge, containing 1228 inhabitants. The living is a donative, in the jurisdiction of the Commissary of London concurrently with the Consistorial Court of the Bishop, and in the patronage of Charles Newdigate Newdigate, Esq. The church, dedicated to the Virgin Mary, contains several memorials of the ancient family of Newdigate, and a splendid monument to the memory of Alice, Countess of Derby, who, about 1637, founded and endowed almshouses for six poor widows. The Knights Hospitallers had here a preceptory, a cell to that of St. John, Clerkenwell, the chapel of which, still standing, is in the early style of English architecture. The parish is bounded on the west by the river Colne, and the Grand Junction canal passes through it.

HARESCOMB, a parish in the middle division of the hundred of DUDSTONE and KING'S BARTON, county of GLOUCESTER, 2¼ miles (W. by N.) from Painswick, containing 104 inhabitants. The living is a discharged rectory with that of Pitchcomb, in the archdeaconry and diocese of Gloucester, rated in the king's books at £6. 8., and in the patronage of—Pernal, Esq. The church, dedicated to St. John the Baptist, has been lately rebuilt, and the expenses defrayed by voluntary contributions.

HARESFIELD, a parish in the upper division of the hundred of WHITSTONE, county of GLOUCESTER 5½ miles (N. W. by N.) from Stroud, containing 662 inhabitants. The living is a discharged vicarage, in the archdeaconry and diocese of Gloucester, rated in the king's books at £17, and in the patronage of the Earl of Hardwicke. The church, dedicated to St. Peter, appears to have been built by the prior of Llanthony; it has a western tower, surmounted by a handsome spire. The Gloucester and Berkeley canal passes through the parish. A trifling sum, the united bequests of Mrs. Capel and Mr. Daniel Niblett, is appropriated to the instruction of children.

HAREUP, or HAREHOPE, a township in the parish of EGLINGHAM, northern division of COQUETDALE ward, county of NORTHUMBERLAND, 10¼ miles (N. W.) from Alnwick, containing 46 inhabitants.

HAREWOOD, a parish in the upper division of the hundred of WORMELOW, county of HEREFORD, 5½ miles (N.W. by W.) from Ross, containing 80 inhabitants. The living is a perpetual curacy, in the peculiar jurisdiction and patronage of the Bishop of Hereford, rated in the king's books at £1. 15. 3. The church is dedicated to St. Denis. The petty sessions for the division are held here every fourth Tuesday. This parish formed part of the ancient Forest of Harewood, in which it is said King Edgar assassinated Earl Ethelwold for his deceitful conduct towards the fair Elfrida. The earl had a castle here, the scene of Mason's dramatic poem " Elfrida."

HAREWOOD, a parish comprising the townships of Dunkeswith and Weeton, in the upper division of the wapentake of CLARO, the township of East Keswick, in the lower division, and the townships of Alwoodley, Harewood, Weardley, Wigton, and Wike, in the upper division of the wapentake of SKYRACK, West riding of the county of YORK, and containing 2348 inhabitants, of which number, 849 are in the township of Harewood, 6½ miles (W. S. W.) from Wetherby. The living is a discharged vicarage, in the archdeaconry and diocese of York, rated in the king's books at £14. 1. 10., endowed with £37 per annum private benefaction, and £200 royal bounty, and in the patronage of the Parishioners and Mr. Wheeler alternately. The church, dedicated to All Saints, was erected in the reign of Edward III., upon the site of an edifice supposed to have been built soon after the Conquest : it contains stately monuments to the memory of several of the ancient possessors of Harewood, and one to the memory of the celebrated Sir William Gascoigne, Knt., Lord Chief Justice in the reign of Henry IV., the upright judge, who, for an insult offered to the dignity of the bench, committed the Prince of Wales (afterwards Henry V.) to prison. There is a place of worship for Wesleyan Methodists. The parish is thought to contain coal, though none is obtained. A charter for a market on Monday was granted to Lord Strafford about 1633, also a fortnight fair in Summer and two other fairs; the latter only are continued, and are held on the last Monday in April, and the second Monday in October. On the acclivity of a hill, at the foot of which winds the river Warf, are the noble ruins of a castle, supposed to have been built about the time of the erection of the original church, by one of the Romellis : it afterwards came into the family of Lascelles, and was neglected as a residence by Edwin Lascelles, Esq., who, before he was raised to the peerage in 1790, fixed upon a spot on the opposite side of the hill, and there built the present splendid seat of the family, at an expense stated to exceed £100,000. Harewood gives the titles of baron and earl to the family of Lascelles.

HARFORD, a parish in the hundred of ERMINGTON, county of DEVON, 6¼ miles (N. by W.) from Modbury, containing 199 inhabitants. The living is a rectory, in the archdeaconry of Totness, and diocese of Exeter, rated in the king's books at £11. 14. 4½., and in the patronage of Sir John Leman Rogers, Bart., and the Heirs of the late Rev. Humphrey Julian, alternately. The river Erme has its source in the parish, and a large paper manufactory has been erected on its banks.

HARGHAM, a parish in the hundred of SHROP-HAM, county of NORFOLK, 3½ miles (S. W. by S.) from Attleburgh, containing 72 inhabitants. The living is a discharged rectory with that of Wilby, in the archdeaconry of Norfolk, and diocese of Norwich, rated in the king's books at £4. 4. 2. The church is dedicated to All Saints.

HARGRAVE, a chapelry in that part of the parish of TARVIN which is in the lower division of the hundred of BROXTON, county palatine of CHESTER, 5¾ miles (E.) from Tarporley. The population is returned with the parish. The living is a perpetual curacy, in the archdeaconry and diocese of Chester, and in the patronage of certain Trustees nominated by the parishioners Tarvin. The chapel is dedicated to St. Michael.

HARGRAVE, a parish in the hundred of HIGHAM-FERRERS, county of NORTHAMPTON, 3½ miles (W. by N.) from Kimbolton, containing 192 inhabitants. The living is a rectory, in the archdeaconry of Northampton, and diocese of Peterborough, rated in the king's books at £13. 6. 8. John Baker, Esq. was patron in 1818. The church is dedicated to All Saints.

HARGRAVE, a parish in the hundred of THINGOE, county of SUFFOLK, 6½ miles (W. S. W.) from Bury-St. Edmund's, containing, with Southwell Park 360 inhabitants. The living is a rectory, in the archdeaconry of Sudbury, and diocese of Norwich, rated in the king's books at £4. 11. 8. The Rev. John White was patron in 1819.

HARKSTEAD, a parish in the hundred of SAMFORD, county of SUFFOLK, 6½ miles (S. by E.) from Ipswich, containing 301 inhabitants. The living is a rectory, in the archdeaconry of Suffolk, and diocese of Norwich, rated in the king's books at £11. 3. 9. The Rev. H. D. Berners was patron in 1803. The church is dedicated to St. Mary, besides which there was formerly a chapel dedicated to St. Clement. The navigable river Stour runs on the southern side of the parish.

HARLAXTON, a parish in the soke of GRANTHAM, parts of KESTEVEN, county of LINCOLN, 3 miles (S. W.) from Grantham, containing 389 inhabitants. The living is a rectory, in the archdeaconry and diocese of Lincoln, rated in the king's books at £25. 6. 10½., and in the alternate patronage of the Prebendaries of North and South Grantham in the Cathedral Church of Salisbury. The church is dedicated to St. Mary and St. Peter ; its tower is surmounted by a spire, and the chancel is separated from the nave by a carved wooden screen. The Nottingham and Grantham canal passes through the parish.

HARLE (KIRK), a parish in the north-eastern division of TINDALE ward, county of NORTHUMBERLAND, comprising the chapelry of Kirkheaton, and the townships of Hawick and Kirk-Harle, and containing 354 inhabitants, of which number, 192 are in the township of Kirk-Harle, including therein Belridge, Greatlaw, Kidlaw, Mirlow-House, Shield-Hill, and Thrivewell, 13½ miles (W. by S.) from Morpeth. The living is a vicarage, in the archdeaconry of Northumberland, and diocese of Durham, rated in the king's books at £3. 8. 4. Sir C. Loraine, Bart. was patron in 1805. The church is dedicated to St. Wilfrid. On an eminence called Chapel Hill, in the township of Hawick, there was formerly a chapel.

HARLE (LITTLE), a township in the parish of KIRKWHELPINGTON, north-eastern division of TINDALE ward, county of NORTHUMBERLAND, 12½ miles (W. by S.) from Morpeth, containing 48 inhabitants. Little Harle

tower, an ancient border fortress, now forms part of a handsome and commodious mansion.

HARLE (WEST), a township in the parish of KIRKWHELPINGTON, north-eastern division of TINDALE ward, county of NORTHUMBERLAND, 14½ miles (W. by S.) from Morpeth, containing 64 inhabitants.

HARLESTON, a market town in the parish of REDDENHALL, hundred of EARSHAM, county of NORFOLK, 19 miles (S.) from Norwich, and 99½ (N. E.) from London. The population is returned with the parish. The original appellation of Herolfston, or Herolveston, of which the present is a corruption, was derived from Herolf, one of the Danish leaders who came over with Sweyn, and settled in this part of the kingdom : in the centre of the town stands a stone, formerly called Herolf's stone, whence probably originated the name of a family to which belonged Sir John Herolvestone, who in the reign of Richard II. quelled a formidable insurrection in Norfolk and the neighbouring counties. The town is situated on the high road from Bury-St. Edmund's to Yarmouth, about one mile from the river Waveney, over which there is a bridge : it is lighted with oil by subscription among the inhabitants, and well supplied with water from springs, but not paved. The manufacture of bombazines has been carried on of late years to a limited extent. The market is on Wednesday : fairs are held on Midsummer-day, and on the 9th and 10th of September ; the latter, which is still a large sheep and cattle fair, formerly continued eight days; on the 1st of December is a fair for Scotch cattle, which continues one month, and which was removed hither many years since from Hoxne in Suffolk. The whole town is under the superior jurisdiction of the Duke of Norfolk, who is lord of the manor, and has the tolls of the markets and fairs, holding courts for the manor occasionally. In the centre of the town is a chapel of ease, dedicated to St. John the Baptist, which was rebuilt in 1726, and enlarged in 1823, at the expense of the parishioners, by taking in the site of the market cross, which stood at the east end : the curate is nominated by the Master and Fellows of Emanuel College, Cambridge, pursuant to the direction of Dr. Sancroft, Archbishop of Canterbury, who in 1688 settled upon that society £54 per annum, in trust, to nominate a chaplain and schoolmaster, and pay him that sum for the performance of daily service in this chapel, and for the education of youth. The chapel has lately received an addition of one hundred and fifty free sittings, towards defraying the expense of which the Incorporated Society for the enlargement of churches and chapels granted £100. There are places of worship for Independents and Wesleyan Methodists. The rents of an estate in the adjoining parish of Rushall, purchased with £200, the gift of Mr. John Dove, who died in 1690; likewise a rent-charge of 20s. on a piece of land called the Fairstead, are appropriated to the same purpose. A National school, supported by voluntary contributions, affords instruction to about one hundred children of both sexes.

HARLESTON, a chapelry in the parish of CLIFTON-CAMPVILLE, northern division of the hundred of OFFLOW, county of STAFFORD, 4¼ miles (N.) from Tamworth, containing 211 inhabitants.

HARLESTON, a parish in the hundred of STOW, county of SUFFOLK, 3 miles (N. W. by W.) from Stow-Market, containing 94 inhabitants. The living is a discharged rectory, in the archdeaconry of Sudbury, and diocese of Norwich, rated in the king's books at £2, and endowed with £200 royal bounty. R. Pettiward, Esq. was patron in 1826.

HARLESTONE, a parish in the hundred of NOBOTTLE-GROVE, county of NORTHAMPTON, 4 miles (N. W.) from Northampton, containing 564 inhabitants. The living is a rectory, in the archdeaconry of Northampton, and diocese of Peterborough, rated in the king's books at £20. 9. 7. R. Andrews, Esq. was patron in 1809. The church is dedicated to St. Andrew. On Delves heath are vestiges of an ancient fortification.

HARLEY, a parish in the hundred of CONDOVER, county of SALOP, 2¼ miles (N. W. by W.) from Much Wenlock, containing 235 inhabitants. The living is a rectory, in the archdeaconry of Salop, and diocese of Lichfield and Coventry, rated in the king's books at £5. 12. 1., and in the patronage of Sir Edward Kynaston, Bart. The church is dedicated to St. Mary. The river Perry, and the Ellesmere canal, pass through the parish.

HARLING (EAST), a market town and parish in the hundred of GUILT-CROSS, county of NORFOLK, 22 miles (S. W.) from Norwich, and 89 (N. E. by N.) from London, containing 867 inhabitants. This place is called East Harling and Market Harling, to distinguish it from the neighbouring parish of West Harling. It is situated on the banks of a rivulet, between the towns of Thetford and Buckenham : the streets are neither lighted nor paved, but the inhabitants are well supplied with water. The manufacture of linen was formerly considerable, but the town is now nearly destitute of trade. A charter for a market and two fairs was granted in the reign of Edward IV.; the market is held on Tuesday, and there are fairs for live stock on May 4th, the first Tuesday after September 19th, a fortnight after Michaelmas-day, and October 24th, and a statute fair for hiring servants a fortnight before Michaelmas-day. The living is a rectory, in the archdeaconry of Norfolk, and diocese of Norwich, rated in the king's books at £12, and in the patronage of John Steward, Esq. The church, dedicated to St. Peter and St. Paul, was erected about the middle of the fifteenth century ; it is a fine uniform edifice, with a south porch, and a square tower surmounted by an open battlement and a small spire : the screen, separating the nave from the chancel, is finely carved, and the chancel windows are adorned with ancient stained glass removed from the dilapidated mansion of Harling hall : adjoining the south aisle is a sepulchral chapel belonging to the family of Harling, in which is an altar-tomb, with the recumbent effigies in marble of Sir Robert Harling and his lady, and various other tombs and memorials of individuals belonging to that family. There are places of worship for the Society of Friends and Wesleyan Methodists.

HARLING (MIDDLE), a hamlet, formerly a parish, in the hundred of GUILT-CROSS, county of NORFOLK. The living has long since been united to the rectory of West Harling, with which parish the population is returned. The church, which was dedicated to St. Andrew the Apostle, has been demolished.

HARLING (WEST), a parish in the hundred of GUILT-CROSS, county of NORFOLK, 2¼ miles (W. S. W.) from East Harling, containing 116 inhabitants. The living is a rectory, in the archdeaconry of Norfolk, and

diocese of Norwich, rated in the king's books at £9. 18. 4. N. W. P. Colborne, Esq. was patron in 1826. The church is dedicated to All Saints.

HARLINGTON, a parish in the hundred of MANSHEAD, county of BEDFORD, 5¼ miles (S.) from Ampthill, containing 398 inhabitants. The living is a discharged vicarage, in the archdeaconry of Bedford, and diocese of Lincoln, rated in the king's books at £11. J. Cooper, Esq. was patron in 1822. The church is dedicated to St. Mary.

HARLINGTON, a parish in the hundred of ELTHORNE, county of MIDDLESEX, 4 miles (N. W. by W.) from Hounslow, containing 472 inhabitants. The living is a rectory, in the archdeaconry of Middlesex, and diocese of London, rated in the king's books at £24. The Rev. E. Davison was patron in 1822. The church, dedicated to St. Peter and St. Paul, has a Norman doorway, and a square embattled tower at the west end. There is a place of worship for Baptists. Harlington, otherwise Arlington, gave the titles of baron and earl to the family of Bennet.

HARLOW, a parish in the hundred of HARLOW, county of ESSEX, 17 miles (W. by N.) from Chelmsford, and 23 (N. N. E.) from London, containing 1928 inhabitants. The living is a vicarage, in the archdeaconry of Middlesex, and diocese of London, rated in the king's books at £15. 7. 11. The Earl of Guilford was patron in 1801. The church, dedicated to St. Mary, was partly destroyed by fire in 1711, but was rebuilt and its windows adorned with stained glass at the expense of the Rev. Mr. Taylor, then vicar, and the gentry in the neighbourhood : the ancient tower, which rose from the centre of the original cruciform structure, has been succeeded by a cupola. There is a place of worship for Baptists. Harlow had formerly a weekly market, also a considerable woollen manufactory, but the chief branch of trade now is spinning. Fairs are held on May 13th for wool, November 28th for horses and cattle ; and one on September 9th, called Harlow-Bush fair, on a common about two miles from the village, which is much resorted to. The petty sessions for the division are held here every Monday. Almshouses for four widows were erected in 1717, agreeably to the will of Francis Reeve, who, in 1637, left £100 for founding them : other almshouses were founded in 1651, by Alexander Stafford, for two widows, towards clothing whom John Wright, in 1659, bequeathed £160, and, in 1728, John Taylor conveyed to trustees two tenements, with certain land, in further aid of both these charities.

HARLOWHILL, a township in the parish of OVINGHAM, eastern division of TINDALE ward, county of NORTHUMBERLAND, 10½ miles (W. N. W.) from Newcastle upon Tyne, containing 124 inhabitants.

HARLTHORPE, a township in the parish of BUBWITH, Holme-Beacon division of the wapentake of HARTHILL, East riding of the county of YORK, 7½ miles (N. by W.) from Howden, containing 93 inhabitants.

HARLTON, a parish in the hundred of WETHERLEY, county of CAMBRIDGE, 6½ miles (S. W.) from Cambridge, containing 221 inhabitants. The living is a rectory, in the archdeaconry and diocese of Ely, rated in the king's books at £14. 9. 7., and in the patronage of the Master and Fellows of Jesus College, Cambridge. The church is dedicated to St. Mary.

HARMBY, a township in the parish of SPENNI-THORN, western division of the wapentake of HANG, North riding of the county of YORK, 2 miles (N. by W.) from Middleham, containing 194 inhabitants.

HARMONDSWORTH, a parish in the hundred of ELTHORNE, county of MIDDLESEX, 2½ miles (E. by N.) from Colnbrook, containing 1076 inhabitants. The living is a vicarage consolidated with that of West Drayton, in the archdeaconry of Middlesex, and diocese of London, rated in the king's books at £12, and in the patronage of J. G. De Burgh, Esq. The church, dedicated to the Virgin Mary, has a Norman door, and a western tower with angular turrets and battlements. On Hounslow heath, within this parish, is a square intrenchment, each side measuring one hundred yards, supposed to have been the work of Cæsar in his war with Cassibelaunus.

HARMSTON, a parish in the higher division of the wapentake of BOOTHBY-GRAFFO, parts of KESTEVEN, county of LINCOLN, 6 miles (S.) from Lincoln, containing 333 inhabitants. The living is a discharged vicarage, in the archdeaconry and diocese of Lincoln, rated in the king's books at £7. 6. 8., endowed with £300 private benefaction, and £200 royal bounty, and in the patronage of Benjamin Thorold, Esq. The church is dedicated to All Saints.

HARNHAM, a township in that part of the parish of BOLAM which is in the north-eastern division of TINDALE ward, county of NORTHUMBERLAND, 12 miles (W.S.W.) from Morpeth, containing 61 inhabitants. Harnham, the site of an ancient fort, has been a place of great strength: it is situated on the brow of a precipice formed of rag-stone, having vast rocks on one side, and a morass on the other; the entrance, which is through a narrow defile to the northward, was formerly defended by an iron gate.

HARNHAM (WEST), a parish in the hundred of CAWDEN and CADWORTH, county of WILTS, 1½ mile (S. W. by W.) from Salisbury, containing 267 inhabitants. The living is a perpetual curacy with the vicarage of Coombe-Bissett, in the peculiar jurisdiction of the Prebendal court of Coombe and Harnham. The church is dedicated to St. George.

HARNHILL, a parish in the hundred of CROW-THORNE and MINETY, county of GLOUCESTER, 4 miles (E.S.E.) from Cirencester, containing 75 inhabitants. The living is a discharged rectory, in the archdeaconry and diocese of Gloucester, rated in the king's books at £5. 16. 5½., and in the patronage of the Rev. Robert Ashe. The church is dedicated to St. Michael.

HARPENDEN, a parish in the hundred of DACO-RUM, county of HERTFORD, 3 miles (N.E. by E.) from Redburn, containing 1693 inhabitants. The living is a perpetual curacy annexed to the rectory of Wheathampstead, in the archdeaconry of Huntingdon, and diocese of Lincoln. The church, dedicated to St. Nicholas, is an ancient cruciform structure, composed of flint and stone: it is in the Norman style, with a square embattled tower. There are places of worship for Independents and Wesleyan Methodists. A fair for horses and cattle is held on May 16th.

HARPFORD, a parish in the eastern division of the hundred of BUDLEIGH, county of DEVON, 3½ miles (N.W. by W.) from Sidmouth, containing 262 inhabitants. The living is a vicarage with that of Fen-Ottery, in
VOL II.

the archdeaconry and diocese of Exeter, rated in the king's books at £18. 11. 3., and in the patronage of Lord Rolle. The church, dedicated to St. Gregory, once belonged to the abbey of St. Michael de Monte, and was subsequently given to Sion College, London.

HARPHAM, a parish in the wapentake of DICKER-ING, East riding of the county of YORK, 5½ miles (N.E. by E.) from Great Driffield, containing 251 inhabitants. The living is a perpetual curacy annexed to the vicarage of Burton-Agnes, in the archdeaconry of the East riding, and diocese of York. The church is the burial-place of the family of St. Quintin, whose founder came over with the Conqueror; their pedigree, from 1080 to 1777, shewing an uninterrupted succession of twenty-eight generations in the male line, is beautifully represented in stained glass in the windows: on the western side of the church-yard are vestiges of the ancient family mansion and fish-ponds. There ·is a place of worship for Wesleyan Methodists.

HARPLEY, a parish in the Lynn division of the hundred of FREEBRIDGE, county of NORFOLK, 8 miles (E. by N.) from Castle-Rising, containing 359 inhabitants. The living is a rectory, in the archdeaconry and diocese of Norwich, rated in the king's books at £22. A. Hamond, Esq. was patron in 1786. The church is dedicated to St. Lawrence: the windows exhibit some fragments of stained glass, of which the insignia of that saint, viz., a gridiron, Or, is the most conspicuous.

HARPOLE, a parish in the hundred of NOBOTTLE-GROVE, county of NORTHAMPTON, 4 miles (W.) from Northampton, containing 687 inhabitants. The living is a rectory, in the archdeaconry of Northampton, and diocese of Peterborough, rated in the king's books at £18. 13. 4. Earl Fitzwilliam was patron in 1803. The church, dedicated to All Saints, is partly Norman, and partly in the early style of English architecture. There is a place of worship for Baptists. In pursuance of an act of parliament passed in 1778 for enclosing land, an allotment was made for the support of a free school; the rental is £50 a year, for which all children who apply are educated.

HARPSDEN, a parish in the hundred of BINFIELD, county of OXFORD, 1¾ mile (S.) from Henley upon Thames, containing, with Bolney, 223 inhabitants. The living is a rectory, in the archdeaconry and diocese of Oxford, rated in the king's books at £12. 10. 5., and in the patronage of the Warden ·and Fellows of All Souls' College, Oxford. The church is dedicated to St. Margaret.

HARPSWELL, a parish in the western division of the wapentake of ASLACOE, parts of LINDSEY, county of LINCOLN, 7¾ miles (E. by S.) from Gainsborough, containing 79 inhabitants. The living is a perpetual curacy, in the archdeaconry of Stow, and diocese of Lincoln, and in the patronage of Sir T. Whichcote, Bart. The church is dedicated to St. Chad.

HARPTON (LOWER), a township in that part of the parish of OLD RADNOR (Wales) which is in the hundred of WIGMORE, county of HEREFORD, 1¼ mile (S.S.E.) from New Radnor, containing 76 inhabitants.

HARPTREE (EAST), a parish in the hundred of WINTERSTOKE, county of SOMERSET, 7 miles (N.by E.) from Wells, containing 627 inhabitants. The living is a discharged vicarage, in the peculiar jurisdiction and patronage of the Prebendary of East Harptree in the

Cathedral Church of Wells, rated in the king's books at £8. 15. The church, dedicated to St. Lawrence, has a northern doorway in the Norman style. There is a place of worship for Wesleyan Methodists. A school-house was erected by John Newton, Esq., and £7. 10. per annum, the gift of William Plumley, Esq., is paid to the schoolmaster for teaching poor children. The village is situated in a rich valley, on the north-eastern side of the Mendip hills, where are several mines of *lapis calaminaris*, in which are also found manganese and chrystal spar; and above the village is a curious cavern, the roof of which, consisting of limestone rock, is splendidly ornamented with concretions of stalactite. Richmond castle, an ancient baronial fortress of the families of Harptree and Gournay, stood about half a mile north-westward from the church. It was garrisoned by the Empress Maud, in 1138, and shortly afterwards besieged and taken by King Stephen, but was not destroyed till the reign of Henry VIII., when its remains were removed for the purpose of erecting a private mansion.

HARPTREE (WEST), a parish in the hundred of CHEWTON, county of SOMERSET, 8 miles (N. by E.) from Wells, containing 528 inhabitants. The living is a discharged vicarage, in the archdeaconry of Bath, and diocese of Bath and Wells, rated in the king's books at £13. 19. 4½., endowed with £200 private benefaction, and £200 royal bounty, and in the patronage of the King, as Prince of Wales. The church, dedicated to St. Mary, has been partly destroyed, and the manor-house, which displays several marks of antiquity, is converted into a farm-house. Ten poor children are instructed for £15 a year, the produce of a bequest by Samuel Lockier, in 1817; and there is a benefaction for apprenticing children, left by John Buckland, in 1673. *Lapis calaminaris* is obtained here to a considerable extent. Ralph Buckland, a Roman Catholic priest and a learned theological writer in the reign of James I., was born here.

HARPURHEY, a township in the parish of MANCHESTER, hundred of SALFORD, county palatine of LANCASTER, 2½ miles (N.N.E.) from Manchester, containing 297 inhabitants. The spinning, manufacturing, and printing of cotton are carried on here.

HARRABY, a township in that part of the parish of St. CUTHBERT, CARLISLE, which is in CUMBERLAND ward, county of CUMBERLAND, 1¾ mile (S. E.) from Carlisle, containing 46 inhabitants.

HARRATON, a township in that part of the parish of CHESTER le STREET which is in the middle division of CHESTER ward, county palatine of DURHAM, 8½ miles (N.N.E.) from Durham, containing 2217 inhabitants. There are valuable and extensive coal mines in the neighbourhood, one of which exploded in 1708, whereby sixty-nine persons were killed; and in 1817 a similar explosion took place in another, by which thirty-eight individuals lost their lives. There are several staiths for shipping coal on the banks of the Wear, across which river is a ferry at the village of Fatfield-Staiths.

HARRIETSHAM, a parish in the hundred of EYHORNE, lathe of AYLESFORD, county of KENT, 7½ miles (E. by S.) from Maidstone, containing 707 inhabitants. The living is a rectory, in the archdeaconry and diocese of Canterbury, rated in the king's books at £11. 10., and in the patronage of the Warden and Fellows of All

Souls' College, Oxford. The church, dedicated to St. John the Baptist, is principally in the early style of English architecture. A fair for cattle, pedlary, and toys, is held on the 5th of July. Almshouses for six poor persons of Harrietsham, and six decayed members of the Fishmongers' Company, were founded in 1642, by Mr. Mark Quested, citizen and fishmonger of London. Sir Charles Booth, in 1792, bequeathed certain stock, now producing upwards of £67 a year, for the support of a schoolmaster and a schoolmistress, who teach thirty-five boys and twenty-six girls on the Madras system.

HARRINGTON, a small sea-port and parish in ALLERDALE ward above Darwent, county of CUMBERLAND, 2½ miles (S.) from Workington, containing 1845 inhabitants. The living is a discharged rectory, in the archdeaconry of Richmond, and diocese of Chester, rated in the king's books at £7. 7. 3½., and in the patronage of H. C. Curwen, Esq. The church is a neat structure, without a tower, standing upon an eminence a little westward from the old village of Harrington, and eastward of the new town, which is a small but thriving sea-port, formerly termed *Bella-port*, situated at the mouth of a small stream called the Wyre, which falls into the Irish sea, and subordinate to the port of Whitehaven. The harbour was considerably improved at the expense of the late J. C. Curwen, Esq., whose father constructed the first quay, from which period its trade has been gradually increasing. In 1760, not a single ship belonged to the port, but there are now upwards of forty, averaging one hundred and twenty-two tons each; they can sail quite into the town, loading and unloading before the houses, and are chiefly employed in conveying large quantities of coal obtained here to Ireland; besides these, about five hundred sloops annually take in lime, which is brought by land from the adjoining parish of Distington, for Scotland. Iron-stone and fire-clay abound in the parish, and much of both was formerly exported to Scotland and Wales. The town now consists of several streets, though seventy years ago not a single house had been erected. There are two shipwrights' yards, a rope-walk, and vitriol and copperas manufactories. The Primitive and Wesleyan Methodists have each a place of worship. A school-house has been recently erected by subscription, to which the late Mr. Curwen was the principal contributor, for teaching children on the Lancasterian plan.

HARRINGTON, a parish in the hundred of HILL, parts of LINDSEY, county of LINCOLN, 5¼ miles (N. N. W.) from Spilsby, containing 105 inhabitants. The living is a discharged rectory, in the archdeaconry and diocese of Lincoln, rated in the king's books at £9. 16. 10½. Mrs. Buckworth was patroness in 1802. The church is dedicated to St. Mary.

HARRINGTON, a parish in the hundred of ROTHWELL, county of NORTHAMPTON, 3 miles (W. by S.) from Rothwell, containing 184 inhabitants. The living is a rectory, in the archdeaconry of Northampton, and diocese of Peterborough, rated in the king's books at £15. 9. 7. The Earl of Dysart was patron in 1801. The church is dedicated to St. Botolph. Harrington gives the titles of baron and earl to the family of Stanhope.

HARRINGWORTH, a parish in the hundred of CORBY, county of NORTHAMPTON, 3¾ miles (E.S.E.)

from Uppingham, containing 350 inhabitants. The living is a discharged vicarage, in the archdeaconry of Northampton, and diocese of Peterborough, rated in the king's books at £11. 15. 10., and in the patronage of the Dean and Canons of Christ Church, Oxford. The church is dedicated to St. John the Baptist.

HARROGATE, a watering-place and joint township with Bilton, in the parish of KNARESBOROUGH, lower division of the wapentake of CLARO, West riding of the county of YORK, 3 miles (S.W.) from Knaresborough, 15 (N.) from Leeds, 21 (W. by N.) from York, and 200 (N.N.W.) from London, containing, with Bilton, 1934 inhabitants. This place, originally called *Heywragate*, derives its appellation from being situated on the direct road from Knaresborough to Heyward park. It comprehends the two villages of High and Low Harrogate, which are half a mile apart, both standing on part of what was formerly the Forest of Knaresborough, now enclosed and cultivated. High Harrogate occupies an eminence which commands the view of an extensive landscape, diversified with woods, fields, towns, and villages, and bounded by the mountains of Craven, Hambleton hills, and the wolds of Yorkshire. Low Harrogate is pleasantly situated in a valley, and is adorned with many handsome stone houses, erected principally for the accommodation of visitors. The rapid increase of buildings renders it probable that the two villages will at no distant period become united. The mineral waters, which have long rendered Harrogate a place of fashionable resort from May to October, are of three kinds, chalybeate, sulphureous, and saline chalybeate, similar to the Cheltenham waters. In High Harrogate is the old spa, a chalybeate spring, which was discovered in 1571, by Captain William Slingsby, surrounded by a terrace sixty yards square in 1656, the sides of which furnish an agreeable promenade, and surmounted by a handsome dome, in 1786, at the expense of Lord Loughborough. About three quarters of a mile to the westward is the Tewit well, the water of which possesses similar properties. These were the only chalybeate wells known for a long time; but in 1819 a saline chalybeate spring was discovered, which is daily increasing in repute: the water is called Cheltenham water, from the similarity of its properties to those of the purgative waters of Cheltenham; and being private property, persons are admitted to the spa on subscribing two shillings and sixpence a week, and also to the grounds, in which are pleasant walks, a large sheet of water, and various ornamental plantations. In Low Harrogate is the old sulphur well, situated at the foot of a hill which rises to the south-west, the water of which is received in a circular stone basin, surmounted by a large cupola covered with lead and supported on stone pillars. In the grounds adjoining the Crown Hotel is a new sulphur well, enclosed in a Chinese octagonal building, and surrounded by walks and shrubberies tastefully arranged: the water is raised by a pump, and resembles the former in its medicinal qualities. The sulphur wells are numerous, but only four are used; and their sanative properties were not discovered till several years after the wells at the upper village were generally frequented. A sulphureous chalybeate spring, called the Crescent water, discovered in 1783, is situated in the garden of the Crescent: it is private property, and the terms of subscription are half a

guinea for the season. The medicinal quality of the chalybeate waters is principally tonic and alterative; that of the sulphureous strongly purgative: the latter are used externally and internally, and are considered particularly serviceable in scorbutic complaints, and disorders of the skin. The principal place of public resort is a large and elegant room near the sulphur wells, called the Promenade room, which is supplied with periodical publications, an appropriate library, and an organ, on which, during the season, an organist plays every morning and evening, and on Sunday evenings there is a performance of sacred music: the terms of subscription are moderate. In High Harrogate are also a good library and a theatre, the latter being open during the months of July, August, and September. Assemblies are held at the different hotels three or four nights in the week during the season; and there are races in summer.

A chapel, dedicated to St. John, was erected in High Harrogate in 1749, by subscription, Lady Elizabeth Hastings having been a liberal contributor: it is a neat edifice of freestone, containing several marble monuments to the memory of visitors who have died here; and it has lately received an addition of two hundred and forty sittings, of which one hundred and eighty-six are free, the Incorporated Society for the enlargement of churches and chapels having granted £2 towards defraying the expense. The living is a perpetual curacy, in the archdeaconry of Richmond, and diocese of Chester, and in the patronage of the Vicar of Knaresborough. In Low Harrogate is a small church or chapel, erected in 1824, and containing about seven hundred and fifty sittings, of which five hundred are free, the Incorporated Society having granted £500 for that purpose. The living is a perpetual curacy, in the archdeaconry and diocese of York, and in the patronage of the Crown. There is a place of worship for Independents in High Harrogate, and one for Methodists midway between the two, villages. There is also an endowed school for the children of the poor of Bilton *cum* Harrogate. The Bath hospital was erected by subscription in 1826, upon a plot of land near the bogs, granted for that purpose by the Earl of Harewood; and here the poor may obtain the benefit of the mineral waters free of expense: at present only twenty-four patients can be accommodated, but it is in contemplation to enlarge the building, and extend the benefits of the institution.

HARROLD, a market town and parish in the hundred of WILLEY, county of BEDFORD, 8 miles (N.W. by W.) from Bedford, and 58 (N.N.W.) from London, containing 939 inhabitants. This small town is situated in a fertile agricultural district, on the banks of the river Ouse, over which there is a stone bridge. The only branch of manufacture carried on is that of lace. There is a small market on Tuesday; and fairs for the sale of cattle and pedlary are held on the Tuesdays preceding May 13th, July 6th, and October 11th. The petty sessions for the hundreds of Barford, Stodden, and Willey, are chiefly held here, but sometimes at Bletsoe. The living is a discharged vicarage, in the archdeaconry of Bedford, and diocese of Lincoln, rated in the king's books at £8, endowed with £200 private benefaction, and £200 royal bounty, and in the patronage of the Countess de Grey. The church, dedicated to All Saints, is a fine structure, with a handsome tower and spire. There is a place of worship for Independents. Six

2 T 2

almshouses for six poor widows were founded in 1723, by Mrs. Anne Jolliffe, and subsequently received a small endowment from a benefaction by her niece, Ann Mead, who also gave £20 per annum to the vicar, for an afternoon lecture every Sunday. A priory was founded here in the reign of Stephen, which afterwards became a convent of Augustine nuns, the revenue of which, at the dissolution, was estimated at £47. 3. 2.: there are no remains of the conventual buildings except the refectory, which has been used as a barn.

HARROW on the HILL, a parish (formerly a market town) in the hundred of Gore, county of Middlesex, 9 miles (N.W. by W.) from London, containing, with the hamlet of Weald with Greenhill, 3017 inhabitants. This place is chiefly distinguished on account of the free grammar school, founded in the reign of Elizabeth, in 1571, which ranks among the most celebrated classical schools in England. The founder was John Lyon, a native of the neighbouring hamlet of Preston, who, in 1590, drew up a set of statutes for the school, in which, among various regulations, he directed that the pupils should be instructed in archery, and it was customary, until about the middle of the last century, for the scholars to hold an annual festival on the 4th of August, when they shot at a mark for a silver arrow: this usage having been abolished, public speeches are now delivered on the anniversary of that day: the school is under the direction of six governors. The head master has a salary of £20 per annum from the funds of the institution, with liberty to take private pupils; the second master has £10 per annum; and there are six assistant masters; but the emoluments of all these gentlemen are principally derived from stipendiary tuition. The school is free for all boys belonging to the parish of Harrow, who are entitled to gratuitous instruction, but very few avail themselves of the privilege. The number of boys not on the foundation is usually between three and four hundred, and they enjoy all the privileges attached to the institution. Two exhibitioners from this school are admitted at Cambridge, and two at Oxford, with pensions allotted by the founder, who directed that £20 per annum should be divided among them, but they now receive £20 per annum each for eight years. The governors have not long since instituted two annual scholarships, with pensions of £52. 10. for four years at either of the Universities. The rents of the estates given for the support of this institution by Mr. Lyon, amounted in 1795 to £669 per annum, which was expended by the governors in paying salaries and exhibitions, educating poor children, relieving decayed housekeepers, repairing roads, &c., agreeably to the directions of the donor: at present the income is much more considerable, part of the estates having been let on building leases. A charter was granted by Henry III. to the inhabitants of Harrow, for a market on Monday, and an annual fair; the former has been discontinued, but a fair is still held on the first Monday in August. No staple manufacture is carried on, the trade of the place depending chiefly on the demand for the necessaries of life for the supply of the school, and of the numerous visitors from the metropolis and its neighbourhood.

The living is a vicarage, in the exempt deanery of Croydon, in the peculiar jurisdiction of the Archbishop of Canterbury, rated in the king's books at £33. 4. 2., and in the patronage of Lord Northwick. The church, dedi-

cated to St. Mary, is a spacious structure, with a tower and lofty spire at the west end; the pillars between the nave and the aisles, and a part of the tower, where there is a curious Norman doorway, probably formed portions of a church recorded to have been founded by Lanfranc, Archbishop of Canterbury, in the reign of William I.; but the remainder of the edifice appears to have been rebuilt in the latter part of the fourteenth century: in this church was interred the celebrated poet and physician, Sir Samuel Garth. There is a chapel of ease at Pinner, in this parish. Here are places of worship for Baptists and Wesleyan Methodists. Besides the grammar school, there is a charity school for twelve poor children, with a small endowment, partly from a bequest by Edward Robinson, in 1711; and also a school on the National plan. At the extremity of the parish, towards Stanmore, was anciently a priory called Benethly, or Bentley, the site of which now forms part of the estate of the Marquis of Abercorn, who has near it a splendid and richly furnished mansion, called Bentley Priory. The learned Dr. Samuel Parr was born, in 1747, at Harrow,)where his father practised as an apothecary,) and died at Hatton, in Warwickshire, in 1825.

HARROWBY, a township in that part of the parish of Grantham which is in the wapentake of Winnibriggs and Threo, parts of Kesteven, county of Lincoln, 1¾ mile (E.) from Grantham, containing 45 inhabitants. Harrowby gives the titles of baron and earl to the family of Ryder.

HARROWDEN (GREAT), a parish in the hundred of Orlingbury, county of Northampton, 2¼ miles (N.N.W.) from Wellingborough, containing 140 inhabitants. The living is a discharged vicarage, with which that of Little Harrowden is united, in the archdeaconry of Northampton, and diocese of Peterborough, rated jointly in the king's books at £13. 3. 8., and endowed with £200 private benefaction, and £200 royal bounty. Earl Fitzwilliam was patron in 1808. The church is dedicated to All Saints.

HARROWDEN (LITTLE), a parish in the hundred of Orlingbury, county of Northampton, 3 miles (N.W. by N.) from Wellingborough, containing 420 inhabitants. The living is a discharged vicarage, united to that of Great Harrowden, in the archdeaconry of Northampton, and diocese of Peterborough, endowed with £200 private benefaction, and £200 royal bounty. The church is dedicated to St. Mary.

HARSLEY (EAST), a parish in the wapentake of Birdforth, North riding of the county of York, 6¾ miles (N.E. by E.) from North Allerton, containing 420 inhabitants. The living is a perpetual curacy, in the archdeaconry of Cleveland, and diocese of York, endowed with £300 private benefaction, and £200 royal bounty. J. C. Maynard, Esq. was patron in 1818.

HARSLEY (WEST), a township in the parish of Osmotherley, wapentake of Allertonshire, North riding of the county of York, 5¼ miles (N.E. by E.) from North Allerton, containing 51 inhabitants.

HARSTON, a parish in the hundred of Thriplow, county of Cambridge, 5½ miles (S.S.W.) from Cambridge, containing 529 inhabitants. The living is a discharged vicarage, in the archdeaconry and diocese of Ely, rated in the king's books at £5. 10. 2½., and in the patronage of the Bishop of Ely. The church is dedicated to All Saints. There is a place of worship for Baptists.

HARSTON, a parish in the hundred of FRAMLAND, county of LEICESTER, 6 miles (S. W. by W.) from Grantham, containing 162 inhabitants. The living is a discharged rectory, in the archdeaconry of Leicester, and diocese of Lincoln, rated in the king's books at £8. 1. 8., and in the patronage of the Crown. The church, dedicated to St. Michael, has lately received an addition of fifty sittings, of which twenty-seven are free, the Incorporated Society for the enlargement of churches and chapels having granted £50 towards defraying the expense.

HARSWELL, a parish in the Holme-Beacon division of the wapentake of HARTHILL, East riding of the county of YORK, 3½ miles (W. by S.) from Market-Weighton, containing 78 inhabitants. The living is a discharged rectory, in the archdeaconry of the East riding, and diocese of York, rated in the king's books at £4. —Slingsby, Esq. was patron in 1816. The church is dedicated to St. Peter.

HART, a parish in the north-eastern division of STOCKTON ward, county palatine of DURHAM, comprising the townships of Dalton-Piercy, Elwick, Hart, and Throston, and containing 590 inhabitants, of which number, 231 are in the township of Hart, 4½ miles (W. N. W.) from Hartlepool. The living is a vicarage, with the perpetual curacy of Hartlepool, in the archdeaconry of Northumberland, and diocese of Durham, rated in the king's books at £11. 17. 1., and in the patronage of the Crown. The church, dedicated to St. Mary Magdalene, has a low massive tower with Norman piers and arches, and contains an enriched font. In the register are recorded the deaths of eighty-nine victims to the plague in 1587. The strata of magnesian limestone extending across the country from Nottingham terminates in this parish.

HARTBURN, a township in the parish of STOCKTON upon TEES, south-western division of STOCKTON ward, county palatine of DURHAM, 1½ mile (S. W. by W.) from Stockton upon Tees, containing 121 inhabitants.

HARTBURN, a parish comprising the townships of High Angerton, Low Angerton, Corridge, Hartburn, Hartburn-Grange, Highlands, Longwitton, North Middleton, South Middleton, Rothley, East Thornton, West Thornton, Todridge, and Whitridge, in the western division of MORPETH ward, and the townships of Cambo, Deanham, Favinley, otherwise Farnlaws, Greenleighton, Hartington, Hartington Hall, Harwood, East Shafto, West Shafto, and Wallington-demesne, in the north-eastern division of TINDALE ward, county of NORTHUMBERLAND, and containing 1474 inhabitants, of which number, 23 are in the township of Hartburn, 7 miles (W.) from Morpeth. The living is a vicarage, to which is annexed the perpetual curacy of Netherwitton, in the archdeaconry of Northumberland, and diocese of Durham, rated in the king's books at £20. 0. 10., and in the patronage of the Bishop of Durham. The rivers Hart and Wanspeck run through the parish, and on the north side of the former are three springs, called the Holy Wells, the water of which is said to possess a medicinal quality. At Rothley is a building, in imitation of a castle, commanding a fine view over an extensive lake. Various kinds of stone are obtained in abundance, and here are lead mines and coal-works.

HARTBURN-GRANGE, a township in that part of the parish of HARTBURN which is in the western division of MORPETH ward, county of NORTHUMBERLAND, 9 miles (W.) from Morpeth, containing 68 inhabitants.

HARTEST, a parish in the hundred of BABERGH, county of SUFFOLK, 7 miles (N. E.) from Clare, containing 740 inhabitants. The living is a rectory with that of Boxted, in the archdeaconry of Sudbury, and diocese of Norwich, rated in the king's books at £29. 14. 2., and in the patronage of the Crown. The church is dedicated to All Saints. Almshouses for four widows were founded in 1646, by Thomas Wright, who left a small rent-charge to keep them in repair. Thomas Sparke, in 1721, bequeathed a house and land, now producing an annual income of £50, for teaching children.

HARTFIELD, a parish in the hundred of HARTFIELD, rape of PEVENSEY, county of SUSSEX, 6 miles (E. S. E.) from East Grinsted, comprising North and South Hartfield, and containing 1440 inhabitants, of which number, 474 are in North Hartfield, and 966 in South Hartfield. The living is a discharged vicarage, in the archdeaconry of Lewes, and diocese of Chichester, rated in the king's books at £10, and in the patronage of the Rector of Hartfield : the rectory is a sinecure, rated at £7, and in the patronage of the Heirs of the Duke of Dorset. The church, dedicated to St. Mary, is partly in the early, and partly in the decorated, style of English architecture. There is a place of worship for Wesleyan Methodists. The rivers Medway, Bole, and Kentwater, run through the parish, which includes part of Ashdown Forest : there are some fields, called Castle fields, probably the site of an ancient fortress. The Rev. Richard Rennes, in 1640, founded a free school, and endowed it with certain property, now producing £27 per annum ; and, in 1725, the Earl of Thanet gave a rent-charge of £10 a year, in augmentation of the master's salary, for which all children who apply are instructed. There is a spring, the water of which possesses similar efficacy to that of Tunbridge Wells.

HARTFORD, a chapelry in that part of the parish of GREAT BUDWORTH which is in the second division of the hundred of EDDISBURY, county palatine of CHESTER, 1½ mile (S. W. by W.) from Northwich, containing 772 inhabitants. The living is a perpetual curacy, in the archdeaconry and diocese of Chester, endowed with £1000 parliamentary grant, and in the patronage of three Trustees on the part of the founders. The chapel is dedicated to St. John. Here is an endowed school, also a Sunday school supported by the profits of a bazaar, which in 1828 amounted to more than £100.

HARTFORD, a parish in the hundred of HURSTINGSTONE, county of HUNTINGDON, 1½ mile (E. by N.) from Huntingdon, containing 371 inhabitants. The living is a discharged vicarage, in the archdeaconry of Huntingdon, and diocese of Lincoln, rated in the king's books at £4. 1. 0½., endowed with £200 royal bounty, and in the patronage of the Crown. The church, dedicated to All Saints, has various portions in the Norman style of architecture.

HARTFORD (EAST), a township in the parish of HORTON, eastern division of CASTLE ward, county of NORTHUMBERLAND, 7½ miles (S. E.) from Morpeth, containing 15 inhabitants.

HARTFORD (WEST), a township in the parish of HORTON, eastern division of CASTLE ward, county of NORTHUMBERLAND, 6½ miles (S. E. by S.) from Morpeth, containing 57 inhabitants. The river Blyth is here crossed by a bridge on the north road.

HARTGROVE, a chapelry in the parish of FONT-MELL-MAGNA, in that part of the hundred of SIXPENNY-HANDLEY which is in the Shaston (West) division of the county of DORSET, 4 miles (S. W. by S.) from Shaftesbury, containing 274 inhabitants. The curacy is annexed to the vicarage of Iwerne-Minster, in the archdeaconry of Dorset, and diocese of Bristol. The chapel is dedicated to St. Peter.

HARTHILL, a parish in the higher division of the hundred of BROXTON, county palatine of CHESTER, 7 miles (S. W.) from Tarporley, containing 147 inhabitants. The living is a perpetual curacy, in the archdeaconry and diocese of Chester, endowed with £200 private benefaction, and £400 royal bounty, and in the patronage of Thomas Tyrwhitt Drake, Esq. The church, dedicated to All Saints, was erected about 1609; it has no tower. There are several quarries of a soft sandstone in the parish.

HARTHILL, or HARTLE, a township in the parish of BAKEWELL, hundred of HIGH PEAK, county of DERBY, 3¼ miles (S.S.E.) from Bakewell, containing 60 inhabitants.

HARTHILL, a parish in the southern division of the wapentake of STRAFFORTH and TICKHILL, West riding of the county of YORK, 9¾ miles (S.S.E.) from Rotherham, containing, with the township of Woodall, 650 inhabitants. The living is a rectory, in the archdeaconry and diocese of York, rated in the king's books at £18. 11. 10½. The Duke of Leeds was patron in 1812. The church is dedicated to All Saints. The Rev. John Hirst, in 1812, bequeathed certain property, producing about £16 a year, for the education of children, in addition to which, £12, the annual donation of the Duke of Leeds, is paid in augmentation of the master's salary.

HARTING, a parish in the hundred of DUMPFORD, rape of CHICHESTER, county of SUSSEX, 7 miles (W. by S.) from Midhurst, containing 1072 inhabitants. The living comprises a rectory and a vicarage, in the archdeaconry and diocese of Chichester, the former rated in the king's books at £26. 13. 4., and in the patronage of Sir H. Fetherstonhaugh, Bart., and the latter at £9, and in the gift of the Rector. The church, dedicated to St./Mary,'is partly in the early, and partly in the decorated, style of English architecture. There is a place of worship for Independents. Harting has the privilege of sending four boys to the school founded by Mr. Oliver Whitby, at Chichester. An hospital for lepers, in honour of St. John the Baptist, was established here by Henry Hoes, in the time of Henry II.

HARTINGTON, a parish in the hundred of WIRKS-WORTH, county of DERBY, 9½ miles (S. W.) from Bakewell, comprising the townships called Town Quarter, Middle Quarter with Earl-Sterndale, Nether Quarter, and Upper Quarter, and containing 2218 inhabitants. The living is a discharged vicarage, in the peculiar jurisdiction of the Dean's court for the manor of Hartington, rated in the king's books at £10, endowed with £400 parliamentary grant, and in the patronage of the Duke of Devonshire. The church, dedicated to St. Giles,

is an ancient cruciform structure. There is a chapel of ease at Earl-Sterndale, in this parish. Here is a place of worship for Wesleyan Methodists. A charity school is supported by subscription. Hartington had anciently a market and a fair, both of which have been long disused, but fairs are held at Newhaven, for cattle, sheep, and hardware, on the 2nd Tuesday in September and October 30th; the latter is also a great pleasure fair. There are lead mines in the parish. Hartington gives the title of marquis to the family of Cavendish, Dukes of Devonshire.

HARTINGTON, a township in that part of the parish of HARTBURN which is in the north-eastern division of TINDALE ward, county of NORTHUMBERLAND, 12½ miles (W. by N.) from Morpeth, containing 55 inhabitants.

HARTINGTON-HALL, a township in that part of the parish of HARTBURN which is in the north-eastern division of TINDALE ward, county of NORTHUMBERLAND, containing 45 inhabitants.

HARTLAND, a parish and sea-port (formerly a market town) in the hundred of HARTLAND, county of DEVON, 14¾ miles (W. by S.) from Bideford, 53 (W.N.W.) from Exeter, and 215¾ (W. by S.) from London, containing 1968 inhabitants. This place probably owed its origin to a convent said to have been originally founded by Githa, wife of Earl Godwin, in the reign of Edward the Confessor; and re-founded for canons regular of the order of St. Augustine, by Geoffrey Dinant, in the reign of Henry II., the revenue of which, at the dissolution, was £306. 13. 2¼.: a modern mansion now occupies the site of the ancient conventual edifice, some portions of which are retained, particularly the cloisters, forming the basement story of the eastern and western fronts of the mansion. The town is bleakly situated on a cape which terminates in the promontory of Hartland point, about three miles to the north-west; and on the south are some marshy heights, among which is the source of the river Torridge: the government is vested in a portreeve. An act of parliament passed in the reign of Queen Elizabeth for completing this port, which is subject to the port of Bideford: there is a pier or quay on the coast, two miles westward from the town, the descent to which is very steep, being by steps cut in the rocky cliff. Coasting-vessels here discharge their cargoes of coal and limestone, and receive their export ladings of corn, &c. Off the coast is a herring fishery, in which the inhabitants of the town are interested, they having advanced money to the fishermen at Bideford to enable them to engage in it. Here is a market-house; but the market has been discontinued for many years. Fairs for cattle are held on the Wednesday in Easter week, and the 25th of September, and there is a great market for cattle on the second Saturday in March. The living is a perpetual curacy, in the archdeaconry of Barnstaple, and diocese of Exeter, endowed with £800 parliamentary grant, and in the patronage of the Governors of the Charter-house, London. The church, dedicated to St. Nectan, is situated on a lofty eminence between the town and the quay, about half a mile from the latter, serving as a land-mark for mariners: it is a large and handsome structure, with a screen between the nave and the chancel. There were anciently eleven chapels in this parish, the remains of two being still visible. Here is a place of worship for Independents. An almshouse for three poor widows was founded in 1618, by William Mill, of London, but it has no endowment. Paul Orchard, Esq., who died in 1812, bequeathed property producing £31 per annum, for distribution among the poor of this parish.

HARTLEBURY, a parish comprising the hamlet of Upper Mitton, in the lower division of the hundred of HALFSHIRE, but chiefly in the lower division of the hundred of OSWALDSLOW, county of WORCESTER, 2 miles (E. by S.) from Stourport, and containing 1857 inhabitants. The living is a rectory, in the peculiar jurisdiction of the Rector, rated in the king's books at £30, and in the patronage of the Bishop of Worcester. The church, dedicated to St. James, has considerable portions in the Norman style of architecture, and some in the decorated style. The free grammar school is one of the five in the county having alternately the right of presentation to six scholarships in Worcester College, Oxford, founded by Sir Thomas Cookes, Bart.: the exact period of its establishment is unknown, but it existed in 1400: in the 1st of Elizabeth it was by charter made a royal foundation, when twenty discreet men of the parish were constituted a body corporate, with a common seal, for the management of its funds, &c.; there are now, however, only seven trustees: its possessions consist of about one hundred and eighty-four acres of land, the rental of which is about £120: the head master and the under master have, in addition to their salary, each a good house, and liberty to take boarders. A school for twelve girls was founded and endowed with £200, by Mrs. Hannah Eyre, in 1726; and a Sunday school, under the patronage of the Bishop, was established in 1824, which is supported by voluntary contributions, and attended by about ninety children. Hartlebury castle has long been the residence of the diocesans, to whom it was given by Burthred, King of Mercia: the present is a neat brick mansion, erected about the time of the Restoration, the ancient castle having been taken by Colonel Morgan in 1646, and destroyed during the great rebellion. The Staffordshire and Worcestershire canal passes through the north-western part of the parish.

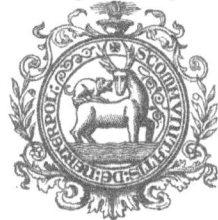

Corporate Seal.

HARTLEPOOL, a seaport, borough, and parish, in the north-eastern division of STOCKTON ward, county palatine of DURHAM, 19 miles (E. S. E.) from Durham, and 257 (N. by W.) from London, containing 1249 inhabitants. In the time of the Normans this place obtained the name of *Hart le pol*, signifying the *pool* or mere of the "*Harts*," or deer, from its situation on the eastern coast, near the mouth of the Tees, on a promontory frequented by deer. The earliest mention of it in history is towards the middle of the seventh century, when Heiu, who is said to have been the first female that took the veil in the Saxon kingdom of Northumberland, founded the monastery of Heruteu at or near this place, of which she became abbess. Retiring soon after, she was succeeded in the abbacy by Hilda, whom the inhabitants subsequently chose for their tutelary saint. No further mention is made of this re-ligious house until the period of its utter demolition by the Danes, which, according to Leland, took place in the year 800. In 1171, Hugh, Earl of Bar, brought his fleet into St. Hilda's bay, with a body of Flemish soldiers, intended to assist William, King of Scotland, in his invasion of England. The family of Bruce were lords of Hartness, but on the accession of Robert Bruce to the throne of Scotland, his estates in England were forfeited, and Hartlepool was conferred on Robert de Clifford. Soon after this it was attacked by Sir James Douglas, whose soldiers committed great devastation in the town, compelling the inhabitants to take refuge on board the vessels in the bay, to preserve their lives and property. During the invasion of Scotland by Edward I. and his immediate successors, the port was frequently visited, and its ships and sailors pressed into the service. In 1346, it furnished five ships and one hundred and forty-five men towards the armament prepared by Edward III. for the invasion of France. It was at this time a place of considerable importance, and on the insurrection of the northern lords it was taken possession of and garrisoned by them. The royalists held it during the early part of the contest between Charles I. and his parliament; but in 1644, when the Scots entered England to assist the parliament a second time, Hartlepool was taken by the Earl of Calender, who threw up intrenchments, placed a garrison in the fortress, and kept possession of it till 1647, when, with other northern towns, it was transferred to the parliament. It appears to have been strongly fortified: within the walls was a basin which served as a harbour; it comprised nearly twelve acres of ground, and was guarded by a range of towers on each side, and at the entrance were two round towers, with a chain capable of being thrown across the mouth of the harbour, which was so capacious that one hundred large ships might anchor in it, secure from storms or the enemy: it is now nearly choked up, and in 1808 it was granted to an individual who enclosed it for cultivation, but an indictment having been brought against him, a verdict was obtained at Durham in 1813, and the undertaking was abandoned. The old walls and forts are in ruins, yet sufficient still remains to convey, probably beyond those of any others in the kingdom, a correct idea of the ancient method of fortification. On the moor near the town are two batteries mounted with cannon and defended by an intrenchment.

The town stands on a kind of peninsula formed by the German ocean, and consists of one principal and several smaller streets; but it is only scantily supplied with water from a few wells. The surrounding scenery is of a romantic character, particularly along the sea-shore, where the shelving precipitous rocks, which the lashing of the waves has hollowed into caverns and recesses, present a wild and picturesque appearance: several good houses have been erected for the accommodation of numerous visitors, who resort to the town for sea-bathing. Without the walls, near Water gate, is a celebrated chalybeate spring, called the Spa Well, which is covered by the tide at high water: it contains iron with Epsom salt, calcareous earth, some sea-salt, and a little sulphur; and near the southern battery is another spring, which contains iron and sulphur. The commerce of the port, now a member of the port of Stockton, was formerly considerable, but it has almost entirely declined. In 1680 the custom-house establishment was removed to Stockton;

and a principal coast officer, two tide waiters, and boatmen, are the only custom-house agents stationed here. The limits of the port extend from the Black shore in the river Tees on the south, to the Blackhalls on the sea-shore northward. The present harbour, which is distinct from the old one, possesses considerable advantages for commerce: it is formed by a pier projecting from a point to the south of the southern wall, which having become greatly dilapidated, application was made to government for assistance towards repairing it, but without success: a subscription was then set on foot with a view to raise £3500, the amount estimated to be necessary for that purpose: in 1811 and the two succeeding years, the sum of £1857 was raised, and expended thereon; but this being wholly insufficient, an act of parliament was passed, April 15th, 1813, authorising a duty to be levied on vessels, and a rate on the householders, for the purpose of completing this desirable object. The pier is nearly straight, and extends one hundred and fifty-four yards from east to west. The Master and Brethren of the Trinity House at Newcastle have the appointment and regulation of the pilots for this port; and here is a life-boat under the management of a local committee. The fishery is now the chief source of employment to the inhabitants, about two-thirds of them being engaged in it: the kinds of fish caught are cod, haddock, ling, skate, whiting, soles, plaice, herrings, and mackerel, and likewise turbot, the fishery for which is very productive, and a considerable quantity is annually sent to London. The market, formerly held on Thursday, is now on Saturday; and the fairs, which were once held on May 14th, August 21st, October 9th, and November 27th, and to which a court of pie-powder was attached, have nearly fallen into disuse. The first charter granted to the borough was by John, in 1230; and Elizabeth, in 1593, gave the inhabitants a new charter, by which the government is vested in a mayor, recorder, and twelve capital burgesses, assisted by a town clerk, two serjeants at mace, and other officers. The mayor is annually chosen from among the aldermen, on the Monday after Michaelmas-day, and is a justice of the peace for the borough. The freedom is obtained by gift of the corporation, patrimony, or servitude; it descends to the eldest son only, or to the eldest surviving son, in case the former die before he has been admitted. Among the privileges of the freemen is the right of pasturage for a cow and a horse on the town moor, the soil of which belongs to the mayor and chief burgesses. Courts leet and baron, the latter of which takes cognizance of debts under 40s., are held twice a year, before the recorder or his deputy. The guildhall, in which the public affairs of the borough are transacted, was built about the year 1750.

The living is a perpetual curacy, in the archdeaconry and diocese of Durham, endowed with £600 private benefaction, £200 royal bounty, and £1600 parliamentary grant, and in the patronage of the Vicar of Hart. The church, dedicated to St. Hilda, is a spacious structure in the early style of English architecture, with some portions in the later Norman character, and having a lofty embattled tower strengthened with bold flying buttresses, and enriched with crocketed pinnacles. The nave is separated from the aisles by a range of light clustered pillars, and pointed arches on each side; the chancel having sustained much injury from high winds,

was rebuilt in 1724, and is the most modern part of the structure. Among the ancient monuments are some belonging to the royal family of Bruce, and a very large altar-tomb to the memory of some individual unknown. There is a place of worship for Wesleyan Methodists. The free school was founded in 1742, by John Crooks, of this town, gent., by whom it was endowed with land producing then £15 per annum, for a master to instruct twenty-four boys, in reading, writing, and arithmetic, and £5 a year for purchasing shoes and shirts for them: the endowment now yields £28 per annum, and the number of boys has consequently been increased to thirty, but the distribution of clothes is discontinued. A Sunday school, established about the year 1810, is supported by subscription. The poor receive the interest on various sums of money bequeathed for their benefit, besides the rent of nineteen acres of land, purchased with a bequest of £500 by Henry Smith, alderman of London, in 1620, and now let for about £110 per annum. A convent of Franciscan friars was founded here prior to the year 1275, the exact site of which is not known, but it is supposed to have been near a house now called the Priory, where the foundations of some ancient building have been discovered. The Rev. William Romaine, a learned divine, and a celebrated Hebrew scholar, was born at Hartlepool in 1714: he was for many years rector of St. Anne's, Blackfriars, London, where he was buried.

HARTLEY, a parish in the hundred of Axton, Dartford, and Wilmington, lathe of Sutton at Hone, county of Kent, 6¾ miles (S. E. by S.) from Dartford, containing 161 inhabitants. The living is a rectory, in the archdeaconry and diocese of Rochester, rated in the king's books at £7. Richard Forrest, Esq. was patron in 1827. The church is dedicated to All Saints.

HARTLEY, a sea-port and township in the parish of Earsdon, eastern division of Castle ward, county of Northumberland, 5 miles (N.) from North Shields, containing 1795 inhabitants, who are chiefly employed in the collieries, fisheries, and salterns, and in the glass and copperas works established here. There are places of worship for Primitive and Wesleyan Methodists. A chapel, dedicated to St. Mary, and a hermitage, formerly stood on Bates' island, opposite to the village of Hartley. The small harbour was made at the expense of Lord Delaval, to shelter fishing-boats in stormy weather. A woodcock was shot near this place in 1765, in the stomach of which was found a very valuable diamond. See SEATON-SLUICE.

HARTLEY, a township in the parish of Kirkby-Stephen, East ward, county of Westmorland, 1½ mile (E.) from Kirkby-Stephen, containing 136 inhabitants. Veins of lead and copper have been wrought here since 1827, but much larger quantities of the former were raised some years ago, and coal has been obtained on Hartley fell. Vestiges of Hartley castle, formerly a stately edifice, may still be traced on a commanding eminence, near which is a petrifying spring, and a cascade falling sixty feet perpendicularly.

HARTLEY-BURN, a township in the parish of Haltwhistle, western division of Tindale ward, county of Northumberland, 4 miles (S. W.) from Haltwhistle, containing 92 inhabitants.

HARTLEY-DAMMER, a liberty in that part of the parish of Shinfield which is in the hundred of

THEALE, county of BERKS, 3½ miles (S. W. by S.) from Reading, containing 323 inhabitants.

HARTLEY-MAUDIT, a parish in the hundred of ALTON, Alton (North) division of the county of SOUTHAMPTON, 2¾ miles (S. E.) from Alton, containing 56 inhabitants. The living is a rectory, in the archdeaconry and diocese of Winchester, rated in the king's books at £10. 1. 10½., and in the patronage of Lord Sherborne.

HARTLEY-ROW, a hamlet in the parish of HARTLEY-WINTNEY, hundred of ODIHAM, Basingstoke division of the county of SOUTHAMPTON, ½ a mile (S. W. by W.) from Hartford-Bridge. The population is returned with the parish. There is a place of worship for Baptists. Fairs are held on Shrove-Tuesday and June 29th, for pedlary.

HARTLEY-WESTPALL, a parish in the hundred of HOLDSHOTT, Basingstoke division of the county of SOUTHAMPTON, 5 miles (W.) from Hartford-Bridge, containing 272 inhabitants. The living is a discharged rectory, in the archdeaconry and diocese of Winchester, rated in the king's books at £6. 16. 8., and in the patronage of the Dean and Canons of Windsor. The church is dedicated to St. Mary. A branch of the river Loddon runs through the parish.

HARTLEY-WINTNEY, a parish in the hundred of ODIHAM, Basingstoke division of the county of SOUTHAMPTON, 1¼ mile (S. by W.) from Hartford-Bridge, containing, exclusively of the tything of Hazely-Heath, a part of which is in this parish, 935 inhabitants. The living is a discharged vicarage, in the archdeaconry and diocese of Winchester, rated in the king's books at £4. 0. 7½., endowed with £300 private benefaction, and £200 royal bounty, and in the patronage of Paulet St. John Mildmay, Esq. The church is dedicated to St. Mary. A Cistercian nunnery, in honour of the Blessed Virgin Mary, St. Mary Magdalene, and St. John the Baptist, was founded here in the reign of William the Conqueror, which at the dissolution contained a prioress and seventeen nuns, whose revenue was £59. 1.

HARTLINGTON, a township in the parish of BURNSALL, eastern division of the wapentake of STAINCLIFFE and EWCROSS, West riding of the county of YORK, 10 miles (N. N. E.) from Skipton, containing 141 inhabitants.

HARTLIP, a parish in the hundred of MILTON, lathe of SCRAY, county of KENT, 6 miles (E. S. E.) from Chatham, containing 300 inhabitants. The living is a vicarage, in the archdeaconry and diocese of Canterbury, rated in the king's books at £9. 10. 10., and in the patronage of the Dean and Chapter of Rochester. The church is dedicated to St. Michael. Mrs. Mary Gibbon, in 1678, bequeathed certain premises, now let for £52. 13. per annum, which, except £1 paid to the vicar, is given to a schoolmaster for teaching sixty children of this and the adjoining parishes : the master resides in a house, the gift of an individual unknown. Quendown, a long tract of land on the north side of the parish, has been for many years a noted rabbit warren. In Lower-Danefield, about a mile from the church, are the remains of a large subterranean building, the rooms and passages of which are rudely constructed, and contain a great quantity of Roman tiles. Other foundations have been also discovered in the contiguous grounds.

HARTOFT, a township in the parish of MIDDLE-

TON, PICKERING lythe, North riding of the county of YORK, containing 134 inhabitants.

HARTON, a township in the parish of JARROW, eastern division of CHESTER ward, county palatine of DURHAM, 2 miles (S. E.) from South Shields, containing 235 inhabitants. Velvet Bed, an island near the sea-shore, covered with soft grass, is much resorted to by pleasure parties from the neighbouring bathing-places ; near it is a remarkable cavern, termed Fairies' Kettle.

HARTON, a township in that part of the parish of BOSSALL which is in the wapentake of BULMER, North riding of the county of YORK, 10 miles (N. E.) from York, containing 190 inhabitants.

HARTPURY, a parish in the lower division of the hundred of DUDSTONE and KING'S BARTON, county of GLOUCESTER, 4¼ miles (E. by S.) from Newent, containing 811 inhabitants. The living is a vicarage, in the archdeaconry and diocese of Gloucester, rated in the king's books at £16. 6. 5½., and in the patronage of the Bishop of Gloucester. The church is dedicated to St. Mary.

HARTS-GROUNDS, otherwise GIBBET-HILLS, an extra-parochial district, though locally in the parish of Gosberton, wapentake of KIRTON, parts of HOLLAND, county of LINCOLN, containing 67 inhabitants.

HARTSHEAD, a township in the parish of ASHTON under LINE, hundred of SALFORD, county palatine of LANCASTER, 9 miles (E.N.E.) from Manchester, containing 9137 inhabitants.

HARTSHEAD, a joint chapelry with Clifton, in that part of the parish of DEWSBURY which is in the wapentake of MORLEY, West riding of the county of YORK, 5½ miles (N. E. by N.) from Huddersfield, containing 2007 inhabitants. The living is a perpetual curacy, in the archdeaconry and diocese of York, endowed with £460 private benefaction, £400 royal bounty, and £800 parliamentary grant, and in the patronage of the Vicar of Dewsbury.

HARTSHILL, a hamlet in the parish of MANCETTER, Atherstone division of the hundred of HEMLINGFORD, county of WARWICK, 3 miles (N.W. by W.) from Nuneaton, containing 662 inhabitants. There is an endowed school in the township, also the remains of an ancient castle. Michael Drayton, the poet, was born here in 1563, and died in 1631.

HARTSHORN, a parish in the hundred of REPTON and GRESLEY, county of DERBY, 3 miles (N.W. by N.) from Ashby de la Zouch, containing 870 inhabitants. The living is a rectory, in the archdeaconry of Derby, and diocese of Lichfield and Coventry, rated in the king's books at £3. 2. 1., and in the patronage of the Earl of Chesterfield. The church, which is dedicated to St. Peter, is in the early style of English architecture. There is a place of worship for Wesleyan Methodists. This parish is in the honour of Tutbury, duchy of Lancaster, and within the jurisdiction of a court of pleas held at Tutbury every third Tuesday, for the recovery of debts under 40s. A school was endowed with lands and tenements by the Rev. William Dethick, in 1624; the annual income is £65. Near the village is a manufactory for screws, and there are mines of coal and iron-stone in the parish.

HARTSIDE, a joint township with Fawdon and Clinch, in the parish of INGRAM, northern division of COQUETDALE ward, county of NORTHUMBERLAND, 8½ miles (S. by W.) from Wooler, containing 80 inhabitants.

HARTSOP, a joint chapelry with Patterdale, in the parish of BARTON, WEST ward, county of WESTMORLAND, 6¼ miles (N.N.E.) from Ambleside, containing 282 inhabitants. A school is supported by charitable donations amounting to about £6 per annum.

HARTWELL, a parish in the hundred of AYLESBURY, county of BUCKINGHAM, 2 miles (W.S.W.) from Aylesbury, containing 133 inhabitants. The living is a rectory, with the perpetual curacy of Little Hampden, in the archdeaconry of Buckingham, and diocese of Lincoln, rated in the king's books at £14. 5. 5. Sir G. Lee, Bart. was patron in 1803. The church, dedicated to St. Mary, was erected by the late Sir William Lee, Bart., in imitation of the early style of English architecture, with two octagonal towers, and a roof highly decorated with tracery. This was the residence of Louis XVIII. and his court during the stay of that monarch in England, prior to his restoration to the French throne.

HARTWELL, a parish in the hundred of CLELEY, county of NORTHAMPTON, 7¼ miles (S. by E.) from Northampton, containing, exclusively of a portion of the hamlet of Old Stratford which is in this parish, 432 inhabitants. The living is a discharged rectory, in the archdeaconry of Northampton, and diocese of Peterborough, endowed with £200 private benefaction, £600 royal bounty, and £200 parliamentary grant. Colonel P. Skeene was patron in 1791. The church is dedicated to St. John the Baptist.

HARTWITH, a joint chapelry with Winsley, in the parish of KIRKBY-MALZEARD, lower division of the wapentake of CLARO, West riding of the county of YORK, 4¼ miles (W. by N.) from Ripley, containing 675 inhabitants. The living is a perpetual curacy, in the peculiar jurisdiction of the Prebendal court of Mashan in the Cathedral Church of York, or in that of the Dean and Chapter of York, being claimed by both, and the matter not yet determined, endowed with £1100 private benefaction, and £800 royal bounty. A small school-room has been erected, and is endowed with an estate by Robert Haxby; the present annual income is £29.

HARTY (ISLE of), a parish in the hundred of FAVERSHAM, lathe of SCRAY, county of KENT, 9 miles (S.E. by E.) from Queenborough, containing 45 inhabitants. The living is a rectory, in the archdeaconry and diocese of Canterbury, rated in the king's books at £20. 6. 0½., endowed with £200 private benefaction, and £600 royal bounty, and in the patronage of S.E. Sawbridge, Esq. The church, dedicated to St. Thomas the Apostle, is a small edifice, comprising a body, chancel, and two side chantries, with a pointed western turret. The isle consists of rich pasture land, on which numerous flocks of sheep are fed. There is no village, only a few small cottages, in which the overseers of different estates reside. The East Swale is navigable on the south side of the parish, which is bounded on the west by Cable creek, and on the east by Muswell creek.

HARVINGTON, a parish in the middle division of the hundred of OSWALDSLOW, though locally in the upper division of the hundred of Blackenhurst, county of WORCESTER, 4 miles (N. by E.) from Evesham, containing 353 inhabitants. The living is a rectory, in the archdeaconry and diocese of Worcester, rated in the king's books at £15. 6. 8., and in the patronage of the Dean and Chapter of Worcester. The church is dedicated to St. James.

HARWELL, a parish in the hundred of MORETON, county of BERKS, 6½ miles (E. by N.) from Wantage, containing 701 inhabitants. The living is a vicarage, in the archdeaconry of Berks, and diocese of Salisbury, rated in the king's books at £12. 4. 2. Sir J. Chetwode, Bart. was patron in 1823. The church is dedicated to St. Matthew. In 1644, Robert Loder bequeathed a messuage and land for a schoolmaster to teach the children of twelve poor men; the total income is £54; the master is appointed by trustees. In 1772, the Rev. Matthew Eaton devised the interest of his estates to trustees, for apprenticing poor children of Harwell, Milton, and Hagbourn, and for the relief of poor widows, or other industrious poor, at the discretion of the trustees: from this fund a sum is paid to the master on Loder's charity, for teaching twenty-five boys reading, writing, and arithmetic; he likewise occupies a house and orchard belonging to the estate rent-free. A benefaction from some person unknown, called the Feoffees' gift, and consisting of fourteen acres of land and an orchard, produces about £26 per annum, which is distributed in money amongst the poor, by the churchwardens and overseers. An almshouse was founded by Frances Geering, or Jennings, in 1715, for six poor widows, who receive six shillings per week, and an annual sum for clothes. In the church is a tablet on which is recorded a singular benefaction by Christopher Elderfield, an eminent divine, and a native of this parish, of £350, vested in land for the purchase of two milch cows, to be given every spring to two of the poorest men in the parish; the proceeds having exceeded the price given for the cows, the surplus is expended in white waistcoats, which are distributed among twenty-five poor men at Christmas.

HARWICH, a sea-port, borough, and market town, having separate jurisdiction, locally in the hundred of Tendring, county of ESSEX, 42 miles (N.E. by E.) from Chelmsford, and 72 (N.E. by E.) from London, containing 4010 inhabitants. The name of this place, which is expressive of circumstances connected with its early history, is, by Camden, derived from the Saxon *Harewic*, signifying a station or harbour for soldiers; and from the same authority it is supposed that, during the time of the Romans, the counts of the Saxon shore had a strong hold or castle here, in which a force was stationed to repel the Saxons and the Danes, who at that time made frequent incursions from the opposite coasts. This opinion is in some degree confirmed by the remains of a Roman camp and tumulus in the vicinity of the town, near which coins and fragments of tesselated pavements have been found at various times, and by the discovery of teeth and bones of large animals in the southern cliff, which are by some antiquaries thought to be the remains of elephants brought into England by the Emperor Claudius. After the departure of the Romans, Harwich,

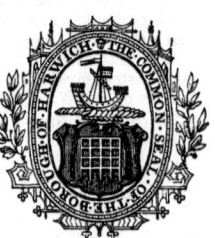

Seal and Arms.

with the district adjoining, was wrested from the Britons by Erehenwine, or Erchwine, a Saxon chief, who held it under Octa, grandson of Hengist, till, with the rest of the kingdom of East Saxony, it fell into the possession of Egbert in 746. In 885, a considerable battle was fought near this port, between the fleet of Alfred and sixteen Danish ships, which terminated in the entire defeat and capture of the latter. In 1326, Prince Edward and his mother, Queen Isabel, landed here from Hainault, with a force of two thousand seven hundred and fifty soldiers, and being joined by several of the nobility, and headed by Thomas de Brotherton, Duke of Norfolk, then lord of the manor and resident in the town, proceeded to Bristol, to make war against the king. In 1338, the same prince, then Edward III., embarked at this port with a fleet of five hundred sail, manned with archers and slingers, on his first expedition against France; and in the year following, the French, in retaliation, made an unsuccessful attempt with eleven galleys to set fire to the town. In 1340, the French navy, consisting of four hundred ships, having been stationed near Sluys, in Flanders, to intercept the king's passage to France, Edward assembled here his naval forces, and sailing on Midsummer-eve, and forming with the northern squadron under the command of Lord Morley, encountered the enemy, destroyed one-half of their ships, and killed or captured nearly thirty thousand of their men. In some of the naval engagements between the English and the Dutch, in the reign of Charles II., the contending parties approached so near to the town as to render their operations visible to spectators on the cliffs. Henry VIII. visited Harwich in 1543, and in 1558 preparations were made there for the reception of Philip, King of Spain, on his arrival to celebrate his nuptials with Mary, Queen of England. Queen Elizabeth was sumptuously entertained here in 1561 by the corporation, who escorted her as far as the windmill on her return. When Harwich was fortified against the Dutch in 1666, Charles II. having proceeded from Newmarket to Landguard fort, sailed hither in his yacht, accompanied by the Dukes of York, Monmouth, Richmond, and Buckingham, and, with others of his suite, attended divine service at the parish church; in the evening the royal party embarked for Aldborough, whence they proceeded by land to Ipswich. William III., George I., and George II., visited Harwich on their respective tours to the continent; and the Princess of Mecklenburgh Strelitz landed at this port on her arrival in England to celebrate her nuptials with King George III. In 1808, the Countess de Lille, consort of Louis XVIII., the Duke and Duchess of Angoulême, the Count and Countess de Demas, and others of the nobility of France, seeking an asylum in this country, in the reign of Napoleon Buonaparte, arrived here in the Euryalus frigate, commanded by the Hon. Captain Dundas. On the 16th of August, 1821, the remains of Queen Caroline, consort of his late majesty, George IV., were brought to this place, whence they were conveyed by the Glasgow frigate to be interred at Brunswick.

Harwich is situated on a peninsular projection on the north-eastern extremity of the Essex coast, bounded on the east by the North sea, and on the west and north by the æstuaries of the Stour and the Orwell, which uniting previously to their influx into the sea, form a spacious and secure harbour nearly three miles

in breadth. The town is in general well built, and consists principally of three streets : an act of parliament was obtained in 1819, for watching, paving, and lighting it, and for supplying the inhabitants with water, under the provisions of which it has been well paved, but is not yet lighted; and, after boring to the depth of four hundred and ninety-five feet, all attempts to procure a supply of fresh water have failed; the inhabitants are consequently supplied with rain water preserved in cisterns, and with spring water brought in carts from Dover-court, and in boats from Landguard fort, and from Arwarton, in the county of Suffolk. The foundations of a castle and fortifications by which the town was defended were seen previously to the encroachment of the sea, at an extraordinary ebb of the tide in 1784; but of its ancient walls and gates, with the exception of a very small portion serving to indicate their former strength, the memorial is preserved only in the record of tolls levied in the reign of Edward III. for their repair. Harwich is much resorted to during the season for sea-bathing, and hot and cold baths, arranged with every accommodation, are supplied from a large reservoir of sea water; there are also bathing-machines on the jetty. The harbour is protected on the east by the isthmus on which the town is built, verging towards the north, and on the west by a similar projection of the coast towards the south : the entrance is defended by Landguard fort, erected on the eastern promontory of the opposite coast, by a large martello tower, and by a number of shoals near the fort, which so much contract the passage as to admit only one large vessel at a time, rendering the harbour difficult of access, except to expert navigators. Though of unequal depth, the harbour and the bay together form a capacious roadstead for the largest ships of war, one hundred of which were assembled here during the war with Holland, in the reign of Charles II., exclusively of their attendant vessels, and three or four hundred sail of vessels carrying coal. To facilitate the entrance into the harbour by night, two light-houses were erected, under letters patent of Charles II., and furnished with patent lamps, previously to building which that object was effected by burning at night a blazing fire of coal, and six one-pound candles, in a room with a glazed front, over the principal gate at the south entrance into the town : on the eastern part of the town, where the light-houses are situated, is a convenient stone quay, and near it is a delightful promenade, called the Esplanade. By means of these lights, vessels are guided off a sand bank called the "Andrews," forming a bar across the entrance to the harbour from Landguard fort into the Rolling grounds, from which the passage leading into good anchorage is safe. The custom-house establishment consists of a collector, comptroller, and other officers. The trade of the port principally arises from its being the station of the post-office packets, by which a constant intercourse is kept up between this country and the continent; four extra packets sail hence every week for Gottingen, and this is the principal place of embarkation for Holland and Germany, from which circumstance, previously to the establishment of steam-packets in so many other places, it derived considerable benefit. The inhabitants are principally employed in maritime pursuits; the North sea fishery, though materially declined, still affords employment to a considerable number of vessels belonging to the port, and a constant traffic is carried on, by means of wherries, with Ipswich and Manningtree. One hundred and three British and ten foreign vessels entered inwards, and fifty-eight British and five foreign vessels cleared outwards, in the year 1826 : the number of ships belonging to the port in 1828 was ninety-one, averaging a burden of sixty-four tons. Shipbuilding is also carried on to a considerable extent; the dock-yard is well provided with launches, storehouses, and other requisites : several third-rate and other large vessels have been built here, and a patent slip has been recently constructed, on which ships of very large burden may be hauled up for repair with great facility. About one hundred small vessels and boats are employed in and near the harbour in dredging for stone for making cement. The manufacture of copperas from stones, which are found in abundance on the shore, was carried on here in the seventeenth century, about which time an attempt was made to obtain potash from various sea-weeds, but it was soon abandoned. The market days are Tuesday and Friday : the fairs, principally for toys, are on May 1st and October 18th, each for three days.

The borough was first incorporated by charter of Edward II., which was renewed, with additional privileges, by James I., through the interest of Sir Edward Coke, and subsequently confirmed by Charles II., by which the government is vested in a mayor, recorder, high steward, eight aldermen, and twenty-four capital burgesses, assisted by a chamberlain, town clerk, and other officers. The mayor is elected annually on the 30th of October, from among the aldermen ; the recorder, high steward, chamberlain, town clerk, water bailiff, and other officers, are elected by the corporation at a court of common council: the mayor, the late mayor, recorder, and steward, are justices of the peace for the borough. The freedom is inherited by the eldest son of a freeman, and obtained by purchase or gift, and, among other privileges, confers an exemption from serving on juries for the county. The mayor and eleven of the corporation possess conjointly the powers of the court of admiralty, with all its privileges and profits, without accounting to the Exchequer ; and at the admiralty sessions, the mayor was usually preceded by a person bearing a silver oar, which was kept for that purpose in the town chest : the extent of their maritime jurisdiction has not been strictly defined, but the corporation have amerced persons for unlawfully fishing at Shotley, about a mile north of the town. The corporation hold quarterly courts of session on the day preceding the sessions for the county, for the trial of all not accused of capital offences ; and a court of record, under the charter of Charles II., every Tuesday, for the recovery of debts not exceeding £100, which from the expensiveness of the proceedings, has almost fallen into disuse. A new guildhall has been recently erected, the lower part of which is used as a prison for the borough, chiefly for the confinement of prisoners previously to their committal to the county gaol, and the upper part is appropriated to the holding of the courts, and to the transaction of the public business of the corporation. In the old guildhall, a small brick building, were several buckets bearing the arms and names of members of the corporation, among which were those of Sir Edward Coke, Attorney-General in the reign of James I.; Christopher Monk,

Duke of Albemarle ; Colonel Sir Charles Lyttleton, Governor of Landguard fort in the reign of Charles II.; Sir Harbottle Grimstone, Master of the Rolls in the same reign ; the Duke of Schomberg ; Lord Bolingbroke ; and Edward, Earl of Oxford ; who were recorders of the borough. The borough first sent members to parliament in the 17th of Edward III., but discontinued till the 12th of James I., since which time it has made regular returns: the right of election is vested in the mayor, aldermen, and capital burgesses, thirty-two in number : the mayor is the returning officer.

The borough comprises the parishes of Dover-court and St. Nicholas, in the archdeaconry of Colchester, and diocese of London. The living of Dover-court is a vicarage, with the perpetual curacy of St. Nicholas, rated in the king's books at £5. 0. 10., endowed with £200 private benefaction, and £200 parliamentary grant, and in the patronage of the Crown. The church, dedicated to All Saints, is an old building : it contains several ancient monuments, and was celebrated for a rood, or crucifix, held in high veneration, for the destruction of which three men from Dedham, who had stolen it from the church and burnt it, were hanged for sacrilege in 1532. The church of St. Nicholas was rebuilt in 1820, at an expense of £18,000: it is a handsome edifice, in the later style of English architecture, with a lofty square embattled tower, and contains one thousand free sittings ; in the chancel are three finely-painted windows, presented by John Hopkins, Esq., and containing severally the arms of that gentleman, those of the town, and of Dr. Howley, then Bishop of London : among the monuments is a well-sculptured bust of Sir William Clarke, Secretary at War to Charles I. and Charles II. There are places of worship for Baptists, Independents, and Wesleyan Methodists. A school-room, with an adjoining house for the master, was built in 1724, by Sir Humphrey Parsons, and given to the corporation, in which thirty-two boys of their nomination are instructed : there is also a National school supported by subscription, in which nearly two hundred children of both sexes are taught. Two almshouses for aged widows were built by the corporation in 1785. A fine spring of clear water formerly issued from the cliff between the beacon and the town ; it was much esteemed for its medicinal properties, and possessed a petrifying quality, turning the blue clay which falls from the cliff into stone, sufficiently hard for paving the streets and for building : it is noticed in the Philosophical Transactions for the year 1669. Quantities of amber, and, according to some, ambergris, are occasionally found on the shore ; and in the vicinity of Landguard fort transparent pebbles are found, which were formerly set in rings by the inhabitants.

HARWOOD, a chapelry in the parish of MIDDLETON in TEASDALE, south-western division of DARLINGTON ward, county palatine of DURHAM, 10½ miles (S. E. by S.) from Aldstone-Moor. The population is returned with the township of Forest with Frith. The chapel was rebuilt in 1802. There are some extensive lead mines in the chapelry and its vicinity. A school-room has been erected on his own land, by the Marquis of Cleveland, who pays a voluntary stipend to the master ; the latter also receiving in addition £4 per annum from a bequest by Robert Brumwell in 1724, and £5 annually from the trustees of Lord Crewe's charities.

HARWOOD, a township in the parish of BOLTON, hundred of SALFORD, county palatine of LANCASTER, 3½ miles (W.) from Bury, containing 1809 inhabitants.

HARWOOD, a township in that part of the parish of HARTBURN which is in the north-eastern division of TINDALE ward, county of NORTHUMBERLAND, 13¼ miles (W. by N.) from Morpeth, containing 39 inhabitants.

HARWOOD (GREAT), a chapelry in the parish and lower division of the hundred of BLACKBURN, county palatine of LANCASTER, 4½ miles (N.E.) from Blackburn, containing 2104 inhabitants. The living is a perpetual curacy, in the archdeaconry and diocese of Chester, endowed with £400 private benefaction, and £400 royal bounty, and in the patronage of the Vicar of Blackburn. The church is dedicated to St. Bartholomew.

HARWOOD (LITTLE), a township in the parish and lower division of the hundred of BLACKBURN, county palatine of LANCASTER, 2 miles (N. E. by N.) from Blackburn, containing 210 inhabitants.

HARWOOD-DALE, a joint chapelry with Silpho, in the parish of HACKNESS, liberty of WHITBY-STRAND, North riding of the county of YORK, 9 miles (N. W.) from Scarborough, containing, exclusively of Silpho, 235 inhabitants.

HARWORTH, a parish in the Hatfield division of the wapentake of BASSETLAW, county of NOTTINGHAM, 2¾ miles (W. S.W.) from Bawtry, containing, exclusively of a portion of the township of Styrrup, which is in this parish, 395 inhabitants. The living is a vicarage, in the archdeaconry of Nottingham, and diocese of York, rated in the king's books at £5. 9. 7. — Hartley, Esq. was patron in 1780. The church is dedicated to All Saints. Robert Brailsford, by will dated October 21st, 1700, devised certain lands for the support of a school, and for distributing clothing among the poor of Harworth, Serlby, and Styrrup: the estate, which is under the superintendence of trustees, consists of a farm-house and about fifty-eight acres of land, now let for a term of years at a rental of £59 per annum, in addition to which the charity possesses stock in the three and a half per cents., producing £9 per annum : of this aggregate amount, the schoolmaster receives £40 per annum (including an annuity of £10 assigned by Mary Saunderson, who died in 1724), and a schoolmistress about £26, the remainder being principally expended in clothing for the poor : the school premises comprise a residence for the master, and separate rooms for the instruction of the children : the school is conducted on the Madras system, and is open to all children of the three abovementioned places. Mary Saunderson also gave £10 per annum towards apprenticing the children. In a part of the parish adjoining the town of Bawtry is an hospital, comprising a chapel and two almshouses, anciently founded by Robert Morton, of Bawtry, Esq., for a master and poor persons, with an endowment in land, and a sum of £5. 6. 8. paid by the receiver-general for the county of York, together with other smaller payments : the master appoints the almspeople, who are poor widows, and allows them 20s. annually : the chapel is in disuse.

HASCOMB, a parish in the first division of the hundred of BLACKHEATH, county of SURREY, 3¾ miles (S. E. by S.) from Godalming, containing 253 inhabitants. The living is a rectory, in the archdeaconry of Surrey, and diocese of Winchester, rated in the king's books at £6. 3. 9., and in the patronage of the Rev. W. Mackenzie, D. D. The church, dedicated to St. Peter, contains portions in the early and decorated styles of English architecture.

HASELBEECH, a parish in the hundred of ROTHWELL, county of NORTHAMPTON, 11½ miles (N. by W.) from Northampton, containing 170 inhabitants. The living is a rectory, in the archdeaconry of Northampton, and diocese of Peterborough, rated in the king's books at £13. 14. 9½. Lady Apreece was patroness in 1822. The church is dedicated to St. Michael.

HASELBURY-BRYAN, a parish forming, with the parish of Fifehead-Neville, a detached portion of the hundred of Pimperne and of the division of Blandford (North), being locally in Cerne sub-division of the county of DORSET, 10 miles (W. N.W.) from Blandford-Forum, containing 574 inhabitants. The living is a rectory, in the archdeaconry of Dorset, and diocese of Bristol, rated in the king's books at £19. 13. 9., and in the patronage of the Duke of Northumberland. The church is dedicated to St. James. Twenty-four acres of land were left by some person unknown, the rental of which is divided amongst the most deserving poor.

HASELEY, a parish in the Snitterfield division of the hundred of BARLICHWAY, county of WARWICK, 3½ miles (N. W. by W.) from Warwick, containing 210 inhabitants. The living is a rectory, in the archdeaconry and diocese of Worcester, rated in the king's books at £4. 9. 4½. Sir E. Antrobus, Bart. was patron in 1827. The church is dedicated to St. Mary. The sum of £4 per annum, the proceeds of the town close, is paid for the instruction of poor children.

HASELEY (GREAT), a parish in the hundred of EWELME, county of OXFORD, 3¼ miles (W.) from Tetsworth, containing, with the township of Little Haseley, and the hamlets of Latchford, Lobb, and Rycote, 628 inhabitants. The living is a rectory, annexed to the deanery of Windsor, in the archdeaconry and diocese of Oxford, rated in the king's books at £30. The church is dedicated to St. Peter,

HASELEY (LITTLE), a township in the parish of GREAT HASELEY, hundred of EWELME, county of OXFORD, 3½ miles (W. by S.) from Tetsworth, containing 153 inhabitants.

HASELOR, a township in that part of the parish of ST. MICHAEL, LICHFIELD, which is in the northern division of the hundred of OFFLOW, county of STAFFORD, 4½ miles (N.) from Tamworth, containing 49 inhabitants. It is within the peculiar ecclesiastical jurisdiction of the Dean of Lichfield. Here was anciently a chapel, which has fallen into ruins.

HASELOR, a parish in the Stratford division of the hundred of BARLICHWAY, county of WARWICK, 2½ miles (E.) from Alcester, containing 387 inhabitants. The living is a vicarage, in the archdeaconry and diocese of Worcester, rated in the king's books at £6. 13. 4., endowed with £100 royal bounty, and in the patronage of the Crown. The church is dedicated to St. Mary and All Saints.

HASELWOOD, or HASLEWOOD, a chapelry in the hundred of PLOMESGATE, county of SUFFOLK, 1¾ mile (N.N. W.) from Aldborough, containing 99 inhabitants. The chapel, which was dedicated to St. Mary, is in ruins. The navigable river Alde runs on the south-east of this chapelry.

HASFIELD, a parish in the lower division of the hundred of WESTMINSTER, county of GLOUCESTER, 6 miles (N.) from Gloucester, containing 237 inhabitants. The living is a rectory, in the jurisdiction of the peculiar court of Deerhurst, within which, however, no ecclesiastical authority is exercised, rated in the king's books at £13. 6. 8. — Miller, Esq. was patron in 1800. The church is dedicated to St. Mary. In 1724 Mrs. Margaret Parker gave £40 for the education of poor children; the present income arising from this benefaction is £8 per annum, which is paid to a schoolmaster for teaching poor children to read. The navigable river Severn runs on the south-east of this parish.

HASKETON, a parish in the hundred of CARLFORD, county of SUFFOLK, 1¾ mile (N. W.) from Woodbridge, containing 530 inhabitants. The living is a discharged rectory, in the archdeaconry of Suffolk, and diocese of Norwich, rated in the king's books at £13. 6. 8., endowed with £200 royal bounty. Mrs. Freeland was patroness in 1819. The church is dedicated to St. Andrew.

HASLAND, a township in the parish of CHESTERFIELD, hundred of SCARSDALE, county of DERBY, 1½ mile (S. S. E.) from Chesterfield, containing 770 inhabitants.

HASLE, a township in that part of the parish of WRAGBY which is in the upper division of the wapentake of OSGOLDCROSS, West riding of the county of YORK, 4 miles (S. W. by S.) from Pontefract, containing 139 inhabitants.

HASLEBURY, a parish in the hundred of CHIPPENHAM, county of WILTS, 6½ miles (S. W.) from Chippenham. The living is a rectory, in the archdeaconry of Wilts, and diocese of Salisbury, rated in the king's books at £1. 15. 5., and in the patronage of the Crown. The church, which was dedicated to All Saints, has fallen to decay, and the inhabitants, consisting only of a few families, attend the church at Box.

HASLEBURY-PLUCKNETT, a parish in the hundred of HOUNDSBOROUGH, BERWICK, and COKER, county of SOMERSET, 2¼ miles (N. E. by E.) from Crewkerne, containing 768 inhabitants. The living is a discharged vicarage, rated in the king's books at £7, endowed with £200 private benefaction, and £200 royal bounty, and in the peculiar jurisdiction and patronage of the Prebendary of Haslebury in the Cathedral Church of Wells. The church is dedicated to St. Michael. St. Walfric, a hermit, had a cell here, and dying in 1154, was interred in the parish church, and his tomb became the resort of pilgrims: a few years prior to his death, a monastery for canons Regular was founded here, but it was destroyed during the war between John and the barons.

HASLEMERE, a borough, market town, and parish, in the second division of the hundred of GODALMING, county of SURREY, 12¼ miles (S. W. by S.) from Guildford, and 43 (S. W.) from London, containing 887 inhabitants. This place is situated in the south-west angle of the county, where it borders on Sussex and Hampshire, whence the termination of its name, *Mere*, signifying a boundary; and the prefix alludes to the numerous coppices of hazel which grow in the vicinity. There is a tradition that the ancient town stood on tne side of a hill to the east of the present, wnere the foundations of buildings have frequently been discovered, its destruction being ascribed to the Danes. It was probably rebuilt before the Conquest, as it is

mentioned as a borough in Domesday-book. In the reign of Henry II. it appertained to the see of Salisbury, and in 1393, the bishop procured a grant for holding a market and a fair, but these had fallen into disuse previously to the grant of the charter by Queen Elizabeth. The town stands on very high ground, and is remarkably clean; it is well supplied with water, but neither lighted nor paved. There is a silk crape manufactory, which formerly afforded employment to more than one hundred persons, but it is at present on the decline; and near the town is a paper-mill, for making fine paper only. The market is on Tuesday; and there are fairs for cattle, May 13th and September 26th. A charter for the re-establishment of the market and fair, which had fallen into disuse, was granted in the 38th of Elizabeth, in which it is also stated that "the burgesses had from time immemorial, at their own costs, sent two members to parliament." This is a borough by prescription, the officers belonging to which, consisting of a bailiff, constable, searchers and sealers of leather, and ale-tasters, are chosen annually at the court leet, in April or May. The privilege of electing representatives has only been regularly exercised since the 27th of Elizabeth: the right of election is vested in the resident freeholders, or burgage tenants: the bailiff is the returning officer; and the patronage of the borough belongs to the Earl of Lonsdale. The living is a perpetual curacy, annexed to the rectory of Chiddingfold, in the archdeaconry of Surrey, and diocese of Winchester. The church, dedicated to St. Bartholomew, is an ancient edifice, situated on an eminence to the north of the town, and consisting of a nave, north aisle, and western tower. Here is a place of worship for Independents. A National school for poor boys of Haslemere and the adjoining parishes is kept in the market-hall. On a common near the town is an unendowed almshouse for eight poor persons, erected in 1676, through the exertions of James Gresham, Esq. A hill, called Blackdown, at a short distance from the town, affords a view of the sea and the surrounding country to a great extent; and in the vicinity is a telegraph.

HASLINGDEN, a market town and chapelry in that part of the parish of WHALLEY which is in the lower division of the hundred of BLACKBURN, county palatine of LANCASTER, 40 miles (S.E.) from Lancaster, 17 (N.) from Manchester, and 203 (N.N.W.) from London, containing 6595 inhabitants. This place, which is situated in the midst of a mountainous district on the border of the Forest of Rossendale, probably took its name from the abundance of hazel trees which formerly grew in its vicinity. The town originally stood on the declivity of a hill, but the modern buildings have been erected at its base; and many old houses of mean appearance have been replaced by new and substantial edifices, which contribute much to the uniformity of the whole. The improvements which have taken place since the beginning of the present century have been greatly facilitated by the abundant supply of stone for building afforded by the neighbouring mountains of granite, and the slate and flags furnished by the quarries of Hutchbank and others. Coal is plentifully produced from mines in the neighbourhood. The woollen manufacture formerly constituted almost the sole occupation of the inhabitants, and it is still carried on to some extent; but the cotton trade has in a great degree superseded it, and the numerous mills on the banks of the Swinnel are principally in the occupation of the manufacturers of cotton goods. The market day has been changed from Wednesday to Saturday, to prevent its interfering with the market of Blackburn; and fairs are held, February 2nd, on Easter Tuesday, May 8th, July 4th, and October 2d; the Easter fair is for the sale of horses, and the others chiefly for cattle. An act of parliament was passed in the 34th of George III., for making a navigable canal from Bury, by Haslingden, to Church Town, to join the Bury, Bolton, and Manchester canal ou the south, and the Leeds and Liverpool canal on the north, but the projected undertaking has not been executed. Here are a public news-room and two subscription libraries. Races were formerly held on Lound-Hey, near the town, but the ground has been recently enclosed for cultivation. The living is a perpetual curacy, with that of Goodshaw, in the archdeaconry and diocese of Chester, endowed with £600 private benefaction, £400 royal bounty, and £1600 parliamentary grant, and in the patronage of the Vicar of Whalley. The church, dedicated to St. James, and standing on an eminence at the north end of the town, is a substantial edifice, rebuilt of stone about fifty years ago, except the tower, which belonged to the preceding church, erected in the reign of Henry VIII.: it has lately received an addition of five hundred and eighteen sittings, of which four hundred and sixty-two are free, the Incorporated Society for the enlargement of churches and chapels having granted £450 towards defraying the expense. There are places of worship for Baptists, Independents, Wesleyan Methodists, Sandemanians, and Swedenborgians. A free grammar school was founded in 1749, for the education of ten poor boys, and subsequently endowed with property producing about £18 per annum.

HASLINGFIELD, a parish in the hundred of WETHERLEY, county of CAMBRIDGE, 5½ miles (S.W. by S.) from Cambridge, containing 544 inhabitants. The living is a vicarage, in the archdeaconry and diocese of Ely, rated in the king's books at £8. 10. 7½. C. Mitchell, Esq. was patron in 1800. The church, which is dedicated to All Saints, was erected in 1352; it is in the early style of English architecture. A charity school was founded by Simon Ertman, a Dane, who died here in 1658; the present income is £28 per annum. In a chapel dedicated to the Virgin, and formerly much resorted to, a pair of huge iron fetters was hung up, as a votive offering, by one Lord Scales, in commemoration of his release from imprisonment.

HASLINGTON, a chapelry in that part of the parish of BARTHOMLEY which is in the hundred of NANTWICH, county palatine of CHESTER, 3¼ miles (S.S.W.) from Sandbach, containing 985 inhabitants. The living is a perpetual curacy, in the archdeaconry and diocese of Chester, endowed with £200 private benefaction, £200 royal bounty, and £1100 parliamentary grant. Sir J. Broughton, Bart. was patron in 1814. There is a place of worship for Independents.

HASSALL, a township in that part of the parish of SANDBACH which is in the hundred of NANTWICH, county palatine of CHESTER, 3 miles (S. by E.) from Sandbach, containing 218 inhabitants.

HASSINGHAM, a parish in the hundred of BLOFIELD, county of NORFOLK, 4 miles (S. W. by S.) from Acle, containing 103 inhabitants. The living is a discharged rectory, consolidated with that of Buckenham,

in the archdeaconry and diocese of Norwich, rated in the king's books at £4, endowed with £200 royal bounty. The church is dedicated to St. Mary.

HASSOP, a hamlet in the parish of BAKEWELL, hundred of HIGH PEAK, county of DERBY, 3 miles (N. by E.) from Bakewell, containing 128 inhabitants. Hassop Hall was garrisoned for the king by Colonel Eyr, in 1643.

HASTINGLEIGH, a parish in the franchise and barony of BIRCHOLT, lathe of SHEPWAY, county of KENT, 6½ miles (E. by N.) from Ashford, containing 194 inhabitants. The living is a rectory, in the archdeaconry and diocese of Canterbury, rated in the king's books at £10. 5., and in the patronage of the Archbishop of Canterbury. The church is dedicated to St. Mary.

HASTINGS, the principal of the cinque-ports, and a borough and market town, having separate jurisdiction, locally in the rape of Hastings, county of SUSSEX, 69 miles (E.) from Chichester, and 64¼ (S.E.) from London, containing, exclusively of that part of the parish of St. Mary in the Castle which is in the hundred of Baldslow, 6085 inhabitants. 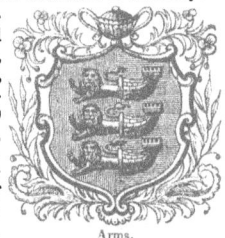 This place, which is of great antiquity, attained considerable importance during the Saxon Heptarchy, and is generally supposed to have derived its name from Hastings, a noted Danish pirate, contemporary with Alfred the Great, who erected a fortress here to secure the retreat of his party after having pillaged the neighbouring country. In 924, Athelstan established a mint at this place, of which some notice occurs in Domesday-book; and William the Conqueror, on his landing at Pevensey, repaired the castle and took up his station in this town, whence he marched to meet Harold, whom he defeated in that decisive battle to which Hastings has given name, but which was fought at the distance of eight miles from the town, on a spot on which he subsequently built the abbey of Battel. Of the castle, which was erected on a high hill to the west of the present town, there are still extensive remains, consisting of a considerable portion of the outer wall, in which are parts of two towers and gateways of Norman architecture, and the foundation of the keep, surrounded by a broad and deep fosse, with vestiges of a draw-bridge and other fortifications. Within, the walls have been cleared from the rubbish, which for more than two centuries had nearly concealed them, and thus have been discovered the remains of the church and conventual buildings of a free college, for a dean and seven prebendaries, probably founded by Henry de Eu, in the reign of Henry I., and dedicated to the Blessed Virgin: at the dissolution, the revenue of the deanery was rated at £20 per annum, and that of the prebends, collectively, at £41. 13. 5. The collegiate church is one hundred and ten feet in length, and adjoining it are the remains of the parish church of St. Mary in the Castle, the chapter-house, and the prebendal buildings, forming an interesting mass of ruins, which have been recently enclosed by the Earl of Chichester. Numerous Saxon coins, fragments of columns, pottery, and other relics of antiquity, have been discovered on the spot. In the reign

Arms.

of Richard I., a priory of Black canons was founded here by Walter Bricet, of which the church and other buildings having been destroyed by the encroachments of the sea, Sir John Pelham, in the reign of Henry IV., gave the brethren lands at Warbilton, for the foundation of a church and monastery, which were finally erected near the town, and of which, at the dissolution, the revenue was £57. 19. By charter of William the Conqueror, this town, together with Hythe, was added to the three previously incorporated ports of Sandwich, Dovor, and Romney, being invested with peculiar privileges; and in the time of Edward I. it was rated at twenty-one ships, with twenty-one mariners in each, for the service of the king for fourteen days, at its own charge: it soon became, and has ever since been considered, the principal of the cinque-ports. In 1377, Hastings was burnt by the French, who made a descent upon this part of the coast; but it was soon afterwards rebuilt.

The town is pleasantly situated in a vale formed into an amphitheatre, open to the sea on the south, by two lofty cliffs, of which one extends to the sea, and the other towards the land, and consists of two principal streets parallel with each other, which, from their declivity towards the sea, are always clean and dry: it is well paved and lighted by act of parliament, the expense being defrayed by a duty of three shillings per chaldron on all coal brought into the port: the houses are in general well built, and the inhabitants are supplied with water from the Bourne, which divides the town into two parts. The salubrity and mildness of the air, arising from the sheltered situation of the town, by which it is defended from the north and east winds, render it peculiarly eligible as a place of residence for invalids, and these advantages concurring with the openness of the coast, and the smoothness of its beach, have long made it a fashionable and well-frequented place for sea-bathing. At low water, the fine level sands afford a healthy and fashionable promenade, and from the high grounds the prospects are richly diversified with scenery of luxuriant cultivation, and of boldly romantic character. Among the more recent improvements are the erection of Pelham-place and crescent, the Bazaar, Wellington-square, and numerous handsome lodging-houses near the sea for the accommodation of visitors: the Pelham baths are well fitted up with hot, cold, vapour, and shower-baths, with every convenience for their use, and numerous bathing-machines are in constant attendance on the beach. There are some good libraries: assemblies and concerts take place during the season at the Swan Inn. A small theatre has been recently erected; and races, established in 1827, which have been highly patronised, are annually held in September. A fine terrace-walk has been formed on the east side of the Castle-hill, where are the ruins already noticed. The town is defended by a strong fort, and the coast by additional batteries and martello towers. The harbour, now called the Stade, formerly afforded safe anchorage for ships, but has fallen into disuse since the reign of Elizabeth, when the pier was destroyed by a storm, since which time the harbour has been inconsiderable, and will not admit vessels of more than one hundred tons' burden. A custom-house, with an establishment of twelve riding officers, is maintained here. The trade of the port is principally in lime, which is burnt near the town; in corn, iron, timber, and coal, which are sent coast-

wise, and in which not more than fifteen vessels are employed; and in the herring and mackerel fishery, which employs about eighty boats for the supply of the London market. The market days are Wednesday and Saturday, the latter for corn: the fairs are on Whit-Tuesday, July 26th and 27th, and November 23rd.

Seal of the Corporation.

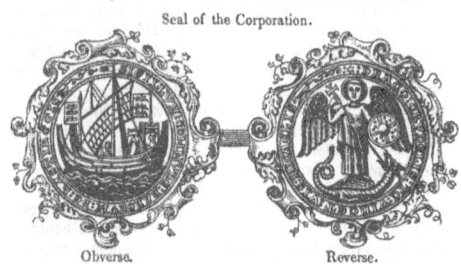

Obverse.   Reverse.

The government, by charter of incorporation granted by Elizabeth in 1588, and confirmed and enlarged by Charles II., is vested in a mayor, recorder, and twelve jurats, who are called barons, assisted by a town-clerk, chamberlain, and other officers, of whom one is pier-warden, and regulates the port, collecting 10s. from every vessel not in ballast which enters it. The mayor is elected from among the jurats by the freemen, on the third Sunday after Easter, and is liable to fine or imprisonment for refusing to serve the office; and the jurats are appointed by the mayor as vacancies occur. The mayor and jurats are justices of the peace, with whom, in respect to the custom and excise laws, the county magistrates have concurrent jurisdiction. The freedom of the borough is inherited by the eldest son of a freeman born within the borough, or obtained by gift from the corporation: the inhabitants are exempt from serving on juries at the assizes or sessions for the county. The corporation hold quarterly courts of session, at which the mayor presides, for determining on offences committed within the borough; but though invested with power to try capital offenders, these are generally tried at the assizes for the county, held at Lewes. They also hold a court of record, for the recovery of debts to any amount, every alternate week, at which the mayor presides. Guestlings and brotherhoods are courts held at uncertain intervals by the corporations of the cinque-ports: a guestling consists of a full assembly, composed of five or six deputies from each port, with plenary powers; the mayor of every port in turn issuing notices for the meetings: a brotherhood consists of one or two deputies from each port, convened to deliberate on affairs of inferior importance. The town-hall, under which the market is held, is a neat edifice, rebuilt in 1823, at the expense of the corporation. The common gaol is a small building divided into two departments, and capable of receiving only eight prisoners. The elective franchise was conferred in the 42nd of Edward III., since which time Hastings has continued to return two members to parliament: the right of election is vested in the mayor, jurats, and freemen resident in the borough, and not receiving alms: the mayor is the returning officer.

The town comprises the united parishes of All Saints and St. Clement, both rectories, in the archdeaconry and diocese of Chichester, the former rated in the king's books at £19. 12. 9., and the latter at £23. 6. 10., each endowed with £200 royal bounty, and in the patronage of the Rev. G. G. Stonestreet. The churches of All Saints' and St. Clement's have been both handsome structures of flint and stone, in the later style of English architecture, but have suffered greatly from mutilation, and repeated repairs and alterations. An episcopal chapel, situated in the centre of Pelham-crescent, a chaste and elegant edifice, was begun by the late, and has been recently completed by the present, Earl of Chichester. There are places of worship for Baptists, Bryanites, Huntingtonians, Independents, and Wesleyan Methodists. A school for the instruction of boys in reading, writing, arithmetic, and navigation, was founded in 1619, by the Rev.William Parker, who endowed it with property producing upwards of £210 per annum; it is open to all the children of the town. A school was founded in 1708, by James Saunders, Esq., who endowed it with estates producing nearly £240 per annum, for teaching seventy boys reading, writing, and the English and Latin languages, and for the payment of £10 per annum to two mistresses, for teaching thirty younger children of each of the parishes of All Saints and St. Clement to read: the schools are under the direction of the corporation. The fourth part of an estate of one hundred and ninety-two acres of land, belonging to the dissolved priory, and producing £270 per annum, was bequeathed, in 1714, by Mr. Richard Ellsworth, for teaching poor children; but the benefaction has not been carried into effect, owing to the property being involved in a suit in Chancery. Mr. J. Spencer Milward, who died intestate in 1760, directed that £10 per annum should be paid for the instruction of poor children; and in consequence of this recommendation a larger sum is now applied by his representative to that purpose. The Magdalene charity, of which the corporation are trustees, was endowed by some unknown benefactor with an estate producing more than £150 per annum. About two miles from Hastings is a large stone, on which it is said that William the Conqueror dined on his landing on this coast. Titus Oates, the ministerial informer in the reign of Charles II., was the officiating clergyman of All Saints' parish, and lived in a house which is still in existence; and Edward Capel, Esq., one of Shakspeare's commentators, resided in a house now called East Cliffe House, in the garden of which is a mulberry tree planted by Garrick. Hastings gives the title of marquis to the noble family of Rawdon-Hastings.

HASWELL, a township in the parish of EASINGTON, southern division of EASINGTON ward, county palatine of DURHAM, 6 miles (E. by N.) from Durham, containing 115 inhabitants.

HATCH, a hamlet in the parish of NORTHILL, hundred of WIXAMTREE, county of BEDFORD, 2¼ miles (W. N. W.) from Biggleswade, containing, with Thorncote, Brookend, Budnor, and a part of Beeston, 241 inhabitants.

HATCH, a hamlet in the parish of KINGSTON upon THAMES, first division of the hundred of KINGSTON, county of SURREY, containing, with Ham, 961 inhabitants.

HATCH (EAST), a chapelry in the parish of TISBURY, hundred of DUNWORTH, county of WILTS, 4 miles (S. S. E.) from Hindon. The population is returned with the parish.

VOL. II.

HATCH (WEST), a parish in the northern division of the hundred of CURRY, county of SOMERSET, 4¼ miles (S. E. by E.) from Taunton, containing 367 inhabitants. The living is a perpetual curacy, annexed to the vicarage of North Curry, in the peculiar jurisdiction of the Dean and Chapter of Wells, endowed with £200 private benefaction.

HATCH-BEAUCHAMP, a parish in the hundred of ABDICK and BULSTONE, county of SOMERSET, 6¾ miles (N. W. by N.) from Ilminster, containing 245 inhabitants. The living is a rectory, in the archdeaconry of Taunton, and diocese of Bath and Wells, rated in the king's books at £13. 5. 2½., and in the patronage of the Rev. W. G. Dymock. The church, dedicated to St. John the Baptist, is a handsome edifice, consisting of a nave, aisle, chancel, and south porch, with an embattled tower at the west end: the altar-piece is a fine painting of the Descent from the Cross. There is a place of worship for Baptists. License for a market and a fair, both long since disused, was obtained by John de Beauchamp, lord of the manor, in 1301.

HATCLIFFE, a parish in the wapentake of BRADLEY-HAVERSTOE, parts of LINDSEY, county of LINCOLN, 6¾ miles (E. by S.) from Caistor, containing 99 inhabitants. The living is a discharged rectory, in the peculiar jurisdiction and patronage of the Collegiate Church of Southwell, rated in the king's books at £5. 4. 2. The church is dedicated to St. Mary.

HATFIELD, a parish in the hundred of WOLPHY, county of HEREFORD, 7 miles (N. W.) from Bromyard, containing 153 inhabitants. The living is a perpetual curacy, in the archdeaconry and diocese of Hereford, endowed with £10 per annum private benefaction, and £600 royal bounty. Sir J. G. Cotterell, Bart. was patron in 1812. The church is dedicated to St. Leonard.

HATFIELD, a parish in the southern division of the wapentake of STRAFFORTH and TICKHILL, West riding of the county of YORK, comprising the townships of Hatfield and Stainforth, and containing 2642 inhabitants, of which number, 1948 are in the township of Hatfield, 3 miles (S. W. by S.) from Thorne. The living is a perpetual curacy, in the archdeaconry and diocese of York, rated in the king's books at £15. 5., endowed with £200 private benefaction, and £1000 royal bounty. Lord and Lady Deerhurst were patrons in 1817. The church, dedicated to St. Lawrence, is in the later English style. Here is a place of worship for Independents. In the reign of Charles I., Thomas Wormeley devised to trustees property for securing an annuity of £10 to a schoolmaster to instruct the children of the inhabitants: in 1682, a school-house was built by John Hatfield, Esq., and in 1716 assigned to trustees for the use of the schoolmaster, but at the time of the inquiry of the Commissioners of Charities, in 1828, the school was discontinued.

HATFIELD (BISHOP'S), a market town and parish in the hundred of BROADWATER, county of HERTFORD, 7 miles (W.S.W.) from Hertford, and 19 (N.N.W.) from London, on the great north road, containing 3215 inhabitants. The manor, which was an ancient demesne of the crown, was given by King Edgar to the monastery of St. Ethelreda, at Ely; and that religious foundation having been converted into a bishoprick by Henry I., in 1108, the parish thence received the prefix to its name. Here the bishops of Ely had a palace,

2 X

which was rebuilt by John Morton, who held the see from 1478 to 1486 ; of this edifice the gateway and the west front are still standing, near the east end of the parish church. Henry VIII. having obtained this manor by exchange, the palace became a royal residence ; and from it Edward VI. and Elizabeth were conducted to London to take possession of the throne, after the death of their respective predecessors, the latter, during the reign of Mary having been kept here in confinement. The town is situated on the declivity of a steep hill, to the west of the river Lea, and consists of one principal street, intersected by a smaller, which are, during the winter months, lighted with oil. A silk-mill, worked by a steam-engine, furnishes employment to about two hundred persons, chiefly children ; and there is a paper-mill on the river Lea. The market is on Thursday : fairs are held on the 23rd of April and the 8th of October. The town is within the jurisdiction of the county magistrates, who hold here a petty session for the division; and a court leet is held by the Marquis of Salisbury, who is lord of the manor. The living is a rectory with the perpetual curacy of Totteridge, in the archdeaconry of Huntingdon, and diocese of Lincoln, rated in the king's books at £36. 2. 1., and in the patronage of the Earl of Salisbury. The church, dedicated to St. Ethelreda, stands on the summit of a hill on which the town is situated; on the north side of the chancel is the sepulchral chapel of the family of the Marquis of Salisbury, in which is a fine marble monument to Robert Cecil, first Earl of Salisbury, and Lord High Treasurer in the reign of James I.; and on the south side is a chapel belonging to the proprietors of Brocket hall, in this parish. There is a place of worship for Independents. A National school for boys is kept in a room over the market-house ; and there is a school of industry for girls, with an endowment given in 1733, by Anne, Countess of Salisbury. There are also six almshouses for widows, founded and endowed by the families of Boteler, Serancke, and Salisbury. Hatfield house, the mansion of the Marquis of Salisbury, is a fine specimen of the domestic style of architecture in the reign of James I.

HATFIELD (GREAT), a township partly in the parish of SIGGLESTHORNE, but chiefly in that of MAPPLETON, northern division of the wapentake of HOLDERNESS, East riding of the county of YORK, 11 miles (E. by N.) from Beverley, containing 127 inhabitants.

HATFIELD (LITTLE), a township in the parish of SIGGLESTHORNE, northern division of the wapentake of HOLDERNESS, East riding of the county of YORK, 10½ miles (E. N. E.) from Beverley, containing 25 inhabitants.

HATFIELD-BROAD-OAK, or HATFIELD-REGIS, a parish in the hundred of HARLOW, county of ESSEX, 6 miles (N. E. by E.) from Harlow, comprising the townships of Brumsend-quarter, Heath-quarter, Town-quarter, and Woodrow-quarter, and containing 1693 inhabitants. The living is a discharged vicarage, in the jurisdiction of the Commissary of Essex and Herts, concurrently with the Consistorial Court of the Bishop of London, rated in the king's books at £7. 11., and in the patronage of the Master and Fellows of Trinity College, Cambridge. The church, dedicated to St. Mary, comprises portions in the later English style, with some of an earlier date. There is a place of worship for Wesleyan

Methodists. Here are some almshouses. Adjoining the church, which was then conventual, stood a priory of Black canons, founded by Albeni de Vere, in 1135, and dedicated to God, St. Mary, and St. Melanius Redenensis, the revenue of which, at the time of the dissolution, was £157. 3. 2.

HATFIELD-PEVERELL, a parish in the hundred of WITHAM, county of ESSEX, 3¼ miles (S. W. by S.) from Witham, containing 1101 inhabitants. The living is a discharged vicarage, in the archdeaconry of Colchester, and diocese of London, rated in the king's books at £8, endowed with £1000 private benefaction, £200 royal bounty, and £2500 parliamentary grant. J. Wright, Esq. was patron in 1823. The church, dedicated to St. Andrew, has received an addition of two hundred sittings, of which one hundred and twenty-one are free, the Incorporated Society for the enlargement of churches and chapels having granted £150 towards defraying the expense. A school was endowed in 1638, by Sir Edward Alleyne, with £5. 10. per annum. Miss Loveman, in 1820, erected four tenements for two aged married couples and two single persons, endowing them with eighteen shillings a week for the former, and twelve shillings for the latter. Here was a college for Secular canons in the time of William Rufus, founded by Ingebrica, wife of Ranulph Peverill, and dedicated to St. Mary Magdalene ; it was converted by her son into a Benedictine monastery. The only remains of the buildings consist of the priory church, now parochial, which has a Norman door. The Chelmar and Blackwater navigation passes along the southern boundary of this parish, where it receives the river Ter.

HATFORD, a parish in the hundred of GANFIELD, county of BERKS, 3½ miles (E. by S.) from Great Farringdon, containing 132 inhabitants. The living is a rectory, in the archdeaconry of Berks, and diocese of Salisbury, rated in the king's books at £12. 17. 6., and in the patronage of Francis Paynter, Esq. The church, dedicated to St. George, presents a few remains of Saxon architecture.

HATHERALL, county palatine of LANCASTER.— See HOTHERSALL.

HATHERLEIGH, a market town and parish in the hundred of BLACK TORRINGTON, county of DEVON, 29 miles (W. N. W.) from Exeter, and 200 (W. by S.) from London, containing 1499 inhabitants. The manor originally belonged to the abbey of Tavistock : one of the abbots bestowed upon the inhabitants the common of Hatherleigh, which is said to comprise an extent of four hundred and sixty acres, and on which are many good springs. Hatherleigh is situated on a branch of the river Torridge, near its confluence with the Oke, and is chiefly remarkable for the peculiar redness of the soil. The town is small, irregularly built, and of very mean appearance, being chiefly composed of low cottages formed of red loam and thatch. The lands in the environs are very fertile ; and about a mile to the north of the town is a handsome and substantial bridge over the river Torridge. The woollen manufacture is carried on to a very limited extent, but the inhabitants are chiefly employed in agriculture. The market days are Tuesday and Saturday : the fairs are, May 21st, June 22nd, September 7th, and November 9th ; and a large cattle market is held on the Friday nearest to the 21st of March. The town is governed by a portreeve annually elected at the court leet of the lord of the manor, at which time constables are also chosen. The living is a vicarage, in the archdeaconry of Totness, and diocese of Exeter, rated in the king's books at £20. The Trustees of James Ireland, Esq. were patrons in 1791. The church, dedicated to St. John the Baptist, is an ancient structure, with a tower surmounted by a neat spire.. There is a place of worship for Independents. A day and Sunday school is supported by subscription. Several houses near the church, and some un-endowed almshouses, are given rent-free for the use of the poor, for whom also there are some small charitable bequests. Jasper Mayne, equally noted as a preacher and as a dramatic writer, was born here in 1604, and died in 1672.

HATHERLEY (DOWN), a parish in the upper division of the hundred of DUDSTONE and KING'S BARTON, county of GLOUCESTER, 3¼ miles (N.E. by N.) from Gloucester, containing 170 inhabitants. The living is a vicarage, in the archdeaconry and diocese of Gloucester, rated in the king's books at £8. 14. 4½., and in the patronage of the Crown. The church is dedicated to St. Mary and Corpus Christi.

HATHERLEY (UP), a joint chapelry with Great Shurdington, in the upper division of the hundred of DUDSTONE and KING'S BARTON, county of GLOUCESTER, 2½ miles (S.W. by S.) from Cheltenham, containing 32 inhabitants.

HATHERN, a parish in the western division of the hundred of GOSCOTE, county of LEICESTER, 2¾ miles (N.W.) from Loughborough, containing 1144 inhabitants. The living is a rectory, in the archdeaconry of Leicester, and diocese of Lincoln, rated in the king's books at £12. C. M. Phillips, Esq. was patron in 1810. The church, dedicated to St. Peter, has received one hundred and seven additional sittings, towards defraying the expense of which the Incorporated Society for the enlargement of churches and chapels contributed £60. There is a place of worship for Wesleyan Methodists.

HATHEROP, a parish in the hundred of BRIGHT-WELLS-BARROW, county of GLOUCESTER, 3 miles (N.) from Fairford, containing 290 inhabitants. The living is a rectory, in the archdeaconry and diocese of Gloucester, rated in the king's books at £10, and in the patronage of the Hon. Mr. Ponsonby. The church is dedicated to St. Nicholas. The river Coln passes through this parish.

HATHERSAGE, a parish in the hundred of HIGH PEAK, county of DERBY, 5¼ miles (N. by E.) from Stoney-Middleton, comprising the chapelries of Darwent and Stoney-Middleton, and the hamlets of Bamford, Hathersage, and Outseats, and containing 1856 inhabitants. The living is a discharged vicarage, in the archdeaconry of Derby, and diocese of Lichfield and Coventry, rated in the king's books at £7. 0. 5., endowed with £200 private benefaction, £400 royal bounty, and £2000 parliamentary grant, and in the patronage of the Duke of Devonshire. The church, dedicated to St. Michael, is an ancient embattled structure in the later style of English architecture, consisting of a nave, side aisles, and chancel, with a lofty spire : ih the chancel are several monuments of the family of Eyre, ancestors of the earls of Newburg ; on an altar-tomb, represented on brass plates, are effigies of Robert Eyre, who fought in the battle of Agincourt, and of his wife and fourteen children. On the south side of the church-yard is a spot shewn as the place of interment of Little John,

the favourite companion of Robin Hood : the body of a Mr. B. Ashton, who was buried here in 1725, was discovered, in 1781, quite perfect and petrified, retaining the flesh colour as when entombed. There is a place of worship for Wesleyan Methodists, and a chapel for Roman Catholics. This parish is in the honour of Tutbury, duchy of Lancaster, and within the jurisdiction of a court of pleas held at Chapel en le Frith every third Tuesday, for the recovery of debts under 40s. In 1718 a school was erected by subscription, on a piece of land given by B. Ashton, Esq., who endowed it with £5 per annum for the schoolmaster ; the premises having become dilapidated, the school has been discontinued, and the arrears of annuity amount to about £100. There are several bequests for the use of the poor. Here are manufactories for needles, buttons, and calico. The river Derwent flows through the parish. Eastward from the church is Camp Green, a circular enclosure encompassed by a single mound and moat, evidently of Danish origin. In the vicinity are some irregular rocks, called rocking stones, or rock basins.

HATHERTON, a township in the parish of WYBUNBURY, hundred of NANTWICH, county palatine of CHESTER, 4¼ miles (S.E. by S.) from Nantwich, containing 418 inhabitants.

HATHERTON, a township in that part of the parish of WOLVERHAMPTON which is in the eastern division of the hundred of CUTTLESTONE, county of STAFFORD, 4 miles (S.E.) from Penkridge, containing 320 inhabitants. This township is within the jurisdiction of the royal peculiar ecclesiastical court of Wolverhampton.

HATLEY (COCKAYNE), a parish in the hundred of BIGGLESWADE, county of BEDFORD, 6 miles (N. by E.) from Biggleswade, containing 117 inhabitants. The living is a rectory, in the archdeaconry of Bedford, and diocese of Lincoln, rated in the king's books at £8. Earl Brownlow was patron in 1806. The church is dedicated to St. John the Baptist.

HATLEY (EAST), a parish in the hundred of ARMINGFORD, county of CAMBRIDGE, 4½ miles (E. by N.) from Potton, containing 108 inhabitants. The living is a rectory, in the archdeaconry and diocese of Ely, rated in the king's books at £7. 16. 8., and in the patronage of the Master and Fellows of Downing College, Cambridge. The church is dedicated to St. Denis.

HATLEY (ST. GEORGE), a parish in the hundred of LONGSTOW, county of CAMBRIDGE, 4 miles (E. N.E.) from Potton, containing 105 inhabitants. The living is a rectory, in the archdeaconry and diocese of Ely, rated in the king's books at £8, and in the patronage of J. W. Quintin, Esq.

HATTERSLEY, a township in the parish of MOTTRAM in LONGDEN-DALE, hundred of MACCLESFIELD, county palatine of CHESTER, 6¼ miles (E. N.E.) from Stockport, containing 563 inhabitants.

HATTON, a township in the parish of WAVERTON, lower division of the hundred of BROXTON, county palatine of CHESTER, 6 miles (S. E.) from Chester, containing 157 inhabitants.

HATTON, a township in the parish of RUNCORN, hundred of BUCKLOW, county palatine of CHESTER, 4¼ miles (S. by W.) from Warrington, containing 397 inhabitants. The Chester canal passes on the east side of this township.

HATTON, a hamlet in the parish of MARSTON upon

Dove, hundred of Appletree, county of Derby, 10 miles (W. S. W.) from Derby, containing 225 inhabitants.

HATTON, a parish in the eastern division of the wapentake of Wraggoe, parts of Lindsey, county of Lincoln, 3¼ miles (E. by S.) from Wragby, containing 165 inhabitants. The living is a rectory, in the archdeaconry and diocese of Lincoln, rated in the king's books at £7. 10. 10., and in the patronage of Col. Sibthorp. The church is dedicated to St. Stephen

HATTON, a hamlet in the parish of East Bedfont, hundred of Spelthorne, county of Middlesex, 3 miles (W.) from Hounslow. The population is returned with the parish.

HATTON, a township in the parish of Shiffnall, Shiffnall division of the hundred of Brimstree, county of Salop, 2½ miles (S. E. by S.) from Shiffnall, containing 588 inhabitants.

HATTON, a parish in the Snitterfield division of the hundred of Barlichway, county of Warwick, 3¾ miles (N. W. by W.) from Warwick, comprising the chapelries of Beausall and Shrewley, and containing 806 inhabitants. The living is a perpetual curacy, in the archdeaconry and diocese of Worcester, endowed with £400 private benefaction, and 400 royal bounty, and in the patronage of Mrs. Baker. The church is dedicated to the Holy Trinity. In 1722, William Edwards bequeathed a rent-charge of £20 for the use of a schoolmaster, to teach male children born within the liberties and precincts of Hatton, Shrewley, and Bursall. The school-house was built by the widow of the testator: the annual stipend of the master is £19, and he occupies the school-house rent free. The parsonage-house was the residence of the late learned Dr. Samuel Parr from 1783, when he obtained the living, until his death in 1825.

HATTON (HIGH), a township in the parish of Stanton upon Hine Heath, Whitchurch division of the hundred of Bradford (North), county of Salop, 7½ miles (E.S.E.) from Wem, containing 193 inhabitants.

HAUGH, an extra-parochial liberty, in the Marsh division of the hundred of Calceworth, parts of Lindsey, county of Lincoln, 2¾ miles (W.) from Alford, containing 7 inhabitants. The living is a perpetual curacy, rated in the king's books at £4, endowed with £1200 royal bounty, and £200 parliamentary grant, and in the patronage of H. Horsfall, Esq. The church is dedicated to St. Leonard.

HAUGHAM, a parish in the Wold division of the hundred of Louth-Eske, parts of Lindsey, county of Lincoln, 3¾ miles (S.) from Louth, containing 100 inhabitants. The living is a discharged vicarage, now sequestrated, in the archdeaconry and diocese of Lincoln, rated in the king's books at £8. 1. 8., and endowed with £400 royal bounty. The church, dedicated to All Saints, has fallen to ruins. Here was an Alien priory, a cell to the Benedictine abbey of St. Mary San Sever, in France, valued at the suppression at twelve marks per annum, and settled upon the Carthusian priory of St. Ann, near Coventry. An intermittent spring, probably connected with some subterraneous reservoir, flows from the side of a hill called Skirbeck, in this parish.

HAUGHLEY, a parish in the hundred of Stow, county of Suffolk, 2¾ miles (N. N. W.) from Stow-Market, containing 854 inhabitants. The living is a discharged vicarage, in the archdeaconry of Sudbury, and diocese of Norwich, rated in the king's books at £7. 9. 2. The Rev. E. Ward was patron in 1812. The church is dedicated to St. Mary.

HAUGHTON, a township in that part of the parish of Bunbury which is in the first division of the hundred of Eddisbury, county palatine of Chester, 5 miles (N. W. by W.) from Nantwich, containing 175 inhabitants.

HAUGHTON, a township in the parish of Simonbourn, north-western division of Tindale ward, county of Northumberland, 6¼ miles (N. by W.) from Hexham, containing 127 inhabitants. Haughton castle is a strong, spacious structure, surmounted by five square turrets: it was formerly surrounded by walls, and there are yet the ruins of a chapel about three hundred yards from it. A paper-mill was built here in 1788, which is now in operation.

HAUGHTON, a parish in the western division of the hundred of Cuttlestone, county of Stafford, 4 miles (S. W. by W.) from Stafford, containing 473 inhabitants. The living is a rectory, in the archdeaconry of Stafford, and diocese of Lichfield and Coventry, rated in the king's books at £9. 11. 3., and in the patronage of James Royds, Esq. The church is dedicated to St. Giles.

HAUGHTON le SKERNE, a parish comprising the townships of Barmpton, Great Burdon, Haughton, and Whessoe, in the south-eastern division of Darlington ward, and the chapelry of Sadberge, and the township of Coatham-Mundeville, in the south-western division of Stockton ward, county palatine of Durham, and containing 1245 inhabitants, of which number, 466 are in the township of Haughton, 1¾ mile (N. E. by E.) from Darlington. The living is a rectory, in the archdeaconry and diocese of Durham, rated in the king's books at £53. 6. 8., and in the patronage of the Bishop of Durham. The church, dedicated to St. Andrew, presents several traces of early Norman architecture. There is a customary manor attached to the benefice, in the township of Haughton, but the ancient services are fallen into desuetude. Several of the inhabitants are employed in weaving coarse linen for the manufacturers at Darlington. A place of worship for Wesleyan Methodists was erected in 1825. A charity school was established by subscription about 1768, which has a small endowment of £7 per annum: in 1816 commodious school premises were erected, comprising separate rooms for boys and girls, and apartments for the master; the latter have since been enlarged into a dwelling-house: the school is chiefly supported by voluntary contributions.

HAUKSWELL, a parish in the western division of the wapentake of Hang, North riding of the county of York, comprising the townships of Barton, Garriston, East Haukswell, and West Haukswell, and containing 334 inhabitants, of which number, 176 are in the townships of East and West Haukswell, 5¼ miles (S.) from Richmond. The living is a rectory, in the archdeaconry of Richmond, and diocese of Chester, rated in the king's books at £20. 14. 4½., and in the patronage of Henry Gale, Esq. The church, dedicated to St. Oswald, stands at a distance from the village, and consists only of one aisle and a narrow choir. Six poor children are instructed for £3 annually, the gift of Mr. Gale.

HAULGH, a joint township with Tonge, in the parish of Bolton, hundred of Salford, county palatine of LANCASTER, 1 mile (E. S. E.) from Bolton le Moors, containing 1678 inhabitants.

HAULT-HUCKNALL, county of DERBY.—— See AULT-HUCKNALL.

HAUNTON, a township in the parish of CLIFTON-CAMPVILLE, northern division of the hundred of OFFLOW, county of STAFFORD, 4½ miles (N. N. E.) from Tamworth. The population is returned with the parish. This township is in the honour of Tutbury, duchy of Lancaster, and within the jurisdiction of a court of pleas held at Tutbury every third Tuesday, for the recovery of debts under 40s.

HAUTBOYS (GREAT), a parish in the southern division of the hundred of ERPINGHAM, county of NORFOLK, ¾ of a mile (N.W. by N.) from Coltishall, containing 102 inhabitants. The living is a discharged rectory, in the archdeaconry and diocese of Norwich, rated in the king's books at £4. 6. 8., and in the patronage of Sir J. W. Lubbock, Bart. The church is dedicated to St. Theobald. A maison Dieu, for a master and poor persons, was founded here about the reign of Henry III., by Sir Peter de Alto Bosco, Knt., and dedicated to the Virgin Mary; it was subordinate to the hospital at Horning.

HAUTBOYS (LITTLE), a parish in the southern division of the hundred of ERPINGHAM, county of NORFOLK, 2 miles (N. W. by N.) from Coltishall, containing, with the parish of Lammas, 284 inhabitants. The living is a discharged rectory with Lammas, in the archdeaconry and diocese of Norwich, rated in the king's books at £7. The Rev. P. Candler was patron in 1764. The church is dedicated to St. Mary.

HAUXLEY, a township in that part of the parish of WARKWORTH which is in the easternd ivision of MORPETH ward, county of NORTHUMBERLAND, 10½ miles (S.E.) from Alnwick, containing 114 inhabitants.

HAUXTON, a parish in the hundred of THRIPLOW, county of CAMBRIDGE, 4½ miles (S. by W.) from Cambridge, containing 236 inhabitants. The living is a discharged vicarage with that of Newton, in the archdeaconry and diocese of Ely, rated in the king's books at £6. 16., and in the patronage of the Dean and Chapter of Ely. The church, dedicated to St. Edmund, is principally in the Norman style.

HAVANT, a market town, parish, and liberty, in the Portsdown division of the county of SOUTHAMPTON, 21¼ miles (E. by S.) from Southampton, and 64 (S. W.) from London, containing 2099 inhabitants. The town, situated on the high road from Southampton and Fareham to Chichester, is neatly built, and consists principally of one long street, intersected by another at right angles : it is partially paved and well supplied with water, but not lighted. There are a subscription newsroom and a book club. The manufacture of parchment is carried on to some extent. The market, granted by King John, but now very inconsiderable, is held on Saturday ; and there are fairs on June 22nd and October 17th. This parish is within the jurisdiction of the Cheyney Court held at Winchester every Thursday, for the recovery of debts to any amount. The living is a rectory, in the peculiar jurisdiction of the incumbent, rated in the king's books at £24. 6. 0½., and in the patronage of the Bishop of Winchester. The church, dedicated to St. Faith, and standing in the centre of the town, is a cruciform structure,

with a tower rising from the intersection : the architecture is of different periods; the chancel has a handsome groined ceiling, and at the east end a painted window has been recently put up, the gift of Sir John Staunton, Bart., of Leigh park, in this parish. The church has lately received an addition of one hundred and seventy free sittings, towards defraying the expense of which, the Incorporated Society for the enlargement of churches and chapels contributed £20. There are places of worship for Independents and Roman Catholics. A National school for about one hundred boys and seventy girls is supported by subscription: there is likewise a school on the Lancasterian system. About four years since a swing-bridge was erected, at an expense of nearly £12,000, across the channel which connects Langston harbour with that of Chichester, thus affording a communication with Hayling Island, which lies about a mile to the south of Havant. Vessels of two hundred tons' burden enter Langston harbour with coal, oysters, &c.

HAVENGORE-MARSH, an extra-parochial liberty, in the hundred of ROCHFORD, county of ESSEX, 7 miles (E. by S.) from Rochford, containing 23 inhabitants.

HAVENINGHAM, a parish in the hundred of BLYTHING, county of SUFFOLK, 5½ miles (S. W. by W.) from Halesworth, containing 411 inhabitants. The living is a discharged rectory, in the archdeaconry of Suffolk, and diocese of Norwich, rated in the king's books at £11. 6. 8., and in the patronage of the Crown. The church is dedicated to St. Margaret.

HAVERAH-PARK, an extra-parochial liberty, in the lower division of the wapentake of CLARO, West riding of the county of YORK, 8 miles (W.S.W.) from Knaresborough, containing 87 inhabitants. It is within the peculiar and exclusive ecclesiastical jurisdiction of the court of the honour of Knaresborough.

HAVERBRACK, a township in the parish of BEETHAM, KENDAL ward, county of WESTMORLAND, 2 miles (S.S.W.) from Milnthorpe, containing 127 inhabitants.

HAVERCROFT, a joint township with Cold Heindley, in the parish of FELKIRK, wapentake of STAINCROSS, West riding of the county of YORK, 6¼ miles (N. E. by N.) from Barnesley, containing 189 inhabitants.

HAVERHILL, a parish (formerly a market town), partly in the hundred of HINCKFORD, county of ESSEX, but chiefly in the hundred of RISBRIDGE, county of SUFFOLK, 28 miles (S. W.) from Bury-St. Edmund's, and 58½ (N.N.E.) from London, containing 1649 inhabitants. This place was formerly of greater extent than it is at present, and had a castle, of which the only memorial is preserved in the name of a farm now occupying the site; and tradition reports the existence of another church, of which there are at present no visible traces. The greater part of the town was destroyed by fire in 1665, from the effects of which, though it has recently experienced some improvements, it has not entirely recovered. The town is pleasantly situated in a valley, and consists of one spacious street, nearly a mile in length, of which the northern extremity is in Essex, and the southern in Suffolk: the houses are in general badly built, and of mean appearance; the inhabitants are amply supplied with water. The principal articles of manufacture are silk (for which two factories have been recently established), and fustian, which is made in private looms. The market, formerly on Wednesday, has been discontinued : the fairs are, May 12th, for cattle and toys, and October 10th, for toys only. Constables, ale-tasters, and other officers, are annually appointed at the court held for the manor. The living is a discharged vicarage, in the archdeaconry of Sudbury, and diocese of Norwich, rated in the king's books at £6. 5., and the patronage of Lady Beaumont. The church, dedi-cated to St. Mary, is a large ancient structure. There are places of worship for Baptists and Independents. A National school for boys, and another for girls, in each of which about sixty children are instructed, are supported by subscription.

HAVERHOLM-PRIORY, an extra-parochial liberty, in the wapentake of FLAXWELL, parts of KESTEVEN, county of LINCOLN, 4 miles (N. E.) from Sleaford. It consists of an island, formed by the river Slea, contain-ing about three hundred acres. Here was a priory of nuns and canons of the strict order of St. Gilbert of Sempringham, founded in 1139, and dedicated to the Virgin Mary, the revenue of which, at the disso-lution, was estimated at £88. 5. 5.

HAVERING atte BOWER, a parish in the liberty of HAVERING atte BOWER, county of ESSEX, 3 miles (N.) from Romford, containing 352 inhabitants. The living is a perpetual curacy, in the peculiar jurisdiction of the court for the liberty, endowed with £400 private bene-faction, and £600 royal bounty. John Heaton, Esq. was patron in 1784. The church is dedicated to St. John the Evangelist. A free school is endowed with £10 per annum, but the house is dilapidated, there being no trus-tees. This place was originally held in ancient demesne by the Saxon kings, and was the favourite residence of Edward the Confessor, who built a palace here, of which there are still some vestiges. The name is derived from a ring given to the Confessor by a pilgrim, according to a legendary tale, the particulars of which are recorded in basso relievo on a screen which separates the chapel of Edward from the altar in Westminster abbey. The liberty comprises also the parishes of Hornchurch and Romford.

HAVERINGLAND, a parish in the hundred of EYNSFORD, county of NORFOLK, 4¼ miles (S.E. by E.) from Reepham, containing 174 inhabitants. The living is a discharged vicarage, now sequestrated, in the archdeaconry of Norfolk, and diocese of Norwich, rated in the king's books at £4. 12. 1., and endowed with £400 royal bounty. The church was dedicated to St. Peter. Here was a chapel dedicated to St. Lawrence, founded by William Gisneto, and afterwards given to the con-vent of Wymondham, to which it became a cell for a prior and Black canons; at the dissolution it is supposed to have been given to Cardinal Wolsey.

HAVERSHAM, a parish in the hundred of NEW-PORT, county of BUCKINGHAM, 3½ miles (W. by S.) from Newport-Pagnell, containing 289 inhabitants. The liv-ing is a rectory, in the archdeaconry of Buckingham, and diocese of Lincoln, rated in the king's books at £15. — Kitelee, Esq. was patron in 1827. The church, dedicated to St. Mary, exhibits portions in the decorated style ; it contains a beautiful altar-tomb, with a recum-bent effigy under a rich canopy, supposed to be that of Elizabeth, Lady Clinton, heiress of the De la Planches, whose fourth husband was Sir John Clinton.

HAVERTHWAITE, a chapelry in the parish of COULTON, hundred of LONSDALE, north of the sands, county palatine of LANCASTER, 5 miles (N. E.) from Ulverstone. The population is returned with the parish. The chapel, recently erected, contains three hundred and forty sittings, of which two hundred are free, and towards defraying the expense of which the Incorporated Society for building and enlarging churches and chapels contributed £200.

HAW, a hamlet in the parish of TIRLEY, lower di-vision of the hundred of DEERHURST, county of GLOU-CESTER, 4 miles (S.W. by S.) from Tewkesbury. The population is returned with the parish.

HAWCOAT (above Town), a township in the parish of DALTON in FURNESS, hundred of LONSDALE, north of the sands, county palatine of LANCASTER, 2¼ miles (S.W. by W.) from Dalton, containing 710 inhabitants.

HAWERBY, a parish in the wapentake of BRAD-LEY-HAVERSTOE, parts of LINDSEY, county of LINCOLN, 10½ miles (N.N.W.) from Louth, containing, with the parish of Beesby, 55 inhabitants. The living is a dis-charged rectory with that of Beesby consolidated, in the archdeaconry and diocese of Lincoln, rated in the king's books at £5. 7. 11., endowed with £200 private benefaction, and £200 royal bounty. The church is dedicated to St. Margaret.

HAWES, a chapelry in the parish of BASSEN-THWAITE, ALLERDALE ward below Darwent, county of CUMBERLAND, 6½ miles (N. N. W.) from Keswick. The population is returned with the parish. The chapel was founded and endowed by the inhabitants in 1471.

HAWES, a market town and chapelry in the pa-rish of AYSGARTH, western division of the wapentake of HANG, North riding of the county of YORK, 17¼ miles (W.) from Middleham, and 251½ (N.W. by N.) from London, containing 1408 inhabitants. This place is pleasantly situated near a branch of the river Ure, and the houses, which are in general built of stone, display the appearance of neatness and respectability. Here is a well-selected subscription library. Hardraw Scarr, or Force, a magnificent cascade, falling perpendicularly one hundred and two feet, is at a short distance from the town. In the neighbourhood are lead mines, which are worked, but are not very productive. The principal articles of manufacture are those of knit hosiery, caps, &c., with some other kinds of woollen goods. A market is held on Tuesday; and there are fairs on Whit-Tuesday and the 28th of September ; besides cattle fairs every alternate Tuesday from the last Tuesday in February until Whitsuntide. The living is a perpetual curacy, in the archdeaconry of Richmond, and diocese of Chester, endowed with £400 royal bounty, and £400 parliament-ary grant, and in the patronage of the Land-owners. The chapel is a low plain edifice. Here are places of worship for the Society of Friends and Sandemanians. A charity school was founded in 1764, with an endow-ment of £10. 10. per annum : the school-room was built by subscription.

HAWICK, a township in the parish of KIRKHARLE, north-eastern division of TINDALE ward, county of NORTHUMBERLAND, 9½ miles (E.) from Bellingham, containing 22 inhabitants.

HAWKCHURCH, a parish comprising the tything of Wyldecourt, in the hundred of CERNE, TOTCOMBE, and MODBURY, Cerne sub-division, and the tything of

Phillyholme, in the hundred of UGGSCOMBE, Dorchester division, of the county of DORSET, 4¼ miles (E. N. E.) from Axminster, containing 856 inhabitants. The living is a rectory, in the archdeaconry of Dorset, and diocese of Bristol, rated in the king's books at £23. 2. 11., and in the patronage of — Newnham, Esq. The church, dedicated to St. John the Baptist, exhibits portions in the Norman style of architecture, with insertions in the early and later English styles, and various modern alterations. This parish is bounded on the north-west by the river Ax: on Lambert's Castle hill are some remains of an ancient fortification.

HAWKEDON, a parish in the hundred of RIS-BRIDGE, county of SUFFOLK, 6 miles (N. N. E.) from Clare, containing 329 inhabitants. The living is a rectory, in the archdeaconry of Sudbury, and diocese of Norwich, rated in the king's books at £7. 10. The Rev. William Gilly was patron in 1788.

HAWKESBURY, a parish in the upper division of the hundred of GRUMBALD'S ASH, county of GLOU-CESTER, comprising the tythings of Little Badminton, Hawkesbury, Hillcott, Hillesley, Saddlewood, Tresham, and Upton, and containing 1834 inhabitants, of which number, 389 are in the tything of Hawkesbury, 3¾ miles (E. S. E.) from Wickwar. The living is a discharged vicarage, in the archdeaconry and diocese of Gloucester, rated in the king's books at £20. 14. 2. The Earl of Liverpool was patron in 1813. The church, dedicated to St. Mary, has portions in the early and later English styles. Here is a small endowment of £6 per annum, being the interest of £100 bequeathed by Daniel Walker, in 1734, which is divided amongst the teachers of two or three small schools. Hawkesbury confers the title of baron on the family of Jenkinson.

HAWKESDALE, a township in the parish of DAL-STON, ward and county of CUMBERLAND, 6¼ miles (S. S. W.) from Carlisle, containing 336 inhabitants.

HAWKESHEAD, a parish in the hundred of LONS-DALE, north of the sands, county palatine of LANCAS-TER, comprising the market town of Hawkeshead, the chapelry of Satterthwaite, and the townships of Claife and Monk-Coniston with Skellwith, and containing 2014 inhabitants, of which number, 829 are in the town of Hawkeshead, 28 miles (N. N. W.) from Lancaster, and 268 (N. N. W.) from London. This place, the origin of which is not satisfactorily known, is in respect of importance, the fourth town in the district of Furness, and during the existence of the abbey of Furness it was governed by a bailiff appointed by the abbots, who dispensed justice, for the whole of that district, in a court-room over the gateway of a house inhabited by some of the monks who officiated in the church, and performed other parochial duties: of this house, which was a quadrangular building belonging to the abbots, there are still some remains in tolerable preservation. In the reign of Elizabeth the tenants of Hawkeshead, in conjunction with those of Colton, petitioned for the suppression of certain iron-works in High Furness, in order to preserve, for the nourishment and protection of their cattle during the winter, those woods and coppices in the neighbourhood which were cut down to supply the furnaces with fuel, and charged themselves with the payment to the queen of £20 per annum, for which the works had been let to the proprietors. In the reign of James I., the

inhabitants obtained the privilege of a market, granted by that monarch to Adam Sandys, of Graithwaite, Esq. The town is pleasantly situated at the head of Esthwaite-water, a smooth lake beautifully indented with richly-wooded promontories, luxuriant meadows, and corn fields, and nearly in the centre of a fertile vale, almost surrounded by the fells of Furness, and defended by those of Coniston from the north and north-west winds. The environs abound with pleasing and picturesque scenery, bordering on the lakes of Winandermere and Coniston to the east and west, and bounded on the north by the river Brathy, which separates the counties of Lancaster and Westmorland. The hills in the vicinity are rich in mineral produce, and extensive iron-works are carried on, affording employment to a considerable number of workmen; there are also very spacious quarries of slate, and some copper mines, the latter of which are not very productive. Several females in the town and parish were formerly employed in spinning yarn; but since the application of machinery to that purpose, the trade has declined, and the wool produced from the numerous flocks which are fed on the neighbouring hills, is sold in the fleece, to be used by distant manufacturers. The market is on Monday; and the fairs are on Easter Monday, the Monday before Ascension-day, Whit-Monday, and Oct. 2nd, chiefly for cattle and pedlary.

Hawkshead, formerly a chapelry to the vicarage of Dalton, was constituted a parish in the reign of Elizabeth, by Archbishop Sandys. The living is a perpetual curacy, in the archdeaconry of Richmond, and diocese of Chester, and in the patronage of the King, as Duke of Lancaster. The church, dedicated to St. Michael, and supposed to have been founded about the time of the Conquest, was repaired and modernised by Archbishop Sandys, in the reign of Elizabeth. The grammar school was founded in 1585, by the same archbishop, who endowed it with houses and lands producing about £150 per annum; it is free to all sons of parishioners, who pay a certain sum per quarter for writing and arithmetic, and open to sons of persons not residing in the parish on payment to the master of four guineas per annum and two guineas entrance: the management is vested in trustees, who appoint the master, subject to the approval of the Bishop of Chester. There is also a sum of about £60 per annum, arising from divers benefactions, which is appropriated to boarding and clothing a proportionate number. The Rev. Thomas Sandys, in 1717, bequeathed a collection of books for the use of the school; and in 1816 the Rev. William Wilson left £100, the interest of which is annually distributed in prizes to the scholars. The Rev. Dr. Wordsworth, Master of Trinity College, Cambridge, received the rudiments of his education in this school.

HAWKHILL, a joint township with Lesbury, in that part of the parish of LESBURY which is in the southern division of BAMBROUGH ward, county of NORTHUMBERLAND, 3 miles (E. by S.) from Alnwick, containing 576 inhabitants.

HAWKHURST, a parish partly in the hundred of HENHURST, rape of HASTINGS, county of SUSSEX, but chiefly in the eastern division of the hundred of BARN-FIELD, lathe of SCRAY, county of KENT, 5 miles (S. S. W.) from Cranbrooke, containing 2250 inhabitants. The living, formerly a vicarage rated in the king's books at

£12. 10., is now a perpetual curacy, in the archdeaconry and diocese of Canterbury, endowed with £1000 private benefaction, £400 royal bounty, and £1100 parliamentary grant, and in the patronage of the Dean and Canons of Christ Church, Oxford. The church, dedicated to St. Lawrence, is a spacious edifice in the early style of English architecture, with portions in the decorated style. In 1718, Sir Thomas Dunk bequeathed land for the site, and £2000 for the erection and endowment, of a school and six almshouses, the former for the instruction of twenty poor boys in reading, writing, and arithmetic, with accommodation for the master, the latter for six inmates : this endowment was subsequently augmented by William Richards : the net annual income of the school is £216. 6. 10. ; thirty boys are instructed, and the stipend of the master is £62 per annum : the surplus of the income is appropriated to the maintenance of the pensioners, and for repairs. A fair is held on August 10th for cattle and pedlary. An estate called Fowlers was the residence of Richard Kilburne, an eminent lawyer and magistrate, and author of the Survey of Kent, in 1659.

HAWKINGE, a parish in the hundred of Folkestone, lathe of Shepway, county of Kent, 2½ miles (N.) from Folkestone, containing 132 inhabitants. The living is a discharged rectory, in the archdeaconry and diocese of Canterbury, rated in the king's books at £7. 7. 10., endowed with £400 private benefaction, and £400 royal bounty, and in the patronage of the Archbishop of Canterbury. The church is dedicated to St. Michael.

HAWKLEY, a parish in the hundred of Selborne, Alton (North) division of the county of Southampton, 3¾ miles (N.) from Petersfield, containing 253 inhabitants. The living is a perpetual curacy, annexed to the vicarage of Newton-Vallence, in the archdeaconry and diocese of Winchester. The church is dedicated to St. Peter and St. Paul. There is a place of worship for Independents.

HAWKRIDGE, a parish in the hundred of Williton and Freemanners, county of Somerset, 4¼ miles (W. N. W.) from Dulverton, containing 50 inhabitants. The living is a rectory, in the archdeaconry of Taunton, and diocese of Bath and Wells, rated in the king's books at £13. 8. 4. Miss Wood was patroness in 1801. The church is dedicated to St. Giles. Castle bridge, so named from its vicinity to an ancient fortress called Monceaux castle, crosses a stream which separates this parish from Dulverton : near it is an old encampment called Hawkridge Castle.

HAWKSWITH, a township in that part of the parish of Arncliffe which is in the western division of the wapentake of Staincliffe and Ewcross, West riding of the county of York, 12¼ miles (N. E. by E.) from Settle, containing 86 inhabitants.

HAWKSWORTH, a parish in the northern division of the wapentake of Bingham, county of Nottingham, 8 miles (S. W. by S.) from Newark, containing 215 inhabitants. The living is a rectory, in the archdeaconry of Nottingham, and diocese of York, rated in the king's books at £8. 13. 9. John Storer, M.D., was patron in 1808. The church, which is dedicated to St. Mary and All Saints, is a neat edifice, having the dedication stone preserved over the west door, bearing a Latin inscription in Saxon characters. This parish is in the honour of Tutbury, duchy of Lancaster, and within the juris-

diction of a court of pleas held at Tutbury every third Tuesday, for the recovery of debts under 40s.

HAWKSWORTH, a township in that part of the parish of Otley which is in the upper division of the wapentake of Skyrack, West riding of the county of York, 3½ miles (S. W.) from Otley, containing 323 inhabitants.

HAWKWELL, a parish in the hundred of Rochford, county of Essex, 1¾ mile (N. W.) from Rochford, containing 362 inhabitants. The living is a rectory, in the archdeaconry of Essex, and diocese of London, rated in the king's books at £13. 6. 8. — Bristow, Esq. was patron in 1791. The church is dedicated to St. Mary.

HAWKWELL, a township in the parish of Stamfordham, north-eastern division of Tindale ward, county of Northumberland, 12 miles (N. W. by W.) from Newcastle upon Tyne, containing 136 inhabitants.

HAWLEY, a tything in the parish of Yately, hundred of Crondall, Basingstoke division of the county of Southampton, 5 miles (E. by N.) from Hartford-Bridge, containing 661 inhabitants.

HAWLING, a parish in the lower division of the hundred of Kiftsgate, county of Gloucester, 4½ miles (S. E. by S.) from Winchcombe, containing, with the hamlet of Rowell, 227 inhabitants. The living is a discharged rectory, in the archdeaconry and diocese of Gloucester, rated in the king's books at £10. 3. 8½. W. Wyndham, Esq. was patron in 1808. The church is dedicated to St. Edward.

HAWNBY, a parish in the wapentake of Birdforth, North riding of the county of York, comprising the townships of Arden with Ardenside, Bilsdale-Westside, Dale-Town, and Hawnby, and containing 620 inhabitants, of which number, 286 are in the township of Hawnby, 6¼ miles (N.W.) from Helmsley. The living is a discharged rectory, in the archdeaconry of Cleveland, and diocese of York, rated in the king's books at £7. 18. 6½. Lord George Cavendish was patron in 1823. The church is dedicated to All Saints. There is a place of worship for Wesleyan Methodists.

HAWORTH, a chapelry in the parish of Bradford, wapentake of Morley, West riding of the county of York, 4 miles (S.W.) from Keighley, containing 4668 inhabitants. This chapelry is situated in a district abounding with manufactories for cloth and worsted. Fairs are held, July 22nd and October 14th. There are places of worship for Baptists and Wesleyan Methodists.

HAWRIDGE, a parish in the hundred of Cottesloe, county of Buckingham, 3 miles (N. by W.) from Chesham, containing 208 inhabitants. The living is a discharged rectory, in the archdeaconry of Buckingham, and diocese of Lincoln, rated in the king's books at £8. 10. 5. —— Sandby, Esq. was patron in 1813. The church is dedicated to St. Mary.

HAWSKER, a joint township with Stainsiker, in the parish of Whitby, liberty of Whitby - Strand, North riding of the county of York, 3 miles (S. E.) from Whitby, containing 634 inhabitants.

HAWSTEAD, a parish in the hundred of Thingoe, county of Suffolk, 4 miles (S.) from Bury-St. Edmund's, containing, with the extra-parochial liberty of Hardwick, 404 inhabitants. The living is a rectory, in the archdeaconry of Sudbury, and diocese of Norwich, rated in the king's books at £11. 16. 10½., and in the patronage of Mrs. Gosling. The church is dedicated to All Saints. At Hawstead Place, now a farm-house, Queen Elizabeth was entertained in one of her progresses.

HAWTHORN, a township in the parish of EASINGTON, southern division of EASINGTON ward, county palatine of DURHAM, 10½ miles (E. by N.) from Durham, containing 140 inhabitants. The village is situated about one mile from the German ocean, on a dangerous rocky shore, broken into deep caverns. A small stream runs through the glen, and forms, at its junction with the ocean, a creek, on the southern side of which is an, eminence called Beacon Hill, where fires were formerly lighted to warn mariners from the rocks. On the northern side of the creek is a bay, called Hawthorn Hive, formed by a projecting rock, termed the Skaw, and capable of being converted into a secure harbour. On the 5th of November, 1824, nearly fifty vessels were wrecked within a short distance of the Hive, and the crews of all, except one, perished. A school for eight children was endowed, in 1738, by Robert Forster, of this place ; the number has been increased to twelve : the master's fixed salary is £12. 12. per annum, and he has a rent-free residence.

HAWTHORP, a chapelry in the parish of IRNHAM, wapentake of BELTISLOE, parts of KESTEVEN, county of LINCOLN, 4½ miles (N. E. by E.) from Corby, containing 58 inhabitants.

HAWTON, a parish in the southern division of the wapentake of NEWARK, county of NOTTINGHAM, 2 miles (S. by W.) from Newark, containing 216 inhabitants. The living is a rectory, in the archdeaconry of Nottingham, and diocese of York, rated in the king's books at £17. 13. 4., and in the patronage of the Duke of Portland. The church, dedicated to All Saints, has portions in the early style of English architecture, with decorated and later insertions ; the tower is lofty, with rich tracery in the later English style : the chancel is wholly in the decorated style ; on the south side are three stone stalls, and on the north a lofty arch, having deep and rich mouldings, fine tracery, and crockets ; beneath is the effigy of a knight in armour.

HAXBY, a parish within the liberty of ST. PETER of YORK, East riding, though locally in the wapentake of Bulmer, North riding, of the county of YORK, 4¾ miles (N.) from York, containing 417 inhabitants. The living is a perpetual curacy, within the peculiar jurisdiction and patronage of the Prebendary of Strensall in the Cathedral Church of York. There is a place of worship for Wesleyan Methodists.

HAXEY, a parish in the western division of the wapentake of MANLEY, parts of LINDSEY, county of LINCOLN, 8 miles (N.N.W.) from Gainsborough, containing 1888 inhabitants. The living is a vicarage, in the archdeaconry of Stow, and diocese of Lincoln, rated in the king's books at £20. 17. 8½., and in the patronage of the Archbishop of York. The church, dedicated to St. Nicholas, is in the later style of English architecture, with a chancel of brick ; on the north side of the nave is a chapel, separated from the aisle by a handsome carved oak screen. There is a place of worship for Wesleyan Methodists.

HAYDOCK, a township in the parish of WINWICK, hundred of WEST-DERBY, county palatine of LANCASTER, 2¾ miles (W.N.W.) from Newton in Mackerfield, containing 916 inhabitants.

HAYDON, a parish in the hundred of SHERBORNE, Sherborne division of the county of DORSET, 3 miles (E. S. E.) from Sherborne, containing 109 inhabitants. The living is a discharged vicarage, in the peculiar jurisdiction of the Dean of Sarum, rated in the king's books at £5. Earl Digby was patron in 1810. The church is dedicated to St. Catherine.

HAYDON, a parish in the hundred of UTTLESFORD, county of ESSEX, 7½ miles (W. by N.) from Saffron-Walden, containing 272 inhabitants. The living is a rectory with that of Little Chishall united, in the jurisdiction of the Commissary of Essex and Herts, concurrently with the Consistorial Court of the Bishop of London, rated in the king's books at £18. The church is dedicated to St. Peter. Here is a small endowment of about £5 per annum for a school.

HAYDON, a chapelry in the parish of WARDEN, north-western division of TINDALE ward, county of NORTHUMBERLAND, 6 miles (W.) from Hexham, containing 358 inhabitants. The village of Haydon-Bridge, situated on both sides of the South Tyne river, is in this chapelry. The chapel was built in 1797, and is dedicated to St. Cuthbert. There is a place of worship for Independents and Wesleyan Methodists. Edward III., in 1344, granted permission to Anthony, Lord Lucy, then owner of the manor, to hold a weekly market here on Tuesday, and an annual fair on St. Mary Magdalene's day, and the three following days, both which have fallen into disuse. The Commissioners of Greenwich Hospital are at present proprietors of a considerable part of the chapelry, and have recently erected a small building, with suitable offices, for the receiver of their revenues. A free school and twenty almshouses were founded and endowed by the Rev. John Shaftoe, in 1685, and school-rooms, dwellings for the masters, and apartments for twenty almspeople born in the chapelry, were erected ; each of the pensioners receives two shillings and sixpence and a supply of coal weekly. The school is extensively endowed, and about one hundred and forty boys and ninety girls, resident in the chapelry of Haydon, or in the constablewick of Wood-Shields, are educated : the salaries of the teachers are discretional with the trustees, but that of the senior master must be at least £250 ; the present stipends are £64 and £63 to the two ushers, and £30 to the mistress. The ruins of the old chapel are situated about a mile north of the bridge.

HAYDOR, a parish partly in the wapentake of As-WARDHURN, consisting of the chapelries of Culverthorpe and Kelby, but chiefly in the wapentake of WINNI-BRIGGS and THREO, parts of KESTEVEN, county of LINCOLN, 6½ miles (E. N. E.) from Grantham, containing 522 inhabitants. The living is a vicarage, in the peculiar jurisdiction and patronage of the Prebendary of Haydor in the Cathedral Church of Lincoln, rated in the king's books at £12. 6. 10½. The church, dedicated to St. Michael, has portions in the early, decorated, and later, styles of English architecture.

HAYES, a parish in the hundred of RUXLEY, lathe of SUTTON at HONE, county of KENT, 2 miles (S.) from Bromley, containing 429 inhabitants. The living is a discharged rectory, in the peculiar jurisdiction of the Archbishop of Canterbury, rated in the king's books at £6. 18., and in the patronage of the Rector of Orpington. The church, dedicated to St. Mary, contains the banners borne at the public funeral of the great Earl of Chatham. A school was endowed, in 1693, by Mrs. Elizabeth Lloyd, with a rent-charge of £3; the school-room was built, in 1791, by the rector: it is further supported by a small bequest from Mrs. Elizabeth Hameson, and by voluntary contributions. A small fair is held on Whit-Tuesday. Hayes-place, near the church, formerly a seat of the family of Scott, was rebuilt by the Earl of Chatham, and was the birthplace of his son, the Right Hon. William Pitt.

HAYES, a parish in the hundred of ELTHORNE, county of MIDDLESEX, 3½ miles (S. E.) from Uxbridge, containing 1530 inhabitants. The living comprises a rectory, which is a sinecure, and a vicarage, with the perpetual curacy of Norwood, in the peculiar jurisdiction of the Archbishop, rated jointly in the king's books at £60, and in the patronage of T. and J. Graham, Esqrs. The church, dedicated to St. Mary, is an ancient edifice, with a low square tower, in the early style of English architecture, with some small Norman portions; the font is unique in form, and sculptured; the altar-piece is a painting of the Adoration of the Shepherds, and in the chancel windows are some armorial bearings in stained glass; the roof of the church is ornamented by carved representations in wood of the sponge and spear used at the Crucifixion. There is a place of worship for Independents. Near this place is the commencement of the Paddington canal.

HAYFIELD, a chapelry in the parish of GLOSSOP, hundred of HIGH PEAK, county of DERBY, 4½ miles (N. by W.) from Chapel en le Frith. The population is returned with the parish. The living is a perpetual curacy, in the archdeaconry of Derby, and diocese of Lichfield and Coventry, endowed with £600 private benefaction, £600 royal bounty, and £500 parliamentary grant, and in the patronage of certain Trustees. The chapel was rebuilt in 1420, at the expense of Robert de Kinder. There are places of worship for Independents at Chinley, and for Methodists at Hayfield, Chinley, and New Mills. The free school, held in the ancient grammar school-house, was endowed, in 1604, by John Hyde, with an annuity of £10; the income, with various augmentations, amounts to £20. 6. 2.; fifteen children are instructed. Eight children are likewise taught by a schoolmistress, for which purpose Mrs. Dorothy Hague bequeathed £16 per ann. Fairs are held on May 11th, for horses and cattle, and July 23rd for sheep and wool.

HAYLING (NORTH), a parish in the hundred of BOSMERE, Portsdown division of the county of SOUTHAMPTON, 2 miles (S. by E.) from Havant, containing 295 inhabitants. The living is a perpetual curacy, in the archdeaconry and diocese of Winchester. The Earl of Albemarle was patron in 1817. The church is dedicated to St. Peter. This parish, with that of South Hayling, constitutes Hayling island, which is bounded on the north and west by Langston harbour, on the east by Emsworth channel, and on the south by the English channel.

HAYLING (SOUTH), a parish in the hundred of BOSMERE, Portsdown division of the county of SOUTHAMPTON, 4½ miles (S.) from Havant, containing 443 inhabitants. The living is a discharged vicarage, in the archdeaconry and diocese of Winchester, rated in the king's books at £8. 10. The Earl of Albemarle was patron in 1817. The church is dedicated to St. Mary.

HAYNES, a parish in the hundred of FLITT, county of BEDFORD, 4 miles (N. E.) from Ampthill, containing 775 inhabitants. The living is a vicarage, in the archdeaconry of Bedford, and diocese of Lincoln, rated in the king's books at £8, and in the patronage of Lord Carteret. The church is dedicated to St. Mary. A Sunday school is endowed with 50s. per annum, the gift of Villiers Fowler in 1708, for the instruction of poor children.

HAYTON, a joint township with Melay, in the parish of ASPATRIA, ALLERDALE ward below Darwent, county of CUMBERLAND, 7 miles (N. by W.) from Cockermouth, containing, with Melay, 241 inhabitants.

HAYTON, a parish in ESKDALE ward, county of CUMBERLAND, comprising the townships of Faugh with Fenton, Hayton, and Talkin, and containing 1102 inhabitants, of which number, 491 are in the township of Hayton, 8 miles (E. by N.) from Carlisle. The living is a perpetual curacy, in the archdeaconry and diocese of Carlisle, endowed with £400 private benefaction, £400 royal bounty, and £1000 parliamentary grant, and in the patronage of the Dean and Chapter of Carlisle. The church, dedicated to St. Mary Magdalene, was rebuilt by subscription in 1780. There are coal mines on Talkin Fells. The rivers which flow through this parish are, the Gelt, the Irthing, and the Carn; there is a lake one mile in circumference, called Talkin tarn. At Talkin is a school endowed, in 1798, by John Nulbourne, with seven or eight acres of land, which produce an income of £9 per annum.

HAYTON, a parish in that part of the liberty of SOUTHWELL and SCROOBY which nearly separates the North-clay from the Hatfield division of the wapentake of BASSETLAW, county of NOTTINGHAM, 3 miles (N. E. by N.) from East Retford, containing 244 inhabitants. The living is a discharged vicarage, in the archdeaconry of Nottingham, and diocese of York, rated in the king's books at £4. 15. 5., endowed with £200 royal bounty, and in the patronage of the Archbishop of York. The church is dedicated to St. Peter. The Chesterfield canal passes through the parish.

HAYTON, a parish in the Holme-Beacon division of the wapentake of HARTHILL, East riding of the county of YORK, comprising the chapelry of Beilby, and the township of Hayton, and containing 416 inhabitants, of which number, 177 are in the township of Hayton, 2 miles (S. E. by S.) from Pocklington. The living is a discharged vicarage, rated in the king's books at £7. 11. 0½., endowed with £200 private benefaction, and £200 royal bounty, and in the peculiar jurisdiction and patronage of the Dean of York. The church is dedicated to St. Martin.

HAYWOOD FOREST, an extra-parochial liberty, partly in the hundred of WEBTREE, and partly in the upper division of the hundred of WORMELOW, county of HEREFORD, 2½ miles (S. S. W.) from Hereford, containing 138 inhabitants.

HAZELEIGH, a parish in the hundred of DENGIE, county of ESSEX, 2¾ miles (S. S. W.) from Maldon, containing 128 inhabitants. The living is a discharged rectory, in the archdeaconry of Essex, and diocese of London, rated in the king's books at £4. 13. 4. Mrs. Irwin was patroness in 1804. The church is dedicated to St. Nicholas.

HAZELY HEATH, a tything partly in the parish

of HARTLEY-WINTNEY, hundred of ODIHAM, but chiefly in the parish of HECKFIELD, hundred of HOLDSHOTT, Basingstoke division of the county of SOUTHAMPTON, 2 miles (W.) from Hartford-Bridge. The population is returned with the chapelry of Mattingley.

HAZLEBADGE, a liberty in the parish of HOPE, hundred of HIGH PEAK, county of DERBY, 5½ miles (N.W. by W.) from Stoney-Middleton, containing 51 inhabitants.

HAZLETON, a parish in the hundred of BRADLEY, county of GLOUCESTER, 4 miles (N.W. by N.) from North Leach, containing, with the chapelry of Yanworth, 265 inhabitants. The living is a rectory, in the archdeaconry and diocese of Gloucester, rated in the king's books at £19. 5. 5., and in the patronage of the Crown. The church is dedicated to St. Andrew.

HAZLEWOOD, a township in the parish of DUFFIELD, hundred of APPLETREE, county of DERBY, 6 miles (N.) from Derby, containing 483 inhabitants. There is a place of worship for Wesleyan Methodists.

HAZLEWOOD, a joint township with Stutton, in that part of the parish of TADCASTER which is in the upper division of the wapentake of BARKSTONE-ASH, West riding of the county of YORK, 3¾ miles (S.W. by S.) from Tadcaster, containing 256 inhabitants.

HAZLEWOOD, a joint township with Storiths, in that part of the parish of SKIPTON which is in the upper division of the wapentake of CLARO, West riding of the county of YORK, 7 miles (E. by N.) from Skipton, containing 209 inhabitants.

HAZON, a township in the parish of SHILBOTTLE, eastern division of COQUETDALE ward, county of NORTHUMBERLAND, 7½ miles (S. by E.) from Alnwick, containing 99 inhabitants.

HEACHAM, a parish in the hundred of SMITHDON, county of NORFOLK, 9 miles (N. by E.) from Castle-Rising, containing 710 inhabitants. The living is a discharged vicarage, in the archdeaconry of Norfolk, and diocese of Norwich, rated in the king's books at £6. 13. 4., and endowed with £200 royal bounty. H. Spelman, Esq. was patron in 1812. The church is dedicated to St. Mary. Here was formerly a cell of Cluniac monks, subordinate to the monastery of Lewes.

HEADBOURN-WORTHY, county of SOUTHAMPTON. — See WORTHY (HEADBOURN).

HEADCORN, a parish in the hundred of EYHORNE, lathe of AYLESFORD, county of KENT, 8½ miles (S.E. by S.) from Maidstone, containing 1191 inhabitants. The living is a discharged vicarage, in the archdeaconry and diocese of Canterbury, rated in the king's books at £15. 13. 4., and in the patronage of the Archbishop of Canterbury. The church, which is dedicated to St. Peter and St. Paul, is principally in the later style of English architecture. There is a place of worship for Wesleyan Methodists. A fair is held on the 12th of June. Headcorn is a decayed market town, situated on a branch of the river Medway.

HEADINGLEY, a joint chapelry with Burley, in the parish of ST. PETER, within the liberty of the town of LEEDS, though locally in the wapentake of Skyrack, West riding of the county of YORK, 2½ miles (N.W.) from Leeds, containing 2154 inhabitants. The living is a perpetual curacy, in the archdeaconry and diocese of York, endowed with £600 private benefaction, and £400 royal bounty, and in the patronage of the Vicar

of Leeds. The chapel is dedicated to St. Michael. An allotment of waste land yields the sum of £6. 5. per annum, which is paid to a schoolmaster for the instruction of a few poor children.

HEADINGTON, a parish in the hundred of BULLINGTON, county of OXFORD, 1½ mile (E.N.E.) from Oxford, containing 1087 inhabitants. The living is a vicarage not in charge, in the archdeaconry and diocese of Oxford, endowed with £400 royal bounty, and in the patronage of the Rev. T. H. Whorwood. The church is dedicated to St. Andrew. A school for children of both sexes is endowed with the interest of £400, the gift of Catherine Mather in 1805 : there is a spacious lunatic asylum. The colleges in Oxford, and other public buildings, have been principally erected with stone dug in Headington quarry: a great quantity of bricks is made here. A field, called Court Close is said to be the site of one of the palaces of King Etheldred.

HEADLAM, a township in that part of the parish of GAINFORD which is in the south-western division of DARLINGTON ward, county palatine of DURHAM, 8 miles (W.N.W.) from Darlington, containing 232 inhabitants.

HEADLEY, a parish, forming a detached portion of the hundred of BISHOP'S SUTTON, Alton (North) division of the county of SOUTHAMPTON, 6½ miles (S. by W.) from Farnham, containing 1093 inhabitants. The living is a rectory, in the archdeaconry and diocese of Winchester, rated in the king's books at £21. 4. 7., and in the patronage of the Provost and Fellows of Queen's College, Oxford. The church is dedicated to All Saints. A school-room was built about 1755, by the Rev. George Holmes, D.D., for the education of twelve children, and endowed by him with a rent-charge on certain lands.

HEADLEY, a parish in the second division of the hundred of COPTHORNE, county of SURREY, 2¾ miles (E.S.E.) from Leatherhead, containing 184 inhabitants. The living is a discharged rectory, in the archdeaconry of Surrey, and diocese of Winchester, rated in the king's books at £8. 7. 6. The Hon. G. Howard was patron in 1819. The church is dedicated to St. Mary.

HEADON, a parish in the South-clay division of the wapentake of BASSETLAW, county of NOTTINGHAM, 4 miles (S.E.) from East Retford, containing, with the hamlet of Upton, 241 inhabitants. The living comprises a rectory and a discharged vicarage, in the archdeaconry of Nottingham, and diocese of York, rated jointly in the king's books at £15. 15. 10., endowed with £200 private benefaction, £200 royal bounty, and £200 parliamentary grant, and in the patronage of A. Eyre, Esq. The church is dedicated to St. Peter.

HEADWORTH, a township in the parish of JARROW, eastern division of CHESTER ward, county palatine of DURHAM, 6 miles (N. W.) from Sunderland. The population is returned with the township of Monkton cum Jarrow.

HEAGE, a chapelry in the parish of DUFFIELD, hundred of APPLETREE, county of DERBY, 5 miles (S.W.) from Alfreton, containing 1742 inhabitants. The living is a perpetual curacy, in the archdeaconry of Derby, and diocese of Lichfield and Coventry, endowed with £1000 royal bounty, and £1000 parliamentary grant, and in the patronage of the Vicar of Duffield. The church contains three hundred and sixty-two free

2 Y 2

sittings, for which purpose the Incorporated Society for the enlargement of churches and chapels, contributed £300. There are places of worship for Baptists, Independents, and Primitive and Wesleyan Methodists. A school was founded, in 1705, by George Storer, in which about thirty children are instructed: the school-room was rebuilt about 1810. Iron-stone has been worked here from a very early period; charcoal was anciently used in the smelting and manufacturing of it, and the neighbourhood abounds with charcoal hearths, but coal is now found in abundance. Headge is partly bounded by the rivers Derwent and Amber.

HEALAUGH, a parish in the ainsty of the city, and East riding of the county, of York, 3¼ miles (N. by E.) from Tadcaster, containing 191 inhabitants. The living is a discharged vicarage, in the archdeaconry and diocese of York, rated in the king's books at £6, endowed with £200 private benefaction, and £800 royal bounty. — Brooksbank, Esq. was patron in 1814. The church is dedicated to St. John the Evangelist. About the year 1218 a convent of Regular canons was established here, which at the dissolution was valued at £86. 5. 9.

HEALY, a joint township with Combe-Hill, in the parish of Netherwitton, western division of Morpeth ward, county of Northumberland, 10 miles (W. N. W.) from Morpeth, containing 43 inhabitants.

HEALEY, a joint township with Sutton, in the parish of Masham, eastern division of the wapentake of Hang, North riding of the county of York, 7¾ miles (S.E. by S.) from Middleham, containing 413 inhabitants.

HEALING, a parish in the wapentake of Bradley-Haverstoe, parts of Lindsey, county of Lincoln, 5½ miles (W.) from Great Grimsby, containing 94 inhabitants. The living is a discharged rectory, in the archdeaconry and diocese of Lincoln, rated in the king's books at £6. 4. 2. The Rev. R. Parkinson was patron in 1793. The church is dedicated to St. Peter and St. Paul. The name of this place is supposed to be derived from the healing or medicinal properties of two mineral springs, the water of which is impregnated with iron and sulphur; notwithstanding their propinquity, being only about a yard apart, their properties are different, one being used for bathing, and the other internally, in cutaneous diseases.

HEALLY, a township in the parish of Bywell-St. Peter, eastern division of Tindale ward, county of Northumberland, 7¾ miles (S. E.) from Hexham, containing 49 inhabitants.

HEANOR, a parish in the hundred of Morleston and Litchurch, county of Derby, comprising the town of Heanor (formerly a market town), and the townships of Codnor with Loscow, and Shipley, and containing, with the liberty of Codnor castle and park, which is extra-parochial, 4981 inhabitants, of which number, 2364 are in the town of Heanor, 9 miles (N. E.) from Derby. This town is pleasantly situated on an eminence on the road from London to Matlock, and in the neighbourhood are several collieries and some extensive ironworks, affording employment to a considerable portion of the inhabitants. A navigable part of the Erewash river, being a continuation of the Erewash canal, passes along the eastern boundary of this parish. It is crossed

by Langley bridge, on the Derby and Mansfield road, near which a railway branches off and extends to the coal pits south of the town. The principal branches of manufacture are cotton goods, hosiery, and bobbin net-lace, in the making of which last several females are employed. The market, formerly on Wednesday, has been discontinued; an attempt was made to revive it some few years since, but without effect. The living is a discharged vicarage, in the archdeaconry of Derby, and diocese of Lichfield and Coventry, rated in the king's books at £9. 10., endowed with £200 private benefaction, £400 royal bounty, and £1800 parliamentary grant, and in the patronage of the Crown. The church is dedicated to St. Michael. There are places of worship for Independents and Wesleyan Methodists. Among the charitable bequests is one of £5 per annum for the instruction of poor children; and this parish has the privilege of sending eight boys to the school at Smalley, in the parish of Morley, founded by John and Samuel Richardson, Esqrs. The ruins of the ancient castle of Codnor, founded by Richard de Grey in the reign of Henry III., may here be traced over a considerable extent of ground, and some of the walls are still standing.

HEANTON-PUNCHARDEN, a parish in the hundred of Braunton, county of Devon, 4½ miles (W.N.W.) from Barnstaple, containing 485 inhabitants. The living is a rectory, in the archdeaconry of Barnstaple, and diocese of Exeter, rated in the king's books at £22. 7. 11., and in the patronage of — Bassett, Esq. The church, dedicated to St. Augustine, contains a handsome monument bearing the arms of the Coffin family; it has also a wooden screen. The navigable river Tor runs on the south of this parish.

HEAP, a chapelry in that part of the parish of Bury which is in the hundred of Salford, county palatine of Lancaster, 3 miles (E.) from Bury, containing 6552 inhabitants. There is a place of worship for Independents and Wesleyan Methodists. A National school for five hundred boys, erected in 1815, is supported by subscription. The spinning and manufacture of cotton is carried on to a considerable extent in the chapelry.

HEAPEY, a chapelry in the parish and hundred of Leyland, county palatine of Lancaster, 2¼ miles (N. N. E.) from Chorley, containing 530 inhabitants. The living is a perpetual curacy, in the archdeaconry and diocese of Chester, endowed with £400 private benefaction, £400 royal bounty, and £600 parliamentary grant, and in the patronage of the Vicar of Leyland.

HEAPHAM, a parish in the wapentake of Corringham, parts of Lindsey, county of Lincoln, 5 miles (E. S. E.) from Gainsborough, containing 112 inhabitants. The living is a discharged rectory, in the archdeaconry of Stow, and diocese of Lincoln, rated in the king's books at £10. Charles Chaplin, Esq. was patron in 1822. The church is dedicated to All Saints.

HEATH, a joint chapelry with Reach, in the parish of Leighton-Buzzard, hundred of Manshead, county of Bedford, 2 miles (N. by E.) from Leighton-Buzzard, containing 726 inhabitants. It is within the peculiar ecclesiastical jurisdiction of the Prebendary of Leighton-Buzzard in the Cathedral Church of Lincoln. The church, dedicated to St. Leonard, has recently received an addition of sixty sittings, of which forty are free, the Incorporated Society for the enlargement of churches and chapels having contributed £100 towards defraying the expense. There is a place of worship for Wesleyan Methodists.

HEATH, a parish in the hundred of SCARSDALE, county of DERBY, 5¼ miles (S. E. by E.) from Chesterfield, containing 411 inhabitants. The living is a vicarage, in the archdeaconry of Derby, and diocese of Lichfield and Coventry, rated in the king's books at £4. 18. 9., and in the patronage of the Duke of Devonshire. The church, dedicated to All Saints, has portions in the Norman style of architecture.

HEATH, a joint township with Jay, in the parish of LEINTWARDINE, hundred of WIGMORE, county of HEREFORD, containing 42 inhabitants.

HEATH, or HETHE, a parish in the hundred of PLOUGHLEY, county of OXFORD, 4 miles (N. by E.) from Bicester, containing 350 inhabitants. The living is a rectory, in the archdeaconry and diocese of Oxford, rated in the king's books at £7. 9. 4½., and in the patronage of the Crown. The church is dedicated to St. George and St. Edmund. There is a place of worship for Wesleyan Methodists.

HEATH, a chapelry in that part of the parish of STOKE-ST. MILBOROUGH which is in the hundred of MUNSLOW, county of SALOP, 9 miles (N. E. by N.) from Ludlow, containing 41 inhabitants.

HEATH, a joint township with Warmfield, in the parish of WARMFIELD, lower division of the wapentake of AGBRIGG, West riding of the county of YORK, 2 miles (E. by S.) from Wakefield. The population is returned with the township of Warmfield.

HEATH (UPPER), a township in the parish of WORTHEN, hundred of CHIRBURY, county of SALOP, containing 504 inhabitants.

HEATHENCOTE, a hamlet in the parish of PAULERS-PURY, hundred of CLELEY, county of NORTHAMPTON, 1¼ mile (S. E.) from Towcester. The population is returned with the parish. Here was formerly a chapel, dedicated to the Blessed Virgin, but it has fallen into ruins.

HEATHER, a parish in the hundred of SPARKENHOE, county of LEICESTER, 5½ miles (N. by W.) from Market-Bosworth, containing 411 inhabitants. The living is a discharged rectory, in the archdeaconry of Leicester, and diocese of Lincoln, rated in the king's books at £7. 17. 8., and in the patronage of the Rev. Paul Belcher. The church is dedicated to St. John. There is a place of worship for Wesleyan Methodists. Here was anciently a preceptory of Knights Hospitallers, granted in the reign of Edward VI. to Oliver St. John and Robert Thornton : about the time of the dissolution the value was computed at £39. 1. 5. per annum. There is a coal mine in the parish.

HEATHERYCLEUGH, a chapelry in the parish of STANHOPE, north-western division of DARLINGTON ward, county palatine of DURHAM, 4 miles (W. N. W.) from St. John's Chapel. The population is returned with the parish.

HEATHFIELD, a parish in the hundred of TAUNTON and TAUNTON-DEAN, county of SOMERSET, 5¼ miles (W. N. W.) from Taunton, containing 131 inhabitants. The living is a rectory, in the archdeaconry of Taunton, and diocese of Bath and Wells, rated in the king's books at £9. 1. 8. — Cornish, Esq. was patron in

1787. The church is dedicated to St. John the Baptist.

HEATHFIELD, a parish in the hundred of HAWKESBOROUGH, rape of HASTINGS, county of SUSSEX, 8¼ miles (N. by E.) from Haylsham, containing 1613 inhabitants. The living is a vicarage, in the archdeaconry of Lewes, and diocese of Chichester, rated in the king's books at £10, and in the patronage of the Prebendary of Heathfield in the Cathedral Church of Chichester. The church, dedicated to All Saints, has recently received an addition of one hundred and twenty free sittings, towards defraying the expense of which the Incorporated Society for the enlargement of churches and chapels contributed £10 : it has portions in the early, with insertions in the decorated, style of English architecture. In a part of this village, called Cadestreet, Jack Cade, the notorious rebel, was slain, by the sheriff of Kent, in 1450; a stone pedestal, with a tablet and inscription, has been erected by Mr. Newbery, to record the event.

HEATHPOOL, a township in the parish of KIRKNEWTON, western division of GLENDALE ward, county of NORTHUMBERLAND, containing 42 inhabitants.

HEATHWAITE, a joint chapelry with Woodland, in the parish of KIRKBY-IRELETH, hundred of LONSDALE, north of the sands, county palatine of LANCASTER, 6 miles (S. W. by W.) from Hawkshead, containing 267 inhabitants.

HEATHY-LEE, a township in the parish of ALLSTONEFIELD, northern division of the hundred of TOTMONSLOW, county of STAFFORD, 2¾ miles (W. by N.) from Longnor, containing 788 inhabitants.

HEATON, a joint township with Oxcliffe, in that part of the parish of LANCASTER which is in the hundred of LONSDALE, south of the sands, county palatine of LANCASTER, 3 miles (W. by S.) from Lancaster, containing 176 inhabitants. This township is situated on the banks of the Lune.

HEATON, a township in the parish of DEAN, hundred of SALFORD, county palatine of LANCASTER, 2½ miles (W. by N.) from Great Bolton, containing 826 inhabitants.

HEATON, a township in that part of the parish of ALL SAINTS, NEWCASTLE, which is in the eastern division of CASTLE ward, county of NORTHUMBERLAND, 1¼ mile (N. E.) from Newcastle upon Tyne, containing 470 inhabitants.

HEATON, a township in that part of the parish of LEEK which is in the northern division of the hundred of TOTMONSLOW, county of STAFFORD, 5 miles (N. W. by N.) from Leek, containing 391 inhabitants.

HEATON, a chapelry in the parish of BRADFORD, wapentake of MORLEY, West riding of the county of YORK, 2 miles (N. W. by N.) from Bradford, containing 1217 inhabitants. Here is a place of worship for Wesleyan Methodists.

HEATON (GREAT), a township in the parish of OLDHAM cum PRESTWICH, hundred of SALFORD, county palatine of LANCASTER, 4½ miles (N. by W.) from Manchester, containing 224 inhabitants.

HEATON (KIRK), a parish in the upper division of the wapentake of AGBRIGG, West riding of the county of YORK, comprising the townships of Dalton, Kirk-Heaton, Lepton, and Upper Whitley, and containing 7968 inhabitants, of which number, 2186 are in the township of Kirk-Heaton, 2 miles (E. by N.) from Huddersfield. The living is a rectory, in the archdeaconry and diocese of York, rated in the king's books at £25. 13. 9. The Duke of Northumberland was patron in 1785. The church is dedicated to St. John the Baptist.

HEATON (LITTLE), a township in the parish of OLDHAM cum PRESTWICH, hundred of SALFORD, county palatine of LANCASTER, 5 miles (N.) from Manchester, containing 630 inhabitants.

HEATON-NORRIS, a chapelry in the parish of MANCHESTER, hundred of SALFORD, county palatine of LANCASTER, 2 miles (N. W. by N.) from Stockport, containing 6958 inhabitants. The living is a perpetual curacy, in the archdeaconry and diocese of Chester, endowed with £800 private benefaction, £400 royal bounty, and £1400 parliamentary grant, and in the patronage of the Warden and Fellows of the Collegiate Church of Manchester. The chapel is dedicated to St. Thomas. There is a place of worship for Independents. Two cottages were built by subscription for the purpose of a school; one is occupied by a schoolmaster, the other is let for £5. 5. per annum. Near the chapel is a building comprising a school-room, with apartments above for the master's residence: it is supposed to have been erected on the waste, about a century ago, by subscription among the inhabitants of the township, who appoint the master, and is endowed with £10 per annum, arising from a bequest of £200 by John Hollingpriest, in 1785. The petty sessions for the Manchester division of the hundred of Salford are held here. This place is separated from Stockport by the river Mersey. At Heaton-Mersey a Sunday school was endowed with £500, in 1815, by Robert Parker, Esq.

HEAVITREE, a parish in the hundred of WONFORD, county of DEVON, 1 mile (E.) from Exeter, containing 1253 inhabitants. The living is a vicarage, with the curacies of St. David and Seidwell, rated in the king's books at £34. 3. 4., and in the peculiar jurisdiction and patronage of the Dean and Chapter of Exeter. The church, dedicated to St. Michael, is in the later style of English architecture. This parish is a suburb of Exeter, including the villages of Whipton, Polsloe, Monkaton, and East and West Wonford. The name is said to have been derived from its having been a place of execution, the gallows being called "heavy (i. e. grievous) tree." It was the western head-quarters of the parliamentary forces during the civil war. At Polesloe was formerly a Benedictine monastery, founded by Lord Brewer, and dissolved in 1538, when its revenue was valued at £164. 8. 11.: some remains of it are yet visible. There was also a monastic cell, of the Cluniac order, dedicated to St. James, the estates of which were given to the Provost and Fellows of King's College, Cambridge, by Henry VI. Here is a small school, wherein sixteen children are educated for £5 per annum, paid out of the proceeds of parish lands. Dennis' almshouses, for twelve aged poor, are endowed with a rent-charge of £45 per annum: there is also an almshouse, founded in 1603 by R. Duck, consisting of four tenements. The river Ex bounds the parish on the south-west.

HEBBURN, a township in the parish of CHILLINGHAM, eastern division of GLENDALE ward, county of NORTHUMBERLAND, 6 miles (E. S. E.) from Wooler, containing 93 inhabitants.

HEBBURN, a parish in the western division of MOR-PETH ward, county of NORTHUMBERLAND, comprising the townships of Causey-Park, Cockle-Park, Earsdon, Earsdon-Forest, Fenrother, Hebburn, and Tritlington, and containing 564 inhabitants, of which number, 93 are in the township of Hebburn, 3 miles (N. by W.) from Morpeth. The living is a perpetual curacy, in the archdeaconry of Northumberland, and diocese of Durham, and in the patronage of the Rector of Bothall.

HEBDEN, a township in the parish of LINTON, eastern division of the wapentake of STAINCLIFFE and EWCROSS, West riding of the county of YORK, 11 miles (N. by E.) from Skipton, containing 377 inhabitants. There are places of worship for Baptists and Wesleyan Methodists.

HECK, or HICK, a township in that part of the parish of SNAITH which is in the lower division of the wapentake of OSGOLDCROSS, West riding of the county of YORK, 4 miles (W. by S.) from Snaith, containing 228 inhabitants. This township is within the peculiar ecclesiastical jurisdiction of the court of Snaith.

HECKFIELD, a parish in the hundred of HOLDSHOTT, Basingstoke division of the county of SOUTHAMPTON, comprising the chapelry of Mattingley, and the tythings of Heckfield, Holdshott, and the greater portion of Hazely Heath, and containing, with the whole of Hazely Heath, 1149 inhabitants, of which number, 636 are in the tything of Heckfield, 3¾ miles (N.W. by W.) from Hartford-Bridge. The living is a vicarage, in the archdeaconry and diocese of Winchester, rated in the king's books at £16. 12. 11., and in the patronage of the Warden and Fellows of New College, Oxford. The church is dedicated to St. Michael. A fair is held on Good Friday. The rivers Loddon and Blackwater skirt this parish on the north-west.

HECKINGHAM, a parish in the hundred of CLAVERING, county of NORFOLK, 6 miles (N. N. W.) from Beccles, containing 146 inhabitants, but including the House of Industry, and the Hospital of Loddon and Clavering, which are in this parish, 541. The living is a perpetual curacy, in the archdeaconry of Norfolk, and diocese of Norwich. Thomas Smyth, Esq. was patron in 1816. The church is dedicated to St. Gregory.

HECKINGTON, a parish in the wapentake of ASWARDHURN, parts of KESTEVEN, county of LINCOLN, 5 miles (E. by S.) from Sleaford, containing 1438 inhabitants. The living is a discharged vicarage, in the archdeaconry and diocese of Lincoln, rated in the king's books at £12. 16. 3., and in the patronage of the Rev. H. B. Benson. The church is dedicated to St. Andrew. Here is a place of worship for Baptists.

HECKMONDWIKE, a chapelry in the parish of BIRSTALL, wapentake of MORLEY, West riding of the county of YORK, 8¼ miles (W. N. W.) from Wakefield, containing 2579 inhabitants. A new chapel is now being erected. There are two places of worship for Independents, and one for Wesleyan Methodists. The manufacture of blankets, carpets, and woollen cloths is here extensive: a blanket hall is open every Monday and Thursday, for the sale of blankets.

HEDDINGTON, a parish in the hundred of CALNE, county of WILTS, 3 miles (S.) from Calne, containing 296 inhabitants. The living is a rectory, in the archdeaconry of Wilts, and diocese of Salisbury, rated in the king's books at £8. 14. 4½. The Rev. S. Rogers was patron in 1800. The church is dedicated to St. Andrew.

HEDDON (BLACK), a township in the parish of STAMFORDHAM, north-eastern division of TINDALE ward, county of NORTHUMBERLAND, 2¾ miles (N.) from Stamfordham, containing 63 inhabitants.

HEDDON (EAST), a township in that part of the parish of HEDDON on the WALL which is in the western division of CASTLE ward, county of NORTHUMBERLAND, 8 miles (N. W. by W.) from Newcastle upon Tyne, containing 44 inhabitants.

HEDDON (WEST), a township in that part of the parish of HEDDON on the WALL which is in the eastern division of TINDALE ward, county of NORTHUMBERLAND, 8½ miles (W. N. W.) from Newcastle upon Tyne, containing 38 inhabitants.

HEDDON on the WALL, a parish comprising the township of East Heddon and a part of Eachwick, in the western division of CASTLE ward, and the townships of Heddon on the Wall, West Heddon, Houghton with Clowhouse, Whitchester, and the other portion of Eachwick, in the eastern division of TINDALE ward, county of NORTHUMBERLAND, and containing 770 inhabitants, of which number, 362 are in the township of Heddon on the Wall, 7 miles (W. by N.) from Newcastle upon Tyne. The living is a discharged vicarage, in the archdeaconry of Northumberland, and diocese of Durham, and in the patronage of the Crown. The church is dedicated to St. Philip and St. James. This parish is bounded on the south by the river Tyne, and on the north by the Font. The Picts', or Roman, wall intersected the parish, from which circumstance it derives its distinguishing appellation; the fosse alone is now visible.

HEDENHAM, a parish in the hundred of LODDON, county of NORFOLK, 3¼ miles (N. N. W.) from Bungay, containing 283 inhabitants. The living is a discharged rectory, in the archdeaconry of Norfolk, and diocese of Norwich, rated in the king's books at £13. 6. 8. N. Chambers, Esq. was patron in 1812. The church is dedicated to St. Mary.

HEDGELEY, a township in the parish of EGLINGHAM, northern division of COQUETDALE ward, county of NORTHUMBERLAND, 9 miles (W. N. W.) from Alnwick, containing 36 inhabitants. On Hedgeley Moor, in 1463, a battle was fought between the forces of Edward IV. and a party in the service of the deposed monarch, Henry VI., in which Sir Ralph Percy was slain; in memory of whose bravery, a stone pillar, called Percy's Cross, was erected upon the spot, being situated a little to the north-east of the twenty-fourth mile-stone on the Morpeth and Wooler road.

HEDGERLEY, a parish in the hundred of STOKE, county of BUCKINGHAM, 3 miles (S. E. by E.) from Beaconsfield, containing 158 inhabitants. The living is a rectory, in the archdeaconry of Buckingham, and diocese of Lincoln, rated in the king's books at £6, and in the patronage of Colonel Way. The church is dedicated to St. Mary.

HEDGERLEY-DEAN, a hamlet in the parish of FARNHAM-ROYAL, hundred of BURNHAM, county of BUCKINGHAM, 3 miles (S. S. E.) from Beaconsfield, containing 199 inhabitants. Near this place are some large and deep intrenchments, where a battle is supposed to have been fought between the Danes and the Saxons.

HEDINGHAM (CASTLE), a parish in the hundred of HINCKFORD, county of ESSEX, 19 miles (N. by E.)

from Chelmsford, and 48 (N. E.) from London, containing 1163 inhabitants. This place was the head of an extensive barony belonging to the Norman family of De Vere, one of whom, Aubrey De Vere, Earl of Oxford, is supposed to have founded a castle here in the reign of Stephen. During the war between King John and the barons, this fortress was taken by the king, in 1216: in the following year it was surrendered to the Dauphin of France, who had been invited to England by the insurgent barons; and soon after the death of John it was recovered by the Earl of Pembroke, regent under Henry III. Many additional buildings were erected by John De Vere, Earl of Oxford, a distinguished partizan of the house of Lancaster, during the civil war in the fifteenth century, who gave a most sumptuous entertainment at Castle-Hedingham to Henry VII.: that king subsequently caused the earl to be prosecuted for giving liveries to a number of his retainers, in breach of the provisions of a statute then recently enacted, for which offence he was fined fifteen thousand marks. The succeeding earl sold the estate, having previously dismantled the castle and razed the surrounding edifices; but the keep, or great central tower, is still standing, and forms an object of considerable interest to antiquaries. Fairs are held at Hedingham, for hops and cattle, May 14th, July 25th, August 15th, and October 25th; and the petty sessions for the division of North Hinckford are held here on Tuesdays. The living is a perpetual curacy, in the archdeaconry of Middlesex, and diocese of London, and in the patronage of Lewis Majendie, Esq. The church, dedicated to St. Nicholas, is an ancient edifice in the early English style, with a mixture of the Norman, except the tower, which was erected about 1616: in the chancel is a superb monument to the memory of John, Earl of Oxford, mentioned above, and his Countess, with recumbent statues, armorial bearings, and inscriptions. Here is a place of worship for Independents. Some small bequests have been left by different persons for the benefit of the poor. At Nunnery-Street, near Hedingham, are the remains of a Benedictine convent for nuns, founded by the De Vere family, in the twelfth century, the revenue of which, at the dissolution, was £29. 12. 10. On the south-east side of the castle was an hospital, founded by one of the same family, about the middle of the thirteenth century, which has been long since destroyed.

HEDINGHAM (SIBLE), a parish in the hundred of HINCKFORD, county of ESSEX, ¾ of a mile (S.W.) from Castle-Hedingham, containing 2060 inhabitants. The living is a rectory, in the jurisdiction of the Commissary of Essex and Herts, concurrently with the Consistorial Court of the Bishop of London, rated in the king's books at £22. C. Stovin, Esq. was patron in 1792. The church is dedicated to St. Mary. There is a place of worship for Baptists.

HEDLEY, a township in that part of the parish of CHESTER le STREET which is in the middle division of CHESTER ward, county palatine of DURHAM, 6 miles (S. W. by S.) from Gateshead, containing 49 inhabitants.

HEDLEY, a township in the parish of OVINGHAM, eastern division of TINDALE ward, county of NORTHUMBERLAND, 3 miles (S.) from Ovingham, containing 168 inhabitants.

HEDLEY - HOPE, a township in the parish of BRANCEPETH, north-western division of DARLINGTON ward, county palatine of DURHAM, 6 miles (E. N. E.) from Wolsingham, containing 51 inhabitants.

HEDLEY-WOODSIDE, a township in the parish of OVINGHAM, eastern division of TINDALE ward, county of NORTHUMBERLAND, 4 miles (S.) from Ovingham, containing 55 inhabitants.

HEDNESFORD, a joint township with Leacroft, in the parish of CANNOCK, eastern division of the hundred of CUTTLESTONE, county of STAFFORD, 4 miles (S.W. by S.) from Rudgeley, containing 442 inhabitants. A great number of race horses is trained here.

HEDON, or HEYDON, a borough, market town, and parish, possessing separate jurisdiction, but locally in the middle division of the wapentake of Holderness, East riding of the county of YORK, 44 miles (E. S. E.) from York, and 179 (N. by E.) from London, containing 902 inhabitants. This town is reputed to have been anciently a very considerable sea-port. A charter was given to the burgesses of Hedon by King Athelstan; and in 1199, King John granted to Baldwin, Earl of Albemarle and Holderness, and to his wife Hawis, free burgage here, by the same tenure, and with the same privileges as at York and Lincoln. Hedon has possessed but little commercial or maritime importance since the foundation of the port of Hull by King Edward I. In the year 1656, a great part of the town was consumed by fire, after which it was rebuilt in a more handsome and substantial manner. It is pleasantly situated in a level, fertile, and well-cultivated country, within a mile and a half of the Humber, and consists chiefly of one street, in the middle of which is the market-place. The members of the Holderness Agricultural Society hold their meetings here, and possess a valuable and select library of the best works that have been written on agriculture, and on subjects connected with it. Assemblies are regularly held during the season. The old haven has long since been choked up, but a canal, cut from the Humber, extends to within a quarter of a mile of the town, only navigable however for small craft. The market is on Saturday; and the fairs, which are considerable, are on August 2nd and September 22nd, for horses, &c., November 17th and December 6th, for cattle, &c., and every second Monday from Shrovetide to Midsummer, for cattle and sheep.

The government of the borough, by charter dated in the 14th of James I., is vested in a mayor, recorder, two bailiffs, and nine aldermen, assisted by a town clerk, coroner, and other officers, with an indefinite number of burgesses: the mayor is annually elected from among the aldermen, and the bailiffs, who during their office are justices of the peace, from the burgesses; the late mayor acts as coroner. The freedom of the borough is inherited by birth, acquired by servitude, or obtained by gift from the corporation, who by their charter hold quarterly courts of session for offences not capital; and a court of record for the determination of pleas, and the recovery of debts to any amount: the court for the wapentake of Holderness is also held here, for the recovery of debts under 40s. The town-hall is a

Corporate Seal.

small edifice, in which one apartment is appropriated as a place of confinement for prisoners, the corporation being bound by their charter to provide a hall and prison within the town for the lords of the manor of Holderness; but no criminal or debtor has been confined there for many years. The borough first sent members to parliament in the 23d of Edward I., but discontinued till the 1st of Edward VI., since which time it has made regular returns. The right of election is vested in the burgesses generally, the number of whom is about three hundred: the mayor is the returning officer.

The living is a perpetual curacy annexed to the vicarage of Preston, endowed with £200 parliamentary grant, and in the peculiar jurisdiction and patronage of the Archbishop of York. There were formerly three churches in the town; of those of St. Nicholas and St. James only traces of the foundations are visible: the remaining church, dedicated to St. Augustine, is a venerable and spacious cruciform structure in the early, with a lofty central tower in the later, style of English architecture; the front of the north transept is a remarkably fine specimen of the early English, and in the south transept is a very beautiful window, though much mutilated; many portions of this edifice display much elegance of design, and richness of detail. There are places of worship for Baptists, Independents, and Wesleyan Methodists, and a Roman Catholic chapel. A school for boys, and another for girls, the children of burgesses, are supported by the contributions of the members for the borough, and by other donations. Almshouses for poor and infirm burgesses and their widows were erected, and are supported, by the corporation; and there are various charitable bequests for the relief of the poor. An hospital, dedicated to the Holy Sepulchre, was founded at Newton, in this parish, in the reign of John, by Alan, son of Oubernus, for a master and several brethren, the revenue of which, at the dissolution, was £13. 15. 10.

HEDSOR, a parish in the hundred of DESBOROUGH, county of BUCKINGHAM, 4¼ miles (E. by S.) from Great Marlow, containing, with the hamlet of Lilliffee, 188 inhabitants. The living is a discharged rectory, in the archdeaconry of Buckingham, and diocese of Lincoln rated in the king's books at £4, endowed with £200 royal bounty, and £200 parliamentary grant. Lord Boston was patron in 1814. The church is dedicated to St. Nicholas. In the church-yard are interred the remains of Nathaniel Hooke, author of the Roman History, who died in 1763; to whose memory a tablet was erected at the expense of Lord Boston.

HEELYFIELD, a township in the parish of MUGGLESWICK, western division of CHESTER ward, county palatine of DURHAM, 8½ miles (N.) from Wolsingham, containing 161 inhabitants. Here was anciently a chapel: there is a school with a small endowment. This township was severed from the parish of Lanchester by order of the parliamentary commissioners in 1648, and annexed to that of Muggleswick.

HEENE, a hamlet in the hundred of BRIGHTFORD, rape of BRAMBER, county of SUSSEX, ¼ of a mile (W.) from Worthing, containing 178 inhabitants. Here was anciently a chapel, which being demolished, the inhabitants attend the church of West Tarring, to the rector and vicar of which parish they pay tithes.

HEIGHAM (POTTER), a parish in the hundred of HAPPING, county of NORFOLK, 7 miles (N. by E.) from Acle, containing 340 inhabitants. The living is a discharged vicarage, in the archdeaconry of Norfolk, and diocese of Norwich, rated in the king's books at £6. 13. 4., and in the patronage of the Bishop of Norwich. The church is dedicated to St. Nicholas.

HEIGHINGTON, a parish in the south-eastern division of DARLINGTON ward, county palatine of DURHAM, comprising the townships of Coastamoor, Heighington, Killerby, Midridge, Redworth, School-Aycliffe, and Walworth, and containing 1383 inhabitants, of which number, 557 are in the township of Heighington, 6½ miles (N. N. W.) from Darlington. The living is a vicarage, in the archdeaconry and diocese of Durham, rated in the king's books at £12. 14. 9½., and in the patronage of the Dean and Chapter of Durham. The church, dedicated to St. Michael, has a Norman tower, but the structure generally is of a later date : the pulpit is ancient and richly carved. There is a place of worship for Wesleyan Methodists. A free grammar school was founded in 1601, by Elizabeth Jennison, of Walworth, and endowed with a rent-charge of £10, which was subsequently augmented by a donation of £70 from Edward Kirby, vicar of this parish : the present income is £55. 11. per annum, and the school is conducted on the Madras system : a new school-house was built in 1812, by subscription, at an expense of £300.

HEIGHINGTON, a chapelry in the parish of WASHINGBOROUGH, second division of the wapentake of LANGOE, parts of KESTEVEN, county of LINCOLN, 4¾ miles (E.S. E.) from Lincoln, containing 396 inhabitants. There is a place of worship for Wesleyan Methodists.

HEIGHLEY, a township consisting of High Heighley and Low Heighley, in that part of the parish of MITFORD which is in the western division of MORPETH ward, county of NORTHUMBERLAND, 2¼ miles (N. N. W.) from Morpeth, containing, with Espley, Heighley-Gate, and Morpeth North-Gate, 76 inhabitants.

HEIGHTINGTON, a chapelry in the parish of ROCK, lower division of the hundred of DODDINGTREE, county of WORCESTER, 4 miles (S. W.) from Bewdley. The population is returned with the parish. The chapel is dedicated to St. Giles.

HEIGHTON, a parish in the hundred of FLEXBOROUGH, rape of PEVENSEY, county of SUSSEX, 1¾ mile (N.N.E.) from Newhaven, containing 71 inhabitants. The living is a rectory united to that of Tarring-Neville, in the archdeaconry of Lewes, and diocese of Chichester, rated in the king's books at £11. 8. 6½. The church is dedicated to St. Martin.

HELBECK-LANDS, a chapelry in the parish of AYSGARTH, western division of the wapentake of HANG, North riding of the county of YORK, 12 miles (W. byN.) from Askrigg. The population is returned with the parish.

HELEN'S (ST.), a market town and chapelry in the township of WINDLE, parish of PRESCOT, hundred of WEST DERBY, county palatine of LANCASTER, 4 miles (N.E. by E.) from Prescot, 48 (S.) from Lancaster, and 198 (N.W.) from London. The population is returned with Windle. This town, originally an inconsiderable village, began to assume some importance about fifty years since ; its enlargement and prosperity are chiefly attributable to the introduction of different branches of

manufacture, but especially to that of glass, which had been established in the vicinity. In 1773, an incorporated company, styled the British Plate-Glass Company, erected an extensive manufactory at Ravenhead, in the township of Sutton, near this town, which having failed, was succeeded by another company, formed in 1794, whose manufactory covers an area of nearly thirty acres, and is surrounded by a lofty stone wall, on the outside of which are the habitations of the workmen : the erection of this building cost nearly £40,000. This establishment is the largest of the kind in England, and affords employment to upwards of three hundred workmen : the first artisans were brought from France, and the glass now produced is in all respects equal, and in many superior, to the French and Venetian plates. In 1789, a steam-engine was constructed for grinding and polishing plate-glass, which performs the work of one hundred and sixty men, and with greater exactness. Plates of glass measuring one hundred and forty inches by seventy-two, and concave and convex mirrors, thirty-six inches in diameter, are made here; the produce of the manufactory, consisting of crown, plate, and flint glass, is chiefly sent to the company's warehouse in London. In the same township, and in that of Eccleston, are three other manufactories for crown and flint glass, and bottles : there are also several potteries, breweries, and a cotton-mill in the neighbourhood; many of which are worked by steam. The cheapness and abundance of good coal, and the proximity of Liverpool, have greatly contributed to the success of these manufactories. About 1780, extensive works for smelting and refining copper were established here by the proprietors of the Parys mine, in Anglesea, who also had one on a smaller scale near the Sankey canal, but both these were discontinued in 1815. A customary-market is held on Saturday ; and there are fairs on the Monday and Tuesday after Easter-week, and on the first Friday and Saturday after September 8th. At the courts leet and baron of the lord of the manor of Windle, held in November, peace officers are annually appointed for this district. The living is a perpetual curacy, in the archdeaconry and diocese of Chester, endowed with £600 private benefaction, £400 royal bounty, and £600 parliamentary grant, and in the patronage of Trustees. The chapel was originally dedicated to St. Helen, but on being enlarged in 1816, it was dedicated anew to St. Mary. There are places of worship for the Society of Friends, Independents, and Wesleyan Methodists, and a chapel for Roman Catholics : to the first of these is attached a liberal endowment, the interest of which is appropriated to charitable purposes. A free school is endowed with property producing £26 per annum, for the gratuitous instruction of twenty-five poor children within the town, in reading, writing, and arithmetic : the appointment of the master and the management of the revenue of the charity are vested in the Trustees of the chapel. A charity school was founded in 1714, by a bequest from Sarah Cowley, who gave an estate at Hardshaw, near St. Helen's, directing the proceeds to be applied towards educating the children of poor parents belonging to Windle : the property includes coal mines, and, under a decree of the court of Chancery in 1826, a fund is in process of accumulation, in order to provide against the time when the coal mines shall be exhausted. There is a Roman Catholic free school ; and it is computed that in the various Sunday schools instruction is afforded to about one thousand two hundred children. The Sunday school in connexion with the established church was erected by subscription and the proceeds of a bazaar, in 1829, at an expense of nearly £1000. In 1823, a charitable fund was established for the relief of poor married women in child-birth, or of widows who have lost their husbands during pregnancy. A savings bank was opened in 1819.

HELEN'S (ST.), a town and parish in the liberty of EAST MEDINA, Isle of Wight division of the county of SOUTHAMPTON, 9 miles (E.) from Newport, containing 804 inhabitants. The living is a perpetual curacy, in the archdeaconry and diocese of Winchester, endowed with £200 private benefaction, £400 royal bounty, and £1200 parliamentary grant, and in the patronage of the Provost and Fellows of Eton College. The ancient church was partly taken down at the commencement of the last century, in consequence of encroachments made by the sea, but the tower was left standing as a land-mark. There is a place of worship for Wesleyan Methodists. Here was a priory of Cluniac monks, the site of which is now occupied by a modern mansion called the Priory : in an adjacent wood are some remains of an ancient watch-tower. This parish is bounded on the east by the English channel, on the north by Spithead, and on the south by Brading harbour.

HELFORD, a small sea-port in the parish of MANACCAN, hundred of KERRIER, county of CORNWALL, 6 miles (S.S.W.) from Falmouth. The population is returned with the parish. This place, which is situated on the southern side of the river Hel, has a haven where some trade is carried on in timber and coal imported from Wales. Here is a place of worship for Independents.

HELHOUGHTON, a parish in the hundred of GALLOW, county of NORFOLK, 4¼ miles (S.W. by W.) from Fakenham, containing 322 inhabitants. The living is a discharged vicarage, united to that of South Rainham, in the archdeaconry and diocese of Norwich, rated in the king's books at £6. 13. 4. The church is dedicated to All Saints.

HELLABY, a township in the parish of STAINTON, southern division of the wapentake of STRAFFORTH and TICKHILL, West riding of the county of YORK, 5¼ miles (E.) from Rotherham. The population is returned with the parish.

HELLAND, a parish in the hundred of TRIGG, county of CORNWALL, 2½ miles (N. by E.) from Bodmin, containing 264 inhabitants. The living is a rectory, in the archdeaconry of Cornwall, and diocese of Exeter, rated in the king's books at £9. 13. 9. William Morshead, Esq. was patron in 1817. The church is dedicated to St. Helena. Here is a place of worship for Wesleyan Methodists. Dr. Richard Glynn Cloberry, an eminent poet and physician, was born at Brodes, or Broads, the seat of the Glynn family, in this parish.

HELLESDON, a parish partly within the city of NORWICH, and partly in the hundred of TAVERHAM, county of NORFOLK, 2¾ miles (N.W. by W.) from Norwich, containing 293 inhabitants. The living is a rectory with that of Drayton, in the archdeaconry and diocese of Norwich, rated in the king's books at £12. The church is dedicated to St. Mary.

HELLIDON, a parish in the hundred of FAWSLEY,

county of NORTHAMPTON, 5 miles (S.W.) from Daventry, containing 408 inhabitants. The living is a perpetual curacy, in the archdeaconry of Northampton, and diocese of Peterborough, endowed with £200 royal bounty. T. and M. Scrafton, Esqrs. were patrons in 1806. The church is dedicated to St. John the Baptist. There is a place of worship for Wesleyan Methodists. In 1618, Mr. John Ball bequeathed £100 for the erection of a school-room, and a rent-charge of £10 a year towards the support of a master; twenty children are educated. The Rev. Sir John Knightly bequeathed £5. 3. per annum towards a Sunday school. The source of the river Leame is near the village.

HELLIFIELD, a township in the parish of LONG PRESTON, western division of the wapentake of STAINCLIFFE and EWCROSS, West riding of the county of YORK, 6 miles (S.S.E.) from Settle, containing 279 inhabitants.

HELLINGHILL, a township in the parish of ROTHBURY, western division of COQUETDALE ward, county of NORTHUMBERLAND, 4 miles (S. by W.) from Rothbury, containing 130 inhabitants.

HELLINGLY, a parish in the hundred of DILL, rape of PEVENSEY, county of SUSSEX, 2¼ miles (N. by W.) from Haylsham, containing 1313 inhabitants. The living is a vicarage, in the archdeaconry of Lewes, and diocese of Chichester, rated in the king's books at £6. 16. 8., and in the patronage of the Earl of Chichester. The church, dedicated to St. Peter and St. Paul, is in the early style of English architecture. There is a place of worship for Wesleyan Methodists.

HELMDON, a parish in the hundred of KING'S SUTTON, county of NORTHAMPTON, 6 miles (N.) from Brackley, containing 486 inhabitants. The living is a rectory, in the archdeaconry of Northampton, and diocese of Peterborough, rated in the king's books at £13. 11. 0½., and in the patronage of the President and Fellows of Corpus Christi College, Oxford. The church is dedicated to St. Mary Magdalene. In 1723, the Rev. — Jones gave £20 towards the establishment and maintenance of a school, which is now supported by voluntary contributions. A court leet is held here by the crown, for the duchy of Lancaster.

HELMINGHAM, a parish in the hundred of BOSMERE and CLAYDON, county of SUFFOLK, 5 miles (S.S.E.) from Debenham, containing 325 inhabitants. The living is a rectory, in the archdeaconry of Suffolk, and diocese of Norwich, rated in the king's books at £18, and in the patronage of the Crown. The church is dedicated to St. Mary.

HELMINGTON, a joint township with Hunwick, in that part of the parish of ST. ANDREW, AUCKLAND, which is in the north-western division of DARLINGTON ward, county palatine of DURHAM, 3½ miles (N.N.W.) from Bishop-Auckland, containing 160 inhabitants.

HELMSLEY, a parish in the wapentake of RYEDALE, North riding of the county of YORK, comprising the market town of Helmsley, the joint chapelry of Bilsdale-Midcable with Bilsdale-Birkham, and the townships of Haram, Laskill-Pasture, Pockley, Rivaulx, and Sproxton, and containing 3458 inhabitants, of which number, 1520 are in the town of Helmsley, 23 miles (N.) from York, and 218 (N. by W.) from London. This place, which was formerly of considerable importance, derives its name from the dark heathy moors in the parish, and belonged, in the reigns of Edward I. and II., to the family of Ross, who built here a strong castle for their baronial residence, which, in the parliamentary war, being garrisoned for the king, was besieged and taken by Fairfax, in 1644, and soon afterwards dismantled by order of the parliament : the remains of this structure, which was erected on an eminence, and surrounded by a double moat, consist principally of detached portions of the state apartments and offices, and part of the keep and gateway. The town is situated on the declivity of a small eminence, sloping gently towards the river Rye, which gives name to the wapentake ; the houses are chiefly built of stone, and roofed with slate, and the inhabitants are supplied with water from springs and from a rivulet called the Boro' Beck, which, after running through the town, disappears at the distance of a mile, and rises again at the distance of four miles. The environs are extremely pleasant, being richly diversified with extensive woods and fertile valleys. The linen manufacture, which was carried on extensively by families at their own houses, has been almost destroyed here by the introduction of machinery. There are mines of coal in the parish. The market is on Saturday : the fairs are, May 19th, July 16th, October 1st and 2nd, and November 5th and 6th, for cattle, sheep, and linen and woollen cloth. A court for the recovery of debts under 40s. is occasionally held. The living is a discharged vicarage, in the archdeaconry of Cleveland, and diocese of York, rated in the king's books at £11. 8. 6½., endowed with £200 private benefaction, and £200 royal bounty, and in the patronage of Charles Duncombe, Esq. The church, dedicated to All Saints, is a large and handsome structure, partly in the Norman, and partly in the early, style of English architecture, with later insertions, having a tower at the west end : the interior contains some elegant screen-work, and an hexagonal font of early English character. At Haram and Pockley are chapels of ease, the latter built, in 1822, at the sole expense of C. Duncombe, Esq., of Duncombe Park (a noble mansion, within a mile of Helmsley, built, in 1718, in the Doric order of architecture, from a design by Vanbrugh), who is proprietor of nearly the whole of the parish, which is about sixteen miles long from north to south, averaging nearly five miles in breadth, and contains about fifty thousand acres. There are places of worship for the Society of Friends and Wesleyan Methodists. A National school for children of both sexes is supported by Mr. Duncombe. George Villiers, Duke of Buckingham, after he had withdrawn from the court and cabinet of Charles II., spent a considerable portion of his time here, this period of his life having been distinguished by the revelries and profligacy, which soon reduced him to a state of indigence : he died at Kirkby-Moor-Side, in April, 1687. About two miles to the north-west are the interesting remains of the abbey of Rivaulx, or Rivall, so called from its situation in the vale of the river Rye : it was the first Cistercian abbey in Yorkshire, and was founded in 1131, and dedicated to the Blessed Virgin Mary, by Walter Espec, who endowed it with ample revenues, which at the dissolution were estimated at £351. 14. 6.

HELMSLEY (GATE), a parish within the liberty of ST. PETER of YORK, East riding, though locally in the wapentake of Bulmer, North riding, of the county of YORK, 6¼ miles (E.N.E.) from York, containing 209

inhabitants. The living is a discharged vicarage, rated in the king's books at £2, endowed with £200 private benefaction, and £800 royal bounty, and in the peculiar jurisdiction and patronage of the Prebendary of Osbaldwick in the Cathedral Church of York. The church is dedicated to St. Mary.

HELMSLEY (UPPER), a parish in the wapentake of BULMER, North riding of the county of YORK, 7½ miles (N.E.) from York, containing 63 inhabitants. The living is a discharged rectory, in the archdeaconry of Cleveland, and diocese of York, rated in the king's books at £4. 19. 2., endowed with £400 royal bounty, and in the patronage of the Crown. The church is dedicated to St. Peter.

HELPERBY, a township in that part of the parish of BRAFFERTON which is within the liberty of ST. PETER of YORK, East riding, though locally in the wapentake of Bulmer, North riding, of the county of YORK, 4¼ miles (N.E. by E.) from Boroughbridge, containing 611 inhabitants. This township is within the peculiar ecclesiastical jurisdiction of the Dean and Chapter of York.

HELPERTHORP, a parish in the wapentake of BUCKROSE, East riding of the county of YORK, 12 miles (E.) from New Malton, containing 157 inhabitants. The living is a discharged vicarage, in the peculiar jurisdiction and patronage of the Dean and Chapter of York, rated in the king's books at £4. 19. 7. The church is dedicated to St. Peter.

HELPRINGHAM, a parish in the wapentake of ASWARDHURN, parts of KESTEVEN, county of LINCOLN, 7½ miles (N.E.) from Falkingham, containing 693 inhabitants. The living is a discharged vicarage, in the archdeaconry and diocese of Lincoln, rated in the king's books at £8. 3. 4., and endowed with £200 royal bounty. Mrs. Andrews and others were patrons in 1799. The church, dedicated to St. Andrew, is principally in the decorated style. Here is a place of worship for Independents.

HELPSTONE, a parish in the liberty of PETERBOROUGH, county of NORTHAMPTON, 3¾ miles (S.S.W.) from Market-Deeping, containing 372 inhabitants. The living is a discharged vicarage, in the archdeaconry of Northampton, and diocese of Peterborough, rated in the king's books at £8. 0. 5., endowed with £200 royal bounty, and in the patronage of the Master and Fellows of Christ's College, Cambridge. The church, dedicated to St. Botolph, has traces of Norman, with insertions in the early, later, and decorated, styles of English architecture.

HELSBY, a township in the parish of FRODSHAM, second division of the hundred of EDDISBURY, county palatine of CHESTER, 2¼ miles (S.W. by W.) from Frodsham, containing 378 inhabitants.

HELSINGTON, a chapelry in that part of the parish of KENDAL which is in KENDAL ward, county of WESTMORLAND, 4¼ miles (S.W. by S.) from Kendal, containing 268 inhabitants. The living is a perpetual curacy, in the archdeaconry of Richmond, and diocese of Chester, endowed with £9. per annum and £400 private benefaction, and £600 royal bounty, and in the patronage of the Vicar of Kendal. The chapel, dedicated to St. John, was founded in 1726, by John Jackson, of Holeslack, who likewise endowed it with an estate. A school, erected by subscription, is supported by annual collections.

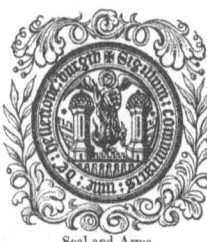

Seal and Arms.

HELSTON, or HELLES-TON, a borough, market town, and chapelry, in the parish of WENDRON, possessing separate jurisdiction, but locally in the hundred of Kerrier, county of CORNWALL, 61 miles (S. W.) from Launceston, and 274 (W. S. W.) from London, containing 2671 inhabitants. This is a place of considerable antiquity, and was one of the original stannary towns, though but little tin is coined here at present. When Domesday-book was compiled it formed part of the royal demesne, and King John granted a charter to the burgesses for the foundation of a guild, which was confirmed by Edward III., who gave the privilege of holding a market and fairs. The town stands on the great road from Plymouth to the Land's End, on the declivity of a hill, to the east of the little river Cober; and it comprises four principal streets arranged in the form of a cross, with a handsome market-house and town-hall near the centre: at the end of the street which takes its name from the building is situated old Coinage-hall. The streets are all paved, and lighted with gas, and a stream of water flows through them, affording an abundant supply to the inhabitants, and giving a neat and agreeable aspect to the place. In the neighbourhood are mines of tin, lead, and copper, which are very productive, especially the famous tin mine of Huel Vor, about three miles westward from the town, the works extending more than a mile and a half under ground. Five large steam-engines are used to pump the water out of the mine, and several smaller ones for raising the ore and other purposes: there are likewise four large stamping-mills worked by steam; and the operations of roasting and smelting are carried on upon the spot. The expense of working this mine has been estimated at £5000 a month, notwithstanding which, the proprietors are said to have obtained a clear profit of £10,000 in three months. Markets are held on Wednesday and Saturday; and there are fairs on the Saturdays before Mid-Lent Sunday and Palm Sunday, on Whit-Monday, July 20th, September 9th, October 28th, and the first, second, and third Saturdays before Christmas-eve.

Notwithstanding the grant of many previous charters, Helston was not made a corporate town till the reign of Elizabeth, who vested the government in a mayor and four aldermen, who constituted the common council, and were to choose twenty-four assistants; and this charter was confirmed by Charles I., who appointed the mayor for the current year to be also recorder, and the mayor for the preceding year to be a justice of the peace within the borough, with power to hold quarter sessions. This charter being forfeited; in consequence of some electioneering intrigues, a new one was obtained in 1774, under which the corporation consists of a mayor and four aldermen, with an indeterminate number of freemen. There is a common gaol within the borough, under the jurisdiction of the mayor and aldermen; but it consists of only a single room, capable of holding only four prisoners, and committals seldom take place. The petty sessions for the west division of the hundred of Kerrier are held here on the first Saturday

in every month. The borough has sent members to parliament ever since the 26th of Edward I.: the right of election is vested in the corporation, and the mayor is the returning officer: the patronage of the borough belongs to the Duke of Leeds.

The living is a perpetual curacy, with the vicarage of Wendron, in the archdeaconry and diocese of Cornwall. The church, dedicated to St. Michael, is a handsome edifice, with a lofty pinnacled tower, standing on an eminence to the north of the town: it was rebuilt in 1762, at the expense of £6000, the benefaction of the Earl of Godolphin. Here are places of worship for Baptists and Wesleyan Methodists. A National school has been established in the town; also a dispensary for the sick poor not receiving parochial relief. In 1704, Charles Godolphin, Esq. gave land producing a considerable income, in trust to the mayor and commonalty "for the education and maintenance of poor scholars, relief of decayed virtuous gentlemen, redemption of prisoners, and apprenticing poor children." Here was anciently a castle, of which some vestiges existed when Leland visited the town, in the reign of Henry VIII.; the site is now a bowling-green. At the village of St. John, adjoining Helston, was a priory, or hospital, dedicated to St. John the Baptist, the revenue of which, at the dissolution, was £14. 7. 4. Near this town is Loo Pool, one of the most considerable lakes in the county, formed by an accumulation of the waters of the river, confined by a sand-bank thrown up by the waves of the sea, through which an opening is made occasionally to drain the lake. This town has from time immemorial been noted for a popular festival, held annually on the 8th of May, called "the Furrey," supposed to have been derived from the Roman Floralia, or games in honour of the goddess Flora: on this occasion persons parade the streets with garlands of flowers, and all ranks partake of the pleasures of dancing and various rural amusements.

HELTON, a township in the parish of ASKHAM, WEST ward, county of WESTMORLAND, 6 miles (S.) from Penrith, containing 162 inhabitants.

HELTON, or HILTON, a township (formerly a chapelry) in the parish of BONGATE, or ST. MICHAEL, APPLEBY, EAST ward, county of WESTMORLAND, 3 miles (E.) from Appleby, containing 300 inhabitants. The London Lead Company work the lead mines here, which are very productive, and they have also a mill for smelting the ore, which yields a considerable quantity of silver. The chapel has long been demolished.

HEMBLINGTON, a parish in the hundred of WALSHAM, county of NORFOLK, 4 miles (W. N. W.) from Acle, containing 255 inhabitants. The living is a perpetual curacy, in the archdeaconry and diocese of Norwich, endowed with £1200 royal bounty, and £200 parliamentary grant, and in the patronage of the Dean and Chapter of Norwich. The church is dedicated to All Saints.

HEMBURY (BROAD), county of DEVON. —— See BROADHEMBURY.

HEMINGBROUGH, a parish in the wapentake of OUZE and DERWENT, East riding of the county of YORK, comprising the chapelry of Barlby, and the townships of Brackenholme with Woodall, Cliff with Lund, South Duffield, Hemingbrough, Menthorp with Bowthorp, and Osgodby, and containing 1855 inhabitants, of which number, 500 are in the township of Hemingbrough, 4¼ miles (E. S. E.) from Selby. The living is a discharged vicarage, in the jurisdiction of the peculiar court of How denshire, endowed with £1800 parliamentary grant, and in the patronage of the Crown. The church, dedicated to St. Mary, is a cruciform structure, principally in the later style of English architecture, with a tower rising from the intersection: it was made collegiate in 1426, the revenue of the society, at the dissolution, having been valued at £84. 11. A small school is endowed with the rent of two acres of land, called the School Close.

HEMINGBY, a parish in the northern division of the wapentake of GARTREE, parts of LINDSEY, county of LINCOLN, 3¾ miles (N. N. W.) from Horncastle, containing 297 inhabitants. The living is a rectory, in the archdeaconry and diocese of Lincoln, rated in the king's books at £17. 8. 6½., and in the patronage of the Provost and Fellows of King's College, Cambridge. There is a place of worship for Wesleyan Methodists. This parish is in the liberty of the duchy of Lancaster.

HEMINGFORD (ABBOTS), a parish in the hundred of TOSELAND, county of HUNTINGDON, 2½ miles (W.) from St. Ives, containing 400 inhabitants. The living is a rectory, in the archdeaconry of Huntingdon, and diocese of Lincoln, rated in the king's books at £26. 13. 4. Lady Olivia Sparrow was patroness in 1811. The church is dedicated to St. Margaret. A school for the education of boys and girls is supported by the rector.

HEMINGFORD (GREY), a parish in the hundred of TOSELAND, county of HUNTINGDON, 1¾ mile (W. by S.) from St. Ives, containing 475 inhabitants. The living is a discharged vicarage, in the archdeaconry of Huntingdon, and diocese of Lincoln, rated in the king's books at £9. 16. 10., and in the patronage of the Master and Fellows of Trinity Hall, Cambridge. The church is dedicated to St. James. The river Ouse passes the village. Cowper, the poet, wrote "The Dog and the Water Lily" when on a visit here.

HEMINGSTONE, or HELMINGSTONE, a parish in the hundred of BOSMERE and CLAYDON, county of SUFFOLK, 4¾ miles (E. S. E.) from Needham, containing 322 inhabitants. The living is a rectory, in the archdeaconry of Suffolk, and diocese of Norwich, rated in the king's books at £8. 11. 5½. Sir W. F. Middleton, Bart. was patron in 1824. The church is dedicated to St. Gregory.

HEMINGTON, a township in the parish of LOCKINGTON, western division of the hundred of GOSCOTE, county of LEICESTER, 8 miles (N. W.) from Loughborough, containing 421 inhabitants. An ancient chapel here is partly in ruins.

HEMINGTON, a parish in the hundred of POLEBROOKE, county of NORTHAMPTON, 5½ miles (E. S. E.) from Oundle, containing 134 inhabitants. The living is a discharged vicarage, in the archdeaconry of Northampton, and diocese of Peterborough, rated in the king's books at £6. 9. 7. Lord Montagu was patron in 1794. The church is dedicated to St. Peter and St. Paul.

HEMINGTON, a parish in the hundred of KILMERSDON, county of SOMERSET, 5¼ miles (N. W. by N.) from Frome, containing 323 inhabitants. The living is a rectory, united to that of Hardington, in the archdeaconry of Wells, and diocese of Bath and Wells, rated

in the king's books at £13. 14. 7. The church is dedicated to St. Mary.

HEMLEY, a parish in the hundred of COLNEIS, county of SUFFOLK, 5 miles (S. by E.) from Woodbridge, containing 80 inhabitants. The living is a discharged rectory, in the archdeaconry of Suffolk, and diocese of Norwich, rated in the king's books at £4. 19. 2., and in the patronage of the Crown. The church is dedicated to All Saints. The navigable river Deben runs on the east of this parish.

HEMLINGTON, a township in the parish of STAINTON, western division of the liberty of LANGBAURGH, North riding of the county of YORK, 4¼ miles (N. by W.) from Stokesley, containing 72 inhabitants.

HEMLINGTON-ROW, a township in the parish of BRANCEPETH, north-western division of DARLINGTON ward, county palatine of DURHAM, 4¼ miles (N. W. by N.) from Bishop-Auckland, containing 154 inhabitants.

HEMPHOLME, a township in the parish of LEVEN, northern division of the wapentake of HOLDERNESS, East riding of the county of YORK, 10½ miles (N. N. E.) from Beverley, containing 93 inhabitants.

HEMPNALL, a parish (formerly a market town) in the hundred of DEPWADE, county of NORFOLK, 3¾ miles (E. by N.) from St. Mary Stratton, containing 1014 inhabitants. The living is a vicarage, in the archdeaconry of Norfolk, and diocese of Norwich, rated in the king's books at £6. 13. 4. John T. Mott, Esq. was patron in 1819. The church is dedicated to St. Margaret. Here is a fair on St. Andrew's day.

HEMPSTEAD, a parish in the hundred of FRESHWELL, county of ESSEX, 5½ miles (N.N.E.) from Thaxted, containing 655 inhabitants. The living is a perpetual curacy annexed to the vicarage of Great Sampford, in the archdeaconry of Essex, and diocese of London. The church is dedicated to St. Andrew.

HEMPSTEAD, a parish in the middle division of the hundred of DUDSTONE and KING'S BARTON, county of GLOUCESTER, 1¾ mile (S. W. by W.) from Gloucester, containing, with South Hamlet, 548 inhabitants. The living is a rectory, in the archdeaconry and diocese of Gloucester, rated in the king's books at £8. Mr. Alderman Jones was patron in 1826. The church is dedicated to St. Swithin. In a field here are vestiges of some earthworks thrown up by the royalists during the civil war. The Gloucester and Berkeley canal passes through this parish, and the navigable river Severn runs along its western boundary.

HEMPSTEAD, a parish in the hundred of HAPPING, county of NORFOLK, 8¾ miles (E. by S.) from North Walsham, containing, with the parish of Eccles, 212 inhabitants. The living is a discharged rectory, with the rectories of Eccles and Lessingham, in the archdeaconry of Norfolk, and diocese of Norwich, rated in the king's books at £9. 6. 8., and in the patronage of the Provost and Fellows of King's College, Cambridge. The church is dedicated to St. Andrew.

HEMPSTEAD, a parish in the hundred of HOLT, county of NORFOLK, 2 miles (S. E.) from Holt, containing 289 inhabitants. The living is a discharged vicarage, in the archdeaconry and diocese of Norwich, rated in the king's books at £7. 2. 6., endowed with £200 royal bounty, and in the patronage of the Dean and Chapter of Norwich. The church is dedicated to All Saints.

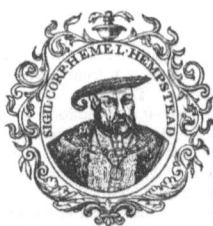

Corporate Seal.

HEMPSTEAD (HE-MEL), a parish in the hundred of DACORUM, county of HERTFORD, comprising the market town of Hemel-Hempstead, and the chapelries of Bovingdon and Flaunden, and containing 5193 inhabitants, of which number, 3962 are in the town of Hemel-Hempstead, 19½ miles (W. by S.) from Hertford, and 23 (N.W.) from London. This place, of which there are no records of a date prior to the Heptarchy, appears from the name to owe its origin to the Saxons, by whom, from its situation among the hills, near the confluence of the rivers Gade and Bulborn, it was called *Hean Hampstede*, implying a dwelling in a high or elevated situation : it was given by Offa, King of Mercia, to the abbey of St. Alban. In Domesday-book it is noticed under the names *Henamstede*, and *Hamelamstede*, from which latter its present appellation is evidently deduced. The town is pleasantly situated on the declivity of a hill, in a fertile valley watered by the river Gade, which has its source within a distance of four miles, and consists principally of one street, nearly a mile in length, partially paved and lighted : the houses are irregularly built, but of neat and respectable appearance, and the inhabitants are amply supplied with water. The principal article of manufacture is straw-plat, which affords employment to nearly all the females and children of the labouring class : there are several corn and paper-mills in the vicinity. The Grand Junction canal, by means of which the neighbourhood is supplied with coal from the Staffordshire mines, passes through Box Moor, within a mile of the town, where extensive docks, wharfs, and warehouses, have been constructed. The market, which is on Thursday, is one of the largest corn markets in the county ; a market is also held on the morning of the same day for straw-plat, a great quantity of which is sold weekly. The fairs are on Holy Thursday, for cattle and sheep, to which a court of piepowder is attached ; the Thursday after Trinity Sunday, and the third Monday in September, which last is a statute fair for hiring servants. The inhabitants received a charter of incorporation from Henry VIII., which was renewed to them by Cromwell on their taking the solemn league and covenant, the copy of which is still preserved. By this charter the government is vested in a bailiff, assisted by a jury of the principal inhabitants, who act as his council : the bailiff is annually chosen from among the principal inhabitants on St. Andrew's day ; he acts as clerk of the market, but possesses no magisterial authority. The court leet of the lord of the manor is, by permission of the bailiff, held in the town-hall ; where also a meeting of the county magistrates takes place every alternate week : the town-hall is a long narrow building, supported on square wooden pillars, of which the upper part contains rooms for the transaction of the business of the corporation, and the lower affords an area for the use of the market.

The living is a vicarage, in the archdeaconry of Huntingdon, and diocese of Lincoln, rated in the king's books at £16. 1. 10½., and in the presentation of the Dean and Chapter of St. Paul's, London, on the nomination of the Bishop of Lincoln. The church, dedicated to St. Mary, is a spacious cruciform structure, partly in the Norman style of architecture, with an embattled tower surmounted by a lofty spire ; the chancel is finely groined, and the east window embellished with painted glass ; there is also a finely-painted window at the west end, presented by Sir Astley Paston Cooper, Bart. In 1809, a large stone coffin was dug up in the church-yard, and in the church is a stone with a brass, bearing the effigy of Robert Albyn, with an inscription in Norman French. There are places of worship for Baptists, the Society of Friends, and Huntingtonians. A charity school for boys, erected by subscription, and endowed with £15 per annum bequeathed, in 1796, by Mr. Thomas Warren, and £10 per annum from a bequest by Francis Combe, Esq., of Hempstead-Bury ; and a charity school for girls, to which Mr. Warren bequeathed £13. 10. per annum, have been consolidated, and are conducted on the National system : there are one hundred boys and eighty girls in the school, which is further supported by subscription. The West Herts Infirmary, at Picott's End, in this parish, is also supported by subscription. The remains of the old manor-house of Bury consist only of a gateway, from a window over which Henry VIII. is said to have delivered the charter; and in Lacker's house are some curious apartments said to have been built by that monarch, in the ceilings of which the royal arms are still preserved : there are also some remains of ancient buildings at a place called Heaven's Gate, at the north-east boundary of the parish, concerning which there are some traditionary records. At Picott's End, and at Poak Mill, in the vicinity of the town, are saline and chalybeate springs, the water of which is said to be similar to that of Cheltenham. Many petrifactions of sponge and other fossils, susceptible of a very high polish, are found in the vicinity, which abounds also with fine specimens of chalcedony. Dr. Hugh Smith, an eminent physician and medical lecturer, was born at Hemel-Hempstead, in 1733 ; Sir Astley Paston Cooper, Bart., pre-eminently distinguished for his skill in surgery, now resides in the vicinity.

HEMPSTON (BROAD), a parish in the hundred of HAYTOR, county of DEVON, 4 miles (S. E.) from Ashburton, containing 789 inhabitants. The living is a vicarage, in the archdeaconry of Totness, and diocese of Exeter, rated in the king's books at £25. 6. 8., and in the patronage of the Crown. There is a place of worship for Wesleyan Methodists. A charity school is supported by donations and subscriptions.

HEMPSTON (LITTLE), a parish in the hundred of HAYTOR, county of DEVON, 1¾ mile (N. by E.) from Totness, containing 323 inhabitants. The living is a rectory, in the archdeaconry of Totness, and diocese of Exeter, rated in the king's books at £19. 15. 2½., and in the patronage of the Crown. The church is dedicated to St. John the Baptist.

HEMPTON, a joint tything with Patchway, in that part of the parish of ALMONDSBURY which is in the lower division of the hundred of LANGLEY and SWINEHEAD, county of GLOUCESTER, 6½ miles (S. by W.) from Thornbury, containing 500 inhabitants.

HEMPTON, a parish in the hundred of GALLOW, county of NORFOLK, 1 mile (S.W.) from Fakenham, containing 299 inhabitants. The living is a perpetual curacy, in the archdeaconry and diocese of Norwich, and in the patronage of the Crown. The church, which was dedicated to St. Andrew, has fallen to decay. Between this place and Fakenham was a priory of canons of the order of St. Augustine, the revenue of which, at the dissolution, was valued at £39. 0. 9.

HEMPTON, a township in the parish of DEDDINGTON, hundred of WOOTTON, county of OXFORD, 1½ mile (W.) from Deddington, containing 172 inhabitants.

HEMSBY, a parish in the western division of the hundred of FLEGG, county of NORFOLK, 4½ miles (N. N. W.) from Caistor, containing 498 inhabitants. The living is a discharged vicarage, in the archdeaconry and diocese of Norwich, rated in the king's books at £4. 6. 8. John T. Hales, Esq. was patron in 1805. The church is dedicated to St. Mary.

HEMSWELL, a parish in the western division of the wapentake of ASLACOE, parts of LINDSEY, county of LINCOLN, 7½ miles (E.) from Gainsborough, containing 271 inhabitants. The living, which was formerly a rectory, rated in the king's books at £27. 13. 4., is now a perpetual curacy, in the archdeaconry of Stow, and diocese of Lincoln, endowed with £400 royal bounty, and in the patronage of the Mayor and Corporation of Lincoln. The church is dedicated to All Saints. There is a place of worship for Wesleyan Methodists. In this parish is the hamlet of Spittal, which derives its name from an ancient hospital, founded for poor widows prior to the 16th of Edward II., which is under the patronage of the Dean and Chapter of Lincoln: attached to it is a small chapel. A sessions-house was built in 1620, by Chief Justice Wray. A fair is held annually in the hamlet on the 22nd of November.

HEMSWORTH, a parish in the wapentake of STAINCROSS, West riding of the county of YORK, 6½ miles (S. S. W.) from Pontefract, containing 963 inhabitants. The living is a rectory, in the archdeaconry and diocese of York, rated in the king's books at £20. 1. 0½. W. Wrightson, Esq. was patron in 1790. The church, dedicated to St. Helen, is principally in the later style of English architecture, with decorated windows at the east end. There is a place of worship for Wesleyan Methodists. A free grammar school was founded about 1548, by Robert Holgate, Archbishop of York, under letters patent of Henry VIII. In the reign of Edward VI., the same archbishop confirmed the foundation and ordinances to John Thurlston, then master, and his successors; the annual income is about £300, which is received by the present master, who does not perform any duty for it: about sixty scholars are instructed in English by an usher, on paying quarterage. In 1813, Robert Duffin, Esq. bequeathed £50, and Mr. Trant £100, for the support of Sunday schools: the dividends of £203. 7. 3., three per cent. consols. are applied according to the direction of the benefactors.

HEMYOCK, a parish in the hundred of HEMYOCK, county of DEVON, 5¼ miles (S.) from Wellington, containing 1159 inhabitants. The living is a rectory, in the archdeaconry and diocese of Exeter, rated in the king's books at £32. 0. 7½. Mrs. Hutton was patroness in 1817. The church is dedicated to St. Mary. Here are the remains of an ancient castle, which is said to have been garrisoned by the parliamentary forces during the civil war: the east entrance has a pointed door-way, and there are the relics of five towers. A

school was endowed by Mrs. Waldron, in 1749, for teaching five poor children to read. At the northern extremity of the parish is a large cairn, called Simon's barrow.

HENBURY, a joint township with Pexall, in the parish of PRESTBURY, hundred of MACCLESFIELD, county palatine of CHESTER, 2½ miles (W.) from Macclesfield, containing, with Pexall, 428 inhabitants.

HENBURY, a parish comprising the tythings of King's Weston and Lawrence-Weston, in the lower division of the hundred of BERKELEY, the joint chapelry of Redwick with Northwick, the township of Henbury, and the tything of Stowick, in the lower division, and the chapelry of Aust, and the tythings of Charlton and Compton, in the upper division, of the hundred of HENBURY, county of GLOUCESTER, and containing 2283 inhabitants, of which number, 431 are in the township of Henbury, 4¼ miles (N. N. W.) from Bristol. The name is derived from the Saxon Hean, or Hen, old, and burie, a fortified place. The living is a discharged vicarage, in the peculiar jurisdiction of the Consistory Court of the Bishop of Bristol, rated in the king's books at £30, and in the patronage of Viscount Middleton, Sir John Smyth, Bart., Edward Francis Colston, Esq., and the Rev. Charles Gore. The church, dedicated to St. Mary, is a spacious and handsome edifice, in the early style of English architecture, with decorated and later insertions: the church-yard is surrounded with ivy-mantled walls and enlivened with numerous evergreens. A free school, or hospital, was founded in 1623, by Mr. Anthony Edmonds, and endowed by him with the proceeds of certain lands, for the instruction of all children born within the parishes of Henbury, Westbury upon Trym, Hafield, Redwick, Northwick, and Aust, in this county; the annual income, augmented in 1736 by a bequest from Christopher Cole, Esq., is about £320: there is appropriate accommodation for the master and usher, with garden and play-ground. The object of this charity has been suspended since 1815, in consequence of great injury done to the property from an inundation of the Severn. In 1756, Robert Sandford bequeathed £1500, the proceeds to be employed in instructing poor children in reading and writing: forty children are educated on this charity, and the present income is £55 per annum. Here are the remains of an old chapel, dedicated to St. Blazius, a Spanish martyr, near which is a castellated summer-house, called Blaize castle, whence there is a most delightful prospect; and on the hill on which it stands is an ancient encampment, with triple ramparts and two deep ditches, having two entrances at the opposite angles, on the line of the ancient "Fosse-way:" this work is usually ascribed to the Britons, but the discovery of Roman coins and other relics evinces its occupation by that people. The Roman *Trajectus Sabrinæ* is usually placed at Aust in this parish. The Severn is navigable on the west, and the Avon on the south-west, the two rivers joining at the Swash.

HENDERSKELF, a chapelry in the parish and wapentake of BULMER, North riding of the county of YORK, 4½ miles (W. S. W.) from New Maltou, containing 159 inhabitants.

HENDON, a parish in the hundred of GORE, county of MIDDLESEX, 7 miles (N. W.) from London, containing 3100 inhabitants. This place was in the tenth century given by Dunstan, Archbishop of Canterbury, to Westminster abbey, the abbots having had a palace here, the remains of which have been converted into a private mansion. The village is pleasantly situated on an eminence, in a small vale watered by the river Brent, over which is an ancient bridge of stone; the houses are irregularly built : in the neighbourhood are many handsome villas, and the environs are pleasant, abounding with rural walks and agreeable scenery. A court leet for the manor is held on the Tuesday before Whitsuntide, and a court baron occasionally. Hendon is within the jurisdiction of a court of requests for the recovery of debts under 40s., held during the summer half-year at Brentford, and during the winter at Uxbridge. The living is a vicarage, in the jurisdiction of the Commissary of London, concurrently with the Consistorial Court of the Bishop, rated in the king's books at £15. The Rev. C. L. Edridge was patron in 1812. The church, dedicated to St. Mary, is a spacious structure in the decorated style of English architecture, with some small remains in the Norman style, and a square embattled tower : the nave is separated from the aisles by octangular pillars and sharply-pointed arches ; the altarpiece is finely sculptured, and the east window is embellished with a well-executed painting of the last Supper, and other subjects ; the interior contains several ancient monuments and a Norman font. A new church is now being erected on Mill Hill, in the later style of English architecture, at the expense of William Wilberforce, Esq. There are places of worship for Independents and Wesleyan Methodists. A school-room for boys was erected by John Bennet, Esq., on a piece of land given by Mr. David Garrick, the celebrated actor, then lord of the manor ; there are fifty-three boys in this school, which is conducted on the National plan, and supported by subscription. A National school is also supported by subscription, in which fifty-one girls are instructed, forty-one of them being also clothed. John Cross, Esq. bequeathed £250 Bank annuities, for clothing four boys and four girls. Robert Daniels, Esq., of London, in 1681, bequeathed £2000 for the erection and endowment of an almshouse for six aged men and four aged women ; with this sum, which had been left in the hands of his executors to accumulate for ten years, one hundred and thirty-two acres of land have been purchased : six almshouses were also erected in 1696, by Thomas Nichol, who endowed them for aged persons, each receiving four shillings per week. At Mill Hill is the Protestant Dissenters' grammar school : it was founded in 1807, and is under the direction of a chaplain, a head master, two assistant classical masters, and masters in the various departments of a liberal education, superintended by a committee : the buildings were erected on the site of the residence of Peter Collinson, Esq., an eminent naturalist, and completed at an expense of £25,000. On Highwood hill is a mansion in which the celebrated Lord William Russel resided previously to his arrest, now inhabited by Lady Raffles ; and near it is a mineral spring impregnated with cathartic salt. Hendon Place, the seat of Lord Tenterden, was a banqueting-house belonging to Queen Elizabeth. At a place called the Hyde, in this parish, a gold coin of one of the Cæsars was found a few years since. William Rawlinson, Esq., one of the masters in Chancery, and keeper of the seals ; Dr. Edward Fowler, Bishop of Gloucester ; Charles Johnson, a dramatic author ; Dr. James Parsons, anatomist and antiquary ; Sir Joseph Ayloffe, Vice-President of the Antiquarian Society ; and other eminent persons, have been interred here.

HENDRED (EAST), a parish in the hundred of WANTAGE, county of BERKS, 4½ miles (E. by N.) from Wantage, containing 863 inhabitants. The living is a rectory, in the archdeaconry of Berks, and diocese of Salisbury, rated in the king's books at £15. 5. 2½., and in the patronage of the Bishop of Salisbury. The church, dedicated to St. Augustine, contains a tomb to the memory of Archbishop Chicheley, formerly rector of the parish. Here is a place of worship for Roman Catholics, which formerly belonged to the chantry of St. Amand. A fair is held on the 11th of October. A branch of the river Isis flows through the parish. The stewardship of this manor is one of the nominal offices given for the purpose of vacating a seat in the House of Commons. Part of an ancient chapel belonging to the monks of Sheen has been converted into a dove-cote. Here are vestiges of a Roman road and a barrow.

HENDRED (WEST), a parish in the hundred of WANTAGE, county of BERKS, 3¾ miles (E.) from Wantage, containing 319 inhabitants. The living is a vicarage, in the archdeaconry of Berks, and diocese of Salisbury, rated in the king's books at £8. 19. 9½., and in the patronage of the President and Fellows of Corpus Christi College, Oxford. The church is dedicated to the Holy Trinity.

HENFIELD, a parish in the hundred of TIPNOAK, rape of BRAMBER, county of SUSSEX, 5¾ miles (N.E. by N.) from Steyning, containing 1404 inhabitants. The living is a vicarage, in the archdeaconry of Lewes, and diocese of Chichester, rated in the king's books at £16, and in the patronage of the Bishop of Chichester. The church, which is dedicated to St. Peter, is in the later style of English architecture. The navigable river Adur flows on the west of the parish.

HENGRAVE, a parish in the hundred of THINGOE, county of SUFFOLK, 3¾ miles (N.N.W.) from Bury-St. Edmund's, containing 168 inhabitants. The living is a rectory, united to that of Flempton, in the archdeaconry of Sudbury, and diocese of Norwich, rated in the king's books at £9. 7. 1. The navigable river Lark passes through this parish, and is crossed by a bridge. Hengrave hall is a fine specimen of the domestic architecture of the time of Henry VIII., and in good preservation.

HENHAM, a parish comprising the hamlet of Pledgon, in the hundred of CLAVERING, but chiefly in the hundred of UTTLESFORD, county of ESSEX, 4 miles (N.N.E.) from Stansted-Mountfitchet, containing 804 inhabitants. The living is a vicarage, in the jurisdiction of the Commissary of Essex and Herts, concurrently with the Consistorial Court of the Bishop of London, rated in the king's books at £17, and in the patronage of Mr. Glynn and Mr. Feake. There is a place of worship for Independents.

HENHAM, a hamlet in the parish of WANGFORD, hundred of BLYTHING, county of SUFFOLK, 5 miles (E. by N.) from Halesworth, containing 131 inhabitants.

HENHEADS, a township in that part of the parish of BURY which is in the higher division of the hundred of BLACKBURN, county palatine of LANCASTER, 1½ mile (E.) from Haslingden, containing 246 inhabitants

HENHULL, a township in the parish of ACTON, hundred of NANTWICH, county palatine of CHESTER, 1¾ mile (N. W. by W.) from Nantwich, containing 90 inhabitants. The Nantwich branch of the Chester canal passes in the vicinity.

HENLEY, a parish in the hundred of BOSMERE and CLAYDON, county of SUFFOLK, 5 miles (N.) from Ipswich, containing 241 inhabitants. The living is a discharged vicarage, in the archdeaconry of Suffolk, and diocese of Norwich, rated in the king's books at £10. 0. 10., and in the patronage of the Dean and Chapter of Norwich. The church is dedicated to St. Peter.

HENLEY (COLD), a chapelry in the parish of WHITCHURCH, hundred of EVINGAR, Kingsclere division of the county of SOUTHAMPTON, 3¼ miles (N. by E.) from Whitchurch, with which the population is returned.

HENLEY in ARDEN, a market town and chapelry in the parish of WOOTTON-WAVEN, Henley division of the hundred of BARLICHWAY, county of WARWICK, 10 miles (W. by N.) from Warwick, and 101 (N.W. by W.) from London, on the road through Oxford to Birmingham, containing 1249 inhabitants. This town takes the. adjunct, by which it is distinguished from other places of the same name, from its situation in the Forest of Arden, a large tract of woodland extending over part of Warwickshire and the adjoining counties. A considerable part of it was burnt at the battle of Evesham, in the reign of Henry III., from which injury, however, it had recovered in that of Edward I. Henry VI., in the 27th of his reign, granted to Sir Ralph Boteler, Knt., lord of the manor, a charter reciting and confirming previous charters, by which it had view of frankpledge, a market, and other privileges, that monarch adding the power to hold courts of pleas of the crown and common pleas, exemption from tolls, and from the jurisdiction of the sheriff for the county, with the right to the chattels of all tenants of the manor wheresoever condemned, with other grants and privileges, which have become obsolete.

The town is pleasantly situated near the confluence of the rivers Arrow and Allen, or Alne, and consists principally of one spacious street extending for more than a mile along the turnpike road; the houses are in general neat and well built, but of ancient appearance, occasionally interspersed with handsome modern buildings; the inhabitants are amply supplied with water from pumps and wells. The only articles of manufacture are nails, needles, and fish-hooks, which afford occupation to not more than fifty persons. The market is on Monday; the fairs are on the Tuesday in Whitsun-week, a pleasure fair; October 29th, a large fair for hops; and March 25th, for cattle and sheep. The market-house is a neat building of stone, supported on pillars; and near it is a handsome ancient cross, of which the shaft, of one entire stone, rises from a pedestal and terminates in a rich canopy at the summit. By charter of Henry VI., the government is vested in a high and low bailiff, appointed at the court leet of the lord of the manor, when constables and other officers are also chosen: a petty session is held weekly by the county magistrates.

The living is a perpetual curacy, in the archdeaconry and diocese of Worcester, endowed with £400 royal bounty, and £1400 parliamentary grant, and in the patronage of the householders in the parish. The church, dedicated to St. John the Baptist, is a small but elegant structure in the later style of English architecture, with a square embattled tower; the porch at the west entrance is a highly enriched and beautiful specimen of the later period of that style : the old roof, of ribbed and carved oak, is still preserved in the chancel; and throughout the whole of the building the traces of a pure and elegant design are discernible. There is a place of worship for Baptists. A charity school was founded by the corporation, to whom George Whateley, Esq., in the 28th of Elizabeth, gave a messuage in trust for that purpose, and it is supported by the appropriation of part of the charitable funds at their disposal, arising from various benefactions: there are thirty boys in the school. A Sunday school, in which from eighty to one hundred children of both sexes are instructed, is supported by subscription. About a quarter of a mile to the east of the town, on the summit of a bold and lofty eminence, called, from its beautiful situation, Bel Desert, or Beau Desert, is the site of a castle, which was erected prior to the reign of Stephen, and demolished during the war between the houses of York and Lancaster; the site of the draw-bridge and some other parts may be traced, and there are faint vestiges of the ancient moat, but no remains of the building. At the base of the castle hill, the parish church of Beaudesert, a small but beautiful edifice, partly in the Norman, and partly in the early English, style of architecture. About two miles to the north-west of the town are the Leveridge hills, where there is a Roman encampment, intrenched with a double moat and high ramparts of earth; and about half a mile to the east is Henley Mount, said to have been thrown up by Cromwell, as an exploratory station during the parliamentary war.

HENLEY upon THAMES, a market town and parish, having separate jurisdiction, locally in the hundred of Binfield, county of OXFORD, on the high road from London to Oxford and Cheltenham, 23 miles (S. E.) from Oxford, and 35 (W.) from London, on the western bank of the river Thames, containing 3509 inhabitants. This is supposed by some antiquaries to have been a town of the ancient Britons; according to others it was the Roman station Calleva, which has with greater probability been fixed at Silchester, in Hampshire. Leland mentions the discovery of gold, silver, and brass coins of the Romans at this place; but no notice of the town occurs in history till after the Norman Conquest. A bridge across the Thames was erected here at an early period, and it is not improbable that the town owed its origin to this circumstance. In the reign of Henry III. the manor belonged to Edmund, Earl of Cornwall, the king's nephew, on whose death it reverted to the crown; and in the 10th of Elizabeth, a charter of incorporation was granted to the town, in which it is denominated Hanleygang, or Hanneburg. In 1643, the parliamentary forces were quartered in the vicinity, when they were attacked by the royalists, who entered the town, but were dispersed

Corporate Seal.

by the firing of a cannon down Duke-street, which did much execution: in the following year the inhabitants sustained considerable damage from the wanton conduct of the parliamentary soldiers, who plundered most of the houses. The town, which is remarkably dry and healthy, is situated on a gentle ascent from the western bank of the Thames, which here takes one of its most agreeable curves: it is surrounded by hills clothed with lofty beech woods and extensive plantations, interspersed with elegant villas; as approached from London, the general appearance is striking, and the scenery remarkably picturesque. At the entrance into the town is a handsome stone bridge over the Thames, erected in 1786, at an expense of £10,000, and consisting of five elliptical arches, surmounted by a balustrade: the key-stone on each face of the central arch is adorned with a sculptured mask, from the chisel of the Hon. Mrs. Damer; that towards the north represents the Genius, or presiding Deity, of the Thames; the mask on the reverse key-stone exhibits the goddess Isis. The hills giving name to the Chiltern hundreds form a ridge extending from Henley, along the southern part of the county of Buckingham, to Tring in Hertfordshire; they were formerly so covered with thickets as to be almost impassable, until, by order of Leofstan, abbot of St. Alban's, these were cut down, on account of the security which they afforded to robbers. The popular appellation is derived from the Saxon words, *cealt*, *cylt*, or *chilt*, signifying chalk, of which substance they are principally composed. The nominal office of steward of the Chiltern hundreds under the crown, by the acceptance of which members of parliament vacate their seats, is derived from these hills. Henley consists of four principal streets, well paved and lighted; at the intersection is a plain stone cross and conduit: the houses, although irregular, are spacious and well built, and some of them handsome. A considerable trade in malt was formerly carried on here: every facility of water carriage to London is afforded by the Thames; and it is stated that so far back as the reign of Anne, there had been sold as much as three hundred cart loads of malt, and various kinds of grain, at the weekly markets: at this period it enjoyed also the manufacture of glass, in the composition of which, a black flint, and a kind of sand which formed part of the soil, essentially contributed. There is a silk-mill on a small scale; and near the town is a paper-mill. The market is on Thursday, for corn (which is pitched), seeds, &c.: fairs are on March 7th, for horses and cattle; Holy Thursday, for sheep; the Thursday in Trinity-week, and the Thursday after September 21st, the last of which is a statute fair. This town was incorporated by Elizabeth, but the charter by which it is now governed was granted by George I., in 1722, to the "mayor, aldermen, portreeves, and burgesses," with power to elect a high steward, "who shall be a baron of this kingdom, or at least a knight," and a recorder. The present corporation consists of a mayor, high steward, ten aldermen, two bridgemen, sixteen burgesses, with a recorder, town clerk, and inferior officers: the mayor, recorder, and the two senior aldermen, are justices of the peace, and have the power of holding a weekly court of record, for the recovery of debts to the amount of £10, at which the mayor presides: quarter-sessions

are also held regularly. One bridgeman is appointed annually by the corporation at Michaelmas, and the junior bridgeman for the preceding year then becomes the senior for the year ensuing: these officers, according to ancient custom, are always the churchwardens of the parish, and each continues in office for two successive years. All the rents received by them on account of the various charities are called "Bridge Rents," and the book in which they are entered, "The Bridge Book," from the ancient title of the officers who collect them. The town-hall, erected by the late Mr. W. Bradshaw, a member of the corporation, in 1796, stands on an elevation in the High-street, and is supported by sixteen Doric columns; it contains a hall and a council-chamber, and on the basement are rooms used on public occasions, and a gaol.

The living is a rectory, in the archdeaconry and diocese of Oxford, rated in the king's books at £21.1.3., and in the patronage of the Bishop of Rochester. The church, dedicated to St. Mary, is a spacious and handsome structure, chiefly in the decorated and later English styles; in the walls are some portions of chequered work in flint and chalk: it has a fine tower, erected at the expense of Cardinal Wolsey, and some good tracery in the east window of the chancel. The present north aisle appears to have formerly constituted the body of the church; in the north part of the chancel are indications of the original altar, with two canopied niches, in one of which is a recess, formerly used for the eucharist. A large sepulchral chapel, or chantry, founded by the family of Elmes, was, in 1820, converted into a vestry-room and library, and contains many valuable works in Greek, Latin, Hebrew, and the oriental languages, with various historical publications, [the liberal bequest of Dean Aldrich, rector of Henley, who died in 1737, and to this library all the inhabitants who pay church rates have free access, being likewise permitted, on certain conditions specified by the donor, to take away the books for perusal. In the chancel is a handsome monument, with a recumbent effigy of Lady Elizabeth Periam, the benefactress to Balliol College, Oxford: there are also monuments to Dr. Cawley, father of Lady Kneller, who died in 1709, and to Mr. William Hayward, of Shrewsbury, the architect of Henley bridge: in a vault on the south side are deposited the remains of General Dumouriez, so celebrated in the revolutionary history of France. Richard Jennings, the "Master Builder of St. Paul's Cathedral," who died at Badgemore, near this town, lies interred in the church-yard. There are places of worship, in the town and environs, for Baptists, the Society of Friends, and Independents. A grammar school was founded, in 1604, by James I., and endowed with the proceeds of certain church lands and other property, partly bequeathed by Augustine Knapp, and its funds were subsequently augmented by a benefaction from William Gravett, in 1664. A Blue-coat school, for educating, clothing, and apprenticing twenty boys, was founded, in 1609, by Lady Elizabeth Periam; and in 1774 these two schools were united by act of parliament, and their incomes consolidated, amounting at present to about £360 per annum, the two foundations to be called the "United Charity Schools in Henley," being placed under the direction of trustees, who were incorporated, and invested with the right of a common seal, and other privileges. The schools are still kept separately: the upper school, for the instruction of twenty-five boys in Latin and Greek, is under a master, who has a salary of £70 per annum; and the lower school, for sixty boys, under a master whose salary is £60, and an usher with £40 per annum. A Green school, for six boys and six girls, was founded in 1717, in consequence of a bequest by Mr. John Stevens, and subsequently endowed with property producing £54 per annum; and there is a National school, supported by voluntary contributions, and at present containing one hundred and eighty boys and one hundred girls. An almshouse for five poor men, and an adjoining house for three poor women, who receive a weekly allowance of three shillings each, were founded and endowed by John Longland, Bishop of Lincoln, in 1547, and are under the management of the corporation. There are ten almshouses for poor persons, founded and endowed with a bequest by Humphrey Newbury, in 1664; and four for poor widows, founded in 1743, by Mrs. Ann Messenger; and numerous other charities are at the disposal of the bridgemen, and the mayor and corporation. A savings-bank was established in 1817.

HENLLIS, a parish in the upper division of the hundred of WENTLLOOG, county of MONMOUTH, 3¾ miles (N. W. by W.) from Newport, containing 209 inhabitants. The living is a perpetual curacy, in the archdeaconry and diocese of Llandaff, endowed with £600 royal bounty, and £200 parliamentary grant, and in the patronage of the Vicar of Bassaleg. The church is dedicated to St. Peter.

HENLOW, a parish in the hundred of CLIFTON, county of BEDFORD, 4¼ miles (S. by W.) from Biggleswade, containing 688 inhabitants. The living is a vicarage, in the archdeaconry of Bedford, and diocese of Lincoln, rated in the king's books at £9. 6. 8., and in the patronage of the Crown. The church is dedicated to St. Mary.

HENNOCK, a parish in the hundred of TEINGBRIDGE, county of DEVON, 3 miles (W. N. W.) from Chudleigh, containing 678 inhabitants. The living is a discharged vicarage, in the archdeaconry of Totness, and diocese of Exeter, rated in the king's books at £16. Francis Garratt, Esq. was patron in 1828. There is a place of worship for Wesleyan Methodists. In the parish register is the following entry: "The eleventh day of October, the yeare of our Lord God, 1537, was borne Prince Edwarde, which was the 29th yeare of our Sovereign Lord, King Henry VIII. &c. God send him good oldinge, and his father a long and prosperous reign. Amen." Pipe and potters' clay, also lead and iron, in the granite rock, are found in this neighbourhood. The North Teign river bounds the parish on the east.

HENNOR, a hamlet in the parish of LEOMINSTER, hundred of WOLPHY, county of HEREFORD, 3¾ miles (E.) from Leominster. The population is returned with the township of Broadward.

HENNY (GREAT), a parish in the hundred of HINCKFORD, county of ESSEX, 2¾ miles (S. by W.) from Sudbury, containing 368 inhabitants. The living is a rectory with that of Little Henny, in the archdeaconry of Essex, and diocese of London, rated jointly in the king's books at £13. 6. 8. N. Barnardiston, Esq. was patron in 1810. The church is dedicated to St. Mary.

The navigable river Stour runs on the east of this parish.

HENNY (LITTLE), a parish in the hundred of HINCKFORD, county of ESSEX, 2¼ miles (S.) from Sudbury, containing 59 inhabitants. The living is a rectory, united with that of Great Henny, in the archdeaconry of Middlesex, and diocese of London. The church is demolished.

HENSALL, a township in that part of the parish of SNAITH which is in the lower division of the wapentake of OSGOLDCROSS, West riding of the county of YORK, 3½ miles (W. by N.) from Snaith, containing 233 inhabitants.

HENSHAW, a township in the parish of HALTWHISTLE, western division of TINDALE ward, county of NORTHUMBERLAND, 11 miles (W.) from Hexham, containing 593 inhabitants.

HENSINGHAM, a chapelry in the parish of ST. BEES, ALLERDALE ward above Darwent, county of CUMBERLAND, 1 mile (S. E.) from Whitehaven, containing 860 inhabitants. The living is a perpetual curacy, in the archdeaconry of Richmond, and diocese of Chester, and in the patronage of the Earl of Lonsdale. The village, occupying an elevated site, commands an interesting view of the town and harbour of Whitehaven: there are some neat villas in the neighbourhood. A school is supported by subscription. There is a manufactory for thread and check; and at Overend a large quantity of limestone is obtained and burnt. Archbishop Grindal was born here in 1519, and died in 1583.

HENSINGTON, a hamlet in the parish of BLADON, hundred of WOOTTON, county of OXFORD, ¼ of a mile (E.) from Woodstock, containing 130 inhabitants.

HENSTEAD, a parish comprising the hamlet of Hulverstreet, in the hundred of WANGFORD, but chiefly in the hundred of BLYTHING, county of SUFFOLK, 5¾ miles (S. E. by E.) from Beccles, containing 509 inhabitants. The living is a rectory, in the archdeaconry of Suffolk, and diocese of Norwich, rated in the king's books at £12. Robert Sparrow, Esq. was patron in 1811. The church is dedicated to St. Mary.

HENSTRIDGE, a parish in the hundred of HORETHORNE, county of SOMERSET, 6½ miles (S. by E.) from Wincanton, containing 911 inhabitants. The living is a vicarage, rated in the king's books at £13. 0. 2½., and in the peculiar jurisdiction and patronage of the Prebendary of Henstridge in the Cathedral Church of Wells. The church is dedicated to St. Nicholas. Here was an Alien priory, a cell to the Benedictine monastery of St. Sever, in Normandy, founded in the eleventh century, by Hugh Lupus, Earl of Chester.

HENTLAND, a parish in the lower division of the hundred of WORMELOW, county of HEREFORD, 4½ miles (N. W. by W.) from Ross, containing 577 inhabitants. The living is a perpetual curacy, annexed to the vicarage of Lugwardine, in the archdeaconry and diocese of Hereford. The chapel is dedicated to St. Dubritius.

HENTON, a liberty in the parish of CHINNOR, hundred of LEWKNOR, county of OXFORD, 4¼ miles (S. E. by E.) from Thame, containing 232 inhabitants.

HEPPLE, a township in the parish of ROTHBURY, western division of COQUETDALE ward, county of NORTHUMBERLAND, 5½ miles (W. by S.) from Rothbury, containing 111 inhabitants.

HEPPLE-DEMESNE, a township in the parish of ROTHBURY, western division of COQUETDALE ward, county of NORTHUMBERLAND, containing, with White-field House, 45 inhabitants.

HEPSCOT, a township in that part of the parish of MORPETH which is in the eastern division of CASTLE ward, county of NORTHUMBERLAND, $2\frac{1}{4}$ miles (S. E.) from Morpeth, containing 164 inhabitants.

HEPTONSTALL, a chapelry in the parish of HALIFAX wapentake of MORLEY, West riding of the county of YORK, $8\frac{1}{4}$ miles (W. by N.) from Halifax, containing 4543 inhabitants. The living is a perpetual curacy, in the archdeaconry and diocese of York, endowed with £800 private benefaction, £600 royal bounty, and £1700 parliamentary grant, and in the patronage of the Vicar of Halifax. The chapel, dedicated to St. Thomas à Becket, has recently been erected, and contains one thousand and thirty-one sittings, of which seven hundred and thirty-three are free, and towards defraying the expense of which the Incorporated Society for enlarging churches contributed £1000. A grammar school was founded and endowed in 1642, by the Rev. Charles Greenwood, the income of which is about £77 per annum; from sixty to seventy children are instructed on moderate terms, seventeen of whom are taught the classics gratuitously: the usher receives £5. 11. 4. per annum, bequeathed by Abraham Wall in 1638, for teaching poor children to read and write. Here are extensive cotton manufactories.

HEPWORTH, a parish in the hundred of BLACKBOURN, county of SUFFOLK, $4\frac{1}{2}$ miles (W. by S.) from Botesdale, containing 523 inhabitants. The living is a discharged rectory, in the archdeaconry of Sudbury, and diocese of Norwich, rated in the king's books at £13. 17. $3\frac{1}{2}$., and in the patronage of the Provost and Fellows of King's College, Cambridge. The church is dedicated to St. Peter.

HEPWORTH, a township in the parish of KIRK-BURTON, upper division of the wapentake of AGBRIGG, West riding of the county of YORK, $7\frac{3}{4}$ miles (S. by E.) from Huddersfield, containing 1048 inhabitants. Here is a place of worship for Wesleyan Methodists.

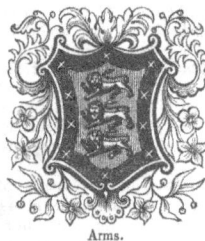

Arms.

HEREFORD, an ancient city, having separate jurisdiction, locally in the hundred of Grimsworth, county of HEREFORD, of which it is the chief town, 135 miles (W. N. W.) from London, containing, exclusively of the townships of Lower Bullingham and Grafton, which are in the hundred of Webtree, 9090 inhabitants. This place is thought to have derived its origin from a Roman station in the neighbourhood, named *Ariconium*, supposed to be the present Kenchester, and its more recent name of *Her-ford*, or *Here-ford*, which is pure Saxon, importing "a military ford," from its having been, previously to the erection of the bridge, a pass over the river Wye, on the bank of which it is situated. Hereford is said to have become the seat of an episcopal see before the invasion of Britain by the Saxons; and, in 655, Oswy, King of Mercia, made it part of the diocese of Lich-

field, which then included the whole Mercian kingdom. At a synod held here by Theodore, Archbishop of Canterbury, in 673, the division of the diocese of Lichfield was decreed, to which Wilford, then bishop of that see, refused assent, and was subsequently deprived of part of his diocese for contumacy; but with the consent of *Sexulph*, his successor, Hereford was disunited from Lichfield, and restored to its original independence as a distinct diocese, and Putta, who previously held the see of Rochester, was made bishop in 680. It was the capital of the kingdom of Mercia, and possessed a large church in the reign of Offa, who, it is stated, founded the cathedral in expiation of the murder of Ethelbert, King of the East Angles, whose body was removed hither from its original place of sepulture in 782. In the reign of Athelstan the city occupied an area of eighteen hundred yards in circuit, and, with the exception of an extent of five hundred and fifty yards guarded by the river, which formed a natural barrier, was surrounded with walls sixteen feet in height, in which were six gates and fifteen embattled towers thirty-four feet high: to these fortifications, which were nearly perfect in Leland's time, a castle was added by Edward the Elder. About 1055, a battle was fought two miles from this place between Ralph, Earl of Hereford, and Griffith, Prince of Wales, in which the former was defeated; and the Welch, having taken the city, massacred the inhabitants, and reduced it to a heap of ruins. Harold, afterwards king, marched against the Welch, whom he attacked and defeated with great slaughter: he then repaired the fortifications and enlarged the castle, to secure the city against the future inroads of the invaders. From the earliest period the citizens have enjoyed a high reputation for loyalty, and Hereford has in consequence become the scene of many sanguinary conflicts and sieges: it held out successfully against the first attack of Stephen, who was opposed by Milo, son of Walter, constable of England, for which service the latter was made Earl of Hereford, by the Empress Maud, in 1141: the patent, which is still extant, was the first ever granted for the creation of an earl: but in the same year Stephen, having again laid siege to the city, reduced it, and divested Milo of his recent honours. The great council of the realm assembled here to decide on the deposition of Edward II.; and here likewise Hugh le Despencer, the Earl of Arundel, and three others, were executed. At the commencement of the parliamentary war, Hereford was garrisoned for the king, but on the approach of an army under Sir William Waller, in April 1643, it surrendered without opposition: on the subsequent retreat of Waller, it was again occupied by a party of royalists, who, under the governorship of Barnabas Scudamore, Esq., made a gallant defence against the Scots, commanded by the Earl of Leven, who was forced to raise the siege. The city was subsequently the scene of some minor transactions during the war, and was ultimately taken by stratagem, when the castle was dismantled, and the fortifications levelled, by order of the parliament. At the Restoration, the inhabitants received from Charles II. a new charter, with extended privileges, also new heraldic bearings, emblematical of fidelity to the royal cause.

The city occupies a gentle eminence on the northern bank of the river Wye, and is surrounded by a fertile tract of country, consisting of orchards, with rich arable and pasture land : the environs, especially along the banks of the river, are celebrated for picturesque beauty. The principal streets are wide and airy ; and, together with the lanes and passages, are well lighted with gas, and paved under the provisions of an act of parliament : the town is also abundantly supplied with water. The houses in general are good, and during the last fifty years considerable improvements have been made in the general appearance of the place. A bridge of six arches was erected over the river Wye, about the end of the fifteenth century, replacing a wooden bridge built in the reign of Henry I. The Hereford reading society was established in 1796 ; and, in 1815, a permanent library, containing a valuable collection of ancient and modern works, was instituted by the late Benjamin Fallows, Esq. : it is under the direction of a president, treasurer, librarian, and a committee ; the subscription is 30s. per annum, and the number of members about one hundred and thirty. An agricultural society was established in 1797, and a horticultural society in 1826. The theatre, a commodious edifice in Broad-street, was erected about 1789. Races are held in August, when a gold cup, three plates of £50 each, and sweepstakes, are run for : the course comprises a circuit of two miles. Assemblies commence in October, and are held generally once a month during the winter season. The triennial music meetings of the choirs of Hereford, Worcester, and Gloucester, established in 1724, take place here during three days in September ; oratorios are performed in the morning at the cathedral, and in the evening miscellaneous concerts and balls are held at the county hall ; the receipts, after payment of the expenses, are appropriated to the benefit of the widows and orphans of the distressed clergy. A bowling-green is supported by subscription.

From the want of greater facility of communication, Hereford has never attained eminence in trade or manufactures : the principal articles of commerce are gloves of the best kinds, which are made in less quantities than formerly ; cider and hops, the latter of which are extensively cultivated in the vicinity ; and oak and oak-bark : a considerable quantity of timber and bark is annually sent to Chepstow, and shipped thence for Ireland, and the different ports and yards for ship-building in England. Salmon of excellent quality are caught in the river Wye, but not in so great abundance as formerly, when here, as elsewhere, a condition was inserted in the indentures of apprentices that they should not be compelled to eat it more than a certain number of days in the week. To remedy the inconvenience arising from the difficulty of navigation in the river, an act of parliament was obtained, in 1791, for cutting a canal to join the Severn at Gloucester ; but it has not been completed, only extending at present to Ledbury, and consequently Hereford derives no benefit from the undertaking. Coal is principally supplied from the Forest of Dean, in Gloucestershire, by conveyance up the Wye, which is navigable for barges of from eighteen to thirty tons (for towing which a path was made by act of parliament in 1809), and from the neighbourhood of Abergavenny, along a rail-road, to Monmouth Cap, thirteen miles hence. In 1826, an act was obtained to extend this rail-road to Hereford, which design having been completed, the supply of coal has been

materially increased, and the price considerably diminished : it is under the direction of three different companies, and is called the Llanfihangel, Grosmont, and Hereford tram-road. In 1668, the late Lord Scudamore left £400 to be lent without interest, in order to establish a woollen manufactory ; but not being applied for, it was put out to interest, and, in 1772, £500 was expended in an attempt to instruct a portion of the poorer class in spinning wool, which however failed : the remainder of this bequest has increased to £3000 three per cents. ; a portion of this trust money is occasionally lent to manufacturers of woollen cloth, flannel goods, &c., for a limited time, without interest, for finding employment for the poor inhabitants, especially women and children. The markets are on Wednesday, Friday, and Saturday ; and fairs are held on the Tuesday after Candlemas-day ; on the Wednesday in Easter week, for cattle and sheep ; May 19th ; July 1st, for wool : October 20th is a great fair for cattle and hops : at the May fair, granted by Henry I. to Bishop Richard, soon after 1120, and commonly known as the "nine days' fair," the bishop's bailiff, or bailiff of the manor called the Barton, or the Bishop's fee, has considerable power, but does not exercise magisterial authority. As lords of this fee the bishops formerly exercised considerable authority in the city ; they administered justice within its limits, and had a prison within the walls of their palace ; they also held courts baron, leet, and pie-powder, but most of these privileges have become obsolete. In 1816, an act of parliament was passed for forming a market-place, and effecting other improvements, which contained a clause providing accommodation for slaughtering cattle ; and, in 1822, fourteen slaughter-houses were erected, on the site of part of the old city wall, northward of the market-place ; the fish-market is well supplied with sea fish from Wales and Bristol.

Corporate Seal.

The city was first incorporated by charter of Richard I., dated at Westminster in 1189, and has since that period received twenty-four confirmatory charters from successive monarchs, under the last of which, the government was vested in a mayor, high steward, deputy steward (who performs the duty of recorder), two chamberlains, six aldermen, and twenty-four chief citizens, assisted by a town clerk, coroner, sword bearer, and four serjeants at mace, and other officers. The mayor is annually chosen from the body corporate, the members of which usually succeed by rotation, on the first Monday in August, and is sworn into office on the first Monday after the festival of St. Michael. The high steward, who is generally a nobleman, holding the office for life, appoints a deputy learned in the law : the chamberlains and the coroner are appointed by the corporation. The mayor (who is keeper of the city gaol and clerk of the market, which offices he may execute by deputy), the late mayor (who acts as escheator for the year after his mayoralty), the high steward, the deputy steward, and the six aldermen, are justices of the peace within the city and liberties. The freedom of the city is inherited by the eldest sons of freemen, acquired by servitude within the city, marriage with a freeman's widow, and with the eldest daughter of a freeman, provided he has no male issue, by gift of the corporation, or by purchase, the usual fee being £33. 11. 9. The corporation hold quarterly courts of session, and meetings daily at the guildhall, for determining on affairs of police ; and a court of record on the Monday and Thursday in every week, for the recovery of debts to any amount, under the charter of James I., confirmed by William III. The county assizes are held here, likewise the petty sessions for the hundred of Grimsworth every Saturday ; and, under certain restrictions, those of Oyer and Terminer for the whole of South Wales. The old town and shire-hall, erected in the reign of James I., is a large edifice of timber and brick, supported on twenty-seven pillars of solid oak : it formerly contained an upper story, in which were chambers for the fourteen different trading companies of the city, but has been much reduced in height and beauty, and, though formerly appropriated, by consent of the corporation, as proprietors of it, to the courts of assize, session, and public meetings for the county, was surrendered to that body in 1817. The new shire-hall was erected by act of parliament passed in the 55th of George III., authorising a sum not exceeding £30,000 to be raised, for the purpose of building courts of justice, county hall, &c., together with a depôt for arms and military clothing, including the purchase of an appropriate site ; also a further sum of £3150, to purchase a house for the accommodation of the judges. This edifice has been completed from a design by Mr. Smirke : the portico in front is a fine specimen of Grecian Doric architecture, copied from the Temple of Theseus at Athens: a subterraneous passage, through which prisoners are brought to the bar, leads to the Crown court, from an apartment beneath the grand jury room, in which they are kept during the trials : the hall is decorated with portraits of George III. and the late Duke of Norfolk, and here the quarter sessions, county meetings, and the triennial musical festivals, are held. The city gaol is an ancient building, the original part containing seven cells for felons, and three sleeping-rooms for debtors ; to which an addition has recently been made, comprising four cells for males, and three for females, with spacious airing-yards. The county gaol was erected in 1798, upon Mr. Howard's plan, and occupies the site of St. Guthlac's priory, at the foot of Aylestone hill, being enclosed by a brick wall : the entrance, over which is the place of execution, is ornamented with Tuscan pillars : the prison contains appropriate apartments for the classification of prisoners of both sexes, with day-rooms, court-yard, inspection-room, a newly-built penitentiary, infirmary, chapel, work-rooms, a room for the meeting of the county magistrates, and apartments for the gaoler and his family : the inspecting-room is about eighteen yards in diameter, nearly circular, and having six windows, which open into each court : the total expense of erecting it was £22,461. 7. 5., and the annual expenditure of the establishment is estimated at from £2000 to £3000. The elective franchise was conferred in the 23d of Edward I., since which time the city has regularly returned two members to parliament : the right of election is vested in the freemen generally, nearly one thousand in number : the mayor is the returning officer.

Arms of the Bishoprick.

The diocese of Hereford includes nearly the whole of the county, with part of Shropshire, four parishes in Monmouthshire, six in Montgomeryshire, six in Radnorshire, and twenty-one in Worcestershire. The ecclesiastical establishment consists of a bishop, dean, two archdeacons, six canons residentiary (of whom the dean is one), a precentor, chancellor, treasurer, twenty-eight prebendaries, twelve priests-vicars, one of whom is custos, four lay clerks, eight choristers, a head and under master of the grammar school, an organist, and other officers. The cathedral, originally erected in expiation of the murder of Ethelbert, and dedicated to St. Mary and St. Ethelbert, was built by Melfrid, a viceroy under Egbert, about 825, principally by means of the propitiating gifts of Offa, but having fallen into decay in less than two centuries, it was rebuilt during the prelacy of Bishop Athelstan, or Ethelstan, between 1012 and 1015 ; it was subsequently destroyed by fire, and lay in ruins till 1079, when Bishop Robert de Lezinga, appointed to this see by William the Conqueror, commenced a new edifice, erected on the model of the church of Aken, now Aix la Chapelle, which was completed by Bishop Raynelm in 1107, with the exception of the tower, that having been built by Bishop Giles de Braos in the following century. It is a noble cruciform structure, with a lofty tower rising from the intersection, formerly surmounted by a spire, which has been taken down. The tower at the west end fell down in 1785, at which time the west front was rebuilt in a style different from the original, and the north porch, built by Bishop Booth in the sixteenth century, and various additions made by his predecessors since its original elevation, have given to the exterior of this edifice a great variety of architectural style. The nave, which is of Norman architecture, is separated from the aisles by massive circular columns and arches, above which are the triforium and clerestory, which were altered at the time of its being repaired. The north transept is a rich specimen of the early English, with large windows in the decorated style, having a triforium of exquisite beauty, and trefoiled circular clerestory windows. The choir, which is handsome and well proportioned, is of the Norman character, intermixed with the early English style: the bishop's throne and the stalls are surmounted by ornamented canopies of tabernacle-work ; and a very rich altar-piece was put up in 1816, the subject of which is Christ bearing the Cross, a copy, by Leeming, from the original picture over the altar in the chapel of Magdalene College, Oxford : the east window, forty feet high and twenty feet wide, representing the Lord's Supper, is considered the largest in this branch of the art since its revival in England : the figures are fifteen feet in height, beautifully painted by Mr. Backler, from West's picture of the Lord's Supper, at an expense of £2000, towards defraying which the late Dr. Cope, canon residentiary, bequeathed £500 : near the choir was the shrine of St. Ethelbert, which was destroyed during the usurpation of Cromwell. The arched roof of the upper transverse aisle is supported by a single column. Eastward of the choir is the Lady chapel, in the early style of English architecture, but of a character different from that of the transept, now used as a library, and containing a valuable collection of books: beneath this chapel is a fine crypt, called Golgotha, from the mass of human bones which it contained; it is supposed to have been originally the parochial church of St. John the Baptist. There are some beautiful chapels in the later style of English architecture, built by Bishop Audley and other prelates. The whole length of the interior of the cathedral, from east to west, is three hundred and twenty-five feet; of the great transept, from north to south, one hundred and forty feet; the height, from the area pavement to the vaulting, ninety-one feet, and the height of the central tower, two hundred and forty-four feet. The cathedral contains monuments to the memory of thirty-four bishops of this see: the most ancient is that of Bishop Walter, who was consecrated by the Pope in the year 1060: there is likewise a splendid monument of Dr. Tyler, Bishop of Llandaff, and Dean of Hereford; and another of Sir Richard Pembridge, Knight of the Garter in the reign of Edward III. On the east side of the transept is a monument to the memory of Bishop Cantelupe, who died in 1282; his heart was brought to Hereford, and buried in the cathedral, and he was canonized in 1310; it is curiously adorned with a number of effigies, but is now somewhat mutilated: this tomb was a place of resort and reputed miraculous efficacy to pilgrims from all parts of Europe, no less than four hundred and twenty-five miracles having, according to monkish story, been performed here: in consequence, the succeeding bishops of this diocese relinquished their ancient arms, which were those of St. Ethelbert, in order to assume the paternal coat of Cantelupe, which is continued at the present time. At the north-eastern extremity of the transept is a monument in memory of Velters Cornwall, Esq., representative in parliament of the county of Hereford for forty-six years; and amongst many others is a plain marble tablet to the memory of John Philips, the well-known author of poems entitled " The Splendid Shilling " and " Cyder." The bishop's palace is an ancient structure westward of the cathedral, containing several elegant apartments, with a fine garden and grounds attached; it has also a handsome chapel, built by Bishop Butler, and completed in 1798. Near the palace was a Saxon edifice of very early date and curious structure, consisting of two stories, which were severally used as chapels, and dedicated to St. Catherine and St. Mary Magdalene: being in a ruinous condition, it was taken down in 1737. Of the chapter-house, only a very small portion remains: the chapter meetings are now held in a building attached to the south aisle of the cathedral, in which is an ancient map of the world upon vellum, illuminated with gilt Saxon characters; in the centre is an inscription in black letter and a representation of the city of Jerusalem: the date of this piece of antiquity is assigned to the reign of Henry III. Here also are preserved, in a neat frame, the ring, crosier, and balla, of Bishop Frilleck, who died in 1360; they were discovered in digging a grave in the choir, in August 1813. The deanery is near the church, and four houses adjacent, in the gift of the bishop, are usually appropriated as residences for the prebendaries. There is also a good house of stone, with a spacious garden, in St. John's street, for the chancellor of the choir; and attached to the bishop's prebend is a very good house in Broad-street. The college is a brick building of the time of Edward IV., forming a quadrangle eastward of the cathedral, with which it communicates by a cloister one hundred feet in length, leading to the south end of the eastern transept: this edifice contains a chapel, a library, a spacious hall, common dining-room, and dormitories: in 1820, several attempts were made by some undiscovered incendiary to destroy this college by fire.

The city comprises the parishes of All Saints, St. John the Baptist, St. Martin, St. Nicholas, St. Owen, and St. Peter, all in the peculiar jurisdiction of the Dean of Hereford. The living of All Saints' is a discharged vicarage, consolidated with that of St. Martin's, rated in the king's books at £8. 10., and in the patronage of the Dean and Canons of Windsor: the church is an ancient structure partly in the Norman style of architecture, with a tower strengthened with buttresses and surmounted by a lofty spire: the nave is separated from the aisles by circular columns and pointed arches; and the interior contains a fine altar-piece, and some ancient stalls supposed to have been appropriated to the brethren of St. Anthony, to whom this church anciently belonged. The living of St. John the Baptist's is a discharged vicarage, rated in the king's books at £7. 12. 1., endowed with £200 private benefaction, and £400 royal bounty, and in the patronage of the Dean and Chapter of Hereford: the north transept of the cathedral was, in 1796, appropriated as a church for this parish. The living of St. Martin's is a discharged vicarage, united to that of All Saints': the church, which stood on the bank of the Wye, near the bridge, was destroyed during the parliamentary war: it is now in contemplation to restore it, through the persevering exertions of the Rev. H. J. Symons, L.L.D., the present vicar, for which purpose a grant has been obtained from the Incorporated Society for building churches, &c., another from government, of £1000, and a donation of £100 from the Bishop of the diocese. The living of the parish of St. Nicholas is a discharged rectory, rated in the king's books at £10, endowed with £200 royal bounty, and £400 parliamentary grant, and in the patronage of the Crown: the church, which previously to the dissolution had two chantries in honour of the Virgin, is an ancient edifice with a tower. The living of St. Owen's is a rectory, united to the vicarage of St. Peter's, and rated in the king's books at £4. 10. 10.: the church was destroyed during the parliamentary war in the reign of Charles I. The living of St. Peter's is a discharged vicarage, with the rectory of St. Owen's, rated in the king's books at £10. 0. 2., and in the patronage of the Rev. H. Gipps: the church, an ancient structure founded in 1070, in the Norman style of architecture, with a tower surmounted by a neat spire, was repaired and partly rebuilt in 1793: the nave is separated from the south aisle by octagonal pillars, and from the north by clustered columns, and the chancel contains stalls which were anciently appropriated to the brethren of St. Guthlac's priory; previously to the dissolution there were four chantries in the church. There are places of worship for the Society of Friends, Independents, those in the late Countess of Huntingdon's Connexion, Wesleyan Methodists, and a Roman Catholic chapel.

The college grammar school is of ancient foundation :

the earliest authentic document extant is the appointment of Ricardus de Cornwaille as master, by Bishop Gilbert, in 1385, owing to the refusal of the chancellor, with whom the appointment then rested. The school was placed under the control of the Dean and Chapter, and a head and under master were appointed, by statute of Queen Elizabeth, in the first year of her reign, which received confirmation from Charles I., when he gave to the cathedral the "Caroline Statutes," by which £4 per annum is payable to a scholar in the University of Oxford. The scholarships attached to this school are, four founded by Dean Langford, of which two are at Brasenose College, Oxford, of the value of £40 per annum each, arising from the rental of a house in High Town, Hereford, devised by Roger Philpotts in 1615; five in St. John's College, Cambridge, founded by deed enrolled in the Exchequer in 1682, by Sarah, Duchess of Somerset, the scholars to be chosen within forty days after each vacancy, by the Master and Fellows of that college, preference being given to natives of Somersetshire, Wiltshire, and Herefordshire. Her Grace likewise bequeathed her manor of Thornhill, in Wiltshire, to Brasenose College, Oxford, and that of Wootton-Rivers, in the same county, to St. John's College, Cambridge, by will dated May 17th, 1686, for founding scholarships; the candidates to be elected alternately from the schools of Marlborough, Hereford, and Manchester, for ever: the value of each is computed at £30 per annum, the number varying according to the revenue: provision is likewise made by the same noble lady for twelve other scholars, who receive £1. 4. per week, and are elected in a similar manner: she also left the valuable living of Wootton-Rivers, in the alternate presentation of the above-mentioned colleges, to one of her aforesaid scholars. The school, erected by the Dean and Chapter, under the statutes of Edward VI. and Elizabeth, stands on part of the decayed cloister, which was rebuilt in 1760, by subscription; it is eighty feet in length, forty wide, and forty in height: there are eleven scholars on the foundation, of whom seven are nominated as choristers by the canons, and four by the dean: the entire number of pupils is about one hundred, half of whom are boarded, the rest having the benefit of tuition only: the senior master receives £40 per annum, with a dwelling-house and other emoluments. Miles Smith, Bishop of Gloucester, the celebrated translator of the Bible; Gwillim, author of a system of Heraldry; John Davis, an eminent writing-master; and his pupil, Gethin, or Gerthinge, were educated in this school. The Blue-coat charity schools were established in 1710, for clothing and educating forty boys and thirty girls, and afterwards making some provision for them on leaving school, by collections and other contributions: the premises have lately been handsomely rebuilt, with houses for the master and the mistress. A school for freemen's sons was established in 1809, and is supported by an annual contribution of £35 from the chief steward, the Rt. Hon. Earl Somers, aided by donations of £10 per annum each from the two city members, and from Sir Robert Price, one of the representatives for the county. A National school for girls is supported by voluntary contributions; there was formerly one for boys, which has been discontinued. A female adult school, established in 1816, affords instruction to about one hundred persons, who assemble twice a week, and are gratuitous-

ly taught to read by ladies. About three hundred and fifty children of the parishes of St. Peter and St. Owen are instructed, partly clothed, and supplied with Bibles and prayer-books, in Sunday schools. There is also an infant school, established in 1825, which contains upwards of one hundred children.

The general infirmary originated in a benefaction of £500 by the late Rev. Dr. Talbot, rector of Ullingswick, in this county, which was followed by ample subscriptions from the nobility, clergy, and gentry, of the city and county, with various donations and legacies: the ground on which the building stands was the gift of the late Earl of Oxford; the late Dr. Harris, Chancellor of this diocese, bequeathed £5000 towards the support of the institution, and the annual subscriptions amount to nearly £700: two physicians. and two surgeons attend daily, an apothecary resides in the house, and the expense of a regular chaplain is defrayed by the contributions of the bishop, the members of the cathedral, and the clergy of the city. The institution commenced March 26th, 1776, but the building was not open for the admission of patients for some years after: it is calculated to accommodate seventy persons, with every appropriate convenience for the requisite attendants, and is under the superintendence of governors, who are subscribers of £2. 2. per annum, or contributors of £20. The lunatic asylum occupies part of the ground given for the infirmary, and is under the direction of the committee of that institution: it was erected by subscription, and opened in 1801: it is calculated for the reception of twenty patients, and is under the superintendence of a physician and a surgeon. There is a charity for assisting the necessitous widows and orphans of clergymen, and likewise clergymen themselves, disabled by age or infirmity, with narrow incomes; it is supported by annual subscriptions both of the clergy and laity of the archdeaconry. A lying-in charity was instituted in 1806. St. Ethelbert's hospital was built and endowed in the reign of Henry III., for the maintenance of ten poor persons, to be nominated and governed by a master, who is the treasurer of the cathedral, if residentiary, but the present master is the senior canon: the inmates receive 1s. 6d. weekly in summer, and 2s. 6d. in winter, and each of them has a garden. St. Giles's hospital, founded by Richard II. in 1290, for monks of the order of Savigny, and afterwards Knights Templars, was rebuilt in 1770, and contains apartments for five poor men, each of whom receives 5s. per week. Williams's hospital was founded about 1601, for six poor men, who have a weekly allowance of 17s. 6d. each. This hospital and St. Giles's are in the patronage of the Corporation; and there is a chapel common to both, in which divine service is performed twice a week. Lazarus', or sick man's, hospital, originally a religious foundation for lazars, is now appropriated to the reception of six poor widows, among whom £17. 10. is annually divided by direction of the mayor and corporation. Price's hospital was founded in 1636, by W. Price, merchant of London, for twelve poor men, and a chaplain, who performs duty thrice a week and has a salary of £10 per annum: each inmate receives 10s. per week: the institution is under the care of the mayor and aldermen. Trinity hospital was founded by Thomas Kerry, Esq., in 1600, for one corporal, two poor unmarried men, and twelve widows, each receiving 5s. per week: the

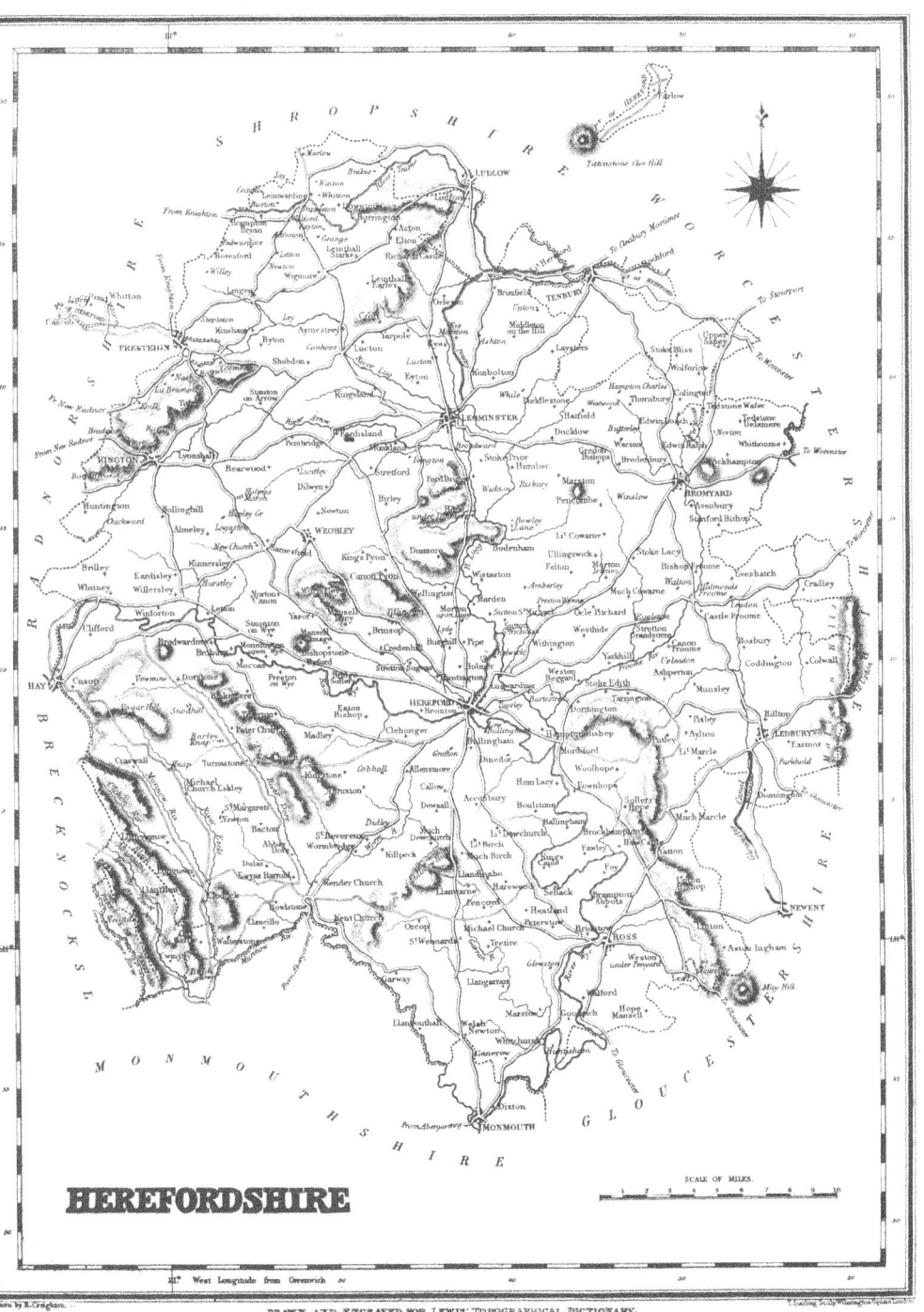

HEREFORDSHIRE

SCALE OF MILES.

Drawn by R. Creighton.

DRAWN AND ENGRAVED FOR LEWIS' TOPOGRAPHICAL DICTIONARY.

present building was erected by subscription in 1825, and contains sixteen dwellings; it is under the superintendence of the mayor and corporation, who are governors. Coningsby's hospital was founded by Sir Thomas Coningsby, Knt., in 1614: it stands on the site of a small building and chapel formerly belonging to the Knights Hospitallers of St. John of Jerusalem, and contains twelve apartments, a chapel, and a hall: the master is styled, according to the founder's will, Corporal Coningsby, and the ten members, servitors: the corporal and five servitors must have performed at least three years' actual service as soldiers, and be natives of the counties of Hereford, Worcester, or Salop; the remaining five to be old men of seven years' service in the ranks: the allowances are £20 per annum to the chaplain, £1. 13. 4. per month to the corporal, £1. 1. 8½. per month to each of the servitors, with a scarlet suit of clothes and a hat every second year, and a scarlet cloak every third year: an excellent garden is attached to the building. The vicarage of Bodenham, in this county, with all its appurtenances, is, by the founder's will, appropriated to the successive chaplains. The Hampton Court estate, in this county, is charged with the support of this hospital, and the holder of it is the governor; the judges of assize are visitors of the institution. Symonds's almshouse was founded in 1695, for four decayed housekeepers, who receive 10s. per quarter each, chargeable on an estate at Breinton, the proprietor of which is patron of the charity. In addition to these are, Weaver's hospital for five poor persons, who receive £2. 13. per annum each; and Shelley's hospital, founded about 1640, and rebuilt in 1801, for six poor widows, who receive £5 per annum each: there are also various other minor charities of different kinds. In the reign of Henry VIII., John Phillips, citizen of Hereford, gave lands and tenements of the clear yearly value of £28. 1. 4., to exempt all persons from the payment of toll at the several gates of the city. In the reign of Mary, Sir Thomas White, alderman of London, gave the sum of £100 to each of twenty-four cities, of which Hereford is one, to be lent to young freemen, and a further sum of £4 to the mayor, for executing this trust. George Cope, D.D., who died in 1821, was an extensive benefactor to this city, having bequeathed £1000 to the Dean and Chapter, in trust to distribute the interest annually among ten aged single women of virtuous character; £500 towards erecting a window of stained glass for the east end of the choir, or west end of the nave, of the cathedral; £200, the interest to provide an eighth chorister under certain conditions; £200 to the general infirmary; £200, the interest to provide fuel for the poor of St. Ethelbert's hospital at Christmas; £300, the interest to be paid to the poor of St. Peter's parish; £1000, for equal division between four benevolent institutions; £300, the interest to be paid to the poor of Madley; £300 to the poor of Bromyard; £200 to those of Allansmore; and £200 to those of Selleck and King's Castle.

Prior to the Reformation, Hereford contained several monastic establishments. A college of Grey friars was founded in the reign of Edward I., by Sir William Pembridge, Knt.: amongst the many distinguished persons buried in it was Owen Tudor, otherwise Meredith, father of Edmund, Earl of Richmond, and grandfather of Henry VII., who, according to tradition, was interred

in the nave of the church, without any monumental memorial. St. Guthlac's priory, originally a college of Prebendaries, afterwards became a cell to the Benedictine abbey of St. Peter, at Gloucester; the revenue, at the dissolution, was £121. 3. 3.: the new county gaol and house of correction now occupies the site. The monastery of Black friars, the largest and most celebrated of all the ancient religious houses, was originally established under the auspices of William, brother of Bishop Cantelupe, and situated in the Portfield, in Bye-street suburb, but afterwards removed to Widemarsh suburb, where a new church and priory were commenced, in the reign of Edward II., and completed in that of Edward III., who, with his son, the Black Prince, two archbishops, and several bishops and nobles, were present at the dedication: it became a flourishing institution, and many persons of distinction were interred in the church. The only remaining vestiges of the ancient buildings are the south side of the prior's lodgings, some decayed offices, and a curious ancient stone pulpit, which has been much admired. About a mile westward from the city is the "White Cross," built by Dr. Lewis Charleton, afterwards bishop of this see, about 1347, as a market-place for the country people, during the ravages of an infectious disorder with which the city was at that time visited. According to tradition, reservoirs of vinegar were placed on each side of the cross, for the purification of articles brought from the city, and suspected to be infectious: the base of the cross consists of an hexagonal flight of seven steps; the lower and only remaining part of the shaft is hexagonal, six feet high, and two feet wide, exclusively of a pillar between each side, in which are as many niches, with shields, and lions rampant: above is an embattled parapet, with mouldings and base of the upper division; the present entire height is fifteen feet. Hereford has given birth to several eminent persons, amongst whom are, John Breton, L.L.D., bishop of the diocese in the thirteenth century, who wrote a celebrated work called "The Laws of England;" David Garrick, the inimitable comedian, who was born at the Angel Inn, Widemarsh-street, in 1716, his father bearing at that time a lieutenant's commission in a regiment of horse quartered here; and the famous Eleanor Gwyn, favourite of Charles II., who was born in an humble dwelling in Pipe-lane, in this city.

HEREFORDSHIRE, an inland county, bounded on the north by the county of Salop, on the north-east and east by the county of Worcester, on the south-east by the county of Gloucester, on the south-west by the county of Monmouth, on the west by the county of Brecknock, and on the north-west by the county of Radnor: it extends from 51° 53′ 7″ to 52° 29′ 43″ (N. Lat.), and from 2° 28′ 30″ to 3° 19′ 32″ (W. Lon.); and contains, with the detached parts, about five hundred and fifty thousand four hundred acres, or eight hundred and sixty square miles. The population, in 1821, amounted to 103,243. At the period when the Romans, under Claudius, penetrated into this part of Britain, the present county of Hereford, or the greater part of it, formed the most easterly portion of the territory inhabited by that warlike tribe the Silures, whose valour, combined with the natural obstacles of a mountainous district, opposed such a powerful impediment to the Roman conquests in this quarter.

The defeat of Caractacus is thought to have taken place in the vicinity of an eminence called Coxwall Knoll, situated near Brampton-Bryan, and on the line of boundary between this county and Shropshire; but it was not until twenty years after that event, and almost one hundred and twenty after the first Roman invasion, that Herefordshire was finally subjugated by Julius Frontinus: it was afterwards included in the Roman province *Britannia Secunda.* For some time after the establishment of the Saxon kingdom of Mercia, this county being situated nearly on the frontier between that kingdom and the territory still possessed by the descendants of the ancient Britons, it was frequently the scene of war and devastation, and appears to have been alternately in the possession of the contending parties. At length Offa, King of Mercia, having repulsed the Britons in one of their invasions, crossed the river Severn, which had hitherto been the boundary between the Britons and the Saxons, and formed a new line of demarcation by his famous dyke, called in the British language *Clawdd Offa* (considerable remains of it being still visible), by which part of the present county of Monmouth, nearly the whole of that of Hereford, and parts of those of Radnor and Salop, were wrested from the Britons, and annexed to the kingdom of Mercia. Soon after its completion, however, the Britons routed Offa's army on the Mercian side of this rampart, but were finally compelled to retire beyond it. At Sutton, about three miles north-east from Hereford, that sovereign erected and fortified a palace, which was afterwards the scene of his treacherous murder of Ethelbert, King of the East-Angles. When the Danish fleet entered the Severn, during the administration of Ethelfleda, Countess of Mercia, the Danes advanced along the banks of the Wye, until they were attacked by a provincial force collected from Hereford and the neighbouring places, when they were defeated with great slaughter, those who escaped being driven into Wales, and made prisoners by the Britons. The Danes and the Saxons, however, continued their occasional hostilities; but King Edward the Elder defeated the former, and frustrated the attempts of the latter upon this county. In the reign of Ethelred, the Danes again desolated this part of the country. In that of Edward the Confessor, the Britons ravaged the English frontier, which had then acquired the name of the Marches, and included a considerable part of this county; they were opposed by the garrison in the castle of Hereford, but carried off much plunder. In this reign also, Gryffyth, a prince of Wales, accompanied by Algar, Earl of Chester, whom the king had banished, proceeded into Herefordshire, and laid it waste; they defeated Ranulph, Earl of Hereford, within two miles of the city, which they afterwards entered, burning the cathedral, and killing seven of the canons, who offered resistance: they also put to death many persons of rank, set the city on fire, levelled its walls, and then retired into Wales laden with spoil. In revenge for this outrage, Edward sent Harold, son of Earl Godwin, against the Britons, who led part of his army to Hereford, which he strongly fortified.

In the reign of William the Conqueror, Edric, surnamed the Forester, son of Alfric, Earl of Mercia, whose lands had been repeatedly ravaged by the Norman garrison of Hereford, having formed an alliance with Blethyn and Rywalhon, princes of Wales, with their assistance laid waste the county as far as the bridge of Hereford. In the contest between Stephen and Matilda, Geoffrey de Talebot and Robert, Earl of Gloucester, who had large possessions here, declared for the Empress. Talebot reduced and totally demolished the castle of Weobley, which had been garrisoned for Stephen; the king soon afterwards invested the city of Hereford, but appears to have speedily raised the siege. King John, when Prince Louis of France had landed with his army in England, retired to Hereford, in the vain hope of procuring succour. During the hostilities of the barons against his son, Henry III., Hereford was selected by them as the place of rendezvous: the king marched against them, but found this county so much impoverished from the continual devastations it had endured, that he was obliged to retreat to Gloucester for want of sustenance for his troops. Humphrey de Bohun, Earl of Hereford, being one of the confederated barons who afterwards rose against the same sovereign, with the Earl of Leicester at their head, Prince Edward, after the capture of himself and his father at Lewes, was conducted to Hereford, and left there in custody by the allied armies of Leicester and Llewellyn, Prince of Wales; and from that city it was that he made his escape previously to the decisive battle of Evesham. After the subjection of Wales to the English crown by Edward I., the Welch still occasionally made predatory incursions; and Edward found it necessary to issue orders for raising a body of infantry in Herefordshire, to check this petty warfare. Isabella, Queen of Edward II., advanced with an army as far as Hereford, when in pursuit of her unfortunate husband, who having been seized in Carmarthenshire, was conveyed to Ledbury in this county. Hereford was also the scene of the execution of his favourite, Hugh le Despencer, together with the Earl of Arundel and others. In the war between Henry IV. and Owen Glyndwr, the latter infesting the estate of the Earl of March amongst others, Sir Edmund Mortimer, uncle to that nobleman, led out the retainers of the family, and gave him battle, but his troops were routed, and himself made prisoner. At the same time, the earl himself, who had been allowed to return to his castle of Wigmore, and who, though yet a boy, led his followers into the field, fell also into Glyndwr's hands, and was carried into Wales, where Henry, from motives of policy, suffered him to remain in captivity; which wilful neglect on the part of the king occasioned the earl to join the league of Glyndwr with the Earl of Northumberland. In the early part of the contest between the houses of York and Lancaster, the Duke of York advancing into this county from Wales, with a force of twenty thousand men, met the Earls of Pembroke and Ormond, who had been detached by Queen Margaret to oppose him, and routed them with great slaughter on Candlemas-eve, in the year 1461, at a place called Mortimer's Cross, in the parish of Kingsland, about four miles south of Wigmore, the seat of the Mortimer family. Owen Tudor, husband of Catherine of France, having been taken prisoner in this castle, was afterwards beheaded at Hereford, with nine other officers. The incorporation of the Welch Marches with the adjoining counties, by act of parliament passed in the 27th of Henry VIII., added, or rather restored, a considerable extent of territory to Herefordshire: Wigmore, Stapleton, and Lugharness, on the northern side of the county, were appointed to constitute the hundred of Wigmore; and on the western side, Ewyas-Lacy was formed into the hundred of that name; Huntington, Clifford, Winforton, Eardisley, and Whitney, into the hundred of Huntington; and Ewyas-Harrold was added to that of Webtree.

From this period no very remarkable event bearing particular relation to this county occurred, until the commencement of the contest between Charles I. and the parliament, when the greater number of the principal Herefordshire families espoused the royal cause. The city of Hereford was garrisoned by the royalists, but surrendered without resistance to a parliamentarian force under Sir William Waller: it was soon after evacuated, and again garrisoned for the king, under Barnabas Scudamore. The Scottish army in the interest of the parliament, and under the orders of the Earl of Leven, was directed to retake it, and previously to the commencement of the siege, attacked and carried away by assault a post occupied by the royalists at Canon-Froome, near Ledbury: for this service the House of Commons ordered a letter of thanks to be written to the general; and a jewel of the value of £500 was presented to him as an earnest of the favour of both houses. After the defeat at Naseby, the king marched towards Hereford, in order to relieve it from the siege, or give battle to the Scots, who, after levying very heavy contributions throughout the county, at length raised the siege on the approach of Charles and his army from Worcestershire. At Hereford, the king assembled all his forces from Worcestershire, Shropshire, and South Wales, to attempt the relief of Bristol. In 1646, Hereford was taken by surprise, and, after considerable resistance from other places, the whole county was reduced by detachments of the parliamentary troops under the command of Sir William Waller, and of Colonel Birch, a very zealous and active officer.

The whole of this county, excepting the parishes of Clodock, Dulas, Ewyas-Harrold, Llancillo, Michael-Church-Eskley, Rowlstone, St. Margaret's, and Walterstone, (which are in the diocese of St. David,) is included in the diocese of Hereford, and province of Canterbury, and forms an archdeaconry, comprising the deaneries of Clun, Froome, Hereford, Irchenfield, Leominster, Ross, Weobley, and Weston, and containing two hundred and eighteen parishes, of which, eighty-three are rectories, eighty-four vicarages, and the remainder perpetual curacies. For civil purposes it is divided into the eleven hundreds of Broxash, Ewyas-Lacy, Greytree, Grimsworth, Huntington, Radlow, Stretford, Webtree, Wigmore, Wolphy, and Wormelow (Lower and Upper). Some detached parts are situated beyond its general outline: the township of Farlow is wholly isolated by Shropshire; that of Rochford by Worcestershire; Litton Hill by Radnorshire; and a considerable tract of land, called the Foothog, and a few acres on the Devaudon-hill, by Monmouthshire. On the other hand, the parish of Edwin-Loch, which forms part of Worcestershire, is surrounded by Herefordshire. This county contains the city of Hereford, the borough and market towns of Leominster and Weobley, and the market towns of Bromyard, Kington, Ledbury, Pembridge, and Ross. Two knights are returned for the shire, two representatives for the city, and two for each of the boroughs. The county members are elected at Hereford. Herefordshire is

included in the Oxford circuit: the assizes and general quarter sessions are held at Hereford, where stands the county gaol and house of correction: there are one hundred and thirty-six acting magistrates. The rates raised in this county for the year ending March 25th, 1827, amounted to £68,731. 17.; the expenditure to £69,433. 5., of which £57,423. 9. was applied to the relief of the poor. The Malvern hills form a kind of natural boundary on the eastern side of the county, and the Halterell, or Black mountains, rise to an equal elevation on its western border; from these and other eminences Herefordshire exhibits a scene of beauty and richness not surpassed by any other county in England. The river Wye, in particular, enriches and adorns a tract of this county, between forty and fifty miles in length, and the scenery on its banks is thought to excel any of a similar kind in the kingdom. The general character of the river, from its entrance into the county down to Hereford, is mild and pleasing, consisting of delightful reaches, with the most luxuriant landscapes on their sides; the bolder and more romantic features of the scenery of this river occur in its course below Hereford.

The climate, on the whole, is favourable to health and longevity; but it varies much in different districts and at different altitudes. The vicinity of Ross is the earliest as regards vegetation: the western and north-western parts of the county are the coldest, on account of their superior elevation, and their exposure to the westerly winds, which, blowing over the bleak mountains of Wales, are, in this part of the county, chill and ungenial. The general character of the soil is a mixture of marl and clay of great fertility, containing also a certain proportion of calcareous earth; below the surface are strata of limestone, often beautifully intersected by red and white veins, bearing some resemblance to calcareous spar: near Snodhill castle, in the hundred of Webtree, it becomes a kind of marble, and was in considerable use and estimation during part of the seventeenth century. Towards the western border of the county the soil is often cold and sterile, but still argillaceous and resting on nodules of impure limestone, or on a base of soft crumbling-stone, which perishes by exposure to air and frost. In many places in the eastern part of the county it is loose and shallow, covering stone of inferior value, provincially called dun-stone, the more favourable portions of which are found suitable to the culture of hops. Deep beds of fine gravel are more especially met with in the centre of the county, in the vicinity of the city of Hereford. The soil of a large portion of the hundred of Wormelow, on the south, consists of a light sand, which has been much improved by the use of lime as a manure. A clayey tract extends from Hereford towards Ledbury, and produces the most abundant crops of wheat in the county. About five hundred and twenty thousand acres of land are in cultivation. On the stiff clays with which Herefordshire abounds wheat is the principal crop, and a very considerable quantity is raised beyond the internal consumption, the surplus being sent every year chiefly to Worcester, Abergavenny, and Bristol. The greatest quantity of oats sown is in those parts approaching the Welch border, and on portions of the eastern border of the county. The average produce of wheat per acre is twenty bushels; that of bar-

3 B 2

ley about eighteen; and of oats and peas about twenty. Hop plantations exist in all parts of the county, but more especially on the Worcestershire side: five hundred weight are esteemed the fair produce of a provincial hop-acre, which contains two thousand poles, there being on an average two poles to each root. The plantations are more generally worked with the plough than with the spade. The most fertile meadow lands are on the banks of the Wye, the Frome, and the Lug; their herbage being of the very best quality. The vicinity of Bromyard produces cheese, which is brought to the market, and rivals the best Shropshire cheese; but this not being a dairy county, it is supplied from Wales with excellent butter, and with cheese from Shropshire and Gloucestershire. The cattle have long been esteemed superior to most breeds in England; they are of large size, sinewy form, and unusual neatness, and the prevailing colour is a reddish brown with white faces. At the Michaelmas fair at Hereford, where the show of oxen in thriving condition is remarkably fine, they are generally sold to the principal graziers of the counties near the metropolis, to be there fattened for the London market. Grazing and cattle-feeding are not generally practised, except for provincial consumption; but the rearing of oxen for the purposes of agriculture prevails. The oxen perform nearly half the ploughing, and the same proportion of the harvest work; and in situations where their labour is frequently required on hard roads they are shod with iron. The Herefordshire cow is comparatively small, and extremely delicate in her appearance. The provincial breed of sheep is termed the Ryeland, from the district so named lying partly in the county of Gloucester, and partly in this county, in the vicinity of Ross, which is particularly favourable to them from the dryness of the soil and the sweetness of the herbage. They are small and white-faced; in symmetry of form, and in the flavour of their flesh, they exceed most English sheep; and in the fineness of their wool they are unrivalled: the ewes weigh from nine to twelve and fourteen pounds per quarter, the wethers from twelve to sixteen and eighteen. The Ryeland sheep have been crossed with the New Leicester, to the advantage perhaps of the breeder who is situated on good land, but to the detriment of the wool. A cross has been advantageously made between the Ryeland and the real Spanish breed. To the barrenness of the pasture on which the Ryeland sheep usually feed, may in some degree be attributed the fineness of their wool, for the quality of it is immediately impaired by a copious supply of food. The sheep-shearing in Herefordshire is performed by women.

Plantations of fruit trees are found in every aspect and on every soil: these orchards, which form so important a part of the produce of Herefordshire, seem to have first acquired celebrity in the reign of Charles I., and the county has long been celebrated for its cider, a large quantity of which is sent to London and the other principal towns in the kingdom. The soil best adapted to the growth of most kinds of apple trees, and the best kinds of pear trees, is a deep rich loam, when under culture by the plough. An Agricultural Society was established in this county in 1797. Considerable quantities of saffron were formerly grown, but the culture of it in this county has long been discontinued. The waste lands form a very inconsiderable

proportion of the extent of Herefordshire; the largest tract is on the east side of the Hatterell, or Black mountains, where the steepness of the hills, and the sterility of the soil, oppose powerful obstacles to improvement. Almost every part of the county abounds with woods and plantations, containing fine oak and elm trees. The northern side of it, including the Forests of Mocktree and Prestwood, has a greater abundance of fine oak than the southern parts, although large and valuable supplies of timber are produced in the latter. Some of the most extensive coppices are situated in the parishes of Fownhope, Woolhope, and Little Birch, and in the vicinity of Ledbury. They consist chiefly of oak, ash, and willow, and are generally cut down once in thirteen years; the ash is converted into hoops, which are in great demand within the county for the cider casks; the oak and the willow furnish hop-poles, while the blackpoles, which are those of larger size, and of oak only, are used as rafters, &c., in building.

Iron-ore is of very ancient discovery in the hundred of Wormelow, where many of the hand-blomeries used by the Romans, and considerable quantities of ore imperfectly smelted, have been found on Peterstow common; of late years, however, no iron has been manufactured in Herefordshire. There have been found red and yellow ochre, fullers' earth, and pipe-clay. The southern part of the county, and the city of Hereford, are supplied with coal from the pits in the Forest of Dean, in Gloucestershire; the Clee hills of Shropshire furnish the northern and eastern parts; and the western procure it occasionally from Abergavenny.

The principal rivers are the Wye, the Lug, the Munnow, the Arrow, the Frome, the Teme, and the Leddon. The Wye, having separated the counties of Brecknock and Radnor, enters Herefordshire between the parishes of Whitney and Clifford, and pursuing a south-easterly course, by Hereford and Ross, quits it at its southern extremity; the latter part of its course in Herefordshire being remarkably circuitous. This river is navigable up to Hereford for barges of from eighteen to thirty tons' burden, but the navigation is frequently interrupted by either a scarcity of water, or by the violence of the stream when swelled by the mountain torrents, which is often such as to make great alterations in the bed of the river, and sometimes occasions it to form new channels. The principal sea fish taken in the Wye is the salmon, which, however, is much less abundant than it was formerly, when it was a common clause in the indentures of children apprenticed in Hereford that they should not be compelled to eat salmon more than twice a week: its chief fresh water fish are pike, graylings, trout, perch, and eels. The Lug rises in Radnorshire, and enters the north-western border of this county near Stapleton castle, in the hundred of Wigmore, then taking a south-easterly direction, by Leominster, it falls into the Wye immediately below the village of Mordiford. In the year 1714 an attempt was made, by private subscription, to render this river navigable, and a few barges ascended it as far as Leominster; but a high flood following soon after, the locks, &c. which had been constructed were so materially injured, that no attempts to repair or renew the works had been made up to the year 1805. The sea fish common to the Wye are seldom found in the Lug; but the river fish are found alike in either. The Munnow rises on the Herefordshire side of the Hatterel mountains, and flowing southward, becomes the boundary between this county and Monmouthshire, and so continues until it passes Llanrothall and quits the county, falling into the Wye immediately below Monmouth : its principal fish are trout, gudgeons, eels, and cray-fish. The Arrow, so called from the swiftness of its stream, rises in Radnorshire, and entering this county near Kington, joins the Lug a few miles below Leominster : its fish are trout, graylings, and cray-fish. The Frome rises near Wolferlow, in the hundred of Broxash, and flowing southward, passes Bromyard, and falls into the Lug near Mordiford. The Teme, or Team, enters Herefordshire from the north-west, near Brampton-Bryan, and passes alternately through parts of this county and Shropshire; it then makes a considerable circuit in Worcestershire, but returns to Whitbourne, below the town of Bromyard, immediately after which it finally quits this county for Worcestershire. The Leadon, or Leddon, rises above Bosbury, in Radlow hundred, and passes the town of Ledbury, to which it gives name, a short distance below which it enters Gloucestershire. In consequence of the precariousness of the navigation of the Wye, an act of parliament was obtained, in the year 1791, for making a navigable canal from the city of Hereford, by the town of Ledbury, to the Severn at Gloucester, with a lateral cut to the collieries at Newent. The expense of constructing this canal, commonly called the Hereford and Glouces-ter canal, was found so much to exceed the original estimate of £69,000, that in 1807, when £105,000 had been expended upon it, the work, though completed on the Gloucestershire side, had made little progress in Herefordshire. Soon after the former, an act was ob-tained for another canal, from Kington to Leominster and Stourport, the chief articles of importation by which were stated to be lime and coal from Shropshire. A part of the line from Leominster to Stourport was completed in 1796; but the expense of this undertaking, like that of the former, was found so much to ex-ceed the estimate as to prevent the further progress of the work. The road from London to New Radnor en-ters the south-western border of the county from Glou-cester, and passes through Hereford and Kington.

The only remarkable Druidical relic in this county is Arthur's stone, in the parish of Dorstone; but British intrenchments are numerous. Two Roman towns are supposed, by the most respectable authorities, to have been situated within the limits of modern Herefordshire, those of *Ariconium* and *Magna* ; and with respect to their situations, the most probable opinion seems to be that of Horsley, that *Magna* was at Kenchester, where the circumvallation may still be traced, and *Ariconium* near Ross, in the parish of Weston *sub* Penyard, where the extent and limits are discernible by a blackness of soil, strikingly different from all around it; and where Roman coins have been occasionally found. Of the four Roman military roads in Britain, only that called Watling-street intersects this county : it enters it from Worcestershire, across the river Teme, at Leintwardine, and passing by Wigmore, Mortimer's Cross, Stretford, Kenchester, Kingstone, Dore-Abbey, and Longtown, en-ters Monmouthshire at a short distance beyond the latter place : the most perfect remains of it are on Four-ways common, near Madley, where it crosses the turnpike-road from Hereford. A vicinal way may also be traced

in a great part of its line, which enters the county from Worcester, and passes by Frome-hill, Stretton-Grand-some, Lugg-bridge, Holmer, and Stretton-Sugwas, to Kenchester. The cathedral of Hereford, and several of the parochial churches, exhibit specimens of Anglo-Saxon architecture. Prior to the Reformation there were twenty-one religious houses in this county, the principal remains of which are those of the abbeys of Dore and Wigmore. The castles were numerous ; the chief re-mains are those of Brampton-Bryan, Clifford, Hunting-ton, Goodrich, Kilpec, Longtown, Lyonshall, Wigmore, and Wilton castles. Several petrifying or encrusting springs exist in such hilly parts as consist of argillaceous marl upon limestone. The custom of decking the grave with flowers after an interment is general in Hereford-shire, as it is throughout Wales. On the first of May it is customary to deck the houses with birchen boughs ; on the 29th of May to celebrate the Restoration with oak boughs ; and on Ascension-day with elm branches. On twelfth-day-eve thirteen small fires are lighted on the growing wheat, and cakes and liquor distributed on the spot, amid the loud invocations of the party for the prosperity of the owner, and for a plentiful crop ; this custom is well known under the name of wassailing. The parish feasts, or wakes, are held in the church-yards, on the Sunday after the festival of the saint to whom the church is dedicated.

HEREFORD (LITTLE), a parish in the hundred of WOLPHY, county of HEREFORD, 3 miles (W.) from Tenbury, containing, with Upton, 353 inhabitants. The living is a discharged vicarage, with the perpetual cu-racy of Ashford-Carbonell, in the peculiar jurisdiction and patronage of the Chancellor of the Choir in the Cathedral Church of Hereford, rated in the king's books at £6. 14. The church is dedicated to St. Mary Magdalene.

HERGESTS (BOTH), a township in the parish of KINGTON, hundred of HUNTINGTON, county of HERE-FORD, 1½ mile (S.W. by W.) from Kington, containing 145 inhabitants.

HERMITAGE, a parish and a detached portion of the liberty of FORDINGTON, situated between the divisions of Cerne and Sherborne, in the Dorchester di-vision of the county of DORSET, 7 miles (S. by E.) from Sherborne, containing 143 inhabitants. The living is a vicarage not in charge, with the rectory of Ryme-Intrinsica, in the peculiar jurisdiction of the Dean of Sarum, and in the patronage of the Crown. The church is dedicated to St. Mary.

HERNE, a parish in the hundred of BLEANGATE, lathe of ST. AUGUSTINE, county of KENT, 5¾ miles (N.E. by N.) from Canterbury, containing 1675 inhabit-ants. The living is a vicarage, in the peculiar juris-diction and patronage of the Archbishop of Canterbury, rated in the king's books at £20. 16. 3. The church, dedicated to St. Martin, has a tower and other portions in the early style of English architecture, with insertions in the later and decorated styles. There is a place of worship for Independents and Wesleyan Methodists. In the channel near the bay, numerous fragments of Roman earthenware have been found, supposed to be the vestiges of a cargo of pottery wrecked whilst the Romans were in Britain. At Herne Sheel is a pleasure fair on Easter Monday.

HERNHILL, a parish in the hundred of BOUGHTON

under BLEAN, lathe of SCRAY, county of KENT, 3½ miles (E. by S.) from Faversham, containing 477 inhabitants. The living is a vicarage, in the peculiar jurisdiction and patronage of the Archbishop of Canterbury, rated in the king's books at £15. The church, dedicated to St. Michael, is a handsome edifice, principally in the later style of English architecture, situated on a lofty eminence; it is divided within by clustered columns of Bethersden marble, of peculiar elegance.

HERRIARD, a parish in the hundred of BERMONDSPIT, Basingstoke division of the county of SOUTHAMPTON, 4¾ miles (S.S.E.) from Basingstoke, containing, with the tything of Southrop, 369 inhabitants. The living is a discharged vicarage, in the archdeaconry and diocese of Winchester, rated in the king's books at £7. 6. 5½., and in the patronage of Lord Bolton. The church is dedicated to St. Mary.

HERRINGBY, a parish in the eastern division of the hundred of FLEGG, county of NORFOLK, 3¼ miles (E. by S.) from Acle, containing, with the parish of Stokesby, 294 inhabitants. The living is a rectory united to that of Stokesby, in the archdeaconry and diocese of Norwich, rated in the king's books at £5. The church is dedicated to St. Ethelbert. A college, or hospital, under the title of God's poor almshouse, was founded here soon after 1475, pursuant to the will of Hugh Attefenne: at the dissolution its revenue was valued at £23. 6. 5.

HERRINGFLEET, a parish in the hundred of MUTFORD and LOTHINGLAND, county of SUFFOLK, 6 miles (N.W. by W.) from Lowestoft, containing 168 inhabitants. The living is a perpetual curacy, in the archdeaconry of Suffolk, and diocese of Norwich. John Leathes, Esq. was patron in 1824. The church is dedicated to St. Margaret. Mrs. Elizabeth Merry bequeathed £20 per annum for the education of poor children, of which the master receives £17, and £3 are appropriated to the purchase of books: twelve children are instructed gratuitously. In the reign of Henry III. here was a priory of Black canons, founded by Roger Fitz-Osbert, and dedicated to St. Mary and St. Olave: at the dissolution its revenue was valued at £49. 11. 7. The navigable river Waveney runs along the south-west boundary of this parish, and is crossed by St. Olave's bridge.

HERRINGSTONE, or WINTERBOURNE-HERRINGSTONE, a chapelry in the parish of WEST CHICKERELL, hundred of CULLIFORD-TREE, Dorchester division of the county of DORSET, 2 miles (S. by W.) from Dorchester, containing, with Winterbourne-Farringdon, 88 inhabitants.

HERRINGSWELL, a parish in the hundred of LACKFORD, county of SUFFOLK, 3¼ miles (S. by E.) from Mildenhall, containing 215 inhabitants. The living is a discharged rectory, in the archdeaconry of Sudbury, and diocese of Norwich, rated in the king's books at £9. 9. 9½. H. Sperling, Esq. was patron in 1812. The church is dedicated to St. Ethelbert.

HERRINGTON (EAST and MIDDLE), a township in the parish of HOUGHTON le SPRING, northern division of EASINGTON ward, county palatine of DURHAM, 3¼ miles (S. W. by S.) from Sunderland, containing 133 inhabitants.

HERRINGTON (WEST), a township in the parish of HOUGHTON le SPRING, northern division of EASINGTON ward, county palatine of DURHAM, 4½ miles (S. W.

by W.) from Sunderland, containing 329 inhabitants. Here was anciently a chapel, dedicated to the Virgin Mary.

HERTFORD, a borough and market town, having separate jurisdiction, locally in the hundred of Hertford, county of HERTFORD, of which it is the chief town 21 miles (N.) from London, containing, exclusively of that part of the parish of All Saints which is within the hundred, 4265 inhabitants. Hertford is supposed by Sir Henry Chauncy to have been the

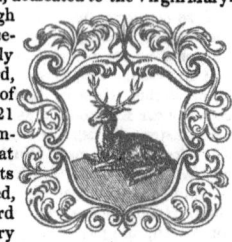

Arms.

Roman station called *Durocobrivæ*, which has by subsequent writers, with greater probability, been referred to Dunstable. The modern name is of somewhat doubtful etymology: according to Bede it is derived from *Herudford*, or red ford, while Salmon deduces it from *Here-ford*, a military ford, whence, by corruption, Hertford. Its antiquity however, is unquestionable, for so early as the year 673, Theodore, a native of Tarsus in Cilicia, then Archbishop of Canterbury, convened a council here; and about 905, Edward the Elder, to protect the inhabitants from the incursions of the Danes, erected a castle, the custody of which, and the government of the town, were given by William the Conqueror to Peter de Valoignes. In the reign of Henry III. William de Valence was governor, and at his death it descended to Aymen de Valence: it was subsequently surrendered to the crown. The town is pleasantly situated on the river Lea, in a dry valley surrounded by hills, and consists of three principal streets meeting obliquely in the centre, parallel with one of which is the high thoroughfare through the town. Over the Lea, which is navigable to Hertford for small vessels, is the toll-bridge; beyond this is an opening leading to Cow-bridge, a structure of brick with two arches across the river Beane, which flows into the Lea, as also does the Mimram, which runs through the castle grounds, and is crossed by a wooden bridge: about a mile above the toll-bridge in this direction are some neat modern cottages, and on the north road is a handsome range of buildings, called the North Crescent. In Castle-street, on the site of the ancient castle, of which little remains except a line of embattled wall and a mound, is a handsome brick edifice, fitted up some years since at considerable expense, by the late Marquis of Downshire, for his own residence: it was afterwards taken by the East India Company, as a temporary college during the erection of one at Haileybury, to which it was subsequently appropriated as a preparatory establishment, but is now occupied as a ladies' boarding-school. "The Herts, Cambridgeshire, and Country Fire Office," established in 1824, is situated at the lower part of Fore-street. At a small distance from the town, on the river Lea, are the gas works, erected in November 1825, formerly under the direction of the International Gas-Light Company, but now the property of private individuals, who have purchased them of the Company. The buildings in general are so irregular that not one street presents an entire row of uniform houses: the inhabitants are amply supplied with excellent water. A considerable trade is carried on in corn, malt, and flour, of which large quantities are annually sent to the metropolis. The market, by charter of Charles II., is held under the shire-hall every Saturday, and the business transacted in grain is scarcely equalled in any other provincial market: another, formerly held on Wednesday, is now disused. Fairs, chiefly for cattle, three of which are by charter of Mary, and one by charter of Charles II., are held on the third Saturday before Easter, May 12th, July 5th, and November 8th, with courts of pie-powder attached. On the north side of Fore-street is the butchers' market, constructed at the sole expense of Alderman Kirby, and forming three sides of a quadrangle.

The inhabitants were first incorporated by Queen Mary, in the year 1554; Elizabeth granted them a new charter in the 31st of her reign, which was confirmed and modified by James I., and further enlarged by Charles II., in the 23rd of his reign. James I. changed the style into mayor, burgesses, and assistants, and by the last charter,

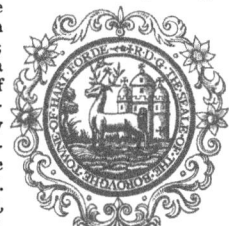

Corporate Seal.

dated in the 32nd of Charles II., the government is vested in a mayor, high steward, recorder, chamberlain, and ten aldermen (who constitute the common council), with sixteen assistants, a town clerk, two serjeants at mace, and inferior officers: the mayor is annually chosen, by the corporation at large, from two aldermen nominated by the mayor, recorder, and aldermen: the mayor, the late mayor, recorder, together with one alderman, or freeman, learned in the laws of England, who is chosen by the mayor and common council, to continue during pleasure, are justices of the peace within the borough and liberties. The county magistrates have concurrent jurisdiction, which however is but rarely exercised. The corporation possess, by virtue of their charter from Charles, the tolls of the market, and are empowered to prevent any but freemen from trading within the borough; they also have authority to hold a court of record for pleas, actions, and suits under the value of £60, every Wednesday, at which the mayor or his deputy, being an alderman, and the recorder or his deputy, preside: this court, after having been discontinued for many years, has very recently been revived. The usual Lent and Summer assizes are held in the shire-hall, and there is a gaol delivery in December. The quarter sessions for the county and the borough are held in the same place, the former always beginning on Monday, and the latter usually two days afterwards. A court leet for the manor is held annually in the townhall. This borough sent two members to parliament from the reign of Edward I. to the 50th of Edward III., from which period elections were discontinued till the time of James I., when, on petition, their ancient right was restored. The members are chosen by the inhabitant householders, by freemen who were resident when their freedom was granted, and by three honorary freemen, who may be non-residents: the number of voters is seven hundred and fifty: the mayor is the returning officer. The shire-hall, a spacious edifice, erected in 1780, and situated in the market-place, contains in addition to the courts of law, a handsome assembly-room: a good clock, with a projecting dial,

has been recently put up in it by public subscription. The common gaol for the borough, and the common gaol and house of correction for the county, are adjacent buildings, and comprehended within the same walls, enclosing an area of about four acres: the borough gaol contains only one division, with one airing-yard and four sleeping-cells: the county gaol contains four wards for male and two for female criminals, and one for male and one for female debtors, and is well adapted to the classification of prisoners: the house of correction, also well fitted for that purpose, contains four wards, four day-rooms, four airing-yards, in which is a tread-wheel, with four divisions and two yards for females: these prisons are all under the same regulations, and under one governor, assisted by turnkeys and other officers appointed annually by the sheriff for the county, and the mayor and corporation.

Hertford comprises the united parishes of All Saints and St. John, and the liberties of Little Amwell and Brickendon within the parish of All Saints, together with the united parishes of St. Andrew, St. Mary, and St. Nicholas, in the archdeaconry of Huntingdon, and diocese of Lincoln. The living of All Saints' is a vicarage with that of St. John's, rated together in the king's books at £10. 8. 6½., and in the alternate patronage of the Crown and the proprietor of the estate of Balls in this parish: the church has been recently repaired, and enlarged with three hundred and four additional sittings, of which one hundred and sixty-three are free, and towards defraying the expense of which the Incorporated Society for enlarging churches and chapels granted £200, and the Governors of Christ's Hospital £100, the latter having previously erected a gallery containing sittings for about two hundred boys, at their own expense: it is a spacious cruciform structure in the later style of English architecture, with a tower surmounted by a spire; within are several ancient monuments, the inscriptions on which are nearly obliterated, and some of modern erection. The living of St. Andrew's is a rectory with the vicarages of St. Mary and St. Nicholas, rated together in the king's books at £12. 7. 3½., and in the patronage of the King, as Duke of Lancaster: the church is a neat edifice, with a low embattled tower surmounted by a small spire: the churches of the other three parishes have fallen into ruins. There are places of worship for Baptists, the Society of Friends, Independents, those in the Countess of Huntingdon's connexion, and Wesleyan Methodists. At the entrance into the town from London is a branch establishment in connexion with Christ's hospital, London, appropriated to the reception of junior boys, who are sent from this to the parent institution, as vacancies arise: it includes three sides of a quadrangle, two opposite sides being occupied by the several wards for the children, and terminated by residences for the steward and the beadle; on the third side are the reading and writing-school, a spacious brick building capable of accommodating upwards of two hundred and fifty boys, and affording a residence for the master: in a line with the writing-school, westward, is the dining-hall, in dimensions about one hundred feet by thirty, and behind it the infirmary for about one hundred patients: eastward of the great gates in front of the buildings is the grammar school, besides the residence for the master; and on the opposite side, the porter's lodge, with a continuation of buildings within the walls for the girls, of whom there are usually from sixty-to seventy, with a residence for the governess and matron. The children are instructed on Dr. Bell's system, and the officers of the establishment are the grammar and writing-masters, a governess, matron, steward, surgeon, nine nurses, three ushers, beadle, porter, &c. A free grammar school for the children of the inhabitants was founded in 1617, by Richard Hale, Esq., of Cheshunt in this county, and endowed by him with £800, to be laid out in lands and tenements in the town and neighbourhood; which direction was carried into effect by Rowland Hale, a descendant of the founder; and an estate in the parish of Tewin is now chargeable with the payment of £40 per annum, of which £20 are appropriated to the master, £10 to his assistant, and the remainder to repairing the school. A commodious house for the master was built in the town, in 1727, by subscription, which has lately undergone a thorough repair by means of the liberal contributions of the nobility, gentry, and inhabitants. The master, who is appointed by Lord Melbourne, or, in the event of his minority, by the mayor and corporation, is allowed to receive boarders; and the boys on the foundation, in consideration of being taught writing and arithmetic, pay half a guinea per quarter. Bernard Hale, D.D., gave £100 per annum to maintain seven poor scholars at St. Peter's College, Cambridge, for seven years, the candidates to be appointed from this grammar school by Lord Melbourne: each scholarship is now of the value of £14 per annum. A Green-coat school, for clothing and educating forty boys, was erected in 1812, and is supported by funds which arise partly from £26 per annum, the gift of Mr. Gabriel Newton, of Leicester, and paid to the corporation for this purpose, and partly from voluntary contributions: there are likewise two other schools supported by subscription. The East India College, instituted in 1806, for the education of young men intended for the civil service of the Hon. East India Company in India, is situated two miles on the London side of the town of Hertford, and will admit one hundred and five students, who are under the tuition of a principal student, and several professors. Lady Harrison, who died in 1706, founded four almshouses, and gave £50 towards clothing the inmates; and there is another almshouse for poor widows. The principal charity, called Grass Money, was formerly at the disposal of the corporation, but is now vested in trustees appointed under a decree of the Court of Chancery: it produces a net income of about £250 per annum. A county dispensary was established in January, 1822. Eastward of the town was formerly a monastery, founded by Ralph de Limesi, a nephew of William the Conqueror, who, afterwards assuming the cowl, became its first prior, and was interred in the church belonging to the convent: at the dissolution it was valued at £86.14.2.: the site is now occupied by a dwelling-house still called the Priory, which, about sixty years ago was inhabited by Thomas Dimsdale, M.D., a native of Thoydon-Garnon, in Essex, who spent the early part of his professional life here, and having received his diploma in 1768, went to Russia, where he inoculated the Empress Catherine, for which he received £12,000 and a pension, with the title of Baron, which descends to his family: he also inoculated the late Emperor and his brother, and wrote a treatise on inoculation: he died here in the year 1800, at the advanced age of eighty-seven, and was interred in the

burial-ground belonging to the Society of Friends, at Bishop's Stortford. His son Nathaniel, who accompanied him to Russia, and also recieved the title of baron, was twice representative of this borough in parliament. Hertford confers the title of marquis on the family of Seymour Conway.

HERTFORDSHIRE, an inland county, bounded on the north by the county of Cambridge, on the north-west by the county of Bedford, on the west by the county of Buckingham, on the south by the county of Middlesex, and on the east by the county of Essex: it extends from 51° 37' to 52° 5' (N. Lat.), and from 13' (E.) to 46' (W. Lon.); and contains three hundred and thirty-seven thousand nine hundred and twenty acres, or five hundred and twenty-eight square miles. The population, in 1821, amounted to 129,714.

The Celtic inhabitants of this part of Britain were the Cassii, or Cattieuchlani, whose country, long before the invasion of Cæsar, was overrun by the Belgæ (who had previously established themselves in the south-western part of England), and their capital city, Verulam, taken possession of by the conquerors. Of the operations of Cæsar in the territory forming the modern county of Hertford, and his capture of Verulam, little more is known than what may be collected from the succinct narrative of this campaign by the conqueror himself; the result of it, however, was, that the British chief Cassivelaunus was obliged to sue for peace; which being granted, Mandubritius, the sovereign of the Cassii, had his dominions restored to him, and Cæsar led back his army, along the Watling-street, to Richborough, where he embarked for the Continent. Shortly after the second invasion of Britain, in the reign of Claudius, in the revolt of the Iceni, under Boadicea, against the Romans, which commenced while the Roman army under Suetonius was engaged in the conquest of the Isle of Anglesey, the Britons, after utterly destroying the Roman colony and garrison of Camalodunum, advanced against Verulam with such an overwhelming force, that the Roman general, who had hastened back along the Watling-street to its relief, was compelled to retire, leaving Verulam to the same disastrous fate which had befallen Camalodunum, the city being sacked, and the inhabitants massacred. It was not long, however, before this important post again fell into the hands of the invaders, who renewed its fortifications, and appear to have erected a new fortress at Cheshunt, on the Ermin-street. In the Roman division of Britain, this territory was included in Flavia Cæsariensis; and under the Saxon octarchy part of it was comprised in the kingdom of Mercia, and part in that of the East Saxons, or Essex. In 794, Offa, the celebrated king of Mercia, died at Offley, in this county; and in 896, near Ware, Alfred captured the Danish ships, by obstructing the channel of the river Lea, so that they could not be brought down it. In his camp at Berkhampstead, in 1066, William the Conqueror took the oath to maintain the laws of Edward the Confessor. At Wheathampstead, in 1312, the barons assembled their forces against Edward II. and his favourite Gaveston. The year 1381 is memorable in this county for the transactions connected with the suppression of Wat Tyler's rebellion, when Richard II. and his chief justice Tresilian, with a guard of a thousand men, came to St. Alban's: a number of the insurgents, brought from the gaol at Hertford,

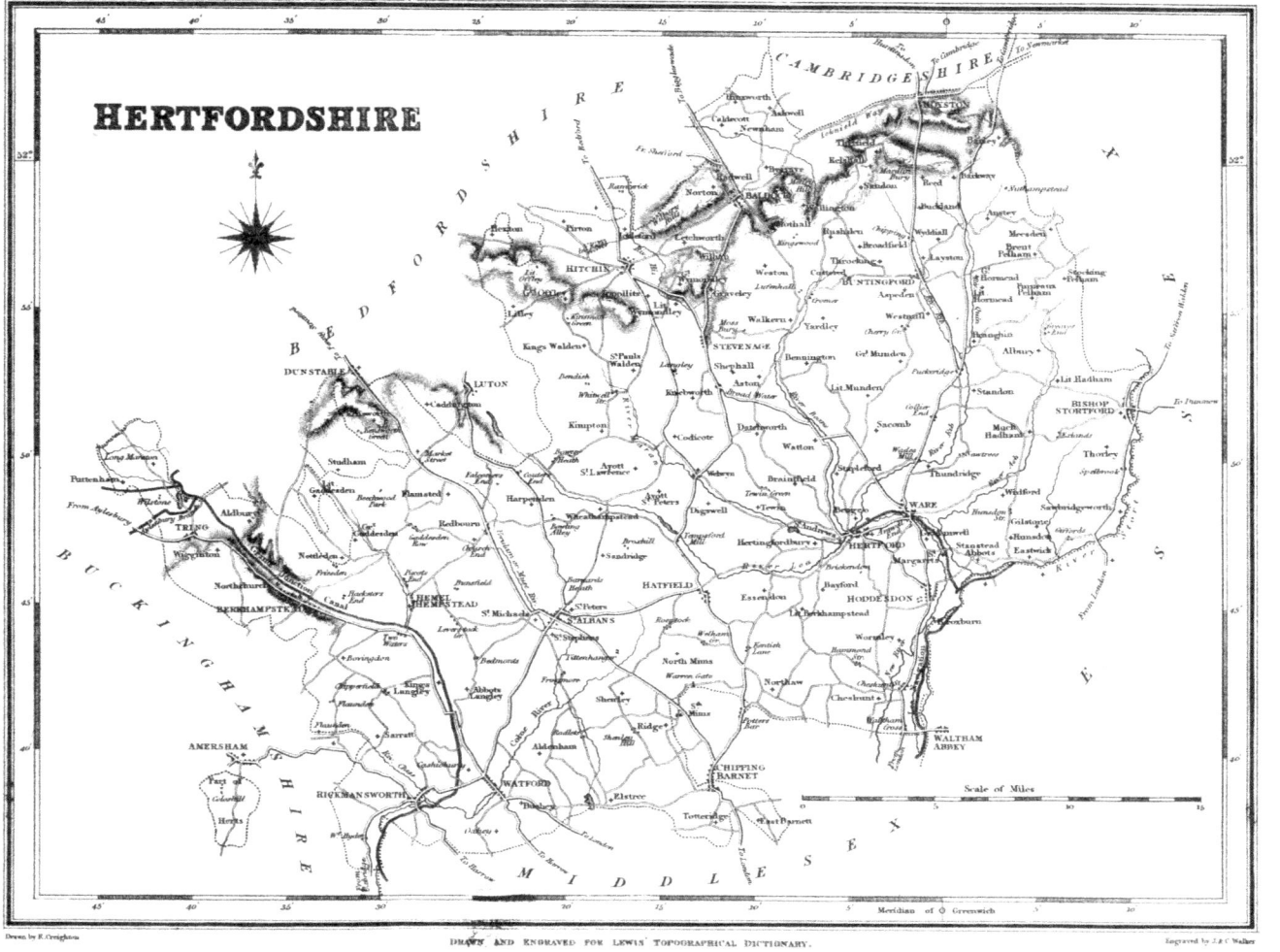

HERTFORDSHIRE

Scale of Miles

Drawn by R. Creighton.   DRAWN AND ENGRAVED FOR LEWIS' TOPOGRAPHICAL DICTIONARY.   Engraved by J. & C. Walker.

were there executed, and the male inhabitants of the county, from fifteen to sixty years of age, were assembled in the great court of the abbey, and swore to be faithful subjects for the future : at Hertford also, Henry, Duke of Lancaster, afterwards Henry IV., kept his court, at the time that Richard II. was deposed. Three of the most important battles, during the war between the houses of York and Lancaster, were fought within the limits of this county, viz., in 1455, the first battle of St. Alban's, in which Henry VI. was wounded and made prisoner; in 1461, the second battle of St. Alban's, in which Margaret of Anjou was defeated by the Earl of Warwick; and in 1468, the decisive battle of Barnet, in which the Earl of Warwick and ten thousand of his army were slain. It was from Theobalds that Charles I., in 1642, after receiving there the petitions of both houses of parliament, departed to place himself at the head of his army.

This county lies partly within the diocese of London, and partly in that of Lincoln, the whole being included in the province of Canterbury. That part which is in the diocese of London comprises the deanery of Braughin, which is in the archdeaconry of Middlesex, and contains thirty-four parishes, and the archdeaconry and deanery of St. Alban, containing twenty-two parishes. The part which is in the diocese of Lincoln is included within the archdeaconry of Huntingdon, and comprises the four deaneries of Baldock, Berkhampstead, Hertford, and Hitchin, containing eighty parishes; the total number of parishes in the county being one hundred and thirty-six, of which, sixty-seven are rectories, fifty-three vicarages, and the remainder perpetual curacies, or consolidated with other parishes. For civil purposes it is divided into the eight hundreds of Braughin, Broadwater, Cashio (or the liberty of St. Alban's), Dacorum, Edwinstree, Hertford, Hitchin, and Pirton, and Odsey, in which are the borough and market towns of Hertford and St. Alban's, and the market towns of Baldock, Berkhampstead, Hatfield, Hemel-Hempstead, Hitchin, Hoddesdon, Rickmansworth, Standon, Stevenage, Bishop's Stortford, Tring, Ware, and Watford, and parts of those of Chipping-Barnet and Royston. Two knights are returned to parliament for the shire, and two representatives for each of the two boroughs. Hertfordshire is included in the home circuit : the assizes are held at Hertford, where also are held the quarter sessions, except for the hundred of Cashio, or liberty of St. Alban's, which are held at St. Alban's. The county gaol is at Hertford. There are ninety - five acting magistrates. The rates raised in the county for the year ending March 25th, 1827, amounted to £109,072. 19.; the expenditure to £108,054. 6., of which £93,064. 12. was applied to the relief of the poor.

The natural features of Hertfordshire are of a gentle character, but it possesses scenes of considerable beauty : the southern parts of the county, the heights of which overlook part of the county of Middlesex, and command a prospect of the distant hills of Surrey, are eminently pleasing; while, for an extensive view over a rich vale, few prospects, without a great river, are more striking than that which is obtained from Lilley-Hoo. Considerable addition is also made to the beauty of this county by the mansions, villas, and ornamented grounds, of rich proprietors, which present themselves in every direction. The scenery of Moor park is particularly beau-

tiful; and the various scenes round Ware, North Mimms, Watford, and the banks of all the streams from Berkhampstead and Hempstead, when viewed from the adjoining hills, are worthy of attention. With respect to the soil, it may be remarked that the vales through which the rivers and brooks flow are invariably composed of rich sandy loam, with the exception only of a small quantity of peat and marshy moor; that the slopes of the hills descending to these vales are inferior qualities of the same loams, and at the same time dry and sound; but that the flatter surfaces of the higher lands are composed of a wet and strong loam, sometimes so much so as to require hollow draining. The late secretary to the Board of Agriculture, Mr. Arthur Young, divides the soil into one district of loams, two of clay, one of chalk, and one of gravel; at the same time observing, that the soils intermingle in a remarkable manner, so that it is sometimes extremely difficult to draw the boundary line between them. The district of the loams includes a very considerable portion of the county, no less than one hundred and forty-seven thousand eight hundred and forty acres, and may properly be divided into flinty and sandy; the flinty loams spread into a considerable tract from the river Beane to the limits of the county beyond Berkhampstead, extending southward to the gravel and clay districts, and northward to that of the chalk : from Berkhampstead towards Chesham they are of a reddish colour : for some miles around Buntingford these loams are strong, and produce heavy crops of wheat; and from St. Alban's to Redbourn, and about Watford, they form a fine mellow turnip land, easily worked, and adapted to the production of almost every kind of grain. Some of the finest loam in the county is the sandy vale of Cheshunt up to Hoddesdon, which produces five quarters of wheat per acre. Some of these loams, more especially where they are wet, are provincially, but improperly, designated clay : the whole of this district is cropped with turnips, which are eaten on the land. The two clay districts are comparatively small; one is in the southern part of the county, adjoining Middlesex, and the soil is stiff, hard, and tenacious, being the same as the bean lands of the north of that county : the other, which is by far the larger of the two, lies on the eastern side of the county, and nearly resembles the contiguous clay lands of Essex, being rather a strong wet loam on a stiff basis of clay marl. Both these tracts are in a great measure free from stone and flint : conjointly they include ninety thousand two hundred and forty acres; the southern tract, by the use of London manure, has been converted into very rich hay ground. The chalk district extends along the whole border of the northern part of the county, and comprehends forty-six thousand seven hundred and twenty acres; this soil is of two kinds, chalk, unmixed with any thing but what ages of cultivation have added; and what is provincially called marme, being a white marl formed by the mixture of a portion of clay; both these soils are fruitful, but the last-mentioned is the best. The gravel tract lies in the south-eastern part of the county, around Hatfield, North Mimms, and Northall, and contains seventeen thousand two hundred and eighty acres; this soil is characterised by wetness, from many springs, most of which are impregnated with sulphur; it abounds with smooth blue pebbles, which, at various depths, and in some places close to the surface, are conglomerated by sulphureous clay into plum-pudding-stones; and the whole district, excepting only some patches of fine loam, which occur more especially on the banks of many of the smaller streams, is among the most unproductive land in the south of England. The substratum of the whole of Hertfordshire is chalk; for obtaining which, pits are sunk all over the county, its use as manure being general throughout its limits; for this purpose, the chalk which lies farthest beneath the surface soil is esteemed the best.

By far the greater part of the county is under tillage. Upon all the turnip land the rotation of crops is, turnips, barley, clover, the first crop mown, the second eaten off, and wheat; some farmers adding oats: on the other soils various systems are practised. Of wheat, the turnip soils produce on an average from seventeen to twenty bushels per acre; the strong land about twenty-five; on the fine rich loams of Buntingford, forty bushels are by no means an uncommon crop; while the average produce of this grain thoughout the county is estimated at twenty-three bushels per acre: the general average produce of barley and oats is about thirty-two bushels per acre. The artificial grasses are, clover (which has probably been cultivated in this county longer than in any other part of the kingdom, and from the vicinity of the metropolis yields a greater profit here than elsewhere), trefoil, sainfoin, and lucerne; the culture of tares is general throughout the county. Besides the chalk already mentioned, and the manures common to other counties, soot and night-soil brought from London, are found very beneficial on the land; about Lilley, peat-ashes are brought as manure from Bedfordshire, where they are burned in heaps, and sold at Tingrith, Flitwick, and Flitton. The grass land is in a great measure confined to a narrow border on the south side of the county, in the vicinity of Barnet, which, being near London, is made productive by means of the manures brought from that city: with this exception, the only grass lands are those belonging to the numerous gentlemen's seats, and those in the flat bottoms of the vales which are watered by rivers; of the last-mentioned, some of the principal are on the Stort, from Hockerill to Hertford, and thence to Hatfeild, on the banks of the same river. In the parishes of the south-western corner of the county are many orchards, rarely exceeding four or five acres in extent, principally of apples and cherries: the former are the most profitable; of the latter, the caroon and the small black cherry are the favourite sorts, and a full grown tree, in a favourable season, will produce six hundred pounds weight. In consequence of so much of Hertfordshire being arable land, and the quantity of clover carried to London being so great, live stock is an object of inferior consideration: the cattle are of various sorts: the sheep are chiefly of the South-down and Wiltshire breeds; there are also some of the new Leicester: the hogs are of different kinds. The quantity of waste lands, compared with those of most other counties, is very inconsiderable: they consist of small commons scattered over the county, the principal being near Berkhampstead. There are large tracts of coppice wood lying to the south of Hertford, in the direction of London: in the tract between Hockerill, Ware, and Buntingford, are also coppice woods; and the Marquis of

Salisbury has one thousand five hundred acres. There is much fine flourishing timber about the different seats of the nobility and gentry, such as oak, ash, elm, beech Spanish chesnut, cedar, larch, spruce, silver fir, Scotch fir, &c.; much of that in Moor park is of great antiquity. The women and children about Stevenage, Hatfield, Redbourn, St. Alban's, Berkhampstead, Hitchin, &c., are much employed in making straw-plat. The manufacture of black lace has been carried on at Berkhampstead time immemorially, but has of late given place to that of straw-plat.

The principal rivers are the Lea and the Colne, formed by the junction of many minor streams, which rise chiefly within the bounds of the county. The Lea rises in Bedfordshire, enters Hertfordshire near Bower heath, and traverses the county in a direction nearly from north-west to south-east, passing the town of Hertford, from which place it has been made navigable to its conflux with the Stort, about a mile east of Hoddesdon, where it takes a southerly course, becoming the boundary of the county on the east, and continuing so until it reaches the border of Middlesex. The Colne rises near Kitt's-end in Middlesex, and running by North Mimms, Watford, and Rickmansworth, it soon after quits the county for Buckinghamshire. The Stort, rising in Essex, becomes navigable at Bishop's Stortford, from which place to its junction with the river Lea it forms the boundary between Essex and Hertfordshire. The Mimram rises near Frogmore, in Hitchin and Pirton hundred, and, with the Beane, which rises near Cromer, in Odsey hundred, joins the Lea near Hertford. The sources of the Rib are near Buntingford, in Edwinstree hundred, and it joins the Lea between Hertford and Ware. The source of the Ash is also in Edwinstree hundred, near Upperwick, and it falls into the Lea about a mile below Ware. The Verulam, Verlam, or Muse river, rises in Dacorum hundred, near Market-street, and on the confines of Bedfordshire, and runs in a south-south-easterly direction to St. Alban's, and thence nearly south until it joins the Colne, then only a small stream. The Gade rises also in Dacorum hundred, near Gaddesden, on the borders of Buckinghamshire, and runs in a direction nearly south, to its conflux with the Colne near Rickmansworth. At Ashwell, in this county, are the nine sister springs of the Cam, which flows by Cambridge. The Grand Junction canal, from Branston wharf on the Coventry canal to Old Brentford, where it opens into the Thames, enters Hertfordshire above Tring, and follows the course of the Bulburn and Gade rivers to Rickmansworth, and from that place the course of the Colne until it leaves the county. An act of parliament was obtained for the construction of another canal from St. Alban's to the Grand Junction canal, below Cashiobury park; but the proposed subscription of £17,000 failing, the design was abandoned. The road from London to Oxford, through Aylesbury, enters Hertfordshire at Bushey Heath, and passing through Watford, Berkhampstead, and Tring, quits the county about half a mile beyond the last place. The road from London to Berwick upon Tweed, through York, after passing through a corner of the county which surrounds East Barnet, re-enters it on Hatfield chase, and passing through Hatfield, Welwyn, and Baldock, enters Bedfordshire about two miles beyond the latter town. The road from London to Holyhead, through Chester, after passing through the same corner and through Chipping-Barnet, re-enters Hertfordshire immediately beyond South Mimms, and passing through St. Alban's and Redbourn, quits the county about a mile before it reaches Dunstable. This line is also part of the road from London to Chester, through Birmingham ; of that from London to Carlisle, through Warrington and Lancaster ; of that from London to Manchester, through Northampton and Derby; of that from London to Whitehaven, through Sheffield, Settle, and Kirkby-Lonsdale ; and of that from London to Manchester and Clitheroe, through Leek, Uttoxeter, and Hinckley. The road from London to Halifax and Clitheroe, through Bedford, Nottingham, and Rotherham, branches off from the last-mentioned road at St. Alban's, and passing through Harpenden, quits the county about two miles before it reaches Luton. The road from London to Scarborough, through the counties of Huntingdon and Lincoln, enters Hertfordshire near Waltham-Cross, and passing through Cheshunt, Ware, Puckeridge, and Buntingford, enters Cambridgeshire at Royston. The road from London to Lynn-Regis, through Cambridge, branches off from the last mentioned road at Puckeridge, and passing through Barkway and Barley, enters Cambridgeshire about a mile beyond the latter place. The road from London to Norwich, through Newmarket, enters Hertfordshire from Essex, where it crosses the river Stort, at Harlow Mills, and passing through Sawbridgeworth and Bishop's Stortford, again crosses that river into Essex near the latter place : this is also the road from London to Lynn-Regis, through Brandon and Newmarket.

The British Watling-street, entering Hertfordshire on the south, passed to St. Alban's, and thence along the line of the present great Irish road, to Dunstable. The Ermin-street, passing near Enfield, entered the south-eastern border of Hertfordshire near Little Hockgate, and passed between Standon and Puckeridge, near Braughin, and through Buntingford to Royston, where it crossed the Iknield-street. The line of the Iknield-street, entering the north-eastern border of the county at Royston, passes through Baldock, and after crossing a small part of Bedfordshire and of Buckinghamshire, re-enters Hertfordshire for a short distance, running a little to the right of Tring. The only Roman station in this county, the situation of which has been precisely ascertained, is the celebrated one of *Verulam*, contiguous to St. Alban's. Excepting the ancient British roads above-mentioned, which appear to have been used and improved by the Romans, the only Roman road (of the many which it is probable once intersected this county) that can now be traced with any degree of distinctness within its limits, is that which connected Verulam with the station at Chesterford, near Sandy, on the banks of the Ivel, which runs in the line of the present great north road, through Stevenage, Graveley, and Baldock. Before the Reformation there were in this county, according to Tanner, thirty-four religious houses and hospitals. The principal ecclesiastical antiquities are St. Alban's abbey church and gate-house. At Waltham-Cross is the well known cross, erected, with several others, by Edward I., to perpetuate the remembrance of those places at which the body of his consort, Queen Eleanor, rested, in its way from Herdeby, in Lincolnshire, for interment in Westminster abbey. There are some remains of the ancient castles of Hertford, Bishop's Stort-

ford, and Berkhampstead ; and Hatfield house is a fine specimen of the style of domestic architecture which prevailed in the reign of James I. On the east side of the village of Great Amwell, at the foot of the steep bank upon which the church is situated, rises a considerable spring, which, together with that of Chadwell, feeds the canal commonly called the New River, commenced in 1609, under the powers of an act of parliament, by Mr. (afterwards Sir) Hugh Myddelton, for supplying the northern side of the metropolis with water, and completed in 1613, its length being nearly thirty-nine miles : about half its course is within the eastern border of this county, and near the line of the road from London to Ware. For a more detailed account of this undertaking, see CLERKENWELL.

HERTINGFORDBURY, a parish in the hundred and county of HERTFORD, 1¾ mile (W. S. W.) from Hertford, containing 827 inhabitants. The living is a rectory, in the archdeaconry of Huntingdon, and diocese of Lincoln, rated in the king's books at £12. 15. 2½., and in the patronage of the King, as Duke of Lancaster. The church is dedicated to St. Mary.

HESKET in the FOREST, a parish in LEATH ward, county of CUMBERLAND, comprising the townships of Calthwaite, Nether and Upper Hesket, Itonfield, Petterell-Crooks, and Plumpton-Street, and containing 1799 inhabitants, of which number, 780 are in the township of Nether and Upper Hesket, 9 miles (N. by W.) from Penrith. The living is a perpetual curacy, in the archdeaconry and diocese of Carlisle, endowed with £800 private benefaction, £200 royal bounty, and £1900 parliamentary grant, and in the patronage of the Dean and Chapter of Carlisle. The church, dedicated to St. Mary, was built about 1530, and rebuilt in 1678, and again in 1760. In 1763, John Brown bequeathed £200 towards the support of a school, in which one hundred children are now educated at a small charge. The courts for the Forest of Inglewood are held in this parish, yearly on St. Barnabas' day, in the open air, under a tree called Court Thorn, on the road between Upper and Nether Hesket, on which occasion the inhabitants of more than twenty townships attend, from whom a jury is ballotted and sworn. Near Aiketgate is a lake called by the general name of Tarn, covering about one hundred acres, and abounding in carp.

HESKET-NEWMARKET, a market town in the township of CALDBECK-HALTCLIFFE, parish of CALDBECK, ALLERDALE ward below Darwent, county of CUMBERLAND, 14 miles (S. S.W.) from Carlisle, and 297 (N.N.W.) from London. The population is returned with the township. This is a small, but neat and compact town, situated in a secluded and romantic district, on the western side of the river Caldew. The surrounding country is mountainous, and contains mines of lead, copper, and manganese. At Carrickbeck, in the neighbourhood, are smelting-works for the lead-ore. The market, which is held on Friday, is but inconsiderable ; but there are well-frequented fairs on the first Friday in May, and every alternate Friday till Whitsuntide, for cattle ; and the last Thursday in August, and the second Thursday in October, for sheep. Here is a place of worship for the Society of Friends. Near the town is a petrifying spring, issuing from a rock on the margin of the river.

HESKETH, a joint township and chapelry with Bec-

3 C 2

consall, in the parish of CROSTON, hundred of LEYLAND, county palatine of LANCASTER, 11 miles (N. by E.) from Ormskirk. The population is returned with Becconsall.

HESKIN, a township in the parish of ECCLESTON, hundred of LEYLAND, county palatine of LANCASTER, 5½ miles (W. S. W.) from Chorley, containing 274 inhabitants. In 1806, Hannah Anderton gave a cottage as a school-room, and £200 in support of it, for the education of poor girls : the annual income is about £10.

HESLERTON (EAST), a chapelry in the parish of WEST HESLERTON, wapentake of BUCKROSE, East riding of the county of YORK, 8¼ miles (E. N. E.) from New Malton, containing 196 inhabitants. Here is a place of worship for Wesleyan Methodists.

HESLERTON (WEST), a parish in the wapentake of BUCKROSE, East riding of the county of YORK, comprising the chapelry of East Heslerton, and the township of West Heslerton, and containing 469 inhabitants, of which number, 273 are in the township of West Heslerton, 8 miles (E. N. E.) from New Malton. The living is a rectory, in the archdeaconry of the East riding, and diocese of York, rated in the king's books at £21. 6. 8., and in the patronage of the Crown. The church is dedicated to St. Andrew.

HESLETON (COLD), a township in the parish of DALTON le DALE, northern division of EASINGTON ward, county palatine of DURHAM, 7 miles (S.) from Sunderland, containing 55 inhabitants.

HESLETON (MONK), a parish in the southern division of EASINGTON ward, county palatine of DURHAM, comprising the townships of Hulam, or Holom Hutton-Henry, Monk-Hesleton, Nesbit, Sheraton, and Thorpe-Bulmer, and containing 503 inhabitants, of which number, 164 are in the township of Monk-Hesleton, 10 miles (E. by S.) from Durham. The living is a vicarage, in the archdeaconry and diocese of Durham, rated in the king's books at £7. 12. 6., and in the patronage of the Dean and Chapter of Durham. The church is dedicated to St. Mary. Petty races are held here on St. Peter's day.

HESLEY-HURST, a township in the parish of ROTHBURY, western division of COQUETDALE ward, county of NORTHUMBERLAND, 4 miles (S. E. by S.) from Rothbury, containing 46 inhabitants.

HESLINGTON, a parish partly in the liberty of ST. PETER of YORK, comprising the greater portion of the township of Heslington, but chiefly in the wapentake of Ouze and Derwent, East riding of the county of YORK, and containing 513 inhabitants, of which number, 221 are in the township of Heslington, a portion of which is in the parish of St. Lawrence, York, 1½ mile (S. E. by E.) from York. The living is a perpetual curacy, in the peculiar jurisdiction and patronage of the Prebendary of Ampleforth in the Cathedral Church of York, endowed with £800 royal bounty. The church is dedicated to St. Peter and St. Paul. Here is an almshouse for eight poor men and one poor woman, endowed with a rent-charge of £50 per annum, and £5 per annum from a rectory in Cleveland.

HESSETT, a parish in the hundred of THEDWESTRY, county of SUFFOLK, 6 miles (E.S.E.) from Bury-St. Edmund's, containing 393 inhabitants. The living is a rectory, in the archdeaconry of Sudbury, and diocese of Norwich, rated in the king's books at £12. 17. 11. The King, for that turn, presented in 1813. The church is dedicated to St. Ethelbert.

HESSEY, a township in the parish of MOOR-MONKTON, ainsty of the city, and East riding of the county, of YORK, 5¾ miles (W. by N.) from York, containing 161 inhabitants.

HESSLE, a parish in the county of the town of KINGSTON upon HULL, locally in the East riding of the county of York, 5¼ miles (W. S. W.) from Kingston upon Hull, containing 1021 inhabitants. The living is a vicarage, in the archdeaconry of the East riding, and diocese of York, rated in the king's books at £10. 7. 1., and in the patronage of the Crown. The church is dedicated to All Saints. There is a place of worship for Wesleyan Methodists, also a National school and an almshouse.

HEST, a joint township with Slyne, in the parish of BOLTON le SANDS, hundred of LONSDALE, south of the sands, county palatine of LANCASTER, 2½ miles (N. by W.) from Lancaster, containing 317 inhabitants.

HESTERCOMBE, a hamlet in the parish of KINGSTON, hundred of TAUNTON and TAUNTON-DEAN, county of SOMERSET, 3¼ miles (N. by E.) from Taunton, containing 16 inhabitants.

HESTON, a parish in the hundred of ISLEWORTH, county of MIDDLESEX, 1½ mile (N. by W.) from Hounslow, containing, with a portion of the town of Hounslow, which is in this parish, 2810 inhabitants. The living is a vicarage, in the archdeaconry of Middlesex, and diocese of London, rated in the king's books at £11, and in the patronage of the Bishop of London. The church, dedicated to St. Leonard, has received an addition of two hundred and fifty-six sittings, of which one hundred and ninety-three are free, the Incorporated Society for building and enlarging churches and chapels having contributed £200 towards defraying the expense : in this church were interred Sir Joseph Banks, President of the Royal Society, and his lady. A parochial school for children of both sexes, under the patronage of the vicar, is supported by voluntary contributions. Here is a manufactory for oil of vitriol ; but the inhabitants are chiefly employed in agriculture. A pleasure fair is held on the 1st of May. This parish is within the jurisdiction of a court of requests for the recovery of debts under 40s., held at Brentford during the summer, and at Uxbridge during the winter. At North Hyde, near Heston, is a large magazine for gunpowder, surrounded by mounds of earth, to protect the neighbourhood from the danger of an explosion. The soil of this parish is remarkable for producing excellent wheat, which, according to Norden and Camden, was used to make bread for the royal table in the reign of Elizabeth.

HESWALL, a parish in the lower division of the hundred of WIRRALL, county palatine of CHESTER, comprising the townships of Gayton and Heswall with Oldfield, and containing 386 inhabitants, of which number, 233 are in the joint township of Heswall with Oldfield, 3¾ miles (N. W. by N.) from Great Neston. The living is a rectory, in the archdeaconry and diocese of Chester, rated in the king's books at £18. 8. 4., and in the patronage of Davies Davenport, Esq. and Mrs. O'Kell, alternately. The church, pleasantly situated on the banks of the Dee, is an ancient structure, and contains several monuments in memory of different members of the Glegg family. There is a small un-endowed school.

HETHEL, a parish in the hundred of HUMBLEYARD, county of NORFOLK, 4½ miles (E. by S.) from Wymondham, containing 209 inhabitants. The living is a rectory, in the archdeaconry of Norfolk, and diocese of Norwich, rated in the king's books at £10. Sir Thomas Beevor, Bart. was patron in 1792. The church is dedicated to All Saints.

HETHERSETT, a parish in the hundred of HUMBLEYARD, county of NORFOLK, 3¾ miles (N. E. by E.) from Wymondham, containing 927 inhabitants. The living is a rectory in medieties, with the rectory of Cantelose, in the archdeaconry of Norfolk, and diocese of Norwich, rated in the king's books at £8, and in the patronage of the Master and Fellows of Caius College, Cambridge. The church is dedicated to St. Remigius.

HETHERSGILL, a township in the parish of KIRK-LINTON, or KIRK-LEVINGTON, ESKDALE ward, county of CUMBERLAND, 6 miles (N. W.) from Brampton, containing 776 inhabitants.

HETT, a township in the parish of MERRINGTON, south-eastern division of DARLINGTON ward, county palatine of DURHAM, 5½ miles (S. by E.) from Durham, containing 233 inhabitants. There is a paper-mill about a mile eastward from the village, also a good freestone quarry at Broom hill.

HETTON, a joint township with Bordley, in the parish of BURNSALL, eastern division of the wapentake of STAINCLIFFE and EWCROSS, West riding of the county of YORK, 6½ miles (N. N. W.) from Skipton, containing 180 inhabitants.

HETTON le HOLE, a township in the parish of HOUGHTON le SPRING, northern division of EASINGTON ward, county palatine of DURHAM, 6¼ miles (N. E. by E.) from Durham, containing 919 inhabitants. Here are places of worship for Baptists, Kilhamites, and Primitive and Wesleyan Methodists. Extensive mines of coal are worked in the vicinity. In a field on the right-hand side of the road from Eppleton to Hetton is a tumulus, consisting of a collection of small stones, at the top of which is a small oblong cavity, called the Fairies' Cradle.

HEUGH, a township in the parish of STAMFORD-HAM, north-eastern division of TINDALE ward, county of NORTHUMBERLAND, 12½ miles (N. W. by W.) from Newcastle upon Tyne, containing 512 inhabitants.

HEVER, a parish in the hundred of SOMERDEN, lathe of SUTTON at HONE, county of KENT, 8½ miles (W. by S.) from Tunbridge, containing 606 inhabitants. The living is a rectory, in the peculiar jurisdiction of the Archbishop of Canterbury, rated in the king's books at £15. 7. 3½. The Rev. T. Streatfeild was patron in 1799. The church, dedicated to St. Peter, contains a magnificent monument of the Boleyne family. The castle, the seat of that illustrious house, is a very ancient building, defended by a moat, drawbridge, portcullis, and tower, and was the residence of Sir Thomas Boleyne, father of Ann Boleyne, queen of Henry VIII., who is stated to have been born here, and here Anne of Cleves died: the chamber of Ann Boleyne is still called by her name, and several other curious mementos are shewn to visitors.

HEVERSHAM, a parish in KENDAL ward, county of WESTMORLAND, comprising the chapelries of Crosthwaite with Lyth and Stainton, and the townships of Hincaster, Levens, Milnthorpe with Heversham, Preston-Richard, and Sedgwick, and containing, including the whole of Levens, a small portion of which township is in Kendal parish, 3996 inhabitants, of which number, 1401 are in the joint township of Milnthorpe with Heversham, 1½ mile (N.) from Milnthorpe. The living is a vicarage, in the archdeaconry of Richmond, and diocese of Chester, rated in the king's books at £36. 13. 4., and in the patronage of the Master and Fellows of Trinity College, Cambridge. The church, dedicated to St. Peter, is a fine edifice in the early style of English architecture. The free grammar school was founded in 1613, by Edward Wilson, Esq., who endowed it with land now producing about £60 per annum, and with two exhibitions to Queen's College, Oxford, one to Trinity College, and one to Magdalene College, Cambridge: attached to the school is a library, founded, in 1766, by the associates of Dr. Wray; and in 1824, £267. 11. was subscribed to rebuild the school-room and a residence for the master. The school is open to all the boys of the parish, and no charge is made but for writing and arithmetic. This parish is bounded on the north and on the west by the river Kent. The learned Dr. Richard Watson, Bishop of Llandaff, was a native of this place.

HEVINGHAM, or HEVENINGHAM, a parish in the southern division of the hundred of ERPINGHAM, county of NORFOLK, 3 miles (S. by E.) from Aylsham, containing 744 inhabitants. The living is a discharged rectory, in the archdeaconry and diocese of Norwich, rated in the king's books at £10. 16. George Anson, Esq. was patron in 1787. The church is dedicated to St. Botolph.

HEWELSFIELD, a parish in the hundred of ST. BRIAVELLS, county of GLOUCESTER, 5½ miles (N.N.E.) from Chepstow, containing 434 inhabitants. The living is a perpetual curacy, annexed to the vicarage of Lydney, in the archdeaconry of Hereford, and diocese of Gloucester. The church is dedicated to St. Mary Magdalene.

HEWICK-BRIDGE, a township in that part of the parish of RIPON which is within the liberty of RIPON, though locally in the lower division of the wapentake of Claro, West riding of the county of YORK, 1¾ mile (E. S. E.) from Ripon, containing 77 inhabitants.

HEWICK-COPT, a township in that part of the parish of RIPON which is within the liberty of RIPON, though locally in the lower division of the wapentake of Claro, West riding of the county of YORK, 2 miles (E.) from Ripon, containing 131 inhabitants.

HEWISH, a parish in the hundred of SWANBOROUGH, county of WILTS, 3 miles (N. N. W.) from Pewsey, containing 112 inhabitants. The living is a rectory, in the archdeaconry of Wilts, and diocese of Salisbury, rated in the king's books at £8. 6. 8., and in the patronage of the Trustees of the Froxfield almshouses. The church is dedicated to St. Nicholas. A college, or almshouses, for thirty widows of laymen and twenty of clergymen, was founded at Froxfield, in 1690, by Sarah, Duchess of Somerset, and endowed with the proceeds of this manor.

HEWORTH, a township in that part of the parishes of ST. CUTHBERT and ST. GILES, YORK, which is in the wapentake of BULMER, North riding of the county of YORK, 1 mile (N.E.) from York, containing 146 inhabitants.

HEWORTH (NETHER), a chapelry in the parish of

JARROW, eastern division of CHESTER ward, county palatine of DURHAM, 2¼ miles (E. S. E.) from Gateshead, containing 3921 inhabitants. The chapel, erected by subscription in 1822, on the site of a former one, at an expense of £2026, contains one thousand four hundred sittings, of which six hundred and eighty-seven are free, the Incorporated Society for the enlargement of churches and chapels having granted £500 towards defraying the expense. In the church-yard is an inscribed obelisk recording the names and ages of ninety-one persons who were killed by explosion of fire damp in Felling colliery, in 1812, and buried here side by side; also a tomb-stone in memory of Richard Dawes, A. M., author of *Miscellanea Critica, &c.*, and head master of the grammar school at Newcastle, who spent a portion of the latter part of his life at this place, where he died. Here are manufactories for copperas, earthenware, paper, and ropes; also many ship-yards, wherein are constructed vessels of large burden. The neighbourhood abounds with coal pits. A few years since an earthen vessel was discovered, containing coins struck by Egfrid, one of the Saxon kings of Northumberland. Here is a school for boys and girls, with apartments for the master and mistress.

HEXGRAVE-PARK, a township in the parish of SOUTHWELL, liberty of SOUTHWELL and SCROOBY, county of NOTTINGHAM, 4 miles (N. W.) from Southwell. The population is returned with the parish. This was formerly an extra-parochial liberty, having been, prior to the Reformation, a park belonging to the archiepiscopal palace of the see of York, at Southwell. On the most elevated part of the township are the remains of a very large camp, supposed to be Roman, including a space of about forty acres, and commanding very extensive prospects : near it a brass celt was found in 1800, and fragments of military weapons have frequently been turned up by the plough.

HEXHAM, a parish in the southern division of TINDALE ward, county of NORTHUMBERLAND, comprising the market town of Hexham, and the wards of Gilligate, Hencoats, Market, and Priestpople, besides a district called Hexhamshire, in which are the townships of High Quarter, Low Quarter, Middle Quarter (North), Middle Quarter (South), and West Quarter, and containing 5436 inhabitants, of which number, 4116 are in the town of Hexham, 21 miles (W.) from Newcastle upon Tyne, and 283 (N.N.W.) from London. The origin of this place, which Camden supposes to have been the *Axelodunum* of the Romans, is, perhaps, with greater probability, referred to the Saxons, by whom it was called *Hextoldesham* and *Halgustad*, from the neighbouring streams Hextol and Halgut, from the former of which its present name is derived. Horsley refers the station of *Axelodunum* to Brough in Cumberland, and the supposition of Camden is not confirmed by any Roman relics, except a few inscribed stones, which have been obviously brought from some other place. About the year 673, Wilfrid, Archbishop of York, having obtained from Ethelreda, wife of Egfrid, King of Northumberland, a grant of the town, and a large adjoining tract, called Hexhamshire, founded a monastery and erected a church, which, according to Richard of Hexham, was the most beautiful and magnificent ecclesiastical edifice in the kingdom. Wilfrid being expelled from the see of York, in 678, that province was divided, and Hexham was erected into a see,

which continued, under a regular succession of bishops, for more than a century, till being united with Lindisfarne, it eventually became a part of the see of Durham. Tilford, the last bishop, was expelled from his bishoprick in 821, by the Danes, who, about fifty years afterwards, destroyed the monastery and plundered the town. The monastery was restored for Augustine canons, in 1112, and Hexham, together with Holme, was appropriated to the endowment of a prebendal stall in the Cathedral Church of York. In 1138, the Scots, under David I., pillaged the monastery, and, in 1296, again attacking the town, burnt the monastery and the nave of the conventual church. In the reign of Henry VIII., the last prior of Hexham having been involved in the insurrection called the Pilgrimage of Grace, was hanged at the gate of the monastery in 1536 : at the dissolution, the revenue was £138. 1. 9.

Hexham possessed all the rights and privileges of a county palatine, which, with the *jura regalia*, were confirmed by Edward I., during whose reign the town was again plundered by an army of forty thousand Scots, under the command of David II., who was taken prisoner by Sir John Copeland, then sheriff of Northumberland, at the battle of Nevil's Cross. In 1463, the decisive battle of Hexham was fought on the plains near the town, between the Yorkists and Lancastrians, in which the former, commanded by Lord Montacute, defeated the latter, under the Duke of Somerset, who was taken prisoner and beheaded at Hexham. A dreadful riot happened here on the 9th of March, 1761, when five thousand persons, principally miners, assembled to obstruct the magistrates, who had met to superintend a ballot for militia men. A party of the North York militia was called in to support the civil authorities, and one of their officers was murdered by some of the infuriated mob, on which, the riot act having been read, the soldiers were ordered to fire, when forty-eight persons were killed, and three hundred wounded. Several of the rioters were subsequently apprehended, and one of them was hanged at Morpeth. Hexham, with its adjoining district, coming into the possession of the Crown by an exchange with the Archbishop of York, was, in the 14th of Elizabeth, annexed to the county of Northumberland.

The town, which is irregularly built, consists of several spacious streets diverging from an extensive market-place in the centre, partially paved, and indifferently lighted by subscription : the inhabitants are supplied with water conveyed from a considerable distance into two reservoirs, provincially called pants, of which one was built by subscription, and the other at the sole charge of Robert Allgood, Esq. The bridge over the river Tyne, a handsome stone structure of nine principal arches, was erected by two country masons, from a design by Mr. Robert Mylne, the architect of Blackfriars' bridge, London ; on the south side are three smaller arches, to afford a speedier passage to the waters during high floods, for want of which precaution four preceding bridges have been carried away. A suspension bridge was constructed in 1826 over the South Tyne, near the western ferry, at an expense of £5000, by Capt. Samuel Brown, R.N. ; the span is three hundred and ten feet, and the breadth twenty feet : the dimensions of the piers at the base, are twenty-eight feet by fourteen, one of them being sunk nine, and the other eight, feet below the bed of the river; and a bridge of two arches has been recently erected at Gilligate, where the Cowgarth and Cockshaw burns unite their streams. A mechanics' institution, with a library of three hundred and fifty volumes, was established in 1825. The principal branches of trade are the dressing of leather and the making of gloves, the town having long been in high repute for the latter : tanning is also carried on to a considerable extent, and there are two woollen factories, a manufactory for hats, and a brewery. The Vale of Hexham presents a rich landscape of picturesque scenery, being beautifully diversified with well-cultivated fields, shrubberies, and pleasure grounds, and is remarkable for producing earlier crops than the surrounding district : a considerable portion of the land belongs to the Commissioners of Greenwich Hospital. The market days are Tuesday and Saturday, the former for corn ; a large cattle market is also held every alternate Tuesday, from the end of February to Midsummer, and from October to Christmas : the market-house is a neat and commodious building, with a piazza. The fairs are on August 6th and November 9th, for horses, cattle, sheep, and swine. Though the town never received a charter of incorporation, there are four trading companies, viz., weavers, shoemakers, glovers, and hatters, exercising, by a kind of prescriptive right, as great a control over those respective trades as is generally practised in towns regularly incorporated. A bailiff, appointed by the lord of the manor, presides at the manorial courts, and holds his office generally for life. A court of record is held twice in the year, within a month after Easter and at Michaelmas, for the recovery of debts to any amount, at which the steward of the manor, who must be a barrister, presides ; its jurisdiction extends over the whole liberty, comprising the parishes of Hexham, Allendale, and St. John Lee, in Northumberland : a side court is also held four times in the year, or oftener, if requisite, for the recovery of debts under 40s., at which the bailiff presides ; the jurisdiction of this court also extends ove, the whole liberty. Courts leet and baron are held here for the manor of Arrick-Grange, which is partly within this parish ; as are also the Midsummer quarter sessions for the county, and a petty session for Tindale ward, on the first Tuesday in the month. The town-hall is an ancient edifice, formerly the court-house of the bishops and priors, in which the manor courts and quarter sessions are held, and prisoners for debt are occasionally confined : at a small distance from it is an ancient tower, supposed to have been built for the defence of the monastery, and now used as the manor office. In Gilligate is a house of correction for the county, which was repaired, with the addition of a new wing, a few years ago. The living is a perpetual curacy with that of Whitley, in the peculiar jurisdiction of the Archbishop of York, endowed with £420 private benefaction, £400 royal bounty, and £800 parliamentary grant, and in the patronage of Colonel and Mrs. Beaumont. In 1623, the corn tithes of Erringside, which formerly belonged to the abbey, were left to the Mercers' Company, by Mr. Richard Fishborne, in trust for the endowment of a lectureship. The church, dedicated to St. Andrew, is part of the conventual church of the monastery, built on the site of the ancient cathedral, a spacious cruciform structure, exhibiting portions in various styles of

English architecture, with a tower rising from the intersection of the transepts and the choir ; the nave, burnt by the Scots in 1296, has not been rebuilt ; the choir is separated from the transepts by a screen of wood richly carved in the lower part, and ornamented in the upper with an allegorical painting of the Dance of Death ; the choir, of which the roof is very lofty and panelled with oak, is separated from its aisles, which are groined, by ranges of clustered columns, above which are the triforium and clerestory, the arches of the former springing from a second tier of clustered columns, and the windows of the latter separated by plain masonry. On the south side of the altar, which is lighted with a large east window of elegant tracery, but disfigured by an incongruous embellishment of Grecian architectural painting, is a gallery of oak, beautifully carved, beneath which are three stalls highly enriched with tabernacle - work, and on the north side is a shrine, or oratory, in the decorated style of English architecture, exquisitely ornamented with foliated arches, tracery, and figures, supposed to have been erected for Prior Richard, of Hexham, to whom also is attributed a recumbent figure on an altar-tomb adjacent ; among the monuments is one said by Pennant and others to be that of Elfwald, a Northumbrian king, who was killed in 788, but its style appears to be of the thirteenth century ; and on an altar-tomb is the figure of an armed knight, cross-legged, with a shield of arms identifying him as one of the baronial family of Umfraville, though the effigy is supposed by Wallis the historian to be that of the Duke of Somerset, executed at Hexham. There are places of worship for Independents and Wesleyan Methodists, besides a Scottish church and two Roman Catholic chapels, in both of which latter the altar-pieces are embellished with fine paintings of the Crucifixion. The grammar school was founded in 1599, by Queen Elizabeth, who placed it under the control of an incorporated body of governors : it has but a trifling endowment, the master being paid by the pupils. A National school, founded in 1813, in which three hundred children of both sexes are instructed, is supported by subscription. Near a spot called St. Mary's Chare are some remains of the ancient church founded by Wilfrid in 678, and dedicated to the Blessed Virgin. John, Prior of Hexham, in the twelfth century, wrote the history of the reign of Henry II. ; and his successor, Richard of Hexham, was the author of several historical works. Joseph Richardson, the dramatist, who died in 1803, was a native of Hexham ; and John Tweddel, born in 1769, at Threepwood, near this place, greatly distinguished himself as a classical scholar and antiquary, and died, in 1799, at Athens, while travelling to qualify himself for a diplomatic employment.

HEXTHORP, a joint township with Balby, in that part of the parish of DONCASTER which is within the soke of DONCASTER, though locally in the northern division of the wapentake of STRAFFORTH and TICKHILL, West riding of the county of YORK, 1¼ mile (S. W.) from Doncaster, containing 392 inhabitants.

HEXTON, a parish in the hundred of CASHIO, or liberty of ST. ALBAN'S, county of HERTFORD, 5¼ miles (W. by N.) from Hitchin, containing 338 inhabitants. The living is a discharged vicarage, in the archdeaconry of St. Alban's, and diocese of London, rated in the king's books at £7. 13. 4., endowed with £400 royal bounty, and in the patronage of Joseph Andrew Lautour, Esq. The church is dedicated to St. Faith. A complete intrenchment, called Ravensburgh castle, occupies a site of about twelve acres, on the south-west side of this parish. The Iknield-street passes through the parish. Springs of water, slightly chalybeate, constantly descend from a hill here, so as to form a river in Hexton park, and turn a mill. Quantities of gold and silver coins, principally Roman and Saxon, have been found. Courts leet and baron are held annually.

HEXWOOD, a tything in the parish of CUMNER, hundred of HORMER, county of BERKS, containing 7 inhabitants.

HEY, a chapelry in the parish of ASHTON under LINE, hundred of SALFORD, county palatine of LANCASTER, 2 miles (E.) from Oldham. The population is returned with the parish. The living is a perpetual curacy, in the archdeaconry and diocese of Chester, endowed with £200 private benefaction, £200 royal bounty, and £800 parliamentary grant, and in the patronage of the Rector of Ashton under Line. The chapel is dedicated to St. John.

HEYBRIDGE, a parish in the hundred of THURSTABLE, county of ESSEX, 1 mile (N. N. E.) from Maldon, containing 868 inhabitants. The living is a vicarage, rated in the king's books at £10, and in the peculiar jurisdiction and patronage of the Dean and Chapter of St. Paul's, London. The church is dedicated to St. Andrew. The Chelmer navigation has much improved the trade of this place, by means of a canal which passes through the parish, and separates it from Northey island, on the Blackwater river; its buildings have likewise considerably increased in number. The bridge was erected by Henry VI. A causeway was constructed between Heybridge and Maldon before the time of Edward II.

HEYDON, a parish in the southern division of the hundred of ERPINGHAM, county of NORFOLK, 3½ miles (N. N. E.) from Reepham, containing 333 inhabitants. The living is a rectory with Irmingland, in the archdeaconry and diocese of Norwich, rated in the king's books at £9. 16. 10½. W. W. Bulmer, Esq. was patron in 1786. The church is dedicated to St. Peter.

HEYFORD (LOWER), a parish in the hundred of PLOUGHLEY, county of OXFORD, 6 miles (W.N.W.) from Bicester, containing 495 inhabitants. The living is a rectory, in the archdeaconry and diocese of Oxford, rated in the king's books at £10. 13. 1½., and in the patronage of the President and Fellows of Corpus Christi College, Oxford. The church is dedicated to St. Mary.

HEYFORD (NETHER), a parish in the hundred of NOBOTTLE-GROVE, county of NORTHAMPTON, 7 miles (W. by S.) from Northampton, containing 422 inhabitants. The living is a rectory, in the archdeaconry of Northampton, and diocese of Peterborough, rated in the king's books at £8. 10. 5. The Rev. J. L. Crawley was patron in 1809. The church is dedicated to St. Peter and St. Paul. A school for the children of Upper and Nether Heyford, and all of the name of Bliss within five miles, was endowed by W. Bliss, with a bequest of £400, but at what period is not known. The Grand Junction canal passes through the parish, and on its southern boundary runs the Watling-street. Dr. John Preston, surnamed the

Patriarch of the Puritans, was born here in 1587.

HEYFORD (UPPER), a parish in the hundred of NOBOTTLE-GROVE, county of NORTHAMPTON, 6¼ miles (W.) from Northampton, containing 122 inhabitants.

HEYFORD (WARREN, or UPPER), a parish in the hundred of PLOUGHLEY, county of OXFORD, 6 miles (N.W. by W.) from Bicester, containing 257 inhabitants. The living is a rectory, in the archdeaconry and diocese of Oxford, rated in the king's books at £13. 16. 0½., and in the patronage of the Warden and Fellows of New College, Oxford. The church is dedicated to St. Mary.

HEYHOUSES, a township in that part of the parish of WHALLEY which is in the higher division of the hundred of BLACKBURN, county palatine of LANCASTER, 3¼ miles (S. E.) from Clitheroe, containing 187 inhabitants.

HEYSHAM, a parish in the hundred of LONSDALE, south of the sands, county palatine of LANCASTER, 5 miles (W.) from Lancaster, containing 540 inhabitants. The living is a rectory, in the archdeaconry of Richmond, and diocese of Chester, rated in the king's books at £8. 9. 2., and in the patronage of the Rev. T. Yates Ridley. The church, dedicated to St. Peter, is an ancient edifice placed on the summit of a rock. A sum was given by Robert Thompson, in 1817, for the instruction of children, which produces £8. 9. per annum. On the hill above the church are the remains of an ancient oratory, dedicated to St. Patrick. In the church-yard are several coffin-like excavations in the solid rock, in the shape of the human body. In High Heysham are the remains of a Roman Catholic chapel, which originally belonged to the Stanley family.

HEYSHOT, a parish in the hundred of EASEBOURNE, rape of CHICHESTER, county of SUSSEX, 2½ miles (S. by E.) from Midhurst, containing 309 inhabitants. The living is a rectory with Stedham, in the archdeaconry and diocese of Chichester. The church has portions in the decorated and later styles of English architecture. The Rother, or Arundel, navigation passes on the north of this parish.

HEYTESBURY, a borough, formerly a market-town, in the hundred of HEYTESBURY, county of WILTS, 3½ miles (E. S. E.) from Warminster, and 93 (W. S. W.) from London, containing 1329 inhabitants. The ancient appellations of this town were *Hegtredesbyrig* and *Heightsbury*, whence is obviously derived its present

Seal and Arms.

name. During the contest between Stephen and Matilda, the empress is said to have occasionally resided here. The town is situated in a pleasant valley, on the south-west verge of Salisbury plain, and on the northern bank of the small river Wily, on the high road from London to Bridg-water. In its vicinity are several bold eminences, which are for the most part crowned with ancient encampments, British, Roman, Saxon, and Danish. It consists principally of ° ne long and irregular street, of which the borough comprises the western extremity, called in ancient records West Heytesbury, or Heytesbury Magna; it is neither paved nor lighted, but is supplied with good water. The manufacture of cloth is carried on to a considerable extent, the vicinity of the river affording a facility for the erection of mills and factories : there are two manufactories, one for broad cloth, the other both for cloth and kerseymere, one of the proprietors having also an extensive establishment at Upton, about a mile and a half distant, where the articles are finished. The number of persons employed in the various branches of the trade amounts to about eight hundred. There is a small fair on May 14th, for cattle, sheep, &c. Heytesbury is a borough by prescription, but not incorporated : it first sent members to parliament in the 28th of Henry VI., since which time two have been regularly returned. The right of election is in the burgage-holders, about thirty-three in number, and the returning officer is the bailiff, who is appointed by Lord Heytesbury, as lord of the manor, his lordship also appointing the bailiff of the hundred, which is co-extensive with the manor. A court leet is held annually at Michaelmas, at which two constables and two tythingmen for the town, and similar officers for the hundred, are appointed. Heytesbury is within the jurisdiction of a court of requests held at Warminster, for the recovery of debts to the amount of £5.

The living is a perpetual curacy, in the peculiar jurisdiction and patronage of the Dean of Sarum, endowed with £1000 private benefaction, £1000 royal bounty, and £600 parliamentary grant. The church, situated in the centre of the town, is a spacious, massive, cruciform structure, with a square tower at the intersection : in the choir are fourteen very ancient oak stalls. It was made collegiate about the year 1165, by Josceline, Bishop of Salisbury, and was rebuilt by Thomas, Lord Hungerford, in 1404; there were formerly two chantries, to which are now attached the prebends of Tytherington, Horningsham, Hill-Deverill, and Swallowcliff. There is a place of worship for Independents. An hospital, begun by Robert, Lord Hungerford, was completed and endowed, pursuant to his will, by his widow Margaret, Lady Hungerford and Botseaux, who, about 1472, amortized the manors of Cheverell-Burnell and Cheverell-Hales for the latter purpose. The design of the institution was to maintain a custos (who was to be a priest in full orders, and to teach grammar), twelve poor men, and one woman, nine of whom are nominated by the Lord of the Manor, and three from the parish of Cheverell. By the 11th of Edward IV. this endowment was confirmed, and the society invested with power to hold lands, to plead and be impleaded, and to use a common seal, &c., by the title of "The Custos, Poor Men and Women of the Hospital of Walter and Robert, late Lords of Hungerford and Heytesbury." At the dissolution, it being discovered that daily prayers were directed for the souls of the founders, it escheated to the crown on the plea of superstitious uses, and was granted, with all its possessions, to Sir John Sharington ; in the reign of Mary it was restored, and afterwards exempted by Elizabeth from the payment of tenths and first fruits. James I., at the request of the Earl of Northampton, fully confirmed all its rights and privileges by his charter of Inspeximus, dated in 1610, since which time its affairs have been and still are regulated by this charter. In 1633, a body of statutes for its government was framed by the Dean and Chapter of Salisbury, who are visitors by appoint-

ment of the foundress, and a revision of them is now in contemplation. The patronage is vested in the Chancellor of Sarum, if resident, otherwise in the Dean and Chapter : the present custos is the incumbent of the collegiate church. The several annual salaries are, £60 to the custos and £40 to the sub-custos, whose offices are now united; that of the schoolmaster is not paid, the school having ceased to exist for nearly a century. All the buildings and furniture of the hospital were destroyed by a fire which occurred in 1765, and which consumed nearly two-thirds of the town; but the whole was rebuilt in a very substantial manner. The original costume of the poor men was a scarlet gown, or cloak, with the greek characters I. H. Σ. in black on the back, and X. P. Σ. on the breast ; and to this has been recently added a complete suit of blue cloth, with a red cross on the left breast of the coat. The hospital possesses the two manors of Cheverell-Burnell and Cheverell-Hales, or Cheverell-Magna, with twenty loads of wood yearly from Southley, which last is now commuted for an annual payment of £14; also certain closes of land in Warminster, and an allowance of wheat yearly from lands in Upton-Scudamore, the gift of another branch of the Hungerford family ; in addition to these are the manor of Churton, purchased many years since with the surplus funds of the hospital, and other more recent but very considerable purchases. On the summit of Cotley hill, north-westward from the town, is a large tumulus, surrounded by a circular ditch and low vallum, and on another hill in the vicinity is the large ancient encampment, called Scratchbury Camp, so named from the British word *Crech*, signifying a hill ; the circuit of its rampart is one mile and eighty-six yards, and its greatest height sixty-six feet, including an area of forty acres. Mr. William Cunnington, an industrious antiquary, was long a resident at this place, where he died and was interred in 1810. Heytesbury confers the title of baron on the family of A'Court.

HEYTHORP, a parish in the hundred of WOOTTON, county of OXFORD, 3¼ miles (E. by N.) from Chipping-Norton, containing, with the hamlet of Dunthorp, 136 inhabitants. The living is a rectory, in the archdeaconry and diocese of Oxford, rated in the king's books at £7. 11. 10½. Mrs. Vernon was patroness in 1800, The church is dedicated to St. Nicholas.

HEYWOOD, a chapelry in that part of the parish of BURY which is in the hundred of SALFORD, county palatine of LANCASTER, 2¾ miles (E.) from Bury, with which the population is returned. The living is a perpetual curacy, in the archdeaconry and diocese of Chester, endowed with £400 private benefaction, £600 royal bounty, and £1200 parliamentary grant. The Rev. G. Hornby was patron in 1823. The chapel contains three hundred free sittings, towards defraying the expense of which the Incorporated Society for the enlargement of churches and chapels contributed £400. There are places of worship for Independents, Wesleyan Methodists, and Swedenborgians. In 1737, James Lancashire bequeathed £50 towards establishing a school for poor children : a school-house and a rent-charge of £5 per annum were likewise conveyed to trustees, by James Starky, as also a bequest of £50, the interest to be applied in aid of the children ; twenty children are taught by a schoolmistress, who has the use of a house rent-free, and a stipend of £5 per annum; 40s. are applied annually for the benefit of the children. A National school is supported by voluntary contributions. Here are extensive manufactories for cotton and woollen goods.

HIBALSTOW, a parish in the eastern division of the wapentake of MANLEY, parts of LINDSEY, county of LINCOLN, 3¾ miles (S. W. by S.) from Glandford-Bridge, containing 522 inhabitants. The living is a discharged vicarage, in the archdeaconry of Stow, and diocese of Lincoln, rated in the king's books at £7. 10. The Rev. J. De Chair was patron in 1814. The church is dedicated to St. Hibald; the chancel and lower part of the tower are in the early English style, and the other parts of more modern architecture. There is a place of worship for Wesleyan Methodists. The Roman road of from Lincoln to the Humber passes through the parish; and about a mile eastward from the church, foundations of buildings, tiles, coins, and other Roman relics, have been discovered.

HIBBURN, county of NORTHUMBERLAND. — See HEBBURN.

HICKLETON, a parish in the northern division of the wapentake of STRAFFORTH and TICKHILL, West riding of the county of YORK, 6 miles (W. by N.) from Doncaster, comprising the township of Hickleton, and containing 153 inhabitants. The living is a perpetual curacy, in the archdeaconry and diocese of York, endowed with £600 private benefaction, and £1200 royal bounty. G. W. Wentworth, Esq. was patron in 1817. The church is dedicated to St. Denis.

HICKLING, a parish in the hundred of HAPPING, county of NORFOLK, 10½ miles (E. N. E.) from Coltishall, containing 679 inhabitants. The living is a discharged vicarage, in the archdeaconry of Norfolk, and diocese of Norwich, rated in the king's books at £5. 3. 4., endowed with £200 private benefaction, and £400 royal bounty. N. Micklethwayte, Esq. was patron in 1811. The church is dedicated to St. Mary. A priory of Black canons, dedicated to the Virgin Mary, St. Augustine, and All Saints, was founded, in 1185, by Theobald de Valentia, or Valoins, the revenue of which at the dissolution was valued at £137. 0. 1.

HICKLING, a parish in the southern division of the wapentake of BINGHAM, county of NOTTINGHAM, 8¼ miles (N. W. by N.) from Melton-Mowbray, containing 497 inhabitants. The living is a rectory, in the archdeaconry of Nottingham, and diocese of York, rated in the king's books at £18. 8. 4., and in the patronage of the President and Fellows of Queen's College, Cambridge. The church, dedicated to St. Luke, is a handsome ancient structure, with a quadrangular tower: the lid of a stone coffin, curiously inscribed with Runic characters, has been discovered in the chancel. Here is a place of worship for Wesleyan Methodists. The Grantham canal passes through the parish, and crosses the northern boundary into Leicestershire. Some years ago several Roman coins were dug up on Standard Hill, so called from a standard, or pole, having been formerly erected on it.

HIDCOATE-BATRIM, a hamlet in the parish of MICKLETON, upper division of the hundred of KIFTS-GATE, county of GLOUCESTER, 2 miles (N. E.) from Chipping-Campden. The population is returned with the parish.

HIDDON, a joint tything with Eddington, in the parish of HUNGERFORD, hundred of KINTBURY-EAGLE, county of BERKS, 2 miles (N. E.) from Hungerford, containing 421 inhabitants.

HIDE (WEST), a parochial chapelry in the parish of STOKE EDITH, hundred of RADLOW, county of HEREFORD, 8 miles (E. N. E.) from Hereford, containing 193 inhabitants. The living is a perpetual curacy, with the rectory of Stoke-Edith, in the archdeaconry and diocese of Hereford.

HIENDLEY (COLD), a joint township with Havercroft, in the parish of FELKIRK, wapentake of STAINCROSS, West riding of the county of YORK, 5½ miles (S. E. by S.) from Wakefield, containing 189 inhabitants.

HIENDLEY (SOUTH), a township in the parish of FELKIRK, wapentake of STAINCROSS, West riding of the county of YORK, 7 miles (N. E.) from Barnesley, containing 166 inhabitants.

HIGHAM, a hamlet in the parish of SHIRLAND, hundred of SCARSDALE, county of DERBY, 16¼ miles (N. by E.) from Derby, containing 591 inhabitants. Higham is a place of great antiquity: it is situated upon the Roman Iknield-street, and had formerly a market; fairs for cattle are held on the first Wednesday after new year's day, and on February 27th. Many of the inhabitants are employed in weaving stockings and in the adjoining bleaching-grounds.

HIGHAM, a parish in the hundred of SHAMWELL, lathe of AYLESFORD, county of KENT, 4½ miles (N. N. W.) from Rochester, containing 568 inhabitants. The living is a vicarage, in the archdeaconry and diocese of Rochester, rated in the king's books at £8. 10., and in the patronage of the Master and Fellows of St. John's College, Cambridge. The church is dedicated to St. Mary. The river Thames bounds the parish on the north, and the Thames and Medway canal is conducted into the adjoining parish of Frindsbury by a tunnel two miles and a quarter in length. One of the pensioners in Cobham College is to be selected from among the inhabitants. Gad's hill, mentioned by Shakspeare in his play of Henry IV., is in this parish. A nunnery of the Benedictine order, dedicated to the Blessed Virgin Mary, was founded here, before 1151, by King Stephen, whose daughter Mary, afterwards abbess of Romsey, became one of the nuns: it was suppressed by Fisher, Bishop of Rochester, in the 13th of Henry VIII., and given by the King to the Master and Fellows of St. John's College, Cambridge.

HIGHAM, a parish in the hundred of SAMFORD, county of SUFFOLK, 4¾ miles (S.) from Hadleigh, containing 262 inhabitants. The living is a discharged vicarage, in the archdeaconry of Sudbury, and diocese of Norwich, rated in the king's books at £5. 6. 8., endowed with £210 private benefaction, and £200 royal bounty, and in the patronage of certain Feoffees. The church is dedicated to St. Mary. The navigable river Stour runs on the south-western side of the parish, where it receives a small stream.

HIGHAM (COLD), a parish in the hundred of TOWCESTER, county of NORTHAMPTON, 3½ miles (N. W. by N.) from Towcester, containing 314 inhabitants. The living is a rectory, in the archdeaconry of Northampton, and diocese of Peterborough, rated in the king's books at £10, and in the patronage of the Earl of Pomfret. The church is dedicated to St. Luke. The parish is bounded on the north-east by the Roman Watling-street.

HIGHAM on the HILL, a parish in the hundred of SPARKENHOE, county of LEICESTER, 3¼ miles (W. by N.) from Hinckley, containing, with the hamlet of Lindley, 533 inhabitants. The living is a rectory, in the archdeaconry of Leicester, and diocese of Lincoln, rated in the king's books at £7. 9. 4½. Thomas Fisher, Esq. was patron in 1792. The church is dedicated to St. Peter. The Ashby de la Zouch canal passes through the parish. In 1607, a great many silver coins of the reign of Henry III. were discovered, on turning up a large stone which lay at the intersection of Watling-street with another road leading to Coventry : several Roman coins, a gold ring with a ruby, another with an agate, and a third of silver, with an Arabic inscription, were found here about the same period.

HIGHAM-BOOTH, a township in that part of the parish of WHALLEY which is in the higher division of the hundred of BLACKBURN, county palatine of LAN-CASTER, 4½ miles (N. W.) from Burnley, containing 891 inhabitants. There is a place of worship for Wesleyan Methodists.

HIGHAM-DYKES, a township in the parish of PONTELAND, western division of CASTLE ward, county of NORTHUMBERLAND, 10 miles (N. W.) from Newcastle upon Tyne, containing 23 inhabitants.

Corporate Seal.

HIGHAM-FERRERS, a borough and parish (former-ly a market town) possessing separate jurisdiction, though locally in the hundred of Higham - Ferrers, county of NORTHAMPTON, 15½ miles (E.N.E.) from Northampton, and 65 (N.N.W.) from London, containing 877 inha-bitants. The town derives its distinguishing appellation from the ancient family of Ferrers, who were its lords, and had a castle here. The name *Higham* is said to be a contraction of *High-ham*, denoting the elevated situation of the place, which stands on a rocky eminence abounding with springs, about half a mile from the north-eastern bank of the navigable river Nen, and consists chiefly of two streets, with a market-place, in which stands a cross ; its elevated site rendering it clean and healthy. It is supposed to have been for-merly much larger than it now is, having possessed, at one period, three weekly markets, not one of which, for the last thirty years, has been held. The chief bu-siness consists in making boots, shoes, and bobbin-lace. There are five annual fairs, viz., on March 7th, June 28th, the Thursday before August 5th, October 11th, and December 6th.

The town was first incorporated in the 2d and 3rd of Philip and Mary, and its privileges were confirmed by a charter granted in the 36th of Charles II., under which the corporation consists of a mayor, recorder, deputy recorder, seven aldermen, and thirteen capital burgesses : the aldermen are chosen from among the bur-gesses, and the mayor is elected annually from among the aldermen. The mayor is lord of a manor called Borough-hold, extending from Stump-cross northward, to Spittle-cross southward : he holds a court leet annu-

ally before the expiration of the term of his office ; and he and his predecessor are justices of the peace. There is a court of record, for the recovery of debts under £40, called the "Three Weeks' court," from the period of its recurrence; but it is now held. and that only for the sake of form, once a year, three weeks after the election of the mayor, when the constables are sworn in. The town-hall was erected by the corporation in 1812, near the site of a prior one, which had fallen into decay. This borough has sent a representative to par-liament since the third year of Philip and Mary : the right of election is vested in the body corporate and the resident freemen of the borough, the freedom of which is inherited by birth, and acquired by servitude, or gift from the corporation. The number of voters is about forty, and the mayor is the returning officer : the pa-tronage of the borough is possessed by Earl Fitzwil-liam.

The living is a vicarage not in charge, with the perpetual curacy of Chelveston, in the archdeaconry of Northampton, and diocese of Peterborough, and in the patronage of Earl Fitzwilliam. The church, dedicated to the Virgin Mary, is a handsome building, displaying the various styles of English architecture : it consists of two naves, with north and south aisles, and a chancel separated by a decorated screen ; on each side of the chancel are stalls, with curious emblematical devices : at the west end is a porch, much ornamented with sculp-ture, also an embattled tower, from which rises a finely-proportioned octagonal crocketed spire ; the latter hav-ing fallen down, with part of the tower, was rebuilt in 1632, by subscription, to which Archbishop Laud was a liberal contributor : the church contains some ancient monuments and sepulchral brasses. There is a place of worship for Wesleyan Methodists. A free grammar school has long existed here : it was founded by Arch-bishop Chichele, in 1420, who left an endowment of about £10 a year, to which Earl Fitzwilliam adds £10 more, as a salary for the master, but the school has of late years fallen into decay : the appointment of the master is vested in the corporation. The school-house is a handsome stone building, situated at the north-west end of the church, and having an embattled parapet. An almshouse, or bead-house, on the south side of the church, was also founded and endowed by Archbishop Chichele, for twelve poor men and one woman : the te-nements are now occupied by men and women, each of whom receives sevenpence a week, and an annual al-lowance of ten shillings, for what was originally termed "shaving and lamp money." Some remains of an ancient college are still discernible, but in a ruinous state : a portion of them was a few years ago converted into a dwelling-house. On the north side of the church is a spot called Castle-yard, the site of an ancient castle; some parts of the moat, and a few traces of the foun-dations, are remaining. Archbishop Chichele, a great patron of literature in the reign of Henry V., was born here in 1362.

HIGHAM-GOBION, a parish in the hundred of FLITT, county of BEDFORD, 2¾ miles (S.E. by S.) from Silsoe, containing 86 inhabitants. The living is a rec-tory, in the archdeaconry of Bedford, and diocese of Lincoln, rated in the king's books at £8. 9. 7. R. Lee, Esq. was patron in 1812. The church, dedicated to St. Margaret, contains a monument to the memory of Dr.

3 D 2

Edmund Castell, a learned orientalist, author of the Lexicon Heptaglotton, and a principal in the publication of the Polyglott Bible; he was born at Hatley, in Cambridgeshire, in 1606, was for several years rector of this parish, and a Prebendary in the Cathedral Church of Canterbury; he died here at the age of seventy-nine, having lost his sight some time previously, caused, as it is related, by incessant study.

HIGHAM-GREEN, a hamlet in the parish of GAZELEY, partly in the hundred of LACKFORD, but chiefly in that of RISBRIDGE, county of SUFFOLK, 6¾ miles (E. by N.) from Newmarket, containing 270 inhabitants.

HIGHAM-PARK, an extra-parochial liberty, in the hundred of HIGHAM-FERRERS, county of NORTHAMPTON, 3½ miles (S. S. E.) from Higham-Ferrers, containing 14 inhabitants.

HIGHAMPTON, county of DEVON.—See HAMPTON (HIGH).

HIGHCLERE, a parish in the hundred of EVINGAR, Kingsclere division of the county of SOUTHAMPTON, 8½ miles (N. by W.) from Whitchurch, containing 457 inhabitants. The living is a rectory, in the peculiar jurisdiction of the incumbent, rated in the king's books at £7. 13. 9. The Earl of Carnarvon was patron in 1825. The church, dedicated to St. Michael, was rebuilt in the time of Charles II. by Sir Robert Sawyer, Attorney General in that and the succeeding reign, who was buried here. A National school has been established, and is supported partly by subscription, and partly from an annuity of about £4. 4., the moiety of certain dividends bequeathed by the Rev. Archibald Gardner. Highclere is within the jurisdiction of the Cheyney Court held at Winchester every Thursday, for the recovery of debts to any amount. It was anciently part of the bishoprick of Winchester, and is recorded as such in Domesday-book. The bishops had a palace here, in which they occasionally resided, until the bailiwick held by them was, in the reign of Edward VI., dismembered by Bishop Poynet, and vested in the crown. Upon the site of the original edifice, which stood in a well-wooded and beautiful park, upwards of thirteen miles in circumference, is a fine mansion, erected by the Hon. Robert Herbert, and greatly enlarged by the Earl of Carnarvon, his descendant; and just without the park gate is Beacon hill, on the level summit of which is an ancient encampment. On a plain, about a mile from this camp, are some tumuli, or barrows, of considerable size, with three smaller ones. A mile and a half eastward from Beacon hill, on an eminence called Ladle Hill, is a circular intrenchment, enclosing an area of about eight acres; southward from this are three barrows; and at a short distance towards the north-north-east, on the declivity of the hill, is another small circular work, pitched entirely with flint-stones. Dr. Jeremiah Miller, a learned antiquary, was born here in 1713; he died in 1784.

HIGHEAD, or IVEGILL, a chapelry in the parish of DALSTON, ward and county of CUMBERLAND, 4 miles (S. by W.) from Dalston, containing 129 inhabitants. The living is a perpetual curacy, in the archdeaconry and diocese of Carlisle, endowed with £600 royal bounty, and £200 parliamentary grant, and in the patronage of sixteen trustees. The chapel, a mean building without a ceiling, and devoid of ornament, was erected by William L'Englise, and anciently belonged to the lords of the manor: near it, situated on the brow of a rocky eminence, are the gateway-tower, a turret, and other remains of Highead castle, the ancient residence of the Richmond family, now a farm-house.

HIGHGATE, a chapelry partly in the parish of ST. PANCRAS, Holborn division of the hundred of OSSULSTONE, but chiefly in the parish of HORNSEY, Finsbury division of the same hundred, county of MIDDLESEX, 4 miles (N.) from London. The population is returned with the respective parishes in which it is situated. This village is said to have taken its name from a toll-gate erected on the brow of the hill, near the site of an ancient hermitage, by one of the bishops of London, on the construction of a new road leading from the metropolis towards the north of England. The hill on which it stands is four hundred feet above the summit of St. Paul's cathedral, and it affords many extensive and beautiful prospects of London and the neighbouring country. In the village and its vicinity are several handsome houses and detached villas: the streets, which are not paved, are lighted with oil, and the inhabitants are supplied with water chiefly from wells. After various attempts to render the ascent up Highgate hill, over which the old road passes, less difficult and dangerous, by raising the road in some parts, and lowering it in others, which produced only a partial improvement, a scheme was projected in the year 1809, by Mr. Robert Vazie, an engineer, for forming a subterraneous arched tunnel, twenty-four feet wide, eighteen high, and three hundred yards in length, through the body of the hill, and an act of parliament was obtained, incorporating the proprietors a body politic, by the style of "The Highgate Archway Company," and authorising them to raise £40,000, by transferable shares of £50 each, with an additional sum of £20,000, if necessary; the work was commenced, and the tunnel constructed to the length of about one hundred and thirty yards, when the whole fell in with a tremendous crash, on the morning of the 13th of April, 1812. The plan was then altered, and a road in the line of the intended tunnel was formed: this road, by which upwards of one hundred yards are saved, and the hill and village both avoided, was opened on the 21st of August, 1813: it passes under an arch, over which Hornsey-lane, an ancient cross road, is continued. The foundation stone of the arch was laid October 31st, 1812: it is built of stone, flanked with brick-work, and surmounted by three semi-arches supporting a bridge, with open battlements of stone, along which the lane passes, and is about thirty-six feet in height, and half as much in width. During the progress of the excavations for the tunnel, various fossils and other geological remains were discovered in the strata, among which were pyrites, fossil teeth, petrified fish and fruit, and a variety of shells, petrified wood, and a peculiar resinous substance, emitting, on being rubbed, an odour similar to that of amber, being also slightly electric, insoluble in water, but soluble in alcohol, spirit of turpentine, and æther. The disastrous issue of the tunnel was made the subject of a dramatic entertainment, called "The Highgate Tunnel, or the Secret Arch," introduced at one of the London theatres. Highgate is within the jurisdiction of a court of requests held in Kingsgate-street, Holborn, for the recovery of debts under 40s.

The chapel, which is dedicated to St. Michael, was

founded as a chapel of ease to the church at Hornsey, prior to 1565, when the Bishop of London, as lord of the manor of Hornsey, and proprietor of the chapel, granted it, with other property, in trust, to Sir Roger Cholmeley, for the endowment of a free grammar school, to which it has ever since been attached, the schoolmaster being the minister of the chapel. An act of parliament has recently been passed for the erection of a new church, and for making Highgate a separate district. Here are places of worship for Baptists, Independents, and Wesleyan Methodists. In 1565, Queen Elizabeth issued letters patent for the foundation of a free grammar school, by Sir Roger Cholmeley, Chief Justice of the Queen's Bench, who endowed it with landed property vested in six wardens, or governors : the present income is about £600 per annum, from which the master receives a salary of £200, but the school is conducted by an assistant with a small stipend : in 1819 a new school-room was erected, at an expense of £697, in which about one hundred boys are instructed on the National system : in 1822, proceedings were instituted in the Court of Chancery against the governors and the master, to compel them to restore the grammar school to its original purpose ; and, in consequence of the decree of the Lord Chancellor, that the institution should be again made a free grammar school, it is expected that the National school will be removed to some other part of the village, and the free school re-established, according to the directions of its founders. A charity school for girls was established in 1719, in which twenty-six girls are educated, twenty of them being also clothed from the funds of the charity, which include £35 per annum, permanent revenue, and about £75 per annum, arising from voluntary contributions : the mistress has a salary of £26 per annum, besides occasional gratuities. In Hornsey-lane is a National school for girls belonging to Highgate and Holloway ; and there is also an infant school. Almshouses for six poor women were founded pursuant to a bequest by Sir John Wollaston, in 1658, and endowed with a rent-charge of £18. 10.; and six more almshouses for poor women, with an endowment of £30 per annum, were founded by Edward Pauncefort, Esq., who rebuilt the preceding almshouses, and by will, in 1723, left property for the support of this charity and the girls' school, with £10 per annum to the minister, which, with other benefactions to the almspeople, is vested in the governors of the free school. An hospital for lepers was founded on the lower part of Highgate hill, by William Poole, yeoman of the crown in the reign of Edward IV., which continued until the time of Henry VIII., and is supposed to have occupied a site now called Lazarets, or Lazarcot-field, near Whittington-stone.

HIGHLAWS, a township in that part of the parish of HARTBURN which is in the western division of MORPETH ward, county of NORTHUMBERLAND, 9½ miles (W. by S.) from Morpeth, containing 27 inhabitants.

HIGHLEY, a parish in the hundred of STOTTESDEN, county of SALOP, 7½ miles (S. by E.) from Bridgenorth, containing 424 inhabitants. The living is a vicarage, in the archdeaconry of Salop, and diocese of Hereford, rated in the king's books at £5. 19. 2. J. Fleming, L.L.D., was patron in 1790. The church is dedicated to St. Mary.

HIGHLOW, a township in the parish of HOPE, hun-

dred of HIGH PEAK, county of DERBY, 3½ miles (N. by W.) from Stoney-Middleton, containing 36 inhabitants.

HIGHNAM, a hamlet in that part of the parish of CHURCHAM which is in the lower division of the hundred of DUDSTONE and KING'S BARTON, county of GLOUCESTER, 2¼ miles (N. W. by W.) from Gloucester, containing, with the hamlets of Linton and Over. 252 inhabitants.

HIGHWAY, a parish in the hundred of POTTERNE and CANNINGS, though locally in the hundred of Calne, county of WILTS, 4½ miles (N. E.) from Calne, containing 108 inhabitants. The living is a perpetual curacy, with the vicarage of Bremhill, in the archdeaconry of Wilts, and diocese of Salisbury. The church is dedicated to St. Peter.

HIGHWEEK, a parish in the hundred of TEINGBRIDGE, county of DEVON, 1 mile (N. by W.) from Newton-Abbots, containing 907 inhabitants. The living is a perpetual curacy with the vicarage of Kingsteington, in the archdeaconry of Totness, and diocese of Exeter. The church is dedicated to All Saints. The Stover canal passes through the parish.

HIGHWORTH, a parish in the hundred of HIGHWORTH, CRICKLADE, and STAPLE, county of WILTS, comprising the market town of Highworth, the chapelries of Broad Blunsdon, South Marston, and Sevenhampton, and the tythings of Fresdon, and Eastrop with Westrop, and containing 3005 inhabitants, of which number, 1888 are in the tything of Eastrop with Westrop, and the town of Highworth, 48 miles (N. by E.) from Salisbury, and 77 (W. by N.) from London. The name is expressive of the elevated situation of the town, and the extensive prospects which it commands. At the time of the Norman survey this was part of the royal demesne, but the only historical event connected with the town, transpired during the parliamentary war, on the 27th of June, 1645, when Major Hen, the governor of a royal garrison here, who had fortified the church, was summoned to surrender by the parliamentary forces, who, on their way to Taunton, had drawn up before it ; after a short resistance, he yielded, and the besiegers took seventy prisoners, with arms and a considerable booty. In the following month a skirmish took place here, in which great slaughter appears to have ensued on both sides ; for, on sinking a fence in a field to the west of the church, about six years since, a vast number of skeletons in high preservation was discovered, imbedded in the sand, at the depth of five feet.

The town is situated between the Thames and Severn canal, which passes about four miles to the north, and the Wilts and Berks canal, about the same distance toward the south : the houses in general are built of stone ; the streets are neither lighted nor paved, but the inhabitants are well supplied with water from springs. There is a small subscription library. Quarries of excellent limestone exist in the neighbourhood, where fossil remains are frequently discovered. The market is on Wednesday : fairs are held on the 13th of August (old Lammas day) for horses, cattle, and sheep, and the 11th of October, a statute fair, for hiring servants. The old market-house was removed about twenty years since ; a fixed pillory is still preserved in the market-place. The precise period when this town was incorporated is unknown : at present there is no corporate body, nor has there been from time immemorial ; it is under the jurisdiction of the county magistrates, who meet weekly at Swindon. A bailiff is appointed annually at the court held by the steward for the "manor of the borough of Highworth;" but his office is only to collect quit-rents : at this court also constables are appointed for the town, and the day following a court for the hundred is usually held by the steward for the manor, when the constables and tything-men for the different parishes and places in the hundred are appointed. He also holds, once in three weeks, a court of pleas, or court baron, for the manor, or borough, and ancient hundred of Highworth, supposed to have been established by charter of Edward I., in which debts under 40s. are recoverable. This town probably sent members to parliament at a very early period, as a writ was addressed to the bailiffs in the 26th of Edward I., to which no return was made, nor does it appear that the elective franchise was ever afterwards exercised, though writs continued to be sent to the bailiffs until the 24th of Edward IV.

The living is a vicarage, rated in the king's books at £44. 8. 4., in the peculiar jurisdiction and patronage of the Prebendary of Highworth in the Cathedral Church of Sarum, the Dean of Sarum possessing ordinary jurisdiction. The church, dedicated to St. Michael, is an ancient building, erected in the reign of Henry VI., with a tower at the west end, which, as well as the other parts of the church, is surmounted by an open parapet : on the south side is a chantry, or monumental chapel, hung round with pieces of ancient armour. There is a place of worship for Independents. A school for about seventy children is held in the vestry-room of the church: the master has a stipend of £27.6, per annum, the produce of various benefactions. There are several charitable donations for apprenticing boys and other purposes; the principal is Batson's charity, producing about £50 per annum, which is expended in clothing the poor, and assisting them with small sums of money.

HILARY (ST.), a parish in the hundred of PENWITH, county of CORNWALL, comprising the market town of Marazion, and containing 2811 inhabitants. The living is a vicarage, in the archdeaconry of Cornwall, and diocese of Exeter, rated in the king's books at £ 11. 6. 0½. Mrs. Beard and others were patrons in 1814. The Rev. John Penneck, in 1723, bequeathed £ 5 per annum for the instruction of four children.

HILBECK, a township in the parish of BROUGH, EAST ward, county of WESTMORLAND, ½ a mile (N.N.E.) from Brough, containing 101 inhabitants. In old records this place is called Hellebeck, Helle, in Saxon, denoting water-falls, of which there are several among the mountains in the neighbourhood. A cotton-mill was erected by John Metcalf Carlton, Esq., but it has been disused for many years. In the neighbourhood is a coal mine ; not far from which, on an eminence commanding an extensive view, is a building called Fox Tower.

HILBOROUGH, a parish in the southern division of the hundred of GREENHOE, county of NORFOLK, 6 miles (S.) from Swaffham, containing 349 inhabitants. The living is a discharged rectory, in the archdeaconry of Norfolk, and diocese of Norwich, rated in the king's books at £13. 6. 8., endowed with £200 private benefaction, and £300 royal bounty. Earl Nelson was patron in 1806. The church, dedicated to All Saints, is built of flints, having a strong square tower, with free-

stone quoins, embattled and crowned with carved pinnacles ; in one of the east windows are some remains of stained glass. At the north-western extremity of the village are the remains of an ancient chapel, dedicated to St. Margaret, called the Pilgrims' chapel, probably from having been visited by them on their way to Walsingham: it was richly endowed, having included among its possessions one hundred acres of land in this parish.

HILCOTT, a tything in the parish of NORTH NEWTON, hundred of SWANBOROUGH, county of WILTS, 3½ miles (W. by S.) from Pewsey. The population is re turned with the parish.

HILDENLEY, a township in the parish of APPLETON le STREET, wapentake of RYEDALE, North riding of the county of YORK, 3 miles (W.S. W.) from Malton, containing 23 inhabitants.

HILDERSHAM, a parish in the hundred of CHILFORD, county of CAMBRIDGE, 1¾ mile (N. W. by N.) from Linton, containing 193 inhabitants. The living is a rectory, in the archdeaconry and diocese of Ely, rated in the king's books at £15. 0. 5. The Rev. Charles Goodwin was patron in 1806. The church is dedicated to the Holy Trinity.

HILDERSTONE, a liberty in the parish of STONE, southern division of the hundred of PIREHILL, county of STAFFORD, 3 miles (E.N.E.) from Stone, containing 1591 inhabitants. R. Bourne, Esq. has recently erected a chapel at his own expense, to which he appoints the minister.

HILDERTHORP, a township in the parish of BRIDLINGTON, wapentake of DICKERING, East riding of the county of YORK, 1½ mile (S.) from Bridlington, containing 51 inhabitants.

HILFIELD, a chapelry in the parish of SYDLING-ST. NICHOLAS, hundred of CERNE, TOTCOMBE, and MODBURY, Cerne subdivision of the county of DORSET, 9 miles (S.) from Sherborne, containing 127 inhabitants.

HILGAY, a parish in the hundred of CLACKCLOSE, county of NORFOLK, 3½ miles (S. by E.) from Downham-Market, containing 968 inhabitants. The living is a rectory, in the archdeaconry of Norfolk, and diocese of Norwich, rated in the king's books at £10. The King presented in 1819. The church is dedicated to All Saints. Near the bank of the Ouse, in this parish, was a small priory of Black monks, a cell to Ramsey abbey.

HILL, a parish in the lower, though locally in the upper, division of the hundred of BERKELEY, county of GLOUCESTER, 3¼ miles (N.N.E.) from Thornbury, containing 259 inhabitants. The living is a perpetual curacy, in the archdeaconry and diocese of Gloucester. Miss Langley was patroness in 1819. The church is dedicated to St. Michael. The navigable river Severn runs through this parish.

HILL, a joint township with Moor, in the parish of FLADBURY, middle division of the hundred of OSWALD-SLOW, county of WORCESTER, 4 miles (N. E. by E.) from Pershore, containing 295 inhabitants.

HILL (CROOM), county of WORCESTER. —— See CROOM-HILL.

HILL-DEVERILL, a parish in the hundred of HEYTESBURY, county of WILTS, 3 miles (S.) from Warminster, containing 135 inhabitants. The living is a perpetual curacy, rated in the king's books at £10. 4. 2., endowed with £200 private benefaction, £400 royal bounty, and £500 parliamentary grant, and in the peculiar jurisdiction and patronage of the Dean of Salisbury, as Dean of the Collegiate Church of Heytesbury. The church is dedicated to St. Mary.

HILL-END, a tything in the parish of CUMNER, hundred of HORMER, county of BERKS, 4 miles (W. S.W.) from Oxford, containing 102 inhabitants.

HILLAM, a township in the parish of MONK-FRYSTON, lower division of the wapentake of BARK-STONE-ASH, West riding of the county of YORK, 3½ miles (N. N. E.) from Ferry-Bridge, containing 269 inhabitants.

HILL-FARRANCE, a parish in the hundred of TAUNTON and TAUNTON-DEAN, county of SOMERSET, 4¼ miles (W.) from Taunton, containing 483 inhabitants. The living is a perpetual curacy, in the archdeaconry of Taunton, and diocese of Bath and Wells, endowed with £200 private benefaction, and £400 royal bounty, and in the patronage of the President and Fellows of Trinity College, Oxford. The church is dedicated to the Holy Cross.

HILL-HAMPTON, county of WORCESTER.—See HAMPTON (HILL).

HILL-TOP, a township in that part of the parish of WRAGBY which is in the upper division of the wapentake of OSGOLDCROSS, West riding of the county of YORK, 5 miles (S. E.) from Barnesley, containing 97 inhabitants.

HILLERSDON, a parish in the hundred and county of BUCKINGHAM, 3¾ miles (S. by W.) from Buckingham, containing 247 inhabitants. The living is a perpetual curacy, in the archdeaconry of Buckingham, and diocese of Lincoln, endowed with £8 per annum private benefaction, and £200 royal bounty, and in the patronage of the Dean and Canons of Christ Church, Oxford. The church, dedicated to All Saints, was rebuilt about 1493, and exhibits some portions in the later style of English architecture, with a profusion of stained glass in one of the eastern windows, representing the legendary history of St. Nicholas. The ancient manor-house, now demolished, was held for the king in the parliamentary war, but its garrison having surrendered in 1643, it was plundered, and its owner, Sir Alexander Denton, committed to prison, where he died of a broken heart.

HILLESLEY, a tything in the parish of HAWKES-BURY, upper division of the hundred of GRUMBALD'S ASH, county of GLOUCESTER, 1¾ mile (S. S. E.) from Wotton under Edge, containing, with Hillcott, Saddle-wood, and Tresham, 800 inhabitants. Here was anciently a chapel dedicated to St. Giles, but it has been demolished.

HILLINGDON, a parish in the hundred of EL-THORNE, county of MIDDLESEX, 13½ miles (W. by N.) from London, comprising part of the market town of Uxbridge, and containing 5636 inhabitants. The living is a dischaged vicarage, in the archdeaconry of Middlesex, and diocese of London, rated in the king's books at £16, and in the patronage of the Bishop of London. The church, dedicated to St. John the Baptist, is principally in the later style of English architecture, with an embattled tower at the west end, and contains among others, a fine monument to the memory of Henry Earl of Uxbridge, who died in 1743 : in the church-yard is the tomb of John Rich, comedian, who died in 1761.

HILLINGTON, a parish in the Lynn division of the hundred of FREEBRIDGE, county of NORFOLK, 4 mile (E.) from Castle-Rising, containing 252 inhabitants. The living is a rectory, in the archdeaconry and diocese

of Norwich, rated in the king's books at £13. 6. 8., and in the patronage of Sir W. B. Folkes, Bart. The church, dedicated to St. Mary, has a Norman door of great beauty.

HILLINGTON, a parish in the hundred of LODDON, county of NORFOLK, 6¾ miles (S. E.) from Norwich, containing 63 inhabitants. The living is a perpetual curacy, in the archdeaconry and diocese of Norwich. Sir Charles Rich, Bart. was patron in 1823. The church is dedicated to St. John the Baptist.

HILLMARTON, a parish in the hundred of KINGS-BRIDGE, county of WILTS, 3¼ miles (N. N. E.) from Calne, containing 787 inhabitants. The living is a vicarage, in the archdeaconry and diocese of Salisbury, rated in the king's books at £20. 6. 8., and in the patronage of the Crown. The church is dedicated to St. Lawrence.

HILLMORTON, a parish in the Rugby division of the hundred of KNIGHTLOW, county of WARWICK, 3 miles (E. S. E.) from Rugby, containing 779 inhabitants. The living is a discharged vicarage, in the archdeaconry of Coventry, and diocese of Lichfield and Coventry, rated in the king's books at £6. 10. 6., endowed with £400 parliamentary grant, and in the patronage of Baroness Grey de Ruthyn. The church is dedicated to St. John the Baptist. There is a place of worship for Wesleyan Methodists. The Oxford canal passes through the parish.

HILPERTON, a parish in the hundred of MELKS-HAM, county of WILTS, 1¼ mile (N. E.) from Trow-bridge, containing 904 inhabitants. The living is a discharged rectory, in the archdeaconry and diocese of Salisbury, rated in the king's books at £16, and in the joint patronage of Richard Godolphin Long, John Long, and Jones Long, Esqrs. The church is dedicated to St. Michael. There are places of worship for Baptists and Wesleyan Methodists. The river Avon, and the Kennet and Avon canal, pass through the parish.

HILSTON, a parish in the middle division of the wapentake of HOLDERNESS, East riding of the county of YORK, 14 miles (E. by N.) from Kingston upon Hull, containing 39 inhabitants. The living is a discharged rectory, in the archdeaconry of the East riding, and diocese of York, rated in the king's books at £5. The Rev. C. Sykes was patron in 1809. The church is dedicated to St. Margaret.

HILTON, a township in the parish of MARSTON upon DOVE, hundred of APPLETREE, county of DERBY, 8½ miles (W. S. W.) from Derby, containing 533 inhabitants. A school-house was erected about 1655, by Arthur and Thomas Hanison, and in 1781 the Commissioners of enclosures allotted land for the support of a schoolmaster, whose annual income is £20, for teaching all the poor children of the parish.

HILTON, a parish in the hundred of WHITEWAY, Cerne sub-division of the county of DORSET, 7½ miles (W. S. W.) from Blandford-Forum, containing 610 inhabitants. The living is a vicarage, in the archdeaconry of Dorset, and diocese of Bristol, rated in the king's books at £8. 10. 5., and in the patronage of the Bishop of Salisbury. The church is dedicated to All Saints. A school-house has been erected by Lady C. Damer, which is supported by subscription. On Bulbarrow hill, the highest in the neighbourhood, is a circular double intrenchment, supposed to be of Danish formation.

Within the parish are some mineral springs, the water of which possesses calcareous and ferruginous properties. Bog iron and bituminous schist, or slate coal, are found in profusion; also good brick-clay of a blue colour, in which are oyster shells nine inches in diameter, large scallop and muscle shells, *cornua ammonis*, mineralised wood, and a quantity of pyrites. Some specimens of iron-ore, dug at Belchalwel, near this place, have been analysed, and found to contain four grains of gold in the pound weight. Curious fossils have been discovered in the flint rocks, with some chalcedony and carmelite: on the side of a chalk hill were found the bones, teeth, and tusks, of the mammoth; the bones were of great size, but mouldered on being touched. In draining some land a few years since, ancient ornaments of fine gold, weighing from eight to nine ounces, consisting of a wreath more than four feet long, with a trumpet-shaped ornament at each end, and at the larger end a ring of gold three inches in diameter, were discovered; these were probably a Druidical collar and armlet, as it is known the Druids adorned their persons with trinkets of this description. Many urns, filled with ashes and burnt bones, have been found from time to time, and in getting gravel on the hills, twenty-four of them were discovered in one barrow.

HILTON, a township in the parish of STAINDROP, south-western division of DARLINGTON ward, county palatine of DURHAM, 6½ miles (S. S. W.) from Bishop-Auckland, containing 113 inhabitants.

HILTON, a parish in the hundred of TOSELAND, county of HUNTINGDON, 3½ miles (S.S.W.) from St. Ives, containing 303 inhabitants. The living is a perpetual curacy, annexed to the vicarage of Fen-Stanton, in the archdeaconry of Huntingdon, and diocese of Lincoln. The church is dedicated to St. Mary Magdalene.

HILTON, a township in that part of the parish of WOLVERHAMPTON which is in the eastern division of the hundred of CUTTLESTONE, county of STAFFORD, 4½ miles (N.E. by N.) from Wolverhampton, containing 55 inhabitants. Here was anciently a chapel, which was dedicated to St. John the Baptist, but it has been demolished. A Cistercian abbey, in honour of the Blessed Virgin Mary, was founded in 1223, by Henry de Audley, the revenue of which, at the dissolution, was estimated at £89. 10. 1.

HILTON, county of WESTMORLAND. — See HELTON.

HILTON, a parish in the western division of the liberty of LANGBAURGH, North riding of the county of YORK, 3¼ miles (E.S.E.) from Yarm, containing 135 inhabitants. The living is a perpetual curacy, in the archdeaconry of Cleveland, and diocese of York, endowed with £1000 royal bounty. Lord G. H. Cavendish was patron in 1818.

HIMBLETON, a parish in the middle division of the hundred of OSWALDSLOW, county of WORCESTER, 4½ miles (S.E.) from Droitwich, containing, with the hamlet of Shell, 482 inhabitants. The living is a discharged vicarage, in the archdeaconry and diocese of Worcester, rated in the king's books at £8. 6. 10½., and in the patronage of the Dean and Chapter of Worcester. The church is dedicated to St. Mary Magdalene.

HIMLEY, a parish in the northern division of the hundred of SEISDON, county of STAFFORD, 3¾ miles (W.) from Dudley, containing 379 inhabitants. The living is a rectory, in the archdeaconry of Stafford, and diocese of Lichfield and Coventry, rated in the king's books at £3. 13. 4. The Earl of Dudley was patron in 1799. The church is dedicated to St. Michael. Courts leet and baron are held annually; there is also a copyhold court. Himley has been long notedfor its blade-mills, which impart a peculiar sharpness to edge-tools.

HINCASTER, a township in the parish of HEVERSHAM, KENDAL ward, county of WESTMORLAND, 2½ miles (N.N.E.) from Milnthorpe, containing 120 inhabitants. The Kendal and Lancaster canal passes through a tunnel north of this township. There are annual donations of about £7 for the support of a school.

HINCHINBROOK, partly in the parish of ST. MARY, borough of HUNTINGDON, and partly in the hundred of HURSTINGSTONE, the latter portion being extraparochial, county of HUNTINGDON, 1 mile (W.) from Huntingdon. A small Benedictine nunnery, dedicated to St. James, was founded here by William the Conqueror, to which the nuns removed from Eltesley, in Cambridgeshire; its revenue, at the dissolution, was £19. 9. 2.: the site is now occupied by Hinchinbrook house, which formerly belonged to Sir Oliver Cromwell, uncle of the Protector, who sumptuously entertained James I. in it, with all his court, on the monarch's arrival from Scotland, also Charles II. at different periods : the mansion, which has recently sustained considerable injury from a fire, now belongs to the Earl of Sandwich, who enjoys the inferior title of Viscount Hinchinbroke.

HINCKLEY, a parish comprising the market town of Hinckley, the chapelries of Dadlington and Stoke-Golding, and the hamlet of Wykin, in the hundred of SPARKENHOE, county of LEICESTER, and the hamlet of Hydes-Pastures in the southern division of the hundred of KNIGHTLOW, county of WARWICK, and containing, exclusively of Hydes-Pastures, 6706 inhabitants, of which number, 5835 are in the town of Hinckley, 13 miles (S. W. by W.) from Leicester, and 100 (N.W. by N.) from London. This place was created a barony soon after the Conquest, and held by Hugh de Grentismenil, seneschal of England in the reigns of William Rufus and Henry I., who erected a stately castle and a church, and founded a small priory of Benedictine monks, which, prior to 1173, was given as a cell to the abbey of Lyra, in Normandy, by Robert Blanchmaines, Earl of Leicester: having fallen into the hands of the crown, Richard II. gave it to the Carthusian priory of Montgrace, in Yorkshire, to which it was finally annexed by Henry V., and, on the dissolution of that priory, it was granted to the Dean and Chapter of Westminster.

Under its ancient lords this town had all the privileges of a borough; but the inhabitants taking part with the house of Lancaster in the civil war of the fifteenth century, their privileges were annulled by Edward IV. Leland mentions the ruins of the castle (which in the time of Henry VIII., the period at which he wrote, belonged to the crown, but which had previously belonged to the Earl of Leicester), as being situated two miles from the town of Leicester, on the borders of the forest, and as being spacious and celebrated. The assizes for the county were formerly held here. The town stands close to the border of Warwickshire, from which county it is separated by the Roman Watling-street; and so elevated is its situation, that it commands a view of fifty churches. It comprises the Borough, within the limits of the ancient town, and the Bond, without those limits. The houses are indifferently built, the town is paved but not lighted, and is well supplied with water : the walks and views are pleasant and extensive. A permanent subscription library, including a news-room, has lately been established. The waste lands were enclosed in 1760, and one-seventh of the lordship allotted to the Dean and Chapter of Westminster. The town has derived great benefit from the introduction of the stocking manufacture, which is now so extensive that a greater quantity of cotton and worsted hose, particularly the former, of the coarser kind, is supposed to be made here than in any other town of equal size in the kingdom: the number of frames in the town and villages adjacent is computed at two thousand five hundred, affording employment to nearly three thousand persons. It possesses a commercial communication with all parts of the kingdom by means of the Ashby canal, which traverses the south-western part of the parish. The market is on Monday; and fairs are held annually on the 1st, 2d, and 3rd Mondays after January 6th, Easter-Monday, the Monday before Whitsuntide, and also on Whit-Monday, on August 26th, and the Monday after October 28th : the last is a cheese fair, and the rest are for horses, cattle, and sheep. The town is under the government of a mayor, or bailiff, a constable, and two headboroughs, chosen at the annual court leet of the lord of the manor : the Bond, or Bound, is under that of a constable and three headboroughs. There is also a town-master, chosen at the church on the Tuesday in Easter week, who is empowered, in conjunction with his predecessor in the office, to audit annually the accounts of the trustees of the feoffment. In 1764, Shuckburgh Ashby, Esq. gave up to the town the tolls on corn and hogs, in order that they might be abolished. The town-hall was rebuilt in 1803, by means of funds arising from what is called the Feoffment benefaction. A bridewell was erected in 1768, the magistrates at the sessions allowing £25 towards the expense, and the remainder being paid by the overseers of the poor.

The living is a vicarage, in the archdeaconry of Leicester, and diocese of Lincoln, rated in the king's books at £9. 9. 9½., and in the patronage of the Dean and Chapter of Westminster. The church, dedicated to St. Mary, is a spacious edifice, erected chiefly in the thirteenth century, with a tower and finely-proportioned spire, the latter built in 1788 : this church underwent a thorough repair, and had new windows inserted, and an organ erected, in 1808, at an expense of £500, raised by subscription, and it has recently received an addition of three hundred and forty free sittings, towards defraying the expense of which, the Incorporated Society for enlarging churches and chapels contributed £200. Of the several chapels of ease which formerly belonged to the church, only that of Dadlington remains, the chapelry having a distinct parochial rate. There are places of worship for General Baptists, the Society of Friends, Independents, Wesleyan Methodists, and Unitarians, and a Roman Catholic chapel. On the dissolution of the Catholic college at Douay, in Flanders, some years ago, the institution was re-established here : it has a library, and there are funds for the support of two clergymen as tutors, several foreign students being now on the establishment. A National school was established in 1821, and is supported

from the funds belonging to the Feoffment benefaction; and an infant school has been recently established, which is supported by subscription. At a short distance from Hinckley, on the road to Lutterworth, is a spring called Holy Well, and in the neighbourhood are good mineral waters, at Cogg's well, Christopher's spa, and the Priest hills.

HINDERCLAY, a parish in the hundred of BLACK-BOURN, county of SUFFOLK, 2 miles (N.W. by W.) from Botesdale, containing 403 inhabitants. The living is a discharged rectory, in the archdeaconry of Sudbury, a and diocese of Norwich, rated in the king's books at £9. 19. 4½., and in the patronage of G. St. Vincent Wilson, Esq. The church is dedicated to St. Mary.

HINDERWELL, a parish in the eastern division of the liberty of LANGBAURGH, North riding of the county of YORK, comprising the townships of Hinderwell and Roxby, and containing 1719 inhabitants, of which number, 1483 are in the township of Hinderwell, 9 miles (N.W. by W.) from Whitby. The living is a rectory, in the archdeaconry of Cleveland, and diocese of York, rated in the king's books at £15. Thomas Smith, Esq. was patron in 1823. The church is dedicated to St. Hilda. In the church-yard is a spring of pure water, called St. Hilda's well, near which it is said she had a retreat that still retains her name. In 1603, a Turkish ship, infected with the plague, was wrecked upon this coast, and communicated the disease to the village, where it raged for six weeks, carrying off several of the inhabitants.

HINDLEY, a chapelry in that part of the parish of WIGAN which is in the hundred of WEST DERBY, county palatine of LANCASTER, 2¼ miles (E. S. E.) from Wigan, containing 3757 inhabitants. The living is a perpetual curacy, in the archdeaconry and diocese of Chester, endowed with £400 private benefaction, £200 royal bounty, and £300 parliamentary grant, and in the patronage of the Rector of Wigan. The chapel was erected in 1651. There are places of worship for Independents and Unitarians. A school-room was built in 1632, by Mrs. Mary Abram : the master has a residence, with certain land attached, £10 a year arising from property vested in the corporation of Liverpool, and two shillings and sixpence entrance money from each pupil; the average number taught is thirty. Three Sunday schools have been built, and are supported by voluntary subscriptions. Here is a rare phenomenon, called "The Burning Well," which attracts many visitors; it is similar to that at Petoa Mela, near Fierenzota in Italy, except that the flame of the Italian spring is perpetual, in the absence of heavy rains, and consists of sulphuric gas; while the inflammable principle of that at Hindley is the decomposition of water acting upon ores and sulphate of iron.

HINDOLVESTON, a parish in the hundred of EYNSFORD, county of NORFOLK, 3¼ miles (N. by W.) from Foulsham, containing 756 inhabitants. The living is a discharged vicarage, in the archdeaconry of Norfolk, and diocese of Norwich, rated in the king's books at £6. 1., endowed with £1200 parliamentary grant, and in the peculiar jurisdiction and patronage of the Dean and Chapter of Norwich. The church is dedicated to St. George.

HINDON, a borough, market town, and parochial chapelry, in the hundred of DOWNTON, though locally in the hundred of Mere, county of WILTS, 16 miles (W. by N.) from Salisbury, and 96 (W. S. W.) from London. This small town consists principally of one street, extending along a gentle declivity on the great western road from London to Exeter : a considerable part of it was consumed by fire in 1754, and at present it contains not more than about two hundred houses. The manufacture of silk twist, for which Hindon was formerly noted, has declined, and is superseded by that of linen, dowlas, and bed-ticking, which is principally carried on in the vicinity. A few women are employed in spinning silk, and at the head of the Fonthill river, about a mile and a half distant, is a large establishment for the manufacture of broad cloth and kerseymere. The market, on Thursday, was formerly considerable for corn, but it has declined since the great fire, and the establishment of a corn market at Warminster : there are fairs on the Monday before Whitsuntide, for cattle and sheep, and on October 29th, for horses, cattle, poultry, &c.; a fair is also held at Berwick Hill, about a mile from the town, on the 6th of November, for horses and sheep. In the 7th of Richard II., a precept was directed to this borough to send burgesses to parliament, but no return was made : it first sent representatives in the 27th of Henry VI., since which period the returns have been regular. The right of election is vested in the inhabitant housekeepers and parishioners not receiving alms, the number of whom is about one hundred and seventy-three. The bailiff, who is appointed by the Bishop of Winchester, and is non-resident, is the returning officer. The petty sessions for the Hindon division are held here on the first Wednesday in every month. The living is a perpetual curacy, in the archdeaconry of Wilts, and diocese of Salisbury, endowed by charter of the 6th of Philip and Mary, renewed in the 19th of George III., with land and houses within the borough, producing about £60 per annum, and £400 parliamentary grant, and in the patronage of the Crown. The chapel, dedicated to St. John the Baptist, is a plain turreted modern edifice, and was repaired in 1814. There is a place of worship for Independents near the town, without the precincts of the borough, buildings not being permitted therein. A school for boys and girls is supported by Lord Calthorpe. In the vicinity of the town, towards the north-west, and near the Roman road which leads to Old Sarum, are Stockton works, occupying an area of sixty-two acres, and supposed to be the remains of an ancient British settlement.

HINDRINGHAM, a parish in the northern division of the hundred of GREENHOE, county of NORFOLK, 3¾ miles (E. by S.) from Little Walsingham, containing 657 inhabitants. The living is a discharged vicarage, in the archdeaconry and diocese of Norwich, rated in the king's books at £9, endowed with £200 private benefaction, and £200 royal bounty, and in the patronage of the Dean and Chapter of Norwich. The church is dedicated to St. Martin.

HINGHAM, a parish (formerly a market town) in the hundred of FOREHOE, county of NORFOLK, 14 miles (W. by S.) from Norwich, and 98 (N. E. by N.) from London, containing 1442 inhabitants. This place, formerly called Hincham, is situated near the source of the river Yare ; and though not so considerable as at the period when it gave name to the deanery, it is yet respectable. About a century ago a fire consumed the greater part of

the town, but it was rebuilt in an improved style, and the market-place is distinguished for neatness : the inhabitants are well supplied with water. There is a book society, the members of which meet monthly, to exchange publications, and manage its concerns. The market, which was formerly held on Saturday, has fallen into disuse, in consequence of its being on the same day as the principal market of Norwich : the fairs are held on the 7th of March, Whit-Tuesday, and October 2nd ; the first is chiefly for horses, and the last for different kinds of live stock. General courts baron and customary courts, for the manors of Hingham, Hingham-Gurney, and Hingham rectory, are held annually on the 25th of October. The town being part of the ancient demesne of the crown, the inhabitants are exempted from serving on juries at the assizes and sessions. The living is a rectory, in the archdeaconry of Norfolk, and diocese of Norwich, rated in the king's books at £24. 18. 4., and in the patronage of Lord Wodehouse. The church, dedicated to St. Andrew, is a fine structure, chiefly in the decorated style of English architecture, with a handsome tower of flint and stone; it was rebuilt in the reign of Edward III., by the rector, Remigius de Hethersete, aided by the then patron, John le Marshall : it had anciently seven chantry chapels, and as many guilds. Against the north wall of the chancel is a noble monument, erected to the memory of Thomas Parker, Lord Morley, who died in 1435; and on the east window of Trinity chapel are emblazoned the arms of Morley : the chapel itself is supposed, from the fragment of an inscription, to have been built at the expense of the young women of the place. The east window of the chancel, presented by Lord Wodehouse in 1812, is of fine ancient stained glass, brought from a nunnery in the Netherlands : it is thirty-six feet high, and eighteen feet wide, and is divided into seven compartments, emblematical of the Crucifixion, Resurrection, and Ascension of our Saviour. The free school was founded by William Parlett, in 1727, for the education of all the sons of the inhabitants of Hingham, and one son of any inhabitant of the adjoining parish of Scoulton, except the minister, in reading, writing, arithmetic, Latin, and Greek; but the English and classical branches now form separate schools : the master of the grammar school has a good house; and the proceeds of an estate at Hingham, amounting to £156 per annum, are divided between the masters of the classical and English schools, in the ratio of two-thirds to the former, and one-third to the latter. A National school, in which fifty boys and fifty girls are taught, is supported by subscription ; the master has a salary of £25 a year.

HINKSEY (NORTH), a parish in the hundred of HORMER, county of BERKS, 1½ mile (W.) from Oxford, containing 182 inhabitants. The living is a perpetual curacy, in the archdeaconry of Berks, and diocese of Salisbury, endowed with £400 private benefaction, £200 royal bounty, and £300 parliamentary grant, and in the patronage of the Earls of Abingdon and Harcourt alternately. The church is dedicated to St. Lawrence Both North and South Hinksey were chapelries in the parish of Cumner till separated from the mother church, to which they still pay sixpence a year, called "smoke money." This place, sometimes called Ferry Hinksey, is situated on the western bank of the Isis.

HINKSEY (SOUTH), a parish in the hundred of

HORMER, county of BERKS, 1½ mile (S.) from Oxford, containing 142 inhàbitants. The living is a perpetual curacy, in the archdeaconry of Berks, and diocese of Salisbury, endowed with £200 private benefaction, and £400 royal bounty, and in the patronage of the Earl of Abingdon. The church is dedicated to St. John. In a field north of the church is a conduit, erected in 1620, for supplying the city of Oxford with water.

HINLIP, a parish in the lower division of the hundred of OSWALDSLOW, county of WORCESTER, 3½ miles (N. E. by N.) from Worcester, containing 129 inhabitants. The living is a discharged rectory, in the archdeaconry and diocese of Worcester, rated in the king's books at £5. 16. 0½. James West, Esq. was patron in 1815. The church is dedicated to St. James. The Birmingham and Worcester canal passes along the southern boundary of the parish. Hinlip, or Hendlip Hall, is a perfect and interesting specimen of the style of building in the time of Henry VIII.; it is also noted as having been the property and residence of Thomas Habingdon, author of copious manuscript collections for the history of Worcestershire.

HINSTOCK, a parish in the Drayton division of the hundred of BRADFORD (North), county of SALOP, 5¾ miles (N. W. by N.) from Newport, containing 671 inhabitants. The living is a discharged rectory, in the archdeaconry of Salop, and diocese of Lichfield and Coventry, rated in the king's books at £5. 16., and in the patronage of the Rev. H. C. Cotton during his lifetime, and afterwards in that of the Trustees of the late Sir C. Corbet, Bart. The church is dedicated to St. Oswald. There is a chalybeate sulphureous spring in the parish ; also vestiges of an ancient castle.

HINTLESHAM, a parish in the hundred of SAMFORD, county of SUFFOLK, 4½ miles (E. by N.) from Hadleigh, containing 562 inhabitants. The living is a rectory, in the archdeaconry of Suffolk, and diocese of Norwich, rated in the king's books at £33. 9. 7., and in the patronage of William Deane, Esq. The church is dedicated to St. Nicholas. Seven children are instructed for £10 per annum, the proceeds of land purchased by subscription ; a house for the master and a spacious play-ground were given by the Misses Lloyd.

HINTON, a tything in the parish and upper division of the hundred of BERKELEY, county of GLOUCESTER, containing 346 inhabitants. There is a place of worship for Wesleyan Methodists.

HINTON, a tything in the parish of DIRHAM, lower division of the hundred of GRUMBALD'S ASH, county of GLOUCESTER. The population is returned with the parish.

HINTON, a hamlet in the parish of WOODFORD, hundred of CHIPPING-WARDEN, county of NORTHAMPTON, 7½ miles (S. S. W.) from Daventry. The population is returned with the parish. Here is a mineral spring.

HINTON, a township in that part of the parish of WHITCHURCH which is in the Whitchurch division of the hundred of BRADFORD (North), county of SALOP, 1¼ mile (N. N. E.) from Whitchurch, with which the population is returned.

HINTON, a tything in the parish and hundred of CHRISTCHURCH, New Forest (West) division of the county of SOUTHAMPTON, 3¾ miles (N. E.) from Christchurch, with which the population is returned.

HINTON (BROAD), a liberty in that part of the parish of HURST which is in the hundred of AMESBURY, county of WILTS, though locally in that of Sonning, county of Berks, 3¾ miles (N. by W.) from Wokingham, containing 489 inhabitants.

HINTON (CHARTERHOUSE), a parish in the hundred of WELLOW, county of SOMERSET, 5 miles (S. S. E.) from Bath, containing 640 inhabitants. The living is a perpetual curacy, in the archdeaconry of Wells, and diocese of Bath and Wells, endowed with £1800 parliamentary grant, and in the patronage of the Rev. James Commeline. The church, dedicated to St. John the Baptist, has two hundred free sittings, the Incorporated Society for the enlargement of churches and chapels having granted £200 towards defraying the expense. Ela, Countess of Salisbury, relict of William Longespee, founded a Carthusian monastery here in 1227, dedicating it to the Blessed Virgin, St. John the Baptist, and All Saints, to which she caused the monks of Hethorp, in Gloucestershire, to be removed in 1232 : its revenue, in the 26th of Henry VIII., was estimated at £262. 12. The manor-house was built from the ruins of the priory ; the other remains are, the chapel, charnel-house, and granary, and are surrounded by a grove of aged oaks. This was anciently a Roman station, considerable vestiges of which are still discernible, the ground being covered with squares, circles, and other earth-works ; and in turning up the soil an abundance of pottery was found, from the finest Samian to the coarsest kind, together with iron, glass, scoriæ of iron, numerous small coins of the lower empire, and the remains of a small Roman amphitheatre : from this place the course of a Roman road may also be traced.

HINTON (CHERRY), a parish in the hundred of FLENDISH, county of CAMBRIDGE, 2¾ miles (E. by S.) from Cambridge, containing 474 inhabitants. The living is a discharged vicarage, in the archdeaconry and diocese of Ely, rated in the king's books at £9. 14. 7., and in the patronage of the Master and Fellows of Peter House, Cambridge. The church, dedicated to St. Andrew, stands near the Gogmagog hills : the valley beneath was formerly noted for an abundance of cherry trees growing in it ; it is now the principal spot in the county where saffron is cultivated. Various fossil teeth, and vertebræ of fish, are found in the chalk pits here.

HINTON (ST. GEORGE), a parish in the hundred of CREWKERNE, county of SOMERSET, 2¼ miles (N. W. by N.) from Crewkerne, containing 737 inhabitants. The living is a discharged rectory, in the archdeaconry of Taunton, and diocese of Bath and Wells, rated in the king's books at £13. 13. 4. Earl Powlett was patron in 1789.

HINTON (GREAT), a tything in the parish of STEEPLE-ASHTON, hundred of WHORWELSDOWN, county of WILTS, 3¾ miles (E. by N.) from Trowbridge, containing 202 inhabitants.

HINTON (LITTLE), a parish forming a distinct portion of the hundred of ELSTUB and EVERLEY, county of WILTS, 5¼ miles (E.) from Swindon, containing 284 inhabitants. The living is a rectory, in the archdeaconry and diocese of Salisbury, rated in the king's books at £13. 6. 8., and in the patronage of the Bishop of Winchester. The church is dedicated to St. Swithin.

HINTON (ST. MARY), a parish in the hundred of STURMINSTER-NEWTON-CASTLE, Sturminster division of the county of DORSET, 8 miles (S. W. by W.) from Shaftesbury, containing 297 inhabitants. The living is a perpetual curacy with the vicarage of Iwerne-Minster, in the archdeaconry of Dorset, and diocese of Bristol. The church is dedicated to St. Peter. Mary Freke, in 1684, gave £6 per annum for teaching poor children.

HINTON (PARVA, or STANDBRIDGE), a parish in the hundred of BADBURY, Shaston (East) division of the county of DORSET, 3 miles (N. by W.) from Wimborne Minster, containing 25 inhabitants. The living is a discharged rectory, in the archdeaconry of Dorset, and diocese of Bristol, rated in the king's books at £4. 12. 1., and in the patronage of Sir Richard Carr Glyn, Bart. The church, dedicated to St. Kenelm, was formerly a chapel to Wimborne-Minster, to which the inhabitants still pay 10s. per annum, and where they bury, there being no church-yard here. The river Allen forms the western boundary of the parish.

HINTON (TARRANT), a parish in the hundred of PIMPERNE, Blandford (North) division of the county of DORSET, 4¾ miles (N. E.) from Blandford-Forum, containing 278 inhabitants. The living is a rectory, in the archdeaconry of Dorset, and diocese of Bristol, rated in the king's books at £12. 17. 1. The Rev. W. Pigott was patron in 1821.

HINTON on the GREEN, a parish in the hundred of TIBALDSTONE, though locally in the lower division of the hundred of Kiftsgate, county of GLOUCESTER, 2¾ miles (S. S. W.) from Evesham, containing 195 inhabitants. The living is a rectory, in the archdeaconry and diocese of Gloucester, rated in the king's books at £8. 13. 11½. J. Baker, Esq. was patron in 1813. The church is dedicated to St. Peter.

HINTON in the HEDGES, a parish in the hundred of KING'S SUTTON, county of NORTHAMPTON, 1½ mile (W.) from Brackley, containing 188 inhabitants. The living is a rectory with that of Stean, in the archdeaconry of Northampton, and diocese of Peterborough, rated in the king's books at £10. Earl Spencer was patron in 1809. The church is dedicated to the Holy Trinity.

HINTON-AMPNER, a parish in the hundred of FAWLEY, Fawley division of the county of SOUTHAMPTON, 4 miles (S. by E.) from New Alresford, containing 325 inhabitants. The living is a rectory, in the archdeaconry and diocese of Winchester, rated in the king's books at £19. 11. 10½., and in the patronage of the Bishop of Winchester. The church is dedicated to All Saints. A charity school was founded and endowed in 1729, by William Blake: the annual income is about £140, for which sum upwards of fifty boys and girls are instructed. This parish is within the jurisdiction of the Cheyney Court held at Winchester every Thursday, for the recovery of debts to any amount.

HINTON-BLEWETT, a parish in the hundred of CHEWTON, county of SOMERSET, 8 miles (N. N. E.) from Wells, containing 264 inhabitants. The living is a discharged rectory, in the archdeaconry of Bath, and diocese of Bath and Wells, rated in the king's books at £9. 8. 1., and in the patronage of Mrs. Johnson. The church is dedicated to All Saints.

HINTON-MARTELL, a parish in the hundred of BADBURY, Shaston (East) division of the county of DORSET, 4¼ miles (N. by E.) from Wimborne-Minster,

containing 257 inhabitants. The living is a rectory, in the archdeaconry of Dorset, and diocese of Bristol, rated in the king's books at £16. 8. 6½., and in the patronage of the Earl of Shaftesbury. The church is dedicated to St. John.

HINTON-WALDRIST, a parish in the hundred of GANFIELD, county of BERKS, 6¼ miles (N. E. by E.) from Great Farringdon, containing 315 inhabitants. The living is a rectory, in the archdeaconry of Berks, and diocese of Salisbury, rated in the king's books at £23. 7. 6. The Rev. J. Loder was patron in 1802. The church is dedicated to St. Margaret. Henry III., in 1217, granted a charter to Henry de St. Valery, for a market to be held here on Wednesday, but it has long been disused. In the neighbourhood are traces of an ancient intrenchment, now an orchard, near which is an eminence called Windmill hill, supposed to have been a signal station.

HINTS, a parish in the southern division of the hundred of OFFLOW, county of STAFFORD, 4 miles (W. by S.) from Tamworth, containing 250 inhabitants. The living is a perpetual curacy, in the peculiar jurisdiction of the Prebendal court of Hansacre and Armitage, endowed with £5 per annum and £100 private benefaction, and £400 royal bounty, and in the patronage of the Prebendary of Handsacre in the Cathedral Church of Lichfield. The church, dedicated to St. Bartholomew, is a handsome modern structure in the Grecian style of architecture. There is a small school founded and supported by the Floyer family. Camwell, a hamlet in this parish, was formerly distinguished for a priory, founded by Gever Riddell, in 1142, for Benedictine monks, which was one of those assigned to Cardinal Wolsey, towards the erection and endowment of his intended colleges. On Hints common, in 1792, a pig of lead was discovered, twenty-two inches and a half long, and weighing one hundred and fifty pounds, on which was inscribed, in bas relief, " IMP. VESP. VII. T. IMP. V. COS.:" it was in high preservation, and is supposed to have been imbedded where it was found, in the year seventy-six.

HINXHILL, a parish in the hundred of CHART and LONGBRIDGE, lathe of SCRAY, county of KENT, 2½ miles (E. by S.) from Ashford, containing 146 inhabitants. The living is a discharged rectory, in the archdeaconry and diocese of Canterbury, rated in the king's books at £7. 16. 8. Sir J. C. Honeywood, Bart. was patron in 1801. The church, dedicated to St. Mary, is principally in the early style of English architecture.

HINXTON, a parish in the hundred of WHITTLESFORD, county of CAMBRIDGE, 5½ miles (W. by S.) from Linton, containing 312 inhabitants. The living is a discharged vicarage, in the archdeaconry and diocese of Ely, rated in the king's books at £8. 5. 2½., and in the patronage of the Master and Fellows of Jesus College, Cambridge. The church is dedicated to St. Mary.

HINXWORTH, a parish in the hundred of ODSEY, county of HERTFORD, 5½ miles (N.) from Baldock, containing 247 inhabitants. The living is a rectory, in the archdeaconry of Huntingdon, and diocese of Lincoln, rated in the king's books at £16, and in the patronage of the Rev. John Lafont. The church, dedicated to St. Nicholas, has a quadrangular tower, embattled and surmounted by a low spire. In the neighbourhood, urns enclosing ashes and burnt bones were discovered in 1724, also several human skeletons, with a glass tribulus, lachrymatories of glass, pateras of red earth, &c.

HIPPENSCOMBE, an extra-parochial liberty in the hundred of KINWARDSTONE, county of WILTS, containing 40 inhabitants.

HIPPERHOLME, a joint township with Brighouse, in the parish of HALIFAX, wapentake of MORLEY, West riding of the county of YORK, 2½ miles (E. N. E.) from Halifax, containing 3936 inhabitants. There is a place of worship for Independents. A court baron is held once a year, at which a constable is chosen. Coal mines and quarries of stone abound in the neighbourhood. A free grammar school was founded, in 1647, by Matthew Broadley, and endowed by him with £5 per an. and part of the annual proceeds of £500; and, for its further maintenance, Samuel Sunderland, in 1671, enfeoffed certain houses and lands for the use of the schoolmaster, subject to the payment of £6 per ann. to an usher : the income is about £90 per annum, for which sum twenty boys are taught the classics.

HIPSWELL, a chapelry in that part of the parish of CATTERICK which is in the eastern division of the wapentake of HANG, North riding of the county of YORK, 2 miles (S. E. by S.) from Richmond, containing 273 inhabitants. The living is a perpetual curacy, in the archdeaconry of Richmond, and diocese of Chester, endowed with £200 private benefaction, £600 royal bounty, and £1000 parliamentary grant, and in the patronage of the Vicar of Catterick. Robert Corkin, in 1757, gave £100 towards the endowment of a free school, the interest of which is paid to the master of a charity school, in which about thirty children are instructed.

HISTON, a parish in the hundred of CHESTERTON, county of CAMBRIDGE, 3½ miles (N. by W.) from Cambridge, containing 678 inhabitants. The living comprises the consolidated discharged vicarages of St. Andrew and St. Etheldreda, in the archdeaconry and diocese of Ely, rated jointly in the king's books at £14. 3. 6½., and endowed with £200 royal bounty. The Heirs of — Mitchell, Esq. were patrons in 1820. The church of St. Andrew is partly in the early, and partly in the later, style of English architecture ; that of St. Etheldreda has been entirely demolished. Here is one of the five schools founded, in 1722, by Mrs. Elizabeth March, who endowed them with lands now producing £100 per annum.

HITCHAM, a parish in the hundred of BURNHAM, county of BUCKINGHAM, 2¼ miles (N. E. by E.) from Maidenhead, containing 172 inhabitants. The living is a rectory, in the archdeaconry of Buckingham, and diocese of Lincoln, rated in the king's books at £11. 5. 7½., and in the patronage of the Provost and Fellows of Eton College. The church is dedicated to St. Mary : the windows of the chancel exhibit a considerable quantity of stained glass of remarkable brilliancy.

HITCHAM, a parish in the hundred of COSFORD, county of SUFFOLK, 1¾ mile (N.N.W.) from Bildeston, containing 965 inhabitants. The living is a rectory, in the archdeaconry of Sudbury, and diocese of Norwich, rated in the king's books at £26. 13. 4., and in the patronage of the Crown. The church is dedicated to All Saints. There are almshouses appropriated by Sir George Waldegrave, in 166°, for two poor persons.

William Burkitt, a biblical writer, though commonly considered a native of Hitcham in the county of Northampton, was born here in 1650 ; he died in 1703.

HITCHENDEN, or HUGHENDEN, a parish in the hundred of DESBOROUGH, county of BUCKINGHAM, 1¾ mile (N.) from High Wycombe, containing, with a portion of the liberty of Brands-Fee, which is in this parish, 1247 inhabitants. The living is a discharged vicarage, in the archdeaconry of Buckingham, and diocese of Lincoln, rated in the king's books at £8. 17. 6., endowed with £200 private benefaction, and £200 royal bounty, and in the patronage of J. Norris, Esq. and others. The church, dedicated to St. Michael, is partly of Norman architecture, and has a curious font. Catherine Pye, in 1713, conveyed certain property towards the endowment of a school.

HITCHIN, a market town and parish, in the hundred of HITCHIN and PIRTON, county of HERTFORD, 15½ miles (N.W.) from Hertford, and 34 (N.N.W.) from London, containing, with the hamlets of Missenden, Preston, and Temple-Dinsley, 4486 inhabitants. This place, which, during the Saxon Heptarchy, formed part of the royal demesne of the King of Mercia, was given by Edward the Confessor to Harold, after whose death, at the battle of Hastings, it was retained by William the Conqueror, and is noticed in Domesday-book under the name of Hiz, a probable modification of its Saxon name, Hicce, or Hitche, from which its present appellation is deduced. It was granted by William Rufus to Bernard de Balliol, on the accession of whose descendant, John Balliol, to the throne of Scotland, it reverted to the crown of England, and was given by Edward III. to his fifth son, Edmund de Langley. The town is situated on a level spot of land environed on every side except the north by rising grounds, and intersected by the small river Hiz, which has its source at the distance of about a mile to the south-west : the streets, with the exception of that which forms the principal thoroughfare to Bedford, are spacious, and partially paved and lighted by subscription : the houses are in general neatly built of brick, but occasionally interspersed with some of less respectable appearance, and the inhabitants are amply supplied with water. The environs are pleasant, a considerable portion of the adjacent grounds being cultivated by market-gardeners, who supply the neighbouring towns with fruit and vegetables. A public subscription library, with a museum in which is a good collection of antiquities and natural curiosities, has been established : there are also several book societies ; and assemblies take place periodically during the winter, in a suite of rooms at the Sun Inn. Hitchin was celebrated at a very early period for its manufacture of woollen goods, and many of the merchants of Calais resided in the town prior to the removal of that branch of business from the towns on the continent. The trade at present is principally in corn and malt, for the latter of which it had obtained a high reputation in the reign of Elizabeth, who used to boast of "the juice of the Hitchin grape." The soil in the vicinity is favourable to the growth of barley and other grain, of which great quantities are sold at the market. The manufacture of strawplat affords employment to a considerable portion of the female inhabitants : a silk-mill, in which about three hundred persons are engaged, has been recently established, and there are some extensive breweries in the town and neighbourhood. The market, which is toll free, is held on Tuesday, and is well supplied with corn : the fairs are on the Tuesdays in Easter and Whitsun-weeks, which are pleasure fairs. The town is divided into Bancroft, Tilehouse, and Bridge wards, for each of which two constables and two head-boroughs are appointed at the court leet of the lord of the manor, held at Michaelmas. The county magistrates hold here a petty session every Tuesday. The bridewell, situated at the extremity of Bancroft-street, is a small brick building, comprising two wards for the classification only of prisoners committed for misdemeanours : the average number of committals is about eighty annually.

The living is a vicarage, in the archdeaconry of Huntingdon, and diocese of Lincoln, rated in the king's books at £25. 6. 8., and in the patronage of the Master and Fellows of Trinity College, Cambridge. The church, originally dedicated to St. Andrew, was, on being rebuilt prior to the reign of Henry VIII., dedicated to the Virgin Mary : it is a spacious structure, principally in the later style of English architecture, with a low massive embattled tower, surmounted by a small spire, and having a turret at one of the angles : the south porch is a beautifully enriched specimen of that style ; and over the entrance is a room which is used as a register office for that part of the archdeaconry of Huntingdon which is in the county of Herts. The interior of the church is very richly ornamented, and on each side of the chancel is a large chapel, separated from it by a handsome screen of carved oak ; over the altar is a fine painting of the Offering of the Wise Men of the East, by Rubens : there are numerous interesting monuments, and a font of singular beauty, with carvings of the twelve Apostles : underneath the eastern part of the chancel is a crypt, communicating by a staircase with the chapel on the north side, which was used by Cromwell as a prison for the royalists. There are places of worship for Baptists, the Society of Friends, those in the late Countess of Huntingdon's connexion, and Independents. The free school was principally founded by John Mattocke, Esq., of Coventry, who, in 1639, endowed it with land in Hitchin for the maintenance of a master : its present endowment, arising from that and subsequent benefactions, consists of nearly fifty-seven acres of land in this and other parishes, a rent-charge of £5, and the school-house, which is a commodious building at the west end of Tylehouse-street: this school has a contingent right to an exhibition to Christ Church College, Oxford, on failure of a candidate from the school at Buntingford. A school for the clothing and instruction of girls is supported partly by the dividends on nearly £1000, the amount of several benefactions vested in the funds, and by subscription. There are also British and foreign schools, in which two hundred boys and one hundred girls are instructed ; and an infant school is supported by subscription. Almshouses for eight poor persons were founded and endowed by Mr. Skinner, in 1668 : there are also almshouses for six poor persons, and others for eighteen women, in a house called the Biggin, said to have been formerly a religious establishment. Various benefactions have also been made for apprenticing poor boys and for other charitable purposes. Near the church was a small priory of Gilbertine nuns, the revenue of which, at the dissolution, was £15. 1. 11.; it was subsequently devised

to the free school by the Rev. Joseph Kemp, A.M.: there are still some remains, which have been converted into dwelling-houses. Towards the western extremity of the town was a house of Carmelite friars, founded by Edward II., and dedicated to the Blessed Virgin, the revenue of which, at the dissolution, was £4. 9. 4.: the cloisters and a small part of the buildings are still existing, and a handsome mansion, called the Priory, has been erected on the site. There was formerly a chapel at Missenden, now nearly demolished, and another at Temple-Dinsley, in this parish, the latter belonging to a preceptory of the Knights Templars, of which there are no vestiges. At Wildberry hill, over which passes the Iknield-street, within a mile of the town, was a Roman exploratory camp, occupying an area of seven acres and a half, and surrounded by a vallum, in which a fine silver coin of Faustina, Consort of the Emperor Marcus Aurelius, was discovered a few years since. Dr. Mark Hildesley, Bishop of Sodor and Man, was formerly vicar of this parish, and a great benefactor to the town.

HITTISLEIGH, a parish in the hundred of Wonford, county of Devon, 7½ miles (W. S. W.) from Crediton, containing 163 inhabitants. The living is a discharged rectory, in the archdeaconry and diocese of Exeter, rated in the king's books at £6. 2. 1., and in the patronage of Mrs. Colmady. The church is dedicated to St. Andrew.

HOARCROSS, a township in the parish of Yoxhall, northern division of the hundred of Offlow, county of Stafford, 3¾ miles (E. by S.) from Abbot's Bromley, containing 611 inhabitants.

HOATH, a parish in the hundred of Bleangate, lathe of St. Augustine, county of Kent, 5¼ miles (N. E.) from Canterbury, containing 348 inhabitants. The living is a perpetual curacy, annexed to the vicarage of Reculver, in the peculiar jurisdiction of the Archbishop of Canterbury. The church, dedicated to the Holy Cross, is principally in the early style of English architecture.

HOATHLY (EAST), a parish in the hundred of Shiplake, rape of Pevensey, county of Sussex, 5 miles (S. E. by S.) from Uckfield, containing 510 inhabitants. The living is a rectory, in the archdeaconry of Lewes, and diocese of Chichester, rated in the king's books at £7. 6. 3., and in the patronage of the Earl of Abergavenny. The church is in the early style of English architecture.

HOATHLY (WEST), a parish in the hundred of Buttinghill, rape of Lewes, county of Sussex, 4¼ miles (S. W. by S.) from East Grinsted, containing 943 inhabitants. The living is a discharged vicarage, in the archdeaconry of Lewes, and diocese of Chichester, rated in the king's books at £9. 16., and in the patronage of the Crown. The church is partly in the early, and partly in the decorated, style of English architecture. There is a place of worship for Dissenters. A fair for pedlary is held on Whit-Monday.

HOBENDRID, a township in the parish of Clun, hundred of Purslow, county of Salop, containing 255 inhabitants.

HOB-LENCH, otherwise ABBOTS-LENCH, a hamlet in the parish of Fladbury, middle division of the hundred of Oswaldslow, county of Worcester, 6¼ miles (N. by W.) from Evesham, containing 102 inhabitants. Here was formerly a chapel, which has gone to decay.

HOBY, a parish in the eastern division of the hundred of GOSCOTE, county of LEICESTER, 5¾ miles (W. by S.) from Melton-Mowbray, containing 352 inhabitants. The living is a rectory, in the archdeaconry of Leicester, and diocese of Lincoln, rated in the king's books at £22. 8. 9. The Rev. H. Browne was patron in 1784. The church is dedicated to All Saints.

HOCKENHULL, a township in that part of the parish of TARVIN which is in the second division of the hundred of EDDISBURY, county palatine of CHESTER, 5 miles (W. N. W.) from Tarporley, containing 38 inhabitants.

HOCKERING, a parish in the hundred of MITFORD, county of NORFOLK, 5¼ miles (E.) from East Dereham, containing 392 inhabitants. The living is a rectory, united to that of Mattishall-Burgh, in the archdeaconry of Norfolk, and diocese of Norwich, rated in the king's books at £7. 3. 4. The church, dedicated to St. Michael, has a round tower. Here was anciently a castle, this having been the principal manor of the Barony of Rye.

HOCKERTON, a parish in the northern division of the wapentake of THURGARTON, county of NOTTINGHAM, 2 miles (N. N. E.) from Southwell, containing 115 inhabitants. The living is a rectory, in the archdeaconry of Nottingham, and diocese of York, rated in the king's books at £9: 9. 4½., and in the patronage of Admiral Sotheron. The church is dedicated to St. Nicholas.

HOCKHAM, a parish comprising Great and Little Hockham, in the hundred of SHROPHAM, county of NORFOLK, 4½ miles (N. W. by N.) from East Harling, containing 525 inhabitants. The living is a discharged vicarage, in the archdeaconry of Norfolk, and diocese of Norwich, rated in the king's books at £8. 17. 11. M. Mallett, Esq. was patron in 1800. The church is dedicated to the Holy Trinity. There was formerly a church, or chapel, at Little Hockham, but it has been demolished.

HOCKLEY, a parish in the hundred of ROCHFORD, county of ESSEX, 2¼ miles (N. E. by N.) from Rayleigh, containing 784 inhabitants. The living is a discharged vicarage, in the archdeaconry of Essex, and diocese of London, rated in the king's books at £16. 3. 9., and in the patronage of the Warden and Fellows of Wadham College, Oxford. The church, dedicated to St. Peter, is of Norman architecture, with a massive octagonal tower surmounted by a shingled spire : it is supposed to have been erected by Canute and Turkil, in commemoration of their victory over Edmund Ironside. The Crouch river is navigable along the northern boundary of the parish. There is a very large barrow in the neighbourhood.

HOCKLIFFE, a parish in the hundred of MANSHEAD, county of BEDFORD, 3½ miles (E. N. E.) from Leighton-Buzzard, containing 393 inhabitants. The living is a rectory, united in 1772 to the vicarage of Chalgrave, in the archdeaconry of Bedford, and diocese of Lincoln, rated in the king's books at £16. 9. 7. Mrs. Robinson was patroness in 1791. The church is dedicated to St. Nicholas. There is a place of worship for Independents. Francis West, in 1690, bequeathed £400 for educating poor children of Hockliffe and Chalgrave : the income is £30 a year, for which nine boys of each parish are instructed. So early as the reign of John here was an hospital, founded for a master and brethren, and dedicated to St. John the Baptist.

HOCKMOOR, a hamlet in the parish of IFLEY, hun-

dred of BULLINGTON, county of OXFORD, 1¾ mile (S. E. by S.) from Oxford. The population is returned with the parish.

HOCKWOLD, a parish in the hundred of GRIMSHOE, county of NORFOLK, 4½ miles (W. by N.) from Brandon-Ferry, containing, with the parish of Wilton, 846 inhabitants. The living is a rectory, in four portions, with which the vicarage of Wilton is united, in the archdeaconry of Norfolk, and diocese of Norwich, rated in the king's books at £9. 13. 11½., and in the patronage of the Master and Fellows of Caius College, Cambridge. The church, dedicated to St. Peter, contains three ancient stalls, for the bishop, priest, and deacon, besides a piscina.

HOCKWORTHY, a parish in the hundred of BAMPTON, county of DEVON, 6 miles (E. S. E.) from Bampton, containing 354 inhabitants. The living is a discharged vicarage, in the archdeaconry and diocese of Exeter, rated in the king's books at £7. 6. 8., and in the patronage of — Comyns, Esq. A considerable traffic in lime is carried on in the parish, which abounds with excellent limestone.

HODDESDON, a market town and chapelry, partly in the parish of GREAT AMWELL, but chiefly in that of BROXBURN, hundred and county of HERTFORD, 4¼ miles (S. E.) from Hertford, and 17 (N. by E.) from London, containing 1354 inhabitants. The name of this place is supposed to have been derived from its having been the residence of Hodo, or Oddo, a Danish chief, or from a tumulus, or barrow, raised here to his memory. The town consists principally of one street, extending along the high road from London to Ware and Hertford : it is supplied with water from a conduit in the market-place, erected by Sir Marmaduke Rawdon in the seventeenth century. A considerable quantity of malt is made here, much of which is conveyed to London by means of the river Lea ; and there is a large brewery. The market, now nearly disused, is on Tuesday ; and a fair is held annually on the 29th of June. In the centre of the town is an ancient market-house, built of wood, and supported on pillars and arches ornamented with curious carving. The site of the old chapel, dedicated to St. Catherine, is marked by a turret, which serves as a clock-house, and which, having become ruinous, was rebuilt about 1730. The present chapel is a handsome brick edifice, standing in the parish of Amwell, but subject to the vicarage of Broxburn : it has received an addition of eight hundred sittings, four hundred of which are free, the Incorporated Society for the enlargement of churches and chapels having granted £700 towards defraying the expense. Here are places of worship for the Society of Friends and Independents. Queen Elizabeth, in the second year of her reign, granted a charter for a free grammar school, with considerable privileges ; and there is a National school for ninety boys and thirty girls, supported by voluntary contributions. Five almshouses, founded in the fifteenth century, are now under the management of the parish officers.

HODDINGTON, a tything in the parish of UPTON-GRAY, hundred of BERMONDSPIT, Basingstoke division, though locally in the hundred of Fawley, Fawley division, of the county of SOUTHAMPTON, 3½ miles (S. W. by W.) from Odiham. The population is returned with the parish.

HODNEL, an extra-parochial liberty, in the Southam division of the hundred of KNIGHTLOW, county of WARWICK, 3 miles (S. by E.) from Southam, containing 9 inhabitants. Here was anciently a chapel dedicated to St. Helen, now in ruins.

HODNET, a parish in the Drayton division of the hundred of BRADFORD (North), county of SALOP, 6 miles (S. W.) from Drayton in Hales, containing, with the joint chapelry of Weston with Wixhill under Red Castle, 2117 inhabitants. The living is a rectory, in the archdeaconry of Salop, and diocese of Lichfield and Coventry, rated in the king's books at £26. 0. 10. Richard Heber, Esq. was patron in 1823. The church is dedicated to St. Peter and St. Paul. Lord Clive, celebrated for his extension of the British empire in India, was born at Styche in this parish, in 1724; Reginald Heber, D.D., an erudite divine and refined scholar, late Bishop of Calcutta, was also born here in 1783 ; he died in India in 1826.

HODSOCK, a lordship in that part of the parish of BLYTH which is in the Hatfield division of the wapentake of BASSETLAW, county of NOTTINGHAM, 2 miles (S. W.) from Blyth, containing 224 inhabitants. Here are a private chapel and the remains of a large and ancient mansion belonging to the Clifton family.

HOE, county of NORFOLK. — See HOO.

HOFFE, a township in the parish of ST. LAWRENCE, APPLEBY, EAST ward, county of WESTMORLAND, 1¾ mile (S. by W.) from Appleby, containing 93 inhabitants. Here was formerly a chapel.

HOGHTON, a chapelry in the parish and hundred of LEYLAND, county palatine of LANCASTER, 5½ miles (S. E. by E.) from Preston, containing 2111 inhabitants. The living is a perpetual curacy, in the archdeaconry and diocese of Chester, endowed with £1600 parliamentary grant, and in the patronage of the Vicar of Leyland. A school, endowed by Sir Charles Hoghton with £26 per annum, is further supported by subscription, and conducted on the National system.

HOGNASTON, a parish in the hundred of WIRKSWORTH, county of DERBY, 5 miles (S.W. by W.) from Wirksworth, containing 292 inhabitants. The living is a perpetual curacy, in the archdeaconry of Derby, and diocese of Lichfield and Coventry, endowed with £800 royal bounty, and in the patronage of the Dean of Lincoln. The church has a Norman south door. Limestone abounds in the parish. An hospital for six poor men was founded and liberally endowed, in 1583, by Anthony Gell. There is also a small endowment for a school, the gift of Temperance Gell, in 1729.

HOGSHAW, a parish in the hundred of ASHENDON, county of BUCKINGHAM, 4 miles (S.W. by S.) from Winslow, containing, with the hamlet of Fulbrook, 68 inhabitants. The church, which was dedicated to St. John the Baptist, being desecrated, the inhabitants attend the church of Quainton. Here was a preceptory of the Knights of St. John of Jerusalem, so early as the reign of Henry II.

HOGSTHORPE, a parish in the Marsh division of the hundred of CALCEWORTH, parts of LINDSEY, county of LINCOLN, 6¼ miles (E. S. E.) from Alford, containing 591 inhabitants. The living is a discharged vicarage, in the archdeaconry and diocese of Lincoln, rated in the king's books at £10, endowed with £200 royal bounty, and £1000 parliamentary grant, and in the patronage of

the Bishop of Lincoln. The church is dedicated to St. Mary. There is a place of worship for Wesleyan Methodists.

HOGSTON, a parish in the hundred of COTTESLOE, county of BUCKINGHAM, 3¾ miles (S. E. by E.) from Winslow, containing 188 inhabitants. The living is a rectory, in the archdeaconry of Buckingham, and diocese of Lincoln, rated in the king's books at £11. 16. 3., and in the patronage of the Provost and Fellows of Worcester College, Oxford. The church is dedicated to St. Peter and St. Paul.

HOLBEACH, a market town and parish, in the wapentake of ELLOE, parts of HOLLAND, county of LINCOLN, 12 miles (S.) from Boston, 42 (S.E.) from Lincoln, and 106 (N. by E.) from London, containing 3621 inhabitants. Its ancient name was Oldbeche, so called from having been built near an old beach which the receding of the waters had left, as it is evident, from the different embankments constructed between the Foss-dyke and the Cross Keys Washes, that all the land in the vicinity of the town has been once covered by the waters of the German ocean. Foundations of walls and pavements have been discovered, and several ancient coins, urns, and seals, dug up at different periods. The town, which is situated in a low marshy district, is indifferently built. The market is on Thursday ; and fairs are held, May 17th and September 17th, for horses and cattle. Holbeach is within the jurisdiction of a court of requests for the recovery of debts under £5, held under the authority of an act passed in the 47th of George III., for the hundred of Elloe.

The living is a vicarage, in the archdeaconry and diocese of Lincoln, rated in the king's books at £20. 5. 10., and in the patronage of the Bishop of Lincoln. The church, dedicated to All Saints, is a noble edifice, consisting of a nave, a chancel, a porch, and a square tower, surmounted by an octangular ornamented spire ; the north porch has two circular towers, with embattled parapets at its extreme angles. In the church are some interesting monuments, and an altar-piece representing our Saviour instituting the Last Supper. The free grammar school was founded in 1669, by George Farmer, Esq., who endowed it with lands and tenements which now let for about £140 per annum : it was formerly held in a part of the church, but in 1807 a new school-room was built, in which about one hundred and forty scholars are instructed on Dr. Bell's plan. An hospital for a warden and fifteen poor persons was founded near the church, about 1351, by Sir John de Kirketon, Knt., which was suppressed at the Reformation. This town is celebrated as the birthplace, or residence, of several eminent literary characters ; amongst whom are, Dr. William Stukeley, the celebrated antiquary ; Henry Rands, otherwise Holbeach, appointed to the bishoprick of Lincoln in 1547, and one of the compilers of the Liturgy. Samuel Frotheringham, a member of the Society of Friends, died here in 1745 : he is said to have been the first in England who invented a clock with hands, denoting both the true and the apparent time at all seasons of the year, according to the eccentricity of the earth's orbit, and the obliquity of the ecliptic.

HOLBECK, a township in the parish of CUCKNEY, Hatfield division of the wapentake of BASSETLAW, county of NOTTINGHAM, 6¾ miles (S.W.) from Worksop, containing 239 inhabitants.

HOLBECK, a chapelry in that part of the parish of St. Peter, Leeds, which is within the liberty of Leeds, though locally in the wapentake of Agbrigg, West riding of the county of York, 1½ mile (S. S. W.) from Leeds, containing 7151 inhabitants. The living is a perpetual curacy, in the archdeaconry and diocese of York, endowed with £400 private benefaction, and £400 royal bounty, and in the patronage of the Vicar of Leeds. The chapel, which was rebuilt in the last century, is mentioned in a bull of the Pope so early as 809. There is a commodious place of worship for Wesleyan Methodists. Holbeck forms a very extensive part of the environs of the town of Leeds, being joined to it by Waterlane, and, like that place, contains many manufactories for linen and woollen goods upon a very large scale. There are warm and cold baths, the water of which possesses properties similar to the Harrogate springs, but weaker, and is considered salutary for every domestic purpose, being daily carried about the streets of Leeds for sale, at a moderate price.

HOLBETON, a parish in the hundred of Ermington, county of Devon, 3¼ miles (W.S.W.) from Modbury, containing 1083 inhabitants. The living is a vicarage, in the archdeaconry of Totness, and diocese of Exeter, rated in the king's books at £24. 1. 8., and in the patronage of the Crown. The church is dedicated to All Saints. Here was formerly a chapel dedicated to St. Leonard. The parish is bounded on the east by the river Erme, and by the English channel on the south. There is an endowed school for the education of ten girls, who are also clothed from the same fund.

HOLBROOK, a chapelry in the parish of Duffield, hundred of Appletree, county of Derby, 5¾ miles (N. by E.) from Derby, containing 563 inhabitants. The living is a perpetual curacy, in the archdeaconry of Derby, and diocese of Lichfield and Coventry, endowed with £200 royal bounty, and £1400 parliamentary grant, and in the patronage of William Evans, Esq. The chapel was built in 1761, by the Rev. S. Bradshaw, and endowed by him with £30 per annum chargeable on the Holbrook estate.

HOLBROOK, a parish in the hundred of Samford, county of Suffolk, 5 miles (S. by E.) from Ipswich, containing 641 inhabitants. The living is a rectory, in the archdeaconry of Stafford, and diocese of Norwich, rated in the king's books at £11. 11. 3., and in the patronage of the Rev. J. B. Wilkinson. The church is dedicated to All Saints. There is a place of worship for Wesleyan Methodists. The river Stour, which at flood tide is two miles across, bounds the parish to the south-east.

HOLCOMB, a tything in the parish of Newington, hundred of Ewelme, county of Oxford, 5⅓ miles (N. by E.) from Wallingford, containing 110 inhabitants.

HOLCOMBE, a chapelry in that part of the parish of Bury which is in the hundred of Salford, county palatine of Lancaster, 4 miles (N.N.W.) from Bury, with which the population is returned. The living is a perpetual curacy, in the archdeaconry and diocese of Chester, endowed with £200 private benefaction, £800 royal bounty, and £1000 parliamentary grant, and in the patronage of the Rector of Bury.

HOLCOMBE, a parish in the hundred of Kilmersdon, county of Somerset, 6¼ miles (N.E. by N. Vol. II.

from Shepton-Mallet, containing 527 inhabitants. The living is a discharged rectory, in the archdeaconry of Wells, and diocese of Bath and Wells, rated in the king's books at £5. 7. 8½., endowed with £200 royal bounty, and £400 parliamentary grant, and in the patronage of John Twyford Jolliffe, Esq. The church, dedicated to St. Andrew, is an ancient edifice, with a fine Norman south porch. There is a place of worship for Wesleyan Methodists. The parish abounds with mines of coal and iron-stone, but there is no iron made here. There is a traditionary report that the inhabitants, at a remote period, deserted the village, then situated in a valley near the church, and settled on the Mendip hills, to avoid the contagion of a malignant fever, thus leaving the church, as it still remains, without an habitation in its immediate vicinity. A canal from the southern part of the parish to Frome was commenced some years since, but has not been completed.

HOLCOMBE-BURNELL, a parish in the hundred of Wonford, county of Devon, 4½ miles (W. by S.) from Exeter, containing 237 inhabitants. The living is a vicarage, in the archdeaconry and diocese of Exeter, rated in the king's books at £8. 9. 2., endowed with £200 private benefaction, and £300 parliamentary grant, and in the patronage of the Prebendary of Holcombe Burnell in the Cathedral Church of Wells. The church, dedicated to St. John the Baptist, has an ornamented doorway in the Norman style, and contains an altar-tomb used before the Reformation to celebrate the festival of Easter. Near the old manorial mansion, built in the reign of Henry VIII., and since converted into a farm-house, there was anciently a chapel.

HOLCOMBE-ROGUS, a parish in the hundred of Bampton, county of Devon, 7 miles (E. S. E.) from Bampton, containing 829 inhabitants. The living is a discharged vicarage, in the archdeaconry and diocese of Exeter, rated in the king's books at £10. 10. 2½. Samuel Wills, Esq. was patron in 1824. The church is dedicated to All Saints. A weekly market and an annual fair were formerly held here; and a branch of the Grand Western canal passes through the parish. One of the free boys in Ayshford's grammar school at Uffculme is appointed from this place.

HOLCOT, a parish in the hundred of Hamfordshoe, county of Northampton, 7½ miles (W. by N.) from Wellingborough, containing 442 inhabitants. The living is a rectory, in the archdeaconry of Northampton, and diocese of Peterborough, rated in the king's books at £13. 6. 8. F. Montgomery, Esq. was patron in 1825. The church is dedicated to St. Mary and All Saints.

HOLCUTT, a parish in the hundred of Manshead, county of Bedford, 4½ miles (N.) from Woburn, containing 62 inhabitants. The living is a rectory, with which the vicarage of Salford was united in 1750, in the archdeaconry of Bedford, and diocese of Lincoln, rated in the king's books at £7. 15. The Rev. E. O. Smith was patron in 1819. The church is dedicated to St. Nicholas.

HOLDENBY, a parish in the hundred of Nobottle-Grove, county of Northampton, 6½ miles (N.W. by N.) from Northampton, containing 149 inhabitants. The living is a rectory, in the archdeaconry of Northampton, and diocese of Peterborough, rated in the king's books at £20. 2. 11., and in the patronage of the Crown. The church is dedicated to All Saints. This is the birth-place of Sir Christopher Hatton, Lord High Chancellor in the reign of Elizabeth, who built the once magnificent mansion of Holdenby House, part of which is still remaining. Here Charles I. was confined, on being surrendered by the Scottish army to the parliamentary commissioners.

HOLDENHURST, a chapelry in the parish of CHRISTCHURCH, liberty of WESTOVER, New Forest (West) division of the county of SOUTHAMPTON, 3 miles (N. W. by W.) from Christchurch, containing 580 inhabitants. The living is a perpetual curacy, annexed to the vicarage of Christchurch, in the archdeaconry and diocese of Winchester. The navigable river Stour bounds the chapelry on the east and north.

HOLDFAST, a hamlet in that part of the parish of RIPPLE which is in the lower division of the hundred of OSWALDSLOW, county of WORCESTER, 1¾ mile (S. by E.) from Upton upon Severn, containing 89 inhabitants. Here was anciently a chapel, which has been demolished.

HOLDGATE, a parish in the hundred of MUNSLOW, county of SALOP, comprising the townships of Bouldon, Brookhampton, and Holdgate, and containing 238 inhabitants, of which number, 77 are in the township of Holdgate, 8¾ miles (S.S.W.) from Much Wenlock. The living is a discharged rectory, in the archdeaconry of Salop, and diocese of Hereford, rated in the king's books at £13. 9. 9½., and in the patronage of the Bishop of Hereford. The church is dedicated to the Holy Trinity.

HOLDINGHAM, a hamlet in the parish of NEW SLEAFORD, hundred of FLAXWELL, parts of KESTEVEN, county of LINCOLN, 1 mile (N. N. W.) from Sleaford, containing 126 inhabitants.

HOLDSHOTT, a tything in the parish of HECKFIELD, hundred of HOLDSHOTT, Basingstoke division of the county of SOUTHAMPTON, 3¼ miles (W. N. W.) from Hartford-Bridge. The population is returned with the parish.

HOLFORD, a parish in, and forming one of five unconnected portions, of the hundred of WHITLEY, county of SOMERSET, 10½ miles (W.N.W.) from Bridgwater, containing 240 inhabitants. The living is a discharged rectory, in the archdeaconry of Taunton, and diocese of Bath and Wells, rated in the king's books at £5. 1. 5½, endowed with £200 private benefaction, and £200 royal bounty, and in the patronage of the Provost and Fellows of Eton College.

HOLGATE, a township in that part of the parish of ST. MARY BISHOPSHILL JUNIOR, which is in the ainsty of the city, and East riding of the county, of YORK, 1¼ mile (W. by S.) from York, containing 88 inhabitants. Lindley Murray, author of a popular English Grammar, and other school books, who was born in Pennsylvania, North America, in 1745, died, in 1826, at this place, where he had long resided.

HOLKER (LOWER), a township in the parish of CARTMEL, hundred of LONSDALE, north of the sands, county palatine of LANCASTER, 1¾ mile (S. W.) from Cartmel, containing 1091 inhabitants.

HOLKER (UPPER), a township in the parish of CARTMEL, hundred of LONSDALE, north of the sands, county palatine of LANCASTER, 1¼ mile (N. by W.) from Cartmel, containing 1120 inhabitants. George Bigland,

in 1685, devised lands which produce £30 a year, for the support of a school.

HOLKHAM, a parish in the northern division of the hundred of GREENHOE, county of NORFOLK, 3 miles (W.) from Wells, containing 810 inhabitants. The living is a discharged vicarage, in the archdeaconry and diocese of Norfolk, rated in the king's books at £8.13.4., endowed with £200 royal bounty, and £200 parliamentary grant, and in the patronage of T. W. Coke, Esq. The church, dedicated to St. Withiburga, is situated on an eminence north of the town ; it has a massive quadrangular embattled tower, serving as a land-mark, which was repaired in 1767, at an expense of £1000, defrayed by the Countess Dowager of Leicester, who also built and endowed almshouses for the support of three aged persons of each sex. A school for boys, and another for girls, with a house and garden attached for the master and mistress, are supported by T. W. Coke, Esq. Holkham was formerly a sea-port of some eminence, and in the reign of Edward II. furnished, conjointly with Burnham-Deepdale, one ship, to assist in the transportation of English troops from Ireland to Scotland.

HOLLACOMBE, a parish in the hundred of BLACK TORRINGTON, county of DEVON, 2½ miles (E. by S.) from Holsworthy, containing 96 inhabitants. The living is a discharged rectory, in the archdeaconry of Totness, and diocese of Exeter, rated in the king's books at £4. 6. 3., endowed with £200 royal bounty, and in the patronage of the Crown. The church is dedicated to St. Petrock.

HOLLAND (DOWN), a township in the parish of HALSALL, hundred of WEST DERBY, county palatine of LANCASTER, 5¼ miles (W.) from Ormskirk, containing 629 inhabitants.

HOLLAND (FEN), a district comprising portions of eleven different parishes, in the wapentake of ELLOE, parts of HOLLAND, county of LINCOLN, 8¼ miles (N. W. by W.) from Boston. The population is returned with the several parishes in which it is situated. A chapel was erected and consecrated in 1812. The living, a perpetual curacy, was endowed, in 1814, with £1400 parliamentary grant.

HOLLAND (GREAT), a parish in the hundred of TENDRING, county of ESSEX, 12½ miles (S. E. by S.) from Manningtree, containing 413 inhabitants. The living is a rectory, in the archdeaconry of Colchester, and diocese of London, rated in the king's books at £17. 13. 9., and in the patronage of the President and Fellows of Corpus Christi College, Oxford. The church is dedicated to All Saints. This parish lies on the coast of the North sea.

HOLLAND (LITTLE), a parish in the hundred of TENDRING, county of ESSEX, 16 miles (S. E. by E.) from Colchester, containing 73 inhabitants. The living, a donative in the jurisdiction of the Commissary of Essex and Herts, concurrently with the Consistorial Court of the Bishop of London, is united to the vicarage of Great Clacton, to the church at which place the parishioners resort, that at Little Holland having been demolished. The parish has the North sea on the southeast, where there are a battery and a signal station. Holland creek marks the boundary between Great and Little Holland, and is crossed by a bridge.

HOLLAND (UP), a chapelry (formerly a market

town) in that part of the parish of WIGAN which is in the hundred of WEST DERBY, county palatine of LANCASTER, 4½ miles (W. by S.) from Wigan, containing 3042 inhabitants. The living is a perpetual curacy, in the archdeaconry and diocese of Chester, endowed with £200 private benefaction, £400 royal bounty, and £1400 parliamentary grant, and in the patronage of the Rector of Wigan. The chapel, dedicated to St. Thomas à Becket, is an ancient edifice, the nave and aisles of which are in the decorated English style, with a large and handsome east window in the chancel: it formerly belonged to a priory of Benedictine monks, founded in the beginning of the fourteenth century, the revenue of which, at the dissolution, was valued at £78. 12. A fair for horses and cattle is held here on the 15th of July.

HOLLESLEY, a parish in the hundred of WILFORD, county of SUFFOLK, 7¼ miles (S. E. by E.) from Woodbridge, containing 575 inhabitants. The living is a rectory, in the archdeaconry of Suffolk, and diocese of Norwich, rated in the king's books at £12. 16. 8. The church is dedicated to All Saints. The parish is bounded on the east by the river Alde, which falls into Hollesley bay.

HOLLETH, a hamlet in the parish of GARSTANG, hundred of AMOUNDERNESS, county palatine of LANCASTER, 5 miles (N. by W.) from Garstang, containing 43 inhabitants.

HOLLINGBOURN, a parish in the hundred of EYHORNE, lathe of AYLESFORD, county of KENT, 6 miles (E.) from Maidstone, containing 1000 inhabitants. The living comprises a rectory and a vicarage, with the perpetual curacy of Hucking, rated jointly in the king's books at £36. 2. 1., and in the peculiar jurisdiction and patronage of the Archbishop of Canterbury. The church, dedicated to All Saints, is a handsome edifice, attached to which is a chapel with a marble floor, containing a superb monument to the memory of Lady Culpepper. There is a place of worship for Wesleyan Methodists. Ann Long, in 1812, bequeathed £7 per annum for teaching six girls, and £3 to poor widows.

HOLLINGFARE, a chapelry in the parish of WARRINGTON, hundred of WEST DERBY, county palatine of LANCASTER, 6 miles (E. N. E.) from Warrington, with which the population is returned. The living is a perpetual curacy, in the archdeaconry and diocese of Chester, endowed with £400 private benefaction, and £400 royal bounty, and in the patronage of the Rector of Warrington.

HOLLINGTON, a township in the parish of LONGFORD, hundred of APPLETREE, county of DERBY, 5½ miles (S. E. by S.) from Ashbourn, containing 314 inhabitants. Joseph Holme, in 1768, bequeathed a small sum for teaching children. Hollington is in the honour of Tutbury, duchy of Lancaster, and within the jurisdiction of a court of pleas held at Tutbury every third Tuesday, for the recovery of debts under 40s.

HOLLINGTON, a parish in the hundred of BALDSLOW, rape of HASTINGS, county of SUSSEX, 2¾ miles (W. N. W.) from Hastings, containing 272 inhabitants. The living is a discharged vicarage, in the archdeaconry of Lewes, and diocese of Chichester, rated in the king's books at £8. 0. 2. W. Eversfield, Esq. was patron in 1812. The church, dedicated to St. Lawrence, is in the early style of English architecture.

HOLLINGWORTH, a township in the parish of MOTTRAM in LONGDEN-DALE, hundred of MACCLESFIELD, county palatine of CHESTER, 8 miles (E. N. E.) from Stockport, containing 1393 inhabitants. About thirty years ago Hollingworth was but an agricultural district with few inhabitants: there are now extensive manufactories for cotton goods, paper, and machinery, also for the printing of calico, and a foundry for smelting metals.

HOLLINSCLOUGH, a township in the parish of ALLSTONEFIELD, northern division of the hundred of TOTMONSLOW, county of STAFFORD, 1¾ mile (N. W. by W.) from Longnor, containing 560 inhabitants.

HOLLOWAY, a hamlet in that part of the parish of ASHOVER which is in the hundred of WIRKSWORTH, county of DERBY, 3 miles (S. E.) from Matlock. The population is returned with the chapelry of Dethwick-Lea.

HOLLOWAY, a district in the parish of ISLINGTON, Finsbury division of the hundred of OSSULSTONE, county of MIDDLESEX, 3 miles (N.) from London. The population is returned with the parish. The village is divided into two parts, Upper and Lower Holloway, consisting principally of detached houses, many of which are handsome buildings, extending along the great north road from London to Liverpool. The place appears to have derived its name from being situated in the hollow way, or vale, between Islington and Highgate. The village is lighted with gas, and supplied with water by the New River Company: it is within the jurisdiction of the court of requests held in Kingsgate-street, Holborn, for the recovery of debts under 40s.; and also under the superintendence of the New Police. A new church, dedicated to St. John, and situated at Upper Holloway, was completed in 1828, at an expense of £11,890. 7. 8., defrayed partly by a grant from the parliamentary commissioners, and partly by a rate on the inhabitants: it is in the decorated English style, with a square tower at the west end: the interior is handsomely fitted up, and lighted with gas; and it contains one thousand seven hundred and eighty-two sittings, of which seven hundred and fifty-three are free. The living is a district incumbency, in the jurisdiction of the Commissary of London, concurrently with the Bishop, and in the patronage of the Vicar of Islington. At Lower Holloway is a chapel of ease to the vicarage of St. Mary's, Islington, which was consecrated in August, 1814, having been erected at an expense (including the site, and a cemetery of five or six acres) of about £32,000, under the authority of an act of parliament passed in 1811, authorising the trustees to raise by annuities £30,000 : it is a large edifice, with a square tower at the west end : the interior is neatly ornamented, and over the altar is a modern painting of the appearance of Christ to Mary Magdalene. Here is a place of worship for Independents, to which is attached a Sunday school. At Upper Holloway is a National school for boys ; there is another for girls belonging to Highgate and Holloway, and also an infant school. Near Highgate archway, but within the limits of Upper Holloway, is situated Sir Richard Whittington's college, or almshouse, originally founded in the parish of St. Michael, Paternoster, London, pursuant to a bequest by Sir Richard Whittington, Knt., alderman and thrice lord mayor of London, who, in 1421, left the residue of his estate, after the payment of debts and legacies, to executors, for the purpose of erecting and endowing almshouses for thirteen poor people, under the conservancy of the Mercers' Company : the funds having received very considerable additions from various benefactors, the conservators, in 1824, erected the present college at Holloway, at an expense of nearly £20,000 : it is a handsome edifice in the later English style, consisting of a front and wings, with a chapel in the centre ; and the grounds before it are tastefully laid out, and planted with flowering shrubs and evergreens : there are tenements for twenty-nine alms-women, who, at the time of admission, must be widows, or spinsters, not less than fifty-five years of age, and not possessing property to the amount of £30 per annum., which sum each of them receives as a pension from the charity. At Upper Holloway was born, in 1649, Sir Thomas Pope Blount, Bart., author of " Censura Authorum Celebriorum," and other learned works ; also, in 1654, his brother, Charles Blount, who became noted as a deistical writer, and who, in August 1693, shot himself in a fit of phrenzy, occasioned by a disappointed attachment to the sister of his deceased wife.

HOLLOWELL, a hamlet in the parish and hundred of GUILSBOROUGH, county of NORTHAMPTON, 8 miles (N. W. by N.) from Northampton, containing 279 inhabitants.

HOLLYM, a parish in the southern division of the wapentake of HOLDERNESS, East riding of the county of YORK, comprising the chapelry of Withernsea, and the township of Hollym, and containing 368 inhabitants, of which number, 260 are in the township of Hollym, 3 miles (N. E.) from Patrington. The living is a discharged vicarage, in the archdeaconry of the East riding, and diocese of York, rated in the king's books at £9. 19. 2., and in the patronage of the Mayor and Corporation of Beverley. The church, dedicated to St. Nicholas, was built in 1814, by the Rev. Charles Barker, then vicar. George Cook, in 1813, bequeathed £300 towards the support of a school, the interest of which is applied to the instruction of eleven poor children.

HOLM, in that part of the parish of BOTTESFORD which is in the eastern division of the wapentake of MANLEY, parts of LINDSEY, county of LINCOLN, 5½ miles (W.) from Glandford-Bridge, containing 39 inhabitants.

HOLM, a joint township with Howgrave, in that part of the parish of PICKHILL which is in the wapentake of ALLERTONSHIRE, though locally in the wapentake of Hallikeld, North riding of the county of YORK, 5¼ miles (W. by S.) from Thirsk, containing 102 inhabitants.

HOLME, a joint hamlet with Stratton, in the parish and hundred of BIGGLESWADE, county of BEDFORD, 1 mile (S. by W.) from Biggleswade, with which the population is returned.

HOLME, a township in the parish of BAKEWELL, hundred of HIGH PEAK, county of DERBY, ¼ of a mile (N.) from Bakewell. The population is returned with the chapelry of Great Longstone.

HOLME, a chapelry in the parish of GLATTON, hundred of NORMAN-CROSS, county of HUNTINGDON, 2¼ miles (E. S. E.) from Stilton, containing 311 inhabitants. The living is a perpetual curacy annexed to the rectory of Glatton, in the archdeaconry of Huntingdon, and diocese of Lincoln. The church is dedicated to St. Giles.

HOLME, a chapelry in that part of the parish of WHALLEY which is in the higher division of the hundred of BLACKBURN, county palatine of LANCASTER, 3½ miles (S. E. by S.) from Burnley. The population is returned with the parish. The living is a perpetual curacy, in the archdeaconry and diocese of Chester, endowed with £400 private benefaction, and £1200 parliamentary grant. — Whittaker, Esq. was patron in 1822. William Whittaker, a controversial divine, was born here in 1548 ; he died in 1595.

HOLME, a chapelry in the parish of NORTH MUSKHAM, northern division of the wapentake of THURGARTON, county of NOTTINGHAM, 4 miles (N. by E.) from Newark, containing 114 inhabitants. This chapelry is in the jurisdiction of the peculiar court of the Chapter of the Collegiate Church of Southwell. The chapel, dedicated to St. Giles, is a spacious edifice.

HOLME, a township in that part of the parish of BURTON in KENDAL which is in LONSDALE ward, county of WESTMORLAND, 1¾ mile (N. by W.) from Burton in Kendal, containing 420 inhabitants. The Lancaster and Kendal canal passes through this place. Here are two extensive flax-mills and a linen manufactory. There is a place of worship for Independents.

HOLME, a township in the parish of ALMONDBURY, upper division of the wapentake of AGBRIGG, West riding of the county of YORK, 9 miles (S. S. W.) from Huddersfield, containing 459 inhabitants. The manufacture of woollen goods is somewhat extensively carried on here. A school has been erected on ground given by James Earnshaw, for the support of which Joshua Earnshaw, in 1691, bequeathed £300.

HOLME (BALDWIN), a township in the parish of ORTON, ward and county of CUMBERLAND, 5¾ miles (S. W. by W.) from Carlisle, containing 234 inhabitants.

HOLME (BENE'T ST.), a hamlet in the parish of HORNING, hundred of TUNSTEAD, county of NORFOLK, 5½ miles (N. by W.) from Acle. The population is returned with Horning. This place is stated to have been given by a petty prince, called Horn, to a religious fraternity, about the year 800, who, with a chapel built here by them, and dedicated to St. Benedict, were destroyed by the Danes, in 870 : the chapel and houses were afterwards rebuilt by a person named Wolfric, and were elevated into a Benedictine abbey by Canute, about 1020, the revenue of which, at the dissolution, was £677. 9. 8.

HOLME (EAST), an extra-parochial liberty, in the hundred of HASILOR, Blandford (South) division of the county of DORSET, 2½ miles (S. W. by W.) from Wareham, containing 42 inhabitants. Here was formerly a cell subordinate to the Cluniac priory of Montacute, in the county of Somerset.

HOLME (NORTH), a township in that part of the parish of KIRKDALE which is in the wapentake of RYEDALE, North riding of the county of YORK, 4½ miles (N. E. by E.) from Helmsley, containing 24 inhabitants.

HOLME (SOUTH), a township in that part of the parish of HOVINGHAM which is in the wapentake of RYEDALE, North riding of the county of YORK, 7¼ miles (N. W. by W.) from New Malton, containing 66 inhabitants.

HOLME next RUNCTON, a parish in the hundred of CLACKCLOSE, county of NORFOLK, 4¼ miles (N.) from Downham-Market, containing 198 inhabitants. The living is a rectory with Wallington, in the archdeaconry of Norfolk, and diocese of Norwich, rated in the king's books at £12. The church is dedicated to St. James.

HOLME next the SEA, a parish in the hundred of SMITHDON, county of NORFOLK, 8½ miles (W. by N.) from Burnham-Westgate, containing 219 inhabitants. The living is a discharged vicarage, in the archdeaconry of Norfolk, and diocese of Norwich, rated in the king's books at £6. 13. 4., endowed with £200 royal bounty, and in the patronage of the Bishop of Norwich. The church, dedicated to St. Mary, was built by Henry de Nottingham, one of the council of the duchy of Lancaster.

HOLME upon SPALDING-MOOR, a parish partly within the liberty of ST. PETER of YORK, but chiefly in the Holme-Beacon division of the wapentake of HARTHILL, East riding of the county of YORK, 5 miles (S. W. by W.) from Market-Weighton, containing 1318 inhabitants. The living is a vicarage, in the archdeaconry of the East riding, and diocese of York, rated in the king's books at £10, and in the patronage of the Master and Fellows of St. John's College, Cambridge. The church, dedicated to All Saints, is an ancient edifice standing on an eminence which commands a fine and extensive prospect, in which York minster is a prominent object. Upon this mount is the beacon from which the division of the wapentake derives its name, and near it is a bed of gypsum, containing also *ammonitæ*, or snake stones. There is a place of worship for Wesleyan Methodists, besides two Roman Catholic chapels. According to tradition, a cell was founded by the Vavasours, or the Constables, on the edge of the moor, for two monks, one of whom acted as a guide to travellers across that extensive waste, the other praying for their safety. The shock of an earthquake was felt here on the night of the 18th of January, 1822.

HOLME on the WOLDS, a parish in the Bainton-Beacon division of the wapentake of HARTHILL, East riding of the county of YORK, 6¼ miles (N.W.) from Beverley, containing 138 inhabitants. The living is a discharged vicarage with that of St. Mary, Beverley, in the archdeaconry of the East riding, and diocese of York, rated in the king's books at £8. 19. 7., endowed with £1000 royal bounty, and £200 parliamentary grant. The church is dedicated to St. Peter.

HOLME-CULTRAM, a parish in ALLERDALE ward below Darwent, county of CUMBERLAND, 6½ miles (W. N. W.) from Wigton, comprising Abbey Quarter, East Waver Quarter, Low Quarter, and St. Cuthbert's Quarter, and containing 2772 inhabitants. The living is a perpetual curacy, with that of Newton-Arlosh, in the archdeaconry and diocese of Carlisle, rated in the king's books at £6. 13. 4., endowed with £600 private benefaction, and £1100 parliamentary grant, and in the patronage of the Chancellor, Masters, and Scholars of the University of Oxford. The church, dedicated to the Virgin Mary, is principally in the early style of English architecture, and was mostly rebuilt in 1606, after the greater part of the old edifice had been destroyed by fire : it was once the conventual church of an abbey of Cistercian monks, founded in 1150, by Prince Henry of Scotland, and so richly endowed,

that at the dissolution its revenue was estimated at £535. 3. 7. ; in the church-yard are various remains of the conventual buildings. The abbots were summoned to several parliaments by Edward I. and II., and the last abbot was instituted to the rectory. The Society of Friends have a meeting-house at Beck-foot, erected in 1745. The parish is bounded on the west by the Irish sea, and on the north by the æstuaries of the Wampool and the Waver, the latter river passing on the eastern side of the village, where it is crossed by a substantial bridge of three arches, erected in 1770, at the expense of the parishioners. Freestone is obtained here. At Newton-Arlosh are the ruins of an ancient chapel, said to have been once the parochial church. Walsey castle, formerly a very strong fort, has dwindled into a small heap of ruins.

HOLME-HALE, a parish in the southern division of the hundred of GREENHOE, county of NORFOLK, 5 miles (N. N. W.) from Watton, containing 422 inhabitants. The living is a discharged rectory, in the archdeaconry of Norfolk, and diocese of Norwich, rated in the king's books at £12. 16. 5½. The Rev. T. P. Young was patron in 1794. The church is dedicated to St. Andrew.

HOLME-PIERREPOINT, a parish in the southern division of the wapentake of BINGHAM, county of Nottingham, 5 miles (E. by S.) from Nottingham, containing, with the hamlet of Adbolton, which was formerly a distinct parish, 205 inhabitants. The living is a rectory, with which the vicarage of Adbolton was united in 1707, in the archdeaconry of Nottingham, and diocese of York, rated in the king's books at £15. 7. 6., and in the patronage of Earl Manvers. The church, dedicated to St. Edmund, was erected in the time of Henry VII. : it is a fine structure, having numerous large windows, with a quadrangular tower surmounted by a lofty handsome spire, and contains the family vault of the dukes of Kingston, several mural monuments, and some ancient brasses. The parish is bounded on the north by the river Trent, and the Grantham canal crosses an angle on the south.

HOLMEFIRTH, a chapelry in the parish of KIRK-BURTON, upper division of the wapentake of AGBRIGG, West riding of the county of YORK, 6½ miles (S.) from Huddersfield. The population is returned with the parish. The living is a perpetual curacy, in the archdeaconry and diocese of York, endowed with £400 private benefaction, and £400 royal bounty, and in the patronage of the Vicar of Kirk-Burton. There are places of worship for Independents and Wesleyan Methodists.

HOLMER, a parish in the hundred of GRIMSWORTH, county of HEREFORD, 2 miles (N.) from Hereford, containing, with the chapelry of Huntington, and the township of Shelwick, 524 inhabitants. The living is a discharged vicarage, in the peculiar jurisdiction of the Dean of Hereford, rated in the king's books at £6. 10. 8., and in the patronage of the Dean and Chapter of Hereford. The church is dedicated to St. Bartholomew.

HOLMESCALES, a hamlet in that part of the parish of KENDAL which is in KENDAL ward, county of WESTMORLAND, 4¾ miles (S. E. by S.) from Kendal. The population is returned with the chapelry of Old Hutton.

HOLMESFIELD, a chapelry in the parish of DRONFIELD, hundred of SCARSDALE, county of DERBY,

2¼ miles (W.) from Dronfield, containing 499 inhabitants. The living is a perpetual curacy, in the archdeaconry of Derby, and diocese of Lichfield and Coventry, endowed with £10 per annum and £200 private benefaction, and £400 royal bounty, and in the patronage of the Vicar of Dronfield. The chapel was rebuilt in 1826. A school was erected, in 1725, on land given by Matthias Webster, previously to which Robert Mower, in 1719, gave certain land toward the maintenance of a schoolmaster, and subsequently, in 1725, Prudence Mower gave £60 : the produce of these endowments, with other subscriptions, amounts to about £18 per annum, for which sum about twenty children receive instruction.

HOLMPTON, a parish in the southern division of the wapentake of HOLDERNESS, East riding of the county of YORK, 3½ miles (E. by N.) from Patrington, containing 256 inhabitants. The living is a discharged rectory, in the archdeaconry of the East riding, and diocese of York, rated in the king's books at £4. 13. 4., and in the patronage of the Crown. The church has lately received an addition of sixty-five free sittings, the Incorporated Society for the enlargement of churches and chapels having granted £30 towards defraying the expense. There is a place of worship for Wesleyan Methodists. The village is situated near the North sea, and is considered a healthy spot. There is a small endowed school.

HOLMSIDE, a township in that part of the parish of LANCHESTER which is in the western division of CHESTER ward, county palatine of DURHAM, 7¼ miles (N.W.) from Durham, containing 228 inhabitants.

HOLNE, a parish in the hundred of STANBOROUGH, county of DEVON, 4 miles (W.) from Ashburton, containing 410 inhabitants. The living is a vicarage, in the archdeaconry of Totness, and diocese of Exeter, rated in the king's books at £8. 5. 5., and in the patronage of the Crown. The church once belonged to the abbey of Buckfastleigh : it contains a stone font in the early English style, and a rood-loft and screen. The river Dart here rapidly pursues its course through a romantic dell of rock, beautifully fringed with wood.

HOLNEST, a parish in the hundred of SHERBORNE, Sherborne division of the county of DORSET, 4¾ miles (S. by E.) from Sherborne, containing 162 inhabitants. The living is a perpetual curacy annexed to the vicarage of Long Burton, in the peculiar jurisdiction of the Dean of Sarum. The church is dedicated to St. Mary.

HOLSWORTHY, a market town and parish in the hundred of BLACK TORRINGTON, county of DEVON, 42 miles (W. by N.) from Exeter, and 214 (W. by S.) from London, containing 1440 inhabitants. The situation of this place is dreary, and it is of little importance, except on account of its fairs and markets. A branch of the Bude and Launceston canal passes at a short distance to the north of the town. The market is on Wednesday ; and there are three fairs: "St. Peter's fair," mentioned in a record of the reign of Edward I., is still a large mart for cattle and various commodities, continuing several days, and commencing on St. Peter's day (July 10th), unless that day falls later in the week than Thursday, in which case the fair begins on the Tuesday following ; the other fairs are, April 27th and Oct. 2nd ; there is also a great market for cattle on the second Wednesday in February. The living is a rectory, in the

archdeaconry of Totness, and diocese of Exeter, rated in the king's books at £32. 0. 5. The Rev. R. Kingdon was patron in 1819. The church, dedicated to St. Peter and St. Paul, is an ancient building with a Norman doorway, and some other portions in the same style. Here are places of worship for Independents and Wesleyan Methodists. A National school is supported by voluntary contributions.

HOLT, a tything in the parish of WIMBORNE-MINSTER, hundred of BADBURY, Shaston (East) division of the county of DORSET, 3 miles (N. E. by N.) from Wimborne-Minster, containing 1180 inhabitants. Here were anciently a forest, chase, and park, and a chapel of ease, dedicated to St. James.

HOLT, a chapelry in the parish of MEDBOURNE, hundred of GARTREE, county of LEICESTER, 4 miles (W.N.W.) from Rockingham, containing, with the hamlet of Bradley, 53 inhabitants. A mineral spring was discovered here in 1728, called the Nevill Holt water, impregnated with iron and aluminous and calcareous salts, and found serviceable in hæmorrhage, scrofula, and other glandular diseases.

HOLT, a market town and parish in the hundred of HOLT, county of NORFOLK, 23 miles (N.N.W.) from Norwich, and 120 (N.N.E.) from London, containing 1348 inhabitants. This place, from the quantity of timber which grew upon its site, or by which it was surrounded, was by the Saxons called Holt, signifying a wood. In the reign of Edward the Confessor it was held in royal demesne, and after the Conquest the lordship belonged to the family of De Vaux, or De Vallibus. The town is pleasantly situated on rising ground, in the midst of a fertile district, remarkable for the purity of its air, and commands a delightful prospect of the surrounding country, which is justly styled " the Garden of Norfolk." The houses are neatly built of brick and stone ; the streets are paved with flint-stones, and the inhabitants are well supplied with water from a spring, and from several wells in the neighbourhood. Here are a circulating library, and two book clubs, supported by subscription ; and assemblies are occasionally held in the sessions-house. The town has undergone great improvement since 1708, in which year a very destructive fire took place on a market day, that consumed a considerable number of houses, the market stalls, &c. In 1810, the commons and heaths that surrounded the town were enclosed for cultivation ; and on the east side, towards Cromer, are now handsome and thriving plantations of forest trees, interspersed with neat dwelling-houses. The market is on Saturday, which is well attended : the fairs, chiefly for live stock, are held on April 25th and November 25th. An adjourned session for the county is held twice a year, in the sessions-house, a handsome and commodious building, in which all public business is transacted ; and constables and other officers are annually chosen at the court leet of the lord of the manor, held on the 21st of December.

The living is a rectory, in the archdeaconry and diocese of Norwich, rated in the king's books at £11. 17. 3½., and in the patronage of the Master and Fellows of St. John's College, Cambridge. The church, dedicated to St. Andrew, had, previously to the fire, a lofty steeple crowned with a spire, which was a useful land-mark ; but this has never been rebuilt. There are places of worship for the Society of Friends and Wesleyan Methodists. The free grammar school was founded in 1556, by Sir Thomas Gresham : annexed to it are a scholarship and fellowship in Sydney Sussex College, Cambridge ; the management is vested in the Fishmongers' Company. Sir Thomas Gresham, born here in 1507, became celebrated as a merchant and financier, and displayed his genius, not only in contriving schemes for paying the debts of the crown, and extending our foreign trade, but also in introducing into the kingdom various new branches of manufacture ; besides other great and charitable endowments, he founded Gresham College and the Royal Exchange ; he died in 1579.

HOLT, a chapelry in the parish of GREAT BRADFORD, hundred of BRADFORD, county of WILTS, 2¼ miles (E. N. E.) from Bradford, containing 846 inhabitants. The chapel, dedicated to St. Catherine, has lately received an addition of one hundred and seventy sittings, of which one hundred and forty are free, the Incorporated Society for the enlargement of churches and chapels having granted £140 towards defraying the expense. There is a place of worship for Independents. A mineral spring, discovered upwards of a century ago, is still resorted to for its sanative properties. Mr. David Arnot, long proprietor of this spa, was the author of the "Commercial Tables" bearing his name.

HOLT, a parish in the lower division of the hundred of OSWALDSLOW, county of WORCESTER, 6 miles (N. N. W.) from Worcester, containing, with the chapelry of Little Witley, 657 inhabitants. The living is a rectory, in the archdeaconry and diocese of Worcester, rated in the king's books at £15. 17. 8½. Lord Foley was patron in 1811. The church, dedicated to St. Martin, is a good specimen of the early style of English architecture. Some remains of a castle, erected by the Beauchamps, are still visible. A bridge of five arches, two hundred and sixty-six feet in length, has been erected over the Severn : the span of the central arch, which is of iron, is one hundred and fifty feet, and its height above the level of the river, at low water, thirty-five feet ; the other arches, two at each end, are of stone.

HOLTBY, a parish in the wapentake of BULMER, North riding of the county of YORK, 5½ miles (E. N E.) from York, containing 170 inhabitants. The living is a rectory, in the jurisdiction of the peculiar court of Howdenshire, rated in the king's books at £8, and in the patronage of Mrs. Nelson. The church, dedicated to the Holy Trinity, is a spacious edifice of brick.

HOLTON, a parish in the western division of the wapentake of WRAGGOE, parts of LINDSEY, county of LINCOLN, 2½ miles (N. N. W.) from Wragby, containing, with the hamlet of Bickering, 142 inhabitants. The living is a rectory, in the archdeaconry and diocese of Lincoln, rated in the king's books at £17. 10. 10. Edmund Turnor, Esq. was patron in 1812. The church is dedicated to All Saints.

HOLTON, a parish in the hundred of BULLINGTON, county of OXFORD, 6 miles (E.) from Oxford, containing 260 inhabitants. The living is a rectory, in the archdeaconry and diocese of Oxford, rated in the king's books at £12. 19. 2., and in the patronage of Elisha Biscoe, Esq. The church, dedicated to St. Bartholomew, is a cruciform structure, having a chapel attached to the north aisle, and another to the south ; the latter, which appears to be the more modern, was built by

William Brome, Esq., who, in 1461, was buried in a vault underneath it. In the parish register is recorded the marriage of Ireton to Bridget, daughter of Oliver Cromwell, June 15th, 1646. A school was built by subscription in 1790, and is partly supported by the interest of £200 left, in 1665, by Dr. Edward Rogers, then rector. A great number of human skeletons has been recently found promiscuously buried just below the surface, it being thought that this was the scene of a battle during the parliamentary war. The ancient manorial mansion, which was surrounded by a moat, was taken down in 1804, and the present built upon its site.

HOLTON, a parish in the hundred of WHITLEY, though locally in that of Horethorne, county of SOMERSET, 2¼ miles (S. W. by W.) from Wincanton. containing 235 inhabitants. The living is a discharged rectory, in the archdeaconry of Wells, and diocese of Bath and Wells, rated in the king's books at £8. 0. 2., endowed with £200 private benefaction, and £200 royal bounty. John Gibbs, Esq. was patron in 1785. The church is dedicated to St. Nicholas.

HOLTON, a parish in the hundred of BLYTHING, county of SUFFOLK, 1¼ mile (E. N. E.) from Halesworth, containing 399 inhabitants. The living is a discharged rectory, in the archdeaconry of Suffolk, and diocese of Norwich, rated in the king's books at £10. 13. 4., endowed with £200 royal bounty, and in the patronage of the Crown. The church is dedicated to St. Peter.

HOLTON le CLAY, a parish in the wapentake of BRADLEY-HAVERSTOE, parts of LINDSEY, county of LINCOLN, 5 miles (S. S. E.) from Great Grimsby, containing 220 inhabitants. The living is a vicarage, in the archdeaconry and diocese of Lincoln, rated in the king's books at £4. 8. 4., and in the patronage of the Crown. The church is dedicated to St. Peter.

HOLTON (ST. MARY), a parish in the hundred of SAMFORD, county of SUFFOLK, 4¾ miles (S. S. E.) from Hadleigh, containing 213 inhabitants. The living is a discharged rectory, in the archdeaconry of Suffolk, and diocese of Norwich, rated in the king's books at £7. 14. 7., and in the patronage of Sir Wm. Rowley, Bart. The church is dedicated to St. Mary. The Rev. Stephen White, in 1756, founded and endowed a school for the instruction of twenty-five children : the annual income is about £35, of which the master receives £12. 12., and the residue is expended in books, &c., and in furnishing each boy with a suit of clothes on his leaving school.

HOLTON le MOOR, a chapelry in that part of the parish of CAISTOR which is in the northern division of the wapentake of WALSHCROFT, parts of LINDSEY, county of LINCOLN, 3½ miles (S. W.) from Caistor, containing 135 inhabitants. Here is a place of worship for Wesleyan Methodists.

HOLVERSTONE, a parish in the hundred of HENSTEAD, county of NORFOLK, 6 miles (S. E.) from Norwich, containing 26 inhabitants. The living is divided into medieties, one of which is held with the rectory of Burgh-Apton, and the other with that of Rockland, in the archdeaconry of Norfolk, and diocese of Norwich. The church, which was dedicated to St. Mary, has been demolished.

HOLWELL, a parish in the hundred of CLIFTON, county of BEDFORD, 3 miles (N. W. by N.) from Hitchin, containing 179 inhabitants. The living is a rectory, in the archdeaconry of Bedford, and diocese of Lincoln, rated in the king's books at £7. 9. 7. — Radcliff, Esq. was patron in 1810.

HOLWELL, a chapelry in the parish of Ab-Kettle-by, hundred of Framland, county of Leicester, 3¼ miles (N. N. W.) from Melton-Mowbray, containing 132 inhabitants. The chapel is dedicated to St. Leonard. There is a chalybeate spring in the neighbourhood.

HOLWELL, a chapelry in the parish of Broadwell, hundred of Bampton, county of Oxford, 2¾ miles (S. W. by S.) from Burford, containing 86 inhabitants. The living is a perpetual curacy, in the archdeaconry and diocese of Oxford, endowed with £400 parliamentary grant, and in the patronage of the Vicar of Broadwell.

HOLWELL, a parish in the hundred of Hore-thorne, county of Somerset, though locally in the hundred of Sherborne, county of Dorset, 5¾ miles (S. E. by E.) from Sherborne, containing, with the hamlet of Backshaw, 342 inhabitants. The living is a rectory, in the archdeaconry of Dorset, and diocese of Bristol, rated in the king's books at £14. 13. 9., and in the pa-tronage of the Provost and Fellows of Queen's College, Oxford. The church is dedicated to St. Lawrence. Here stood the principal lodge of the ancient Forest of Blackmore, which William de Bret and his successors held by service as the King's Forester in Blackmore : the office became extinct when the district was disaf-forested.

HOLWICK, a township in the parish of Romald-Kirk, western division of the wapentake of Gilling, North riding of the county of York, 12½ miles (N. W.) from Barnard-Castle, containing 201 inhabitants.

HOLYBOURNE, a parish in the hundred of Al-ton, Alton (North) division of the county of South-ampton, 1½ mile (N. E.) from Alton, containing 482 inhabitants. The living is a perpetual curacy, in the archdeaconry and diocese of Winchester, and in the pa-tronage of the Dean and Chapter of Winchester. The church is dedicated to the Holy Rood. Thomas Andrews, in 1719, devised estates for the erection and support of a free school for all the children of the parish, for twelve of Alton, five of Binsted, and three of Froyle, and for apprenticing them : the net annual income is nearly £200, and the number receiving instruction is about eighty, of whom twenty are clothed.

HOLY CROSS, a hamlet in the parish of Clent, southern division of the hundred of Seisdon, county of Stafford, locally in the county of Worcester, 3½ miles (S. S. E.) from Stourbridge. The population is re-turned with the parish. Fairs are held on April 11th and Sep. 12th, chiefly for horned cattle and cheese. There is a place of worship for Baptists.

HOLYFIELD, a hamlet in the parish of Waltham-Abbey, or Holy-Cross, hundred of Waltham, county of Essex, 2½ miles (N. by E.) from Waltham-Abbey, containing 293 inhabitants.

HOLY-ISLAND, or LINDISFARN, a parish in Islandshire, county palatine of Durham, though lo-cally to the north of the county of Northumberland, 5½ miles (N. by E.) from Belford, and 10 (S. E.) from Ber-wick upon Tweed, containing 760 inhabitants. It is situated in the German ocean, a mile and a half from the Northumbrian coast, and derives its name from an abbey founded by Oswald, King of Northumberland, which became the seat of a bishop's see ; but after a suc-

cession of fourteen prelates, the cathedral church was destroyed by the Danes, in 893, and the bishoprick was removed to Chester le street. After the Norman Con-quest a Benedictine priory was established here, as a cell to that of Durham, the revenue of which at the dissolution was £60. 5.: its foundations may be traced over a space of nearly four acres, but the only consider-able remains are those of the church, a noble cruciform structure, displaying in the nave, choir, and a part of the central tower, the Norman and early English styles of architecture. Holy Island was invaded and plun-dered by Malcolm I., King of Scotland, in 941. In the great civil war it was the station of a parliamentary garrison ; and in 1715 it was seized by the adherents of the Pretender, who were however soon dislodged by a detachment from the king's troops at Berwick. Besides the principal island, the parish comprises the Farn islands, and the hamlets of Fenham and Goswick on the main land. At the south-western angle of Holy Island is situated the village of Lindisfarn, distinguished for its romantic scenery and the ruins of the monastery. It is a place of considerable resort for sea-bathing, and there are several fishing-boats belonging to the village, employed in catching cod, ling, haddock, and lobsters, which are very abundant in the neighbouring seas, and are sent in large quantities to the London market. The south-eastern extremity of the island rises in a conical peak, sixty feet in height, on the summit of which is a small castellated fort: the north side abounds with lime-stone ; and there are also a small seam of coal, and a stratum of slate, the latter containing a considerable quantity of iron-ore, with which are found the en-trochi, or fossils popularly termed St. Cuthbert's beads. The living is a perpetual curacy, in the archdeaconry of Northumberland, and diocese of Durham, endowed with £400 private benefaction, and £400 royal bounty, and in the patronage of the Dean and Chapter of Dur-ham. The church, dedicated to St. John the Evangelist, is a small neat building, constructed out of the remains of the ancient priory.

HOLY-OAKES, a liberty in that part of the parish of Dry-Stoke which is in the hundred of Gartree, county of Leicester, 3 miles (S. W. by S.) from Up-pingham, containing 7 inhabitants.

HOLYWELL, a parish in the hundred of Hurst-ingstone, county of Huntingdon, 2 miles (E. by S.) from St. Ives, containing, with the hamlet of Need-ingworth, 782 inhabitants. The living is a rectory, in the archdeaconry of Huntingdon, and diocese of Lincoln, rated in the king's books at £30. 6. 3. The Duke of Manchester was patron in 1804. The church, dedicated to St. John the Baptist, stands on a hill, at the foot of which is a spring of clear and excellent water, called the Holy Well, formerly held in great veneration, but now neglected. The river Ouse runs through the parish.

HOLYWELL, a joint chapelry with Awnby, in the parish of Castle-Bytham, wapentake of Beltisloe, parts of Kesteven, county of Lincoln, 7 miles (N. N. W.) from Stamford, containing 116 inhabitants.

HOLYWELL, a township in the parish of Earsdon, eastern division of Castle ward, county of Northum-berland, 5 miles (N. N. W.) from North Shields, con-taining 100 inhabitants. There is a medicinal spring, called St. Mary's Well, the water of which becomes pure by the infusion of galls.

HOMERSFIELD, a parish in the hundred of WANGFORD, county of SUFFOLK, 4¼ miles (S. W.) from Bungay, containing 201 inhabitants. The living is a discharged rectory, in the archdeaconry of Suffolk, and diocese of Norwich, rated in the king's books at £5. 6. 8., and in the patronage of Alexander Adair, Esq. The church is dedicated to St. Mary. The parish is bounded on the north by the river Waveney, which separates it from Norfolk.

HOMINGTON, a parish in the hundred of CAWDEN and CADWORTH, county of WILTS, 3½ miles (S. W. by S.) from Salisbury, containing 177 inhabitants. The living is a perpetual curacy, endowed with £200 royal bounty, and in the peculiar jurisdiction and patronage of the Dean and Chapter of Salisbury. The church is dedicated to St. Mary.

HOM-LACY, a parish in the hundred of WEBTREE, county of HEREFORD, 6 miles (S. E.) from Hereford, containing 389 inhabitants. The living is a vicarage, in the archdeaconry and diocese of Hereford, rated in the king's books at £8, and in the patronage of Sir E. F. Scudamore Stanhope, Bart. The church is dedicated to St. Cuthbert. An abbey for Premonstratensian canons, in honour of the Blessed Virgin and St. Thomas à Becket, was founded and endowed with divers manors, by William Fitzwain, in the time of Henry III. In the manorial mansion Pope wrote his poem entitled "The Man of Ross."

HONEYBOURNE (CHURCH), a parish in the upper division of the hundred of BLACKENHURST, county of WORCESTER, 4 miles (N. W. by N.) from Chipping-Campden, containing, with Poden, 136 inhabitants. The living is a perpetual curacy, with that of Cow-Honeybourne, in the archdeaconry and diocese of Worcester, rated in the king's books at £6. 4. 4½., and in the patronage of Mrs. Williams. The church, dedicated to St. Egwin, has a plain tower surmounted by a spire: it was esteemed the mother church in the Vale of Evesham at the dissolution of the abbey There is a place of worship for Wesleyan Methodists.

HONEYBOURNE (COW), a parish in the upper division of the hundred of KIFTSGATE, county of GLOUCESTER, 4 miles (N. W.) from Chipping-Campden, containing 333 inhabitants. The living was annexed to the perpetual curacy of Church-Honeybourne at the dissolution. The church, long in ruins, has been converted into houses for the poor, but the tower is still entire. A free school was established by subscription in 1806, when a school-room was erected, with a residence for the master, whose salary, amounting to £23 per annum, arises from the interest of certain stock purchased with the overplus, and the liberal contribution of Cotterill Corbet, Esq.

HONEYCHURCH, a parish in the hundred of BLACK TORRINGTON, county of DEVON, 6¾ miles (E. by S.) from Hatherleigh, containing 66 inhabitants. The living is a discharged rectory, in the archdeaconry of Totness, and diocese of Exeter, rated in the king's books at £6. 7. 8., endowed with £200 private benefaction, and £200 royal bounty, and in the patronage of the Hon. Newton Fellowes. The church is dedicated to St. James.

HONILY, a parish in the Snitterfield division of the hundred of BARLICHWAY, county of WARWICK, 6¾ miles (N. N. W.) from Warwick, containing 63 inhabitants.

The living is a rectory, in the archdeaconry of Coventry, and diocese of Lichfield and Coventry. Court Granville, Esq. was patron in 1814. The church is dedicated to St. John the Baptist.

HONING, a parish in the hundred of TUNSTEAD, county of NORFOLK, 3¾ miles (S. E. by E.) from North Walsham, containing 268 inhabitants. The living is a discharged vicarage, united with that of Dilham, in the archdeaconry of Norfolk, and diocese of Norwich, rated in the king's books at £4. 4. The church is dedicated to St. Peter and St. Paul.

HONINGHAM, a parish in the hundred of FOREHOE, county of NORFOLK, 7½ miles (W. N. W.) from Norwich, containing 321 inhabitants. The living is a discharged vicarage united with that of East Tudenham, in the archdeaconry of Norfolk, and diocese of Norwich, rated in the king's books at £8. 12. 6. The church is dedicated to St. Andrew.

HONINGHAM, county of WARWICK. — See HUNNINGHAM.

HONINGTON, a parish in the wapentake of WINNIBRIGGS and THREO, parts of KESTEVEN, county of LINCOLN, 5 miles (N. N. E.) from Grantham, containing 156 inhabitants. The living is a discharged vicarage, in the archdeaconry and diocese of Lincoln, rated in the king's books at £4. 0. 5., endowed with £200 private benefaction, and £200 royal bounty, and in the patronage of Sir Thomas Apreece. The church is dedicated to St. Wilfrid. There is a square double-trenched camp eastward of the village, within the area of which two urns, full of Roman coins, with some fragments of bridles and warlike weapons, were discovered in 1691. In the valley between Honington and Carleton is a large flat tumulus.

HONINGTON, a parish in the hundred of BLACKBOURN, county of SUFFOLK, 2¾ miles (N. N. W.) from Ixworth, containing 250 inhabitants. The living is a discharged rectory, in the archdeaconry of Sudbury, and diocese of Norwich, rated in the king's books at £7. 13. 4., and in the patronage of the Crown. The church is dedicated to All Saints. Robert Bloomfield, the poet, author of the "Farmer's Boy," &c., was born here in 1788.

HONINGTON, a parish in the Brails division of the hundred of KINGTON, county of WARWICK, 1½ mile (N. by E.) from Shipston upon Stour, containing 337 inhabitants. The living is a discharged vicarage, in the archdeaconry and diocese of Worcester, rated in the king's books at £9. 6. 8. The Rev. H. Townsend was patron in 1817. The church is dedicated to All Saints.

HONITON, a borough, market town, and parish, in the hundred of AXMINSTER, county of DEVON, 16½ miles (E. N. E.) from Exeter, and 156½ (W. S.W.) from London, containing 3296 inhabitants. This place is situated on rising ground in a fertile vale on the south side of the river Otter, and on the line of the great western road, from London to Plymouth. It possesses claims to high antiquity, having probably originated from a Roman settlement at Hunbury Fort, contiguous to the present

Corporate Seal.

town, where there are traces of an extensive intrenched camp, supposed to have been the *Moridunum* of Antoninus. During the civil war, Charles I. passed and repassed through the town, which was subsequently visited by the parliamentary general, Fairfax, after his successful campaign in the west of England, in 1645. The town has repeatedly suffered from fire: especially in 1747 and 1765, on which latter occasion, one hundred and fifteen houses were destroyed, together with a part of the chapel, the damage having been estimated at nearly £11,000. It consists chiefly of one very wide street, about a mile in length, lighted and paved, and is plentifully supplied with water: it has a gentle declivity towards the west, and in the central part are some well built brick houses and shops, the principal inn and the town-hall. This part of the town, with the exception of a few old houses, is of modern erection, the buildings having been raised subsequently to the last great fire, and with so much attention to uniformity as to render Honiton one of the neatest towns in the county. The manufacture of serge was established here at an early period; and the place was also noted for the large quantity of valuable lace made, some kinds of which were sold for more than five guineas a yard, being woven of thread, imported from the Netherlands, and rivalling in fineness and beauty the genuine Brussels lace. But the serge trade has long since declined, and the lace-making is not carried on to any considerable extent. Sprigs for the decoration of the Tiverton patent net are however still made here, and retain their former celebrity. Shoes and coarse earthenware are likewise manufactured, but not extensively. Honiton is famous as a mart for butter and cheese, a large quantity of the former article being sent weekly to the metropolis. In the vicinity of the town are quarries producing a peculiar kind of stone, used for making whet-stones for scythes, the trade in which is by no means inconsiderable. The markets, held by prescription, are on Tuesday, Thursday, and Saturday, the last of which is the principal market day. An annual fair takes place on the Wednesday after the 19th of July; and there are great markets on the second Saturday in April, and the Saturday before October 18th. The municipal affairs of the town are under the direction of a portreeve, bailiff, and two ale-tasters, who together with three constables, two tything-men, and other officers, are appointed at the manor court held on Michaelmasday. Under an ancient charter granted to the lord of the manor, the portreeve possessed magisterial power to hold monthly courts, and to make by-laws for the government of the borough; but at present the sole jurisdiction is vested in the county magistrates, who hold petty sessions here every month. This town sent members to parliament in the reigns of Edward I. and Edward II., after which the elective franchise was suspended till the sixteenth of Charles I., since which it has been regularly exercised. The right of election belongs to the inhabitant housekeepers within the borough, not receiving alms, commonly called "potwallopers," about four hundred and fifty in number: the portreeve, or, in his absence, the bailiff, is the returning officer.

The living is a rectory, in the archdeaconry and diocese of Exeter, rated in the king's books at £40. 4. 2., and in the patronage of the Trustees of Viscount Courtenay. The church, dedicated to St. Michael, which stands on an eminence about half a mile from the town, is a fine edifice, with aisles and a transept, in the later English style, having been built or enlarged about 1484, by Courtenay, Bishop of Exeter, who erected the beautiful screen, ornamented with carving and gilding, which separates the nave from the chancel: among several ancient monuments which it contains, is one to the memory of Dr. Thomas Marwood, physician to Queen Elizabeth, who died in 1617, at the age of 105. In the town is Allhallows chapel, a neat structure erected by subscription about 1765, on the site of a preceding chapel. Sir John Kirkham, Knt., and Elizens Harding, clerk, in the 15th of Henry VIII., gave land and tenements in the parishes of Honiton and Yarcombe, for the repair and maintenance of this chapel. Here are places of worship for Baptists, Independents, Wesleyan Methodists, and Unitarians. A free grammar school was founded pursuant to a bequest from the Rev. John Fley, in 1614, and endowed with various benefactions amounting to £12 per annum, but the number of free scholars of late years, has been very small. There is a National school, the master of which has a salary of £25 per annum, partly arising from the dividends of £300 stock in the four per cents., the bequest of the Rev. James How, in 1816. St. Margaret's hospital, about half a mile westward from the town, is an ancient foundation originally intended for lepers, and now consisting of houses for a governor, and eight poor persons, who have small stipends arising from lands producing about £85 per annum: connected with it is a chapel, in which the governor reads prayers twice a week. A mile to the north of Honiton is St. Cyre's Hill, on which a battery has been erected; and races are occasionally held here. Ozias Humphry, a Royal Academician, and eminent as a painter, was a native of this town.

HONLEY, a chapelry in the parish of ALMONDBURY, upper division of the wapentake of AGBRIGG, West riding of the county of YORK, 3½ miles (S. by W.) from Huddersfield, containing 3501 inhabitants. The living is a perpetual curacy, in the archdeaconry and diocese of York, endowed with £200 private benefaction, and £200 royal bounty, and in the patronage of the Vicar of Almondbury. There are places of worship for Independents and Wesleyan Methodists; also a National school erected by subscription in 1816.

HOO, a parish in the hundred of LAUNDITCH, county of NORFOLK, 2½ miles (N. N. E.) from East Dereham, containing 228 inhabitants. The living is a perpetual curacy, annexed to the vicarage of East Dereham, in the archdeaconry of Norfolk, and diocese of Norwich. In the east window of the church is a representation of the Crucifixion in stained glass.

HOO, a parish in the hundred of LOES, county of SUFFOLK, 4¼ miles (N.W.) from Wickham-Market, containing 174 inhabitants. The living is a perpetual curacy, in the archdeaconry of Suffolk, and diocese of Norwich, endowed with £200 private benefaction, and £800 royal bounty, and in the patronage of the Bishop of Ely. The church is dedicated to St. Andrew and St. Eustachius.

HOO, otherwise ST. WERBURGH, a parish in the hundred of Hoo, lathe of AYLESFORD, county of KENT, 4½ miles (N.E.) from Rochester, containing 960 inhabitants. The living is a discharged vicarage, in the archdeaconry and diocese of Rochester, rated in the king's books at £18. 6., and in the patronage of the Dean and Chapter of Rochester. The church is a handsome stone structure, with a lofty spire, conspicuous for many miles round. The parish is bounded on the south by the river Medway, which is here very broad, and deep enough to float first-rate ships of war. Abbey court, now a farm-house, was formerly a monastery subordinate to Leeds abbey, Kent. This parish possesses the right of sending three poor persons to Cobham College.

HOO (ST. MARY), a parish in the hundred of Hoo, lathe of AYLESFORD, county of KENT, 6¾ miles (N.E.) by N.) from Rochester, containing 286 inhabitants. The living is a rectory, in the archdeaconry and diocese of Rochester, rated in the king's books at £16. 12. 1., and in the patronage of the Rev. R. Burt. It possesses the right of nominating one poor person to Cobham College.

HOOD, a township in that part of the parish of KILBURN which is in the wapentake of BIRDFORTH, North riding of the county of YORK, 4½ miles (E.) from Thirsk, containing, with Osgoodby Grange, 30 inhabitants.

HOOE, a parish in the hundred of NINFIELD, rape of HASTINGS, county of SUSSEX, 8 miles (S.W.) from Battle, containing 600 inhabitants. The living is a vicarage, in the archdeaconry of Lewes, and diocese of Chichester, rated in the king's books at £7. 2. 6. Sir G. Webster, Bart. was patron in 1797. The church, dedicated to St. James, is principally in the later style of English architecture. An Alien priory of Benedictine monks, belonging to the abbey of Bec, in Normandy, was erected here about the commencement of the twelfth century; it was given by Henry VI. to Eton College, and subsequently by Edward IV. to Ashford College, in Kent.

HOOK, a hamlet in the parish of KINGSTON upon THAMES, first division of the hundred of KINGSTON, county of SURREY, 3½ miles (S. by W.) from Kingston upon Thames, containing 222 inhabitants. Here is a National school, supported by subscription.

HOOKE, a parish in the hundred of EGGERTON, Bridport division of the county of DORSET, 4¼ miles (E. by S.) from Beaminster, containing 234 inhabitants. The living is a discharged rectory, in the archdeaconry of Dorset, and diocese of Bristol, rated in the king's books at £9. 18. 10., and in the patronage of the Dowager Countess of Sandwich and the Marquis of Cleveland. The church is dedicated to St. Giles.

HOOKE, a chapelry in that part of the parish of SNAITH which is in the lower division of the wapentake of OSGOLDCROSS, West riding of the county of YORK, 2½ miles (S.S.E.) from Howden, containing 363 inhabitants. The living is a perpetual curacy, in the jurisdiction of the Peculiar court of Snaith, endowed with £400 royal bounty, and in the patronage of — Starkie, Esq. The chapel is dedicated to St. John. There is a place of worship for Wesleyan Methodists. Twelve children are instructed for £6 a year, the bequest of Joshua Jefferson in 1721.

HOOLE, a township in that part of the parish of PLEMONSTALL which is in the lower division of the hundred of BROXTON, county palatine of CHESTER, 2½ miles (N.E.) from Chester, containing 237 inhabitants. A court leet is held here annually.

HOOLE, a parish in the hundred of LEYLAND, county palatine of LANCASTER, comprising the townships of Much Hoole and Little Hoole, and containing 860 inhabitants, of which number, 644 are in the township of Much Hoole, 8 miles (S.W.) from Preston, and 216 in that of Little Hoole, 7 miles (S.W. by W.) from Preston. The living is a discharged rectory, in the archdeaconry and diocese of Chester, rated in the king's books at £6. 14., and in the patronage of the Rev. Miles Barton. The church is dedicated to the Holy Trinity : the body is built of bricks, but the west end and the tower, which latter is much admired, are of stone. Hoole was separated from the parish of Croston, and made a distinct parish, in 1642. A school was erected in 1774, and endowed with land purchased by subscription, producing about £16 a year, for which all poor children of the parish, who apply, are taught to read ; the average number is eighty.

HOON, a township in the parish of MARSTON upon DOVE, hundred of APPLETREE, county of DERBY, 9¼ miles (W.S.W.) from Derby, containing 40 inhabitants.

HOOSE, a township in the parish of WEST KIRBY, lower division of the hundred of WIRRALL, county palatine of CHESTER, 9½ miles (N.N.W.) from Great Neston, containing 114 inhabitants.

HOOTON, a township in the parish of EASTHAM, higher division of the hundred of WIRRALL, county palatine of CHESTER, 9 miles (N. by W.) from Chester, containing 112 inhabitants.

HOOTON-LEVETT, a township in the parish of MALTBY, southern division of the wapentake of STRAFFORTH and TICKHILL, West riding of the county of YORK, 5¼ miles (W.S.W.) from Tickhill, containing 95 inhabitants.

HOOTON-PAGNELL, a parish comprising the townships of Bilham and Hooton-Pagnell in the northern, and the township of Stotford in the southern, division of the wapentake of STRAFFORTH and TICKHILL, West riding of the county of YORK, and containing 409 inhabitants, of which number, 326 are in the township of Hooton-Pagnell, 7¼ miles (N.W. by W.) from Doncaster. The living is a discharged vicarage, in the archdeaconry and diocese of York, rated in the king's books at £5. 10. 2½., endowed with £200 royal bounty, and in the patronage of the Governors of Wakefield school. The church is dedicated to All Saints. There is a small endowed school.

HOOTON-ROBERTS, a parish in the southern division of the wapentake of STRAFFORTH and TICKHILL, West riding of the county of YORK, 4½ miles (N.E.) from Rotherham, containing 190 inhabitants. The living is a discharged rectory, in the archdeaconry and diocese of York, rated in the king's books at £7. 11. 8., endowed with £200 private benefaction, and £200 royal bounty. Earl Fitzwilliam was patron in 1796. The church, dedicated to St. John the Baptist, is mostly in the later style of English architecture.

HOPE, a parish (formerly a market town) in the hundred of HIGH PEAK, county of DERBY, comprising the chapelry of Fairfield, the townships of Fernilee, Grindlow, Highlow, Hope, and Stoke, the hamlets of Abney, Aston with Thornton, Bradwell, Brough with Shatton, Great Hucklow, Nether Padley, Offerton, Thornhill, and Woodland-Hope, and the liberties of Hazlebadge and

Little Hucklow, and containing, exclusively of a portion of the township of Wardlow, which is in this parish, 4102 inhabitants, of which number, 518 are in the township of Hope, 6 miles (N. by E.) from Tidswell. The living is a discharged vicarage, in the peculiar jurisdiction and patronage of the Dean and Chapter of Lichfield, rated in the king's books at £13. 13. 4., and endowed with £10 per annum private benefaction. The church, dedicated to St. Peter, is an embattled edifice in the later style of English architecture, with a tower supporting a spire. A charity school for ten children is endowed with about £10 per annum, and a house and garden for the master. The market, anciently held here, and renewed by a grant in 1715, was discontinued about twelve years ago. There are fairs, chiefly for cattle, on March 28th, May 13th, the day before the second Wednesday in September, and October 11th.

HOPE, a township in the parish of BARNINGHAM, western division of the wapentake of GILLING, North riding of the county of YORK, 5½ miles (S.W.) from Greta-Bridge, containing 44 inhabitants.

HOPE under DINMORE, a parish in the hundred of WOLPHY, county of HEREFORD, 4¾ miles (S. by E.) from Leominster, containing 528 inhabitants. The living is a perpetual curacy, in the archdeaconry and diocese of Hereford, endowed with £400 private benefaction, and £1200 royal bounty, and in the patronage of the Bishop of Hereford. The church, dedicated to St. Mary, contains the remains of several members of the Coningsby family, one of whom, Sir Thomas, founded Coningsby's hospital, in Hereford. On the western brow of Dinmore hill is the site of a commandery of the Knights of St. John of Jerusalem.

HOPE (ALL SAINTS), a parish within the liberty of ROMNEY-MARSH, though locally in the hundred of Langport, lathe of SHEPWAY, county of KENT, 1 mile (N. W. by W.) from New Romney, containing 48 inhabitants. The living is a rectory, in the archdeaconry and diocese of Canterbury, rated in the king's books at £10. 1. 0½., and in the patronage of the Crown. The chapel has been demolished.

HOPE (SOLLERS), a parish in the hundred of GREYTREE, county of HEREFORD, 7½ miles (N. by E.) from Ross, containing 187 inhabitants. The living is a discharged rectory, united to that of How-Caple, in the archdeaconry and diocese of Hereford, rated in the king's books at £4. 3. 4. The church is dedicated to St. Michael.

HOPE - BAGGOT, a parish in the hundred of STOTTESDEN, county of SALOP, 6¼ miles (E. by S.) from Ludlow, containing 71 inhabitants. The living is a discharged rectory, in the archdeaconry of Salop, and diocese of Hereford, rated in the king's books at £3. 6. 8., and endowed with £200 royal bounty. The Marquis of Cleveland was patron in 1817. The church is dedicated to St. John the Baptist.

HOPE-BOWDLER, a parish in the hundred of MUNSLOW, county of SALOP, 2 miles (E. S.E.) from Church-Stretton, containing, with the township of Chilmick with Ragdon, 179 inhabitants. The living is a discharged rectory, in the archdeaconry of Salop, and diocese of Hereford, rated in the king's books at £6. 13. 4. C. P. Stainier, Esq. was patron in 1806. The church is dedicated to St. Andrew.

HOPE-MANSELL, a parish in the hundred of GREYTREE, county of HEREFORD, 5 miles (S. E. by S.) from Ross, containing 146 inhabitants. The living is a rectory, in the archdeaconry and diocese of Hereford, rated in the king's books at £6. 5., and in the patronage of the Crown. The church is dedicated to St. Michael. Limestone abounds in the parish. Courts leet are occasionally held here.

HOPESAY, a parish in the hundred of PURSLOW, county of SALOP, 6 miles (S. E.) from Bishop's Castle, containing 612 inhabitants. The living is a rectory, in the archdeaconry of Salop, and diocese of Hereford, rated in the king's books at £16. 12. 6. M. Pilkington, Esq. was patron in 1803. The church is dedicated to St. Mary.

HOPLEY'S GREEN, a township in that part of the parish of ALMELEY which is in the hundred of WOLPHY, county of HEREFORD. The population is returned with the parish.

HOPPEN, a township in the parish and ward of BAMBROUGH, county of NORTHUMBERLAND, 4½ miles (S. E. by E.) from Belford, containing 29 inhabitants.

HOPPERTON, a joint township with, and in the parish of, ALLERTON-MAULEVERER, upper division of the wapentake of CLARO, West riding of the county of YORK, 5½ miles (N. by E.) from Wetherby. The population is returned with the township of Allerton-Mauleverer.

HOPSFORD, a hamlet in the parish of WITHYBROOK, Kirby division of the hundred of KNIGHTLOW, county of WARWICK, 7¼ miles (N. E. by E.) from Coventry. The population is returned with the parish.

HOPTON, a township in that part of the parish of WIRKSWORTH which is in the hundred of WIRKSWORTH, county of DERBY, 1¾ mile (W. by S.) from Wirksworth, containing 116 inhabitants, many of whom are employed in working the lead mines here. Hopton was the property and residence of the zealous parliamentary officer, Sir John Gell, who, when Charles I. had raised the royal standard at Nottingham, proceeded to Derby, assembled a strong body of troops for the parliament, and performed a conspicuous part throughout the war. Almshouses consisting of two rooms each, for four poor persons, were erected, in 1719, by Sir Philip Gell, Bart., and endowed by him with a rent-charge of £22. 6.; which is paid to the inmates by weekly instalments of two shillings each. Military weapons and some other relics of antiquity have been discovered here.

HOPTON, a joint liberty with Coton, in that part of the parish of ST. MARY, LICHFIELD, which is in the southern division of the hundred of PIREHILL, county of STAFFORD, 2½ miles (N.E. by N.) from Stafford, containing 517 inhabitants. There is a lunatic asylum within the liberty, containing upwards of one hundred patients.

HOPTON, a parish in the hundred of BLACKBOURN, county of SUFFOLK, 7½ miles (N.E.) from Ixworth, containing 524 inhabitants. The living is a discharged rectory, in the archdeaconry of Suffolk, and diocese of Norwich, rated in the king's books at £13. 5., and in the patronage of the Crown. The church is dedicated to All Saints.

HOPTON, a parish in the hundred of MUTFORD and LOTHINGLAND, county of SUFFOLK, 4¾ miles (N. by W.) from Lowestoft, containing 274 inhabitants. The living is a perpetual curacy, in the archdeaconry of Suffolk;

and diocese of Norwich, and in the patronage of the Dean and Chapter of Norwich. The church is dedicated to St. Mary. The parish is bounded on the east by the North sea.

HOPTON (CASTLE), a parish in the hundred of PURSLOW, county of SALOP, 9 miles (S. S. E.) from Bishop's Castle, containing 150 inhabitants. The living is a rectory, in the archdeaconry of Salop, and diocese of Hereford, rated in the king's books at £5, and in the patronage of Thomas Beale, Esq. The church is dedicated to St. Mary. Hopton castle, of which there are now but slight remains, was given by Henry II. to Walter de Clifford; it was held for the king during the parliamentary war, but surrendered after a fortnight's siege, upon which most of the royalists who formed the garrison were put to the sword, and the governor was conveyed to Ludlow castle, and there imprisoned.

HOPTON in the HOLE, a parish in the hundred of MUNSLOW, county of SALOP, 5 miles (N.E. by N.) from Ludlow, containing 24 inhabitants. The living is a perpetual curacy, in the archdeaconry of Salop, and diocese of Hereford, endowed with £115 private benefaction, and £1000 royal bounty. Sir C. N. Broughton, Bart. was patron in 1818.

HOPTON (MONK), a parish within the liberty of the borough of WENLOCK, county of SALOP, 4½ miles (S.) from Much Wenlock, containing 168 inhabitants. The living is a perpetual curacy, annexed to the vicarage of Much Wenlock, in the archdeaconry of Salop, and diocese of Hereford, endowed with £800 royal bounty. Sir R. Lawley, Bart. was patron in 1820. The church is dedicated to St. Peter.

HOPTON-WAFERS, a parish in the hundred of STOTTESDEN, county of SALOP, 2¾ miles (W.N.W.) from Cleobury-Mortimer, containing 459 inhabitants. The living is a rectory, in the archdeaconry of Salop, and diocese of Hereford, rated in the king's books at £5. 16. 5½. Thomas Botfield, Esq. was patron in 1820. The church is dedicated to St. Mary. At an early period here was a castle of great strength, which, in 1643, during the parliamentary war, was seized for the king.

HOPWAS-HAYES, an extra-parochial liberty, locally in that part of the parish of Tamworth which is in the southern division of the hundred of OFFLOW, county of STAFFORD, 2 miles (W. by N.) from Tamworth, containing 3 inhabitants. The Birmingham and Fazeley canal passes through this liberty. Thomas Barnes, in 1724, gave a messuage and croft for the residence of a schoolmaster, or mistress : the annual value is £14, for which twenty children are instructed by a schoolmistress.

HOPWELL, a liberty in the parish of SAWLEY, hundred of MORLESTON and LITCHURCH, county of DERBY, 7 miles (E.) from Derby, containing 34 inhabitants.

HOPWOOD, a township in the parish of MIDDLETON, hundred of SALFORD, county palatine of LANCASTER, 2 miles (N. by E.) from Middleton, containing 1384 inhabitants.

HORBLING, a parish in the wapentake of AVELAND, parts of KESTEVEN, county of LINCOLN, 3¾ miles (E. by N.) from Falkingham, containing 491 inhabitants. The living is a discharged vicarage, in the archdeaconry and diocese of Lincoln, rated in the king's books at £6. 10., endowed with £200 private be-

nefaction, and £200 royal bounty, and in the patronage of the Bishop of Lincoln. The church, which is dedicated to St. Andrew, combines portions in the Norman, early, decorated, and later English styles, of architecture : the font is richly sculptured in the decorated style.

HORBURY, a chapelry in the parish of WAKEFIELD, lower division of the wapentake of AGBRIGG, West riding of the county of YORK, 3 miles (S.W. by W.) from Wakefield, containing 2475 inhabitants. The living is a perpetual curacy, in the archdeaconry and diocese of York, endowed with £15 per annum and £200 private benefaction, and £400 royal bounty, and in the patronage of the Vicar of Wakefield. The church, dedicated to St. Peter, is a handsome edifice, erected by Mr. J. Carr, a respectable architect, at an expense of £8000, defrayed by himself: one hundred and fifty-two free sittings have recently been added, by means of a grant of £150 from the Incorporated Society for the enlargement of churches and chapels. The manufacture of cloth is considerable in this chapelry. A school for ten children has an income of £15. 15. per annum, appropriated from the town lands : the master has a residence rent-free, likewise a rent-charge of £2, the gift of Richard Wormald in 1731.

HORDERLEY, an extra-parochial liberty, in the hundred of PURSLOW, county of SALOP, 6 miles (E. by S.) from Bishop's Castle, containing about 150 inhabitants.

HORDLE, a parish in the hundred of CHRISTCHURCH, New Forest (West) division of the county of SOUTHAMPTON, 4½ miles (W.S.W.) from Lymington, containing 517 inhabitants. The living is a perpetual curacy, annexed to the vicarage of Milford, in the archdeaconry and diocese of Winchester. The church is dedicated to All Saints. The parish is bounded on the south by the English channel.

HORDLEY, a parish in the hundred of PIMHILL, county of SALOP, 3 miles (S.S.W.) from Ellesmere, containing 308 inhabitants. The living is a rectory, in the archdeaconry of Salop, and diocese of Lichfield and Coventry, rated in the king's books at £3. 19. 2. J. K. Powell, Esq. was patron in 1803. The church is dedicated to St. Mary. The Ellesmere canal passes through the parish.

HORFIELD, a parish in the lower division of the hundred of BERKELEY, county of GLOUCESTER, 2½ miles (N.) from Bristol, containing 198 inhabitants. The living is a perpetual curacy, endowed with £1000 private benefaction, £1200 royal bounty, and £600 parliamentary grant, and in the peculiar jurisdiction and patronage of the Bishop of Bristol. In this parish are stone quarries and some mineral springs.

HORHAM, a parish in the hundred of HOXNE, county of SUFFOLK, 4¼ miles (E.S.E.) from Eye, containing 423 inhabitants. The living is a rectory, in the archdeaconry of Suffolk, and diocese of Norwich, rated in the king's books at £12. 7. 1. Lord Huntingfield was patron in 1803. The church is dedicated to St. Mary. There is a place of worship for Baptists.

HORKSLEY (GREAT), a parish in the Colchester division of the hundred of LEXDEN, county of ESSEX, 1¾ mile (S.S.W.) from Nayland, containing 623 inhabitants. The living is a rectory, in the archdeaconry of Colchester, and diocese of London, rated in the king's books at £15. The Countess de Grey was patroness in 1817. The church is dedicated to All Saints. The navigable river Stour runs on the northern side of this parish.

HORKSLEY (LITTLE), a parish in the Colchester division of the hundred of LEXDEN, county of ESSEX, 2½ miles (S.W. by S.) from Nayland, containing 238 inhabitants. The living is a perpetual curacy, in the archdeaconry of Colchester, and diocese of London, endowed with £1200 royal bounty. Mrs. Warren and E. C. Warren, Esq. were patrons in 1825. The church is dedicated to St. Peter and St. Paul. Here was a priory of Cluniac monks, subordinate to the monastery of Thetford in Norfolk, founded in the reign of Henry I. by Robert Fitz-Godebold, and Beatrix his wife, and valued at the dissolution at £27. 7. 11. per annum. The navigable river Stour runs along the northern side of this parish.

HORKSTOW, a parish in the northern division of the wapentake of YARBOROUGH, parts of LINDSEY, county of LINCOLN, 4½ miles (S.W. by W.) from Barton upon Humber, containing 200 inhabitants. The living is a discharged vicarage, in the archdeaconry and diocese of Lincoln, rated in the king's books at £4. 18. 4., and in the patronage of Lord Yarborough. The church is dedicated to St. Maurice. This village is pleasantly situated beneath a range of hills: in 1796 fragments of three tesselated pavements were discovered near Horkstow hall, the largest of which is divided into three compartments, one of them exhibiting a curious representation of a chariot race. Roman coins have been discovered here.

HORLEY, a parish in the hundred of BLOXHAM, county of OXFORD, 3¾ miles (N.W.) from Banbury, containing, with the chapelry of Hornton, 846 inhabitants. The living is a vicarage with that of Hornton, in the jurisdiction of the peculiar court of Banbury, belonging to the Dean and Chapter of Lincoln, rated in the king's books at £16. 13. 4., and in the patronage of the Crown. The church is dedicated to St. Ethelreda. Here is a place of worship for Wesleyan Methodists. A free school was endowed by Michael Harding, in the reign of Charles I., with houses and land: the present income is £42 per annum.

HORLEY, a parish in the first division of the hundred of REIGATE, county of SURREY, 5¼ miles (S.S.E.) from Reigate, containing 1063 inhabitants. The living is a discharged vicarage, in the archdeaconry of Surrey, and diocese of Winchester, rated in the king's books at £14. 1. 0½., and in the patronage of the Governors of Christ's Hospital. The church is dedicated to St. Bartholomew.

HORMEAD (GREAT), a parish in the hundred of EDWINSTREE, county of HERTFORD, 2½ miles (E.) from Buntingford, containing 564 inhabitants. The living is a discharged vicarage, in the archdeaconry of Middlesex, and diocese of London, rated in the king's books at £6. 3. 9., endowed with £200 royal bounty, and in the patronage of the Master and Fellows of St. John's College, Cambridge. The church is dedicated to St. Nicholas.

HORMEAD (LITTLE), a parish in the hundred of EDWINSTREE, county of HERTFORD, 2¾ miles (E. by S.) from Buntingford, containing 112 inhabitants. The living is a rectory, in the jurisdiction of the Commissary of Essex and Herts, concurrently with the Consistorial Court of the Bishop of London, rated in the

king's books at £10, and in the patronage of the Master and Fellows of St. John's College, Cambridge. The church is dedicated to St. Mary.

HORN, a parish in the hundred of ALSTOE, county of RUTLAND, 6 miles (N.W. by W.) from Stamford, containing 10 inhabitants. The living is a rectory, united to the vicarage of Exton, in the archdeaconry of Northampton, and diocese of Peterborough, rated in the king's books at £1. 6. 8. Sir Gerard Noel, Bart. was patron in 1825. The church, which was dedicated to All Saints, is supposed to have been destroyed by Oliver Cromwell : the inhabitants resort to the church at Exton.

HORNBLOTTON, a parish in the hundred of WHITESTONE, county of SOMERSET, 4½ miles (N.W. by W.) from Castle-Cary, containing 111 inhabitants. The living is a rectory, in the archdeaconry of Wells, and diocese of Bath and Wells, rated in the king's books at £7. 2. 1. John Roberts, Esq. was patron in 1825. The church is dedicated to St. Peter. The old Roman Fosse-way skirts the north-west boundary of this parish.

HORNBY, a chapelry (formerly a market town) in the parish of MELLING, hundred of LONSDALE, south of the sands, county palatine of LANCASTER, 9¼ miles (N. E.) from Lancaster, containing 477 inhabitants. The living is a perpetual curacy, in the archdeaconry of Richmond, and diocese of Chester, endowed with £7 per annum and £400 private benefaction, £800 royal bounty, and £800 parliamentary grant, and in the patronage of the Heirs of John Marsden, Esq. The chapel, dedicated to St. Margaret, has a window with a fine painting representing the Ascension of Our Saviour. Hornby castle, originally founded soon after the Norman Conquest, was subsequently the baronial residence of the Stanleys, Lords Monteagle, and is now fitted up as a modern mansion. In this chapelry are also the ruins of a fortress ascribed to the Saxons. The ancient weekly market on Friday is disused ; but a market for cattle, held every Tuesday fortnight, is well frequented ; and there is likewise an annual cattle fair on the 30th of July. A charity school was established here in consequence of a bequest of £20 per annum by David Murray, in 1822 ; but the property devised having been since claimed by the heir of the testator, the school has been discontinued. There are some remains of a priory, dedicated to St. Wilfrid, which was a cell to the Premonstratensian abbey of Croxton, and the revenue of which, at the dissolution, was valued at £26.

HORNBY, a township in that part of the parish of GREAT SMEETON which is in the wapentake of ALLERTONSHIRE, North riding of the county of YORK, 7¼ miles (N.) from North Allerton, containing 238 inhabitants. There is a place of worship for Wesleyan Methodists.

HORNBY, a parish in the eastern division of the wapentake of HANG, North riding of the county of YORK, comprising the townships of Ainderby-Myers with Holtby, Hackforth, and Hornby, and containing, exclusively of portions of the townships of Arrowthorne and Hunton, which are in this parish, 315 inhabitants, of which number, 102 are in the township of Hornby, which is partly within the liberty of ST. PETER of YORK, 4 miles (S.S.W.) from Catterick. The living is a discharged vicarage, in the peculiar jurisdiction and patronage of the Dean and Chapter of York, rated in the king's books at £6. 15. 6. The church is dedicated to St. Mary. There is a small endowment for the instruction of children. In Hackforth is a school for twenty poor boys, to which the Duke of Leeds allows £20 per annum, as a salary for the master. Hornby castle, anciently the seat of the family of St. Quintin, and now belonging to his Grace the Duke of Leeds, is a spacious mansion in different styles of architecture, containing superb apartments, and, by its situation, commanding a fine view of the rich valley of Bedale.

HORNCASTLE, a market town and parish in the soke of HORNCASTLE, parts of LINDSEY, county of LINCOLN, 21 miles (E.) from Lincoln, and 134 (N.) from London, containing 3058 inhabitants. From its situation, and the circumstance of a very extensive castle having been erected here (a portion of the remains of which is still visible,) this place has, with great probability, been considered the *Bannovallum* of the Romans, mentioned by the geographer of Ravenna. Its present name is evidently a corruption of *Hyrncastre*, as it was denominated by the Saxons, from *hyrn*, an angle, or corner (the town being situated within an angle formed by the confluence of the rivers Bane and Waring), and *castrum*, a fort, or castle. The *vallum*, or fortification constructed by the Romans having been considerably strengthened by Horsa, soon after the arrival of the two Saxon brothers, was afterwards demolished by Vortimer, the brave king of the Britons, and the castle was taken and destroyed, after a victory obtained by one of his generals over the Saxon prince, at the neighbouring village of Tetford. At the period of the Norman survey, the manor and soke (the latter comprising, besides the town, the parishes of West Ashby, Coningsby, Haltham, Langrick Ville, Mareham le Fen, Mareham on the Hill, Moorby, Roughton, Thimbleby, Thornton le Fen, High Toynton, Low Toynton, Wilksby, and Wood-Enderby,) belonged to the king, previously to which they had formed part of the possessions of Editha, Queen of Edward the Confessor. It does not appear at what time the manor first came into private hands, but, after various grants and reversions, it was sold, in the reign of Henry III., to Walter Mauclerke, Bishop of Carlisle; to whom that monarch granted three charters, conferring various immunities on the inhabitants of the town and soke, whereby Horncastle, from an insignificant village, became the general mart for the surrounding district : with the exception of a short interval during the reign of Edward VI., it has continued to belong to that see ever since.

The town, which is neat and well built, occupies a low but pleasant situation at the foot of the Wolds. From a plan made by Dr. Stukeley, in 1722, it appears to have been scarcely half so large as it is at present; and the houses, then built with clay-walls, and covered with thatch, have been succeeded by respectable brick edifices : the general appearance of the neighbourhood has also been greatly improved by the enclosure of lands, under the authority of an act obtained in 1803. Here is a subscription library, formed in 1790, and containing about one thousand volumes; and the clerical library, in High-street, comprises some respectable standard works. Formerly, many of the inhabitants were employed in tanning leather, but about fifty years

ago this branch of trade here experienced a rapid decline, so that there are now but two tan-yards remaining. The prosperity of the town has been in a great degree advanced by an act obtained in 1792, under the powers of which a canal was constructed, communicating with the river Bane, which was thus made navigable to the Witham ; and by this means a junction has been formed with the Trent and its numerous ramifications. Since the completion of this undertaking, in 1801, considerable commerce has been carried on in corn and wool, about thirty thousand quarters of the former, and three thousand packs of the latter, having been annually sent from this place to different parts of England. The market is on Saturday ; and the fairs are, one concluding on the 22nd of June, which is chartered for eight days, but seldom lasts more than three : the second terminates on the 21st of August, after having continued about ten days, although the charter limits its duration to seven : it is the largest fair for horses in the kingdom, many thousands being exhibited for sale during its continuance, and it is resorted to by dealers from all parts of the country, from the continent, and from America. The third fair, held on the 28th and 29th of October, was removed hither from Market-Stainton, in 1768, for a consideration of £200 paid to the lord of that manor. In the 47th of George III., an act was passed for establishing a court of requests for the recovery of debts under five pounds, which is held here every fourth Thursday, its jurisdiction extending over "the sokes of Bolingbroke and Horncastle, and the wapentake of Candleshoe, (except the parishes of Hagnaby, Welton in the Marsh, Steeping-Magna, and Firsby,) in the county of Lincoln, and for the wapentakes of Gartree, Louth-Eske, Ludborough, Calceworth, Hill, and Walshcroft, the north and south divisions of the wapentake of Yarborough, such parts of the wapentake of Manley as lie east of the river Trent, and the parishes of Faldingworth, Buslingthorpe, Snarford, Friesthorpe, and Hanworth." The charter granted by Henry III. to the bishop, as lord of the manor, gave authority to try felons and to hold a court leet, and exempted the inhabitants from toll and several other payments and services, besides protecting them from arrest by the officers of the king or the sheriff. On the eastern boundary of the parish is a spot called Hangman's Corner, where criminals capitally convicted in the court of the manor were executed : but these manorial rights and privileges, except the court leet, have been long disused.

The living is a vicarage, in the archdeaconry and diocese of Lincoln, rated in the king's books at £14. 4. 2., and in the patronage of the Bishop of Carlisle. The church, dedicated to St. Mary, appears, from the few remaining portions of the original edifice, to have been erected about the time of Henry VII. : it comprises a north and a south aisle, continued on each side of the chancel : the aisle north of the chancel was rebuilt in 1820, and part of the aisle south of the nave, in 1821 : the interior is exceedingly neat, and there are several interesting monuments to different members of the family of Dymoke, of Scrivelsby, holding the office of hereditary champion of England. Baptists, Independents, and Primitive and Wesleyan Methodists, have each a place of worship. The free grammar school was founded by Edward, Lord Clinton and Saye, Lord High

Admiral of England, by virtue of letters patent granted in 1562: its endowment consists of houses and land at Horncastle, Hemingby, Sutton, Huttoft, and Winthorpe, the average rental of which is about £200 per annum; £80 per annum is paid to a master and £30 to an usher; in addition to this, each boy pays two guineas a year for instruction in writing and arithmetic. The management of the affairs of this school is entrusted to ten individuals, who are a body corporate, possessing a common seal. They are also trustees of another charity school, founded by Mr. Richard Watson, in 1784, wherein poor children are instructed to read, sew, and knit, by a teacher whose stipend is £17 per annum, with a residence rent-free. A National school for boys and girls, and a school on the Lancasterian plan, are supported by subscription, and afford the means of education to about four hundred children. A general dispensary was opened in 1789. The poor in general derive considerable assistance from numerous benefactions recorded on a mural tablet in the church. The remains of the ancient fortress of Horncastle merely serve to exhibit its form and magnitude: it appears to have enclosed an area of about six hundred feet in length, and in breadth three hundred and fifty on the east, and three hundred on the west. A little south-westward from the town, near the union of the rivers, was one of those Roman labyrinths called the Julian bower. Many urns, coins, fibulæ, and other vestiges of that people, have been discovered at different periods.

HORNCHURCH, a parish within the liberty of HAVERING atte BOWER, county of ESSEX, 14½ miles (E. N. E.) from London, containing 1938 inhabitants. The living is a vicarage not in charge, in the jurisdiction of the peculiar court of Hornchurch and Havering atte Bower, and in the patronage of the Warden and Fellows of New College, Oxford. The church is dedicated to St. Andrew. Here is a small endowment for the instruction of children. An iron-foundry has been recently established; and a considerable quantity of bricks is made here. A priory, dedicated to St. Nicholas and St. Bernard, a cell to the hospital of Monte Jovis in Savoy, was founded here about the reign of Henry II., and was purchased in that of Richard II., by William of Wickham, for his foundation of New College, Oxford. This parish extends from the great London road between Romford and Brentwood on the north, to the Thames on the south.

HORNCLIFFE, a township in the parish of NORHAM, otherwise Norhamshire, county palatine of DURHAM, though locally to the northward of the county of Northumberland, 5 miles (W.S.W.) from Berwick upon Tweed, containing 351 inhabitants. From Horncliffe hall is a fine prospect of the extensive plain of Merse, and the luxuriant banks of the Tweed.

HORNDON (EAST), a parish in the hundred of BARSTABLE, county of ESSEX, 4 miles (S. E.) from Brentwood, containing 459 inhabitants. The living is a rectory, in the archdeaconry of ESSEX, and diocese of London, rated in the king's books at £10. Earl Brownlow and others were patrons in 1795. The church, dedicated to All Saints, is a small irregular structure, with several chapels, which contain portions in different styles of architecture: the font is in the Norman style.

HORNDON on the HILL, a parish in the hundred of BARSTABLE, county of ESSEX, 16½ miles (S. by W.)

from Chelmsford, containing 420 inhabitants. The living is a discharged vicarage, in the archdeaconry of Essex, and diocese of London, rated in the king's books at £14. 6. 8., endowed with £225 private benefaction, and £200 royal bounty, and in the patronage of the Dean and Chapter of St. Paul's, London. The church is dedicated to St. Peter. Here was formerly a market on Saturday. A fair for wool is held on the 29th of June.

HORNDON (WEST), a parish in the hundred of BARSTABLE, county of ESSEX, 3½ miles (S. S. E.) from Brentwood, containing 45 inhabitants. The living is a rectory, united to that of Ingrave, in the archdeaconry of Essex, and diocese of London, rated in the king's books at £14. 13. 4. Thomas Newman, Esq. was patron in 1797. The church is dedicated to St. Nicholas.

HORNE, a parish in the first division of the hundred of TANDRIDGE, county of SURREY, 5½ miles (S. S. W.) from Godstone, containing 585 inhabitants. The living is a rectory, in the archdeaconry of Surrey, and diocese of Winchester, rated in the king's books at £4. 17. 11. Thomas Poynder, Esq. was patron in 1818. The church is dedicated to St. Mary. This parish participates in the benefits of Evelyn's school at Godstone.

HORNING, a parish in the hundred of TUNSTEAD, county of NORFOLK, 6 miles (N. N. W.) from Acle, containing 440 inhabitants. The living is a discharged vicarage, in the archdeaconry of Norfolk, and diocese of Norwich, endowed with £800 royal bounty, and in the patronage of the Bishop of Norwich. In the reign of Henry III. here was an hospital, dedicated to St. James, and under the government of the almoner of St. Benedict's abbey; it was given to the Bishop of Norwich. The mitred abbey of St. Benedict was only a hermitage in the year 800, and was raised into a monastery of Black monks before 1020, by Canute: the barony and reversion were given in exchange to the Bishop of Norwich, in 1535; its revenue was valued at £583. 17.

HORNINGHOLD, a parish in the hundred of GARTREE, county of LEICESTER, 4½ miles (W. S. W.) from Uppingham, containing 97 inhabitants. The living is a discharged vicarage, in the archdeaconry of Leicester, and diocese of Lincoln, rated in the king's books at £6. 16. 8., and endowed with £400 royal bounty. Mrs. Holland was patroness in 1813. The church, dedicated to St. Peter, is ancient and curious, exhibiting specimens of pure Saxon architecture. There is a chapel of ease at Blaston, in this parish.

HORNINGLOW, a township in that part of the parish of BURTON upon TRENT which is in the northern division of the hundred of OFFLOW, county of STAFFORD, 1¾ mile (N. W. by N.) from Burton upon Trent, containing 341 inhabitants. The Grand Trunk canal passes through this township.

HORNINGSEA, a parish in the hundred of FLENDISH, county of CAMBRIDGE, 4¼ miles (N. E.) from Cambridge, containing 285 inhabitants. The living is a perpetual curacy, in the peculiar jurisdiction of the Bishop of Ely, and in the patronage of the Master and Fellows of St. John's College, Cambridge. The church is dedicated to St. Peter. At an early period here was a considerable monastery of royal foundation, but it was destroyed by the Danes about 870.

HORNINGSHAM, a parish in the hundred of HEY-

TESBURY, county of WILTS, 4¼ miles (S. W.) from Warminster, containing 1267 inhabitants. The living is a perpetual curacy, endowed with £400 private benefaction, £200 royal bounty, and £2400 parliamentary grant, in the peculiar jurisdiction of the Dean of Salisbury, as Dean of the church of Heytesbury, and in the patronage of the Prebendary of Horningsham in the collegiate church of Heytesbury. The church is dedicated to St. John the Baptist. There is a place of worship for Independents.

HORNINGSHEATH, a parish comprising the consolidated parishes of Great and Little Horningsheath, in the hundred of THINGOE, county of SUFFOLK, 2 miles (S. W. by W.) from Bury-St. Edmund's, and containing 539 inhabitants. The living is a rectory, in the archdeaconry of Sudbury, and diocese of Norwich, rated jointly in the king's books at £13. 13. 9., and in the patronage of the Marquis of Bristol. The church is dedicated to St. Leonard, and although much modernised, retains portions in the decorated and later styles of English architecture: that of Little Horningsheath has gone to ruins. Fifty children are educated in an endowed school, which is supported chiefly by a rent-charge on lands in Denston : the school-house was built by the Marquis of Bristol.

HORNINGTOFT, a parish in the hundred of LAUNDITCH, county of NORFOLK, 5 miles (S. by E.) from Fakenham, containing 254 inhabitants. The living is a discharged rectory, in the archdeaconry and diocese of Norwich, rated in the king's books at £6. 17. 8½. F. R. Reynolds, Esq. was patron in 1826. The church is dedicated to St. Edmund.

HORNSEA, a market town and parish, in the northern division of the wapentake of HOLDERNESS, East riding of the county of YORK, 42 miles (E. by S.) from York, and 190 (N.) from London, containing, with the hamlet of Burton, 790 inhabitants. This place, which is situated within less than a mile of the German ocean, was formerly more than ten miles distant from it, but by the encroachment of the waters, which is still in regular progression, the village of Hornsea Beck was not many years since totally destroyed. The town consists of four irregular streets, and contains some good inns, and respectable lodging-houses for the accommodation of visitors who frequent this place for sea-bathing during the season. There is a fine chalybeate spring in the town : the environs are pleasant, abounding with picturesque scenery. On the western side is a beautiful and extensive lake, covering nearly five hundred acres, containing fresh-water fish of every description, and beautifully interspersed with wooded islands, the resort of numerous aquatic birds; the banks are in many places planted with alders, and form a delightful promenade: races are held here annually, between the 17th and 24th of July. The market is on Monday, but it is rapidly falling into disuse : the fairs are, August 13th and December 18th, for horses and cattle. The living is a vicarage with the rectory of Long Reston, in the archdeaconry of the East riding, and diocese, of York, rated in the king's books at £13. 3. 4., and in the patronage of the Crown. The church, dedicated to St. Nicholas, is a spacious structure in the decorated style of English architecture, with insertions of a later date ; the spire, which was a conspicuous land-mark, was blown down

more than a century since. There are places of worship for Independents and Wesleyan Methodists.

HORNSEY, a parish in the Finsbury division of the hundred of OSSULSTONE, county of MIDDLESEX, 5½ miles (N. by;W.) from London, comprising the greater part of the village of Highgate, and the hamlets of Crouch-End, Muswell Hill, and Stroud Green, and containing 4122 inhabitants. The manor of Hornsey, anciently called *Haringay*, has from a remote period belonged to the see of London, and the bishops had formerly a park, which was a lodge, or fort, memorable as the place where, in 1386, Thomas of Woodstock, Duke of Gloucester, and other noblemen, assembled to form a league against the favourites of Richard II.; and here Edward V. and Henry VII., on their succeeding to the crown, respectively, were met by deputations from the citizens of London. The village is agreeably situated in a vale, through which passes the New River, and is encircled by hills commanding varied and beautiful views of London and the adjoining country : it contains many elegant mansions and detached villas, with gardens and pleasure grounds, rendering it one of the most agreeable places of residence, or occasional resort, in the vicinity of the metropolis. Lands held under the lord of the manor descend, according to the custom of gavelkind, in common to all the sons or daughters of a customary tenant. The parish is within the jurisdiction of the court of requests held in Kingsgate-street, Holborn, for the recovery of debts under 40s. The living is a rectory, within the jurisdiction of the Commissary of London, concurrently with the Consistorial Episcopal Court, rated in the king's books at £22, and in the patronage of the Bishop of London. The church, dedicated to St. Mary, is a plain structure, with an embattled western tower, and is said to have been built about the year 1500, from the ruins of the fortress in the bishop's park. A new church is about to be erected, in pursuance of an act of parliament, at Highgate, which will be separated from Hornsey, and converted into a district parish. At Crouch-End there is a place of worship for Baptists. Here is a National school for about fifty boys, who also receive clothing ; and another for fifty girls. Several benefactions have been made for apprenticing poor boys, and for other charitable purposes. At Muswell Hill, to the north of Hornsey, was anciently a chapel, dedicated to Our Lady of Muswell, much resorted to by pilgrims before the Reformation, on account of a mineral spring called Mousewell, or Muswell, famed for the supposed miraculous cure of a king of Scotland, and still in repute for its medicinal properties : the chapel was an appendage to the priory of Clerkenwell; and the manor of Muswell, though locally in the parish of Hornsey, is subordinate to that of Clerkenwell.

HORNTON, a parish in the hundred of BLOXHAM, county of OXFORD, 6½ miles (N. W. by W.) from Banbury, containing 529 inhabitants. The church is dedicated to St. John the Baptist. The living is a vicarage not in charge, with that of Horley, in the jurisdiction of the Dean and Chapter of Lincoln in the peculiar court of Banbury. Here is a school wherein about thirty children are educated : the master's stipend arises from a rent-charge on land given by John Fox, amounting to £12. 12. per annum.

HORSEHEATH, a parish in the hundred of CHIL-

3 H

FORD, county of CAMBRIDGE, 3½ miles (E. by N.) from Linton, containing 413 inhabitants. The living is a rectory, in the archdeaconry and diocese of Ely, rated in the king's books at £13. 6. 8., and in the patronage of the Governors of the Charter-house, London. The church is dedicated to All Saints.

HORSEHOUSE, a chapelry in the parish of COVERHAM, western division of the wapentake of HANG, North riding of the county of YORK, 7 miles (S. W.) from Middleham. The population is returned with the parish. The living is a perpetual curacy, in the archdeaconry of Richmond, and diocese of Chester, endowed with £200 private benefaction, and £800 royal bounty. The Rev. S. Hardcastle was patron in 1809.

HORSELEY, a township in the parish of ECCLESHALL, northern division of the hundred of PIREHILL, county of STAFFORD, 2½ miles (S. W.) from Eccleshall, containing 487 inhabitants.

HORSELL, a parish in the first division of the hundred of GODLEY, county of SURREY, 4½ miles (N. W. by W.) from Ripley, containing 617 inhabitants. The living is a perpetual curacy, in the archdeaconry of Surrey, and diocese of Winchester, endowed with £400 royal bounty, and £1400 parliamentary grant, and in the patronage of certain Trustees. The church is dedicated to St. Mary.

HORSEMONDEN, a parish in the hundred of BRENCHLEY and HORSEMONDEN, lathe of AYLESFORD, county of KENT, 2¾ miles (N. E. by N.) from Lamberhurst, containing 1224 inhabitants. The living is a rectory, in the archdeaconry and diocese of Rochester, rated in the king's books at £26. 3. 9. Sir J. W. Smith, Bart., W. A. Morland, and J. P. Ince, Esqrs., were patrons in 1825. The church, situated at the extremity of the parish, is dedicated to St. Margaret. A school for the instruction of poor children in reading and writing was endowed, in 1792, by means of a bequest of £1000 from Sir Charles Booth, vested in trustees, and now producing £44. 15. 6. per annum : an additional benefaction of £200 was made by Dr. Marriott, the late rector, which produces £8. 11. 4. per annum, making a total of £53. 6. 10.: a school on Dr. Bell's system affords the means of instruction to about fifty boys and forty girls. A fair for cattle and toys is held on the 26th of July. This parish is bounded on the east by the river Tair.

HORSENDON, a parish in the hundred of AYLESBURY, county of BUCKINGHAM, 7 miles (W. by N.) from Great Missenden, containing 50 inhabitants. The living is a discharged rectory, in the archdeaconry of Buckingham, and diocese of Lincoln, rated in the king's books at £6. 17. — Grubb, Esq. was patron in 1811. The church is dedicated to St. Michael. During the parliamentary war the manor-house, then the property of Sir John Denham, was occupied by a garrison for the king.

HORSEPATH, a parish in the hundred of BULLINGTON, county of OXFORD, 4 miles (E. by S.) from Oxford, containing 264 inhabitants. The living is a perpetual curacy, in the archdeaconry and diocese of Oxford, endowed with £400 private benefaction, and £400 royal bounty, and in the patronage of the President and Fellows of Magdalene College, Oxford. The church is dedicated to St. Giles.

HORSEPOOL, a township in the parish of THORN-

TON, hundred of SPARKENHOE, county of LEICESTER, 7½ miles (N. W. by W.) from Leicester. The population is returned with the chapelry of Stanton under Bardon.

HORSEY next the SEA, a parish in the hundred of HAPPING, county of NORFOLK, 8¾ miles (N. N. W.) from Caistor, containing 95 inhabitants. The living is a discharged vicarage, in the archdeaconry of Norfolk, and diocese of Norwich, rated in the king's books at £3. 1. 5½., endowed with £800 royal bounty, and in the patronage of the Governors of North Walsham school. The church, now in ruins, was dedicated to All Saints. This parish principally consists of low marshes and bogs : it is nearly insulated by the sea on the east ; the Hundred stream, or river, which separates Happing from East Flegg, on the south ; and Eelfleet dyke and Horsey mere on the west and north.

HORSFORD, a parish in the hundred of TAVERHAM, county of NORFOLK, 5 miles (N. N. W.) from Norwich, containing 512 inhabitants. The living is a discharged vicarage, in the archdeaconry and diocese of Norwich, rated in the king's books at £4. 5. 2¼., endowed with £200 royal bounty. Viscount Ranelagh was patron in 1812. The church is dedicated to All Saints.

HORSFORTH, a chapelry in the parish of GUISLEY, upper division of the wapentake of SKYRACK, West riding of the county of YORK, 5½ miles (N. W. by W.) from Leeds, containing 2824 inhabitants. The living is a perpetual curacy, in the archdeaconry and diocese of York, endowed with £200 private benefaction, £600 royal bounty, and £1400 parliamentary grant, and in the patronage of the Vicar of Guisley. A chapel was erected on the site of the ancient structure, in 1758, chiefly by the Stanhope family. There are places of worship for Baptists and Wesleyan Methodists. In 1819 a bridge was built over the Aire, at an expense of £1500, by John Pollard, Esq. Special sessions are held here once a fortnight. The manufacture of cloth is carried on to a considerable extent in this chapelry, and there are some bleaching-mills.

HORSHAM, a borough, market town, and parish, in the hundred of FISHERGATE, rape of BRAMBER, county of SUSSEX, 29 miles (N.E.) from Chichester, and 35½ (S. S. W.) from London, containing 4575 inhabitants. This place is supposed to have derived its name from Horsa, the brother of Hengist, who is said to have been

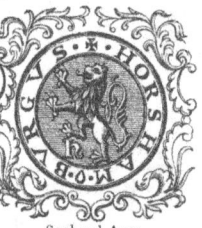

Seal and Arms.

interred in the immediate vicinity, after the battle with Vortimer, near Aylesford, in 457, in which he was slain. The town is pleasantly situated on a branch of the river Adur, and in the centre of a fertile district surrounded by varied and interesting scenery : it consists principally of one spacious street, from which others branch off in various directions : the houses are in general well built, and those in the street leading to the church are agreeably sheltered by rows of trees : the town is well paved with stone found in the neighbourhood, and amply supplied with water. A mechanics' institution has been recently established, to which a useful library is attached and in which lectures on mechanics and scientific subjects are periodically delivered. The approaches to the town are formed by excellent turnpike roads from London, Worthing, Brighton, Guildford, Arundel, and Chichester, and its situation as a thoroughfare is the principal source from which its trade arises. A great quantity of poultry is reared in the neighbourhood, for the supply of the London market. There are quarries of excellent stone in the vicinity, which is used for paving, flooring, and roofing. The market days are Monday for poultry, and Saturday chiefly for corn: the fairs, principally for sheep and lambs, are April 5th and July 18th, and for horses and cattle on the Monday before Whitsuntide and November 27th; on the Saturday after the July fair is a fair for pedlary and toys, and on November 17th is a large fair for Welch cattle, called St. Leonard's fair, from its having been formerly held in an adjoining forest of that name. The town is governed by a steward and two bailiffs, chosen annually at the court leet for the lord of the manor, at which constables and other officers are also appointed. The Lent assizes for the county, and the Midsummer quarter sessions for the division, are held here. The town-hall and sessions-house is a handsome building with a stone front; it has been recently enlarged by the Duke of Norfolk, for the accommodation of the judges of assize. The county gaol, a spacious and commodious building near the south-eastern extremity of the town, is adapted to the classification of prisoners, and comprises fifty-six wards, seven day-rooms, and four airing-yards. Horsham is a borough by prescription, and has returned two members to parliament since the 23rd of Edward I.: the right of election is vested in the burgage-holders, of whom there are twenty-four, in the interest of the Duke of Norfolk: the bailiffs are the returning officers.

The living is a vicarage, in the archdeaconry and diocese of Chichester, rated in the king's books at £25, and in the patronage of the Archbishop of Canterbury. The church, dedicated to St. Mary, is a spacious and venerable structure in the early style of English architecture, with a lofty tower surmounted by a spire: the east window of the chancel is of beautiful design, and the interior, which preserves its original character nearly throughout, contains several ancient and interesting monuments. There are places of worship for Baptists, the Society of Friends, Independents, and Wesleyan Methodists, and a Roman Catholic chapel. The free school was founded in 1532, by Richard Collier, citizen and mercer of London, who endowed it with houses and tenements producing more than £500 per annum, for the instruction of sixty boys of this parish in reading, writing, and arithmetic, of whom some of the upper class are taught Latin: the master has a salary of £110, and the usher one of £73. 6. 8. per annum: the school is under the direction of the Master and Wardens of the Mercers' Company, and the boys are nominated by the vicar and the churchwardens, and by two school-wardens annually elected by the parishioners. The premises comprise a good school-room, and dwelling houses with gardens for the masters. Lancasterian schools, in which two hundred boys and one hundred girls are instructed, and an infant school, are supported by subscription; and there are several small charitable bequests for distribution among the poor.

HORSHAM (ST. FAITH), a parish in the hundred of TAVERHAM, county of NORFOLK, 4¾ miles (N. by W.) from Norwich, containing 735 inhabitants. The living is a vicarage, in the archdeaconry and diocese of Norwich, endowed with £400 royal bounty, and £1200 parliamentary grant. Viscount Ranelagh was patron in 1812. A priory of Black monks, dedicated to St. Faith, was founded here in 1105, by Robert Fitzwalter and Sibell de Cayneto, his wife; it was at first a cell to the abbey de Cenchis, in Normandy: at the dissolution its revenue was estimated at £193. 2. 3. Attached to this institution was an hospital, formerly belonging to the Knights of St. John of Jerusalem.

HORSINGTON, a parish in the southern division of the wapentake of GARTREE, parts of LINDSEY, county of LINCOLN, 4¾ miles (W.) from Horncastle, containing 322 inhabitants. The living is a discharged rectory, in the archdeaconry and diocese of Lincoln, rated in the king's books at £9. 11. 3., endowed with £200 private benefaction, and £200 royal bounty, and in the patronage of the President and Fellows of Magdalene College, Oxford. The church is dedicated to All Saints.

HORSINGTON, a parish in the hundred of HORETHORNE, county of SOMERSET, 4 miles (S. by W.) from Wincanton, containing 925 inhabitants. The living is a rectory, in the archdeaconry of Wells, and diocese of Bath and Wells, rated in the king's books at £18. 6. 0½. G. Whitchurch, Esq. and others were patrons in 1798. The church is dedicated to St. John the Baptist: two hundred free sittings have recently been added, towards defraying the expense of which the Incorporated Society for the enlargement of churches and chapels contributed £150. There is a place of worship for Baptists. Martha Wickham bequeathed an annuity of £5 for the education of twelve poor children.

HORSLEY, a parish in the hundred of MORLESTON and LITCHURCH, county of DERBY, comprising the townships of Horsley, Horsley-Woodhouse, and Kilbourne, and containing 1714 inhabitants, of which number, 624 are in the township of Horsley, 6¼ miles (N. N. E.) from Derby. The living is a discharged vicarage, in the archdeaconry of Derby, and diocese of Lichfield and Coventry, rated in the king's books at £7. 5. 5., endowed with £200 royal bounty, and £800 parliamentary grant, and in the patronage of the Earl of Chesterfield. The church, dedicated to St. Clement, is spacious and handsome, and is surmounted by a spire of curious workmanship: over the south door is a very antique crucifix in a perfect state. Six boys of the township of Horsley are eligible as scholars and pensioners to Richardson's school at Smelley. A National school was erected in 1828, and is supported by voluntary contributions. At Denby, in this parish, is a school founded and endowed, about the year 1739, by Mrs. Jane Massey, with land now producing £30 per annum. The Little Eaton railway passes through this parish. On the summit of a hill, about a mile from the church, are the ruins of the ancient baronial castle of Horestan, or Horston, said to have been built in the twelfth century. In the time of Elizabeth this edifice was in the possession of the Stanhope family, and was then in "neatly good repair."

HORSLEY, a parish in the hundred of LONGTREE, county of GLOUCESTER, 3 miles (S. W. by W.) from Minchin-Hampton, containing, with a small portion of the chapelry of Nailsworth, 3565 inhabitants. The living is a discharged vicarage, in the archdeaconry and diocese of Gloucester, rated in the king's books at £7. 11. 5½., endowed with £200 private benefaction, and £600 royal bounty, and in the patronage of the Bishop of Gloucester. The church is dedicated to St. Martin. There are places of worship for Baptists and Wesleyan Methodists. Edward Webb, in 1744, gave £200 in trust for endowing a school, to which, in 1775, Elizabeth Castleman added £30, and Ann Wright £100 : the present income is £60 per annum; and one hundred children are instructed on Dr. Bell's plan : the school-room was erected, in 1823, at an expense of £230, defrayed by subscription, aided by contributions from the National School Society in London, and from the Diocesan Society in Gloucester. Here is a house of correction, containing a tread-mill and forty fire-proof cells, or sleeping-rooms, for prisoners, who are divided into five classes. The petty sessions for the district of Longtree are held at Tetbury, Rodborough, and Horsley, in rotation.

HORSLEY, a township in the parish of Ovingham, eastern division of Tindale ward, county of Northumberland, 9¾ miles (W. by N.) from Newcastle upon Tyne, containing 257 inhabitants. There is a place of worship for Presbyterians, with an endowment of £37. 5. per annum, also one for Independents.

HORSLEY (EAST), a parish in the second division of the hundred of Woking, county of Surrey, 5½ miles (S. W. by W.) from Leatherhead, containing 192 inhabitants. The living is a rectory, in the peculiar jurisdiction and patronage of the Archbishop of Canterbury, rated in the king's books at £12. 16. 5½. The church, dedicated to St. Martin, has portions in the early style of English architecture.

HORSLEY (LONG), a parish in the western division of Morpeth ward, county of Northumberland, 6¾ miles (N. W. by N.) from Morpeth, comprising the townships of Bigge's Quarter, Freeholders' Quarter, Longshaws, Riddle's Quarter, Stanton, Todburn, Wingates, and Witton-Shiels, and containing 1006 inhabitants. The living is a vicarage, in the archdeaconry of Northumberland, and diocese of Durham, rated in the king's books at £7. 13. 4., and in the patronage of the Crown. The church, dedicated to St. Helen, is a neat edifice of stone, situated nearly half a mile from the village, and was rebuilt in 1783 : the communion table and rails were made out of an oak tree that was found buried in a neighbouring peat-moss a few years ago. There are both coal and lime works in the parish. A strong ancient tower, near the western extremity of the village, has been converted into a Roman Catholic chapel, with a residence for the priest. A National school, partly supported by subscription, was established in 1826.

HORSLEY (WEST), a parish in the second division of the hundred of Woking, county of Surrey, 6½ miles (W. S. W.) from Leatherhead, containing 611 inhabitants. The living is a rectory, in the archdeaconry of Surrey, and diocese of Winchester, rated in the king's books at £22. 17. 1. H. P. Weston, Esq. was patron in 1816. The church is dedicated to St. Mary. A Sunday school was founded in 1813, and endowed by the Rev. Weston Fullerton, with £600 ; the children are taught on the National system.

HORSLEY-WOODHOUSE, a township in the parish of Horsley, hundred of Morleston and Litchurch, county of Derby, 6½ miles (N. N. E.) from Derby, containing 592 inhabitants.

HORSTEAD, a parish in the hundred of Taverham, county of Norfolk, ½ a mile (W.) from Coltishall, containing, with Staininghall, 492 inhabitants. The living is a rectory, in the archdeaconry and diocese of Norwich, rated in the king's books at £7. 10. The church is dedicated to All Saints. Here was an Alien priory, a cell to the convent of the Holy Trinity at Caen in Normandy, the revenue of which, at the suppression, was appropriated as part of the endowment of King's College, Cambridge.

HORSTED (LITTLE), a parish in the hundred of Rushmonden, though locally in that of Loxfield-Dorset, rape of Pevensey, county of Sussex, 2 miles (S.) from Uckfield, containing 286 inhabitants. The living is a rectory, in the archdeaconry of Lewes, and diocese of Chichester, rated in the king's books at £7. The Rev. John Hubbard was patron in 1823.

HORSTED-KEYNES, a parish in the hundred of Danehill-Horsted, rape of Pevensey, county of Sussex, 6 miles (E. N. E.) from Cuckfield, containing 713 inhabitants. The living is a rectory, in the archdeaconry of Lewes, and diocese of Chichester, rated in the king's books at £13. 6. 8. F. M. Austen, Esq. was patron in 1812. The church, dedicated to St. Giles, has portions in the early and decorated styles of English architecture. The free school was founded and endowed with an estate and £400, by Edward Lightmaker, in 1708, for twenty children ; there being no salary the master teaches twelve children for his rent-free residence. Here is a small school on the National system.

HORTON, a hamlet in the parish of Ivinghoe, hundred of Cottesloe, county of Buckingham, 2½ miles (N. N. W.) from Ivinghoe, containing, with Seabrook, 139 inhabitants.

HORTON, a parish in the hundred of Stoke, county of Buckingham, 1¼ mile (S. S. W.) from Colnbrook, containing 796 inhabitants. The living is a rectory, in the archdeaconry of Buckingham, and diocese of Lincoln, rated in the king's books at £22. 9. 4½. The Rev. W. Browne was patron in 1796. The church, dedicated to St. Michael, contains a doorway with a circular arch, enriched with Saxon mouldings, and is surrounded by a Roman wall. A large paper-mill on the banks of the Coln affords employment to between forty and fifty persons. The Colnbrook cattle fair is held in this parish. The parents of Milton the poet resided here, and his mother, who died in 1637, is interred in the church ; a few of the juvenile years of the poet himself were passed at this place.

HORTON, a township in the parish of Tilston, higher division of the hundred of Broxton, county palatine of Chester, 2½ miles (N.W. by W.) from Malpas, containing 141 inhabitants.

HORTON, a joint township with Peele, in that part of the parish of Tarvin which is in the second division of the hundred of Eddisbury, county palatine of Chester, 7½ miles (E. N. E.) from Chester, containing 36 inhabitants.

HORTON, a parish in the hundred of Badbury, Shaston (East) division of the county of Dorset, 5 miles (S. S. W.) from Cranborne, containing 420 inhabitants. The living is a discharged vicarage, with the curacy of Knowlton, in the archdeaconry of Dorset, and diocese of Bristol, rated in the king's books at £7.13.10. The Earl of Shaftesbury was patron in 1816. The church is dedicated to St. Wolfrida. An abbey, founded here in 970, by Ordgar, Earl of Devonshire, became a cell to Sherborne Abbey in 1122. At Knowlton, formerly a hamlet in this parish, now depopulated, but still giving name to a hundred, are the remains of a chapel, which, with the cemetery, are surrounded by a deep circular intrenchment, comprising one acre of ground within its area, and containing several tumuli; in the vicinity are several other works of this kind. A fair formerly held at Knowlton was removed to the adjoining parish of Woodlands, about the year 1730, where it takes place on the 5th of July, for horses, cheese, and toys.

HORTON, a parish in the upper division of the hundred of GRUMBALD'S ASH, county of GLOUCESTER, 3¾ miles (N. E.) from Chipping-Sodbury, containing 385 inhabitants. The living is a rectory, in the archdeaconry and diocese of Gloucester, rated in the king's books at £16, and in the patronage of Thomas Brooks, Esq. The church is dedicated to St. James.

HORTON, a chapelry in that part of the parish of CHARTHAM which is in the hundred of BRIDGE and PETHAM, lathe of ST. AUGUSTINE, county of KENT, 3 miles (S. W. by W.) from Canterbury. The population is returned with the parish.

HORTON, a parish in the hundred of WYMERSLEY, county of NORTHAMPTON, 6½ miles (S.E.) from Northampton, containing 87 inhabitants. The living is a vicarage with the curacy of Piddington, in the archdeaconry of Northampton, and diocese of Peterborough, rated in the king's books at £7. 17. 1., and endowed with £400 parliamentary grant, and in the patronage of Sir R. Gunning, Bart. The church is dedicated to St. Mary. Charles Montague, first earl of Halifax, was born at Horton house in 1661.

HORTON, a parish in the eastern division of CASTLE ward, county of NORTHUMBERLAND, comprising the townships of Bebside, Cowpen, East Hartford, West Hartford, and Horton, and containing 2099 inhabitants, of which number, 139 are in the township of Horton, 7¼ miles (S. E.) from Morpeth. The living is a perpetual curacy, in the archdeaconry of Northumberland, and diocese of Durham, endowed with £200 private benefaction, and £600 royal bounty, and in the patronage of the Vicar of Woodhorn. The church was rebuilt in 1828, at an expense of upwards of £500, raised by subscription. Horton formed part of the parish of Woodhorn until the year 1768, when it was severed from it. There are mines of coal in the parish. Here was formerly a strong castle belonging to the Delaval family, which was razed to the ground in 1809, and the intrenchments levelled. This parish is bounded on the north by the river Blyth.

HORTON, a hamlet in that part of the parish of BECKLEY which is in the hundred of BULLINGTON, county of OXFORD, 7¼ miles (N. E.) from Oxford. The population is returned with the chapelry of Studley.

HORTON, a township in that part of the parish of WEM which is in the Whitchurch division of the hundred of BRADFORD (North), county of SALOP, 1¾ mile (W. by N.) from Wem, containing 99 inhabitants.

HORTON, a parish in the northern division of the hundred of TOTMONSLOW, county of STAFFORD, 2¼ miles (W. by N.) from Leek, containing, with the township of Blackwood with Croborough, and Horton-Hay, 942 inhabitants. The living is a perpetual curacy, in the archdeaconry of Stafford, and diocese of Lichfield and Coventry, endowed with £200 private benefaction, £200 royal bounty, and £200 parliamentary grant, and in the patronage of G. C. Antrobus, Esq. The church, dedicated to St. Michael, is a stone edifice with a tower. A considerable quantity of cheese is made in this neighbourhood. Near Horton is the reservoir belonging to the Caldon canal; it is a mile and three quarters in length, and a quarter of a mile in breadth, and will contain two million four hundred and forty thousand cubic yards of water.

HORTON, a chapelry in the parish of BRADFORD, wapentake of MORLEY, West riding of the county of YORK, 2 miles (S. W. by W.) from Bradford, containing 7192 inhabitants. The living is a perpetual curacy, in the archdeaconry and diocese of York, endowed with £200 royal bounty, and £1800 parliamentary grant, and in the patronage of the Vicar of Bradford. There is a place of worship for Wesleyan Methodists. The manufacture of cotton and woollen goods is carried on here. The free grammar school was founded and endowed by Christopher Scott, in the reign of Charles I., with a school-house and an annuity of £18, since augmented to £68 per annum: all applicants are admitted, and about two hundred children are instructed here; but classical education has been discontinued. A school-room and dwelling-house were erected in 1805, and endowed with £600, raised by contributions, for the education of children and young persons residing in the hamlets of Stanbury and Haworth: the income is £30 per annum, and there are sixty free scholars.

HORTON, a township in the parish of GISBURN, western division of the wapentake of STAINCLIFFE and EWCROSS, West riding of the county of YORK, 9½ miles (W. by S.) from Skipton, containing 187 inhabitants.

HORTON (KIRBY), a parish in the hundred of AXTON, DARTFORD, and WILMINGTON, lathe of SUTTON at HONE, county of KENT, 4 miles (S.S.E.) from Dartford, containing 537 inhabitants. The living is a discharged vicarage, in the archdeaconry and diocese of Rochester, rated in the king's books at £5. 7. 6., endowed with £200 private benefaction, and £200 royal bounty, and in the patronage of the Rev. P. Rashleigh. The church, dedicated to St. Mary, is a cruciform structure, with a tower rising from the intersection, and surmounted by a spire. Here are extensive remains of a castle, founded by the family of Ros about the time of the Conquest, which have been partially converted into the manorial farm-house. This village is situated upon the eastern bank of the river Darent.

HORTON (MONKS), a parish in the hundred of STOUTING, lathe of SHEPWAY, county of KENT, 5 miles (N. N. W.) from Hythe, containing 186 inhabitants. The living is a discharged rectory, consolidated with the vicarage of Brabourne, in the archdeaconry and diocese of Canterbury, rated in the king's books at £7. 10. 8. The church, dedicated to St. Peter, is principally in the early style of English architecture. Here was a cell of Cluniac monks, founded in the reign of Henry II., subordinate to the priory of Lewes, and dedicated to St. Mary, St. John the Evangelist, and St. Pancras: its revenue, at the dissolution, was valued at £111. 16. 11.: the remains of the priory are in the Norman style, with later insertions, and have been converted into a dwelling-house: a large circular arch, a short distance, curiously ornamented, is supposed to have been the entrance into the church.

HORTON in RIBBLESDALE, a parish in the western division of the wapentake of STAINCLIFFE and EWCROSS, West riding of the county of YORK, 5½ miles (N.) from Settle, containing 558 inhabitants. The living is a perpetual curacy, in the archdeaconry and diocese of York, endowed with £400 private benefaction, £600 royal bounty, and £1200 parliamentary grant. The Rev. G. Holden, L.L.D., was patron in 1798. The church is dedicated to St. Oswald. A free grammar school was endowed, in 1725, by John Armitshead, with land and £200 for the support of a schoolmaster: the present income is £160 per annum, and the average number of scholars is fifty, some of whom are taught the classics.

HORTON-GRANGE, a township in the parish of PONTELAND, western division of CASTLE ward, county of NORTHUMBERLAND, 9 miles (N.N.W.) from Newcastle upon Tyne, containing 66 inhabitants.

HORTON-HAY, a township in the parish of HORTON, northern division of the hundred of TOTMONSLOW, county of STAFFORD, 5¼ miles (N.W. by W.) from Leek. The population is returned with the parish.

HORWICH, a chapelry in the parish of DEAN, hundred of SALFORD, county palatine of LANCASTER, 4¾ miles (W. N. W.) from Great Bolton, containing 2873 inhabitants. The living is a perpetual curacy, in the archdeaconry and diocese of Chester, endowed with £400 private benefaction, and £400 royal bounty, and in the patronage of the Vicar of Dean. A new district church, or chapel, has been recently erected by the commissioners for building churches. There are places of worship for Independents, Presbyterians, and Wesleyan Methodists. Bleaching and cotton-spinning are carried on here to a considerable extent. Two stone pillars on Wildersmoore hill are intended, according to tradition, to record the death of two boys in the snow, on going to the grammar school at Rivington.

HORWOOD, a parish in the hundred of FREMINGTON, county of DEVON, 3½ miles (E. N. E.) from Bideford, containing 144 inhabitants. The living is a discharged rectory, in the archdeaconry of Barnstaple, and diocese of Exeter, rated in the king's books at £7. 8. 4., and in the patronage of the Rev. J. Dene. The church is dedicated to St. Michael.

HORWOOD (GREAT), a parish in the hundred of COTTESLOE, county of BUCKINGHAM, 2¼ miles (N.) from Winslow, containing, with the hamlet of Singleborough, 688 inhabitants. The living is a rectory, in the archdeaconry of Buckingham, and diocese of Lincoln, rated in the king's books at £14. 4. 2., and in the patronage of the Warden and Fellows of New College, Oxford. The church is dedicated to St. James. There is a place of worship for Independents. Here was formerly a weekly market on Wednesday, granted to the Society of New College in 1447, with a fair for three days at the festival of St. James.

HORWOOD (LITTLE), a parish in the hundred of COTTESLOE, county of BUCKINGHAM, 2¼ miles (N. E. by N.) from Winslow, containing 429 inhabitants.

The living is a discharged vicarage, in the archdeaconry of St. Alban's, and diocese of London, rated in the king's books at £5. 6. 8., endowed with £400 private benefaction, and £600 royal bounty, and in the patronage of the Bishop of London. The church is dedicated to St. Nicholas.

HOSE, a parish in the hundred of FRAMLAND, county of LEICESTER, 6¾ miles (N. by W.) from Melton-Mowbray, containing 325 inhabitants. The living is a discharged vicarage, in the archdeaconry of Leicester, and diocese of Lincoln, rated in the king's books at £7. 2. 6., and endowed with £200 royal bounty. The King presented by lapse in 1801. The church is dedicated to St. Michael.

HOSPITAL, a tything in that part of the parish of FARRINGDON which is in the hundred of FARRINGDON, county of BERKS. The population is returned with Wadley.

HOTHAM, a parish in the Hunsley-Beacon division of the wapentake of HARTHILL, East riding of the county of YORK, 1½ mile (N. N. E.) from North Cave, containing 293 inhabitants. The living is a rectory, in the archdeaconry of the East riding, and diocese of York, rated in the king's books at £10. 0. 7½., and in the patronage of the Crown. The church is dedicated to St. Oswald. Near this village is a Roman road, passing in a direction towards North and South Newbald.

HOTHERSALL, a joint township with Alston, in that part of the parish of RIBCHESTER which is in the hundred of AMOUNDERNESS, county palatine of LANCASTER, 7 miles (N. E. by E.) from Preston. The population is returned with Alston.

HOTHFIELD, a parish in the hundred of CHART and LONGBRIDGE, lathe of SCRAY, county of KENT, 3¼ miles (W. N. W.) from Ashford, containing 438 inhabitants. The living is a rectory, in the archdeaconry and diocese of Canterbury, rated in the king's books at £17. 5., and in the patronage of the Earl of Thanet. The church is dedicated to St. Mary. A school for girls was endowed, in 1720, by Thomas, Earl of Thanet, and his Countess, with a rent-charge of £15 per annum, for a schoolmistress, and a tenement for her residence; likewise with £100 in the four per cents.: twelve boys and twelve girls are taught gratuitously. In this parish is "Jack Cade's field," said to have been the hiding-place of that rebel in the reign of Henry VI., whence he was dragged to execution by Alexander Iden, Esq., sheriff of Kent.

HOTHORPE, a hamlet in that part of the parish of THEDDINGWORTH which is in the hundred of ROTHWELL, county of NORTHAMPTON, 4½ miles (W. S. W.) from Market-Harborough, containing 62 inhabitants.

HOTON, a chapelry in the parish of PRESTWOULD, eastern division of the hundred of GOSCOTE, county of LEICESTER, 3 miles (N. E. by E.) from Loughborough, containing 412 inhabitants. There is a place of worship for Wesleyan Methodists.

HOUGH, a township in the parish of WYBUNBURY, hundred of NANTWICH, county palatine of CHESTER, 4 miles (E. by S.) from Nantwich, containing 202 inhabitants.

HOUGH on the HILL, a parish in the wapentake of LOVEDEN, parts of KESTEVEN, county of LINCOLN, 7 miles (N.) from Grantham, containing, with the hamlets of Brandon and Gelston, 533 inhabitants. The living is a vicarage, in the archdeaconry and diocese of Lincoln, rated in the king's books at £15. 6. 8., and in the patronage of the Crown. The church is dedicated to All Saints. Here was an Alien priory of Augustine canons, a cell to the abbey of St. Mary de Voto, at Cherburgh in Normandy, the revenue of which was valued at £20, when it was granted by Richard II. to the Carthusians at Coventry: at the dissolution it was a cell to the priory of Montgrace in Yorkshire.

HOUGHAM, a parish partly in the hundred of BEWSBOROUGH, lathe of ST. AUGUSTINE, and partly within the jurisdiction of the Cinque-port liberty of DOVOR, though locally in the hundred of Folkstone, lathe of Shepway, county of KENT, 2½ miles (W.S.W.) from Dovor, containing 834 inhabitants. The living is a vicarage, in the archdeaconry and diocese of Canterbury, rated in the king's books at £6. 13. 4., and in the patronage of the Archbishop of Canterbury. The church, dedicated to St. Lawrence, is principally in the early style of English architecture. This parish is bounded on the east by high chalk cliffs, which command a fine view of the hills of Boulogne, across the channel. A great number of persons who died of the plague in London, in 1665, was buried here, at a place called the Graves.

HOUGHAM, a parish in the wapentake of LOVE-DEN, parts of KESTEVEN, county of LINCOLN, 6¼ miles (N.N.W.) from Grantham, containing 290 inhabitants. The living is a rectory with that of Marston, in the archdeaconry and diocese of Lincoln, rated in the king's books at £33. 8. 6½. The church is dedicated to All Saints.

HOUGHTON, a township in that part of the parish of STANWIX which is in ESKDALE ward, county of CUMBERLAND, 2 miles (N. by E.) from Carlisle, containing 288 inhabitants.

HOUGHTON, a parish in the hundred of HURST-INGSTONE, county of HUNTINGDON, 2 miles (W. by N.) from St. Ives, containing 427 inhabitants. The living is a rectory with the curacy of Witton, in the archdeaconry of Huntingdon, and diocese of Lincoln, rated in the king's books at £34. 17. 8½. Mrs. Peck was patroness in 1811. The church is dedicated to St. Mary.

HOUGHTON, a township in the parish of MAN-CHESTER, hundred of SALFORD, county palatine of LANCASTER, 3¾ miles (N.E.) from Stockport, containing 2084 inhabitants. The name is probably a corruption of High Town, from the district being the most elevated part of the parish of Manchester. There is a place of worship for Wesleyan Methodists. The manufacture of cotton goods and hats affords employment to about seven hundred and fifty persons. An abundance of coal is obtained in this township.

HOUGHTON, a joint township with Middleton and Arbury, in the parish of WINWICK, hundred of WEST DERBY, county palatine of LANCASTER, 4 miles (S. E. by E.) from Newton in Mackerfield, containing 280 inhabitants.

HOUGHTON, a joint township with Clowhouse, in that part of the parish of HEDDON on the WALL which is in the eastern division of TINDALE ward, county of NORTHUMBERLAND, 7½ miles (W. by N.) from Newcastle upon Tyne, containing 100 inhabitants.

HOUGHTON, a parish in the Hatfield division of

the wapentake of BASSETLAW, county of NOTTINGHAM, 3¾ miles (N. W. by W.) from Tuxford, containing, with the township of Serlby, and exclusively of Styrrup, a portion of which is in this parish, 40 inhabitants. The church is in ruins. There is a small endowment for the instruction of children.

HOUGHTON, a parish partly in the hundred of KING's SOMBOURN, Andover division, but chiefly in that of BUDDLESGATE, Fawley division, of the county of SOUTHAMPTON, 2¼ miles (S. W. by S.) from Stockbridge, containing, with the tything of Houghton-Drayton, 365 inhabitants. The living is a rectory, in the peculiar jurisdiction of the incumbent, rated in the king's books at £28. 2. 8½., and in the patronage of the Bishop of Winchester. The church is dedicated to All Saints. The river Test passes on the verge of this parish. Courts leet and baron are held once a year. In this parish is Stockbridge race-course, considered to be one of the finest in the kingdom; the races, held annually in June, are well attended: near the down are extensive training-stables.

HOUGHTON, a parish in the hundred of BURY, rape of ARUNDEL, county of SUSSEX, 3½ miles (N.) from Arundel, containing 162 inhabitants. The living is a vicarage, united to that of Amberley, in the archdeaconry and diocese of Chichester, and in the patronage of the Bishop of Chichester. The church is in the early style of English architecture, with later insertions. The navigable river Arun runs through the parish.

HOUGHTON, East riding of the county of YORK. —See SANCTON with HOUGHTON.

HOUGHTON (ST. GILES in the HOLE), a parish in the northern division of the hundred of GREENHOE, county of NORFOLK, ¾ of a mile (S.W.) from Little Walsingham, containing 206 inhabitants. The living is a discharged vicarage, in the archdeaconry of Norfolk, and diocese of Norwich, rated in the king's books at £8, and endowed with £400 royal bounty. D. H. Lee Warner, Esq. was patron in 1807.

HOUGHTON (GLASS), a township in the parish of CASTLEFORD, upper division of the wapentake of Os-GOLDCROSS, West riding of the county of YORK, 2¾ miles (N. W.) from Pontefract, containing 412 inhabitants.

HOUGHTON (GREAT), a parish in the hundred of WYMERSLEY, county of NORTHAMPTON, 2¼ miles (E.S.E.) from Northampton, containing 249 inhabitants. The living is a rectory, in the archdeaconry of Northampton, and diocese of Peterborough, rated in the king's books at £22, and in the patronage of the President and Fellows of Magdalene College, Oxford. The church is dedicated to St. Mary.

HOUGHTON (GREAT), a township in that part of the parish of DARFIELD which is in the northern division of the wapentake of STRAFFORTH and TICKHILL, West riding of the county of YORK, 7½ miles (E. by N.) from Barnesley, containing 287 inhabitants. A small school, in which ten poor children are instructed gratuitously, was founded and endowed with £3. 5. per annum, and a house for the master, by a member of the family of Rhodes.

HOUGHTON (HANGING), a hamlet in the parish of LAMPORT, hundred of ORLINGBURY, county of NORTHAMPTON, 8 miles (N.) from Northampton, containing 111 inhabitants. Here was anciently a chapel.

HOUGHTON on the HILL, a parish in the hundred of GARTREE, county of LEICESTER, 6½ miles (E. by S.) from Leicester, containing 374 inhabitants. The living is a rectory, in the archdeaconry of Leicester, and diocese of Lincoln, rated in the king's books at £16. 1. 0½., and in the patronage of the Rev. Sherrard Coleman. The church is dedicated to St. Catherine.

HOUGHTON on the HILL, a parish in the southern division of the hundred of GREENHOE, county of NORFOLK, 4¼ miles (N.W.) from Watton, containing 34 inhabitants. The living is a rectory, with that of North Pickenham, in the archdeaconry of Norfolk, and diocese of Norwich, rated in the king's books at £4. 18. 9. The church is dedicated to St. Mary.

HOUGHTON (LITTLE), a parish in the hundred of WYMERSLEY, county of NORTHAMPTON, 3½ miles (E. by S.) from Northampton, containing 501 inhabitants. The living is a vicarage with that of Brafield on the Green, in the archdeaconry of Northampton, and diocese of Peterborough, rated in the king's books at £6. 9. 2. The Rev. J. Johnson was patron in 1825. The church is dedicated to St. Mary.

HOUGHTON (LITTLE), a township in the parish of LONG HOUGHTON, southern division of BAMBROUGH ward, county of NORTHUMBERLAND, 3¾ miles (N.E. by E.) from Alnwick, containing, with the township of Little Mill, 77 inhabitants.

HOUGHTON (LITTLE), a township in that part of the parish of DARFIELD which is in the northern division of the wapentake of STRAFFORTH and TICK-HILL, West riding of the county of YORK, 6½ miles (E.) from Barnesley, containing 112 inhabitants.

HOUGHTON (LONG), a parish in the southern division of BAMBROUGH ward, county of NORTHUMBERLAND, comprising the townships of Boulmer with Seaton-House, Little Houghton, Long Houghton, and Little Mill, and containing 650 inhabitants, of which number, 469 are in the township of Long Houghton, 3¾ miles (E.N.E.) from Alnwick. The living is a discharged vicarage, in the archdeaconry of Northumberland, and diocese of Durham, rated in the king's books at £9. 9. 4., and in the patronage of the Duke of Northumberland. The church is dedicated to St. Peter. A little westward of the village is a romantic and lofty eminence, called Ratcheugh Cray. Boulmer bay, in this parish, is a natural basin, eight hundred yards in length, and four hundred in breadth, with a commodious entrance twelve feet deep at low water, and being already environed by the rocks, it is capable of being formed into an excellent harbour : at present only fishing-boats are moored here.

HOUGHTON (NEW), a parish in the hundred of GALLOW, county of NORFOLK, 9¼ miles (W. by S.) from Fakenham, containing 209 inhabitants. The living is a discharged vicarage, in the archdeaconry of Norfolk, and diocese of Norwich, rated in the king's books at £5, and endowed with £200 parliamentary grant. The Marquis of Cholmondeley was patron in 1822. The church is dedicated to St. Martin.

HOUGHTON le SPRING, a parish in the northern division of EASINGTON ward, county palatine of DURHAM, comprising the market town of Houghton le Spring, the chapelries of Painshaw and West Rainton, and the townships of South Bidick, Bourn-Moor, Cocken, Great Eppleton, Little Eppleton, East and Middle Herrington,

West Herrington, Hetton le Hole, Moorhouse, Moorsley, Morton-Grange, Newbottle, Offerton, East Rainton, and Warden-Law, and containing 12,550 inhabitants, of which number, 2905 are in the market town of Houghton le Spring, 6¾ miles (N.E.) from Durham, and 266 (N.N.W.) from London. This place, which, according to some antiquaries, takes the adjunct to its name from a family who resided here after the Norman Conquest, and according to others, from the chalybeate springs in the parish, is pleasantly situated at the head of a rich and fertile vale, which expands towards the west, and is sheltered by a range of hills to the north and east. The town has been rapidly improving within the last twenty years, and contains several large and handsome houses. A mechanics' institution was established in 1825. The trade of this place arises chiefly from its numerous mines, producing the finer sorts of coal, which command the highest prices in the London market : these are conveyed from the mines by railroads to the river Wear, which flows within four miles of the town, and forms the northern boundary of the parish, and thence by keels or barges to Sunderland. The adjoining district, which is rich in mineral produce, contains extensive quarries of limestone and freestone, in which many of the inhabitants of the surrounding villages find employment. The market, established in 1825, is on Friday, but, from its proximity to those of Durham and Sunderland, it is not well attended. A fair, or wake, on the festival of the saint to whom the church is dedicated, commences on the Sunday after New Michaelmas day, and continues for three or four days, during which, races and other amusements take place in the town and the several villages in the parish. The county magistrates hold a petty session for the division every alternate Thursday, at the White Lion Inn, and the seneschal, or deputy of the Bishop of Durham, the lord of the manor, holds a halmote court for petty cases of assault, and suits for the recovery of debts under 40s.

The living is a rectory, in the archdeaconry and diocese of Durham, rated in the king's books at £124, and in the patronage of the Bishop of Durham. The church, dedicated to St. Michael, is a spacious cruciform structure, in the early and decorated styles of English architecture, with a tower rising from the intersection : the interior contains several ancient monuments, among which is one to the memory of the Rev. Bernard Gilpin, many years rector of the parish, who, during the reigns of Mary and Elizabeth, was styled the Apostle of the North, and was equally distinguished for his great learning and benevolence. There are places of worship for Baptists, Independents, and Wesleyan Methodists. The free grammar school was founded in 1574, by the Rev. Bernard Gilpin, and John Heath, of Kepyer, Esq., who jointly endowed it with lands and tenements; the endowment has been augmented by subsequent benefactions, but there are at present no scholars on the foundation. Hugh Broughton, an eminent Hebrew scholar, and Dr. George Carleton, Bishop of Chichester, and biographer of Gilpin, received the rudiments of their education in this school, under the superintendence of the founder, who also erected an almshouse for the maintenance of the poor scholars and for three aged men or women. This hospital, which was rebuilt and endowed by George Lilburne, Esq., and the Rev. George Davenport, rector of the parish, consists of a centre and two wings. The Blue-coat school for girls was founded by Sir George Wheeler, Knt., who bequeathed £600 for that purpose, which has been since invested in land; the building was enlarged for an additional number of girls in 1803 : there are at present forty instructed, twelve of whom are also clothed. On the south side of the town is a field, called Kirk Ley, where some religious establishment formerly existed, of which there are no distinct records. Several coins, carved stones, and other vestiges of antiquity, have been discovered here; and a few years since a large oak, more than sixty feet in length, and a cart load of nuts, were dug up at Warden-Law hill; and several human skeletons and bones, together with the horns of deer, were found near the township of Newbottle. Dr. Samuel Ward, an eminent divine, and master of Sydney Sussex College, Cambridge, who died in 1643, was born in this parish.

HOUGHTON (WEST), a chapelry in the parish of DEAN, hundred of SALFORD, county palatine of LANCASTER, 4¾ miles (E.) from Wigan, containing 4211 inhabitants. The living is a perpetual curacy, in the archdeaconry and diocese of Chester, endowed with £400 private benefaction, £600 royal bounty, and £200 parliamentary grant, and in the patronage of the Vicar of Dean. The church is dedicated to St. Mary. There is a place of worship for Wesleyan Methodists. A free school was built by subscription in 1742, and enlarged in 1784 : the present income is about £20 per annum, and thirteen children are educated free. The manufacture of muslin and jaconet prevails to a considerable extent : in 1812, a manufactory was burnt down here by the rioters on the Luddite system, four of whom were executed.

HOUGHTON-CONQUEST, a parish in the hundred of REDBORNESTOKE, county of BEDFORD, 2½ miles (N. by E.) from Ampthill, containing 651 inhabitants. The living is a rectory, with which that of Houghton-Gildable was united in 1637, in the archdeaconry of Bedford, and diocese of Lincoln, rated jointly in the king's books at £25. 18. 9., and in the patronage of the Master and Fellows of St. John's College, Cambridge. The church, dedicated to All Saints, contains several monuments to the Conquest family; besides one to the memory of Thomas Archer, rector of the parish, who made a curious entry in the register respecting his own coffin, dated in 1623; and another to that of Dr. Zachary Grey, editor of Hudibras, and a commentator on Shakspeare, also incumbent of this parish. There is a place of worship for Wesleyan Methodists. This place derives the adjunct to its name from the family of Conquest, lords of the manor prior to the thirteenth century, whose mansion, ornamented with grotesque carvings, is now a farm-house : here James I. sojourned two days, in 1605, on a visit to Sir Edmund Conquest. A free school and almshouses for six poor persons were founded and endowed by Sir Francis Clerke, in 1632 : the salary of the master is £16, and the almspeople receive £8 per annum, which is divided amongst them. In 1691, Edmund Wylde, Esq. bequeathed £140 to be expended in land, desiring the rental to be applied to the repair of these premises, and the surplus to be given to the poor people : there are twenty-two scholars. Houghton Park house, now destroyed, was a celebrated seat of the family of Bruce, Earls of Elgin and Aylesbury.

VOL. II.

HOUGHTON-LEE-SIDE, a township in that part of the parish of GAINFORD which is in the southeastern division of DARLINGTON ward, county palatine of DURHAM, 6¼ miles (N.W. by N.) from Darlington, containing 122 inhabitants.

HOUGHTON-REGIS, a parish in the hundred of MANSHEAD, county of BEDFORD, 1¾ mile (N.) from Dunstable, containing 1283 inhabitants. The living is a discharged vicarage, in the archdeaconry of Bedford, and diocese of Lincoln, rated in the king's books at £11. 3. 4. The Duke of Bedford was patron in 1819. The church, dedicated to All Saints, contains an ancient monument, with the statue of a man in armour beneath a highly decorated arch, in the early style of English architecture. A free school was founded and endowed, in 1654, by Thomas Whitehead, with an estate and £250, for the education of twenty poor children : the annual income is £50, and sixteen boys are instructed. This place, as its name imports, was anciently held in royal demesne.

HOUGHTON-WINTERBORNE, a parish in the hundred of PIMPERNE, Blandford (North) division of the county of DORSET, 4½ miles (W. S. W.) from Blandford-Forum, containing 203 inhabitants. The living is a rectory, in the archdeaconry of Dorset, and diocese of Bristol, rated in the king's books at £13. 13. 4. E. M. Pleydell, Esq. was patron in 1823. The church is dedicated to St. Andrew.

HOUND, a parish in the hundred of MANSBRIDGE, Fawley division of the county of SOUTHAMPTON, 3¾ miles (S. E. by E.) from Southampton, containing 387 inhabitants. The living is a discharged vicarage, in the archdeaconry and diocese of Winchester, rated in the king's books at £5. 4. 7., and in the patronage of the Warden and Fellows of Winchester College. The church is dedicated to St. Mary. This parish lies on the verge of the Southampton water, at a short distance from the banks of which, and surrounded by well-wooded and gently-rising grounds, are the celebrated ruins of Netley abbey, founded, in 1239, for monks of the Cistercian order, the revenue of which was valued at the dissolution at £160. 2. 9. : the remains of the chapel, which is cruciform, are particularly beautiful ; the length is two hundred feet, the breadth sixty, and the length of the transept one hundred and twenty. Here is also an ancient crypt, forty-eight feet long, and eighteen wide, commonly called the Abbot's Kitchen : the additional ruins are, parts of the chapter-house and refectory, the richly-ornamented east window, with a circular compartment, an arch of the west window, richly mantled with ivy, and the south transept. Near the abbey, and more contiguous to Southampton water, are the remains of a small fort, called Netley Castle, erected by Henry VIII.

HOUNDSTREET, a tything in the parish of MARKSBURY, hundred of KEYNSHAM, county of SOMERSET, 2¼ miles (S. E. by E.) from Pensford, containing 73 inhabitants.

HOUNSLOW, a chapelry (formerly a market town) partly in the parish of ISLEWORTH, but chiefly in that of HESTON, hundred of ISLEWORTH, county of MIDDLESEX, 9½ miles (W. S. W.) from London. The population is returned with the respective parishes. This place, anciently called Hundeslawe, is situated on the principal road to the West of England : it consists chiefly of a long

3 I

street, extending from east to west, irregularly paved, but lighted with gas; and the inhabitants are well supplied with water. A priory of friars, of the order of the Holy Trinity, was founded here in the thirteenth century, the revenue of which, at the dissolution, was £80. 15. 0¼. In 1296, a charter was granted to the prior, for a weekly market on Thursday, and an annual fair: the former has been discontinued for more than thirty years; but fairs are held on Trinity Monday and Tuesday, and the Monday following Michaelmas-day, for the sale of horses, cattle, &c. Adjoining to the town, on the west, was formerly an extensive heath, which had been the site of ancient encampments, and was at different periods a military station, or place of rendezvous for troops, especially in the reigns of Charles I. and James II.: the latter monarch was visiting his army encamped here, in June 1688, when he was alarmed by the acclamations of the soldiers, on the arrival of the news of the acquittal of the "seven bishops," who had been tried for a supposed libel against the government. On this heath, about forty years since, barracks for cavalry were erected, which afford accommodation for three hundred and sixty men, with their horses. The buildings consist of a centre forming the officers' apartments, and east and west wings, with some additional erections, within an enclosure of nearly four acres in extent; and at a short distance is the ground for military exercise. The heath has been enclosed, in pursuance of an act of parliament passed in the 53rd of George III., since which many buildings have been erected here. About two miles to the south-west of Hounslow are the extensive gunpowder-mills of Messrs. Curtis and Harvey, which have been very much improved within the last few years, and where a curious pump, worked by wind-sails, raises from thirty to fifty tons of water in a minute. Here is also another gunpowder-mill, and a mill for dressing flax. Hounslow is within the jurisdiction of a court of requests for the recovery of debts under 40s., held at Brentford during the summer half year, and at Uxbridge during winter. The living is a perpetual curacy, in the archdeaconry of Middlesex, and diocese of London, and in the alternate patronage of the Bishop of London, and the Dean and Canons of Windsor. The ancient chapel of the priory, which, since the Reformation, had been used as a chapel of ease to Heston, was taken down, and in June 1828, the erection of a new church on its site was commenced, which was completed in December 1829, at an expense of £5310. 10., defrayed partly by the parliamentary commissioners, and partly by voluntary contribution: it is a fine edifice in the later style of English architecture, with a low spire and two turrets; and it contains one thousand and thirty-five sittings, of which, four hundred and eighteen are free. Hounslow is about to be constituted a distinct parish, so far as regards ecclesiastical affairs. There are places of worship for Independents and Wesleyan Methodists.

HOUSHAM, a township in the parish of CADNEY, southern division of the wapentake of YARBOROUGH, parts of LINDSEY, county of LINCOLN, 4 miles (S. E. by E.) from Glandford-Bridge. The population is returned with the parish.

HOVE, a parish in the hundred of PRESTON, rape of LEWES, county of SUSSEX, 2 miles (W. by N.) from Brighton, containing 312 inhabitants. The living is a vicarage not in charge, with that of Preston, in the archdeaconry of Lewes, and diocese of Chichester. The church, dedicated to St. Andrew, is in the early style of English architecture. This was a considerable village for a long time subsequently to the Norman Conquest, but is now almost swallowed up by the encroachments of the sea.

HOVERINGHAM, a parish in the southern division of the wapentake of THURGARTON, county of NOTTINGHAM, 5 miles (S.) from Southwell, containing 335 inhabitants. The living is a perpetual curacy, in the archdeaconry of Nottingham, and diocese of York, endowed with £200 royal bounty, and £400 parliamentary grant, and in the patronage of the Master and Fellows of Trinity College, Cambridge. The church, dedicated to St. Michael, has a Norman porch.

HOVETON (ST. JOHN), a parish in the hundred of TUNSTEAD, county of NORFOLK, 2½ miles (E. S. E.) from Coltishall, containing 270 inhabitants. The living is a discharged vicarage, united with that of Hoveton St. Peter (neither of them rated in the king's books), in the archdeaconry and diocese of Norwich, endowed with £200 royal bounty.

HOVETON (ST. PETER), a parish in the hundred of TUNSTEAD, county of NORFOLK, 2½ miles (E. by S.) from Coltishall, containing 117 inhabitants. The living is a discharged vicarage, with which that of Hoveton St. John is united, in the archdeaconry and diocese of Norwich, and in the patronage of the Bishop of Norwich.

HOVINGHAM, a parish comprising the township of Scackleton, in the wapentake of BULMER, and the townships of Aryholme with Hawthorpe, Cotton, Fryton, Hovingham, South Holme, and Wath, in the wapentake of RYEDALE, North riding of the county of YORK, and containing 1115 inhabitants, of which number, 649 are in the township of Hovingham, 8 miles (W. N. W.) from New Malton. The living is a perpetual curacy, in the archdeaconry of Cleveland, and diocese of York, endowed with £200 private benefaction, £400 royal bounty, and £1500 parliamentary grant, and in the patronage of the Earl of Carlisle. The church is dedicated to All Saints. There is a place of worship for Wesleyan Methodists. A small sum was bequeathed, in 1716, by Mrs. Frances Arthington, for the instruction of six poor children: the income is £2. 8. per annum, and four children are educated. A school was endowed in 1804, by a bequest of £200 from the Rev. James Graves, by means of the dividends upon which twelve children are educated. In a field about one mile from the village are three springs of sulphureous, chalybeate, and clear water: the medicinal properties of the first have attracted many visitors. Hovingham-hall, anciently the seat of Roger de Mowbray, is now the property of the Worsley family: in 1745, a Roman hypocaust and bath, with a piece of tesselated Roman pavement, were discovered in the garden, and near the bath some coins from Antoninus Pius to Constantine: on the side of an adjoining hill is a breast-work, supposed to be of Roman origin. A vicinal way is believed to have passed through the village, from Malton to Aldborough.

HOW-BOUND, a township in the parish of CASTLE-SOWERBY, LEATH ward, county of CUMBERLAND, 3¾ miles (S. E. by E.) from Hesket-Newmarket, containing 279 inhabitants. On the summit of How-hill, in this parish, is an enclosure surrounded by a mound of stone and earth, and crowned with several large oaks.

HOW-CAPLE, a parish in the hundred of GREY-TREE, county of HEREFORD, 6 miles (N. N. E.) from Ross, containing 117 inhabitants. The living is a rectory, united to that of Sollers-Hope, in the archdeaconry and diocese of Hereford, rated in the king's books at £9. The church is dedicated to St. Andrew.

HOWDEN, a parish in the wapentake of HOWDEN-SHIRE, East riding of the county of YORK, comprising the market town of Howden, the chapelries of Barmby on the Marsh, and Laxton, and the townships of Asselby, Balkholme, Belby, Cotness, Kilpin, Knedlington, Metham, Saltmarsh, Skelton, Thorpe, and Yorkfleet, and containing 4443 inhabitants, of which number, 2080 are in the town of Howden, 21 miles (S. E. by S.) from York, and 184 (N. by W.) from London. This place, which is of considerable antiquity, was chiefly distinguished for its collegiate establishment, founded by Robert, Bishop of Durham, in 1266, for secular clerks, and dedicated to St. Peter and St. Paul: there were originally five prebends, to which a sixth was subsequently added: the aggregate revenue, at the dissolution, was £101. 18. A palace was erected here in the fourteenth century, by Walter Skirlaw, Bishop of Durham, as a summer residence for the prelates of that see, the remains of which have been converted into farm-buildings. The town is pleasantly situated in a richly-cultivated and level tract of country, about a mile from the north side of the river Ouse: the houses are in general built of brick, but of mean appearance; the streets are roughly paved, partially lighted with oil, and the inhabitants are but indifferently supplied with water. There is no particular branch of trade carried on, the labouring class being principally employed in agriculture: there is a ferry over the river about a mile from the town, also a small harbour for boats. The market is on Saturday: the fairs are on the second Tuesday in January, April 15th, the second Tuesday after the 13th of July, and every fourth Tuesday in the year, for horses and cattle. Courts leet and baron are held occasionally, in a room belonging to the ancient episcopal palace; and a court of requests for the recovery of debts under 40s., was formerly held, but has fallen into disuse. The living is a vicarage not in charge, in the jurisdiction of the peculiar court of Howdenshire, and diocese of York, endowed with £200 parliamentary grant, and in the patronage of the Crown. The church, dedicated to St. Peter, and formerly collegiate, is a spacious and stately cruciform structure, partly in the early, but principally in the decorated, style of English architecture, with a lofty square embattled tower rising from the intersection, of which the upper part, raised by Bishop Skirlaw, is in the later English style; the west front of the church is of bold and simple character, but a fine composition, and the east end, now in ruins, was one of the richest specimens of the decorated style in the kingdom: the chancel having fallen into decay, the nave was fitted up for the performance of divine service in 1636; the roof is supported by finely-clustered columns and pointed arches, and in the north aisle of the choir, and in a chapel near the south transept, are two finely-executed monuments in the decorated style. The chapter-house, the roof of which has fallen, was a superb octagonal edifice, inferior only in dimensions to the chapter-house at York: it contains thirty canopied stalls richly ornamented with tabernacle-work, and exhibiting a considerable degree of perfection in the principal details, which are extremely beautiful. There are places of worship for Independents, Wesleyan Methodists, and Sandemanians. A free school, in which sixteen children are instructed, is supported by a bequest from Robert Jefferson, of £21 per annum, which is paid to the master, and by a rent-charge of £2. 8. A National school, in which three hundred children of both sexes are instructed, is supported by subscription; and there are Sunday schools in connexion with the established church and the dissenting congregations. Some considerable benefactions have been made for apprenticing poor children, and for other charitable purposes.

HOWDEN-PANS, a township in the parish of WALLSEND, eastern division of CASTLE ward, county of NORTHUMBERLAND, 2¼ miles (S. W.) from North Shields. The population is returned with the parish. Here are places of worship for Wesleyan Methodists and those in the New Connexion. This village is situated on the river Tyne, at the foot of some lofty eminences. Glass-works were in operation here in the sixteenth and seventeenth centuries, afterwards numerous salt-pans, but at present the coal trade chiefly prevails, large quantities being shipped for London and other places from the staiths. Frigates and vessels for India were built here during the American war, but now only those employed in the exportation of coal are built or repaired. Here is an extensive rope-walk; and at East Howden is a large manufactory for lamp-black and coal-tar.

HOWE, a parish in the hundred of CLAVERING, though locally in that of Henstead, county of NORFOLK, 6½ miles (S. S. E.) from Norwich, containing 99 inhabitants. The living is a discharged rectory with Little Poringland, in the archdeaconry of Norfolk, and diocese of Norwich, rated in the king's books at £8. 13. 4., and in the patronage of Mrs. Wheler. The church, dedicated to St. Mary, has a circular tower.

HOWE, a township in that part of the parish of PICKHILL which is in the wapentake of HALLIKELD, North riding of the county of YORK, 5¼ miles (W. S. W.) from Thirsk, containing 32 inhabitants.

HOWELL, a parish in the wapentake of ASWARD-HURN, parts of KESTEVEN, county of LINCOLN, 5 miles (E. by N.) from Sleaford, containing 67 inhabitants. The living is a rectory, in the archdeaconry and diocese of Lincoln, rated in the king's books at £13. 10. Mrs. Reynolds was patroness in 1812. The church, dedicated to St. Oswald, has portions in the Norman, with insertions in the early and decorated styles of English architecture; the font is in the later style.

HOWGILL, a chapelry in the parish of SEDBERGH, western division of the wapentake of STAINCLIFFE and EWCROSS, West riding of the county of YORK, 5 miles (N. W. by N.) from Sedbergh. The population is returned with the parish. The living is a perpetual curacy, in the archdeaconry of Richmond, and diocese of York, endowed with £800 royal bounty, and in the patronage of the Vicar of Sedbergh.

HOWGRAVE, a joint township with Sutton, in the parish of KIRKLINGTON, wapentake of HALLIKELD, North riding of the county of YORK, 5¼ miles (W.S.W.) from Thirsk, containing 122 inhabitants.

HOWGRAVE, a joint township with Nunwick, in that part of the parish of RIPON which is within the liberty of RIPON, though locally in the lower division of the wapentake of Claro, West riding of the county of YORK, 5 miles (N.) from Ripon, containing 28 inhabitants.

HOWICK, a township in the parish of PENWORTHAM, hundred of LEYLAND, county palatine, of LANCASTER, 2¾ miles (W. S. W.) from Preston, containing 136 inhabitants. A free school was built in 1729, by Christopher Walton and others : the income is £29. 5. per annum, and about thirty children are instructed.

HOWICK, an extra-parochial liberty, in the upper division of the hundred of CALDICOTT, county of MONMOUTH, 3¼ miles (N. W. by W.) from Chepstow, containing 34 inhabitants. The tithes of this liberty are claimed by the rector of Itton.

HOWICK, a parish in the southern division of BAMBROUGH ward, county of NORTHUMBERLAND, 5½ miles (N. E. by E.) from Alnwick, containing 234 inhabitants. The living is a rectory, annexed to the archdeaconry of Northumberland, diocese of Durham, rated in the king's books at £36. 13. 4., and in the patronage of the Bishop of Durham. The church is dedicated to St. Mary. A free school was founded and built by the first Sir Henry Grey, Bart., who endowed it with £10 per annum charged on the Howick estate, with a house and garden for the master: the endowment was augmented by Mrs. Magdalen Grey, of Durham, with a rent-charge of £13. The school-room has been recently rebuilt, and the master receives £5 per annum from Earl Grey, in addition to the previous endowment. In the park of Howick hall, the seat of Earl Grey, is a fine trout stream, crossed by a bridge of ashlar work : on the eastern side are the remains of a Roman encampment, where, more than half a century ago, spears, swords, coins, gold rings linked together in the form of a gorget, were discovered. In the vicinity were also found several large urns and some human bones, four feet beneath the surface of the earth. Howick confers the inferior title of viscount upon the family of Grey.

HOWSHAM, a township in the parish of SCRAYINGHAM, wapentake of BUCKROSE, East riding of the county of YORK, 7½ miles (S. S. W.) from New Malton, containing 225 inhabitants.

HOWTELL, a township in the parish of KIRKNEWTON, western division of GLENDALE ward, county of NORTHUMBERLAND, 8 miles (N. W. by W.) from Wooler, containing 190 inhabitants.

HOXNE, a parish in the hundred of HOXNE, county of SUFFOLK, 3¼ miles (N. E.) from Eye, containing 1066 inhabitants. The living is a vicarage, annexed to that of Denham, in the archdeaconry of Suffolk, and diocese of Norwich, rated in the king's books at £12. 3. 6½. The church is dedicated to St. Peter and St. Paul. A free school was founded and endowed by Lord Maynard, in 1761 : the premises consist of schoolrooms and residences for the master and the mistress : about forty boys and twenty girls are instructed, and some of the children are occasionally apprenticed: the master's salary is £42 per annum, and that of the mistress £12. Here was a priory of Benedictine monks, subordinate to that at Norwich, the revenue of which, at the dissolution, was valued at £18. 10. per annum.

HOXTON, a district parish in the Tower division of the hundred of OSSULSTONE, county of MIDDLESEX, ½ a mile (N.E.) from London. The population is returned with the parish of St. Leonard, Shoreditch. This place, formerly a hamlet in the parish of St. Leonard, has been greatly enlarged within the last few years, and having become an extensive and populous district, was constituted a parish by act of parliament in 1830. It is divided into Hoxton Old Town, and Hoxton New Town ; the former containing many ancient and spacious houses, some of which have fallen into decay, and others have been converted into private lunatic asylums ; and the latter, consisting of numerous well-formed streets and neat ranges of modern buildings, occasionally interspersed with pleasant cottages. The town is well paved, lighted with gas, and amply supplied with water. The principal manufactories are for machinery of various kinds, pins, vinegar, &c.: there are an extensive saw-mill, and numerous lime and coal wharfs on the banks of the Regent's canal, which passes through the northern part of the parish. Hoxton is within the jurisdiction of a court of requests held at Whitechapel, for the recovery of debts under 40s.

The living is a vicarage not in charge, in the archdeaconry of Middlesex, and diocese of London, and in the patronage of the Dean of St. Paul's. The church, dedicated to St. John the Baptist, and containing one thousand nine hundred and ninety-five sittings, of which one thousand are free, was erected, in 1826, by grant from the parliamentary commissioners, at an expense of £13,000 : it is a handsome edifice of light brick, with a cornice and ornaments of stone, and a steeple consisting of successive stages of campanile turrets crowned with a dome. There are places of worship for Independents, Wesleyan Methodists, and Methodists of the New Connexion. The ancient cemetery of the Jews is in this parish. A spacious National school is supported by subscription, in which about five hundred children are instructed ; and an infant school, in which are two hundred children, was established in 1829. Lady Viscountess Lumley founded almshouses, and endowed them for three aged persons of the parish of St. Botolph, Aldgate, and three of the parish of St. Botolph, Bishopsgate : they were rebuilt in 1822. The Haberdashers' almshouses were founded, in 1692, by Robert Aske, who endowed them with estates in this parish and at Ashford in Kent, for the residence and support of twenty poor members of that company, and for the clothing, maintenance, and education of twenty boys, sons of freemen of the company : the old buildings were taken down in 1825, and the present handsome structure erected on the site. The premises occupy three sides of a quadrangular area, in the centre of which is a statue of the founder : the centre comprises a handsome chapel, with a portico of the Grecian Doric order, on each side of which are apartments for the chaplain and schoolmaster, schoolroom and dormitory for the boys, and domestic offices ; the wings, in front of which is a colonnade, are appropriated to the aged men, who have each a separate house, and are in other respects comfortably provided for. William Fuller, Esq., in 1795, founded and endowed almshouses for twelve aged women, who have a weekly allowance of money, and a chaldron of coal annually ; and also other almshouses in Gloucester-street, for sixteen aged women, who receive a similar allowance

Almshouses near Gloucester-terrace were founded in 1749, by Mrs. Mary Westby, who endowed them for ten aged women.

HOYLAND (HIGH), a parish in the wapentake of STAINCROSS, West riding of the county of YORK, comprising the townships of West Clayton and High Hoyland, and containing, exclusively of a portion of the township of Skelmanthorpe which is in this parish, 1122 inhabitants, of which number, 268 are in the township of High Hoyland, 5½ miles (N.W. by W.) from Barnesley. The living is a discharged rectory, formerly in medieties, now united, in the archdeaconry and diocese of York, each rated in the king's books at £5. 3. 4., the first endowed with £200 private benefaction, and £200 royal bounty, and in the patronage of T. W. Beaumont, Esq. The church is dedicated to All Saints.

HOYLAND (NETHER), a chapelry in the parish of WATH upon DEARN, northern division of the wapentake of STRAFFORTH and TICKHILL, West riding of the county of YORK, 5 miles (S.S.E.) from Barnesley, containing, with Upper Hoyland, 1229 inhabitants. The living is a perpetual curacy, in the archdeaconry and diocese of York, endowed with £800 private benefaction, £200 royal bounty, and £1300 parliamentary grant, and in the patronage of the Vicar of Wath upon Dearn. A new church is being erected by means of a grant from the parliamentary commissioners. Ten poor boys and ten poor girls are educated for £10 per annum, paid by Earl Fitzwilliam.

HOYLAND-SWAINE, a township in the parish of SILKSTONE, wapentake of STAINCROSS, West riding of the county of YORK, 2 miles (N.E.) from Penistone, containing 738 inhabitants.

HUBBERHOLME, a chapelry in that part of the parish of ARNCLIFFE which is in the eastern division of the wapentake of STAINCLIFFE and EWCROSS, West riding of the county of YORK, 18 miles (N.E. by N.) from Settle. The population is returned with the parish. The living is a perpetual curacy, in the archdeaconry and diocese of York, endowed with £200 private benefaction, and £800 royal bounty, and in the patronage of the Vicar of Arncliffe. The church is dedicated to St. Michael.

HUBY, a township in the parish of SUTTON on the FOREST, wapentake of BULMER, North riding of the county of YORK, 9 miles (N.N.W.) from York, containing 497 inhabitants. Here are places of worship for the Society of Friends, and Primitive and Wesleyan Methodists.

HUCKING, a parish in the hundred of EYHORNE, lathe of AYLESFORD, county of KENT, 7 miles (E. by N.) from Maidstone, containing 158 inhabitants. The living is a perpetual curacy, with the vicarage of Hollingbourn, in the archdeaconry and diocese of Canterbury. The church is dedicated to St. Margaret. The village stands on the ridge of a line of chalk hills, and was anciently called *Honkynge*, from its elevated situation.

HUCKLE-COT, a hamlet in the parish of CHURCHDOWN, upper division of the hundred of DUDSTONE and KING'S BARTON, county of GLOUCESTER, 2½ miles (E. S. E.) from Gloucester, containing 439 inhabitants.

HUCKLOW (GREAT), a hamlet in the parish of HOPE, hundred of HIGH PEAK, county of DERBY, 2¼ miles (N. E.) from Tidswell, containing 274 inhabitants.

There are places of worship for Presbyterians, Wesleyan Methodists, and Unitarians.

HUCKLOW (LITTLE), a liberty in the parish of HOPE, hundred of HIGH PEAK, county of DERBY, 2 miles (N. N. E.) from Tidswell, containing 218 inhabitants.

HUCKNALL under HUTHWAITE, a hamlet in the parish of SUTTON in ASHFIELD, northern division of the wapentake of BROXTOW, county of NOTTINGHAM, 5 miles (W. by S.) from Mansfield, containing 712 inhabitants. This place is within the ecclesiastical jurisdiction of the peculiar court of the manor of Mansfield. There is a place of worship for Wesleyan Methodists.

HUCKNALL-TORKARD, a parish in the northern division of the wapentake of BROXTOW, county of NOTTINGHAM, 6½ miles (N. N. W.) from Nottingham, containing 1940 inhabitants. The living is a discharged vicarage, in the archdeaconry of Nottingham, and diocese of York, rated in the king's books at £4. 18. 1½., endowed with £400 royal bounty, and £200 parliamentary grant, and in the patronage of the Duke of Portland. The church, dedicated to St. Mary Magdalene, is an ancient edifice, containing several monuments in memory of different members of the Byron family: here lie the remains of the late celebrated poet, George Gordon, Lord Byron; he died at Missolonghi, in Western Greece, in 1824, and was interred here, on the 16th of July in that year, in the family vault, which is beneath the communion table, and contains twelve leaden coffins: in the chancel is a neat mural monument, with an appropriate inscription, to his memory, placed there by his lordship's sister, the Hon. Augusta Mary Leigh. In the church is a book wherein the names of several hundred visitors to the poet's tomb are entered. There is also a monument to his ancestor Richard, Lord Byron, who, with the rest of his family, being seven brothers, faithfully served Charles I. during the civil war, and sustained great losses and hardships on account of his loyalty to that monarch; he died in 1679. Here are places of worship for General Baptists, and Primitive and Wesleyan Methodists. A Sunday school is endowed with £13 per annum, being a third portion of the proceeds of a bequest for charitable purposes by John Byron, in 1571: a parochial schoolroom was built by subscription in 1815. Frame-work knitting is carried on to a great extent in the parish. On the enclosure of the waste lands twenty-five acres were allotted for the benefit of poor housekeepers, now yielding the sum of £22. 10. per annum.

HUDDERSFIELD, a parish in the upper division of the wapentake of AGBRIGG, West riding of the county of YORK, comprising the market town of Huddersfield, the chapelries of Lindley, Longwood, Scammonden, and Slaithwaite, and a portion of Marsden, and the township of Golcar, and containing 24,220 inhabitants, of which number, 13,284 are in the town of Huddersfield, 40 miles (S. W.) from York, and 189 (N. N. W.) from London. The town possesses no claim to antiquity, having sprung up within the last century, almost entirely in consequence of the progress of the woollen manufacture, of which it is one of the principal marts in the county. The origin of its name is uncertain, though Gough, in his additions to Camden, is of opinion that it is derived from *Hudard*, a Saxon, whom he supposes to have gained a victory here. The town is situated on the river Colne, on the high road between Leeds and Manchester, partly on the declivity, and partly on the summit, of an eminence, which is surrounded by others of superior height. The streets are regular and well paved, and contain several houses of considerable respectability; but the chief ornaments of the town are the churches and chapels, which are principally constructed of stone: there are also several extensive mills, erected lately, for the manufacture of woollen cloth. In 1765, Sir John Ramsden, of Byram, near Ferrybridge, to whom nearly the whole of the town belongs, erected a hall for the accommodation of the manufacturers, in which they expose their goods for sale : it is a large circular building, consisting of two stories, and the interior is divided into two courts, or semicircular areas : the light is admitted through windows fronting the inner areas, the outer wall being a perfect blank : the hall is divided into avenues, and the cloth exposed for sale upon stalls. Above the entrance door is a handsome cupola, in which are placed a clock and a bell, the market opening and closing at the sound of the latter. The town is lighted with gas, under the management of a joint-stock company; and supplied with water from reservoirs at Longwood and Nettleton hill, an act of parliament appointing commissioners for that purpose having been recently obtained. The chief articles of manufacture are woollen cloth (broad and narrow), serge, kerseymere, and corduroy, with a variety of fancy goods to a very considerable extent : the fancy manufacture of this town and neighbourhood has been established within the present century, and, besides the articles already referred to, includes a great variety intended for waistcoats and pantaloons, made of worsted and cotton. The silk valentias, now so commonly exposed in the shops of the drapers throughout the kingdom, are the produce of this neighbourhood, and, for beauty of design and texture, possess superior merit. An immense quantity of these articles is exported to the continent, and their manufacture affords employment to several thousand individuals. The manufacture of shawls, toilinets, capinets, &c., has also been introduced with success, and the shawls are acknowledged to equal the French merinos, though fabricated from British wool. The town is advantageously situated for commerce, and the inhabitants enjoy the benefit of that line of inland navigation which extends across the kingdom from the Atlantic to the German ocean. The Huddersfield canal, constructed pursuant to an act of parliament obtained in 1774, commences here, and, taking a south-westerly course, enters a tunnel near Marsden, which is about three miles and a half in length, under Pule hill and Standage, and emerges near Digloe mill, in Saddleworth, about two miles and a half from Dobcross; and after crossing the winding course of the Tame, in several places, it leaves the county near Lydgate, and joins the Ashton and Oldham canal near Ashton under Line, whence the line extends to Manchester and Liverpool. The Ramsden canal, which commences at the King's mills, close to the town, unites with the Calder at Cooper's bridge; then, by means of that river, the Aire, the Ouse, and the Humber, a navigable line extends to the German ocean; embracing in its direction the trading towns of Halifax, Wakefield, Leeds, and Hull. The market is on Tuesday, when the doors of the hall are opened early in the morning, and closed at half past

eleven; but are again opened at three, for the removal of cloth, &c. There are three fairs, viz., on the 31st of March, 4th of May, and 1st of October, chiefly for cattle. A constable for the town, and a deputy constable, are chosen annually. The petty sessions for the upper division of Agbrigg are held here : and there is a court baron for the liberty and honour of Pontefract, for the recovery of debts under £5; also a court of requests, instituted under an act of parliament passed in the 33rd of George III., for the recovery of debts under 40s. Besides these there are courts leet and baron for the manor of Almondbury, the former of which is held here, and the latter at Almondbury, Huddersfield being within its jurisdiction.

The living is a discharged vicarage, rated in the king's books at £17. 13. 4., in the peculiar jurisdiction of the manorial court of Marsden, and in the patronage of Sir John Ramsden. The church, dedicated to St. Peter, is an ancient and spacious, but plain, cruciform edifice, having a tower with battlements and pinnacles rising from the intersection. There is also a chapel dedicated to the Holy Trinity, an elegant structure, occupying an elevated situation on the north-western side of the town : it was begun in 1817, and consecrated on the 10th of October, 1819, having been built at the expense of B. Haigh Allen, Esq., and contains more than one thousand five hundred sittings, of which one third are free. The living is a perpetual curacy, endowed with £1000 parliamentary grant, and in the patronage of B. Haigh Allen, Esq. Christ church, at Woodhouse, consecrated on the 28th of October, 1824, was built by John Whitacre, Esq., who holds the presentation. There are also three chapels of ease, viz., at Longwood, Deanhead, and Slaithwaite; and three new churches have been recently built at Paddock, Golcar, and Lindley, by grants from the parliamentary commissioners, all of which are within the parish, and in the presentation of the Vicar. Besides these, another church is now being erected in Huddersfield, to be dedicated to St. Paul. Here are places of worship for Baptists, the Society of Friends, Independents, Primitive and Wesleyan Methodists, and Methodists in the New Connexion, Southcotians, and Roman Catholics ; those of the Independents and the Wesleyan Methodists are large and handsome buildings. A National school, built in 1820, on ground given for the foundation of a school by John Ramsden, Esq., in 1681, is supported by voluntary contributions, and about five hundred children at present are educated in it. There is also a school of industry for girls, recently established by the ladies of Huddersfield ; and two infant schools are about to be erected. A mechanics' institute, with a library attached to it, was founded in 1825, and a savings bank in 1818. A dispensary was established in 1814 ; and an infirmary is now being erected at the estimated expense of between £4000 and £5000. Sulphureous and chalybeate springs have been discovered at Erringden and Slaithwaite, in this parish, and at other places in the neighbourhood ; and public baths, called Lockwood spa, have lately been established about three quarters of a mile from Huddersfield. These elegant and commodious baths were first opened to the public in May 1827 : they are built of stone, and embrace every desirable convenience ; they are abundantly supplied with the spa water, and the charges and direction of the whole are regulated by a committee of shareholders, under the management of an experienced steward. The spa water is said to possess qualities highly beneficial in glandular, rheumatic, gouty, and dyspeptic complaints.

HUDDINGTON, a parish in the middle division of the hundred of OSWALDSLOW, county of WORCESTER, 4¾ miles (S. S. E.) from Droitwich, containing 125 inhabitants. The living is a perpetual curacy, in the archdeaconry and diocese of Worcester, endowed with £600 royal bounty, and £200 parliamentary grant, and in the patronage of the Earl of Shrewsbury. The church is dedicated to St. Michael.

HUDDLESTON, a joint township with Lumby, in that part of the parish of SHERBURN which is in the upper division of the wapentake of BARKSTONE-ASH, West riding of the county of YORK, 7 miles (N. N. W.) from Ferry-Bridge, containing 184 inhabitants. Here is a quarry of fine stone, which, although soft at first, acquires considerable hardness by exposure to the atmosphere : the chapel of Henry VII., in Westminster abbey, was partly built of this stone.

HUDNALL, a hamlet in the parish of EDDLESBOROUGH, hundred of COTTESLOE, county of BUCKINGHAM, containing 91 inhabitants.

HUDSWELL, a chapelry in that part of the parish of CATTERICK which is in the western division of the wapentake of HANG, North riding of the county of YORK, 2¼ miles (W. S. W.) from Richmond, containing 305 inhabitants. The living is a perpetual curacy, in the archdeaconry of Richmond, and diocese of Chester, endowed with £600 royal bounty, and in the patronage of the Vicar of Catterick. A free school is supported by the proceeds of an allotment assigned on the enclosure of waste lands, now amounting to £18 per annum, for which twelve children are educated gratuitously. Here are an extensive lead mine and a colliery.

HUELSFIELD, county of GLOUCESTER. — See HEWELSFIELD.

HUGGATE, a parish in the Wilton-Beacon division of the wapentake of HARTHILL, East riding of the county of YORK, 7½ miles (N. E.) from Pocklington, containing 413 inhabitants. The living is a rectory, in the archdeaconry of the East riding, and diocese of York, rated in the king's books at £15, and in the patronage of the Crown. The church is dedicated to St. Mary. There is a place of worship for Wesleyan Methodists. The inhabitants are supplied with water from a well one hundred and sixteen yards in depth. Races are held in July.

HUGGLESCOTE, a joint chapelry with Donnington, in the parish of IBSTOCK, hundred of SPARKENHOE, county of LEICESTER, 6 miles (S. E. by E.) from Ashby de la Zouch, containing 683 inhabitants.

HUGHLEY, a parish within the liberty of the borough of WENLOCK, county of SALOP, 4¼ miles (W. S. W.) from Much Wenlock, containing 101 inhabitants. The living is a discharged rectory, in the archdeaconry of Salop, and diocese of Hereford, rated in the king's books at £4. 11. 3., endowed with £200 private benefaction, and £200 royal bounty, and in the patronage of the Earl of Bradford. The church is dedicated to St. John the Baptist. The woods in this parish anciently afforded a secure retreat to robbers, since, in the reign of Richard II., a special commission was issued to enquire as to the malefactors in the woods of Hughley.

HUGIL, a chapelry in that part of the parish of KENDAL which is in KENDAL ward, county of WESTMORLAND, 6¼ miles (N. W.) from Kendal, containing 300 inhabitants. The living is a perpetual curacy, in the archdeaconry of Richmond, and diocese of Chester, endowed with £200 private benefaction, and £600 royal bounty, and in the patronage of the Landowners. The chapel, rebuilt in 1743, by Robert Bateman, stands in the village of Ings, which is in this chapelry. The free school was endowed with land, in 1650, by Rowland Wilson, producing at present £12 per annum : the average number of boys is twenty-five : this endowment was augmented with £8 per annum, by Robert Bateman, who also gave £1000 for purchasing an estate, and erecting eight almshouses for as many poor families, besides a donation of £12 per annum to the curate. This worthy benefactor was born here, and, from a state of indigence, succeeded in amassing considerable wealth by mercantile pursuits : he is stated to have been poisoned in the straits of Gibraltar, on his voyage from Leghorn, with a valuable cargo, by the captain of the vessel. Bobbin-turning and the manufacture of woollen cloth are carried on here. On the summit of High Knott is a circular obelisk, erected by the Rev. Thomas Williamson, to the memory of his father.

HUISH, a parish in the hundred of SHEBBEAR, county of DEVON, 4¾ miles (N.) from Hatherleigh, containing 118 inhabitants. The living is a discharged rectory, in the archdeaconry of Barnstaple, and diocese of Exeter, rated in the king's books at £7. 19. 10., and in the patronage of Lord Clinton. The church is dedicated to St. James.

HUISH (NORTH), a parish in the hundred of STANBOROUGH, county of DEVON, 4¾ miles (N. E.) from Modbury, containing 440 inhabitants. The living is a rectory, in the archdeaconry of Totness, and diocese of Exeter, rated in the king's books at £29. 18. 11½., and in the patronage of Sir John Perring, Bart. Here is an almshouse, endowed, in 1517, by T. Tremayne, Esq. The river Avon separates this parish from that of Diptford.

HUISH (SOUTH), a parish in the hundred of STANBOROUGH, county of DEVON, 3¾ miles (S. W.) from Kingsbridge, containing 383 inhabitants. The living is a perpetual curacy, annexed to the vicarage of West Allington, in the archdeaconry of Totness, and diocese of Exeter. On the rocks near the sea are the remains of an old castle, which, according to tradition, suffered from Cromwell's party during the civil war : a cannon ball and a curious antique key were found, about seven years since, within the walls. At Woodville, in this parish, lemons, oranges, citrons, and olives, flourish against the garden walls, with only a temporary protection from the weather : about seven years since the Mediterranean aloe blossomed in open ground, and attained the height of twenty-seven feet, but died immediately, though not twenty years of age, leaving numerous suckers. The fishing cove in Bigbury bay called Outer Hope, is in this parish.

HUISH-CHAMPFLOWER, a parish in the hundred of WILLITON and FREEMANNERS, county of SOMERSET, 2¾ miles (W. by N.) from Wiveliscombe, containing 317 inhabitants. The living is a rectory, in the archdeaconry of Taunton, and diocese of Bath and Wells, rated in the king's books at £13. 9. 4½.   Sir J.

Trevelyan, Bart, was patron in 1823. The church is dedicated to St. Peter.

HUISH-EPISCOPI, a parish in the eastern division of the hundred of KINGSBURY, though locally in the hundred of Somerton, county of SOMERSET, ½ a mile (E.) from Langport, containing 472 inhabitants. The living is a discharged vicarage with that of Langport, in the peculiar jurisdiction and patronage of the Archdeacon of Wells, as Prebendary of Huish in the Cathedral Church of Wells, rated in the king's books at £14. 10. 5., endowed with £200 private benefaction, and £200 royal bounty. The church, dedicated to St. Mary, has a handsome western tower ornamented with battlements and pinnacles. The navigable rivers Parret and Yeo, or Ivel, unite in this parish.

HUISH-ROAD, a chapelry in the parish and hundred of CARHAMPTON, county of SOMERSET, 4 miles (S.E.) from Dunster. The population is returned with the parish.

HULAM, or HOLOM, a township in the parish of MONK-HESLETON, southern division of EASINGTON ward, county palatine of DURHAM, 12¾ miles (N.) from Stockton upon Tees, containing 16 inhabitants.

HULCOTE, a hamlet in the parish of EASTON-NESTON, hundred of CLELEY, county of NORTHAMPTON, 1½ mile (N.E. by E.) from Towcester. The population is returned with the parish.

HULCOTT, a parish in the hundred of AYLESBURY, county of BUCKINGHAM, 3 miles (N.E. by E.) from Aylesbury, containing 139 inhabitants. The living is a rectory, in the archdeaconry of Buckingham, and diocese of Lincoln, rated in the king's books at £10. 0. 2½. John Brereton, Esq. was patron in 1819. The church, dedicated to All Saints, is a small structure with a wooden steeple. The river Thames runs through the parish.

HULL, a joint township with Appleton, in that part of the parish of GREAT BUDWORTH which is in the hundred of BUCKLOW, county palatine of CHESTER, containing 1435 inhabitants.

HULL (County of the town of).—See KINGSTON upon HULL.

HULL (BISHOP'S), a parish in the hundred of TAUNTON and TAUNTON-DEAN, county of SOMERSET, 1½ mile (W.) from Taunton, containing 928 inhabitants. The living is a perpetual curacy, in the archdeaconry of Taunton, and diocese of Bath and Wells, endowed with £200 private benefaction, £400 royal bounty, and £200 parliamentary grant, and in the patronage of the Rev. H. W. Rawlins. The church is dedicated to St. Peter and St. Paul.

HULLAND, a township in that part of the parish of ASHBOURN which is in the hundred of APPLETREE, county of DERBY, 4½ miles (E.) from Ashbourn, containing 221 inhabitants.

HULLAND-WARD, a hamlet in that part of the parish of ASHBOURN which is in the hundred of APPLETREE, county of DERBY, 5 miles (E. by N.) from Ashbourn, containing 289 inhabitants.

HULLAND-WARD-INTACKS, a township in that part of the parish of ASHBOURN which is in the hundred of APPLETREE, county of DERBY, 6½ miles (E. by S.) from Ashbourn, containing 39 inhabitants.

HULLAVINGTON, a parish partly in the hundred of CHIPPENHAM, comprising the tything of Surren-

dral, but chiefly in the hundred of MALMESBURY, county of WILTS, 4¾ miles (S. W. by S.) from Malmesbury, containing 506 inhabitants. The living is a discharged vicarage, in the archdeaconry of Wilts, and diocese of Salisbury, rated in the king's books at £6. 13., endowed with £200 private benefaction, and £200 royal bounty, and in the patronage of the Provost and Fellows of Eton College. The church is dedicated to St. Mary.

HULME, a joint township with Kinderton, in that part of the parish of MIDDLEWICH which is in the hundred of NORTHWICH, county palatine of CHESTER, 2¼ miles (S.E. by E.) from Middlewich, containing 469 inhabitants.

HULME, a chapelry in the parish of MANCHESTER, hundred of SALFORD, county palatine of LANCASTER, 2½ miles (S.E. by S.) from Manchester, containing 4234 inhabitants. The chapel is dedicated to St. George.

HULME, a joint township with Weston-Coyney, in the parish of CAVERSWALL, northern division of the hundred of TOTMONSLOW, county of STAFFORD, 4½ miles (W. by N.) from Cheadle, containing 527 inhabitants.

HULME (CHURCH), a chapelry in that part of the parish of SANDBACH which is in the hundred of NORTHWICH, county palatine of CHESTER, 3½ miles (E. by N.) from Middlewich, containing 397 inhabitants. The living is a perpetual curacy, in the archdeaconry and diocese of Chester, endowed with £200 private benefaction, and £200 royal bounty, and in the patronage of the Vicar of Sandbach. Thomas Hall, Esq., in 1708, gave a rent-charge of £14 for the instruction of boys and girls, which, in 1713, he augmented with another of £4. 10., for clothing them. There is also a small sum, the gift of Josiah Dean, for teaching and apprenticing one boy.

HULME (LEVENS), a township in the parish of MANCHESTER, hundred of SALFORD, county palatine of LANCASTER, 3¾ miles (S.E.) from Manchester, containing 768 inhabitants.

HULME-WALFIELD, a township in that part of the parish of ASTBURY which is in the hundred of NORTHWICH, county palatine of CHESTER, 2¼ miles (N. by W.) from Congleton, containing 108 inhabitants.

HULSE, a township in that part of the parish of GREAT BUDWORTH which is in the hundred of NORTHWICH, county palatine of CHESTER, 4 miles (E. by S.) from Northwich, containing 54 inhabitants.

HULTON (LITTLE, or PEEL), a chapelry in the parish of DEAN, hundred of SALFORD, county palatine of LANCASTER, 4½ miles (S.) from Great Bolton, containing 2465 inhabitants. The living is a perpetual curacy, in the archdeaconry and diocese of Chester, endowed with £800 private benefaction, £400 royal bounty, and £2100 parliamentary grant. Lord Kenyon was patron in 1814. The chapel is dedicated to St. Paul.

HULTON (MIDDLE), a township in the parish of DEAN, hundred of SALFORD, county palatine of LANCASTER, 3 miles (S.S.W.) from Great Bolton, containing 938 inhabitants.

HULTON (OVER), a township in the parish of DEAN, hundred of SALFORD, county palatine of LANCASTER, 3¾ miles (S.W.) from Great Bolton, containing 591 inhabitants.

HULTON-ABBEY, a township in the parish of

BURSLEM, northern division of the hundred of PIRE-HILL, county of STAFFORD, 1½ mile (E. by N.) from Hanley, containing 477 inhabitants. There is a place of worship for Wesleyan Methodists at Sneyd Green. Coal is obtained in the neighbourhood. An abbey of Cistercian monks, in honour of the Blessed Virgin Mary, was founded in 1223, by Henry de Audley, the revenue of which, at the dissolution, was £76. 14. 11.: its remains have been converted into a farm-house.

HULVERSTREET, a hamlet in that part of the parish of HENSTEAD which is in the hundred of WANG-FORD, county of SUFFOLK, containing 241 inhabitants.

HUMBER, a parish in the hundred of WOLPHY, county of HEREFORD, 4 miles (S.E. by E.) from Leominster, containing, with the township of Risbury, 219 inhabitants. The living is a discharged rectory, in the archdeaconry and diocese of Hereford, rated in the king's books at £5. 16. 3., endowed with £200 private benefaction, and £200 royal bounty, and in the patronage of the Crown. The church is dedicated to St. Mary.

HUMBERSHOE, a hamlet in that part of the parish of STUDHAM which is in the hundred of MANSHEAD, county of BEDFORD, containing 363 inhabitants.

HUMBERSTON, a parish in the wapentake of BRADLEY-HAVERSTOE, parts of LINDSEY, county of LINCOLN, 4½ miles (S.E.) from Great Grimsby, containing 217 inhabitants. The living is a discharged vicarage, in the archdeaconry and diocese of Lincoln, rated in the king's books at £5. 18. 4., endowed with £1000 royal bounty, and £200 parliamentary grant, and in the patronage of Lord Carrington. The church, dedicated to St. Peter, was rebuilt, except the tower, in the early part of the last century, at the expense of £1000, the bequest of Matthew Humberston, Esq., who died in 1709, and being interred here, a splendid monument was erected to his memory. He is said to have been a foundling from Homerton, in the parish of Hackney, who having been educated at Christ's Hospital, obtained a situation in the Custom-house, and acquiring a large fortune, purchased the manor of Humberston, from which he took his name. He also left £1100, to build and endow a school and almshouses here, which sum remained unappropriated till 1821, when the school-house and six almshouses were completed, and a residence for the vicar, to whose stipend Mr. Humberston made an addition. There is a place of worship for Wesleyan Methodists. A Benedictine monastery was founded here in the reign of Henry II., the revenue of which, at the dissolution, was £42. 11. 3.

HUMBERSTONE, a parish in the eastern division of the hundred of GOSCOTE, county of LEICESTER, 2¾ miles (E.N.E.) from Leicester, containing 415 inhabitants. The living is a discharged vicarage, in the archdeaconry of Leicester, and diocese of Lincoln, rated in the king's books at £8, endowed with £200 private benefaction, and £200 royal bounty. The Rev. John Dudley was patron in 1794. The church is dedicated to St. Mary. There is a place of worship for Wesleyan Methodists.

HUMBERTON, a joint township with Milby, partly in the parish of KIRBY on the MOOR, wapentake of HALLIKELD, North riding, and partly in that part of the parish of ALDBOROUGH which is in the lower division of the wapentake of CLARO, West riding, of the

county of YORK, 2½ miles (N.N.E.) from Boroughbridge, containing 143 inhabitants.

HUMBLETON, a township in the parish of DODDINGTON, eastern division of GLENDALE ward, county of NORTHUMBERLAND, 1 mile (W.N.W.) from Wooler, containing 184 inhabitants. On a rising ground near Humbleton-Bourn is an ancient encampment, called Green Castle; and on a hill in the vicinity is a circular intrenchment, with a large cairn: the declivity of the hill forms several terraces, each twenty feet deep, rising one above another. A pillar of stone has been set up on the plain, in commemoration of a great battle fought in 1402, when ten thousand Scots under Earl Douglas, who had previously plundered the country as far as Newcastle, were totally defeated by Lord Percy and the Earl of March: the field is still termed Redriggs, a name derived from the sanguinary nature of the conflict. A stone coffin, enclosing the remains of a gigantic skeleton and an urn, was discovered here in 1811.

HUMBLETON, a parish in the middle division of the wapentake of HOLDERNESS, East riding of the county of YORK, comprising the chapelry of Elstronwick, and the townships of Danthorpe, Fitling, Flinton, and Humbleton, and containing 586 inhabitants, of which number, 136 are in the township of Humbleton, 9¼ miles (N.E. by E.) from Kingston upon Hull. The living is a discharged vicarage, in the archdeaconry of the East riding, and diocese of York, rated in the king's books at £10. 1. 0½., endowed with £600 royal bounty, and in the patronage of the Crown. The church is dedicated to St. Peter. Francis Heron, in 1718, devised certain houses and lands, now producing an annual income of £70, for teaching and apprenticing eighteen children of both sexes. At Elstronwick is a school, towards the support of which, £11. 10. is paid annually to a schoolmistress from the poor's estate.

HUMBY (GREAT), a hamlet in the parish of SOMERBY, wapentake of WINNIBRIGGS and THREO, parts of KESTEVEN, county of LINCOLN, 6 miles (W. by S.) from Falkingham. The population is returned with the parish.

HUMBY (LITTLE), a hamlet in the parish of ROPSLEY, wapentake of WINNIBRIGGS and THREO, parts of KESTEVEN, county of LINCOLN, 5½ miles (W. by S.) from Falkingham, containing 65 inhabitants.

HUMSHAUGH, a chapelry in the parish of SIMONBURN, north-western division of TINDALE ward, county of NORTHUMBERLAND, 5 miles (N. by W.) from Hexham, containing 334 inhabitants. The living is a perpetual curacy, in the archdeaconry of Northumberland, and diocese of Durham, and in the patronage of the Vicar of Simonburn. The chapel and parsonage-house were erected, and a cemetery formed, in 1818, at an expense of about £4000.

HUNCOAT, a township in that part of the parish of WHALLEY which is in the higher division of the hundred of BLACKBURN, county palatine of LANCASTER, 5 miles (W.S.W.) from Burnley, containing 629 inhabitants. There is a place of worship for Baptists.

HUNCOTE, a hamlet in the parish of NARBOROUGH, hundred of SPARKENHOE, county of LEICESTER, 7 miles (S.W.) from Leicester, containing 289 inhabitants. Here was anciently a chapel, which has long since been demolished.

HUNDERSFIELD, a chapelry comprising four distinct townships, in that part of the parish of ROCHDALE which is in the hundred of SALFORD, county palatine of LANCASTER, 4 miles (N. E.) from Rochdale, with which the population is returned. The living is a perpetual curacy, in the archdeaconry and diocese of Chester, endowed with £200 private benefaction, and £200 royal bounty, and in the patronage of the Vicar of Rochdale. The chapel, dedicated to St. Mary, was consecrated in 1768. Theophilus Halliwell, in 1688, devised a messuage and lands, and Richard Halliwell, in 1699, an annual rent-charge of £6, together producing about £17 per annum, for the support of a free school, in which eleven children are educated.

HUNDERTHWAITE, a township in the parish of ROMALD-KIRK, western division of the wapentake of GILLING, North riding of the county of YORK, 5¾ miles (N. W. by W.) from Barnard-Castle, containing 313 inhabitants.

HUNDLEBY, a parish in the eastern division of the soke of BOLINGBROKE, parts of LINDSEY, county of LINCOLN, 1 mile (N. W. by W.) from Spilsby, containing 348 inhabitants. The living is a discharged vicarage held by sequestration, in the archdeaconry and diocese of Lincoln, rated in the king's books at £7. 19. 4., and endowed with £200 royal bounty. The church is dedicated to St. Mary.

HUNDON, a parish in the hundred of RISBRIDGE, county of SUFFOLK, 3¼ miles (N.N.W.) from Clare, containing 956 inhabitants. The living is a discharged vicarage, in the archdeaconry of Sudbury, and diocese of Norwich, rated in the king's books at £7. 13. 4., endowed with £200 private benefaction, and £200 royal bounty, and in the patronage of the Master and Fellows of Jesus College, Cambridge. The church is dedicated to All Saints : in a building attached to it is a noble marble pyramidal monument to the memory of Arethusa, daughter of Lord Clifford, wife of James Vernon, Esq.,and the mother of the Earl of Shipbrooke : she died in 1728. A variety of Saxon coins of Athelstan, Eadred, and Edmund, was found in a grave here, in 1687.

HUNGERFORD, a parish comprising the market town of Hungerford, and the tythings of Eddington with Hiddon, and Sandon-Fee, in the hundred of KINTBURY-EAGLE, county of BERKS, and the township of Charnham-Street in the hundred of KINWARDSTONE, county of WILTS, and containing 2373 inhabitants, of which number, 1478 are in the town of Hungerford, 26 miles (W. by S.) from Reading, and 64 (W. by S.) from London. This place was anciently called *Ingleford Charman Street*, a name signifying the ford of the Angles on the Ermin-street, a Roman road which crossed the site of the town ; the adjunct is still preserved in one of its avenues, now called Charnham-Street. The town stands on the road from London to Bath, partly on the declivity of a hill, and is considered to be particularly salubrious : the houses in general have a mean appearance, the streets are neither paved nor lighted, but the inhabitants are plentifully supplied with water from wells. At the entrance into the town, the river Kennet, which flows through it, is crossed by a handsome bridge of five arches ; and the Kennet and Avon canal affords a line of communication with Bath and Bristol, for the conveyance of corn, coal, and other heavy articles. Near the centre of the principal street is the market-house, a neat structure of brick, erected in 1787, which contains a spacious room for the transaction of public business. The market is on Wednesday; and fairs are held on the last Wednesday in April and the 10th of August for cattle; and on the Wednesdays before and after New Michaelmas, which are statute fairs. The town is under the government of a chief constable, assisted by twelve burgesses, a steward, and town clerk: the constable, who is lord of the manor, and holds his office immediately under the crown, is annually chosen on Hock-Tuesday, by the inhabitants of the town, who are convened on that occasion by the sound of a brazen horn, said to have been presented to the townsmen by John of Gaunt.

The benefice is a vicarage, in the peculiar jurisdiction and patronage of the Dean and Canons of Windsor, rated in the king's books at £9. 13. 4. The church, dedicated to St. Lawrence, is a handsome edifice, surmounted by a square embattled tower : it was erected on the site of the former church, in 1814, at the extremity of a pleasant walk, shaded by lofty trees, on the western side of the town. A window of painted glass, representing the figure of the tutelar saint, was presented by Mr. Collins, of London, on the completion of the building : in the north aisle is a circular stone, with a brass plate, to the memory of Robert de Hungerford, who was the first of that family settled in this county. There are places of worship for Independents and Wesleyan Methodists. A free grammar school for boys and girls was founded, in 1636, by the Rev. Dr. Sheaff, and endowed by Mr. Hamblen in 1729, and Mrs. Cummins in 1735 ; and Edward Capps, an old servant of the Hungerford family, bequeathed £50 for the erection of a new school-room, and £4 per annum as an addition to the master's salary. The National school, a handsome brick building erected in 1814, for an unlimited number of children, is supported by voluntary contributions. Hungerford park, situated at the extremity of the town, formerly the residence of the barons of Hungerford, is now the property of Charles Delbiac, Esq., who has erected a neat mansion in the Italian style, on the site of the old house, which was built by Queen Elizabeth, and given by her to the Earl of Essex. Dr. Samuel Chandler, a learned dissenting minister and theological writer, was born here in 1693.

HUNGERTON, a parish comprising the chapelry of Ingarsby, and the liberty of Baggrave, in the hundred of GARTREE, and the hamlet of Quenby in the eastern division of the hundred of GOSCOTE, county of LEICESTER, 7 miles (E. by N.) from Leicester, and containing 292 inhabitants. The living is a discharged vicarage, united in 1732 to that of Twyford, in the archdeaconry of Leicester, and diocese of Lincoln, rated in the king's books at £9. 8. 1½. The church is dedicated to St. John the Baptist.

HUNGERTON, a parish in the wapentake of WINNIBRIGGS and THREO, parts of KESTEVEN, county of LINCOLN, 4¾ miles (S. W. by S.) from Grantham, containing, with the parish of Wyvill, 124 inhabitants. The living is a discharged rectory with Wyvill, in the archdeaconry and diocese of Lincoln, rated in the king's books at £2. 3. 4., endowed with £400 royal bounty, but held by sequestration. The church being demolished, the inhabitants repair to Harlaxton.

HUNMANBY, a parish in the wapentake of DICK-ERING, East riding of the county of YORK, 8¼ miles (S. S. E.) from Scarborough, containing 1018 inhabitants. The living is a vicarage, in the archdeaconry of the East riding, and diocese of York, rated in the king's books at £20. 1. 8. H. Osbaldeston, Esq. was patron in 1796. The church, dedicated to All Saints, contains a splendid monument to different members of the Osbaldeston family who died within the last century. There are places of worship for Baptists and Wesleyan Methodists. A market, formerly on Tuesday, has been long disused ; but a monthly cattle market, and fairs on May 26th and October 29th, are still held here. A library was founded by the associates of Dr. Bray, for the use of the neighbouring clergy, and a parochial library, for the benefit of the poor. A National school was established, in 1810, by H. Osbaldeston, Esq., the master of which receives £60 per annum. On an eminence, called Castle hill, are vestiges of an ancient fortification.

HUNNINGHAM, a parish in the Southam division of the hundred of KNIGHTLOW, county of WARWICK, 5½ miles (N. W. by N.) from Southam, containing, exclusively of the hamlet of Hydes-Pastures, 193 inhabitants. The living is a vicarage, in the archdeaconry of Coventry, and diocese of Lichfield and Coventry, rated in the king's books at £5, endowed with £300 private benefaction, £200 royal bounty, and £200 parliamentary grant. Chandos Leigh, Esq. was patron in 1820. The church is dedicated to St. Margaret.

HUNSDON, a parish in the hundred of BRAUGHIN, county of HERTFORD, 5 miles (W. by S.) from Sawbridgeworth, containing 584 inhabitants. The living is a rectory, in the archdeaconry of Middlesex, and diocese of London, rated in the king's books at £12. N. Calvert, Esq. was patron in 1777. The church has a chapel attached on the south side, belonging to the family of Cary, Barons Hunsdon, and at the west end an embattled tower surmounted by a spire. The parish is bounded on the south by the river Stort, which separates it from Essex.

HUNSHELF, a township in the parish of PENISTONE, wapentake of STAINCROSS, West riding of the county of YORK, 3¼ miles (S. E.) from Penistone, containing 436 inhabitants.

HUNSINGORE, a parish in the upper division of the wapentake of CLARO, West riding of the county of YORK, comprising the townships of Cattal, Hunsingore, and Great Ribston with Walshford, and containing 599 inhabitants, of which number, 237 are in the township of Hunsingore, 4 miles (N. N. E.) from Wetherby. The living is a vicarage, in the peculiar jurisdiction of the Lord of the Manor, rated in the king's books at £5. 17. 3½. Sir H. Goodricke was patron in 1801. The church is dedicated to St, John the Baptist.

HUNSLET, or HUNFLEET, a chapelry within the parish and liberty of the town of LEEDS, though locally in the wapentake of Morley, West riding of the county of YORK, 2 miles (S. S. E.) from Leeds, containing 8171 inhabitants. The living is a perpetual curacy, in the archdeaconry and diocese of York, endowed with £220 private benefaction, and £200 royal bounty, and in the patronage of the Vicar of Leeds. The chapel, dedicated to St. Mary the Virgin, was erected in 1636, and enlarged to twice its first dimensions in 1744 : it has

lately received an addition of five hundred and seventy sittings, of which five hundred and fifty-five are free, the Incorporated Society for the enlargement of churches and chapels having granted £300 towards defraying the expense. A little to the eastward of it are the remains of an old building, encompassed by a moat. There are places of worship for Wesleyan Methodists and those in the New Connexion. This place, formerly the seat of the Gascoignes and Nevilles, has of late years, from its vicinity to Leeds, and the establishment of manufactories similar to those in that town, become superior in extent and importance to many of the market towns in the kingdom.

HUNSONBY, a township in the parish of ADDINGHAM, LEATH ward, county of CUMBERLAND, 7 miles (N. E.) from Penrith, containing, with the township of Winskill, 151 inhabitants. There is a place of worship for Wesleyan Methodists. Mr. Joseph Hutchinson, in 1726, devised an estate at Gartree, now let for £40 a year, for teaching children.

HUNSTANTON, a parish in the hundred of SMITHDON, county of NORFOLK, 10 miles (W.) from Burnham-Westgate, containing 433 inhabitants. The living is a discharged vicarage, in the archdeaconry of Norfolk, and diocese of Norwich, rated in the king's books at £12, and in the patronage of the Bishop of Ely. The church, dedicated to St. Mary, is a large edifice with a strong tower rising from the west end of the north aisle : it contains several memorials of the Le Stranges, to which family belonged the celebrated political writer, Sir Roger le Strange, who was born here in 1616 : on the breaking out of the civil war he espoused the royal cause, and intending to surprise Lynn, was betrayed by two of his associates, seized, and condemned to death, which sentence was afterwards commuted for imprisonment in Newgate. Escaping from prison he fled to the continent, but returned prior to the Restoration, and afterwards published a newspaper, called " The Public Intelligencer and the News," which was suppressed, and the London Gazette substituted, the first number of which was published, February 4th, 1666. Subsequently he was appointed licenser of the press, wrote " The Observator" in defence of Government, and on the accession of James II. was knighted ; he died in 1704. There are vestiges of an ancient chapel on St. Edmund's Point, a high cliff overlooking the North sea.

HUNSTERTON, a township in the parish of WYBUNBURY, hundred of NANTWICH, county palatine of CHESTER, 6 miles (S. E.) from Nantwich, containing 239 inhabitants.

HUNSTON, a parish in the hundred of BLACKBOURN, county of SUFFOLK, 8½ miles (N. W. by N.) from Stow-Market, containing 178 inhabitants. The living is a perpetual curacy, in the archdeaconry of Sudbury, and diocese of Norwich, endowed with £16 per annum private benefaction, and £600 royal bounty. J. Heigham, Esq. was patron in 1792. The church is dedicated to St. Michael.

HUNSTON, a parish in the hundred of Box and STOCKBRIDGE, rape of CHICHESTER, county of SUSSEX; 2½ miles (S.) from Chichester, containing 166 inhabitants. The living is a vicarage, in the archdeaconry and diocese of Chichester, rated in the king's books at £9. 4. 7. W. Brereton, Esq. was patron in 1803. The church, dedicated to St. Leodegar, is in the early style of English architecture. The Arundel and Portsmouth canal passes through the parish.

HUNSTONWORTH, a chapelry in the parish of EDMONDBYERS, western division of CHESTER ward, county palatine of DURHAM, 8 miles (N. N. W.) from Stanhope, containing 411 inhabitants. The living is a perpetual curacy, in the archdeaconry and diocese of Durham, endowed with £200 private benefaction, and £600 royal bounty. John Ord, Esq. was patron in 1811. The river Derwent is formed here by the union of two rivulets, called Beldon-Beck and Nuckton-Beck. The Derwent lead mines are principally in this parish, and produce annually about thirty-five thousand pigs of lead.

HUNSWORTH, a township in the parish of BIRS-TALL, wapentake of MORLEY, West riding of the county of YORK, 4¼ miles (S. S. E.) from Bradford, containing 870 inhabitants. The manufacture of woollen goods is carried on here.

Seal and Arms.

HUNTINGDON, a borough and market town, having separate jurisdiction, locally in the hundred of Hurstingstone, county of HUNTINGDON, 59 miles (N. by W.) from London, containing 2806 inhabitants. This place, called by the Saxons *Huntantun*, and in the Norman survey *Hunters dune*, appears to have derived its name from its situation in a tract of country which was anciently an extensive forest abounding with deer, and well suited for the purposes of the chase. A castle was built here by Edward the Elder, in 917, and afterwards enlarged by David, Earl of Huntingdon, and King of Scotland, to whom King Stephen gave the borough, but having become a retreat for the disaffected in the reign of Henry II., it was, by that monarch's order, levelled with the ground. This fortress, of which there are no remains, is generally supposed, from the form of its outworks, which may still be traced, to have been the site of *Duroliponte*, a station of the Romans. A mint was established here at a very early period, and coins of Edwy and of his successors until the time of William Rufus, have been struck and issued from this place. Huntingdon has been honoured with many royal visits: James I., on his arrival from Scotland, with all his court, was sumptuously entertained by Sir Oliver Cromwell, uncle of the Protector, in his princely mansion of Hinchinbrooke, a spacious quadrangular building in the Elizabethan style, in which also Charles I. frequently partook of the liberal hospitality of its possessor. Prior to the commencement of the parliamentary war, that monarch kept his court at Huntingdon, where he carried on his negociations with the parliament then sitting in London, and during the subsequent contests it was frequently the head-quarters of his army. Not long after the breaking out of the war, however, it appears to have fallen into the hands of the parliament; for it is stated to have been plundered, in August 1645, by the royalists, commanded by the king in person. In 1646, the king, on his route from Holmby to Hampton Court, in the care of Cornet Joyce and the parliamentary commissioners, was lodged at Hinchinbrook house, then be-

longing to Colonel Montague, an officer in the army of the parliament, and afterwards, on his joining Charles II. at the Restoration, created Earl of Sandwich, from whose lady the captive monarch received every tribute of sympathising loyalty, and by whose courage he was protected from the insults of a factious mob. In 1745, the inhabitants, assisted by the surrounding gentry, came forward to support the reigning dynasty against the claims of the Pretender, and raised a large sum of money by subscription for that purpose.

The town is pleasantly situated on a gentle acclivity on the northern bank of the river Ouse, over which an ancient stone bridge of six arches connects it with Godmanchester: it consists of one principal street, extending a mile in length, and intersected at right angles by several smaller streets: the houses are in general large, well built, and of handsome appearance; the town is well paved, lighted during the winter season, and amply supplied with water. The environs are pleasant, and from the Castle hill the prospect is rich, varied, and extensive. Within a quarter of a mile of the town is a luxuriant meadow, called Portholm, more than two miles in circumference, and preserving an entire and beautiful level, environed by the river, which is of considerable breadth, and shaded in its course by ranges of stately poplars and graceful willows. On this extensive plain, which forms one of the finest courses in the kingdom, races take place annually, commencing on the first Tuesday in August, and continuing three days, during which, and usually for a fortnight after, the theatre, a small edifice erected in 1800, is open. There are three literary institutions, or reading-societies, and a public subscription reading-room; and, in 1821, an horticultural society was established, the members of which award prizes at their meetings in April and July. Monthly assemblies are held, during the season, in a suite of rooms in the town-hall, and public balls take place twice in the race week. The trade is principally in wool and corn: there are also two public breweries. The river Ouse is navigable for small vessels from Lynn, whence the inhabitants are supplied with coal and timber, and other articles of merchandise, and for barges from this town to Bedford. The market, on Saturday, is plentifully supplied with corn and provisions: the fairs are on the Tuesday before Easter, and the second Tuesday in May, for cattle of all sorts; and there is a statute fair about two weeks before Michaelmas, on a day fixed by the mayor: there are also large cattle markets on the Saturday before Old Michaelmas-day, and on the third Saturday in November. The market-place, which is conveniently arranged, occupies a spacious square in the centre of the town.

Huntingdon was first incorporated in 1206, by charter of King John, confirmed and extended by Henry III. and succeeding sovereigns until the 6th year of the reign of Charles I., when it was renewed with modifications; under which charter the government is vested in a mayor, high steward, recorder, twelve aldermen, and twelve burgesses, assisted by a town clerk, two serjeants at mace, and subordinate officers. The mayor, recorder, and aldermen, form the common council. The mayor, who is also coroner and clerk of the market, the late mayor, the high steward, the recorder, and the senior alderman, if he has passed the chair, are justices of the peace. The mayor, assisted by the recorder, holds quarterly courts of session for the trial of all offenders within the borough; and a court of record, for the recovery of debts to any amount, is held once in three weeks : the county court is held every fourth Saturday, and there are courts leet and baron for the manor. The assizes for the county, and the general quarter sessions of the peace, are also held in this town. The town-hall is a handsome modern building of brick, coated with stucco, erected in 1745, by voluntary subscription, on the site of the old courthouse, and surrounded with piazzas, under which the market for eggs, poultry, meat, and butter, is kept: the ground-floor contains the courts for criminal and civil causes, each accommodated with a gallery, and a room in which the grand jury assemble, and the borough magistrates sit weekly, for the dispatch of business : above these is a suite of assembly-rooms, handsomely fitted up; the ball-room, sixty-three feet in length, and twenty-four in width, is ornamented with portraits of George II. and George III., and with those of their queens, by Sir Joshua Reynolds; also of John, Earl of Sandwich, by Gainsborough. A new prison has been erected on the western side of the great north road, combining a common gaol and house of correction for the county, and comprising eight wards for the classification of prisoners, with the same number of day-rooms and airing-yards (in one of which is a tread-wheel for supplying the prison with water), and fifty-one separate cells. The old gaol, with the yards and appurtenances, has been surrendered to the use of the corporation, and the county bridewell has been purchased to be converted into a workhouse.

Huntingdon was formerly much more extensive than it is at present, and contained fifteen parish churches, the greater number of which had fallen into decay before Leland's time, when only four were remaining, and two of these were destroyed during the parliamentary war. The borough at present comprises the parishes of All Saints, St. Benedict, St. John the Baptist, and St. Mary, all in the archdeaconry of Huntingdon, and diocese of Lincoln. The living of All Saints' is a rectory, united with that of St. John the Baptist, the former rated in the king's books at £6. 11. 10½., and the latter at £6. 7. 6., and in the patronage of the Crown : the church of All Saints is a venerable and handsome structure, partly in the early, and partly in the later, style of English architecture, with a fine square embattled tower in the later style, strengthened with buttresses, ornamented with niches, and crowned with pinnacles ; the sides of the tower are enriched with foliage, flowers, heads, and other devices, among which are the Tudor rose and portcullis ; the chancel is in the early English style, and has a remarkably fine doorway, now walled up ; the nave is separated from the chancel by a lofty and finely-pointed arch, and from the aisles by pointed arches resting upon clustered columns ; the oak roof is richly carved, and decorated with full-length figures, with various musical instruments : there are several ancient monuments, among which are some to the ancestors of Oliver Cromwell, who were interred in the church. The living of St. Benedict's is a rectory, united with the discharged rectory of St. Mary's, rated in the king's books at £10. 0. 5., endowed with £400 royal bounty, and £1200 parliamentary grant, and in the patronage of the Crown. The church of St. Mary

was rebuilt in 1620 : it is a handsome structure in the later style of English architecture, with a fine square embattled tower, strengthened with buttresses, and profusely ornamented with niches and sculpture ; the nave is separated from the aisles by finely-pointed arches and octangular and circular columns alternately ; the font is of an octagonal form, and supported on a column encircled by small pillars : in the chancel are several handsome monuments, and in other parts of the church are some mural tablets highly finished, together with several marble slabs, from which the brasses were torn away by the parliamentary soldiers. There are places of worship for Baptists, the Society of Friends, Independents, and Wesleyan Methodists. The free grammar school, which is of uncertain origin, is endowed with part of the revenue of the ancient hospital of St. John, in the chapel of which it is kept : the number of scholars is not limited, and they are instructed on the Eton plan. There is a scholarship for a boy from this school at Peter House, Cambridge, founded by Thomas Miller, who gave for that purpose land now producing £20 per annum, tenable from admission until obtaining the degree of M.A.: there is also a scholarship founded in Christ's College, Cambridge, for a native of Huntingdon. A charity school is supported partly by the surplus benefactions of Mr. Richard Fishborn, Mr. Lionel Walden, and Mr. Gabriel Newton, and by subscription, for the maintenance, clothing, and education of thirty boys, of whom six go out every year, receiving £10 as an apprentice fee : twelve girls are also clothed and instructed from the proceeds of Mr. Fishborn's charity. National schools, under the patronage of the Bishop of the diocese, were established in 1813, and are supported by subscription: the boys' school-room, in which one hundred boys are instructed, is a neat building at the northern extremity of the town ; opposite to which is that for the girls, of whom about seventy are taught. Mr. Richard Fishborn, in 1625, gave £2000 in trust to the Company of Mercers, in London, for the maintenance of a lecture, a grammar school, and an almshouse, in this town ; which sum, together with £4560 arising from other donations, was, in 1630, vested in the purchase of the manor of Chalgrave, in the county of Bedford, now producing £700 per annum, of which £60 is paid to a lecturer, £175 per annum to the corporation for charitable uses, of which £35 per annum is appropriated to the clothing and education of twelve poor girls, £90 per annum for apprenticing six poor children of the charity school, and £5 each to ten aged men or women: there are various other charitable bequests for distribution among the poor. Of the monastic establishments which formerly existed here, was a priory of Black canons, dedicated to St. Mary, founded prior to the year 973, and removed by Eustace de Lovetot in the reign of Stephen, or that of Henry II., to the eastern part of the town, the revenue of which, at the dissolution, was £232. 7. ; there are no remains. A priory for nuns of the Benedictine order was removed from Eltesley, in the county of Cambridge, to this town, the revenue of which, at the dissolution, was £19. 9. 2. : the site was granted by Henry VIII. to Sir Richard Cromwell, who erected the mansion of Hinchinbrook house with part of the materials. A convent of Augustine friars was founded in the parish of St. John, in the reign of Edward I., which subsisted until the Reformation; and in the latter part of the sixteenth century, the site of the friary belonged to Robert Cromwell, whose son Oliver became Lord Protector of England. Here was also an hospital dedicated to St. Margaret, for a master and leprous brethren, to which Malcolm, Earl of Huntingdon, and King of Scotland, was a benefactor, and which was, in 1445, annexed to Trinity Hall, Cambridge, by letters patent of Henry VI.; besides an Hospital dedicated to St. John the Baptist, founded in the reign of Henry II., by David, Earl of Huntingdon, the revenue of which, at the dissolution, was £9. 4.: the chapel, which is all that remains of the ancient building, is appropriated to the use of the free grammar school. A stone coffin, containing a human skeleton, was dug up on the castle hills, about twenty years since. The learned Henry of Huntingdon, author of a History of England continued to the reign of Stephen; and the noted Oliver Cromwell; were natives of this town. Huntingdon gives the title of earl to the family of Rawdon-Hastings.

HUNTINGDONSHIRE, an inland county, bounded on the north and west by the county of Northampton, on the south-west and south by the county of Bedford, and on the east by the county of Cambridge: it extends from 52° 7′ to 52° 32, (N. Lat.), and from 0° 2′ (E. Lon.) to 0° 31′ (W. Lon.), in its broadest part; and it contains about two hundred and thirty-six thousand eight hundred acres, or about three hundred and seventy square miles. The population, in 1821, amounted to 48,771. Before the Romans obtained possession of this part of Britain, the territory now included in the small county of Huntingdon formed the western extremity of the country of the Iceni: it subsequently became part of the great division of Roman Britain, called *Flavia Cæsariensis*, and on the establishment of the Saxon octarchy, it was at first included in the kingdom of East-Anglia, but was afterwards annexed, by conquest, to the more powerful one of Mercia. The early annals of this county afford no materials for history, but such as relate to the acquisition and possession of its earldom by the royal family of Scotland, which furnished the two crowns with an additional object of contention and mutual annoyance. A short time before the Norman Conquest, the earldom, or governorship, of this shire (being then an office granted at pleasure, and not an hereditary honour) was held by one Siward, who was in consequence styled Earl of Huntingdon, but who, having afterwards the earldom of Northumberland conferred upon him, was then called Earl of Northumberland. William the Conqueror, having taken into favour Waltheof, the son of Siward, gave him his own niece Judith in marriage. After the execution of Waltheof, on the charge of treason, his widow was offered in marriage to Simon de St. Liz, a Norman soldier, but she refusing him, from dislike to his person, was deprived of her estates, which were conferred upon her eldest daughter, the latter being at the same time given in marriage to the Norman whom her mother had rejected. Simon de St. Liz thus became Earl of Huntingdon; but dying in the beginning of the reign of Henry I., his widow was married to David, brother to Alexander, King of Scotland, and afterwards his successor on the throne, who, in her right, inherited the possessions of Waltheof, and was made Earl of Huntingdon and Northumberland. After his death, according to the fluctuations in the tide of political

events, or in the favour of the English monarchs, this earldom was sometimes in the hands of the descendants of Matilda by Simon de St. Liz, and sometimes in those of her posterity by her marriage with the Scottish prince. Henry, son of the latter, was at first admitted earl; but on his father's refusal to acknowledge Stephen, Count of Blois, as sovereign of England, to the exclusion of the Empress Matilda, Stephen, seizing all his possessions in England, restored this earldom to the young Simon de St. Liz. When the subsequent war between the two countries (in which both King David, and his son, Prince Henry, invaded England, at the head of a large army,) was terminated by the mediation of the Empress, one of the conditions of the peace then concluded was, that the counties of Northumberland and Huntingdon should remain in the government of Prince Henry, as heir to them by maternal right, and that for these lands, he and his successors, Princes of Scotland, should do homage to Stephen and his successors, Kings of England. Nevertheless, the possession of these counties was afterwards the object of frequent disputes between the two crowns. On the accession of Henry's grandson, Malcolm, to the Scottish throne, at the age of thirteen, he was summoned to London by Henry II., to do homage to him for the lands of Cumberland, Northumberland, and Huntingdon, on pain of losing them; and not long afterwards, Henry sent him a second summons, commanding him to repair to York where he had assembled a parliament, by which, on the charge of having in the late campaign in France, whither King Henry had carried him, betrayed to the French the plans of the English army, he was condemned to forfeit his English possessions. A war between the two countries ensued, but it terminated by a treaty concluded near Carlisle, in which it was stipulated, that Malcolm should receive back Cumberland and Huntingdon, but should make a full surrender of Northumberland to Henry and his successors for ever. On the breaking out of the war with Malcolm's successor, William, surnamed the Lion, in which the Scottish monarch was made prisoner, this earldom was seized, together with the rest of his possessions in England, which were afterwards held in pledge for that king's ransom, until delivered up by Richard I., on condition that all the castles and fortified places within the earldoms of Huntingdon and Cumberland should be garrisoned by his own officers and soldiers. In the subsequent wars occasioned by the rival claims to the Scottish crown, between the families of Bruce and Balliol, this earldom was finally seized by the kings of England; since which it has been granted to several successive families. A portion of the lands, however, was still retained by the Bruces, and from them descended to the family of Cotton. The ancient celebrity of this part of the country for the purposes of the chase has found a lasting evidence in the name of the shire and of the county town. According to Leland, the shire was in former times very woody, and the deer resorted to the fens: it was not entirely disafforested until the reign of Edward I. In later times, the only events of political importance that have happened within its limits, occurred in the course of the great civil war. The first of these was the plundering of the town of Huntingdon, in August 1645, by the king's troops, which, commanded by the king in person, and taking advantage of the absence of

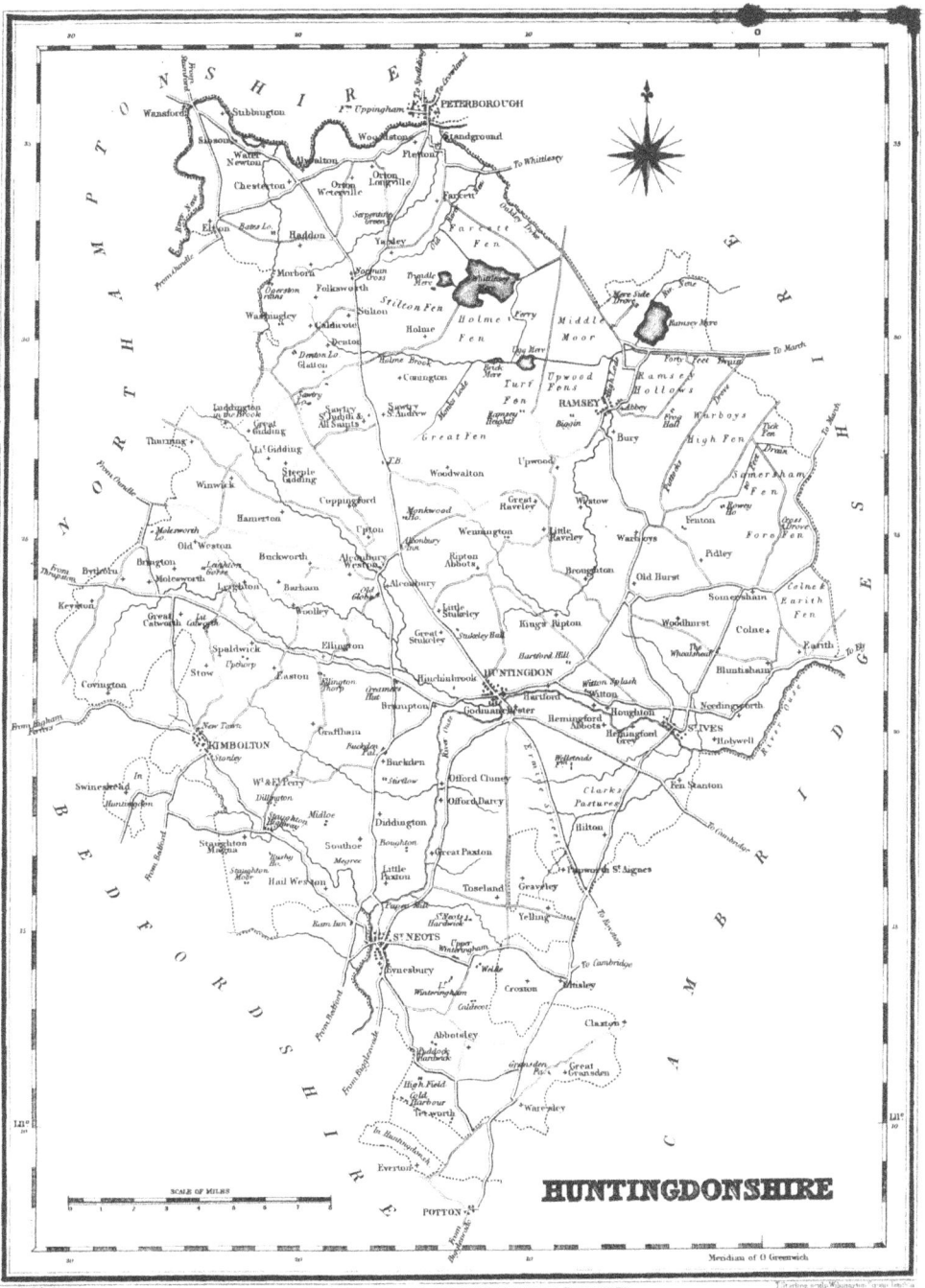

HUNTINGDONSHIRE

SCALE OF MILES

Meridian of 0 Greenwich

Drawn by R. Creighton.

DRAWN AND ENGRAVED FOR LEWIS' TOPOGRAPHICAL DICTIONARY.

the parliamentary army in the west, had suddenly entered the associated eastern counties. Again Huntingdonshire was the scene of a part of the hostilities occasioned, in 1648, by the appearance in arms of the Earl of Holland, the Duke of Buckingham, and others in the royal cause, with an immediate view to the relief of Colchester. The Earl of Holland, after being driven by some of the parliamentary troops from his quarters at Kingston upon Thames, and wandering over the country with about a hundred horse, came to St. Neots, in this county, where he was beset by his pursuers, and surrendered himself without resistance, two of his officers at the same time being killed upon the spot, and the Duke of Buckingham making his escape by forcing his way through the enemy.

Huntingdonshire is included in the diocese of Lincoln, and province of Canterbury, and forms an archdeaconry, comprising the deaneries of Huntingdon, St. Ives, Leightonstone, St. Neots, and Yaxley, and containing ninety-three parishes, of which fifty-seven are rectories, twenty-nine vicarages, and the remainder perpetual curacies, or united with other parishes. For civil purposes it is divided into the four hundreds of Norman-Cross, which includes the northern part of the county; Toseland, the southern; Hurstingstone, the eastern; and Leightonstone, the western. It contains the borough and market town of Huntingdon, and the market towns of Kimbolton, Ramsey, St. Ives, and St. Neots. Two knights are returned for the shire, and two representatives for the borough of Huntingdon. This county is included in the Norfolk circuit: the assizes and the quarter sessions are held at Huntingdon, where stands the county gaol: there are twenty-two acting magistrates for the county. A peculiarity in the civil government of Huntingdonshire is, that it is included under the same shrievalty with Cambridgeshire; the sheriff being chosen, in rotation, one year from the county of Cambridge, another year from the Isle of Ely, and the third year from this county. The rates raised in the county for the year ending March 25th, 1827, amounted to £49,518. 13; the expenditure to £48,276. 12., of which, £42,127. 6. was applied to the relief of the poor. It has been observed that the temperature of the air varies nearly as much in this county as in any district in the kingdom of the same extent. The upland parts are very salubrious, while the fenny tract in the north-east is much less healthful, in consequence of the effluvia arising from the marshes, and the broad, shallow, and stagnant meres: this district, however, has been rendered much more healthy by the recent improvements in the draining of it. The soils consist chiefly of clay and loam of various qualities, sand, gravel, and peat-earth; of these, the clay mostly predominates, being found all over the county; the sandy and light soils, and the loams, are dispersed in small tracts in different parts; and the peat-earth belongs almost wholly to the fens, in the north-eastern part of the county. These fens, including the lakes, the chief of which are Whittlesea Mere and Ramsey Mere, comprise about forty-four thousand acres, and form about one-seventh of the great Bedford Level: eight or ten thousand acres of this may be considered as productive; but, as stated in the last agricultural survey of this county, drawn up for the Board of Agriculture, it requires a sum equal to two-thirds of their rental to preserve even these from

inundation; for although they have a more elevated surface than those which lie between them and the sea, yet they are much worse drained, in consequence, as it is asserted in the report of the survey, of some defect in the original plan of the dykes. The county is rather bare of timber, which is owing to the very great demand for it in the fens. Turf is used as fuel in nearly half the parishes; but the inhabitants generally use wood and coal also, though in many places very little of the latter is burnt: in the cottages of the lower class, stubble, bean straw, reeds, and dried dung, are also used as fuel. The only rivers of magnitude are the Ouse and the Nene. The Ouse enters the county at St. Neots, whence it flows northward to Huntingdon: in the vicinity of that town it takes an easterly course by St. Ives, and having formed the boundary between this county and that of Cambridge, it enters Cambridgeshire near Earith, being navigable in the whole of its course through this county. The Nene forms the northern boundary of the county, separating it from Northamptonshire, and is navigable in all that part of its course. The greater part of the county, owing to the want of springs, is supplied with water from ponds. The great north road from London to Edinburgh enters the southern border of the county near St. Neots, and passing through Buckden, Stilton, and Yaxley, enters Northamptonshire at Wansford bridge. The turnpike roads are numerous, and most of them very good and well formed: in consequence of the scarcity of materials in many parts, a power is given to the commissioners to pick off all the stones that can be found on any of the farmers' lands.

The principal Roman stations in Huntingdonshire were *Duroliponte* and *Durobrivæ*, the sites of which are respectively at Godmanchester, or Huntingdon, and near Dornford Ferry. Of the ancient roads the three principal were as follows: — The British Ermin-street appears to have entered the county from the neighbourhood of Cæsar's Camp, in Bedfordshire, and to have run by Crane hill, in the track since known by the name of Hell lane, whence, passing through Toseland, Godmanchester, and Huntingdon, and by Alconbury, Weston, and Upton, and falling into the line now called the Bullock road, it entered Northamptonshire at Wansford. The Roman Ermin-street entered this county from Cambridgeshire, in the vicinity of Papworth-St. Agnes, and proceeding, nearly in the line of the present high road, to Godmanchester, thence followed the course of the British Ermin-street, to the vicinity of Alconbury, where branching off to the eastward, it resumed the line of the present high road, through Sawtry, Stilton, and Chesterton, to the station of *Durobrivæ*, where it entered Northamptonshire. The *Via Devana* entered the county from Cambridgeshire, in the neighbourhood of Fen-Stanton, and proceeded, in the line of the present turnpike-road, to Godmanchester, whence pursuing the track of the British Ermin-street to Alconbury, it passed to the north of Buckworth and Old Weston, and entered Northamptonshire in the vicinity of Clapton. Numerous Roman coins have been discovered at Godmanchester: coins, coffins, urns, lachrymatories, &c., have been found near the site of the station *Durobrivæ*; urns and coins near Somersham; urns in Sawtrey field; and Roman pottery at Holywell. The celebrated Cars-dyke, supposed to have been originally a work of the Romans, enters Huntingdonshire at Earith, crosses

Huntingdon river, passes by Littleport, and proceeds northward to the stream called the West Water, by Benwick, and then by that called the Old River Nene, to Whittlesea dyke. At the time of the Reformation, the number of religious houses in this county, according to Bishop Tanner, was nine, including one hospital: the principal monastic remain is the ruinous gateway of the ancient and mitred abbey of Ramsey, and the most remarkable churches are those of Bluntisham, St. Ives, St. Neots, Godmanchester, and All Saints, Huntingdon. Among the ancient mansion-houses, the most interesting, from their antiquity and other circumstances, are, Buckden palace, the residence of the Bishops of Lincoln; Kimbolton castle, the seat of the Dukes of Manchester; and Hinchinbrook house, anciently the seat of the Cromwell family, and subsequently that of the Montagues, Earls of Sandwich, and Viscounts Hinchinbroke. There is a mineral spring at Somersham, but it is now in but little repute.

HUNTINGFIELD, a parish in the hundred of BLYTHING, county of SUFFOLK, 4 miles (W. S. W.) from Halesworth, containing 386 inhabitants. The living is a rectory with that of Cookley, in the archdeaconry of Suffolk, and diocese of Norwich, rated in the king's books at £13. 6. 8., and in the patronage of Lord Huntingfield. The church is dedicated to St. Mary. Berry Snelling, in 1725, left a rent-charge of £4 a year for the instruction of children. Huntingfield gives the title of baron to the family of Vanneck.

HUNTINGFORD, a tything in the parish of WOTTON under EDGE, upper division of the hundred of BERKELEY, county of GLOUCESTER. The population is returned with the parish.

HUNTINGTON, a township in that part of the parish of St. OSWALD, CHESTER, which is in the lower division of the hundred of BROXTON, county palatine of CHESTER, 3 miles (S. S. E.) from Chester, containing 133 inhabitants. The township is bounded on the west by the river Dee, which is crossed by a ferry to Ecclestone.

HUNTINGTON, a chapelry in the parish of HOLMER, hundred of GRIMSWORTH, county of HEREFORD, 2½ miles (W. N. W.) from Hereford, containing 82 inhabitants. The living is a perpetual curacy with the vicarage of Holmer, in the peculiar jurisdiction of the Dean of Hereford.

HUNTINGTON, a chapelry in the parish of KINGTON, hundred of HUNTINGTON, county of HEREFORD, 4½ miles (W. S. W.) from Kington, containing 215 inhabitants. The chapel is dedicated to St. Mary Magdalene. There is a place of worship for Independents.

HUNTINGTON, a township in the parish of CANNOCK, eastern division of the hundred of CUTTLESTONE, county of STAFFORD, 3¼ miles (E.) from Penkridge, containing 138 inhabitants.

HUNTINGTON, a parish in the wapentake of BULMER, North riding of the county of YORK, comprising the township of Huntington, and a portion of the townships of Earswick and Towthorpe, and containing 517 inhabitants, of which number, 346 are in the township of Huntington, which is partly within the liberty of St. Peter of York, 3 miles (N. N. E.) from York. The living is a discharged vicarage, in the archdeaconry of Cleveland, and diocese of York, rated in the king's books at £5, endowed with £7 per annum private benefaction, and £200 royal bounty, and in the patronage of the

Subchanter and Vicars Choral of the Cathedral Church of York. The church is dedicated to All Saints. The parish is bounded on the west by the navigable river Foss.

HUNTISHAM, a township in the parish of GOODRICH, lower division of the hundred of WORMELOW, county of HEREFORD. The population is returned with the township of Goodrich.

HUNTLEY, a parish in the Duchy of LANCASTER, county of GLOUCESTER, 4¼ miles (S. by W.) from Newent, containing 405 inhabitants. The living is a discharged rectory, in the archdeaconry of Hereford, and diocese of Gloucester, rated in the king's books at £7. 5. 10., and in the patronage of the Rev. John Morse. The church, dedicated to St. John the Baptist, has lately received an addition of one hundred and five free sittings, the Incorporated Society for the enlargement of churches and chapels having granted £30 toward defraying the expense. There is a trifling endowment for teaching two children.

HUNTON, a parish in the hundred of TWYFORD, lathe of AYLESFORD, county of KENT, 6 miles (S. W. by S.) from Maidstone, containing 683 inhabitants. The living is a rectory, rated in the king's books at £16. 13. 1½., and in the peculiar jurisdiction and patronage of the Archbishop of Canterbury. The church, dedicated to St. Mary, is a neat edifice, containing some handsome monuments of the Fanes, whose old family seat at Burston is now used as a farm-house, and its chapel desecrated. The river Beult runs through the parish, and falls into the Medway at Yalding. Here are extensive plantations of hops. In the 41st of Henry III., Nicholas de Lenham, then proprietor of Hunton, obtained grants of free warren, a weekly market, and a fair for five days annually, which have long since fallen into disuse. The manor afterwards passed to the Gyffords, and, in the reign of Edward III., to the noble family of Clinton, the site of whose ancient mansion, encompassed by a moat, is visible near the church. Beilby Porteus, twenty-two years rector of this parish, successively Bishop of Chester and London, and celebrated for his universal benevolence, bequeathed £1000 three per cent. consols. for teaching children. A stratum of petrified shells in marl, of the sort called conchites, was discovered in 1683. On Midsummer-day, 1746, and on August 19th, 1763, two of the most awful and destructive storms ever recorded in this country occurred in this and the neighbouring parishes.

HUNTON, a chapelry in the parish of CRAWLEY, hundred of BUDDLESGATE, Fawley division of the county of SOUTHAMPTON, 5½ miles (S. by E.) from Whitchurch, containing 122 inhabitants. This chapelry is within the peculiar jurisdiction of the Rector of Crawley. The chapel is dedicated to St. James.

HUNTON, a chapelry partly within the liberty of ST. PETER of YORK, East riding, and partly in the parish of HORNBY, eastern division, but chiefly in the parish of BROMPTON-PATRICK, western division, of the wapentake of HANG, North riding of the county of YORK, 6 miles (S. by E.) from Richmond, containing 496 inhabitants. The living is a perpetual curacy, with that of Brompton-Patrick, in the archdeaconry and diocese of Chester, endowed with £200 private benefaction, £800 royal bounty, and £1000 parliamentary grant. The chapel has been demolished.

HUNTSHAM, a parish in the hundred of TIVERTON, county of DEVON, 3 miles (E. S. E.) from Bampton, containing 153 inhabitants. The living is a rectory, in the archdeaconry and diocese of Exeter, rated in the king's books at £10. 12. 11. William Troyte, Esq. was patron in 1799.

HUNTSHAW, a parish in the hundred of FREMINGTON, county of DEVON, 3 miles (N. N. E.) from Great Torrington, containing 291 inhabitants. The living is a rectory, in the archdeaconry of Barnstaple, and diocese of Exeter, rated in the king's books at £11. 7. 1. The Earl of Orford was patron in 1787. The church is dedicated to St. Mary Magdalene. John Lovering, in 1671, bequeathed £200 to purchase lands, a moiety of the proceeds of which, viz., £16, is applied in teaching sixteen children. Huntshaw has also the right of sending two poor boys to the school at Weare-Giffard.

HUNTSPILL, a parish comprising the tything of Aston-Morris, in the hundred of BEMPSTONE, but chiefly in the hundred of HUNTSPILL and PURITON, county of SOMERSET, 7½ miles (N. by E.) from Bridgwater, and containing 1337 inhabitants. The living is a rectory, in the archdeaconry of Wells, and diocese of Bath and Wells, rated in the king's books at £72. 5. 5., and in the patronage of the Master and Fellows of Balliol College, Oxford. The church is dedicated to All Saints. Here is a place of worship for Baptists. This parish borders on the Bristol channel, and is situated at the mouth of the river Parret, which is navigable for vessels of considerable burden up to Highbridge, at which hamlet it is crossed by a bridge. A market formerly held here has been long discontinued. There are three fairs, toll free; one at Huntspill on June 29th, and two at Highbridge, on August 10th and December 17th. The Rev. Thomas How, in 1817, bequeathed a trifling sum for the instruction of ten children. Beautiful marine shells, of the Wentletrap and Helix species, abound among the sedge by the sea-side.

HUNWICK, a joint township with Helmington, in that part of the parish of ST. ANDREW, AUCKLAND, which is in the north-western division of DARLINGTON ward, county palatine of DURHAM, 2¼ miles (N. W. by N.) from Bishop-Auckland, containing 160 inhabitants. It is situated on the northern bank of the Wear. The water of a spring here, called Furnival Well, possesses some medicinal properties.

HUNWORTH, a parish in the hundred of HOLT, county of NORFOLK, 2½ miles (S. S. W.) from Holt, containing 220 inhabitants. The living is a discharged rectory, united to that of Stody, in the archdeaconry and diocese of Norwich, rated in the king's books at £4. Lord Suffield was patron in 1801. The church is dedicated to St. Lawrence.

HURDSFIELD, a township in the parish of PRESTBURY, hundred of MACCLESFIELD, county palatine of CHESTER, 1¾ miles (E. N. E.) from Macclesfield, containing 1082 inhabitants.

HURLESTON, a township in the parish of ACTON, hundred of NANTWICH, county palatine of CHESTER, 2½ miles (N. W.) from Nantwich, containing 191 inhabitants. A branch of the Chester canal passes through the township.

HURLEY, a parish in the hundred of BEYNHURST, county of BERKS, 4¾ miles (W. N. W.) from Maidenhead, containing 1065 inhabitants. The living is a discharged

vicarage, in the archdeaconry of Berks, and diocese of Salisbury, rated in the king's books at £6. 13. 6½., and in the patronage of the Hon. Mr. Flower. The church, dedicated to St. Mary, has portions in the Norman style of architecture, the supposed remains of a chapel belonging to a priory of Black monks, dedicated to the Virgin Mary, a cell to the abbey of Westminster, which was founded, in the reign of William the Conqueror, by Godfrey de Mandevill, and the revenue of which, at the dissolution, was valued at £134. 10. 8. : its site is now occupied by a mansion called Lady Place, in a vault beneath which were held the meetings of the confederate lords for promoting the Revolution, in 1688, among whom Lord Lovelace distinguished himself in bringing about the abdication of James II., and the elevation of William and Mary to the throne. On a tablet at one end are recorded the visits of William III., George III. and his Royal Consort, and of the celebrated General Paoli, to this dark recess. The adjoining stable was once the refectory of the priory, the windows of which are still remaining. The river Thames runs through the parish.

HURN, a joint tything with Parly, in the parish and hundred of CHRISTCHURCH, New Forest (West) division of the county of SOUTHAMPTON, 3¾ miles (N. W. by N.) from Christchurch, with which the population is returned.

HURSLEY, a parish in the hundred of BUDDLESGATE, Fawley division of the county of SOUTHAMPTON, 4½ miles (S. W. by W.) from Winchester, containing 1302 inhabitants. The living is a vicarage, with the perpetual curacy of Otterbourne, in the peculiar jurisdiction of the incumbent, rated in the king's books at £9, and in the patronage of Sir W. Heathcote, Bart. The church is dedicated to All Saints. Hursley is within the jurisdiction of the Cheyney Court held at Winchester every Thursday, for the recovery of debts to any amount. At Merdon, in this parish, are some remains of a palace of the bishops of Winchester, which was erected by Bishop De Blois, and became ruinous so long ago as the fourteenth century. It was at this place, called by the ancient chroniclers Merantune, that Kynewulph, King of the West Saxons, was murdered by Kyenard, brother to Sigebert, whom he had succeeded on the throne, but who had afterwards been driven into exile. Merdon belonged to the Protector, Richard Cromwell, in right of his wife Dorothy, eldest daughter of Richard Maijor, Esq., of Hursley. In the old mansion at Hursley park Richard resided during a great part of the time that his father held the Protectorate : hither, also, he retired for a short period prior to the Restoration and to his voluntary exile on the continent: on his death, in 1712, he was interred in the parish church. In pulling down the ancient manor-house, in the early part of the last century, to erect the present mansion, the identical seal that Oliver took from the parliament was discovered in one of the walls.

HURST, a parish comprising the liberty of Whistley-Hurst in the hundred of CHARLTON, the liberties of Newland and Winnersh in that of SONNING, county of BERKS, and the liberty of Broad-Hinton in the hundred of AMESBURY, county of WILTS, 3½ miles (N. N. W.) from Wokingham, and containing 2091 inhabitants. The living is a perpetual curacy, annexed to the vicarage of Sonning, in the peculiar jurisdiction and patronage of the Dean of Salisbury. The church, dedicated to

St. Nicholas, contains, among other handsome monuments, one to the memory of Margaret, wife of Sir Henry Savile, founder of the Savilian Professorship at Oxford, and another to Sir Richard Harrison, who twice raised, at his own expense, a troop of cavalry for the service of Charles I. An hospital was founded here by William Barker, Esq., who died in 1685, for eight poor persons, to each of whom he gave three shillings and sixpence weekly. Dame Dorothy Harrison, in 1690, gave £7 per annum for the instruction of eight boys; and Edward Polehampton, in 1721, erected a chapel, school-room, and dwelling-house, which he endowed with £40 a year, for a clergyman to officiate in the chapel and teach ten boys.

HURST, a parish partly within the liberty of ROMNEY-MARSH, but chiefly in the hundred of STREET, lathe of SHEPWAY, county of KENT, 5½ miles (W.) from Hythe, containing 30 inhabitants. The living is a rectory, in the archdeaconry and diocese of Canterbury, rated in the king's books at £4. 18. 4. Miss Carter was patroness in 1818. The church, dedicated to St. Leonard, being in ruins, the inhabitants attend divine worship at Aldington. The Grand Military canal passes through the parish.

HURST, a township in the parish of WOODHORN, eastern division of MORPETH ward, county of NORTHUMBERLAND, 5½ miles (E. by N.) from Morpeth, containing 42 inhabitants. Hurst castle was one of the fortresses erected in this part of the kingdom to repel the incursions of the Scots.

HURST (LONG), a township in that part of the parish of BOTHALL which is in the eastern division of MORPETH ward, county of NORTHUMBERLAND, 2½ miles (N. E.) from Morpeth, containing 176 inhabitants.

HURST (OLD), a parish in the hundred of HURSTINGSTONE, county of HUNTINGDON, 4¼ miles (N. by W.) from St. Ives, containing 156 inhabitants. The living is a perpetual curacy with that of Woodhouse, in the archdeaconry of Huntingdon, and diocese of Lincoln, and in the patronage of the Vicar of St. Ives. The church is dedicated to St. Peter.

HURST (TEMPLE), a township in the parish of BIRKIN, lower division of the wapentake of BARKSTONE-ASH, West riding of the county of YORK, 3½ miles (N.W.) from Snaith, containing 141 inhabitants. The Knights Templars founded a preceptory here about 1152.

HURST-COURTNEY, a township in the parish of BIRKIN, lower division of the wapentake of BARKSTONE-ASH, West riding of the county of YORK, 3 miles (N.W.) from Snaith, containing 145 inhabitants.

HURST-MONCEAUX, a parish in the hundred of FOXEARLE, rape of HASTINGS, county of SUSSEX, 4 miles (E.) from Haylsham, containing 1318 inhabitants. The living is a rectory, in the archdeaconry of Lewes, and diocese of Chichester, rated in the king's books at £20, and in the patronage of Francis Hare Naylor, Esq. The church, dedicated to All Saints, is an ancient and spacious edifice in the early style of English architecture, containing some curious sepulchral monuments. There is a place of worship for Independents. The house of Hurst-Monceaux, erected by Lord Dacre, treasurer to Henry VI., was formerly one of the finest castellated brick buildings in England; but in 1777 the roof was taken down, and a great part destroyed, though a con-

siderable part of the walls, and the towers and gateway, are still standing.

HURST-PIERREPOINT, a parish in the hundred of BUTTINGHILL, rape of LEWES, county of SUSSEX, 11 miles (W.N.W.) from Lewes, containing 1321 inhabitants. The living is a rectory, in the archdeaconry of Lewes, and diocese of Chichester, rated in the king's books at £15. 9. 4½., and in the patronage of Sir E. Winnington, Bart. The church, erected in the reign of Edward III., and dedicated to St. Lawrence, comprises two chancels, one being a continuation of the south aisle; and there is a very ancient font, besides several interesting monuments. Henry Campion, in 1750, bequeathed a rent-charge of £5, and William and Ann Lindfield, in 1806, left certain stock producing annually about £50, for which sums one hundred children are instructed at different schools in the parish. A fair formerly held in August was changed, about sixty years ago, to the 1st of May.

HURSTBOURN-PRIORS, a parish in the hundred of EVINGAR, Kingsclere division of the county of SOUTHAMPTON, 2 miles (W. S.W.) from Whitchurch, containing 404 inhabitants. The living is a discharged vicarage, in the peculiar jurisdiction of the incumbent, rated in the king's books at £12. 19. 4½., endowed with £300 private benefaction, and £200 royal bounty, and in the patronage of the Bishop of Winchester. The church is dedicated to St. Andrew. Hurstbourn is within the jurisdiction of the Cheyney Court held at Winchester every Thursday. for the recovery of debts to any amount.

HURSTBOURN-TARRANT, a parish in the hundred of PASTROW, Kingsclere division of the county of SOUTHAMPTON, 5½ miles (N. by E.) from Andover, containing 766 inhabitants. The living is a vicarage, with the perpetual curacy of Vernhams-Dean, in the archdeaconry and diocese of Winchester, rated in the king's books at £8. 12. 6., and in the patronage of the Prebendary of Hurstbourn and Burbage in the Cathedral Church of Salisbury. The church is dedicated to St. Peter. The river Swift has its source in this parish. Peter Dore and William Jones, in 1756, bequeathed together £7. 10. per annum, for teaching eighteen children.

HURSTLEY, a township in that part of the parish of LETTON which is in the hundred of WOLPHY, though locally in that of Stretford, county of HEREFORD, 5 miles (W. S. W.) from Weobley, containing 68 inhabitants.

HURSTWICK, a joint township with Nostal, in that part of the parish of WRAGBY which is in the upper division of the wapentake of OSGOLDCROSS, West riding of the county of YORK, 3½ miles (S. W. by W.) from Pontefract, containing 49 inhabitants.

HURWORTH, a parish in the south-western division of STOCKTON ward, county palatine of DURHAM, comprising the townships of Hurworth and Neasham, or Nysam, and containing 1124 inhabitants, of which number, 811 are in the township of Hurworth, 3¾ miles (S. S. E.) from Darlington. The living is a rectory, in the archdeaconry and diocese of Durham, rated in the king's books at £27. 5. 5. W. Hogg and R. H. Williamson, Esqrs. were patrons alternately in 1784. The church, dedicated to All Saints, stands in the centre of the village, which consists of a spacious, well-built street, situated on the brow of a steep hill, at the foot of which flows the Tees, and commanding a fine and extensive view of the windings of that river through Teesdale, and of its opposite banks, which, rising abruptly to a great height, form an amphitheatre several miles in circuit. A place of worship for Wesleyan Methodists was opened in 1827. The manufacture of linen is carried on in the parish. A school-house was erected in 1825, by subscription, aided by a grant of £30 from the National Society, in which about one hundred children receive daily instruction, and forty attend on Sundays. William Emmerson, a self-taught mathematician, was born and resided here; he died in 1782, aged eighty-one years.

HUSBORN-CRAWLEY, a parish in the hundred of MANSHEAD, county of BEDFORD, 2½ miles (N. by E.) from Woburn, containing 572 inhabitants. The living is a discharged vicarage, in the archdeaconry of Bedford, and diocese of Lincoln, rated in the king's books at £9, endowed with £200 private benefaction, and £200 royal bounty, and in the patronage of the Duke of Bedford. The church, dedicated to St. Mary Magdalene, occupies an elevated situation, and has a tower eighty feet high.

HUSTHWAITE, a parish within the liberty of ST. PETER of YORK, East riding, though locally in the wapentake of Birdforth, North riding, of the county of YORK, comprising the chapelry of Carlton, and the township of Husthwaite, and containing 493 inhabitants, of which number, 324 are in the township of Husthwaite, 4 miles (N. by W.) from Easingwould. The living is a perpetual curacy with Carlton, in the peculiar jurisdiction of the Dean and Chapter of York, endowed with £200 private benefaction, and £200 royal bounty, and in the patronage of the Prebendary of Husthwaite in the Cathedral Church of York.

HUTTOFT, a parish in the Marsh division of the hundred of CALCEWORTH, parts of LINDSEY, county of LINCOLN, 4 miles (E.) from Alford, containing 401 inhabitants. The living is a discharged vicarage, in the archdeaconry and diocese of Lincoln, rated in the king's books at £6. 11. 8., endowed with £600 royal bounty, and in the patronage of the Bishop of Lincoln by sequestration. The church is dedicated to St. Margaret. There is a place of worship for Wesleyan Methodists.

HUTTON, a parish in the hundred of BARSTABLE, county of ESSEX, 2½ miles (W.) from Billericay, containing 418 inhabitants. The living is a rectory, in the archdeaconry of Essex, and diocese of London, rated in the king's books at £8, and in the patronage of the Dean and Chapter of St. Paul's, London. The church is dedicated to All Saints.

HUTTON, a township in the parish of PENWORTHAM, hundred of LEYLAND, county palatine of LANCASTER, 4 miles (S. W. by W.) from Preston, containing 613 inhabitants. The free grammar school of Penwortham is situated in this township.

HUTTON, a township in the parish of WARTON, hundred of LONSDALE, south of the sands, county palatine of LANCASTER, 9½ miles (N. N. E.) from Lancaster, containing 213 inhabitants.

HUTTON, a parish in the hundred of WINTERSTOKE, county of SOMERSET, 7 miles (N. W. by W.) from Axbridge, containing 325 inhabitants. The living

is a rectory, in the archdeaconry of Wells, and diocese of Bath and Wells, rated in the king's books at £14. A. G. H. Battersby, Esq. was patron in 1825. The church is dedicated to St. Mary: in the interior is a fine groined ceiling, and the pulpit is of stone, richly ornamented with sculpture. The manorial court-house is a curious edifice, comprising an antique hall, with a fine old oak ceiling, and a large square tower on one side. Some ores of copper, lapis calaminaris, and yellow ochre, have been dug out of a hill southward of the church : here are also curious subterraneous caverns communicating with the shafts of old mines, in which have been discovered considerable quantities of the bones of elephants, tigers, hyenas, boars, wolves, horses, and other animals, and of birds, supposed to be of antediluvian origin.

HUTTON, a township in the parish of LONG MARSTON, ainsty of the city, and East riding of the county, of YORK, 4¾ miles (N. N. E.) from Tadcaster, containing 125 inhabitants. Here were formerly a market and a fair for three days.

HUTTON, a township in the parish of RUDBY in CLEVELAND, western division of the liberty of LANGBAURGH, North riding of the county of YORK, 4¼ miles (W. S. W.) from Stokesley, containing 919 inhabitants.

HUTTON in the FOREST, a parish in LEATH ward, county of CUMBERLAND, comprising the townships of Hutton in the Forest and Thomas-Close, and containing 252 inhabitants, of which number, 157 are in the township of Hutton in the Forest, 5½ miles (N. W.) from Penrith. The living is a discharged rectory, in the archdeaconry and diocese of Carlisle, rated in the king's books at £18. 12. 8½., and in the patronage of the Dean and Chapter of Carlisle. The church is dedicated to St. James. A school was founded in 1715, by Thomas Fletcher, Esq. and others, and endowed with land producing about £30 per annum. There are thirty-five scholars, each of whom pays quarterage.

HUTTON (HANG), a township in the parish of FINGALL, western division of the wapentake of HANG, North riding of the county of YORK, 3¼ miles (E. N. E.) from Middleham, containing 25 inhabitants.

HUTTON i' th' Hay, a joint township with Scathwaiterigg-Hay, in that part of the parish of KENDAL which is in KENDAL ward, county of WESTMORLAND, 3½ miles (S. E. by E.) from Kendal, containing 348 inhabitants.

HUTTON le HOLE, a township in the parish of LASTINGHAM, wapentake of RYEDALE, North riding of the county of YORK, 9 miles (N. W. by W.) from Pickering, containing 304 inhabitants.

HUTTON (NEW), a chapelry in that part of the parish of KENDAL which is in KENDAL ward, county of WESTMORLAND, 4 miles (E. S. E.) from Kendal, containing 127 inhabitants. The living is a perpetual curacy, in the archdeaconry of Richmond, and diocese of Chester, endowed with £200 private benefaction, £600 royal bounty, and £200 parliamentary grant, and in the patronage of the Vicar of Kendal. The chapel, built in 1739, is now being rebuilt. In 1778, Miles Tarn gave £40 in aid of a school for poor children : £4 per annum is given to a master, the boys paying also a small quarterage. A large reservoir, which supplies the Kendal and Lancaster canal, is situated partly in this township.

HUTTON (OLD), a chapelry in that part of the parish

of KENDAL which is in KENDAL ward, county of WEST-MORLAND, 2 miles (S.) from Burton in Kendal, containing, with the hamlet of Holmescales, 424 inhabitants. The living is a perpetual curacy, in the archdeaconry of Richmond, and diocese of Chester, endowed with £200 private benefaction, and £600 royal bounty, and in the patronage of the Vicar of Kendal. The chapel, dedicated to St. John the Baptist, was built in 1628, and rebuilt in 1699. A school was built by Edward Milner, who in 1613 gave land towards the support of a schoolmaster: the income is £19. 11. per annum, and twenty children are educated: the school was rebuilt by the inhabitants and others in 1753, and in 1757 a parochial library was established in it.

HUTTON (SAND), a chapelry in the parish of THIRSK, wapentake of BIRDFORTH, North riding of the county of YORK, 4 miles (W. by S.) from Thirsk, containing 273 inhabitants. The living is a perpetual curacy, with that of Thirsk, in the archdeaconry of Cleveland, and diocese of York, endowed with £800 royal bounty. The chapel is dedicated to St. Mary. Here is a place of worship for Wesleyan Methodists.

HUTTON (SAND), a township in that part of the parish of BOSSALL which is in the wapentake of BULMER, North riding of the county of YORK, 8 miles (N.E.) from York, containing 202 inhabitants.

HUTTON (SHERIFF), a parish in the wapentake of BULMER, North riding of the county of YORK, comprising the chapelry of Farlington, and the townships of Cornbrough, Lillings-Ambo, Sheriff-Hutton, and Stittenham, and containing 1278 inhabitants, of which number, 756 are in the township of Sheriff-Hutton, 11 miles (N. N. E.) from York. The living is a discharged vicarage, in the archdeaconry of Cleveland, and diocese of York, rated in the king's books at £10, endowed with £200 private benefaction, and £200 royal bounty, and in the patronage of the Archbishop of York. The church is dedicated to St. Helen. There are places of worship for Primitive and Wesleyan Methodists. A school is endowed with a rent-charge upon land given for charitable purposes, in which more than twenty boys are educated gratuitously in reading, writing, and arithmetic, under two masters. A castle erected here in the time of Stephen, by Bertram de Bulmer, was seized by Edward IV., and subsequently became the prison of Edward Plantagenet, wherein he remained till the death of Richard at the battle of Bosworth field: the Princess Elizabeth, afterwards consort of Henry VII., was also confined here.

HUTTON-BONVILLE, a chapelry in the parish of BIRKBY, wapentake of ALLERTONSHIRE, North riding of the county of YORK, 4¼ miles (N. W. by N.) from North Allerton, containing 107 inhabitants. The living is a perpetual curacy, in the peculiar jurisdiction of the Bishop of Durham, for Allerton and Allertonshire, endowed with £800 royal bounty. H. Piers, Esq. was patron in 1791. The chapel is dedicated to St. Lawrence.

HUTTON-BUSHELL, a parish in PICKERING lythe, North riding of the county of YORK, comprising the townships of West Ayton and Hutton Bushell, and containing 648 inhabitants, of which number, 419 are in the township of Hutton-Bushell, 6 miles (S. W. by W.) from Scarborough. The living is a vicarage, in the archdeaconry of Cleveland, and diocese of York, rated in the king's books at £14. 17. 6., and in the patronage

of Earl Fitzwilliam. The church is dedicated to St. Matthew. Here is a free school, endowed with £14 per annum arising from various bequests, for which fourteen children are instructed.

HUTTON-CONYERS, an extra-parochial liberty, in the wapentake of ALLERTONSHIRE, though locally in that of Hallikeld, North riding of the county of YORK, 1¾ mile (N. N. E.) from Ripon, containing 127 inhabitants.

HUTTON-CRANSWICK, a parish in the Bainton-Beacon division of the wapentake of HARTHILL, East riding of the county of YORK, comprising the townships of Hutton-Cranswick, Rotsea, and Sunderlandwick, and containing 1000 inhabitants, of which number, 917 are in the township of Hutton-Cranswick, 3½ miles (S.) from Great Driffield. The living is a discharged vicarage, in the archdeaconry of the East riding, and diocese of York, rated in the king's books at £15. 8. 6½., endowed with £200 private benefaction, and £1100 parliamentary grant, and in the patronage of Lord Hotham. The church is dedicated to St. Peter.

HUTTON-HENRY, a township in the parish of MONK-HESLETON, southern division of EASINGTON ward, county palatine of DURHAM, 12¾ miles (N. by W.) from Stockton upon Tees, containing 174 inhabitants. Here is a place of worship for Roman Catholics.

HUTTON-JOHN, a township in the parish of GREY-STOCK, LEATH ward, county of CUMBERLAND, 6 miles (W. S. W.) from Penrith, containing 30 inhabitants. This township consists of two estates only.

HUTTON-LOCRAS, a township in the parish of GUILSBROUGH, eastern division of the liberty of LANG-BAURGH, North riding of the county of YORK, 1½ mile (S. W. by S.) from Guilsbrough, containing 56 inhabitants. Here was an hospital for lepers, dedicated to St. Leonard, afterwards given to the priory of Guisburn.

HUTTON-MAGNUM, a parish in the western division of the wapentake of GILLING, North riding of the county of YORK, comprising the townships of Hutton-Magnum with Lane-Head, and West Layton, and containing 317 inhabitants, of which number, 248 are in the township of Hutton-Magnum with Lane-Head, 3¼ miles (E. by S.) from Greta-Bridge. The living is a perpetual curacy, in the archdeaconry of Richmond, and diocese of Chester, endowed with £800 royal bounty, and in the patronage of the Vicar of Gilling. The church is supposed to have been built before the reign of Edward III.

HUTTON-MULGRAVE, a township in the parish of LYTHE, eastern division of the liberty of LANG-BAURGH, North riding of the county of YORK, 4¾ miles (W.) from Whitby, containing 90 inhabitants.

HUTTON-ROOF, a township in the parish of GREYSTOCK, LEATH ward, county of CUMBERLAND, 3¾ miles (S. E.) from Hesket-Newmarket, containing 214 inhabitants. Here is a good freestone quarry.

HUTTON-ROOF, a chapelry in the parish of KIRK BY-LONSDALE, LONSDALE ward, county of WESTMORLAND, 3¼ miles (W. by S.) from Kirkby-Lonsdale, containing, with the hamlet of Newbiggin, 257 inhabitants. The living is a perpetual curacy, in the archdeaconry of Richmond, and diocese of Chester, endowed with £200 private benefaction, and £800 royal bounty, and in the patronage of the Vicar of Kirkby-Lonsdale. The chapel, a small edifice, was built in 1757. A school-room was erected by subscription in 1773, and endowed by Thomas Chamney with £100 : the income is £10 per annum. Here are several quarries of limestone.

HUTTON - SESSAY, a township in the parish of SESSAY, wapentake of ALLERTONSHIRE, though locally in that of Birdforth, North riding of the county of YORK, 5¾ miles (N.W.) from Easingwould, containing 129 inhabitants.

HUTTON-SOIL, a township in the parish of GREYSTOCK, LEATH ward, county of CUMBERLAND, 6 miles (W. by S.) from Penrith, containing 280 inhabitants.

HUTTONS-AMBO, a parish in the wapentake of BULMER, North riding of the county of YORK, 3 miles (S.W.) from New Malton, consisting of High and Low Hutton, and containing 445 inhabitants. The living is a perpetual curacy, in the archdeaconry of Cleveland, and diocese of York, endowed with £400 private benefaction, £400 royal bounty, and £300 parliamentary grant, and in the patronage of the Archbishop of York. The church is dedicated to St. Margaret. There is a place of worship for Wesleyan Methodists.

HUXHAM, a parish in the hundred of WONFORD county of DEVON, 3¾ miles (N.N.E.) from Exeter, containing 172 inhabitants. The living is a rectory, united to that of Poltimore, in the archdeaconry and diocese of Exeter, rated in the king's books at £8. 6. 8., and in the patronage of the Rev. Richard Bampfylde. There are mines of manganese in this parish.

HUXLEY, a township in the parish of WAVERTON, lower division of the hundred of BROXTON, county palatine of CHESTER, 3¾ miles (W. by S.) from Tarporley, containing 247 inhabitants. The Chester canal passes on the south side of this parish.

HUYTON, a parish in the hundred of WEST DERBY, county palatine of LANCASTER, comprising the townships of Huyton, Knowsley, Roby, and Tarbock, and containing 3046 inhabitants, of which number, 863 are in the township of Huyton, 1½ mile (S.W. by W.) from Prescot. The living is a discharged vicarage, in the archdeaconry and diocese of Chester, rated in the king's books at £6. 9., endowed with £200 private benefaction, and £1700 parliamentary grant, and in the patronage of the Earl of Derby. The church, dedicated to St. Michael, has portions in the later style of English architecture : one hundred free sittings have been added, towards defraying the expense of which the Incorporated Society for enlarging churches and chapels contributed £100. Here is a small school, in which four free boys are instructed for £10 per annum, arising from an endowment of £200, and payable by the corporation of Liverpool. There are veins of coal in this parish.

HYCKHAM (NORTH), a parish in the lower division of the wapentake of BOOTHBY-GRAFFO, parts of KESTEVEN, county of LINCOLN, 4¾ miles (S. W. by S.) from Lincoln, containing 296 inhabitants. The living is a rectory, in the archdeaconry and diocese of Lincoln, rated in the king's books at £19. 16. 3., and in the patronage of the Crown. The church, which was dedicated to All Saints, has fallen into ruins.

HYCKHAM (SOUTH), a parish in the lower division of the wapentake of BOOTHBY-GRAFFO, parts of KESTEVEN, county of LINCOLN, 6 miles (S.W. by S.) from Lincoln, containing, exclusively of a portion of the township of Haddington which is in this parish, 102 inhabitants. The living is a perpetual curacy, in the archdeaconry

and diocese of Lincoln, and in the patronage of the Bishop of Lincoln. The church is dedicated to St. Michael.

HYDE, a hamlet, consisting of East and West Hyde, in the parish of LUTON, hundred of FLITT, county of BEDFORD, 3¾ miles (S. E.) from Luton, containing 508 inhabitants.

HYDE, a chapelry in the parish of STOCKPORT, hundred of MACCLESFIELD, county palatine of CHESTER, 4 miles (N. E. by E.) from Stockport, containing 3355 inhabitants. The living is a perpetual curacy, in the archdeaconry and diocese of Chester, and in the patronage of the Rector of Stockport. A chapel is in progress of erection, towards defraying the expense of which, the commissioners for building churches have granted £4500 ; the site was given by George Clarke, Esq. There are places of worship for Independents, Wesleyan Methodists, and Unitarians. Several large Sunday schools are attached to these places of worship, supported by voluntary contributions, and another on an extensive scale is now being erected by subscription, as an appendage to the Independent chapel. So early as the reign of John, this township was in part owned by a family bearing the name of Hyde, a descendant of which was the great Lord Chancellor Hyde, Earl of Clarendon. It remained until within a few years since a mere agricultural district, thinly inhabited, but has since, by the establishment of the cotton manufacture, become a rapidly increasing township, which has also been greatly facilitated by a new communication with Manchester, effected by means of an act of parliament obtained in 1818. In this village and neighbourhood are some of the largest spinning and power-loom establishments in the kingdom, giving employment to nearly five thousand persons ; an additional conveyance has also been made to Manchester by water, by the Peak Forest canal, which passes through this place, and unites with the Ashton canal: there are extensive coal mines in the vicinity. One of the county magistrates sits twice a week for the transaction of business : constables and other officers are appointed at the court leet of the King's Forest and manor of Macclesfield. The court baron of Hyde and Haughton is held at Hyde Hall. A literary and scientific institution was established in May, 1821, and a mechanics' institute in 1827.

HYDE - ASH, a hamlet in the parish of LEOMINSTER, hundred of WOLPHY, county of HEREFORD, 6 miles (S. W) from Leominster. The population is returned with the township of Ivington.

HYDE-PASTURES, an extra-parochial liberty, in the Southam division of the hundred of KNIGHTLOW, county of WARWICK, 2¼ miles (E.) from Nuneaton. The population is returned with the parish of Hinckley, county of Leicester.

HYLTON, a township in the parish of MONK-WEARMOUTH, eastern division of CHESTER ward, county palatine of DURHAM, 3 miles (W.N.W.) from Sunderland, containing 320 inhabitants. The castle, an ancient baronial mansion, has been greatly modernised, the centre only possessing any claim to antiquity : a little to the northward there is a small but elegant private chapel. It was the residence of the ancient family of Hylton from the time of King Athelstan to the year 1746 : the building has the arms of the Hyltons and their alliances engraven on it in numerous places.

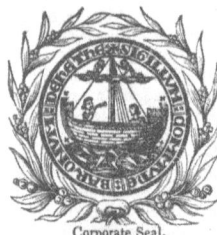

Corporate Seal.

HYTHE, a borough, parish, and one of the cinque-ports, having separate jurisdiction, locally in the hundred of Hythe, lathe of SHEPWAY, county of KENT, 33 miles (S.E. by E.) from Maidstone, and 67 (S.E. by E.) from London, containing 2181 inhabitants. This place, which is of great antiquity, was noted for the security of its haven, from which circumstance it appears to have derived its Saxon name, signifying harbour. In 456, a sanguinary battle took place on this part of the coast, between the Britons and the Saxons, and many were slain on both sides: their bones, whitened by long exposure on the sea-shore, having been collected, were deposited in one large pile, twenty-eight feet long, eight feet broad, and eight feet high, in the crypt under the chancel of the parish church: in many of the skulls are deep incisions, probably made by a battle-axe, or other heavy military weapon. Hythe, from its maritime importance, was constituted one of the cinque-ports, rated at five ships, with a complement of twenty-one men each, for the service of the king, and invested with ample privileges. In 1036, the town, with the manor of Saltwood, was given to the see of Canterbury, the archbishops of which had a castle at Saltwood, about a mile to the northward. In the early part of the reign of Henry IV., according to Lambard, "Hythe was grievously afflicted, in so much, beside the furie of the pestilence which raged all over, there were in one day two hundred of the houses consumed by fire, and five of the ships with one hundred men drowned:" the inhabitants, impoverished and dispirited by this calamity, had thoughts of abandoning the town, but were prevented by the interposition of the king, who released them for a time from their services as inhabitants of a cinque-port. At the Reformation, Archbishop Cranmer exchanged the manor of Saltwood, and the town of Hythe, with Henry VIII., and they continued vested in the crown until the 17th of Elizabeth, who granted the town at a fee farm rent of £3 to the inhabitants, whom she incorporated, by the style of "the mayor, jurats, and commonalty, of the town and port of Hythe." Since the maritime survey made in that reign, the haven has been entirely choked up with sand, and the beach is at present nearly three quarters of a mile from the town.

Hythe consists principally of one long street, running parallel with the sea, and intersected nearly at right angles by several smaller streets: the houses are irregularly built, but those on the higher grounds command a fine view of the sea, Romney Marsh, and the adjacent country, which abounds with romantic scenery, and affords numerous pleasing walks and rides. At the entrance into the town from the London road are the barracks of the royal staff corps, which is permanently stationed here. The theatre, a small but neat and well-arranged building, is opened occasionally, and the public library and reading-rooms are under good regulations and well attended. The town is much frequented during the season for sea-bathing, and there are several machines on the beach. The coast is defended by a range of strong forts and a line of martello towers, erected during the late war with France. The Royal Military canal from Hythe to Appledore affords a facility of conveyance for goods and merchandise; and a passage-boat plies daily between this place and Rye. The market is on Saturday: the fairs are, July 10th and December 1st. The government, by charter of Elizabeth, is vested in a mayor, two chamberlains, twelve jurats, and twenty-four common council-men, assisted by a town clerk and other officers: the mayor and jurats are justices of the peace within the borough and liberties, and hold a general court of session and gaol delivery in July, which is continued by adjournment on the Saturday in every month. The corporation have power to try for all offences except high treason, and to determine all pleas and civil actions; they also hold a court of record monthly, for the recovery of debts to any amount. The county magistrates for the division hold a meeting in the town on the third Monday in every month. The court-hall is a convenient building in the centre of the town; and the market-place was formed by Viscount Strangford in the reign of Charles II. The borough gaol and house of correction is a small building, containing three wards for the classification of prisoners. The borough has returned two members to parliament since the 42nd of Edward III., who are called barons: the right of election is vested in the corporation and burgesses generally, of whom the number is about one hundred and thirty: the mayor is the returning officer.

The living is a perpetual curacy annexed to the rectory of Saltwood, in the peculiar jurisdiction and patronage of the Archbishop of Canterbury. The church, dedicated to St. Leonard, is a spacious and handsome structure, partly in the Norman, and partly in the early English, style of architecture, with a tower at the west end in the former style, and a central tower of the latter character: the whole building displays remarkably good and well-executed designs in each of these styles, and under the chancel is a very fine crypt, beautifully groined, and having a door on each side, with highly enriched mouldings: over the porch is a large apartment used as the town-hall, in which the mayor and other officers of the corporation are annually chosen. There are places of worship for Independents and Wesleyan Methodists. National schools are supported by subscription, and there are also Sunday schools in connexion with the established church and the dissenting congregations. St. Bartholomew's hospital, for five poor men and five women, natives of Hythe, was founded by Haimo, Bishop of Rochester, about 1336, and is endowed with land near the town, producing a considerable revenue, which is vested in the corporation. Another almshouse, for six poor persons, called St. John's hospital, is endowed with landed property, vested in six trustees, usually members of the corporation: there are some other charitable benefactions for the relief of the poor. Near the end of Stane-street, the Roman road from Canterbury, is the ancient port Lemanus, or Limne, where the remains of the walls of that station are still visible.

HYTHE, a chapelry in the parish of FAWLEY, in that part of the hundred of BISHOP'S WALTHAM which is in the New Forest (East) division of the county of SOUTHAMPTON, 3 miles (S.) from Southampton. The population is returned with Fawley. This place is very agreeably situated on the bank of the Southampton water, opposite to that town, with which a constant communication is kept up by means of passage-boats. Here are numerous respectable houses, and an extensive yard for ship-building. The chapel, which was built a few years ago, contains four hundred and fifty-seven sittings, of which two hundred and forty-six are free, the Incorporated Society for the enlargement of churches and chapels having granted £300 towards defraying the expense.

HYTHE (WEST), a parish within the liberties of the town and port of HYTHE, of which it is a member, hundred of HYTHE, lathe of SHEPWAY, county of KENT, 2 miles (W. by S.) from Hythe, containing 119 inhabitants. The living is a vicarage, in the archdeaconry and diocese of Canterbury, rated in the king's books at £8. 14. 4½., and in the patronage of the Archbishop of Canterbury. The church, dedicated to St. Mary, has been demolished. The Grand Military, or Shorncliffe and Rye, canal passes through this parish.

I.

IBBERTON, a parish in the hundred of WHITEWAY, Cerne sub-division of the county of DORSET, 7 miles (W. by N.) from Blandford-Forum, containing 222 inhabitants. The living is a rectory, in the archdeaconry of Dorset, and diocese of Bristol, rated in the king's books at £19. 13. 9. Lord Rivers was patron in 1813. The church is dedicated to St. Eustache.

IBLE, a township in that part of the parish of WIRKSWORTH which is in the hundred of WIRKSWORTH, county of DERBY, 4½ miles (N. W.) from Wirksworth, containing 135 inhabitants. This township is in the honour of Tutbury, duchy of Lancaster, and within the jurisdiction of a court of pleas held at Tutbury every third Tuesday, for the recovery of debts under 40s.

IBSLEY, a chapelry in the hundred and parish of FORDINGBRIDGE, New Forest (West) division of the county of SOUTHAMPTON, 2½ miles (N. by E.) from Ringwood, containing 317 inhabitants. The chapel is dedicated to St. Martin.

IBSTOCK, a parish in the hundred of SPARKENHOE, county of LEICESTER, 4¾ miles (N.) from Market-Bosworth, containing, with the joint chapelry of Hugglescote with Donnington, 1741 inhabitants. The living is a rectory, in the archdeaconry of Leicester, and diocese of Lincoln, rated in the king's books at £19. 8. 11½., and in the patronage of the Bishop of Rochester. The church is dedicated to St. Denis. There is a place of worship for Wesleyan Methodists.

ICCOMB, a parish partly in the upper division of the hundred of SLAUGHTER, county of GLOUCESTER, but chiefly in the upper division of the hundred of OSWALDSLOW, county of WORCESTER, 3 miles (S. E.) from Stow on the Wold, containing 164 inhabitants. The living is a rectory, in the archdeaconry and diocese of Worcester, rated in the king's books at £8, and in the patronage of the Dean and Chapter of Worcester. The church is dedicated to St. Mary. There is a chalybeate spring in this parish. An Alien priory was founded by Gervaise Paganel, as a cell to Wenlock priory, the revenue of which, at the suppression, was £36. 3. Here

are the remains of an encampment supposed to be Danish.

ICKBOROUGH, a parish in the hundred of GRIMSHOE, county of NORFOLK, 6 miles (N. N. E.) from Brandon-Ferry, containing 154 inhabitants. The living is a discharged rectory, with that of Langford, in the archdeaconry of Norfolk, and diocese of Norwich, rated in the king's books at £10. 2. 8½. The church is dedicated to St. Bartholomew. Here was an hospital for lepers, with a free chapel dedicated to St. Mary and St. Lawrence : its revenue, at the dissolution, was valued only at £3. 7. 6.

ICKENHAM, a parish in the hundred of ELTHORNE, county of MIDDLESEX, 2¾ miles (N. E.) from Uxbridge, containing 281 inhabitants. The living is a rectory, in the jurisdiction of the Commissary of London, concurrently with the Consistorial Court of the Bishop, rated in the king's books at £13. 6. 8., and in the patronage of T. Truesdale Clarke, Esq. The church is dedicated to St. Giles.

ICKFORD, a parish partly in the hundred of EWELME, county of OXFORD, but chiefly in that of ASHENDON, county of BUCKINGHAM, 4¼ miles (W. by N.) from Thame, containing 324 inhabitants. The living is a rectory, in the archdeaconry of Buckingham, and diocese of Lincoln, rated in the king's books at £9. 9. 7. R. Townsend, Esq. was patron in 1808. The church is dedicated to St. Nicholas. Here is a place of worship for Baptists. In 1733, £10 per annum was given by Thomas Phillips, for the use of a schoolmaster. Ickford is supposed by some writers to have been the place where the treaty between Edward and the Danes was signed, in 907. Calybute Downing, a celebrated divine in the seventeenth century, was rector of this parish.

ICKHAM, a parish in the hundred of DOWNHAMFORD, lathe of ST. AUGUSTINE, county of KENT, 1¼ mile (N.W. by W.) from Wingham, containing 521 inhabitants. The living is a rectory with the curacy of Weld, in the exempt deanery of Shoreham, which is in the peculiar jurisdiction of the Archbishop of Canterbury, rated in the king's books at £29. 13. 4., and in the patronage of the Archbishop of Canterbury. The church, dedicated to St. John the Evangelist, is principally in the early style of English architecture, with insertions in the decorated style.

ICKLEFORD, a parish in the hundred of HITCHIN and PIRTON, county of HERTFORD, 1¾ mile (N.) from Hitchin, containing 442 inhabitants. The living is a rectory with the vicarage of Pirton, in the archdeaconry of Huntingdon, and diocese of Lincoln, rated in the king's books at £8. C. Peers, Esq. was patron in 1773. The church is dedicated to St. Catherine. A fair is held on the 2nd of August. The village is situated on the line of the ancient Iknield-street.

ICKLESHAM, a parish in the hundred of GUESTLING, rape of HASTINGS, county of SUSSEX, 2 miles (W. by S.) from Winchelsea, containing 585 inhabitants. The living is a vicarage, in the archdeaconry of Lewes, and diocese of Chichester, rated in the king's books at £13. 1. 8., and in the patronage of the Bishop of Chichester. The church, dedicated to St. Nicholas, is in the early style of English architecture. The manorial courts are held at Icklesham Place house. The Brede canal passes on the north side of this parish.

ICKLETON, a parish in the hundred of WHITTLES-

FORD, county of CAMBRIDGE, 4¾ miles (W. S. W.) from Linton, containing 602 inhabitants. The living is a vicarage, in the archdeaconry and diocese of Ely, rated in the king's books at £8. 6. 8., endowed with £200 private benefaction, £200 royal bounty, and £200 parliamentary grant, and in the patronage of the Bishop of Ely. The church is dedicated to St. Mary Magdalene. A Benedictine nunnery was founded in the reign of Henry II., the revenue of which, at the dissolution, was valued at £80. 1. 10. A market, now disused, was granted to the Prioress by Henry III., together with a fair, which is still held on the 22nd of July.

ICKLINGHAM, a parish comprising the consolidated parishes of All Saints and St. James, in the hundred of LACKFORD, county of SUFFOLK, 3½ miles (E. S. E.) from Mildenhall, containing 424 inhabitants. The living is a rectory, in the archdeaconry of Sudbury, and diocese of Norwich, rated jointly in the king's books at £24. 8. 11½. The Rev. D. Gwilt was patron in 1820. The navigable river Lark passes through the parish. Here are several tumuli and other relics of antiquity.

ICKWELL, a hamlet in the parish of NORTHILL, hundred of WIXAMTREE, county of BEDFORD, 2¾ miles (W. by N.) from Biggleswade. The population is returned with the parish.

ICKWORTH, a parish in the hundred of THINGOE, county of SUFFOLK, 2½ miles (S. W.) from Bury-St. Edmund's, containing 82 inhabitants. The living is a discharged rectory, united to that of Chedburgh, in the archdeaconry of Sudbury, and diocese of Norwich, rated in the king's books at £7. 11. 5½., and in the patronage of the Marquis of Bristol. The church has a chancel in the early style, and some windows in the decorated and later styles, of English architecture.

IDBURY, a parish in the hundred of CHADLINGTON, county of OXFORD, 5½ miles (N. by W.) from Burford, containing 193 inhabitants. The living is a perpetual curacy, in the archdeaconry and diocese of Oxford, endowed with £16 per annum private benefaction, and £600 royal bounty, and in the patronage of F. F. Turville, Esq. There are vestiges of a large military camp near the turnpike-road from Stow on the Wold to Burford.

IDDESLEIGH, a parish in the hundred of SHEBBEAR, county of DEVON, 3¾ miles (N. E. by N.) from Hatherleigh, containing 482 inhabitants. The living is a rectory, in the archdeaconry of Barnstaple, and diocese of Exeter, rated in the king's books at £17. 1. 3., and in the patronage of H. Harris, Esq. The church, dedicated to St. James, contains a monumental effigy of a crusader, supposed to represent Sir J. Sully, whose family once possessed this manor. The Rev. William Tasker, a poet and dramatist, was born here in 1740; he died in 1800.

IDE, a parish in the hundred of EXMINSTER, county of DEVON, 2¼ miles (S. W.) from Exeter, containing 724 inhabitants. The living is a perpetual curacy, in the peculiar jurisdiction of the Dean and Chapter of Exeter. The church is dedicated to St. Ida.

IDEFORD, a parish in the hundred of TEINGBRIDGE, county of DEVON, 2½ miles (S. E.) from Chudleigh, containing 356 inhabitants. The living is a rectory, in the archdeaconry of Totness, and diocese of Exeter, rated in the king's books at £17. 13. 9. The Rev. J. Heywood was patron in 1811. The church is dedicated to St. Mary.

IDE-HILL, a chapelry in the parish of SUNDRIDGE, hundred of CODSHEATH, lathe of SUTTON at HONE, county of KENT, 3¾ miles (W. S. W.) from Sevenoaks. The population is returned with the parish. The living is a perpetual curacy, in the peculiar jurisdiction and patronage of the Archbishop of Canterbury, endowed with £400 private benefaction, and £600 parliamentary grant. The chapel was erected and endowed in 1807, by the Rt. Rev. Beilby Porteus, Bishop of London.

IDEN, a parish in the hundred of GOLDSPUR, rape of HASTINGS, county of SUSSEX, 2¼ miles (N.) from Rye, containing 542 inhabitants. The living is a rectory, in the archdeaconry of Lewes, and diocese of Chichester, rated in the king's books at £18. 8. 6½. Thomas P. Lamb, Esq. was patron in 1807. The church is dedicated to All Saints. Here is a place of worship for Wesleyan Methodists. The Royal Military canal and the river Rother pass through this parish.

IDLE, a chapelry in the parish of CALVERLEY, wapentake of MORLEY, West riding of the county of YORK, 4 miles (N. N. E.) from Bradford, containing 4666 inhabitants. The living is a perpetual curacy, in the archdeaconry and diocese of York, endowed with £250 private benefaction, £400 royal bounty, and £400 parliamentary grant, and in the patronage of the Vicar of Calverley. A chapel is in progress of erection, according to the provisions of the act of parliament for building additional churches. There are places of worship for Baptists, Independents, and Wesleyan Methodists. An academy for the education of students preparing for the ministry, in connexion with the Independents, was founded here in 1800, and subsequently endowed with £150 per annum, by Edward Hanson, Esq., of Clapton in Middlesex, a native of this county; it is additionally supported by voluntary contributions.

IDLICOTE, a parish in the Brails division of the hundred of KINGTON, county of WARWICK, 3¼ miles (N. E.) from Shipston upon Stour, containing 88 inhabitants. The living is a rectory, in the archdeaconry and diocese of Worcester, rated in the king's books at £13. 6. 8. Samuel Peach, Esq. was patron in 1800. The church is dedicated to St. James.

IDMISTON, a parish in the hundred of ALDERBURY, county of WILTS, comprising the chapelry of Porton, and the tythings of Ford, Gomeldon, Idmiston, and Shripple, and containing 438 inhabitants, of which number, 177 are in the tything of Idmiston, 5¼ miles (N. E. by N.) from Salisbury. The living is a vicarage, in the archdeaconry and diocese of Salisbury, rated in the king's books at £15. 6. 0½., and in the patronage of the Bishop of Salisbury. The church is dedicated to All Saints. The Rev. John Bowle, celebrated for his critical knowledge of Spanish literature, who published one of the best editions of the Spanish Don Quixote, was vicar of this parish.

IDRIDGEHAY, a joint township with Allton, in that part of the parish of WIRKSWORTH which is in the hundred of APPLETREE, county of DERBY, 3½ miles (S.) from Wirksworth, containing 160 inhabitants. In 1752, H. Jackson left £15, for teaching two poor children.

IDSTONE, a tything in the parish of ASHBURY, hundred of SHRIVENHAM, county of BERKS, 5½ miles

(W. N. W.) from Lambourn, containing 154 inhabitants. The ancient Iknield-street intersects this village.

IDSWORTH, a chapelry in the parish of Chalton, hundred of Finch-Dean, Alton (South) division of the county of Southampton, 7½ miles (S. by W.) from Petersfield, containing 310 inhabitants.

IFIELD, a parish in the hundred of Tolting-trough, lathe of Aylesford, county of Kent, 2½ miles (S. by E.) from Gravesend, containing 55 inhabitants. The living is a discharged rectory, in the exempt deanery of Shoreham, which is in the peculiar jurisdiction of the Archbishop of Canterbury, rated in the king's books at £4. 7., and in the patronage of H. Edmeads, Esq. The church, dedicated to St. Margaret, is the smallest in the diocese; it was rebuilt in 1596. This village being comprehended in the hamlet of Shinglewell, is usually called Shinglefield-street, it being situated on the line of a Roman road, traces of which are yet visible.

IFIELD, a parish in the hundred of Burbeach, though locally in that of Singlecross, rape of Bramber, county of Sussex, 7 miles (N. E.) from Horsham, containing 758 inhabitants. The living is a vicarage, in the archdeaconry of Lewes, and diocese of Chichester, rated in the king's books at £6. 8. 4., and in the patronage of the Rev. Spencer James Lewin. The church, dedicated to St. Margaret, has portions in the early and decorated styles of English architecture, and contains recumbent statues of a Knight Templar and his lady. The river Mole runs through this parish. Two farm-houses in the parish are each surrounded by a wide moat.

IFLEY, a parish in the hundred of Bullington, county of Oxford, 1¾ mile (S.E. by S.) from Oxford, containing, with the hamlet of Hockmoor, and a portion of the liberty of Littlemoor, 881 inhabitants. The living is a vicarage, in the archdeaconry and diocese of Oxford, rated in the king's books at £8, endowed with £200 private benefaction, £600 royal bounty, and £500 parliamentary grant, and in the patronage of the Archdeacon of Oxford. The church, dedicated to St. Mary, is principally of Norman architecture, having a low square tower between the nave and the chancel, with a handsome south porch, and a fine western doorway, embellished with chevron mouldings and other decorations : the chancel is partly in the early English style, and there are some windows of a later date. In 1805, a school for educating and clothing ten girls was founded, in pursuance of the will of Thomas Nowell, D. D., who left property producing £39 per annum for this purpose. Mrs. Alice Smith, in 1678, gave lands and tenements, producing about £100 per annum, for apprenticing poor boys and other purposes.

IFORD, a parish in the hundred of Swanborough, rape of Lewes, county of Sussex, 2¼ miles (S. by W.) from Lewes, containing 157 inhabitants. The living is a vicarage, united to that of Kingston near Lewes, in the archdeaconry of Lewes, and diocese of Chichester, rated in the king's books at £10. 10. 2½. The church, dedicated to St. Nicholas, is in the early style of English architecture. In the Saxon times here was a shrine or statue of a Pagan deity, called Niorde, of which the present name of the parish is a corruption.

IFORD, a hamlet in the parish of Westwood, hundred of Elstub and Everley, county of Wilts, 2¼ miles (S. W. by W.) from Bradford. The population is returned with the parish.

IFTON, a parish in the lower division of the hundred of Galdicott, county of Monmouth, 6 miles (S.W.) from Chepstow, containing 50 inhabitants. The living is a rectory not in charge, united to the rectory of Roggiet, in the archdeaconry and diocese of Llandaff. The church has been demolished.

IFTON-RHYN, a township in the parish of St Martin, hundred of Oswestry, county of Salop, containing 935 inhabitants.

IGHTENHILL-PARK, a township in that part of the parish of Whalley which is in the higher division of the hundred of Blackburn, county palatine of Lancaster, containing 208 inhabitants. There are coal-works in this township.

IGHTFIELD, a parish in the Whitchurch division of the hundred of Bradford (North), county of Salop, 4¼ miles (S.E. by E) from Whitchurch, containing 261 inhabitants. The living is a rectory, in the archdeaconry of Salop, and diocese of Lichfield and Coventry, rated in the king's books at £7. 14. 9½. P. Justice, Esq. was patron in 1780. The church is dedicated to St. John the Baptist.

IGHTHAM, a parish in the hundred of Wrotham, lathe of Aylesford, county of Kent, 1¼ mile (S. W.) from Wrotham, containing 867 inhabitants. The living is a rectory, within the exempt deanery of Shoreham, which is in the peculiar jurisdiction of the Archbishop of Canterbury, rated in the king's books at £15. 16. 8., and in the patronage of the Rev. S. Cobb. The church is dedicated to St. Peter. In 1720, Elizabeth James gave a rent-charge for the instruction of children, and bequeathed £50 to be placed at interest, directing ten shillings per annum to be given in books to the children, and the surplus to the poor. On Old Berry hill are the remains of a Roman Castra œstiva, which occupied a space of one hundred and thirty seven acres : in the centre of this ancient enclosure are two fine springs. A fair is held annually in Whitsun-week. The ancient name of this parish was Eight ham, it having contained eight hams or villages.

IKEN, a parish in the hundred of Plomesgate, county of Suffolk, 5 miles (N. by W.) from Orford, containing 363 inhabitants. The living is a discharged rectory, in the archdeaconry of Suffolk, and diocese of Norwich, rated in the king's books at £6. 13. 4. Thomas Syer, Esq. was patron in 1793. The church is dedicated to St. Botolph. The navigable river Alde runs on the north of this parish, which on the east is bounded by the North sea.

ILAM, a parish in the northern division of the hundred of Totmonslow, county of Stafford, 4¼ miles (N. W.) from Ashbourn, containing, with the hamlets of Casterton and Throwley, 253 inhabitants. The living is a vicarage, in the archdeaconry of Stafford, and diocese of Lichfield and Coventry, rated in the king's books at £6. 13. 4. J. Watts Russell, Esq. was patron in 1814. The church is dedicated to the Holy Cross. Here is a National school, in which fifty boys and thirty girls are instructed at the expense of Jesse Watts Russell, Esq., with the exception of a benefaction of £4 per annum, left by Lady Bellot for the education of eight children, which is now applied towards the support of this school. Congreve, the dramatic poet, retired to this secluded and romantic spot, after his return from Ireland, and here composed his first comedy, The Old Bachelor.

Seal and Arms.

ILCHESTER, a borough, parish, and formerly a market town, locally in the hundred of Tintinhull, county of SOMERSET, 4 miles (S. S. E.) from Somerton, and 122 (W. S. W.) from London, containing 994 inhabitants. This place, called by the Britons *Pont Ivel Coit*, signifying the bridge over the Ivel in the wood, was the *Ischalis* of Ptolemy, and, from having been a Roman station on the river Ivel, obtained the Saxon appellation of *Ivelceastre*, of which its present name is an obvious contraction. It was anciently a town of much greater extent and importance than it is at present, and was encompassed by walls, and defended by a deep moat: of the former, the foundations are plainly discernible in various places, and of the latter there are still vestiges at Belles-Pool and also in Yard-lane, to the north of the town. The ancient gates are supposed to have occupied the site of the present entrances from Ilminster and Yeovil, and near the bridge may be traced the stones of a ford across the river. The Roman Fosse-way from London to Exeter, which passed through the town, still forms the principal turnpike-road, and there are some remains of a fortification, which is supposed to have been built by the Romans. At the time of the Norman Conquest it appears to have been a place of importance, as it had then one hundred and seven burgesses; and in 1088, during a rebellion against William Rufus, Ilchester was successfully defended against Robert Mowbray, a leader of the insurgents, who had laid siege to it.

The town is pleasantly situated on the south bank of the river Ivel, in a rich vale almost embosomed in mountains, and is connected with the parish of Northover by a stone bridge of seven arches, on which formerly were two ancient buildings: the houses, with few exceptions are indifferently built, and there are extensive piles of building, consisting of several stories, and comprising, on each, different small tenements inhabited by burgage tenants at a nominal rent, and erected for their accommodation by the parliamentary patrons of the borough. The market-place is a commodious area, at the lower end of which is the town-hall, and at the upper a handsome pillar of the Doric order, supporting a vertical sun-dial with four faces directed to the four cardinal points. An ancient building, now used as a workhouse, was formerly the residence of a family of the name of Masters, and the then owner, having entertained Richard Cœur de Lion as his guest, was honoured with that surname by the monarch, and it remained with the family until within the last few years, when it became extinct by the marriage of the last female descendant. Assemblies occasionally take place in the townhall: the races, which were formerly held on Kingsmoor, have been discontinued. There are no particular branches of manufacture: some of the female inhabitants are employed in making gloves for the Yeovil manufacturers; but the town derives its chief trade from its situation as a thoroughfare. The market, formerly on Wednesday, is now disused: the fairs are on the Monday before Palm-Sunday, July 2nd, and August 2nd,

for cattle and pigs; but the two last fairs are rapidly falling into neglect. Ilchester, a borough by prescription, was incorporated by charter of King John, by which the government is vested in a bailiff and twelve capital burgesses: the corporation have power to hold courts of assize, which privilege they have not exercised for a very considerable length of time; and the assizes for the county, formerly held in this town, are now held at Taunton, Wells, and Bridg-water. A county court, called the Sheriff's court, for the recovery of debts under 40s., is held here monthly, besides the court leet of the lord of the manor, at which constables and other officers are appointed. The town-hall is a neat modern structure, commodiously adapted to the discharge of the public business of the town, and containing a large assembly-room. The county gaol is a spacious building, on the northern bank of the Ivel, comprising twelve wards, or divisions, with a day-room and airing-yard to each, including two for debtors: it is well adapted to the classification of prisoners, of whom it is calculated to receive from one hundred and seventy to one hundred and eighty. The borough first exercised the elective franchise in the 26th of Edward I., and made regular returns till the 34th of Edward III., from which time it omitted until the 12th of Edward IV., when it resumed its privileges; it again discontinued until the 19th of James I., since which time it has regularly returned two members to parliament: the right of election is in the bailiff and burgesses, and the inhabitants of the burgage tenements not receiving alms, the number of whom is about one hundred and twenty; for whose accommodation, Lord Huntingtower, the patron, has erected cow-sheds in a large field, in which they have the privilege of depasturing cows, for a small nominal payment. The election of the members for the county takes place in the town.

The living is a rectory, in the archdeaconry of Wells, and diocese of Bath and Wells, rated in the king's books at £7. 16. 10½., endowed with £200 private benefaction, and £200 royal bounty, and in the patronage of the Bishop of Bath and Wells. The church, dedicated to St. Mary, is an ancient building with a small octagonal tower; in the chancel is a monument to the memory of the daughter of William Evers, Esq., servant to Henry VIII., Edward VI., and Queen Mary, and serjeant at arms to Queen Elizabeth. There is a place of worship for Independents. Here are almshouses which appear to have been founded in the reign of Henry VI., by Mr. Robert Veal, who endowed them with lands producing upwards of £100 per annum, for the residence and maintenance of aged men and women; they were, in 1810, commodiously rebuilt of stone, on the site of the ancient tenements, by the bailiff and burgesses, who are the trustees of this charity, and there are thirteen men who receive four shillings, and one woman, officiating as nurse, who receives three shillings and sixpence, per week, with an allowance of coal and other necessaries. A school, in which the children of the parish are instructed in reading, writing, and arithmetic, is held in a room in the town-hall, under the patronage of the corporation. A few years since, in removing part of the old wainscoting in the house anciently occupied by the family of Masters, a beautiful specimen of carved ivory was found, enclosed in a wooden frame in two compartments, representing the Annunciation of the Virgin: the figures, about six inches in height, are exquisitely carved in alto relievo, probably a present from Richard Cœur de Lion to his host ; and in digging a garden nearly opposite the house, an ancient ring of massy gold was discovered, in which was set a coin of the Emperor Severus, in excellent preservation. Among the monastic institutions anciently existing here, was a nunnery, originally founded, about 1220, by William Dacres, as an hospital for poor travellers, and dedicated to the Blessed Trinity, which, prior to the Reformation, had dwindled into a free chapel. Here was also a convent of preaching friars, in which the celebrated Roger Bacon (who is usually stated to have been a native of Ilchester, but his birthplace is uncertain) was educated. The eminent Mrs. Rowe, author of "Devout Exercises of the Heart," and other works, was a native of this parish. Ilchester gives the title of earl to the family of Fox.

ILDERTON, a parish in the northern division of COQUETDALE ward, county of NORTHUMBERLAND, comprising the townships of Ilderton, Middleton-Hall, North Middleton, South Middleton, Roddam, and Rosedon, and containing 579 inhabitants, of which number, 157 are in the township of Ilderton, 4¼ miles (S. S. E.) from Wooler. The living is a discharged rectory, in the archdeaconry of Northumberland, and diocese of Durham, rated in the king's books at £4, endowed with £200 royal bounty, and £600 parliamentary grant, and in the patronage of the Duke of Northumberland. The church is dedicated to St. Michael. The river Bredmish flows on the southern side of this parish, which is intersected by the Caldgate, Lilburn, Roddam, and several minor streams. On Rosedon-Edge are the remains of a square encampment. Between this village and Hedgehope is an ancient temple of the Druids, consisting of ten large unequal stones, placed in an oval form, thirty-eight yards in diameter from east to west, and thirty-three from north to south.

ILFORD (GREAT), a chapelry in the parish of BARK-ING, hundred of BECONTREE, county of ESSEX, 8 miles (N. E. by E.) from London, containing 2972 inhabitants. The living is a perpetual curacy, in the archdeaconry of Essex, and diocese of London, endowed with £200 private benefaction, £600 royal bounty, and £800 parliamentary grant. James H. Leigh, Esq. was patron in 1815. A new chapel is about to be erected by the parliamentary commissioners. There are places of worship for Baptists and Wesleyan Methodists. The petty sessions for the division are held here every Saturday. In the reign of Stephen, the abbess of Barking founded an hospital at Ilford for thirteen lepers : the present buildings are appropriated to the use of six poor persons, and comprise an ancient chapel.

ILFORD (LITTLE), a parish in the hundred of BECONTREE, county of ESSEX, 7 miles (E. N. E.) from London, containing 87 inhabitants. The living is a rectory, in the archdeaconry of Essex, and diocese of London, rated in the king's books at £11. 13. 9. James H. Leigh, Esq. was patron in 1815. The church is dedicated to St. Mary. In this parish, with those of East and West Ham, Leyton, and Wansted, a great mart is annually held for cattle brought from Wales, Scotland, and the North of England, from February until May.

ILFRACOMBE, or ILFORDCOMBE, a sea-port, market town, and parish, in the hundred of BRAUNTON,

county of DEVON, 12 miles (N. W. by N.) from Barnstaple, and 204 (W. by S.) from London, containing 2622 inhabitants. In the latter part of the thirteenth century, a grant was obtained for holding a market and a fair at this place, which, as a sea-port, furnished six ships and eighty-two men towards the armament of Edward III., against Calais. During the parliamentary war, the royalists under Sir F. Doddington took possession of the town. The situation of this port is near the northern extremity of the county, bordering on the Bristol channel, opposite to the coast of Wales. The town is irregularly built on the side of a hill, and consists principally of a long narrow street, some parts of which are very steep, extending from the church to the harbour : it is in contemplation to widen a portion of this street. At the outskirts of the town are several good houses, particularly a range of buildings called Constitution Terrace, in the centre of which are the public rooms, with a handsome front of the Ionic order. A new road passing through a winding valley has lately been formed between this place and Barnstaple. Westward from the town are seven hills, called Torrs, which form a noted land-mark, the descent from which terminates in an opening to the sea, called Wildersmouth ; and on the east is the rock of Hilsborough, its summit being five hundred feet above the level of the sea. The entrance to the harbour is between this rock and a smaller eminence to the west, on which is a lighthouse. The harbour, which is completely environed by a series of rocks, is protected towards the sea by an artificial pier built by the family of Bourchier, lords of the manor, which having been greatly injured by the violence of the sea, an act of parliament was procured, in 1731, for repairing and enlarging it, and improving the harbour ; and it has recently undergone further improvement at the expense of the present proprietor of the manor. Ilfracombe is chiefly of importance as a haven for windbound vessels ; and a great quantity of corn is occasionally shipped from the port, but the vessels belonging to it are principally employed in conveying goods from Bristol, and coal from South Wales. During summer, a packet sails every Monday and Thursday to Swansea, and a steam-packet every Saturday ; and there is a steam-packet to Bristol every Tuesday and Thursday. A market for provisions is held on Saturday ; and there are cattle fairs on April 14th and the Saturday next after August 23rd. Ilfracombe is rapidly increasing in repute as a watering-place, its beach affording the greatest facility for sea-bathing, and there are some convenient lodging-houses. A regatta was established in the summer of 1828. Courts leet are held annually for the manor, at which a portreeve and constables for the town and parish are appointed.

The living is a discharged vicarage, in the archdeaconry of Barnstaple, and diocese of Exeter, rated in the king's books at £50. 4., and in the patronage of the Prebendary of Ilfracombe in the Cathedral Church of Salisbury. The church, dedicated to the Holy Trinity, is an ancient building situated on a hill, at a short distance from the town. Here is a place of worship for Independents. A school for twelve poor children is endowed with £6 per annum, and another for fourteen children, with £4 per annum, both from a benefaction by Mrs. Gertrude Pyncombe, in 1730 ; and there are also charity schools, supported by subscription, a school of industry, and Sunday schools on the plans of Bell and Lancaster.

ILKESTON, a market town and parish, in the hundred of MORLESTON and LITCHURCH, county of DERBY, 9½ miles (N.E. by E.) from Derby, and 128 (N.W. by N.) from London, containing 3681 inhabitants. This place, anciently called *Elchestane*, obtained a grant for a market and a fair in 1251. Its ancient importance may be inferred from a tradition that the assizes were formerly held here, having been transferred from Nottingham on account of the plague; in consequence of which, the inhabitants of Ilkeston were privileged to pay but half toll at fairs and markets, on condition of their keeping in repair a gallows for the execution of criminals, which stands at the southern extremity of the parish, on the border of Nottinghamshire. From time immemorial the people of Ilkeston have claimed this privilege at the neighbouring fairs, but being unable to produce any charter in support of their claim, they have been resisted on some occasions. The town stands on a hill, near the river Erewash, commanding beautiful prospects in every direction, and the situation is healthy; but though there are several springs, the supply of water is not abundant. Considerable advantage is anticipated from the recent discovery of a mineral spring, the properties of which are said to be different from those of any other spa in England, resembling the Seltzer water from Germany. The Ilkeston water appears to contain carbonates of lime and soda, muriate of lime, sulphates of magnesia and soda, a small quantity of iron, and a large portion of carbonic acid gas; and it has been found an efficacious remedy, both internally and externally, in cases of indigestion, diseases of the liver, gravel, gout, scrofula, and cutaneous affections. The spa is at the north end of the town, where a building with a neat front has been erected, comprising every accommodation for bathing. The Old bath, so called because it was the first discovered, was built in September 1829; and there are two slipper-baths, lined with marble, having a shower-bath over each of them, together with convenient dressing-rooms: a cistern for water, heated by steam, contains three thousand gallons, and the cold cistern contains fifteen hundred gallons; these supply the baths with water of any required temperature. Since the discovery of the medicinal spring, Ilkeston has been much frequented: it is in contemplation to form a public library; and there is a choral society, under the direction of which an annual performance of sacred music takes place in the parish church. The principal branches of manufacture carried on are those of stockings and lace; the former affords employment to about four hundred persons, but it is said to be declining; the latter, which is flourishing, employs one hundred and twenty men, and a great number of women and children. The parish abounds with various and extensive veins of coal and iron-stone. In a stratum of hard coal, now in operation, there is a vein of lead-ore, spar, martial pyrites, and coal intermingled, but the ore, though fine, exists only in small quantities. Both the Erewash and the Nutbrook canals pass through this parish, affording a communication with the rivers Trent and Mersey. The market, chiefly for fruit and vegetables, is held on Thursday; and there are fairs, March 6th, Whit-Thursday, and the first Thursday after Christmas-day, for horses, cattle, sheep, and hogs. Courts leet and

baron for the manor are held under the Duke of Rutland. The living is a discharged vicarage, in the archdeaconry of Derby, and diocese of Lichfield and Coventry, rated in the king's books at £5. 7. 9., endowed with £600 royal bounty, and in the patronage of the Duke of Rutland. The church, dedicated to St. Mary, is an ancient structure, with a lofty tower of modern date; and in the interior is a stone screen in the early English style, together with some interesting ancient monuments. An application has recently been made to the parliamentary commissioners, for a grant for the erection of a new church or chapel. There are places of worship for General and Particular Baptists, Independents, Wesleyan Methodists, and Unitarians. In 1704, the Rev. Mr. Courtman bequeathed land producing £2 per annum for the education of poor children, the proceeds being now paid to the account of a Sunday school, which is principally supported by subscription. A charity school for thirty children is endowed with £10 per annum, from a benefaction by Richard Smedley, who, in 1744, gave a rent-charge of £60 for the establishment of this and other schools, and for the foundation and endowment of almshouses for six poor women, who receive £5 per annum each: there are likewise four unendowed almshouses.

ILKETSHALL (ST. ANDREW), a parish in the hundred of WANGFORD, county of SUFFOLK, 3¾ miles (S. E. by E.) from Bungay, containing 472 inhabitants. The living is a discharged vicarage, in the archdeaconry of Suffolk, and diocese of Norwich, rated in the king's books at £5. 13. 4., and in the patronage of the Master and Fellows of Emanuel College, Cambridge.

ILKETSHALL (ST. JOHN), a parish in the hundred of WANGFORD, county of SUFFOLK, 2 miles (S. E.) from Bungay, containing 66 inhabitants. The living is a vicarage, in the archdeaconry of Suffolk, and diocese of Norwich, rated in the king's books at £8. 13. 4., and in the patronage of the Crown.

ILKETSHALL (ST. LAWRENCE), a parish in the hundred of WANGFORD, county of SUFFOLK, 3¼ miles (S. E. by S.) from Bungay, containing 255 inhabitants. The living is a perpetual curacy, in the archdeaconry of Suffolk, and diocese of Norwich, endowed with £800 royal bounty, and £200 parliamentary grant, and in the patronage of the Rev. Henry Stebbing.

ILKETSHALL (ST. MARGARET), a parish in the hundred of WANGFORD, county of SUFFOLK, 2¾ miles (S. S. E.) from Bungay, containing 269 inhabitants. The living is a discharged vicarage, in the archdeaconry of Suffolk, and diocese of Norwich, rated in the king's books at £5. 13. 9., and in the patronage of the Duke of Norfolk.

ILKLEY, a parish comprising the townships of Middleton with Stockhill, and Nesfield with Langbar, in the upper division of the wapentake of CLARO, and the township of Ilkley in the upper division of the wapentake of SKYRACK, West riding of the county of YORK, and containing 911 inhabitants, of which number, 496 are in the township of Ilkley, 5¼ miles (W. N. W.) from Otley. The living is a discharged vicarage, in the archdeaconry and diocese of York, rated in the king's books at £7. 13. 9., endowed with £200 royal bounty, and £1000 parliamentary grant. L. W. Hartley, Esq. was patron in 1813. The church is dedicated to All Saints: in the church-yard are three Saxon crosses.

This place is much frequented in the summer, for the benefit of a cold bath, which is supplied from a spring issuing out of a neighbouring hill. Here is a free school, endowed with a rent-charge arising from a gift of £100, by — Marshall, in the reign of James I., and a bequest of £200 by Reginald Heber, in 1696. The school-room is a very old building, and about forty children are instructed. Ilkley is supposed to have been the *Olicana* of the Romans : here is a Roman fortress, with three sides entire ; and at Middleton Lodge is an altar to Verbeia, the Nymph of the Wharf ; there are also three summer camps and outposts, called Castleburg, Counter-hill, and Woofa Bank.

ILLINGTON, a parish in the hundred of SHROPHAM, county of NORFOLK, 3½ miles (N. W. by W.) from East Harling, containing 96 inhabitants. The living is a discharged rectory, in the archdeaconry of Norfolk, and diocese of Norwich, rated in the king's books at £6. 19. 2. Mrs. Kellett was patroness in 1787. The church is dedicated to St. Andrew.

ILLINGWORTH, a chapelry in the parish of HALI-FAX, wapentake of MORLEY, West riding of the county of YORK, 2¼ miles (N. W. by N.) from Halifax, with which the population is returned. The living is a perpetual curacy, in the archdeaconry and diocese of York, endowed with £450 private benefaction, £600 royal bounty, and £200 parliamentary grant, and in the patronage of the Vicar of Halifax. The chapel is dedicated to St. Mary. Here is a place of worship for Wesleyan Methodists.

ILLMIRE, a parish in the hundred of ASHENDON, county of BUCKINGHAM, 4½ miles (E. by S.) from Thame, containing 68 inhabitants. The living is a discharged vicarage, in the archdeaconry of Buckingham, and diocese of Lincoln, rated in the king's books at £6. 10. 8., endowed with £200 royal bounty, and in the patronage of the Earl of Chesterfield. The church is dedicated to St. Peter.

ILLOGAN, a parish in the hundred of PENWITH, county of CORNWALL, 2¾ miles (N. W.) from Redruth, containing 5170 inhabitants. The living is a rectory, in the archdeaconry of Cornwall, and diocese of Exeter, rated in the king's books at £22. 7. 6., and in the patron-age of Lord de Dunstanville. The church is dedicated to St. Illogan. There is a place of worship for Wesleyan Methodists. Here is a small endowed school. An almshouse for four poor aged women was founded in 1806. At Trevenson, in this parish, a new chapel has been erected, and endowed with lands producing about £42 per annum, by Lord de Dunstanville. At Basset's Cove is a small haven for the importation of coal and lime, and the exportation of copper-ore to the copper works in Wales. A pier was erected in 1760, and has since been greatly improved by a Joint Stock Company, at an expense of £10,000. Cook's Kitchen, one of the principal mines in Cornwall, is in this parish : on the east a railway passes from the various mines in the neighbourhood to Portreath, on the Bristol channel. On the summit of Carn Bre Hill, the supposed site of a Druidical temple, are the remains of a baronial castle, which belonged to Sir John Basset, in the reign of Edward IV. On the side of this hill Roman coins and British gold coins have been discovered. The plague raged at Illogan in 1591, and swept off about one hundred persons.

ILMINGTON, a parish comprising the small hamlet of Lark-Stoke in the upper division of the hundred of KIFTSGATE, county of GLOUCESTER, but chiefly in a detached part of the Kington division of the hundred of KINGTON, county of WARWICK, 4 miles (N.W. by W.) from Shipston upon Stour, and containing, with the hamlet of Compton-Scorpion, 727 inhabitants. The living is a rectory, in the archdeaconry and diocese of Worcester, rated in the king's books at £30. The Rev. H. Townsend was patron in 1807. The church is dedicated to St. Mary.

ILMINSTER, a market town and parish, in the hundred of ABDICK and BULSTONE, county of SOMER-SET, 13 miles (S. W. by W.) from Ilchester, and 136 (W. S. W.) from London, containing 2156 inhabitants. This place, which is of considerable antiquity, and prior to the Conquest had the privilege of a weekly market, is situated within a mile of the river Ile, from which, and from its church, it derived its name : it was formerly more extensive than it is at present, having been repeatedly damaged by conflagrations, of which that in 1491 destroyed the greater part of the town. The Duke of Monmouth, on the day before the battle of Sedgemoor, dined in public under an ancient chesnut tree in White Lackington park, the seat of Colonel Speke, whose son was afterwards executed in this town, for his adherence to the interests of that nobleman, and for the part he took in the rebellion. The town consists principally of two streets, the larger of which is more than a mile in length : the houses are neat and well built, and the general appearance of the place is cleanly and prepossessing. The neighbourhood abounds with interesting scenery : from an eminence in the vicinity there is an extensive prospect, comprehending a view of not less than thirty parish churches, and of the course of the river, over which, to the west of the town, is a neat stone bridge of four arches. The woollen manufacture formerly flourished here to a considerable extent, but at present there is only one factory : a silk-mill has been recently established : there are some tanneries, and a considerable trade in malt is carried on. The market is on Wednesday ; and there is a fair on the last Wednesday in August : the market-house is a neat and commodious building. The town is within the jurisdiction of the county magistrates, who hold a petty session for the division every month during the winter, and constables or tythingmen are annually appointed at the court leet of the lord of the manor. The living is a vicarage, in the jurisdiction of the peculiar court of the manor of Ilminster, rated in the king's books at £25. 5., and in the patronage of William Hanning, Esq. The church, dedicated to St. Mary, is a venerable and spacious cruciform structure, in the decorated style of English architecture, with a fine tower of light and beautiful design rising from the centre, and crowned with twelve pinnacles : within are several ancient and interesting monuments, among which are those of Nicholas and Dorothy Wadham, the munificent founders of Wadham College, Oxford. There are places of worship for Independents, Wesleyan Methodists, and Unitarians. The free grammar school was founded by Edward VI., in the third year of his reign, and endowed with lands and tenements producing an income of £490 per annum, of which a part is appropriated to the repairs of the bridge and the high roads ; there are about ten free scholars on the foundation, appointed by the trustees, who elect the master, whose salary is £100 per annum, with a house, and the privilege of taking stipendiary pupils: in 1824, William Hanning, Esq. gave premises and lands for the establishment of four exhibitions to the University, for boys of this school. A secondary establishment, supported by the same funds, has been recently added, in which forty boys are taught reading, writing, and arithmetic, and forty girls receive evening instruction, under a master who has, according to the number of free scholars, a salary varying from £30 to £50 per annum: a third school is also supported from the same funds, in which young children are taught to read by a female; and £15 per annum are also paid by the trustees towards the support of a Sunday school. There are also various charitable bequests for distribution among the poor.

ILSINGTON, a parish in the hundred of TEING-BRIDGE, county of DEVON, 4¾ miles (N. N. E.) from Ashburton, containing 1122 inhabitants. The living is a vicarage, in the archdeaconry of Totness, and diocese of Exeter, rated in the king's books at £17. 9. 7., and in the patronage of the Dean and Canons of Windsor. The church, which is dedicated to St. Michael, contains some modern screen-work. In 1663, Jane Ford devised a rent-charge for the education of poor children: the present income is about £26 per annum, and fifty children are educated. Pipe and potters' clay, and lead-ore, may be obtained in this parish: the Stover railway passs through the north-eastern part of it.

ILSLEY (EAST), a market town and parish, in the hundred of COMPTON, county of BERKS, 16 miles (E. S. E.) from Reading, and 56 (W.) from London, containing 676 inhabitants. This town is pleasantly situated on rising ground forming a part of the chalk hills, or downs, which extend across the county from east to west, and on the road from Newbury to Oxford: it is neither paved nor lighted, but is sufficiently supplied with water from wells. The inhabitants are principally employed in agriculture; and the town is noted for its sheep market, which, with the exception of that of the metropolis, is the largest in the kingdom, the number of sheep and lambs sold in one day sometimes amounting to twenty-five thousand. The weekly market is on Wednesday, and great sheep markets are held on the Wednesday in Easter week and every alternate Wednesday till Midsummer: there are fairs, August 6th, and on the Wednesdays next after September 29th, October 17th, and November 12th. The county magistrates meet here to dispense justice generally once a fortnight. The living is a rectory, in the archdeaconry of Berks, and diocese of Salisbury, rated in the king's books at £22. 13. 4., and in the patronage of the President and Fellows of Magdalene College, Oxford. The church is dedicated to St. Mary. There is a place of worship for Wesleyan Methodists.

ILSLEY (WEST), a parish in the hundred of COMPTON, county of BERKS, 2 miles (N. W. by N.) from East Ilsley, containing 328 inhabitants. The living is a rectory, in the archdeaconry of Berks, and diocese of Salisbury, rated in the king's books at £22. 7. 1., and in the patronage of the Dean and Canons of Windsor. The church is dedicated to All Saints. Here are two extensive breweries, the beer of which has obtained great celebrity. The learned Mark Antonio de Dominis, Archbishop of Spalatro, was presented to this rectory

by James I.; and, in the reigns of Charles I. and II., Calybute Downing, a celebrated divine, was rector.

ILSTON on the HILL, a chapelry partly in the parish of CARLTON-CURLIEU, and partly in that of KING'S NORTON, hundred of GARTREE, county of LEICESTER, 9 miles (E. S. E.) from Leicester, containing 125 inhabitants. The chapel is dedicated to St. Michael.

ILTON, a parish in the hundred of ABDICK and BULSTONE, county of SOMERSET, 2¼ miles (N. N. W.) from Ilminster, containing 460 inhabitants. The living is a discharged vicarage, rated in the king's books at £6. 19. 4½., endowed with £5 per annum and £500 private benefaction, £400 royal bounty, and £300 parliamentary grant, and in the patronage of the Prebendary of Ilton in the Cathedral Church of Wells. The church is dedicated to St. Peter.

ILTON, a joint township with Pott, in the parish of MASHAM, eastern division of the wapentake of HANG, North riding of the county of YORK, 3 miles (S. W.) from Masham, containing 266 inhabitants.

IMBER, a parish partly in the hundred of HEYTESBURY, and partly in that of SWANBOROUGH, county of WILTS, 4¼ miles (S. S. W.) from East Lavington, containing 414 inhabitants. The living is a perpetual curacy, in the archdeaconry and diocese of Salisbury, endowed with £200 private benefaction, and £300 parliamentary grant, and in the patronage of the Marquis of Bath. The church is dedicated to St. Giles.

IMINGHAM, a parish in the eastern division of the wapentake of YARBOROUGH, parts of LINDSEY, county of LINCOLN, 10 miles (N. W.) from Great Grimsby, containing 207 inhabitants. The living is a discharged vicarage, in the archdeaconry and diocese of Lincoln, rated in the king's books at £7. 18. 4. W. Amcotts, Esq. and others were patrons in 1782. The church is dedicated to St. Andrew.

IMPINGTON, a parish in the hundred of NORTHSTOW, county of CAMBRIDGE, 3¼ miles (N.) from Cambridge, containing 149 inhabitants. The living is a discharged vicarage, in the archdeaconry and diocese of Ely, rated in the king's books at £8. 7., and in the patronage of the Dean and Chapter of Ely. The church, dedicated to St. Andrew, has portions in the decorated, with insertions in the later, style of English architecture. This place had anciently a market and a fair.

INCE, a parish in the second division of the hundred of EDDISBURY, county palatine of CHESTER, 6 miles (W. by S.) from Frodsham, containing 460 inhabitants. The living is a perpetual curacy, in the archdeaconry and diocese of Chester, endowed with £600 private benefaction, £400 royal bounty, and £600 parliamentary grant, and in the patronage of Edmund Yates, Esq. The church, dedicated to St. James, has some traces in the Norman style of architecture, but the greater part of the building is of later date. Near it is the ancient manor-house of the abbots of St. Werburgh, and a barn, called the monastery barn, the only vestige remaining of a religious house which is thought to have formerly existed here. Edmund Yates, Esq. erected and supports a free school for poor children. The parish is bounded on the north by the river Mersey, where a pier has been constructed, at the distance of half a mile from the village.

INCE, a township in that part of the parish of WIGAN which is in the hundred of WEST DERBY, county palatine of LANCASTER, 1½ mile (E. S. E.) from Wigan, containing 1362 inhabitants. There are various coal works and cotton-factories in the vicinity.

INCE-BLUNDELL, a township in the parish of SEPHTON, hundred of WEST DERBY, county palatine of LANCASTER, 8½ miles (N. by W.) from Liverpool, containing 472 inhabitants. Attached to Ince hall, the family seat of the Blundells, is a building called "The Pantheon," erected by the late Henry Blundell, Esq., precisely similar in its architecture and proportions to the Pantheon at Rome, but one third less: it contains a splendid collection of paintings, statuary, sarcophagi, urns, and other relics of antiquity, procured by the founder, and said to be unequalled by any similar collection in the kingdom. Henry Blundell, Esq., in 1808, gave a rent-charge of £10 for teaching ten children.

INGARSBY, a chapelry in that part of the parish of HUNGERTON which is in the hundred of GARTREE, county of LEICESTER, 6½ miles (E.) from Leicester, containing 14 inhabitants.

INGATESTONE, a parish (formerly a market town) in the hundred of CHELMSFORD, county of ESSEX, 6 miles (S. W.) from Chelmsford, and 23 (N. E. by E.) from London, containing 747 inhabitants. This place was anciently called Ing-atte-stone, a name derived from the Saxon word Ing, a meadow, and a Roman military column which stood here. The town, which extends into the adjoining parish of Fryerning, is lighted with oil, by subscription. A considerable market was formerly held for cattle, but within the last sixty years it has been entirely discontinued: there is a large fair for Scotch and Welch cattle on the 1st and 2nd of December. The living is a rectory, in the archdeaconry of Essex, and diocese of London, rated in the king's books at £16. 13. 4., and in the patronage of Lord Petre. The church, dedicated to the Virgin Mary, has a lofty embattled tower of brick at the west end: adjoining the chancel is a sepulchral chapel belonging to the Petre family, which contains several handsome monuments, especially a fine altar-tomb to the memory of Sir William Petre, Treasurer to Edward VI., and his lady, with their statues in Parian marble; and a sumptuous monument for John, the first Lord Petre, with his lady. There is a place of worship for Independents. An almshouse for seven men and three women was founded and endowed by Sir William Petre, in 1557.

INGBIRCHWORTH, a township in the parish of PENISTONE, wapentake of STAINCROSS, West riding of the county of YORK, 9½ miles (W. by S.) from Barnesley, containing 367 inhabitants.

INGERTHORPE, a township in that part of the parish of RIPON which is within the liberty of RIPON, though locally in the wapentake of Claro, West riding of the county of YORK, 4 miles (S. S. W.) from Ripon, containing 44 inhabitants.

INGESTRIE, a parish in the southern division of the hundred of PIREHILL, county of STAFFORD, 3¾ miles (E.N.E.) from Stafford, containing 125 inhabitants. The living is a rectory, in the archdeaconry of Stafford, and diocese of Lichfield and Coventry, rated in the king's books at £10. 16. 8., and in the patronage of Earl Talbot. The church, dedicated to St. Mary, was erected in 1676, by Walter Chetwynd, Esq., on a more convenient site than that occupied by the ancient and decayed edifice: the chancel is paved with black and white marble, and many of the windows are ornamented with stained glass, exhibiting the armorial bearings of the Chetwynds, to which family belonged Ingestrie hall, built in the reign of Edward III., and now the residence of Earl Talbot, though the principal part is more modern, and in the style of architecture prevailing in the reign of Elizabeth. From the grounds, which are extensive and laid out with much taste, there is an extremely picturesque view, embracing the ruins of Chartley castle. The river Trent runs through the parish; and there is a brine spring, the water of which is raised by a steam-engine, conveyed to Weston, and there manufactured into table salt. Ingestrie gives the inferior title of viscount to Earl Talbot.

INGHAM, a parish in the western division of the wapentake of ASLACOE, parts of LINDSEY, county of LINCOLN, 8¼ miles (N. by W.) from Lincoln, containing 287 inhabitants. The living is a discharged vicarage, in the archdeaconry of Stow, and diocese of Lincoln, rated in the king's books at £6. 13. 4. C. Neville, Esq. was patron in 1824. The church is dedicated to All Saints.

INGHAM, a parish in the hundred of HAPPING, county of NORFOLK, 8½ miles (E. S. E.) from North Walsham, containing 418 inhabitants. The living is a discharged perpetual curacy, in the archdeaconry of Norfolk, and diocese of Norwich, endowed with £200 royal bounty, and £400 parliamentary grant. The King, by lapse, was patron in 1825. The church, dedicated to the Holy Trinity, has a very handsome tower, principally in the decorated style, and contains some ancient tombs with effigies, and grave-stones curiously ornamented: annexed to it was a college, or priory of the order of the Holy Trinity, for the Redemption of captives, founded in 1360, by Sir Miles Stapleton, who rebuilt the church, and procured it to be made collegiate, for a prior, sacrist, and six canons, whose revenue, at the dissolution, was estimated at £74. 2. 7. There is a place of worship for Baptists.

INGHAM, a parish in the hundred of BLACKBOURN, county of SUFFOLK, 4¼ miles (N.) from Bury-St. Edmund's, containing 185 inhabitants. The living is a rectory, with the rectories of Culford and Timworth, in the archdeaconry of Suffolk, and diocese of Norwich, rated in the king's books at £12. 16. 0¼. The church, dedicated to St. Bartholomew, is mostly in the later style of English architecture.

INGLEBY, a township in the parish of FOREMARK, hundred of REPTON and GRESLEY, county of DERBY, 7 miles (S.) from Derby, containing 141 inhabitants.

INGLEBY, a township in the parish of SAXELBY, wapentake of LAWRESS, parts of LINDSEY, county of LINCOLN, 6¾ miles (N. W.) from Lincoln. The population is returned with the parish.

INGLEBY-ARNCLIFFE, county of YORK. — See ARNCLIFFE (INGLEBY).

INGLEBY-BERWICK, a township in the parish of STAINTON, western division of the liberty of LANGBAURGH, North riding of the county of YORK, 3¾ miles (N. E.) from Yarm, containing 175 inhabitants.

INGLEBY-GREENHOW, a parish in the western division of the liberty of LANGBAURGH, North riding of the county of YORK, comprising the townships of Battersby, Greenhow, and Ingleby-Greenhow, and containing 347 inhabitants, of which number, 158 are in the township of Ingleby-Greenhow, 4½ miles (E. S. E.)

from Stokesley. The living is a perpetual curacy, in the archdeaconry of Cleveland, and diocese of York, endowed with £400 private benefaction, and £400 royal bounty. Sir William Foulis, Bart. was patron in 1787. The church was rebuilt in 1741. In 1766, John Rowland gave £100 towards the instruction of poor children.

INGLESHAM, a parish partly in the hundred of FARRINGDON, county of BERKS, but chiefly in that of HIGHWORTH, CRICKLADE, and STAPLE, county of WILTS, 3¼ miles (N.) from Highworth, containing 129 inhabitants. The living is a vicarage, in the archdeaconry of Wilts, and diocese of Salisbury, rated in the king's books at £8, and in the patronage of the Bishop of Salisbury. The church is dedicated to St. John the Baptist.

INGLETON, a township in that part of the parish of GAINFORD which is in the south-western division of DARLINGTON ward, county palatine of DURHAM, 8¼ miles (N.W. by W.) from Darlington, containing 295 inhabitants. The school-room, rebuilt by subscription in 1816, is used on Sundays as a place of worship for Primitive Methodists.

INGLETON, a chapelry in the parish of BENTHAM, western division of the wapentake of STAINCLIFFE and EWCROSS, West riding of the county of YORK, 9¾ miles (N. W.) from Settle, containing 1302 inhabitants. The living is a perpetual curacy, in the archdeaconry of Richmond, and diocese of Chester, endowed with £600 private benefaction, £400 royal bounty, and £800 parliamentary grant, and in the patronage of the Rector of Bentham. Six children are instructed for about £8 a year, the united bequests of Jennet Rose, in 1710, and of Henry Bouet. In the neighbourhood are many romantic objects, amongst which are Raven Roe, a rocky promontory covered with evergreens, Thornton Scar, and Thornton Froe, a curious water-fall; but the most striking of all is Yordas cave, in the vale of Kingsdale, under a mountain called Gray Gareth; the excavation, which is carried through a solid rock of black marble, somewhat resembles the interior of a cathedral, having on the right what is called the Bishop's Throne, and on the left the Chapter House, with petrifactions hanging from the roof. From the roof and sides issue numerous rills, forming fantastic cascades, which contribute to the general beauty and sublimity of the whole. The report of a pistol here causes reverberations similar to those produced by the discharge of a park of artillery.

INGLISH-COMBE, county of SOMERSET. — See COMBE (ENGLISH).

INGOE, a township in the parish of STAMFORDHAM, north-eastern division of TINDALE ward, county of NORTHUMBERLAND, 11 miles (N. E.) from Hexham, containing 239 inhabitants.

INGOL, a township in the parish of PRESTON, hundred of AMOUNDERNESS, county palatine of LANCASTER, 2½ miles (N.N.W.) from Preston, containing, with Lea, Ashton, and Cottam, 658 inhabitants.

INGOLDESTHORPE, a parish in the hundred of SMITHDON, county of NORFOLK, 5¾ miles (N.N.E.) from Castle-Rising, containing 247 inhabitants. The living is a discharged rectory, in the archdeaconry of Norfolk, and diocese of Norwich, rated in the king's books at £12. The Rev. Lovick Cooper was patron in 1828. The church is dedicated to St. Michael.

INGOLDMELLS, a parish in the Marsh division of the wapentake of CANDLESHOE, parts of LINDSEY, county of LINCOLN, 9¾ miles (S.E. by E.) from Alford, containing 155 inhabitants. The living is a discharged rectory, in the archdeaconry and diocese of Lincoln, rated in the king's books at £23. 10. 2½. Miss Hutton was patroness in 1817. The church is dedicated to St. Peter and St. Paul.

INGOLDSBY, a parish in the wapentake of ASWARDHURN, though locally in that of Beltisloe, parts of KESTEVEN, county of LINCOLN, 5¼ miles (N. by E.) from Corby, containing 360 inhabitants. The living is a rectory, in the archdeaconry and diocese of Lincoln, rated in the king's books at £21. 6. 10½., and in the patronage of the Master and Fellows of Christ's College, Cambridge. The church is dedicated to St. Andrew. On the verge of a wood within the parish is an ancient circular camp, five hundred feet in diameter, called Round Hills.

INGRAM, a parish in the northern division of COQUETDALE ward, county of NORTHUMBERLAND, comprising the townships of Fawdon and Clinch with Hartside, Ingram and Linop with Greenside-hill, and Reaveley, and containing 228 inhabitants, of which number, 74 are in the township of Ingram with Linop and Greenside-hill, 7½ miles (S. by E.) from Wooler. The living is a rectory, in the archdeaconry of Northumberland, and diocese of Durham, rated in the king's books at £24. 16. 8., and in the patronage of Prideaux John Selby, Esq. The church is dedicated to St. Michael.

INGRAVE, a parish in the hundred of BARSTABLE, county of ESSEX, 2 miles (E. S.E.) from Brentwood, containing 427 inhabitants. The living is a rectory, united to that of West Horndon, in the archdeaconry of Essex, and diocese of London, rated in the king's books at £7. 13. 4. The church, dedicated to St. Nicholas, is a plain brick edifice, erected by Lord Petre after the union of the two livings; it stands about midway between the sites of the two ancient churches.

INGTHORP, a hamlet in the parish of TINWELL, East hundred, county of RUTLAND. The population is returned with the parish.

INGWORTH, a parish in the southern division of the hundred of ERPINGHAM, county of NORFOLK, 2 miles (N.) from Aylsham, containing 161 inhabitants. The living is a discharged rectory, in the archdeaconry and diocese of Norwich, rated in the king's books at £5. W. Wyndham, Esq. was patron in 1788. The church is dedicated to St. Lawrence.

INHURST, a hamlet in the parish of BAUGHURST, hundred of EVINGAR, Kingsclere division of the county of SOUTHAMPTON, 8¼ miles (N.W. by N.) from Basingstoke. The population is returned with the parish.

INKBERROW, a parish in the middle division of the hundred of OSWALDSLOW, county of WORCESTER, 5¼ miles (W.) from Alcester, containing 1667 inhabitants. The living is a vicarage, in the archdeaconry and diocese of Worcester, rated in the king's books at £16. 2. 1. The Earl of Abergavenny was patron in 1792. The church, dedicated to St. Peter, contains numerous monuments. At Cokehill are some remains of a nunnery founded in 1260, by Isabella, Countess of Warwick, who assumed the veil here: at the dissolution the establishment consisted of a prioress and six nuns, whose revenue was estimated at £34. 15. 11.

INKPEN, a parish in the hundred of KINTBURY-EAGLE, county of BERKS, 4 miles (S. E. by S.) from Hungerford, containing 617 inhabitants. The living is a rectory, in the archdeaconry of Berks, and diocese of Salisbury, rated in the king's books at £11. 14. 7., and in the patronage of J. Butler, Esq. The church is dedicated to St. Michael. There is a place of worship for Wesleyan Methodists.

INSKIP, a joint township with Sowerby, in the parish of St. MICHAEL, hundred of AMOUNDERNESS, county palatine of LANCASTER, 4¾ miles (N. N. E.) from Kirkham, containing 739 inhabitants. There is a place of worship for Baptists.

INSTOW, a parish in the hundred of FREMINGTON, county of DEVON, 4¾ miles (N. N. E.) from Bideford, containing 353 inhabitants. The living is a discharged rectory, in the archdeaconry of Barnstaple, and diocese of Exeter, rated in the king's books at £12. 17. 3½., endowed with £200 private benefaction, and £300 parliamentary grant, and in the patronage of C. W. Sibthorp, Esq. The church is dedicated to St. John the Baptist. The navigable river Torr runs on the north, and the Torridge on the west, of the parish. A trifling endowment was given by John Tucker for teaching poor children.

INTWOOD, a parish in the hundred of HUMBLE-YARD, county of NORFOLK, 4 miles (S. W.) from Norwich, containing 44 inhabitants. The living is a rectory, united to that of Keswick, in the archdeaconry of Norfolk, and diocese of Norwich, rated in the king's books at £5. The church, dedicated to All Saints, has a tower round at the base and octangular above.

INWARDLEIGH, a parish in the hundred of BLACK TORRINGTON, county of DEVON, 3¾ miles (N. W. by N.) from Oakhampton, containing 540 inhabitants. The living is a rectory, in the archdeaconry of Totness, and diocese of Exeter, rated in the king's books at £16. 11. 3.. and in the patronage of the Rev. Richard Holland.

INWORTH, a parish in the Witham division of the hundred of LEXDEN, county of ESSEX, 1½ mile (S. E.) from Kelvedon, containing 437 inhabitants. The living is a rectory, in the archdeaconry of Colchester, and diocese of London, rated in the king's books at £10. Thomas Poynder, Esq. was patron in 1802. The church, dedicated to All Saints, is remarkable for a small ancient porch on the south side, composed of a mixture of Roman bricks and flints.

IPING, a parish in the hundred of EASEBOURNE, rape of CHICHESTER, county of SUSSEX, 2¾ miles (N. W. by W.) from Midhurst, containing 305 inhabitants. The living is a rectory with Chithurst, in the archdeaconry and diocese of Chichester, rated in the king's books at £7, and in the patronage of the Earl of Egremont. The church is partly in the Norman style of architecture. The river Rother runs through the parish.

IPPLEPEN, a parish in the hundred of HAYTOR, county of DEVON, 3¾ miles (S. S. W.) from Newton-Abbot's, containing, with the chapelry of Woodland, 1048 inhabitants. The living is a discharged vicarage, in the archdeaconry of Totness, and diocese of Exeter, rated in the king's books at £26. 2. 3½., endowed with £200 private benefaction, and £1100 parliamentary grant, and in the patronage of the Dean and Canons of
VOL. II.

Windsor. The church, dedicated to St. John the Baptist, has a handsome screen and an enriched wooden pulpit : it formerly belonged, with some adjoining lands, to the priory of St. Peter de Fulgeriis in Brittany, and attached to it was a cell to that establishment. Ipplepen had the privilege of a market and fairs before 1320. The Wesleyan Methodists have a place of worship here.

IPPOLITTS, a parish in the hundred of HITCHIN and PIRTON, county of HERTFORD, 1½ mile (S. E. by S.) from Hitchin, containing 671 inhabitants. The living is a vicarage, united to that of Great Wymondley in 1685, in the archdeaconry of Huntingdon, and diocese of Lincoln, rated in the king's books at £11. The church, dedicated to St. Hippolytus, has at the western end a square tower, embattled, and surmounted by a short spire : adjoining the church-yard are two almshouses, endowed by a person unknown.

IPSDEN, a chapelry in the parish of NORTH STOKE, hundred of LANGTREE, county of OXFORD, 3½ miles (S. E. by S.) from Wallingford, containing, with the liberty of Stokerow, 583 inhabitants. The chapel is dedicated to St. Mary.

IPSLEY, a parish in the Alcester division of the hundred of BARLICHWAY, county of WARWICK, 6¼ miles (N. by W.) from Alcester, containing 745 inhabitants. The living is a rectory, in the archdeaconry and diocese of Worcester, rated in the king's books at £11. 10. 7½., and in the patronage of the Rev. T. Dolben Dolben. The church is dedicated to St. Peter.

IPSTONE, a parish partly in the hundred of PIRTON, county of OXFORD, but chiefly in the hundred of DESBOROUGH, county of BUCKINGHAM, 7 miles (N. W. by W.) from Great Marlow, containing 272 inhabitants. The living is a discharged rectory, in the archdeaconry and diocese of Oxford, rated in the king's books at £9. 9. 4½., endowed with £200 private benefaction, and £200 royal bounty, and in the patronage of the Warden and Fellows of Merton College, Oxford. The church, dedicated to St. Nicholas, stands in Oxfordshire, the boundary line of the two counties passing through a room in the manor-house. Two boys of this parish are educated, clothed, and apprenticed, from funds vested in the Governors of Goring Hospital.

IPSTONES, a parish partly in the northern, and comprising the joint township of Morrage with Foxt, in the southern, division of the hundred of TOTMON-SLOW, county of STAFFORD, 5 miles (N. by E.) from Cheadle, containing 1425 inhabitants. The living is a perpetual curacy, in the archdeaconry of Stafford, and diocese of Lichfield and Coventry, endowed with £1000 private benefaction, £600 royal bounty, and £1400 parliamentary grant, and in the patronage of the Freeholders. The church, dedicated to St. Leonard, is a handsome structure with a pinnacled tower, erected in 1790. The entire parish occupies a very elevated situation, but a great portion of it is composed of moors and peat mosses : it abounds, in several places, with rugged projecting rocks, which, overhanging their bases, in many instances, appear as if they would momentarily fall : at a place called Sharp Cliffs, this appearance is particularly striking. The soil is generally barren, but the face of the country has of late been greatly improved by plantations. The Uttoxeter canal and the river Churnet run parallel to each other through the parish.

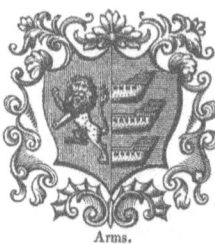

Arms.

IPSWICH, a borough, port, and market town, in the liberty of IPSWICH, county of SUFFOLK, 25 miles (S. E. by E.) from Bury-St. Edmund's, and 69 (N.E.) from London, containing, exclusively of that part of the parish of Westerfield which extends into the borough, 17,186 inhabitants. This place had a mint in the early period of the Heptarchy, and was fortified with walls and surrounded by a moat: of the former there are still some remains in a garden near the church of St. Nicholas, and of the latter the memorial is preserved in the name of the northern suburb, called the Ditches. Though of considerable antiquity, it is not distinguished by any event of historical importance prior to the Conquest : in Domesday-book it is named *Gyppeswid* and *Gyppeswic*, from the river Gyppen, or Gipping, which falls into the Orwell, near the town, and from which its present appellation is immediately deduced. The walls, which were greatly damaged in 991 and 1000, when the town was plundered by the Danes, were repaired in the reign of John, and had four gates, called from their situation respectively, the North, South, East, and West gates ; of these, two were remaining within the last few years, but in the more recent improvement of the town have been totally removed. Soon after the Conquest a castle was erected here, which Hugh Bigod, Earl of Norfolk, defended against Stephen, to whom he at length surrendered it, and which was afterwards demolished by Henry II., insomuch, that scarcely a vestige can be seen. Isabel, Queen of Edward II., who had made a visit to France, landed here on her return, with a force of nearly three thousand men, and being joined by the discontented barons, laid siege to Bristol, where she put the elder Spencer to death, and compelled the king to take refuge in Wales. In the 26th of Henry VIII., Ipswich was made the seat of a suffragan bishop, who was consecrated by Archbishop Cranmer, and had a mansion in the parish of St. Peter, the remains of which are now used as a malt-house. During the persecutions in the reign of Mary, several individuals suffered martyrdom in this town, for their adherence to the Protestant religion. Queen Elizabeth, in her progress through Norfolk and Suffolk, visited this borough, where she remained for four days, and sailed down the Orwell in great pomp, attended by the corporation in their robes of office. Charles II., after his retreat from the battle of Worcester, is traditionally said to have been for some time concealed in an ancient house in the parish of St. Lawrence, erected in 1567, by Robert Sparrow, and still occupied by his descendants : the walls are profusely ornamented with emblematical devices, and in the roof is an apartment fitted up as a private oratory, and ingeniously screened from observation : the family still possess portraits of several of the Stuarts, and a miniature portrait of Charles himself, splendidly set in gold, and stated to have been presented by that monarch to his host on quitting his hospitable asylum ; but notwithstanding this presumptive evidence, it is very doubtful whether Charles was in this county at all after that decisive battle. Among the

sovereigns who have visited Ipswich are, George II., on his way from Lowestoft, upon which occasion a congratulatory address was presented to him by the corporation ; and his late majesty, George IV., when Regent. The town is pleasantly situated on an acclivity bordered on the west and south by the river Orwell, over which is a handsome iron bridge, and another at the entrance into the town from the London road : the streets are irregularly formed, and were formerly inconveniently narrow. Under an act passed in 1816 the town was paved, and is now lighted with gas, and a fund has been raised for its general improvement : the houses, many of which are ancient and ornamented with carved work, are in general well built, and the recent erection of several ranges of building and the construction of some handsome streets, have added much to the regularity of its appearance : the inhabitants are amply supplied with water from the river and from springs ; the air is salubrious and the temperature mild, the town being sheltered from the colder winds by the hills which rise to the north and north-east. The environs are pleasant ; the higher grounds command a fine view of the town, the river, and the adjacent country, which abounds with pleasingly diversified scenery, and with extensive rides and walks, including Christchurch park, the property of the Rev. Charles Fonnereau, in which are some of the finest Spanish chesnut and beech trees in the kingdom, and which, from its extent and the beauty and variety of its scenery, forms a delightful promenade : it is open during the summer to the public, for whose entertainment a military band frequently attends. The barracks, in various parts of the town, which during the war were adapted for the reception of eight or nine thousand troops, have been taken down since the peace, or converted to other purposes, with the exception of the cavalry barracks, a neat range of building at the entrance from the London road, which contains complete accommodations for six troops of cavalry, but only three are usually stationed here. A Philosophical Society was established in 1818 : there is a library for the use of the free burgesses, founded by Mr. W. Smart in 1612, and originally attached to the free grammar school, but recently removed to Christ's Hospital in this town ; and there are a public subscription library, three subscription news-rooms, a mechanics' institution, with a good library and museum, established in 1824, and also a horticultural society. The theatre, a neat and commodious building, is opened twice in the year for a few weeks by the Norwich company of comedians ; it was, at Ipswich that Garrick made his first appearance on the stage, in 1739. The subscription assembly-rooms are extensive and elegantly fitted up ; and races take place annually in the first week in July. There are commodious public baths of all kinds on the quay.

The port of Ipswich has a jurisdiction extending for a considerable distance on both sides of the Suffolk coast, and beyond Harwich on the coast of Essex : it carries on a small foreign, and a very considerable coasting, trade ; the latter consisting chiefly in corn and malt, and in timber for ship-building, with which it supplies the dock-yards : the number of vessels belonging to the port is one hundred and twenty-nine, averaging a burden of sixty-three tons' each ; twenty-six British and nine foreign vessels entered inwards, and nineteen British and five foreign vessels cleared.

outwards, at this port in 1826. The river Orwell is navigable from this town to Harwich, and the Stowmarket canal, constructed in 1793, at an expense of £26,380, affords great facility for inland navigation. The quay, which is accessible to ships of two hundred tons' burden, is commodiously adapted to the loading and unloading of vessels: the custom-house is a neat building of brick. Boats sail with every tide to Harwich, affording an aquatic excursion of twelve miles, which derives much interest from the beauty and variety of the scenery on the banks of the river. The principal articles of manufacture are snuff and tobacco, paper made by steam, patent ploughs and ploughshares, and yarn for the weavers at Norwich: the town was formerly celebrated for the manufacture of broad cloth and Ipswich doubles, and the best canvas for sail-cloth, now transferred to the West of England. Ship-building is carried on to a considerable extent; fourteen vessels were built in 1826: there are different rope-walks for the supply of the shipping. A manufactory for stays affords employment to upwards of seven hundred women and girls: there are an extensive pottery, and a manufactory for Roman cement. There are also several ale and porter breweries: a great quantity of grain and malt is sent to the London market; and there are extensive chalk pits in the neighbourhood. The market days are Wednesday and Saturday, the latter for corn: the fairs are, May 4th, called St. George's fair, for toys and lean cattle; August 26th, for lambs, of which one hundred and thirty thousand were sold in 1828; and September 25th, for butter and cheese, which last has almost fallen into disuse. The corn market is held in the corn exchange, a large building commodiously arranged, erected on the site of the old shambles said to have been built by Cardinal Wolsey. The new market-place, constructed in 1811, at an expense of £10,000, comprises two spacious quadrangular ranges of building, supported on columns of stone, adjoining which is an enclosed cattle market.

Corporate Seal.

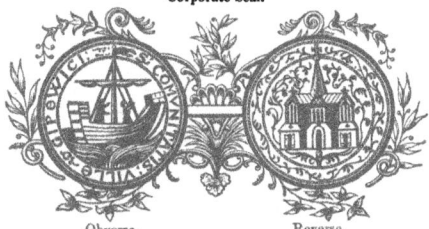

Obverse.   Reverse.

Ipswich was a borough at the time of the Norman survey, and obtained a grant for a free market from William the Conqueror: the burgesses were first incorporated by King John, who granted them extensive privileges; since that time the inhabitants have received seventeen charters, of which the most important are those of Edward IV. and Charles II., under which latter the government is vested in two bailiffs, a high steward, recorder, twelve portmen, and twenty-four common council-men, assisted by a town clerk, two coroners, and other officers. The bailiffs are chosen annually from among the portmen, or common council-men, by a majority of the burgesses, and sworn into office on the 29th of September: the portmen and common council-men are elected by a majority of their own body, as vacancies occur. In consequence of the corporation having omitted to fill up vacancies in the body of portmen, the number has been reduced to five, which is insufficient to constitute a great court; so that the present charter will very soon expire. The freedom of the borough is inherited by all the sons of a free burgess born after the parent has taken up his freedom, acquired by servitude to a freeman, whether resident or not, or obtained by gift from the corporation. Among the privileges which it confers are, exemption from all tolls and other customs, and, for the resident burgesses, from serving on juries at the assizes or sessions for the county. The bailiffs and the recorder, with four assistants chosen from the portmen, are justices of the peace within the borough and liberties, and are also entitled to waifs, estrays, and goods cast on shore within their admiralty jurisdiction. Heirs are considered of age when fourteen years old. The corporation hold quarterly courts of session for the determination of all civil and criminal causes, except such as relate to capital offences, the cognizance of which is reserved for the judges travelling the circuit: these sessions, from the small number of prisoners, are held only twice in the year, a short time prior to the assizes for the county. They also hold a court of record every alternate Monday, under their charter, for the recovery of debts to any amount. A court of requests is held every Tuesday, by commissioners appointed by an act passed in the 47th of George III., for the recovery of debts not exceeding £5. The town-hall was built on the site and partly with the materials of the ancient parochial church of St. Mildred, which was a building of extraordinary beauty: it is principally appropriated to the public business of the corporation, and the sessions are held in the shire-hall, a large brick building commodiously adapted to the purpose, but possessing no peculiar claim to notice. The borough gaol comprises six divisions for the classification of prisoners, exclusively of two solitary cells; and the house of correction for the borough contains two wards. The common gaol and house of correction for the county, in the parish of St. Helen, is spacious building of brick, and one of the first erected on the plan of Mr. Howard: it is well adapted to the classification of prisoners, and comprises eleven divisions, each containing a dayroom, and an airing-yard, radiating from the keeper's house in the centre: this is the first prison into which the tread-mill was introduced, it having been the invention of Mr. William Cubitt, an inhabitant of the town. This borough obtained the elective franchise in the 23rd of Edward I., since which time it has continued to return two members to parliament: the right of election is vested in the burgesses generally not receiving alms, of whom there are about eleven hundred, but not more than four hundred are resident: the bailiffs are the returning officers.

Ipswich comprises the parishes of St. Clement, St. Helen, St. Lawrence, St. Margaret, St. Mary at Elms, St. Mary at the Quay, St. Mary Stoke, St. Mary at the Tower, St. Matthew, St. Nicholas, St. Peter, St. Stephen, the parish of Whitton with Thurleston, and part of the parish of Westerfield, all in the archdeaconry of Suffolk, and diocese of Norwich. The living of St. Clement's is a rectory not in charge, held with that of St. Helen's, rated in the king's books at £8. 13. 9., and in the patronage of the Rev. J.T. Nottidge: the church of St. Clement is a neat edifice of freestone, and that of St. Helen is an ancient structure. The living of St. Lawrence is a perpetual curacy, endowed with £600 royal bounty, and in the patronage of the Parishioners: the church was erected in the early part of the fifteenth century, by John Bottold, and the chancel built by John Baldwyn: in 1808, Sir Robert Kerr Porter, in six days, executed a painting of our Saviour disputing with the doctors in the temple, which he presented to the parishioners. The living of St. Margaret is a perpetual curacy, endowed with £200 private benefaction, £400 royal bounty, and £1500 parliamentary grant, and in the patronage of the Rev. Charles Fonnereau: the church is a handsome and spacious structure, but was materially defaced and stripped of its decorations by the parliamentary visitors, who destroyed the paintings, and removed the statues of the Twelve Apostles: in this church the bishop of the diocese holds his confirmation. The living of the parish of St. Mary at Elms is a perpetual curacy, endowed with £400 private benefaction, and £400 royal bounty, and in the patronage of the parishioners: the church is a small edifice of brick, erected on the spot where St. Saviour's church formerly stood. The living of the parish of St. Mary at the Quay is a perpetual curacy, endowed with £200 private benefaction, £1000 royal bounty, and £1100 parliamentary grant, and in the patronage of the Parishioners: the church was rebuilt soon after 1448, of stone given for that purpose by Richard Gowty, whose will is dated in that year. The living of the parish of St. Mary Stoke is a rectory, rated in the king's books at £12, and in the patronage of the Dean and Chapter of Ely: the church is an ancient edifice, on the south side of the Orwell, and from a hill near the church-yard is an extensive and delightful view. The living of St. Mary at the Tower is a perpetual curacy, endowed with £1000 royal bounty, and £200 parliamentary grant, and in the patronage of the Parishioners; there is also a lectureship, endowed by the corporation, who attend divine service here upon all public occasions: the church is spacious, and had formerly a lofty spire, for the rebuilding of which, Mr. William Edgar bequeathed £200; but, from the apparent want of strength in the tower, the design has not been carried into effect. A handsome marble tablet has been recently erected by subscription among the parishioners, to the memory of Mrs. Elizabeth Cobbold, a lady distinguished for her literary talents. The living of St. Matthew's is a discharged rectory, rated in the king's books at £5, endowed with £200 royal bounty, and £600 parliamentary grant, and in the patronage of the Crown: the church contains the tomb of John, Lord Chedworth, many years chairman of the quarter sessions, who devised property to the amount of £183,050 in legacies to various persons, several of them inhabitants of this town, but not related to him. The living of St. Nicholas is a perpetaul curacy, endowed with £800 royal bounty, and in the patronage of the Parishioners: the church, an ancient structure, sustained considerable injury from the parliamentary visitors, in 1648, who destroyed the paintings and removed several brasses. The living of St. Peter is a perpetual curacy, endowed with £600 private benefaction, £600 royal bounty, and

£1500 parliamentary grant, and in the patronage of the Rev. Charles Fonnereau: the church is an ancient edifice, and contains a large font of great antiquity and curious design. The living of St. Stephen's is a discharged rectory, rated in the king's books at £4. 12. 8½., endowed with £200 private benefaction, £800 royal bounty, and £1100 parliamentary grant, and in the patronage of the Rev. William Marsh, with reversion to the Rev. Charles Fonnereau. Within the precincts of the borough are the churches of Whitton and Westerfield, and the remains of that of Thurleston, which have been converted into a barn. There are places of worship for General and Particular Baptists, the Society of Friends, Independents, Wesleyan Methodists, and Unitarians, a Roman Catholic chapel, and a synagogue.

The free grammar school is of uncertain foundation: it was endowed by Henry VIII., with £38. 13. 4. per annum, from the fee-farm rent of the borough, which endowment was confirmed by a charter of Elizabeth, in the eighth year of her reign, and augmented with £11 per annum from a benefaction by Richard Felaw, who in 1482 bequeathed lands and tenements, the produce of which is now principally appropriated to the support of Christ's hospital. The school is kept in an apartment of the hospital, and there are thirty-five scholars on the foundation. There are two scholarships at Pembroke College, Cambridge, for boys educated in this school, with pensions of £3 per annum each, given by William Smart, in 1598; four scholarships with £5 per annum each, founded by Ralph Scrivener, in 1601; and two exhibitions to the University of Cambridge, one of £14 and the other of £6 per annum, founded, in 1621, by Richard Martin, for boys educated in this school, who are also entitled to share with the school of Bury-St. Edmund's, in a scholarship founded at Trinity College, by Dr. Mopted, in 1558. The master is appointed by the corporation, subject to the approval of the Bishop of Norwich. The Blue-coat school was established in 1709, and is supported by subscription and donations, among which is one of £500 by Dudley North, Esq.: the income amounts to £500 per annum, and is expended in the clothing and education of seventy boys and fifty girls; on leaving school, the boys receive £8 each, as an apprentice fee, and the girls £2 in addition to what they may have earned whilst in it. The Red-sleeve school, established in 1752, for the clothing and education of thirty-six boys, is supported by subscription. A school of industry for females, in which one hundred are educated, was established and is supported by Mr. Henry Alexander, a member of the Society of Friends. A charity school for eighty girls; the ladies' association for the education of African children; a central school on the National plan, in which one hundred and eighty boys and one hundred and twenty girls are taught; and a Lancasterian school, in which are two hundred children, are supported by subscription; and a school for ten boys and eight girls is supported by the congregation of Independents. Mr. Henry Tooley, portman of Ipswich, bequeathed estates, in 1550, for the erection and endowment of almshouses for ten aged persons: the revenue at present arising from these estates is nearly £1000, and, in addition to those maintained in the almshouses, there are sixty out-pensioners, who are relieved from the funds of this institution, which is under the direction and superintendence of the corporation. Mr. William Smart, in 1598, bequeathed, in trust to the corporation, lands producing at present about £480 per annum, for the maintenance and education of poor children, for the employment of the poor and other charitable purposes, which are under the management of the wardens of Mr. Tooley's charity: Christ's hospital, founded by the corporation in 1569, has an endowment of about £400 per annum, arising from a portion of Mr. Felaw's gift, and from other benefactions, which is applied to the maintenance, education, and apprenticing of poor children: the building, which is near the site of a monastery of Black friars, is also appropriated as a bridewell or house of industry for the employment of the poor. Twelve almshouses were founded in the parish of St. Mary at Elms, for twelve aged women, who receive a weekly allowance in money and other supplies, in pursuance of the will of Mrs. Ann Smyth, who, in 1729, bequeathed property now vested in Old South Sea annuities, producing £132. 19. per annum. Fifteen almshouses were built, in 1515, by Mr. Daundy, in the parish of St. Matthew, to which two more were added, in 1680, by Mr. Sheppard; they are kept in repair by the parish and are let rent-free to the poor, as are also five almshouses in the church-yard of St. Clement's. Mr. John Pemberton, in 1718, bequeathed estates in this county for the purpose of establishing a fund for paying £25 per annum each to widows and orphans of clergymen of the established church : these funds have been so far increased by donations and subscriptions, as to enable the trustees to distribute annually the sum of £1500, in sums of £30 each. A similar institution, called the Suffolk Benevolent Society, was formed in 1799, by the dissenters, the funds of which at present have accumulated to £4000. A public-dispensary, a society for the relief of married women in child-birth, a society for clothing the infant poor, and numerous other charitable institutions, have been established, and are liberally supported.

Among the monastic establishments formerly existing here were, a priory of Black canons of the order of St. Augustine, originally founded in 1177, in Christchurch, which, being destroyed by fire, was re-founded soon after, by John, Bishop of Norwich, for a prior and six canons, the revenue of which, at the dissolution, was £88. 6. 9.; a priory of Black canons, founded in the reign of Henry II., by Thomas Lacey and Alice his wife, in honour of St. Peter and St. Paul : Cardinal Wolsey suppressed this, and erected on the site his college for a dean, twelve secular canons, eight clerks, and eight choristers, with a grammar school intended as a nursery for his college at Oxford : upon that statesman's fall, this was demolished; only the gateway, an elegant edifice of brick, now remains. A monastery of Black friars, in the parish of St. Mary at the Quay, was founded here in the reign of Henry III., of which the existing portions present the most perfect relic of antiquity in the town; it is appropriated to the use of Christ's hospital, and for the purpose of Mr. Tooley's endowment. An hospital for lepers was also founded here in the reign of John, and dedicated to St. Mary Magdalene and St. James. There was a monastery of White friars in the centre of the town, of which there are no remains; and a house of Grey friars, founded in the reign of Edward I.,

by Sir Robert Tiptot, of which some portions of the walls are still remaining.

There are several mineral springs in the neighbourhood; and an ancient warm spring, called Ipswich Spa, was in great repute during the last century, though now not used. Cardinal Wolsey was born in the parish of St. Nicholas, and received the rudiments of his education in the grammar school of this town; a considerable part of the house in which his father lived is still standing, but the front has been modernised. Among other distinguished natives of Ipswich are Dr. William Butler, physician to James I.; Dr. Laney, successively Bishop of Peterborough, Lincoln, and Ely; Ralph Brownrig, Bishop of Exeter, of which see he was deprived at the commencement of the parliamentary war; Clara Reeve, authoress of "The Old English Baron," and other works, whose father was for many years minister of St. Nicholas' parish; Mrs. Sarah Trimmer, the ingenious authoress of elementary works for young people; and Thomas Green, author of "Extracts from the Diary of a Lover of Literature," and a liberal and enlightened critic. Among eminent persons who have resided here are, Sir Christopher Hatton, Lord High Chancellor; Sir Harbottle Grimstone, Speaker of the House of Commons during the Long Parliament; Nathaniel Bacon, grandson of the Lord Keeper Sir Nicholas Bacon, and author of the Annals of Ipswich, now in the possession of the corporation; Jeremy Collier, master of the free grammar school, and author of an Ecclesiastical History of Great Britain; and Mr. Capel Lofft, a learned civilian, elegant writer, and patron of literature. Ipswich gives the title of viscount to the Duke of Grafton.

IRBY, a township in the parish of WOODCHURCH, lower division of the hundred of WIRRALL, county palatine of CHESTER, 5 miles (N. by W.) from Parkgate, containing 145 inhabitants.

IRBY upon HUMBER, a parish in the wapentake of BRADLEY-HAVERSTOE, parts of LINDSEY, county of LINCOLN, 6 miles (S. W. by W.) from Great Grimsby, containing 217 inhabitants. The living is a rectory, in the archdeaconry and diocese of Lincoln, rated in the king's books at £18. Lord Yarborough was patron in 1814. The church is dedicated to St. Andrew.

IRBY in the MARSH, a parish in the Wold division of the wapentake of CANDLESHOE, parts of LINDSEY, county of LINCOLN, 5 miles (E. by S.) from Spilsby, containing 78 inhabitants. The living is a perpetual curacy, in the archdeaconry and diocese of Lincoln, endowed with £1000 royal bounty, and in the patronage of the Dean and Chapter of Lincoln. The church is dedicated to All Saints.

IRCHESTER, a parish in the hundred of HIGHAM-FERRERS, county of NORTHAMPTON, 3 miles (E. S. E.) from Wellingborough, containing 689 inhabitants. The living is a discharged vicarage, with that of Wollaston, in the archdeaconry of Northampton, and diocese of Peterborough, rated in the king's books at £8. The church, dedicated to St. Catherine, is partly in the early, and partly in the later, style of English architecture. There is a place of worship for Wesleyan Methodists. Within the parish are vestiges of a Roman fortification, the area of which includes about eighteen acres.

IREBY, a parish in ALLERDALE ward below Darwent, county of CUMBERLAND, comprising the townships of High Ireby and Low Ireby, and containing 457 inhabitants, of which number, 164 are in the town of High Ireby, and 293 in that of Low Ireby, in which is the decayed market town of Ireby, 6½ miles (S. by W.) from Wigton. This place is supposed by Camden to have been the Roman station called *Arbeia*, but no vestiges have been discovered to support this conjecture, nor any other evidence except the similarity of the ancient and modern names. The town, which is irregularly built, is situated in a secluded vale, on the western side of the small river Ellen, which takes its rise in the neighbouring lake of Overwater, and in a hilly part of the county. The market, which was formerly on Thursday for provisions, is now but little attended : fairs are held, February 24th and October 18th. The living is a perpetual curacy, in the archdeaconry and diocese of Carlisle, endowed with £600 royal bounty, and £200 parliamentary grant, and in the patronage of the Dean and Chapter of Carlisle. Here is a school, founded in consequence of a benefaction by Matthew Caldbeck, in 1749, endowed with £7 per annum for eight free scholars, and open to all the children in the parish on payment of a small stipend.

IREBY, a township in the parish of TATHAM, hundred of LONSDALE, south of the sands, county palatine of LANCASTER, 3½ miles (S.E. by E.) from Kirkby-Lonsdale, containing 115 inhabitants.

IRELETH, a chapelry in the parish of DALTON in FURNESS, hundred of LONSDALE, north of the sands, county palatine of LANCASTER, 3 miles (N.) from Dalton, containing 513 inhabitants. ' The living is a perpetual curacy, in the archdeaconry of Richmond, and diocese of Chester, endowed with £800 royal bounty, and in the patronage of the Vicar of Dalton and the Landowners.

IRETON (KIRK), a parish in the hundred of WIRKSWORTH, county of DERBY, 2½ miles (S.S.W.) from Wirksworth, containing, with the township of Wood-Ireton, 826 inhabitants. The living is a rectory, in the archdeaconry of Derby, and diocese of Lichfield and Coventry, rated in the king's books at £7. 10. 10., and in the patronage of the Dean of Lincoln. The church, dedicated to the Holy Trinity, has portions in the Norman style. There is a place of worship for Independents. A school was erected and endowed by John Slater, in 1686; the income is about £15 a year. An annuity of £5, arising from a bequest by John Bower, is also paid for the instruction of seven girls. This parish is in the honour of Tutbury, duchy of Lancaster, and within the jurisdiction of a court of pleas held at Tutbury every third Tuesday, for the recovery of debts under 40s.

IRETON (WOOD), a township in the parish of KIRK-IRETON, hundred of WIRKSWORTH, county of DERBY, 4½ miles (S. by W.) from Wirksworth, containing 165 inhabitants.

IRMINGLAND, a parish in the southern division of the hundred of ERPINGHAM, county of NORFOLK, 5¼ miles (W.N.W.) from Aylsham, containing 16 inhabitants. The living is a discharged rectory, with that of Heydon, in the archdeaconry and diocese of Norwich, rated in the king's books at £5. The church, now in ruins, was dedicated to St. Andrew.

IRNHAM, a parish in the wapentake of BELTISLOE, parts of KESTEVEN, county of LINCOLN, 2½ miles (N.E.

by E.) from Corby, containing, with the chapelries of Bulby and Hawthorp, 413 inhabitants. The living is a rectory, in the archdeaconry and diocese of Lincoln, rated in the king's books at £13. 13. 9. The Rev. F. Burton was patron in 1804. The church is dedicated to St. Andrew.

IRON-BROCK-GRANGE, a hamlet in that part of the parish of WIRKSWORTH which is in the hundred of HIGH PEAK, county of DERBY, containing 34 inhabitants.

IRSTEAD, a parish in the hundred of TUNSTEAD, county of NORFOLK, 6½ miles (E.) from Coltishall, containing 152 inhabitants. The living is a discharged rectory, with the vicarage of Barton-Turf, in the archdeaconry of Norfolk, and diocese of Norwich, rated in the king's books at £6. 13. 4., and in the patronage of the Bishop of Norwich. The church is dedicated to St. Michael.

IRTHINGTON, a parish in ESKDALE ward, county of CUMBERLAND, comprising the townships of Irthington, Leversdale, Newby, and Newtown, and containing 1020 inhabitants, of which number, 251 are in the township of Irthington, 3 miles (W. by N.) from Brampton. The living is a discharged vicarage, in the archdeaconry and diocese of Carlisle, rated in the king's books at £6. 1. 5., endowed with £200 royal bounty. Mrs. Dacre was patroness in 1811. The church, dedicated to St. Kentigern, is in the Norman style of architecture. Jane Hetherington, in 1792, left £100 for the endowment of a school, in aid of which Mr. James Boustead contributes £5 per annum. Near the church is the keep of a castle, said to have been the chief seat of the barony of Gilsland before the erection of Naworth castle. Castle-steads, within this parish, is the site of the Roman fort *Petriana*, where numerous inscribed stones have been found. A little to the southward is a place now called Watch Cross, where Horsley fixes the *Aballaba* of the Romans, but others incline to the opinion that it was only an exploratory post : Roman inscriptions have been discovered here also.

IRTHLINGBOROUGH, a parish comprising the consolidated parishes of All Saints and St. Peter, in the hundred of HUXLOE, county of NORTHAMPTON, 2 miles (N.W.) from Higham-Ferrers, containing 1072 inhabitants. The living is a rectory, in the archdeaconry of Northampton, and diocese of Peterborough, rated in the king's books at £5. 6. 8., jointly endowed with £800 private benefaction, and £800 royal bounty. Earl Fitzwilliam was patron in 1803. The church, dedicated to St. Peter, has a steeple in the early style of English architecture, surmounted by a lofty octagonal lantern of later date ; in the reign of Richard II. it was made collegiate, and endowed by John Pyel, lord mayor of London, for a dean and five secular canons, or prebendaries, besides four clerks, and at the dissolution it possessed a revenue of £64. 12. 10. : there are some remains of the collegiate buildings. The church of All Saints has been demolished. There are places of worship for Baptists and Wesleyan Methodists. In the middle of the village stands a stone cross, the shaft of which, raised upon steps, is thirteen feet high, and is the standard for adjusting the provincial pole, by which the portions of the adjacent meadows are measured.

IRTON, a parish in ALLERDALE ward above Darwent, county of CUMBERLAND, 4½ miles (N. by E.)

from Ravenglass, containing, with the joint township of Santon with Melthwaite, 566 inhabitants. The living is a perpetual curacy, in the archdeaconry of Richmond, and diocese of Chester, endowed with £1000 royal bounty, and in the patronage of Lord Muncaster. The church is dedicated to St. Paul. The rivers Irt and Mite run through the parish. A great variety of granite is obtained near Irton hall. Henry Caddy, in 1716, gave £150 towards the foundation of a free school; which sum, with accumulations and an allotment of land assigned at the time of the enclosure, produces about £12 per annum for the master.

IRTON, a township in the parish of Seamer, Pickering lythe, North riding of the county of York, 4½ miles (S. W.) from Scarborough, containing 105 inhabitants.

ISALL, a parish in Allerdale ward below Darwent, county of Cumberland, comprising the townships of Blindcrake with Isall and Redmain, Isall Old Park, and Sunderland, and containing 449 inhabitants, of which number, 311 are in the township of Isall with Blindcrake and Redmain, 3¾ miles (N. E. by E.) from Cockermouth. The living is a vicarage, in the archdeaconry and diocese of Carlisle, rated in the king's books at £8. 13. 6½., and in the patronage of Wilfrid Lawson, Esq. The church, dedicated to St. Michael, is in the Norman style of architecture. The parish is bounded on the south by the Derwent, which is crossed by a bridge built, in 1691, at an expense of £500. White freestone is obtained on Moothay hill, and coal and copper mines were formerly wrought within the parish. There is a school for seventeen children, supported by subscription, the chief contributors to which are W. Lawson and J. T. Thompson, Esqrs. Isell hall is of great antiquity, and has been fortified ; one of the original towers is still standing, but the rest of the building has been much modernised. At Chapel Guards are vestiges of an extensive monastery.

ISALL-OLD-PARK, a township in the parish of Isall, Allerdale ward below Darwent, county of Cumberland, 4½ miles (N. E.) from Cockermouth, containing 90 inhabitants.

ISFIELD, a parish in the hundred of Loxfield-Dorset, rape of Pevensey, county of Sussex, 3¼ miles (S.W.) from Uckfield, containing 569 inhabitants. The living is a rectory, in the peculiar jurisdiction and patronage of the Archbishop of Canterbury, rated in the king's books at £9. 12. 8½. The church, dedicated to St. Margaret, is principally in the decorated style of architecture. The parish is bounded on the west by the river Ouse, on which there is considerable traffic in coal, marl, and chalk, for some miles up the country. Here are several hop plantations, and an extensive paper manufactory ; also the remains of an ancient castle.

ISHAM, a parish in the hundred of Orlingbury, county of Northampton, 3½ miles (S. S. E.) from Kettering, containing 322 inhabitants. The living is a rectory in two portions, Inferior and Superior, in the archdeaconry of Northampton, and diocese of Peterborough, each rated in the king's books at £7. 10. Isham Inferior is in the patronage of the Bishop of Lincoln, and Isham Superior in that of Edward Henry Hoare, Esq. The church is dedicated to St. Peter.

ISHLAWREOED, a hamlet in the parish of Bedwelty, lower division of the hundred of Wentlloog, county of Monmouth, containing 978 inhabitants.

ISLE-ABBOTTS, a parish in the hundred of Abdick and Bulstone, county of Somerset, 4¾ miles (N. by W.) from Ilminster, containing 342 inhabitants. The living is a discharged vicarage, in the archdeaconry of Taunton, and diocese of Bath and Wells, rated in the king's books at £8, and in the patronage of the Dean and Chapter of Bristol. The church is dedicated to St. Mary. There is a place of worship for Baptists.

ISLE-BREWERS, a parish in the hundred of Abdick and Bulstone, county of Somerset, 5¼ miles (S. W.) from Langport, containing 219 inhabitants. The living is a discharged vicarage, in the archdeaconry of Taunton, and diocese of Bath and Wells, rated in the king's books at £7. 10. D. R. Mitchell, Esq. was patron in 1793. The church is dedicated to All Saints.

ISLEHAM, a parish in the hundred of Staploe, county of Cambridge, 4¼ miles (W.) from Mildenhall, containing 1716 inhabitants. The living is a discharged vicarage, in the peculiar jurisdiction and patronage of the Bishop of Rochester, rated in the king's books at £13. 3. 1½. The church, dedicated to St. Andrew, is in the plain Norman style of architecture, and belonged to a priory dedicated to St. Margaret, founded here as a cell to the abbey of St. Jagitto in Brittany, and granted by Henry VI. to Pembroke Hall, Oxford, at which period its revenue was valued at £10. 13. 4. There are places of worship for Baptists and Independents. An Hospital for five widowers and five widows was founded by the Lady of Sir Robert Peyton, who died in 1518, the annual income of which is now about £108.

ISLEWORTH, a parish in the hundred of Isleworth, county of Middlesex, 9 miles (W. S. W.) from London, containing, with that part of the town of Hounslow which is within the parish, 5269 inhabitants. This place was principally distinguished for a splendid monastery, founded originally at Twickenham, in 1414, by Henry V., and dedicated to Our Holy Saviour, the Blessed Virgin, and St. Bridget, for sixty sisters, thirteen priests, four deacons, and eight lay brethren of the order of St. Augustine, as reformed by St. Bridget : in 1432, the community removed to Isleworth, where was erected a spacious edifice called the monastery of Sion, the revenue of which, at the dissolution, was £1944.11.8. The site was granted, in the 1st of Edward VI., to Edward, Duke of Somerset, Lord Protector, who erected the superb mansion of Sion house, which, in the seventh year of the same reign, was granted to John Dudley, Duke of Northumberland. In the reign of Mary, the convent was re-founded for an abbess and nuns, but was finally suppressed in that of Elizabeth, and continued vested in the crown till the reign of James I., when it was given to Henry Percy, the ninth Earl of Northumberland. The Dukes of York and Gloucester, sons of Charles I., and their sister, the Princess Elizabeth, were placed here by the parliament, under the care of the countess, in 1646. This mansion, which about the middle of the seventeenth century underwent several alterations and repairs, and received considerable additions, under the superintendence of Inigo Jones, is a spacious quadrangular and embattled structure, with towers at the angles. The entrance from the western road is through a handsome gateway, on each side of which is an open colonnade, into a spacious lawn, ornamented with clusters of stately trees, and shelving to the margin of the Thames, which pursues its winding course along the border of the park and grounds. A noble flight of steps leads to the great hall, which is decorated with colossal statues and a fine bronzed cast of the dying gladiator : the hall opens into a handsome vestibule, the floor of which is of scagliola marble, and the walls richly ornamented in relievo, and embellished with gilt trophies; twelve columns of verd antique, supporting gilt statues, and sixteen pilasters of the same rare and costly marble, impart an air of sumptuous magnificence to this part of the building, from which there is an entrance into the dining-room : this apartment is characterised by a chaste simplicity of style, and ornamented with marble statuary and paintings in chiaro-oscuro ; at each end is a semicircular recess, separated by columns of graceful proportion, and the ceiling is elegantly worked in stucco, and enriched with gilding. The drawing-room is splendidly furnished; the walls are hung with rich tri-coloured damask; the mirrors are nine feet high, and nearly six feet in breadth, and the tables are of costly mosaic, found in the baths of Titus, and purchased at Rome; the ceiling, which is coved, is divided into small compartments richly gilt, and displaying designs from the antique, executed by Italian artists. The gallery, which contains the library and museum, is one hundred and thirty-three feet in length, and is finished after the antique style, in stucco, of the most light and elegant design : the ceiling is embellished with paintings, and ornamented with various devices, harmonising with the general character of the whole; and immediately below it are paintings in medallions exhibiting a series of portraits of the Earls of Northumberland, of the Percy and Seymour families. At the west end are folding-doors opening into the gardens and pleasure grounds, which are laid out with a degree of taste and skill that has rendered them in every respect worthy of the splendid mansion to which they are an appendage.

The village is pleasantly situated on the northern bank of the Thames, and consists of one principal street, well lighted with gas; the houses are in general respectable and well built, and the inhabitants are amply supplied with water : the environs are profusely rich in beautiful scenery, on both banks of the river, being adorned with elegant mansions and villas, with their appendant pleasure grounds and shrubberies. A considerable portion of land in the neighbourhood is cultivated by market-gardeners, who supply the London markets. Among the various fruits for the perfection of which the soil is peculiarly favourable, are raspberries and strawberries, of which great quantities are carried to Covent Garden market; of the latter, a new species, called the Scarlet Emperor, has within the last year been grown here, which for beauty and flavour is unequalled. Calico-printing was formerly carried on here to a considerable extent, but within the last three years it has been discontinued : there are two extensive corn-mills, one of which formerly belonged to the monastery; and there is also a large brewery. A branch of the Paddington canal joins the Thames at the eastern extremity of the parish, near Brentford. A pleasure fair is held here on the first Monday in July, and at Hounslow are two annual fairs. Isleworth is within the jurisdiction of the county magistrates, and within that of a court of requests held at Brentford

during the summer half-year, and at Uxbridge during winter, for the recovery of debts under 40s. The Duke of Northumberland holds courts leet and baron in April and October, and the Dean and Canons of Windsor hold an annual court leet.

The living is a vicarage, in the archdeaconry of Middlesex, and diocese of London, rated in the king's books at £18, and in the patronage of the Dean and Canons of Windsor. The church, dedicated to All Saints, occupies an elevated situation near the margin of the river, and forms a conspicuous and interesting feature in the landscape ; the venerable tower, overspread with ivy, and surmounted by a belfry-steeple, in the early style of English architecture, has a picturesque appearance : the body of the church was taken down and rebuilt of brick in 1704, and repaired and beautified in 1829. The interior, which consists of a nave with north and south aisles and a chancel, contains many handsome monuments, among which are, one of white marble, with a finely-sculptured bust, to the memory of Mrs. Ann Tolson, who founded almshouses here ; one to Sir Orlando Gee, registrar of the court of Admiralty after the Restoration; and one to George Keate, Esq., F.R.S. and F.S.A., author of an account of Captain Wilson's Shipwreck among the Pelew Islands. A small brass plate, with the effigy of a nun, belonging to the original convent, has been inlaid in the door of the Duke of Northumberland's pew. There are places of worship for the Society of Friends, Independents, and Wesleyan Methodists, and a Roman Catholic chapel. The charity school, or Blue school, since united with the National school, was first established in 1715, and is endowed with funds which had accumulated from savings invested in the three per cent. consols, arising from a bequest of lands at Langley-Morris, in the county of Buckingham, by Lady Elizabeth Hill, in 1630; and from houses and tenements left, in 1672, by Mrs. Ann Oliver, and exchanged for lands at Orpington, in the county of Kent, by William Chelcott, Esq., who, in 1658, bequeathed a rent-charge of £20 on lands at Nettlebed, in the county of Oxford, for apprenticing boys, and other benefactions, producing in the aggregate more than £280 per annum : one hundred boys and sixty girls are instructed in this school, of which number forty of each sex are clothed, the boys being apprenticed and the girls placed out as servants. An infant school, established in 1829, in which eighty children are instructed ; and a Sunday school, which has also a small endowment, are principally supported by subscription. Almshouses were founded, in 1671, by Sir Thomas Ingram, Knt., for six aged widows, to each of whom he assigned a pension of £4 per annum, secured upon his house at Isleworth; and for the further endowment of which, his wife, Frances, gave, in lieu, a sum of money for the purchase of land ; to which several benefactions having been added, the inmates now receive £10 per annum, with other allowances. There are almshouses for six aged unmarried men and six aged widows, or maidens, founded and endowed with the sum of £5000, given by Mrs. Ann Tolson, in consequence of having unexpectedly succeeded to property of the value of £40,000, after having been obliged to keep a boarding-school for her support : she died in 1750, having married a third husband, who survived her, and contested the validity of the donation, which, by a decree of the court of Chancery, he was at length compelled to pay, with interest, amounting in 1756 to £6125.2.9. Mrs. Gosling subsequently left £210 three per cents. to these almshouses, the whole income belonging to which is £171. 6. per annum, the inmates receiving each an allowance of £9. 4. per annum, with clothing, coal, and other assistance. An almshouse for six aged women was built, in 1764, by Mrs. Mary Bell, who endowed it with lands producing an income of more than £60 per ann., which is distributed among the inmates, after defraying the expenses of repairs, in money, bread, clothes, and firing. There are numerous charitable bequests for distribution among the poor. Anthony Collins, a deistical writer, and the correspondent and friend of Locke, was born here in 1676.

ISLEY-WALTON, a chapelry in the parish of KEGWORTH, western division of the hundred of GOSCOTE, county of LEICESTER, 7 miles (N. E.) from Ashby de la Zouch, containing 65 inhabitants.

ISLINGTON, a parish in the Finsbury division of the hundred of OSSULSTONE, county of MIDDLESEX, 2 miles (N. by W.) from London, the population of which, according to the census of 1821, amounted to 22,417, since which it is supposed to have increased to about 33,000. This place, called anciently *Isendune*, and in Domesday-book *Iseldone*, appears to have derived its name either from fortifications erected here during the time of the Romans, or from the discovery in the neighbourhood of some mineral springs, the waters of which were strongly impregnated with iron. In the fields to the north-west of White Conduit house was a large enclosure, called Redmote, supposed to have been the camp of Paulinus Suetonius, after his retreat from London, and the rendezvous of his forces prior to his battle with Boadicea, Queen of the Iceni, from which event the hamlet of Battle Bridge is said to have derived its name: in the south-east angle is a moated mansion, supposed to have been the prætorium of the Roman general. At Highbury also, in this parish, was another fort surrounded by a moat, the site of which was subsequently occupied by a mansion, which becoming the property of Alexander Aubert, Esq., was by him fitted up as an observatory, and furnished with astronomical instruments of various descriptions. From its proximity to London, and the salubrity of the air, Islington at a very early period became the residence of the more opulent citizens, and was inhabited also by many illustrious and distinguished families. Among the numerous mansions erected there in ancient times, exclusively of a royal palace, of which some part is still remaining, was Canonbury House, the palace of the prior of St. Bartholomew's monastery in Smithfield, of which, though the site is for the greater part occupied by modern dwelling-houses, there are still considerable remains; of these, Canonbury tower, a lofty square structure of brick, commanding an extensive view of the surrounding country, is still entire, and of various other parts many vestiges are preserved in the stables and out-buildings of the houses that have been erected near the spot: the tower has long been occupied as a lodging-house, and deserves notice as having been the temporary residence of several literary characters, particularly Ephraim Chambers, author of the Cyclopædia, and Dr. Oliver Goldsmith. The seat of the Prior of St. John's, at Highbury, was demolished in the reign of Richard II., during the insurrection of Wat Tyler and Jack Straw; in memory of which outrage the small portion of it that remained was denominated Jack Straw's castle, but it has been taken down within the last few years. Mildmay house, at Newington Green, was occupied by Henry VIII. Of the numerous ancient houses which formerly distinguished the village, and which had for a great number of years been occupied as inns, the last possessing any characteristic features of the age in which they were erected (the Queen's Head inn, Lower-street) was taken down in 1829. The greater portion of the village is pleasantly situated on the great north road, along which it extends nearly two miles: it consisted formerly of two principal streets, called the Upper and Lower street; but within the last few years it has been almost connected by continuity of building in every direction with the metropolis, a very considerable portion of the fields in the vicinity having been laid out in streets, and covered with buildings. A new line of road from the city through Hoxton, called the New North road, joining the high road near Highbury; the Liverpool road, branching from the turnpike at Islington, and uniting with the high road at Lower Holloway; and a road from Battle Bridge, joining the main road at Upper Holloway; have recently been formed, on the two former of which, numerous and extensive ranges of building have been erected. The village is well paved and lighted with gas, and the inhabitants are amply supplied with water by the New River Company. Notwithstanding the numerous alterations and extensive additions that have taken place, many parts of Islington still retain much of their original pleasant and rural character; and the windings of the New river give an interesting and in some places a picturesque appearance to the various grounds through which it passes. Highbury Place and Terrace are fine ranges of respectable houses, commanding, in one direction, pleasing views of Holloway and the Hampstead and Highgate hills, and in the other, of Shooter's hill, Greenwich park, and the winding of the Thames: beyond is Highbury Park, consisting of handsome houses detached from each other, on the crest of the hill, and on the opposite side a noble terrace has recently been erected. Barnsbury Park, leading from the Liverpool road into the Copenhagen fields, is a pleasant range of neat villas, commanding extensive and varied prospects, and there are several interesting and agreeable walks in other parts of the parish. The land in the neighbourhood is principally occupied by cow-keepers, who have very extensive dairies for supplying the inhabitants of the metropolis with milk. In that part of the parish which borders on Kingsland is an extensive white lead manufactory, affording employment to from thirty to forty persons; on the road leading to Ball's Pond is a manufactory for floor-cloth; and on the banks of the Regent's canal, which is conducted under the Liverpool road, the Upper-street, and the bed of the New River, by means of a tunnel, are numerous coal and lime wharfs. Courts leet and baron are held for several manors in the parish, which is within the jurisdiction of the court of requests in Kingsgate-street, Holborn, for the recovery of debts under 40s., and within the limits of the new police establishment.

The living is a vicarage, in the jurisdiction of the Commissary of London, concurrently with the Consistorial Court of the Bishop, rated in the king's books at £30, and in the incumbency of the Rev. Daniel Wilson in his own right. The church, dedicated to St. Mary, and erected on the site of the ancient structure, in 1751, is a handsome edifice of brick, with a tower of the same materials, ornamented with quoins and cornices, and surmounted by a spire of stone, for the repair of which, in 1787, scaffolding was constructed of wicker-work by an ingenious basket-maker. In the chancel is a monument to the memory of Dr. William Cave, vicar of the parish, and a learned writer on divinity and ecclesiastical history, who died in 1713: in the churchyard were interred the Rev. John Lindsay, an eminent nonjuring clergyman; John Hyacinth de Magelhaens, F.R.S., an ingenious natural philosopher, who died in 1790; and the celebrated Dr. William Hawes, the founder of the Royal Humane Society, who was a native of this parish; as was also John Nichols, Esq., F.S.A., the editor of the Gentleman's Magazine, and author of several works on antiquities and topography. The chapel of ease at Lower Holloway was erected in 1814, under the authority of an act of parliament which provided also additional burying-ground : it is a spacious and handsome building of brick, with a low square tower ; the interior is very neatly and appropriately fitted up, and the altar is embellished with a good painting of the " *Noli me tangere :*" the cemetery belonging to this chapel comprises from five to six acres, and is planted with avenues of trees. Three churches have been built by the parliamentary commissioners, at an aggregate expense of more than £35,000, towards which sum the parishioners contributed £12,000. St. John's church at Upper Holloway, erected, in 1827, at an expense of £11,890. 7. 8., and containing one thousand seven hundred and eighty-two sittings, of which seven hundred and fifty-three are free, is a handsome structure in the later style of English architecture, with a square embattled tower crowned with pinnacles : the interior is beautifully arranged; the nave, which is very lofty, is lighted by a fine range of clerestory windows, and separated from the aisles by pointed arches and pillars of graceful proportion : the whole of this edifice forms an elegant specimen of beautiful design and correct embellishment. St. Paul's church at Ball's Pond, erected in the same year, at an expense of £10,947. 16. 6., and containing one thousand seven hundred and ninety-three sittings, of which eight hundred and seventeen are free, is a building of similar character with St. John's, though differing in its minuter details ; and the church in Cloudesley-square, dedicated to the Holy Trinity, erected at an expense of £11,535, and containing two thousand and nine sittings, of which, eight hundred and fifty-eight are free, differs from the others principally in the substitution of turrets and minarets in lieu of a tower : the architect of the three churches was Mr. Charles Barry. The living of each will be a district incumbency, in the gift of the patron of the vicarage. There are four places of worship for Independents, and one for Wesleyan Methodists.

The Church Missionary Society, in 1827, purchased the house and grounds formerly occupied by a Mr. Sabine, opposite Tyndal-place, on the site of the back premises of which they have erected a spacious and handsome building, for the residence and preparation of young men intended for foreign missions : it is capable of affording accommodation for forty students, who are in-

structed in Latin, Greek, Hebrew, the Mathematics, &c. : the theological and classical tutors are resident, and a professor of Arabic and other oriental languages, attends two terms in the year. The students usually remain from three to four years, according to circumstances ; and ten, on an average, are annually fitted out for the several stations they are required to occupy abroad. Highbury College, established at Mile-End in 1783, removed to Hoxton in 1791, and thence to Highbury in 1826, is an institution for bestowing a liberal education on young men intending to become dissenting ministers : the building, which is a handsome brick edifice, consists of a centre with a fine portico, and two wings, and was erected at an expense of £22,000, for the reception and accommodation of the students, who must be single men, eighteen years of age and upwards, producing testimonials of their piety, and being able to translate Virgil, having also some acquaintance with the Greek grammar, fractional arithmetic, and the elements of geography : the institution is under the management of a committee chosen from among the subscribers, by whose contributions it is supported : the course of studies, conducted under two tutors, comprises the Latin, Greek, Hebrew, Chaldee, and Syriac languages, the belles lettres, intellectual and moral philosophy, the mathematics, history, biblical criticism, the composition of sermons, theology, Hebrew antiquities, &c. A proprietary grammar school, in connexion with the church of England, was instituted in 1830, for the use of which handsome premises have been erected in the later English style, in Barnsbury-street, at an expense of £1400, to be defrayed by shares of £15 each.

The parochial charity schools, established by subscription about the beginning of the last century, have been re-modelled on the Madras system; two school-rooms, with dwelling - houses for the master and the mistress, have been built in the Liverpool road, at an expense of £3000, defrayed partly by a legacy bequeathed by Mrs. Ann May, and other sums, the produce of donations, amounting in the whole to £1977, which had been vested in the funds, and partly by subscription : three hundred and ninety boys and two hundred and thirty girls are instructed in these schools, of which number, fifty boys and fifty girls are completely clothed, and, when they leave school, are apprenticed, or put to service; a premium of £5 is given with the boys, and one of £2 with the girls. Lady Temple, in 1696, bequeathed, to the vicar and churchwardens, lands at Potter's Bar, producing upwards of £50 per annum, in trust for the education of children of the parish, which sum is, by the vicar and the churchwardens, appropriated to the board and education of three female children. Mr. John Westbrook bequeathed £300 South Sea annuities, to which was subsequently added a legacy of £100 three per cents. reduced, by Mr. Isaac Needham, for the instruction of children in reading and in the catechism of the church of England; the income arising from these funds, amounting to £15 per annum, is paid to a schoolmistress for that purpose. A charity school belonging to Union chapel, in which upwards of one hundred children of both sexes are educated, the majority of them being also clothed; and another for girls, in connexion with Islington chapel, are supported by subscription. The Royal British school, in which one hundred and eighty-five girls are instructed, was established in 1817, and is supported by subscription : there are also Sunday schools in connexion with the established church and the several dissenting congregations, and several infant schools, have been recently established. The parish has the right of sending twenty-four scholars to the free school founded by Lady Alice Owen, under the superintendence of the Brewers' Company, and endowed by her with an estate producing more than £60 per annum, for the education of boys of this parish and of the parish of Clerkenwell, in which latter it is situated.

There are ten almshouses, founded by Lady Alice Owen, adjoining the school under the management of the Brewers' Company, for aged widows of this parish and of that of Clerkenwell, who receive each an allowance of money, coal, and clothes. Ten almshouses in Queen's Head lane were founded, in 1640, by Mr. John Heath, who endowed them with £1500, for decayed members of the Company of Cloth-workers, who receive annually from the trustees of that company £20 each in money, a suit of clothes, and a chaldron of coal. On the opposite side of the lane are eight neat almshouses, erected, in 1794, by Mrs. Jane Davis, in pursuance of the will of her husband, who, in 1793, bequeathed £2000 three per cent: consols. for their endowment ; they are open to the poor of both sexes, who receive £10 per annum each, and are admitted on the nomination of the trustees. In Frog-lane are eight almshouses for widows of decayed members of the Cloth-workers' Company, who have each an allowance of £20 per annum, a gown, and a chaldron of coal, founded, in 1538, by Margaret, Countess of Kent. The Caledonian asylum, for the maintenance and education of the children of soldiers, sailors, and marines, natives of Scotland, who have died or been disabled in the service of their country, and of the children of indigent Scottish parents resident in London and not entitled to parochial relief, was incorporated by act of parliament in 1815. This institution, which is under the patronage of His Majesty, is governed by a president, ten vice-presidents, and a committee of twenty-four directors, elected triennially ; children are admitted from seven till ten years of age, and are maintained in it till they are fourteen, when they are placed out as apprentices. The premises were erected at an expense of £10,000, including the site, and occupy an airy situation in the Copenhagen fields : the building, which is spacious and handsome, is of Suffolk brick, with a fine portico of four fluted columns of the Doric order, surmounted by a statue of St. Andrew; it contains spacious school-rooms and dormitories for one hundred children, and the requisite apartments and offices for the master and superintendents of the institution : there are at present fifty boys on the establishment, who wear the national costume, or highland dress, which, on leaving school, they exchange for a plain suit of clothes. A dispensary, instituted in 1821, and supported by subscription, is attended by two physicians, two surgeons, and a resident apothecary. There are various charitable bequests for distribution among the poor ; and the churchwardens are in the receipt of considerable funds arising from the Stone-field estate, bequeathed by Richard Cloudesley, in 1517, for superstitious uses, but, by an act passed in 1811, the trustees were empowered to let the land, and apply the proceeds to keeping in repair the parish church and chapel

of ease : the land, comprising upwards of sixteen acres, was, in 1814, let on lease for eighty-one years, at a rental amounting in the aggregate to £668. 11. per annum, of which sum, four marks are annually paid to the New River Company, formerly to the Crown, the property having been seized under the statute for suppressing superstitious endowments.

ISLINGTON, a joint parish with Tilney, in the Marshland division of the hundred of FREEBRIDGE, county of NORFOLK, 3¾ miles (S. W. by W.) from Lynn-Regis, containing, with Tilney, 236 inhabitants. The living is a discharged vicarage, in the archdeaconry and diocese of Norwich, rated in the king's books at £6. 13. 4., and in the patronage of the Crown. The church is dedicated to St. Mary.

ISLIP, a parish in the hundred of HUXLOE, county of NORTHAMPTON, 1 mile (W. N. W.) from Thrapston, containing 551 inhabitants. The living is a rectory, in the archdeaconry of Northampton, and diocese of Peterborough, rated in the king's books at £15. 6. 8., and in the patronage of the Duke of Dorset. The church, dedicated to St. Nicholas, is a small but beautiful specimen of the later style of English architecture. There is a place of worship for Baptists.

ISLIP, a parish (formerly a market town) in the hundred of PLOUGHLEY, county of OXFORD, 5½ miles (N. by E.) from Oxford, containing 655 inhabitants. This place, now an insignificant village, is chiefly noted as the birthplace of Edward the Confessor, whose father, Ethelred II., had a palace here, of which Dr. Plot mentions some traces as existing in the latter part of the seventeenth century ; and a building, supposed to have been the royal chapel, was then entire, and used as a barn, but has since been destroyed. The living is a rectory, in the archdeaconry and diocese of Oxford, rated in the king's books at £16. 13. 6½., and in the patronage of the Dean and Chapter of Westminster. The church, dedicated to St. Nicholas, is a plain edifice, the chancel of which was rebuilt in 1618. Here is a school for educating, clothing, and supporting twenty-one poor boys, with a provision for apprenticing two of them annually, founded and endowed by the Rev. Dr. South, in 1712, with landed property vested in the minister and churchwardens, and subject to the visitation of the Dean and Chapter of Westminster. Another charity school has been recently established, with a small endowment from a benefaction by William Auger, in 1668.

ISSEY (ST.), a parish in the hundred of PYDER, county of CORNWALL, 3½ miles (S. S. E.) from Padstow containing 660 inhabitants. The living is a vicarage, in the jurisdiction of the Consistorial Court of the Bishop of Exeter, rated in the king's books at £9, and in the patronage of Sir F. Buller, Bart. There is a place of worship for Methodists. This parish lies at the head of Padstow harbour.

ITCHENOR (WEST), a parish in the hundred of MANHOOD, rape of CHICHESTER, county of SUSSEX, 6½ miles (S. W. by W.) from Chichester, containing 181 inhabitants. The living is a discharged rectory, in the archdeaconry and diocese of Chichester, rated in the king's books at £6. 14. 2., and in the patronage of the Crown. The church, dedicated to St. Nicholas, is in the early style of English architecture. The parish is bounded on the north-west by Chichester harbour.

ITCHIN-ABBAS, a parish in the hundred of BOUNTISBOROUGH, Fawley division of the county of SOUTHAMPTON, 3½ miles (W. N. W.) from New Alresford, containing 254 inhabitants. The living is a rectory, in the archdeaconry and diocese of Winchester, rated in the king's books at £14. 1. 5½., and in the patronage of the Rev. Robert Wright : there is also a sinecure prebend, rated at £4. 6. 8., and in the gift of the Crown. The church is dedicated to St. John. The river Itchin runs through the parish. Nathaniel Bailey, in 1823, gave the interest of £400 three per cents. for teaching six boys and six girls. The foundations of an old abbey may still be traced ; part of it has been converted into a private mansion.

ITCHIN-STOKE, a parish in the hundred of BOUNTISBOROUGH, Fawley division of the county of SOUTHAMPTON, 2 miles (W. by N.) from New Alresford, containing, with the parish of Abbotston, 248 inhabitants. The living is a vicarage not in charge, with which the rectory of Abbotston is united, in the archdeaconry and diocese of Winchester, and in the patronage of Alexander Baring, Esq. The church, dedicated to St. Mary, is in the early style of English architecture. There are the remains of an abbey at Abbotston.

ITCHINGFIELD, a parish in the hundred of EAST EASWRITH, rape of BRAMBER, county of SUSSEX, 3¼ miles (W. S. W.) from Horsham, containing 349 inhabitants. The living is a rectory, in the archdeaconry and diocese of Chichester, rated in the king's books at £8. N. Tredcroft, Esq. was patron in 1822. The church is dedicated to St. Nicholas. The interest of £400, bequeathed by Elizabeth Merlot, is applied to the instruction of twelve children.

ITCHINGSWELL, county of SOUTHAMPTON.—See ECCHINSWELL.

ITCHINGTON, a tything in that part of the parish of TYTHERINGTON which is in the upper division of the hundred of HENBURY, county of GLOUCESTER, containing 144 inhabitants.

ITCHINGTON (BISHOP'S), a parish comprising the hamlets of Upper and Lower Itchington, in the Southam division of the hundred of KNIGHTLOW, and the chapelries of Chadshunt and Gaydon, in the Kington division of the hundred of KINGTON, county of WARWICK, 3¾ miles (S.W.) from Southam, and containing 430 inhabitants. The living is a vicarage, in the peculiar jurisdiction of the Prebendary of Colwich and Bishop's Itchington in the Cathedral Church of Lichfield, rated in the king's books at £10, and in the patronage of the Bishop of Lichfield and Coventry. The Precentor of Lichfield cathedral is rector of this parish, and was entitled to the presentation to the vicarage until 1796, when, by virtue of an act of parliament, it was transferred to the Bishop, with the right of presentation to other livings also. The church, dedicated to All Saints, stood in Lower, or Bishop's, Itchington, but there are now no traces of it, and the chapel in Upper Itchington, dedicated to St. Michael, is now used as the parish church. The Itchen, a small stream, rises in the parish, the substratum of which is chiefly a blue limestone.

ITCHINGTON (LONG), a parish in the Southam division of the hundred of KNIGHTLOW, county of WARWICK, 2 miles (N. by W.) from Southam, containing 836 inhabitants. The living is a vicarage, in the archdea-

conry of Coventry, and diocese of Lichfield and Coventry, rated in the king's books at £7. 1. 8., and in the patronage of Sir R. Newdigate, Bart. and Chandos Leigh, Esq. The church is dedicated to the Holy Trinity. There is an endowment of £10 per annum, the bequest of John Bosworth, for teaching poor children. The Warwick and Napton canal and the river Watergall run through the parish. This was the birthplace of Wulfstan, Bishop of Worcester, in 1062 ; and here, in 1575, Queen Elizabeth was entertained by Dudley, Earl of Leicester, when on her progress to Kenilworth.

ITTERINGHAM, a township in the parish of HESKET in the FOREST, LEATH ward county of CUMBERLAND, 8¾ miles (N.W. by N.) from Penrith, containing 210 inhabitants.

ITTERINGHAM, a parish in the southern division of the hundred of ERPINGHAM, county of NORFOLK, 4¼ miles (N.W.) from Aylsham, containing 334 inhabitants. The living is a discharged rectory in medieties, in the archdeaconry and diocese of Norwich, rated in the king's books at £5. 17. 1. The Earl of Orford was patron in 1809. The church is dedicated to St. Mary.

ITTON, a parish in the upper division of the hundred of CALDICOTT, county of MONMOUTH, 3¼ miles (W. by N.) from Chepstow, containing, exclusively of the extra-parochial liberty of Howick, 123 inhabitants. The living is a discharged rectory, in the archdeaconry and diocese of Llandaff, rated in the king's books at £4. 10. 10., endowed with £200 private benefaction, and £400 royal bounty. W. Curre, Esq. was patron in 1810.

IVE (ST.), a parish in the middle division of the hundred of EAST, county of CORNWALL, 4¼ miles (W.S.W.) from Callington, containing 601 inhabitants. The living is a rectory, in the archdeaconry of Cornwall, and diocese of Exeter, rated in the king's books at £26, and in the patronage of the Crown. Two sums have been bequeathed by Mr. Morshead and the Rev. Mr. Question, for teaching children.

IVEGILL, county of CUMBERLAND.—See HIGHEAD.

IVER, a parish in the hundred of STOKE, county of BUCKINGHAM, 2½ miles (N.N.E.) from Colnbrook, containing 1663 inhabitants. The living is a perpetual curacy, in the archdeaconry of Buckingham, and diocese of Lincoln, rated in the king's books at £13. 6. 8., endowed with £800 parliamentary grant. The Rt. Hon. J. Sullivan was patron in 1805. The church is dedicated to St. Peter. A market to be held here was granted to Lord Neville in 1351, and confirmed to the Dean and Canons of Windsor in 1461, together with two fairs : the market has been long disused, but a small fair is still held on July 10th. Courts leet and baron are held every two years. The river Colne runs through the parish, to the eastward of which passes the Grand Junction canal, upon which there is a continual traffic, principally in coal and grain : here is also a paper-mill. Upwards of a century ago Robert Bowyer founded a free school, and endowed it with money, now producing about £21 per annum ; it was enlarged in 1823, when the National system of instruction was introduced. Oliver Cromwell resided at Thorney, and Queen Elizabeth at Rycots ; the latter is now a farmhouse, surrounded by a moat. There is also a house at Richings, in this parish, formerly in the possession of the Duchess of Somerset, and the resort of Pope with the wits of that age: an adjoining walk is known by the name of Pope's walk.

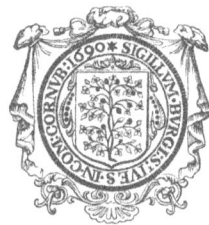

Seal and Arms.

IVES (ST), a borough, sea-port, market town, and parish, possessing separate jurisdiction, though locally in the hundred of Penwith, county of CORNWALL, 8 miles (N. E. by N.) from Penzance, and 278 (W.S.W.) from London, containing 3526 inhabitants. The ancient name of this place was *Porth-Ia*, derived from St. Hya, or Ia, the daughter of an Irish chieftain, who, about the middle of the fifth century, visiting Cornwall with some Christian missionaries, died and was buried here, and being afterwards canonized, the parish church was originally dedicated to her. In the beginning of the reign of Edward VI., the portreeve of this town, whose name was Payne, was hanged, by order of the Provost-marshal, Sir Anthony Kingston, on account of having been engaged in the rebellion under Humphrey Arundel, the governor of St. Michael's Mount. The town is situated on the western side of a bay to which it gives name, and which opens to the Bristol channel. At the entrance to it from Redruth most of the houses are well built and roofed with slate; but in the lower part of the town the streets are narrow and uneven; they are not lighted, nor regularly paved, but there is a good supply of water. The general appearance is mean, except when viewed from the surrounding heights, whence the prospect is extremely picturesque. A good pier was erected for the improvement of the harbour, in 1770, by Mr. Smeaton, the builder of Eddystone lighthouse. The pier originally belonged to the corporation, who still receive a rent of £25 per annum from the proprietors of the new pier. This port, like most of those on the northern coast of the county, is incommoded by the constant accumulation of sand, driven in by the northwest winds; to prevent which it has been proposed to extend the pier, and construct a breakwater: the latter was commenced a few years ago, but was discontinued after an expenditure of about £5000. Ship-building and rope and sail-making are carried on here; but the trade depends chiefly on the neighbouring mines and fisheries; the commercial imports consisting almost wholly of articles for the use of the miners and fishermen, and the exports being derived from the produce of their industry. The number of vessels which entered this port in 1826, was five British and six foreign, and the number that cleared outwards was twelve British and six foreign: the number of vessels belonging to the port in 1828, was, seven of more than one hundred tons' burden, and seventy-seven below that rate. By means of this shipping, commercial intercourse is extensively maintained with the merchants of Bristol, to whom is consigned the produce of the neighbouring mines by agents residing at St. Ives. Off the coast the pilchard fishery is carried on upon a very large scale; and during the season, which lasts from July till the end of November, in some years, the quantity of fish taken and cured has been sufficient to fill

three thousand five hundred hogsheads, which are chiefly exported to Italy, and other parts bordering on the Mediterranean. The valleys in the vicinity of the town are watered by small streams, the currents of which work the machinery used in preparing for the market copper and tin ores, and they also turn several corn-mills. On a peninsular promontory extending northwards from the town was formerly a light-house, now used for preserving government stores; and near it is a battery for the defence of the harbour. Markets are held by charter on Wednesday and Saturday, but that on the former day is inconsiderable: there were anciently four fairs, but those only deserving notice are, on the 29th of May and the Saturday before Advent Sunday. The town is said to have been anciently governed by a portreeve: it was first incorporated by a charter dated in the 16th of Charles I., and under a subsequent charter granted by James II., in 1685, the corporation consists of a mayor, recorder, ten aldermen (exclusively of the mayor), and an unlimited number of common council-men, with a town-clerk and other officers. The mayor is elected by a majority of the aldermen and assistants, or common council-men, from two persons nominated by the aldermen, who are chosen by their own body from the assistants, and the latter by the mayor, recorder, and aldermen: the recorder is elected by the aldermen, who also form a select vestry, and manage the affairs of the parish. The mayor, the late mayor, the recorder, and the senior alderman, are justices of the peace, and hold quarterly courts of session for misdemeanors committed within the borough. No courts of record are now held, though it appears the justices have power to take cognizance of suits for sums to an unlimited amount: courts baron for the manor are held annually. The borough has sent members to parliament since the 5th of Philip and Mary: the right of election is vested in the inhabitants paying scot and lot, between three and four hundred in number; and the mayor is the returning officer: the patronage of the borough belongs to the Marquis of Cleveland.

The living is a perpetual curacy, annexed to the vicarage of Uny Lelant, in the archdeaconry of Cornwall, and diocese of Exeter, endowed with £2000 four per cents., royal bounty. The church, dedicated to St. Andrew, is a handsome edifice with a lofty tower, erected as a chapel of ease to Uny Lelant, in the early part of the fifteenth century. Here are places of worship for the late Countess of Huntingdon's Connexion, and for Wesleyan Methodists. An endowed grammar school was formerly established here, but the property belonging to it has been lost. There is a charity school for boys, which was founded and supported by the late Sir Christopher Hawkins, Bart. Almshouses for six poor widows were founded by Mrs. Cheston Hext, in 1649, which, having become ruinous, were sold by the corporation, and the produce applied to the building of a poor-house. A whimsical custom was established here by John Knill, Esq., a bencher of Gray's Inn, and some time collector for the port of St. Ives, who died in 1811: he directed that, every five years, two old women, and ten girls under ten years old, dressed in white, should walk in procession, with music, from the market-house at St. Ives, to a pyramid which he erected on the summit of a lofty hill near the town, and which he designed for his burial-place ; they were to dance round the pyramid, singing the hundredth psalm ; and for the purpose of keeping up this custom he gave an annuity charged on freehold lands, which are vested in the trust of the officiating minister, the mayor of St. Ives, and the collector, who are allowed £10 for a dinner. At St. Ives was born, in 1713, the Rev. Jonathan Toup, a celebrated critic, who published an edition of Longinus, and other learned works.

IVES (ST.), a market town and parish, in the hundred of HURSTINGSTONE, county of HUNTINGDON, 6 miles (E.) from Huntingdon, and 59 (N. by W.) from London, containing 2777 inhabitants. The Saxon name of this place was *Slepe*, by which it is also distinguished in Domesday-book. It belonged to the abbot of Ramsey, who, in the beginning of the eleventh century, founded a church here in honour of St. Ivo, or Ives, a Persian archbishop, who travelled in England as a Christian missionary, and died about 660, and from whom the place derived its present appellation. The town is situated on the north side of the river Ouse, over which there is a good stone bridge, and the approach to it from the London road has recently been greatly improved by the construction of a causeway on arches, reaching a considerable distance, and affording a free passage for the water during the overflowings of the river. The streets are well paved and lighted, and the inhabitants are amply supplied with water. There is no particular branch of manufacture, but the trade of the town has become very considerable, especially in corn and coal ; and, by means of the navigable river Ouse, an extensive commercial intercourse is carried on with Bedford, Lynn, and other places. A market is held on Monday, for corn and cattle, and it is said to be one of the largest cattle markets in the kingdom : there are fairs on Whit-Monday and Michaelmas-day, the former chiefly for cattle and horses, and the latter for horses, cheese, &c. St. Ives comprises two manors, Slepe and Burstellars, for which a court baron and a customary court are held twice a year : the principal part of these manors is in the tenure of copyholders, who possess the unusual privilege of cutting timber not only for repairs but also for sale. A meeting of the magistrates is held every Monday. The living is a vicarage with the curacies of Oldhurst and Woodhurst, in the archdeaconry of Huntingdon, and diocese of Lincoln, rated in the king's books at £6. 15., and in the patronage of John Ansley, Esq., and the Trustees under the will of Henry Grace, Esq. The church, dedicated to St. Ivo, is a handsome edifice, with a tower supporting a lofty spire, and various parts of the building appear to be of ancient construction. Here are places of worship for Baptists and Wesleyan Methodists. Some remains exist of the Benedictine priory, which was a cell to the abbey of Ramsey. Slepe hall, in this parish, now a boarding-school, was for some time the residence of Oliver Cromwell, who is said to have carried on the trade of a brewer here before he attained political celebrity.

IVESTONE, a township in that part of the parish of LANCHESTER which is in the western division of CHESTER ward, county palatine of DURHAM, 10½ miles (N. W. by W.) from Durham, containing 238 inhabitants.

IVINGHOE, a parish in the hundred of COTTESLOE, county of BUCKINGHAM, comprising the market town of Ivinghoe, and the hamlets of Aston, Horton with Seabrook, and St. Margaret, and containing 1665 inhabitants, of which number, 551 are in the town of Ivinghoe, 9 miles (E. by N.) from Aylesbury, and 33 (N. W.) from London. This small town is situated on the side of a chalk hill, near the ancient British and Roman road called Iknield-street ; it consists principally of two streets extending in the form of the letter T, contains but few good houses, and is neither lighted nor paved, but is abundantly supplied with water from wells. The Grand Junction canal, which passes within the distance of a mile, affords a communication with the northern and western counties of England, and enables the inhabitants to obtain coal from Staffordshire. The only manufacture is that of straw-plat, which furnishes employment for the lower class of the female inhabitants. A small market is held on Thursday for the sale of straw-plat, butchers' meat, and vegetables ; and there are fairs, chiefly for cattle, pigs, and sheep, on May 6th and October 17th. The living is a discharged vicarage, in the archdeaconry of Buckingham, and diocese of Lincoln, rated in the king's books at £12. 16. 1., endowed with £1000 parliamentary grant, and in the patronage of the Trustees of the late Earl of Bridgewater. The church, dedicated to St. Mary, is an ancient building, with a square tower and a small spire ; and in the chancel is an altar-tomb with a recumbent statue, which has been ascribed, perhaps erroneously, to Henry de Blois, Bishop of Winchester, the brother of King Stephen, who is supposed to have had a seat near the town. There are places of worship for Baptists and Wesleyan Methodists. In the hamlet of St. Margaret are some remains of a convent of Benedictine nuns, founded about 1160, by Bishop de Blois, the revenue of which, at the dissolution, was estimated at £22. 6. 7.

IVINGTON, a chapelry in the parish of LEOMINSTER, hundred of WOLPHY, county of HEREFORD, 3 miles (S. W. by W.) from Leominster, containing, with the hamlets of Cholstrey, Hideash, Newtown, Stagbatch, and Wintercott, 674 inhabitants.

IVY-BRIDGE, a chapelry partly in the parishes of CORNWOOD, ERMINGTON, HARFORD, and UGBOROUGH, hundred of ERMINGTON, county of DEVON, 6 miles (E.) from Plympton-Earle. The population is returned with the respective parishes. The living is a perpetual curacy, in the archdeaconry of Totness, and diocese of Exeter, and in the patronage of the Impropriators. The chapel was erected by subscription in 1799. The Wesleyan Methodists have a place of worship here. There are manufactories for paper and ship blocks. A priory, dedicated to the Virgin Mary, was founded by Henry II., for four canons of the order of St. Augustine, which, by the favour of succeeding sovereigns, rose to considerable opulence and distinction.

IVY-CHURCH, a parish in the hundred of MARTIN-POUNTNEY, and within the liberty of ROMNEY-MARSH, lathe of SHEPWAY, county of KENT, 3 miles (N. W.) from New Romney, containing 252 inhabitants. The living is a rectory, in the archdeaconry and diocese of Canterbury, rated in the king's books at £44. 16. 8., and in the patronage of the Archbishop of Canterbury. The church is dedicated to St. George.

IVY-CHURCH, a chapelry in the parish and hundred of ALDERBURY, county of WILTS, 2¼ miles (E. S. E.) from Salisbury. The population is returned with the parish.

IWADE, a parish in the hundred of MILTON, lathe of SCRAY, county of KENT, 2 miles (N. by W.) from Milton, containing, with Chetney Hill, 145 inhabitants. The living is a perpetual curacy, in the archdeaconry and diocese of Canterbury, endowed with £200 private benefaction, and £600 royal bounty, and in the patronage of the Archbishop of Canterbury. The church, dedicated to All Saints, has a low steeple. The parish is bounded on the north-west by Stangate creek, and on the north-eastern side is King's ferry, on the way to the Isle of Sheppy : this ferry is crossed by means of a cable one hundred and forty fathoms long, made fast from shore to shore, which enables the ferrymen to pull the boat over by hand. The public works at Chetney Hill are in an incomplete state, having been neglected for several years past. There are vestiges of ancient military earthworks on Swaines-down, a name evidently of Danish origin.

IWERNE-COURTNAY, otherwise SHROTON, a parish in the hundred of REDLANE, Sturminster division of the county of DORSET, 5¼ miles (N. N. W.) from Blandford-Forum, containing, with the chapelry of Farringdon, 512 inhabitants. The living is a rectory, in the archdeaconry of Dorset, and diocese of Bristol, rated in the king's books at £25. 8. 1½. Lord Rivers was patron in 1810. The church, dedicated to St. Mary, has a tower surmounted by battlements and pinnacles. Lady Elizabeth Freke, in 1640, founded a free school here, and endowed it with a rent-charge of £20. The river Ewern runs through the parish, and gives name to it, the adjunct being derived from the Courtneys, its ancient proprietors.

IWERNE-MINSTER, a parish in that part of the hundred of SIXPENNY-HANDLEY which is in the Shaston (West) division of the county of DORSET, 7 miles (S.) from Shaftesbury, containing 622 inhabitants. The living is a discharged vicarage, in the archdeaconry of Dorset, and diocese of Bristol, rated in the king's books at £10. 1. 0½., endowed with £200 private benefaction, and £200 royal bounty, and in the patronage of the Dean and Canons of Windsor. The church, dedicated to the Virgin Mary, is a large and handsome structure, partly in the Norman, and partly in the early English, style, having a tower and spire one hundred and sixty-two feet high. The small river Ewern has its source here, from which, and the church, the parish derives its name.

IXWORTH, a parish (formerly a market town) in the hundred of BLACKBOURN, county of SUFFOLK, 7 miles (N. E.) from Bury-St. Edmund's, and 77 (N. E. by N.) from London, containing 952 inhabitants. This place, anciently called Gisworth, at the time of the Norman survey belonged to the family of Le Blund ; and about the year 1100 a priory of Augustine canons, dedicated to the Virgin Mary, was founded here by Gilbert le Blund, the revenue of which, at the dissolution, was £204. 9. 5¼. The town derived its principal importance, if not its origin, from this convent, on the site of which has been erected the manor house, in which some of the arches and other parts of the priory crypt may still be traced. The town is pleasantly situated on the high road from Bury to Norwich and Yarmouth, and is a considerable thoroughfare : it is neither lighted nor paved, but is sufficiently supplied with water from wells. The market, now disused, was held on Friday : a small fair is still held on May 13th. The magistrates hold

petty sessions here weekly ; and courts leet and baron are held occasionally for the manor. The living is a perpetual curacy, in the archdeaconry of Sudbury, and diocese of Norwich, and in the patronage of Richard Norton Cartwright, Esq. The church, dedicated to St. Mary, is a small structure, chiefly in the early style of English architecture ; within is an altar-tomb under an arch, with sculptured brasses and an inscription. A charity school for boys, and another for girls, are endowed with the moiety of a benefaction of £1000 three per cent. consols., by William Varey, Esq., who appropriated the other moiety to the poor : there are also some minor charitable benefactions.

IXWORTH-THORPE, county of SUFFOLK.—See THORPE by IXWORTH.

J.

JACOBSTOW, a parish in the hundred of STRATTON, county of CORNWALL, 8 miles (S. S. W.) from Stratton, containing 571 inhabitants. The living is a rectory, in the archdeaconry of Cornwall, and diocese of Exeter, rated in the king's books at £19, and in the patronage of the Earl of St. Germans. The church is dedicated to St. James. Degory Wheare, the first Camden Professor of History at Oxford, and author of a Treatise on the Method of Studying History, was born here in 1573.

JACOBSTOWE, a parish in the hundred of BLACK TORRINGTON, county of DEVON, 3½ miles (S. E. by E.) from Hatherleigh, containing 269 inhabitants. The living is a rectory, in the archdeaconry of Totness, and diocese of Exeter, rated in the king's books at £11. 4. 4½. L. Burton, Esq. was patron in 1814. The church is dedicated to St. James.

JAMES (ST.), a parish partly in the hundred of BARTON-REGIS, county of GLOUCESTER, but chiefly within the city of BRISTOL. That part which is without the city contains, with the out-portion of the parish of St. Paul, 3605 inhabitants.

JAMES (ST.) a chapelry in the parish of BISHOP'S CANNINGS, hundred of POTTERNE and CANNINGS, county of WILTS, containing 1265 inhabitants.

JARROW, a parish in the eastern division of CHESTER ward, county palatine of DURHAM, comprising the chapelries of Heworth, and South Shields, and the townships of Harton, Monkton with Jarrow, and Westoe, and containing 24,189 inhabitants, of which number, 3530 are in the joint township of Monkton and Jarrow, with Headworth and Hebburn included, 2¾ miles (S. W. by W.) from South Shields. The living is a perpetual curacy, in the archdeaconry and diocese of Durham, endowed with £400 private benefaction, and £1000 parliamentary grant. Cuthbert Ellison, Esq. was patron in 1808. The church, dedicated to St. Paul, was partially rebuilt in 1783, but retains some Norman traces, particularly the tower on the north side : the original church, according to an inscription on a stone, was built in 685. There are two places of worship for Wesleyan Methodists. This parish, which is situated on the southern bank of the Tyne, abounds with coal, and the Jarrow pit is one of the deepest in the coal district ; the shaft sinks one hundred and seventy fathoms, but the workings have been carried to the depth of two hundred. Here are numerous manufactories connected with the trade of the port of Newcastle. In a ruined haven, called the *Slake*, which covers about four hundred and sixty acres of ground, the royal navy of Ecgfrid is supposed to have anchored. The village, about one mile in length, is inhabited almost solely by pitmen and their families. The early importance of Jarrow may be attributed to a monastery founded by Benedict, and built on a piece of ground granted by King Ecgfrid : it was completed in 685, and dedicated to St. Paul, of which event there exists a memorial on a stone in the arch of the tower of the present church, which is inscribed in Roman characters. On the establishment of this religious house, Venerable Bede, a native of Monkton in this parish, entered it at the age of nine years, received the rudiments of his education here, and, subsequently becoming an ecclesiastic, spent his useful and literary life within its walls, where he died in 735, and was buried "in a porch built to his honour on the north side of the church." In the vestry-room of the church is his celebrated chair, rudely formed of oak, which was invested by the superstitious devotees of those days with various miraculous powers. This monastery is stated to have been destroyed by the Danes in 870, and again by the Conqueror in 1070 : it was afterwards re-established, and became a cell to the monastery of St. Cuthbert, at Durham, and at the dissolution its revenue was valued at £40. 7. 8. The remains are adjacent to the church, but now consist of little more than a few short Saxon columns and tombs. Numerous Roman relics have been discovered at various times : when the church was rebuilt, an inscribed tablet and the fragment of an altar were found ; and, on the alteration of the road near Jarrow Row, two square pavements of Roman brick were uncovered.

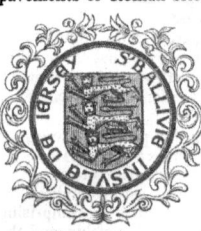

Seal and Arms.

JERSEY (ISLE of), the largest of a cluster of islands in the English channel, dependent on the British crown, 10 leagues (S. S. W.) from Cape de la Hogue, and 7 (S. W.) from the Isle of Guernsey, containing 28,600 inhabitants. This island, the *Cæsarea* of Antoninus, is supposed to retain its ancient name in the modern appellation into which it has been corrupted. That it was occupied by the Romans, at least as a military station, seems more than probable, from the name of part of Gorey, or Mount Orgueil, castle, being still called "*Le Fort de César*," from the vestiges of a camp at Dilament, an immense rampart of earth near Rosel, and from numerous Roman coins having been found in various parts of the island. After the conquest of the western part of Gaul by the Franks, Jersey and the neighbouring islands became part of the province of Neustria, and, about the middle of the sixth century, were annexed, by Childebert, King of France, to the see of Dol in Armorica (Brittany), of which St. Sampson, who had emigrated from Britain, was at that time bishop. St. Magliore, his successor in that see, anxious to convert the inhabitants to the Christian faith, left the administration of his diocese to his disciple, St. Budoc, and retiring to Sark, founded there a small monastery : from that island he proceeded to Jersey, where, by his powerful exhortations and the sanctity of his life, he induced the inhabitants to renounce idolatry, and receive the rites of baptism. The progress of Christianity was greatly accelerated by the exertions of Prætextatus, Archbishop of Rouen, who, being banished to Jersey in 577, lived there in exile for ten years. In the ninth century, a band of Normans having made a descent upon the island, committed great depredations, and murdered St. Helier, a venerable anchoret, whose cell is still to be seen on a rock near Elizabeth Castle. In 912, these islands, as part of the ancient province of Neustria, were, by treaty, ceded to Rollo, by Charles IV., King of France, on the establishment of the duchy of Normandy ; and the Normans having been, about that time, converted to Christianity, one of the principal nobles, a descendant of one of the party who put St. Helier to death, founded an abbey here, and dedicated it to that martyr, from which the principal town in the island derives its name.

From this period nothing important occurs in the history of these islands till the time of the Conquest, when, as forming part of the duchy of Normandy, they became dependent on the British crown. In the reign of John, the French having obtained possession of Normandy, attempted to reduce these islands also, but were vigorously repulsed by the inhabitants ; and King John, having visited them in person, bestowed various privileges, franchises, and immunities, which have formed the basis of all subsequent charters to the present time. On their separation from Normandy, such landowners as had possessions in both were compelled to make their election, and, confining themselves to those on which they preferred to reside, were obliged to abandon the other : the greater number became subjects of that prince in whose territory they had the larger possessions ; but the Seigneur de St. Ouen, of the name and family of Carteret, remaining fixed in his allegiance to the crown of England, abandoned his lordship of Carteret in Normandy, and retained possession of his smaller estates in Jersey. In the reign of Edward I., that monarch incorporated the inhabitants, and gave them a common seal. In that of Henry III., Philip D'Aubigny, Governor of Jersey, intercepted a fleet conveying French troops to England ; and in this and the following reigns the French made frequent attempts upon the island, in which they were invariably defeated. During the reign of Edward II., the judges of assize, who were sent over from England for the administration of justice, flagrantly invaded the most valuable privileges of the inhabitants, and violated their acknowledged rights ; but these abuses were amply redressed by Edward III., on petition from the two principal islands. In this reign, the French again attempting to take possession of Jersey, were vigorously repulsed before *Le Chasteau de Gouray*, which, in commemoration of that event, has been since distinguished by the name of *Mont Orgueil* castle ; they were more successful in their attack upon Guernsey, of which they gained possession, and continued masters for three years : on the arrival of a fleet from England, the inhabitants of Jersey raised a contribution of six thousand four hundred marks, to assist the English in recovering that island. On a sub-

*

JERSEY

Drawn and Engraved for Lewis' Topographical Dictionary.

sequent invasion, under the conduct of the celebrated Bertrand de Guesclin, Constable of France, the castle of Mont Orgueil was saved from falling into the hands of the French, by an English fleet, which, being sent to its relief, compelled the assailants to raise the siege. In the reign of Henry IV., the French renewed their attempts on the island, and ravaged the open country, but could make no impression on the castle.

During the war between the houses of York and Lancaster, Margaret of Anjou having gone over to France, in order to raise troops for the assistance of Henry, entered into a treaty with Pierre de Brezé, Count de Maulevrier et de la Screrme, one of the courtiers of Louis XI., who agreed to raise a body of troops, and make a descent upon England in favour of her party, on condition of having these islands assigned over to him and his heirs, to hold independently of the English crown; and secret orders were sent to the governor of Mont Orgueil, who was an adherent of the Lancastrian party, to deliver up that fortress to Surdeval, a Norman, whom the count had sent to take possession of the island. The count himself soon afterwards arrived, but in all his public acts styling himself Pierre de Brezé, &c., Lord of the islands of Jersey, Guernsey, Alderney, and others adjoining, and adding to his titles that of Counsellor and Chamberlain of our Sovereign Lord the King of France, the inhabitants were so exasperated, that all his endeavours to reconcile them to his government were unavailing; and, influenced by Philip de Carteret, Seigneur de St. Ouen, ancestor of the present Lord Carteret, who held the castle of Grosnez, as a place of defence against the French and Normans, they set his power at defiance, and refused submission to his authority. In the reign of Edward IV., Sir Richard Harleston, Vice-Admiral of England, arriving off Guernsey with a squadron, the seigneur applied to him for assistance, and having previously concerted their plan, the castle of Mont Orgueil was so closely invested both by sea and land, that, after a spirited but unavailing defence, the garrison surrendered at discretion, and the vice-admiral was invested with the government of the island, which he held for sixteen years. The king, to reward the islanders for their conduct upon this occasion, granted them a new charter, in which their loyalty was highly extolled, and the phrase "in perpetuam rei memoriam," expressive of the royal approbation, has been inserted in all subsequent charters. The arbitrary conduct of Matthew Baker, who succeeded Sir Richard, induced Henry VII. (who, while Earl of Richmond, had here found an asylum, on his passage to the continent) to issue an order, restraining any governor from appointing a dean, or bailiff, in the island, and from interfering either in the civil or ecclesiastical courts; and ordered all differences, in which the governor might be interested, to be submitted to the king in council. He also issued ordinances, comprised in thirty-three articles, for the government of the island, which continued in force till superseded by a regular code of laws, in 1771. The harsh measures of Sir Hugh Vaughan, governor in the reign of Henry VIII., who was protected in his tyranny by Cardinal Wolsey, induced Helier de Carteret, bailiff of the island, to seek redress by a personal application to the king; and in the court of Star chamber, in presence of the cardinal, he so powerfully pleaded the cause of his countrymen,

that he obtained the removal of the governor, who had for more than thirty years abused his authority. Jersey suffered not only from the arbitrary tyranny of its governors and their deputies for many years, but also from the continual broils that were kept up between its seigneurs under the feudal system, which prevailed in the island till a very late period. After frequent attempts on the part of the kings of England to put an end to these internal dissensions, by which the peace of the island was continually disturbed, they were finally suppressed by a comminatory bull, obtained from the pope by the influence of Henry VII. In the reign of Edward VI., the French having taken Sark, and made an unsuccessful attack upon Guernsey, anchored in Boulay bay, and disembarked their troops, with a view to effect the reduction of this island; but they were promptly driven back to their vessels, with the loss of a thousand men. To guard more effectually against these external attacks, an additional fortress was erected, in the reign of Elizabeth, in honour of whom it was named Elizabeth Castle. Two commissioners were sent by the queen to remedy some abuses in the island, which, notwithstanding the continued anxiety of successive sovereigns, was distracted by the unequal distribution of justice, and the oppression of the wealthy and the powerful, in whose favour sentence was almost invariably pronounced, by commissioners of their own appointment. To destroy this undue influence, the queen issued an order in council, directing all appeals from the royal court of Jersey to be brought before the privy council, and not before any other tribunal. During the latter period of this reign, Sir Walter Raleigh was appointed governor; and in that of James I., the canons and constitutions forming the basis of the ecclesiastical polity of Jersey (which are noticed in that department of its history) were framed.

In the reign of Charles I., the islanders repulsed another attack of the French; and, to secure them still more effectually from the repeated assaults to which they were exposed, that monarch, at his own charge, added the lower ward to Elizabeth Castle, and repaired and strengthened the other fortifications. On the breaking out of the parliamentary war, Captain George de Carteret, comptroller of the navy, having refused the appointment of vice-admiral under the parliament, retired with his family to Jersey, and openly declaring for the king, equipped a fleet of ten light vessels, to intercept merchantmen trading under the parliamentary banners, which, from its activity and spirit, soon spread alarm around the coast. Prince Charles, eldest son of the king, being no longer able to maintain a contest with the parliamentarians in the West of England, repaired to this island, attended by many of the nobility, among whom was Sir Edward Hyde, afterwards Earl of Clarendon, who, with several of the prince's retinue, remained for a considerable time after the prince had departed, on a visit to his mother, at that time in France. A plan was organised here for delivering the king from his confinement in Hurst castle; but, from some cause not distinctly known, it was rendered abortive. After the decapitation of Charles, his son, being obliged to leave Holland, where he had been residing, landed with a numerous retinue in Jersey, and was joyfully received and proclaimed king. Soon after his arrival, Sir George de Carteret assembled the states, in order to raise a sum of money for the service of his majesty, when about £633 sterling was contributed for that purpose. The king, after staying for several months, retired to Scotland: during his stay, an additional outwork was erected for the defence of Elizabeth Castle, which he named Charles Fort. The parliament, enraged that an asylum had been afforded to the king, and indignant at the numerous captures made by the squadron of Sir George de Carteret, resolved on the reduction of these islands, and for that purpose despatched a fleet, under the command of Admiral Blake, together with a formidable land force, under Major General Haines. After fruitless attempts, for three days, to disembark on the western shore of this island, in which they were driven back by Sir George and the natives, the admiral, dividing his fleet into squadrons, and favoured by a dark night, effected a landing in St. Ouen's bay. On the day following, a violent gale arose, by which one of the largest of the vessels in the parliamentary squadron was driven on the rocks, where it went to pieces, and every soul on board perished. The inhabitants, unable to meet in the field the overwhelming force which was sent against them, and determined on resistance to the last extremity, retreated into their fortresses, and for some time held out against the assailants; but the enemy having made themselves masters of the fort of St. Aubin, and of Mont Orgueil castle, the fortifications of which, after the erection of Elizabeth Castle, had been neglected, and were not in a condition to withstand a siege, they were ultimately obliged to yield. Sir George, having retired into Elizabeth Castle, with a garrison of three hundred and fifty men, continued to defend that post with heroic valour; but having applied in vain to the king, who was then in France, for assistance, and finding all hopes of relief vain, he capitulated upon honourable terms, and went over to join the king. The parliamentarians having thus become victors, gave free quarter to their troops, amounting to five thousand men, who committed dreadful havoc, defacing the churches, which they converted into barracks and stables. On the Restoration, Charles II., after conferring upon Sir George de Carteret many marks of distinction, presented the corporation with a silver gilt mace, with the appropriate motto *" Tali haud omnes dignantur honore,"* which is borne before the bailiff and magistrates, upon all public occasions of importance.

The circumstances which led to the abdication of James II., the troubles which arose in Ireland in consequence of that event, and the subsequent rebellions and commotions which were excited in favour of the exiled family, had no influence on the tranquillity of Jersey, which, from the revolution of 1688 to the reign of George III., enjoyed uninterrupted peace. In 1779, the Prince of Nassau, commanding a force of six thousand men, appeared with a fleet off St. Ouen's bay, destined for the reduction of the island, which at that time was ill provided with regular troops; but the enemy, on attempting to disembark, was repulsed with loss by the regiment then stationed here, assisted by the militia, and supported by artillery, who, after a forced march, arrived in time to prevent their landing. Frustrated in this attempt, the prince sailed to St. Brelade's bay, where he hoped to effect a landing; but there finding adequate preparations made to oppose him, the design was for that time abandoned. After much recrimination among the officers of the fleet, another effort was resolved

upon; but before it could be carried into execution, the squadron appointed to cover the attack was met by a British naval force, under Sir James Wallace, and almost annihilated. The last attempt made by the French to obtain possession of the island was in 1781. On the night of the 25th of December, 1780, when no British ship was on the station, a fire was observed between Rozel and La Coupe, which continued to burn for about eight minutes, and was immediately answered by a similar fire on the French coast, which blazed for about a quarter of an hour. On the following morning, the Baron de Rullicourt embarked with two thousand French troops, thinking to surprise the inhabitants while engaged in celebrating their Christmas festivities, and carry the island by a *coup de main.* The tempestuous state of the weather was unfavourable to his enterprise; several of his vessels were dispersed, and he was obliged to put back for shelter into the small rocky island of Chauzey, and postpone the attempt, after losing several of his ships and men. On the 5th of January, however, he again put to sea with the remainder of his ships, and with the rest of his troops, which had decreased to one thousand two hundred men, and towards midnight arrived off the island. At day-break, on the 6th, the market-place of St. Helier, which now forms the royal square, was filled with their troops, which, under the command of the Baron de Rullicourt, had effected a landing, during the night, at a small point near La Rocque, in the parish of St. Clement. Several of their vessels having been dispersed by the severity of the weather, and the difficulties experienced in landing having greatly diminished their numbers, scarcely more than seven hundred reached the shore; but these proceeding unobserved, secured a small battery of four guns, in which they left a company for the protection of their ships and, in case of necessity, to cover their retreat, established themselves in the town of St. Helier, and took prisoner Major Corbet, the lieutenant-governor. Having induced him to make a promise of surrendering the island, they extorted from him a signature of capitulation, by representing that they had landed four thousand troops, and made prisoners the guard which protected the coasts near La Rocque; and compelled him to sign an order to the commanding officers of the several stations to remain in their quarters; but this order was disregarded, and the troops stationed in various parts, in defiance of repeated injunctions to the contrary, continued to advance upon the town. Part of the French troops left St. Helier to take possession of Elizabeth Castle, the garrison of which they summoned to surrender, according to the terms of the extorted capitulation; but the commander answering only by a discharge of artillery, they prudently retired into the town, and concentrated their forces, in order to sustain a conflict, which now appeared inevitable. On the capture of the lieutenant-governor, the command of the troops devolved on Major Pierson, to whom Rullicourt despatched a messenger, exhorting him to accede to the capitulation, in order to prevent the effusion of blood. Major Pierson had much difficulty in restraining the ardour of the militia, till the various troops had reached their respective destinations, which was not fully accomplished before an impetuous attack was made on the enemy, who, hopeless of escape, fought with desperate obstinacy ; the major was killed at the commencement of the action, but his troops, by no means discouraged, maintained the conflict with determined valour, and obtained a triumphant victory. Rullicourt, and the greater number of his men, were slain, a small number escaped to their ships, and the remainder surrendered : only about eighty of the militia and regulars were killed, or wounded, in this action. Since that period, Jersey, though subject to many alarms, has not been again assaulted. From the year 1779 to 1793, it was distracted by internal dissensions, the most inveterate animosity being cherished by the parties into which the islanders were unhappily divided ; and notwithstanding these feuds have subsided, their effects may still be traced in the acrimony displayed in more recent disputes. In 1814, the Duke de Berri, nephew of Louis XVIII. of France, took up his abode in the island, where he remained till the peace with that country, which ·was joyfully proclaimed, on the 12th of the following July, at St. Helier's and at St. Aubin's.

The island of Jersey is about ten miles in length from south-east to north-west, of an average breadth of five miles (in no part exceeding seven), and about sixty miles in circumference, measuring the indentations of the bays. It is greatly elevated on the north side, and shelves considerably towards the south-east ; the cliffs on the northern coast are in general about one hundred feet in height, though in some places they rise to more than double that elevation : the whole of this side is indented with small coves and bays, and a precipitous ridge of granitic rocks stretches for a considerable distance from east to west : the remainder of it consists of rocks of sienite, of various elevation, exhibiting broad and perpendicular masses towards the sea, every where intersected by perpendicular veins of granite to the north and south, and, where they have been exposed to the action of the waves, forming numerous caverns of remarkable appearance. The rocks of Mont Mado, in the centre of this coast, are particularly abundant in felspar of a flesh colour, and susceptible of a high polish. The west, east, and south sides of the island are formed of shelving shores, with wide sand bays, separated by lofty rocks, with which they are thickly studded. About four leagues to the south are the Minquais, a dangerous group of rugged rocks of considerable elevation, reaching more than ten miles from east to west ; the passage between them and the island is always hazardous, even at high water, as the flood tide sets in upon them with a direct current. A little further to the south-east is an extended chain of rocks, the largest forming the barren island of Chausez, or Chozé. The bay of St. Ouen, a large flat tract of sand, occupies the principal part of the western side of the island, and is bounded by an extensive ridge of sienitic rocks, terminating in the Corbieres, a cluster which stems the current of the Atlantic tide, and is rendered extremely dangerous, from the number of sunken reefs lying near it to the north-west. From this point to the bay of St. Aubin, by which the south side of the island is deeply indented in the centre, and to the westward of which is the smaller bay of St. Brelade, is a succession of points of the same sienitic rocks, their sides every where covered with schistus : the castle of St. Aubin, to the west of the bay, and Elizabeth Castle,

to the east of it, are built on rocks of similar composition. On the eastern side of the island is Mont Orgueil, where the rocks of granite become continuous, and on one of the most prominent of which the castle of that name is built. From Mont Orgueil the coast, with the exception only of a flat shore in the centre of St. Catherine's bay, is an uninterrupted cliff, extending to Rosel harbour, at the northern extremity of the island. At this point a rock of very singular appearance commences, which seems to occupy the whole of Boulay bay ; it is an argillaceous breccia, consisting of large and small masses of schistus, cemented by a basis of the same nature.

The sea around Jersey varies more in depth than round any of the other islands, from the greater number of banks and shoals by which the coast is environed. The tides are not influenced by others in the channel ; they flow, in a direction east-south-east, to the bay of Mont St. Michel, where the declivity of the shore is so inconsiderable, that the bay is filled in the course of two hours ; they then take a northerly direction along the Norman coast, and having encircled the islands in the course of twelve hours, return, after a course of from twelve to sixteen miles, to the spot where they began to flow. These tides rise from forty to forty-five feet round the islands, and at St. Malo's their height exceeds fifty feet. It is high water at Jersey at six o'clock every new and full moon ; but as the flood commences by rushing full against the rocks on the northern shore, it is high water half an hour earlier on that and on the western shores, than on the southern and eastern. The currents, in consequence of being frequently intersected, succeed each other with extreme rapidity, and are in perpetual motion. The principal bays are those of St. Ouen, St. Aubin, Grouville, St. Catherine, and Boulay. St. Ouen's is the most capacious, and the stupendous rocks of L'Etac, which form its northern extremity, are exposed to all the violence of the great wave that breaks upon them from the Atlantic. St. Aubin's opens exactly to the south, and is equally admirable for its extent and for the variety and beauty of its scenery. Grouville bay stretches from La Rocque to the venerable castle of Mont Orgueil, and is inferior only in extent to those already described ; the picturesque harbour of Gorey adds greatly to its beauty. St. Catherine's, though comparatively small, is rich in every variety of picturesque and pleasing scenery ; a few farm-houses, half concealed by woods extending to the edge of the beach, are scattered round its shores, and the points forming its boundaries are composed of lofty and irregular rocks. Boulay bay is surrounded by rocks of bolder elevation than are found in any other part of the island, but they are destitute of wood, and of every kind of vegetation. The stupendous barriers which form the northern coast contrast finely with the interior of the island, which is richly clothed with wood, and studded with cottages, built of stone and thatched, with orchards attached, and inhabited by the proprietors, who are far removed from poverty, many of them, by a long course of industry, having even acquired a degree of comparative wealth. The island is intersected, in every direction, by beautiful vallies, watered by numerous streams, which issue from their wood-crowned banks, and, after irrigating the meadows and turning many mills, empty themselves into the sea. The coasts abound with a great variety of fish: most of those known in England are found here, but the haddock, the smelt, and the muscle, are rarely seen, nor is the cod found to any great extent; the fish most esteemed are the red mullet and the ormer, the latter being highly prized by the natives; the rocks swarm with conger-eels, of which some are fourteen feet in length.

The climate, though tending to humidity, may be considered as temperate and mild; the westerly and south-westerly winds, which prevail generally for three-fourths of the year, convey an abundance of vapour from the Atlantic, a large proportion of which is arrested in its progress by the high lands: no observations have been made to ascertain the quantity of rain that falls during the year, but it is supposed to be about the same as in the western part of Ireland. The dews are also heavy in summer and autumn, and are favourable to vegetation; and though the weather is more variable than in England, the temperature of the air is more genial. The heat of the sun is mitigated in summer by the sea breezes, and the frosts in winter are neither intense nor of long continuance; the snow seldom remains on the ground more than two or three days. Shrubs, which in Devonshire and Cornwall require to be sheltered during the winter months, flourish here in the open air; and carnations, and various other flowers, in a favourable aspect, blossom in the winter. Plants, which cannot be raised in Guernsey, will thrive here in the greatest luxuriance, this being ascribed to the inclination of the shore, which gradually slopes towards the south, while Guernsey, on the contrary, shelves to the north. This island also derives great protection from its proximity to the French coast, which breaks the force of those winds to which Guernsey is constantly exposed. The climate and soil are extremely favourable to the growth of the apple-tree, which is extensively cultivated, and forms a fruitful source of profit to the farmer: thriving orchards are seen in every part of the island, of which they form a distinguishing feature. The Chaumontel pear, cultivated in almost every garden, attains a degree of perfection, both in flavour and size, not elsewhere to be found: it not unfrequently weighs nearly a pound, and so highly is it esteemed, that a hundred of the finest sort will readily sell for £5. 5. Melons are produced in great perfection, the strawberries are remarkable for the richness of their flavour, and the peach and apricot attain a very large size.

The whole of the western end of Jersey consists of light land; the subsoil, in the neighbourhood of Grosnez Point, is chiefly formed of granite in a state of decomposition; on approaching the bay of St. Ouen, the schistose rock may be observed rising nearly to the surface, and the soil is consequently light and thin; but nearer the bay are small fertile glens, which produce the earliest corn in the island. The *mielles*, or hillocks of sand, by which the bay is skirted, extend for about three miles and a half in length, and are about a mile and a half in breadth; and a tract of high land of nearly seven hundred acres, communicating with them to the south and east, and being completely open to the western gales, is inundated with sand drifted from these hillocks, which, in some places, rise to the height of one hundred feet above the level of the shore, whereby a constant sterility is produced. In this tract, called

Les Quenvoais, vegetable mould is found, at irregular depths below the surface, interspersed with fragments of granite, chrystalized quartz, and schistus. Fragments of coarse French earthenware have been dug up here, but there are few traces of ancient dwellings, or of fences. A few acres of this land have been enclosed by order of General Don, the natural soil having been reached by deep trenching. The soil of the island generally is so fertile, that the produce of ten vergees, less than four acres and a half, is sufficient for the maintenance of a large family; but from the difficulty of procuring labourers, from the dislike of innovation, and the propensity in the possessors of small estates to manage their lands without other assistance than what they obtain from their own families, a less efficient system of agriculture prevails here than in the neighbouring islands. The practice of stacking hay, and cutting it in trusses, is seldom observed, it being loosely stowed away in barns. Jersey formerly produced more corn than was sufficient for the supply of its inhabitants, but at present it does not yield more than two-thirds of the quantity consumed: this decay in the tillage of the lands may be attributed to the improvement of navigation and foreign commerce, which, by furnishing employment to an additional number of the inhabitants, has increased the price of labour; and to the introduction and growth of the stocking manufacture, which has withdrawn considerable numbers from agricultural pursuits. Owing to the increase of the population, a greater number of oxen and sheep were imported from England and France, a greater number of horses became necessary for the military stationed here, and the vast number of cows (of the Alderney breed) exported to England, have led to the conversion of considerable quantities of arable into pasture land. A blue and a yellow clay is met with occasionally, but neither limestone, chalk, nor any calcareous substance has been discovered, except in very trifling portions, nor is either marl or gravel to be found: the walks in gardens and pleasure grounds are laid with fragments of broken rock, which being of a very argillaceous nature, binds well, and serves instead of gravel, sometimes even resembling it in colour. Near the town of St. Helier is a superstratum of brick earth, which, though of inferior quality, has been greatly in demand since the improvement of the town, many of the buildings having been erected with that material. The principal manure is a species of sea-weed, called vraic, which from time immemorial has been highly esteemed, its growth being protected by the laws of the island, which allow it to be cut from the rocks only at one particular time of the year on the western, and at two different periods on the eastern, coast. It is either, in its natural state, dug in with the spade, or burnt to ashes and spread thickly over the surface of the land; when burnt, its efficacy is supposed to be so much increased, that one measure of wheat is willingly exchanged for eight measures of the ashes.

The mode of agriculture very much resembles that of Guernsey, being greatly inferior to the system practised in England; it has been invariably pursued by many succeeding generations, without the smallest deviation, or any attempt at improvement. The large plough is generally used, but neither drilling, nor the horse or hand hoe, is used; and the necessary operation of weeding is but little practised: parsnips and potatoes, of which there are abundant crops, are kept tolerably clean, but the corn is in general greatly intermixed with weeds. Fallowing is seldom, if ever, practised. From the most accurate calculations, the Jersey wheat is ascertained to be lighter than that produced in England, in the ratio of fifty-two pounds thirteen ounces to sixty-two pounds ; but the produce per acre exceeds the English wheat, in a ratio of seven hundred and twenty-seven to four hundred and ninety-six, and the average crop of potatoes, in a ratio of twenty-nine to twenty nearly. The *Coteaux*, or slopes, yield timber, broom, gorse, and fern ; and, where neither too steep nor too rocky, afford good pasturage. Most kinds of forest trees thrive well, particularly the chesnut, the elm, and the white oak ; but these and other species of timber would attain a much greater height and girth, were it not for the circumscribed area of the enclosures round which they are planted : some fine beech and ash trees are occasionally seen, and in the parish of St. Clement there is an ever-green oak of extraordinary growth. The fields are enclosed with high banks of great breadth, which, on the side towards the roads, are faced with stone, and most of them are planted with hedge-row trees. The approach to most houses of respectability is by a long narrow avenue, called " *Une Chasse*," the number of which, from the minute subdivisions of property, is exceedingly great. The highways were formerly of various widths, and in that respect were under very strict regulations : in each parish, one of these, called " *Perquage*," led directly from the church to the sea-coast, and was privileged to enable such persons as, for any capital crime, had taken sanctuary in the church, to reach the sea in safety to embark for exile. Along most of the old roads is a paved foot-path, which, as well as the carriage road, is extremely rugged ; and, as the breadth of the road will not admit of quartering, the ruts are very deep : the high banks, planted with trees, afford a pleasant shade, and preserve a refreshing coolness in the summer ; but in the winter the roads are generally damp and muddy : some fine military roads have been made across the island, which are not inferior to those of England. The horses are small, and not remarkable for beauty ; but they are strong, capable of bearing fatigue, and require but little attention, being therefore well adapted for agricultural purposes. The cows, in England distinguished as the Alderney breed, are too generally known and appreciated to require any description ; they are common to all these islands, but at least ten times more, are exported from Jersey than from Alderney ; the number sent annually to England is about one thousand seven hundred. The sheep are of an inferior breed ; they are hardy, but the flesh is indifferent, and the wool coarse and of comparatively little value : the degeneration of the breed is attributed to the discontinuance of the manufacture of knit woollen stockings, which formerly prevailed here to a great extent, but has been superseded by the more profitable pursuits of agriculture and commerce. The island affords various kind of game, but the liberty of shooting, which is now denied to no person, has very much contributed to reduce the quantity. Formerly the jurats, the king's officers, and the lords of the manors, were the only persons privileged to shoot game, in which were included even pigeons and rabbits. The red-legged partridge, which formerly abounded, is now rarely seen ;

and it is remarkable, that the pheasant is not found in this island, which is thickly wooded, although it occasionally frequents the small island of Herm, which is destitute of timber ; the wheatear is common, and, in cold seasons, the woodcock is frequently met with. The coasts are frequented by many species of sea-fowl, and the bernacle is occasionally seen in the winter. Toads, for which Jersey has always been remarkable, are found in every variety of species, some of enormous size, and lizards of every hue may be seen basking in the sun, during the summer.

The only branch of manufacture which ever prevailed was that of knit-stockings, which had attained to such perfection, that laws were framed to preserve its reputation by inflicting penalties on such as, by deteriorating the quality, might injure the sale, of the article; but the extent to which it was carried on being found injurious to the agricultural interest, by withdrawing the labourer from the cultivation of the soil, a law was passed, in 1608, to compel all persons above the age of fifteen to relinquish that employment, and assist the farmers during the seasons of vraicking and harvest : the manufacture still exists, but is confined to females, and to the aged and infirm.

The civil government is vested in the royal court of Jersey, and in the assembly of the states ; and the military command is entrusted to a governor appointed by the crown. The royal court is composed of the bailiff, who is appointed by the crown, and, as the king's representative in the court, occupies a seat elevated above that of the governor ; and of twelve jurats, who must be Protestants of the church of England, and are elected by the people. The bailiff presides ; in all the debates he sums up the opinions, and pronounces the sentence of the court, but has no deliberative voice, unless on an equality of votes of the jurats, in which case he has a casting vote ; in every other instance he is bound by the majority, and decides accordingly. The dignity and prerogatives of his office are very great ; he is the keeper of the public seal, which, however, he cannot affix to any act without the concurrence of three of the jurats : the duties of his office require a thorough knowledge of the laws, and an almost constant attendance at his post. The jurats are appointed for life, but are removable at the pleasure of the sovereign, or may be dismissed on their own petition : their office is honorary and without emolument, and the few privileges attached to it are by no means commensurate to the labour of discharging its duties. There can be no proceedings unless the bailiff, or his lieutenant, be present, but neither of them can sit in judgment on any matter in which he is personally interested. The court is attended by the following officers ; *Le Procureur du Roi*, or attorney-general ; *Le Vicomte*, or high sheriff ; *L'Avocat du Roi*, or solicitor-general ; *Le Greffier*, or clerk, who has the custody of the rolls and records ; two *Denonciateurs*, or under-sheriffs, who publish the injunctions of the court ; six *Avocats du Burreau*, or pleaders at the bar ; and *l'Huissier*, or usher, whose business it is to preserve order. To constitute a court, there must be present the bailiff, two jurats, the procureur, or the avocat du roi, the vicomte, or his deputy, or one of the denonciateurs, and the greffier, and, though not essentially a member of the court, *L'Enregistreur*, or keeper of the register for hereditary contracts. The royal court has cognizance of all pleas, suits, and actions, whether real, personal, or criminal, arising within the island, treason alone excepted ; some other matters are also reserved for the decision of the king in council, to whom alone this tribunal is immediately subordinate. The courts of Westminster have no authority within the island : even prior to the reign of John, by whom the court was in a great degree modelled, the governor held the pleas, and, in extraordinary cases, appeals were made to Normandy, but never to England. Subsequently to that time, appeals were sometimes made to the English courts, but the practice was discontinued in the reign of Edward III., and Lord Chief Justice Coke admits, " that the king's writ runneth not in these isles," but maintains, " that the king's commission under the great seal does operate." After the hearing of a cause before a *Corps de Cour,* or a full court, an appeal may be made to the king in council, under certain regulations, and by consent of the court ; but in every case these appeals must be determined according to the laws and customs of the island. Should the court refuse to grant an appeal, a *doleance,* or complaint to the king, may be preferred : in criminal cases there is no appeal, nor can the governor even suspend the execution of a sentence till the king's pleasure be known.

The assembly of the states is composed of the bailiff, who is perpetual president ; the twelve jurats, representing the inhabitants of the first class ; and the clergy and the twelve constables, representing the several parishes : the procureur and avocat du roi, or attorney and solicitor general, and the vicomte, or sheriff, are also admitted, but have no vote ; and the greffier of the royal court is, by virtue of his office, clerk of the assembly of the states. The assembly is convened by the bailiff, or his lieutenant, but the governor's assent is necessary to authorise the meeting ; if, however, he postpone their assembling for more than fourteen days, he is bound to assign a reason. To constitute a meeting of the assembly, it is requisite that seven from each body should be present, unless upon occasions of very sudden emergency ; foreigners preferred to benefices are not admissible till they have been naturalized. The principal business brought before the assembly of the states is, the granting of supplies for the public service, and the naturalization of foreigners ; the governor possesses a veto on all their deliberations. The constables, who are the principal magistrates in every parish, are chosen in the same manner as the jurats ; their appointment is triennial, but they may be re-elected, and their office is similar to that of mayors in corporate towns in England ; besides being members of the assembly of the states, they preside at all parochial meetings on secular business. Under each of the constables are two *centeniers,* who preside over one hundred families, and, in the absence of the constable, the senior centenier performs his duty, and represents him in the assembly of the states. There are several *vintainiers,* each of whom has the charge of one of the vintaines, or double tythings, into which every parish is divided, except the parish of St. Ouen, of which the divisions are called *cuillettes.* There are also *Officiers du Connetable,* officers of the constable, whose duties are similar to those of constables in England, and two *pro-*

cureurs du bien publique, whose office it is to conduct any parochial lawsuits.

The laws may be comprised under two general heads ; first, the ancient customs of Normandy, together with municipal and local usages ; secondly, ordinances made by different sovereigns, and acts passed by the states and confirmed by the king ; together with such orders as have been, at various times, transmitted from the council board. Acts of parliament, in which the island is particularly named, have no force unless transmitted from the king in council, and registered in due form. A code of laws was compiled by the states in 1771, and sanctioned by the king, which superseded the laws previously enacted by the court ; and though the assembly of the states, or legislative body, can still make provisional statutes, yet they do not remain in force longer than three years, unless sanctioned and rendered permanent by an order of council ; neither can any alteration be made in laws previously established, unless under the sanction of the same authority. As there is but one tribunal before which a great variety of causes requiring different kinds of process must be brought, the court necessarily assumes four distinct characters, and, according to the functions which it has to discharge, is termed, *La Cour d'Heritage, La Cour de Catel, La Cour du Billet,* and *La Cour Extraordinaire,* or *La Cour de Samedi.* La Cour d'Heritage takes cognizance only of hereditary causes, such as the partition of estates, differences concerning boundaries, trespasses, &c.; La Cour de Catel takes cognizance of rents and decrees ; La Cour du Billet is chiefly for arrears of rents and the recovery of small debts ; and La Cour Extraordinaire determines all personal actions. The procureur du roi is the prosecutor in all criminal cases, and every accusation is first examined by a petty jury, termed *la petite enquete,* composed of the parochial constable and twelve of his officers, of whom it is necessary that seven should concur in opinion to find a prisoner guilty : should the prisoner disapprove of the verdict, he may appeal to a grand jury, termed *la grande enquete,* composed of twenty-four persons chosen from the three neighbouring parishes, any of whom, on substantial grounds, may be objected to by him, but a peremptory challenge is not allowed : five concurrent voices are sufficient to acquit the accused party, to whom, if he cannot afford to employ counsel, one of the advocates of the bar is assigned by the court to plead his cause. A prisoner is seldom fettered while in confinement, and never while on his trial, as the laws of these islands, in harmony with the spirit of English law, presume every accused person to be innocent, till he has been pronounced guilty. Prisoners are not, as in England, found either guilty or not guilty; but, according to circumstances, are pronounced either *plutot coupable qu' innocent* (rather guilty than innocent), or *plutot innocent que coupable* (rather innocent than guilty) ; should the former of these verdicts be returned, his indictment is declared to be legal. When sentence of death is pronounced, the bailiff and the jurats put on their hats, and the prisoner kneels to receive it. Forgery is not punished with death, but is considered a fraud : in 1814, an individual convicted of this crime was sentenced to the pillory, and to have the tip of his right ear cut off ; but mutilation of the person appears to be now exploded : the crime of forgery is here of very rare occurrence.

In cases of insolvency, the insolvent makes a public cession of his property for the benefit of his creditors, which is termed "*renoncer*," and his estate is said to be "*en decret*." The creditors who have sued take precedence according to the date of their actions; arrears of rents, if registered, have a preference over simple contract debts, but they cannot be recovered after a lapse of five years. When the creditors are all assembled, those whose debts have not been sued for and registered are first applied to, with an offer of the insolvent's estate, subject to the condition of paying the claims of all the other creditors: should one or more accept the offer, the estate is adjudged to them ; but should they refuse, their own claims are annulled : should they all decline the condition, the estate is offered to the last on the list of registered creditors, on the same terms ; and, on his refusal, to the next in priority before him, till some one accepts the terms. It sometimes thus happens that the party accepting the estate will obtain, after paying the other creditors whose debts have not been cancelled by a refusal, more than the sum due to him ; but if it should be less, it is, notwithstanding, a dividend upon his debt, which he would otherwise have forfeited. The property of those debtors not privileged, that is, of those who do not possess rents in the island, is immediately, upon an arrest being made, placed in the hands of the sheriff, for the benefit of such creditors as have sued, who, if the property be sufficient, are paid in full ; but should there be a deficiency, the creditors are paid in the order in which they have sued, those on the first day in full, and the next day in full, if sufficient assets, if not, the whole is divided amongst them. Should a privileged debtor wish to have his effects secured, with a view to gain time for making an arrangement with his creditors, he may apply to the court, and, upon an assurance of his solvency, two jurats are appointed to superintend the collection of his debts and rents ; a reasonable sum is allowed him for the maintenance of his family, and a year and a day are granted for the liquidation of his debts. In cases of imprisonment for debt, the prisoner is not entitled to the writ of Habeas Corpus, which, though said to extend to Jersey, is not registered in the island, nor allowed by the court. No proprietor of lands or rents can be imprisoned for debt, unless by order of the court. Ten years is the term of limitation on actions of debt, bonds, and other simple contracts. Rents are considered as mortgages on estates, and were formerly paid either in corn or in money, varying according to the value of grain. In all deeds the term corn rent is still retained, and the custom, though anciently originating in the poverty of the inhabitants, and in the scarcity of money, has been found so salutary in its effects, that it has been continued, and extended to every species of real property. Landlords may attach for rent accruing, though not actually due, and prevent the removal of any articles thus attached ; and, should they be perishable articles, they may proceed to sell. The real and personal property of a person dying insolvent are equally liable to the liquidation of his debts.

In the division of property, the eldest son, or, in failure of male issue, the eldest daughter, is entitled to one out of every ten vergees of land in the estate, and to the principal house and all the avenues leading to it, to enable him to discharge the seigneurial services and ground-rent, payable in corn to the original lord of the soil ; and to indemnify him for those military supplies which every estate, in proportion to its extent, is bound to furnish, should the defence of the island require it ; and for the payment of all ground-rents now payable in money, which may have been due upon the estate for forty years. When these claims have been discharged, two-thirds of the remainder of the estate are divided among the other sons, and one-third among the daughters, each being charged with a due proportion of any other mortgages that may be due upon the property. No real property is devisable by will. A wife, on the death of her husband, may claim one-half of his personal property, if he have no children; if he have, she can claim only one-third ; one-third becomes the portion of the children, and the remaining third may be disposed of according to the will of the testator. A widower, having no children, may dispose of his property as he thinks fit : a widow can claim, as her dower, one-third of her husband's estate. A widower, on the death of his wife, if there be issue, enjoys the whole of her real estate till he marries again, in which case, as also if there be no issue, it reverts to her next of kin. A wife, on her husband's death, may reclaim her estate, if it has been sold, or encumbered, by him, without her sanction being expressed by becoming a party to the deed ; and should she die first, her heirs have the same privilege. A father cannot give to any one of his children a greater portion of his landed property than is specified by law ; should he do so, his donation may be annulled by an action brought within a year and a day after his decease. The personal property of persons dying intestate is divided equally among all the children, if they be all sons or all daughters ; but if there be both, two-thirds are divided equally among the sons, and the remaining third among the daughters. All sales of land belonging to minors may be revoked by them, on coming of age. Holders of estates owe homage to the lord of the manor, and, when required, are obliged to deliver into the baronial court an account of all the lands they possess, under a penalty of seizure of their property, till the contempt of court is cleared. In cases of collateral succession, the lords enjoy the estates of the deceased for one year : the undisturbed possession of an estate for forty years is equivalent to a title. Title deeds and mortgages must be inserted in a register, which is kept by a registrar duly appointed ; the neglect of this insertion invalidates the mortgage. If an estate is overcharged with mortgages, the *cessio bonorum*, or relinquishment of property, is allowed to the mortgager, in the same manner as in cases of insolvency ; the mortgagees institute proceedings to establish their claims, which last for a year, and during that time the lord of the manor enjoys the estate of the mortgager. At the end of that time, it is demanded of the last mortgagee whether he will take the estate and make good all the preceding claims upon it ; if he refuses to do so, his own claim is cancelled, and the same offer is made to the next in succession, and continued, as in insolvency, till some one of the mortgagees is found who will accept the estate, and discharge all claims upon it which remain uncancelled.

The tenure of land purchased with money only cannot be considered stable till the expiration of a year and a day, within which time, the next of kin to the seller, or the lord of the manor, is privileged, by the law of *Retraite*, or pre-emption, to take the estate from the buyer, on returning the purchase money : if the estate be purchased with rents, the sale cannot be set aside, as the transaction is considered rather as an exchange of real property than as a 'purchase. All encroachments on property, and civil injuries, which require a prompt redress, may, as in Guernsey, be visited by the *Clameur de Haro*, after which an action is brought : this singular exclamation, of which the form is "*Haro! haro! haro! à l'aide mon Prince!*" was anciently made use of in the duchy of Normandy, on occasions of great peril or importance, and was an appeal to Rollo, the first duke, for justice and protection : the word *Haro* is compounded of *Ha*, an earnest ejaculation, and *Ro*, a contraction of Rollo; and it operates as an instantaneous check, not to be disregarded. There are two regular terms in every year, in which the court meets for the dispatch of business, and they are fixed at such times as not to interfere with the seasons of vraicking or harvest ; the court occasionally holds sittings out of term, for the decision of admiralty causes, and actions on bills of exchange, notes of hand, and commercial matters, which require a prompt decision. The processes are conducted, and all public acts and deeds are recorded, in the French language, which is spoken by the upper classes, but the general language of the island is what is called the Jersey French, a kind of *patois*, which differs in every parish, and also from the *patois* used in Guernsey.

The military government is vested in a governor, appointed by the crown, who enjoys the whole of the revenue arising from the royal demesnes : this revenue has varied at different times, and the privileges and prerogatives of the governor have also been subject to repeated fluctuation. In the earlier periods of the history of Jersey, the governor had not only the entire direction of military operations, but was also at the head of civil affairs, and was then styled bailiff ; his office was of very considerable importance, and the name of it was adopted from the French, among whom it designated an officer invested with high judicial functions, being in Spelman's Glossary thus noticed, " *Ballivus apud Gallos splendidus Magistratus est*." These offices were separated in the reign of Edward I., in 1301 ; and the appointment of the bailiff was vested in the governor, but this privilege was abolished in the reign of Henry VII., since which time the appointment of the bailiff has been exercised solely by the crown. The governor still retains a small degree of civil authority, and has a negative voice in the assembly of the states ; but his duties are principally confined to the military defence of the island. The lieutenant-governor, who is always a military officer, discharges all the duties of the governor, has under his immediate command the garrison of regular troops stationed in the island, and grants commissions to the officers of the militia, which is under his superintendence and control. The militia is a very numerous and efficient force ; every native of the island, between the ages of seventeen and sixty-five, is liable to serve in it, and strangers, after a year's residence, are equally bound to contribute their personal service. Each regiment is composed of a certain number of men, furnished, in proportion to their extent, by a

district consisting of a certain number of parishes. To each regiment is attached a company of artillery, and such as are judged least fit for actual service are appointed to man the coast batteries of their respective districts. The whole of the militia are provided with arms and clothing from the British government, but, with the exception of the adjutants and drill-serjeants, neither officers nor privates receive pay. During war the duty of the militia is very severe ; detachments from the different regiments are successively employed in mounting guard round the island, and, in cases of alarm, they assemble with great celerity. In time of peace their discipline is by no means neglected : during winter they are frequently drilled in companies, and in summer as often exercised in brigade. They are annually inspected by the lieutenant-governor, and boys, who have not attained the age of admission into the ranks, are instructed in the use of arms, and rewarded with prizes, according to their proficiency. Exclusively of the regular force under the more immediate command of the lieutenant-governor, there are five regiments of militia, at all times ready to assemble for the defence of the island. Besides its natural barriers, Jersey is strongly defended by forts at all those points where it is most easy of access, and consequently most liable to assault : of these, the principal are Fort Regent, the castles of Mont Orgueil and St. Aubin, and Elizabeth Castle.

The public revenue of the island is principally derived from a new impost on wine and spirits, and from the sums paid for licenses by the keepers of taverns and public houses : though small, it is sufficient for the general expenditure, and is levied in such a manner as to press lightly upon all classes of the inhabitants. The harbours are kept in repair by the dues of anchorage paid by every vessel entering them, for shelter or for commercial purposes, and by an ancient impost upon the importation of wine, which has been levied for that purpose almost from time immemorial. The great military roads are kept in repair by the several parishes, but a grant is generally made by the assembly of the states, when any important or extensive improvement is to be accomplished. The various parochial expenses are defrayed by a rate levied on the landholders, of which the proportion for each parish is previously fixed by an assembly, consisting of the principal landed proprietors in the island. When any extraordinary works are undertaken, which might draw too largely on the funds of the parish, the expense is generally provided for by lotteries, and in no instance are the needy required to contribute to the supply of the revenue, or to the public expenditure, of the island.

The ecclesiastical government is vested in a dean, appointed by the crown, who is also rector of one of the parishes. The dean holds an ecclesiastical court, in which he is assisted by the rectors of the several parishes : an appeal from his judgment lies to the Bishop of Winchester, and, in the event of a vacancy in that see, to the Archbishop of Canterbury : in these appeals the parties must attend in person, and the decision is irreversible. The ecclesiastical laws, which are regulated by the canons of James I., give the dean the power of granting special licenses for marriage ; the probate of wills, which must be registered in his office, and approved by his seal ; and letters of administration of the goods of intestates dying without heirs, to the next of kin. The early inhabitants were followers of the Druids till the sixth century, when they were converted to Christianity by St. Magliore, who had previously established the Christian faith in the island of Sark; and the efforts of Prætextatus, who, being banished from Rouen, remained for ten years in the island, completed the conversion of the inhabitants. The Normans, to expiate their former cruelty, erected, after their conversion to Christianity, numerous religious edifices in the island, and endowed them with ample revenues. After the alienation of the Norman isles from the parent state, the inhabitants remained under the spiritual control of its bishop, till after the Reformation, when the island was annexed to the see of Winchester, in the reign of Elizabeth. Edward VI. presented them with a copy of the English liturgy, in the French language, which was used in the several churches till the mass and the Roman Catholic religion were revived, in the reign of Mary. Paulet, the last papistical dean, was dismissed by Queen Elizabeth, and the reformed religion was restored, in 1565; but from that time till the year 1620, there was neither a book of common prayer, nor a professed form of liturgy in the island, nor were the churches under the superintendence of any spiritual head. Several French Protestants, disciples of Calvin, having arrived, they began to introduce their own principles, and to overturn the whole system of church government; and a species of discipline, formed upon their own model, was established in the place of episcopal jurisdiction, which was no longer acknowledged; all ecclesiastical affairs were regulated by their councils of consistories, colloquies, and the synod. The church remained in this state till the reign of James I., who ordered that the liturgy should be re-established, but with certain qualifications, adapted to the prejudices of the people at the time, and tending to their gradual eradication. From this period the influence of the presbytery declined, and David Bandinel being appointed dean, the powers of ecclesiastical jurisdiction were restored to the spiritual court. Bandinel continued to discharge the duties of his office till 1643, when, being suspected of encouraging the distraction of the times, he was confined, and, in attempting to escape from Mont Orgueil castle, was killed by falling from the ramparts. From the commencement of the parliamentary war till the Restoration, the liturgy was discontinued, and the office of dean abolished; but, in 1661, the dean was re-appointed, and the regular service of the church restored; since which time the ecclesiastical affairs of the island have remained without any interruption. The revenue of the church is inconsiderable: the corn tithes of the parish of St. Saviour, which had previously belonged to the crown, were annexed to the deanery by James I. The income of the rectors of the other parishes is derived from the small tithes, to which is added that portion of the great tithes which, in some of the parishes, was granted by the Norman abbots to their subordinate ministers. The incumbents of some of the benefices receive also the tithe on waste lands recently brought into cultivation, which were formerly claimed by the clergy, under the designation of "Novels, or Deserts." A parsonage-house is attached to each living, and is kept in repair at the expense of the parishioners: each parish has a fund, arising from

donations and benefactions, for repairing the church and the parsonage-house; and the poor are supported by donations, collections at the churches, and by rates.

The island of Jersey comprises the parishes of St. Brelade; St. Clement; Grouville; St. Helier, or La Ville; St. Jean, or St. John; St. Laurent, or St. Lawrence; St. Marie, or St. Mary; St. Martin; St. Ouen; St. Pierre, or St. Peter; St. Sauveur, or St. Saviour; and La Trinité, or the Holy Trinity; the livings are all rectories, in the deanery of Jersey. Of these, the principal, or, as it is called, the Town parish, is that of St. Helier, which includes the town of that name, the principal in the island, and contains 10,118 inhabitants. The town occupies a very considerable portion of the parish, and is rapidly increasing in extent: it is pleasantly situated, and is completely sheltered from the northerly winds by an extensive range of hills; the streets are spacious and well paved, and the inhabitants are amply supplied with water. The public subscription library was erected in 1736, and furnished with a valuable collection of books by the Rev. Phillip Falle, the venerable historian of the island; the collection was considerably augmented by the late Rev. Dr. Dumaresq; it is open to the inhabitants upon very moderate terms: there is also a circulating library, with a handsome reading-room in the Royal square. The theatre royal, built by subscription in 1827, at an expense of £3000, is a handsome edifice, one hundred feet in length, forming the central compartment of a spacious crescent: in the front is a noble portico of six Doric columns, supporting a handsome pediment, the cornice of which is continued to the extremities of the range: the internal arrangements are complete, and the decorations tastefully splendid. Some commodious and elegant public baths have been recently constructed opposite to the post-office, in Minden-place. The commercial intercourse with other countries having greatly increased, it became necessary, for the protection of the vessels frequenting the harbour, which carry an aggregate burden of twenty thousand tons, to enlarge the pier, which was accordingly accomplished, at an expense of £61,000: it is entirely constructed of the sienite rock, from the quarries of St. John's, and is faced with blocks weighing nearly two tons each.

The town and harbour are defended by Fort Regent and Elizabeth Castle; the former, built on the Mount de la Ville, a solid rock, rising to the height of one hundred and fifty feet above the level of the sea at high water, and commanding the bay of St. Aubin: the whole expense of erecting this extensive and massive fortress, which exceeded one million sterling, was defrayed by the British government; of that sum £11,280 was paid for the purchase of the site, and the interest is appropriated annually to the improvement of the town: the garrison is supplied with water from a well excavated in the solid rock, to the depth of two hundred and thirty-three feet. Elizabeth Castle is situated three quarters of a mile from the town, upon an eminence surrounded by the sea at high water, and, on the reflux of the tide, is connected with the town by a line of loose stones on the sands, called the bridge: it was originally built in 1586, greatly improved by Queen Elizabeth, from whom it took its name, and considerably enlarged by Charles I.; it comprises three wards, defended by strong batteries of heavy ordnance, and con-

**

tains barracks for a very considerable number of troops. The custom-house, a commodious building, is under the superintendence of a collector, comptroller, and subordinate officers ; but, as few articles of merchandise are contraband or prohibited, the import duties are trifling, and the chief business is the registering of the exports. There are several banking establishments in the island, of which the Old Bank, the Commercial Bank, and the Jersey Banking Company, are the principal; they have many notes in circulation : the legal tender is three-shilling and eighteen-penny pieces, of silver coin, issued by the states. The market is on Saturday, and is well supplied with butchers' meat and with provisions of every kind, and, during the winter, with abundance of game from France ; but the supply of fish is not very plentiful. The present market-place combines beauty of appearance with convenience of arrangement : it occupies three sides of a spacious quadrangle, of which the internal fronts are ornamented with piazzas, affording a convenient shelter for the sale of eggs, poultry, and vegetables; and the central buildings comprise two double ranges of shops for butchers, who are not allowed to expose meat for sale in any other place; the fourth side of the quadrangle is parted off from Halkett-place, a spacious handsome street, by iron palisades, in which are the principal entrances to the market. Adjoining the principal market-place is a smaller for the sale of fish ; and a cattle market has been recently formed on a similar plan.

The court-house, a substantial and handsome building, erected in 1647, occupies one side of the Royal square, formerly the old market-place, a spacious area, in the centre of which is a bronze statue of George II., in the Roman costume, elevated on a lofty stone pedestal. The interior of the court-house is conveniently arranged for the holding of the several courts, and the transaction of public business ; and the court-room is decorated with a portrait of George III., by an artist named Jean, and a full-length portrait of Marshal Conway, Governor of the island, by Gainsborough. The prison, which is situated at the extremity of the town, is a substantial and not inelegant building of sienite stone ; the front is ornamented with an arcade, one hundred and twenty feet in length, which supports the upper range of the building : it contains spacious and airy cells for confining criminals, and light and commodious apartments for the debtors : every indulgence of exercise, consistent with security and the nature of their offence, is permitted. The church of St. Helier is supposed to have been built about the year 1341, and its original character has been almost effaced by alterations and repairs ; the exterior possesses few attractions, and the interior, which preserves some traces of original beauty, has been materially deformed by injudicious additions made without any regard to its original style : there are several monuments, among which is that of Major Pierson, who fell at the head of the troops, in the defence of the island against the French, in 1781 : it was erected by a vote of the states, as a just tribute to his valour. The chapels of St. James, in St. James'-street, and St. Paul's, in New-street, the former an elegant structure in the later English style, and the latter a handsome edifice in the Grecian style of architecture, with a noble portico of four Doric columns of Jersey granite, are

proprietary chapels; in both divine service is performed, in the English language, by a clergyman of the established church. There are various places of worship for dissenters : at the Calvinistic chapel, in Upper Halkett Place, service is performed in the French language ; and at the chapel in Zion-place in the English language, morning and evening. The Baptists and Wesleyan Methodists have each two places of worship, in one of which, respectively, the services are performed in the French, and in the other in the English, language. The Bryanites have a chapel in the Hémies ; and there are two Roman Catholic chapels, one in Hue-street for an English, and one in Castle-street for a French, congregation. The Jersey National school, the St. Helier parochial Sunday school and lending library, and several benevolent and charitable associations are supported by subscription. The hospital is a neat and commodious building, in every respect well adapted to the comfort of patients ; it is supported partly by an income arising from donations and bequests, the deficiency being supplied by the several parishes.

The parish of St. Brelade, containing 1717 inhabitants, comprises the town of St. Aubin, situated on the margin of the bay, three miles from St. Helier's : the town is remarkably clean, and, though irregularly built, contains several excellent houses : it was formerly inhabited by many of the most opulent merchants in the island, most of whom, on the completion of the more commodious harbour of St. Helier's, removed to that town, where they found greater advantages for commerce. The bay has the benefit of a good pier, and is protected by St. Aubin's tower, a fortress surrounded by the sea at high water, and defended with a battery of fourteen pieces of heavy ordnance, and a proportionate number of troops. In this parish are the Quenvais, the most unproductive tract of land in the island. The church, which is the most ancient in the island, is beautifully situated on one side of the bay of St. Brelade, and at high tide the water flows up to the church-yard : it resembles in character the church of St. Sampson in Guernsey ; both were consecrated in the year 1111. The parish of St. Clement, containing 938 inhabitants, is the smallest in the island. The church, from its situation, is an interesting and picturesque object : the surrounding scenery is richly diversified, and many of the high grounds in the vicinity afford extensive and delightful prospects. The parish of Grouville, containing 1917 inhabitants, abounds with richly-wooded eminences, and with much picturesque and beautiful scenery. The church, which is in the centre of the village, differs from the general style of the Jersey churches in the extension of the nave, both towards the east and the west, beyond the aisles, and has a lofty spire rising from the centre, which forms a good land-mark. The coast is defended by Seymour tower, which, at high water, is two miles distant from the shore, but may be approached at low water : it is exposed to a very heavy sea, which, during winter, dashes against its base with tremendous force. The parish of St. John, containing 1657 inhabitants, is characterised by the same bold line of coast that distinguishes the northern side of the island, and is chiefly noted for its extensive quarries of a fine kind of sienite, much resembling granite in appearance and hardness, and highly esteemed for architectural purposes ; it is procured from a cliff, called Mont Mado, which is entirely composed of it. The parish of St. Lawrence, containing 1872 inhabitants, is remarkable for its beautiful vallies, its numerous flourishing orchards, and its high state of cultivation : the church has been more defaced than any, by repeated enlargements and alterations. The parish of St. Mary, containing 1020 inhabitants, is bounded towards the sea by high rugged rocks, and contains a great portion of undulating ground. The beautiful bay of *Gréve de Lecq*, partly in this parish, is situated at the bottom of a deep ravine : the sands, on the reflux of the tide, are dry, firm, and of a beautiful colour : the church is unique in its style of architecture, and romantically situated : here are numerous mineral springs of great medicinal virtue. The parish of St. Martin, containing 1691 inhabitants, abounds with objects of interest : among these Mont Orgueil castle is the most remarkable ; though its origin is not distinctly known, it was a fortress of great strength and importance in the reign of John ; the greater part of it is of more modern erection, as is evident from the armorial bearings of several who have contributed to its enlargement : the chapel of St. George, in which many distinguished characters have been interred, is now in ruins, and almost choked up with rubbish. At a place called Anne Ville, on the neighbouring heights, are the remains of a Druidical temple, or *Poquelaye*, consisting of one large stone, fifteen feet long and ten broad, formerly resting transversely upon five smaller masses, but, by the removal of some of them, now reclining on the ground. At *Le Couperon*, on a small cliff not far distant, is the largest monument of this kind in the island : it consists of twenty-one stones, three feet high, enclosing, within an elliptical area, other masses that appear to have formed a cromlech of considerable dimensions ; three slabs, each six feet in length, which were probably united, are supposed to have rested upon fourteen supporting masses. The parish of St. Ouen, containing 2081 inhabitants, is bounded towards the sea by large masses of rock, in which the tide has worn numerous excavations of considerable depth and of singular form. This parish contains a greater number of enclosures than any other ; the church possesses little claim to architectural notice, but the ancient manor-house is an interesting object. The parish of St. Peter, containing 1854 inhabitants, displays much interesting and beautiful scenery ; the lands are fertile, and in a very high state of cultivation. St. Peter's valley is the most extensive and the most picturesque in the island, and the soil is distinguished for its produce : the church is spacious, but has no particular claim to architectural description. The parish of St. Saviour, containing 1687 inhabitants, abounds with pleasing and varied scenery : the church is not devoid of architectural beauty, but has been much disfigured by the various additions and alterations which have been made, without due regard to uniformity of character ; the cemetery contains many stately oak and beech trees, and commands an extensive view : the parish contains several mineral springs of considerable efficacy. Trinity parish, containing 2048 inhabitants, is rich in varied and romantic scenery : the view from the heights above Boulay bay is remarkably interesting and extensive ; the shores of France, bounding the ocean on one side, are distinctly visible, and, on the other, the islands of Guernsey, Alderney, and Sark, present

themselves. The church does not claim particular notice : the ancient manor-house is an interesting object, and there are several remains of antiquity, of which the most important is *La Petite Cesarée*, or Cæsar's wall, which is still visible, and, though now of limited extent, is said to have reached to the harbour of Rosel. The churches generally are cruciform structures in the Norman style of architecture ; the walls are of great thickness, and strengthened with buttresses, many of which have a considerable projection ; the roofs are generally vaulted, and no timber appears to have been used in their construction ; the windows are usually distinguished by the pointed arch, which prevails also in the internal arrangement, and the doorways have the semicircular arch, with mouldings and ornaments of the most simple character. Eight of the churches have steeples, of which that of St. Peter's is the highest ; those of St. Brelade's and St. Lawrence's either had no towers originally rising from the intersection of the nave and transepts, or they have been removed. In most of them a second, and in some a third, aisle has been introduced, the roofs of which are supported upon low massive circular columns ; the windows in many instances have been altered by the introduction of tracery, and in the course of enlargement which most of the churches have undergone, for the accommodation of the increasing population, they have been materially divested of their original character. Divine service is, in all of them, invariably performed in the French language.

Two free grammar schools were founded in 1498, St. Magliore's, or St. Manlier's, and St. Athanasius', the former in the parish of St. Saviour, and the latter in that of St. Peter, each being intended for the accommodation of six parishes ; but the endowments are insufficient to render them at all subservient to the design of their foundation. Lawrence Baudain, of the parish of St. Martin, bequeathed a rent-charge of thirty-two quarters of wheat, for the maintenance, at either of the Universities, of such poor scholars of Jersey as might be desirous of improvement, and deserving of encouragement ; and Charles I. founded three fellowships respectively in the colleges of Pembroke, Exeter, and Jesus, in the University of Oxford, to be held, in alternate succession, by natives of Jersey and Guernsey designed for holy orders : three scholarships for boys from the free schools have been subsequently founded in Pembroke College, Oxford, by Bishop Morley. Jersey formerly contained the magnificent abbey of St. Helier, founded in the early part of the tenth century, for canons regular of the order of St. Augustine, and endowed with an ample revenue. In the reign of Stephen, the Empress Matilda, having engaged its abbot to superintend the erection of a monastery at Cherbourg, appointed him, on its completion, to the abbacy, to maintain which with greater splendour he alienated the principal property of the abbey of St. Helier, which subsequently dwindled into a priory, and continued in that impoverished state till its final suppression, in the reign of Henry V. Among other religious establishments were the priories of Noirmont, St. Clement, Bonne Nuit, and De Lecq ; and several ancient chapels, of a date much earlier than any of the churches. Of these there are remains only of La chapelle des Pécheurs at St. Brelade's, of St. Marguerite at Grouville, of Notre Dame des Pas at Havre des Pas, and of La Hogue Bie, a mile to the west of Mont Orgueil. Some trifling vestiges of other chapels may still be traced in different parts of the island, in one of which at St. Saviour's, St. Magliore, who visited Jersey in 565, was interred. Upon Mont de la Ville, where Fort Regent now stands, a very perfect Druidical temple was discovered, in 1785, on the removal of, an artificial mound of earth, by which it had been concealed : it was presented by the assembly of the states to Marshal Conway, then governor, who removed it to his seat in Berkshire, where it has been carefully re-constructed, with a rigid adherence to its original arrangement. Jersey is the birthplace of many eminent literary characters, among whom may be noticed, Durell, Dean of Windsor ; Brevint, Dean of Lincoln ; Falle, the historian of the island; D'Auvergne, ancestor of the late Prince de Bouillon, and author of the Campaign of William III.; Morant, the celebrated antiquary; Dr. Durel, Principal of Hertford College, Oxford; Dr. Bulkeley Bandinel, Bodley's librarian in that University ; Dr. Dumaresq, the munificent contributor to the public library founded by the Rev. Phillip Falle ; the Rev. Mr. Le Couteur ; Dr. Valpy, author of many valuable classical works, and of a revised edition of the classics ; the Rev. Dr. Lempriere, compiler of the Classical Dictionary ; and Phillpot Payn, seigneur de Samares, from whose manuscript chronicles the history of the island was principally compiled. Among the eminent natives who have been most distinguished in its naval and military annals may be mentioned, Philip de Carteret, seigneur de St. Ouen, who flourished in the reigns of Henry VI. and Edward IV.; Sir George de Carteret, who signalized himself during the parliamentary war; and, in modern times, Admirals Hardy, Durel, and Kempenfeldt. Jersey gives the title of earl to the family of Villiers.

JESMOND, a township in that part of the parish of St. Andrew, Newcastle, which is in the eastern division of Caslte ward, county of Northumberland, 2 miles (N. N. E.) from Newcastle upon Tyne, containing 467 inhabitants. Here are the remains of a chapel and hospital, dedicated to the Virgin Mary, and granted, in the reign of Edward VI., to the corporation of Newcastle : near to these is St. Mary's well, approached by "as many steps as there are articles of the Creed," formerly a place much resorted to. At the southern extremity of the township is Lambert's Leap, a rocky and dangerous precipice forty-five feet in depth. At Villa Real a stone coffin of six slab stones, containing a skeleton and an urn, were found in 1828.

JEVINGTON, a parish in the hundred of Willingdon, rape of Pevensey, county of Sussex, 3 miles (N. W.) from East Bourne, containing 300 inhabitants. The living is a rectory, in the archdeaconry of Lewes, and diocese of Chichester, rated in the king's books at £20, and in the patronage of Lord George Cavendish. The church, dedicated to St. Andrew, has portions in the Norman style of architecture.

JOHN (ST.), a parish in the southern division of the hundred of East, county of Cornwall, 6 miles (S. E. by E.) from St. Germans, containing 178 inhabitants. The living is a rectory, in the archdeaconry of Cornwall, and diocese of Exeter, rated in the king's books at -£12. 12. 6., and in the patronage of the

Rt. Hon. R. P. Carew. Almshouses for six poor persons were founded, in 1680, by Alice Brooking. This village is situated at the head of the æstuary called St. John's lake, opposite to Devonport ; and the parish extends southward to the English channel, part of which, though locally situated on the Cornish side, belongs to the county of Devon.

JOHN (ST.), a parish adjacent to the city, and within the liberty of the soke, of Winchester, Fawley division of the county of Southampton, containing 705 inhabitants. The living is a discharged rectory, united to that of St. Peter, Southgate, endowed with £300 private benefaction, £400 royal bounty, and £800 parliamentary grant, and in the patronage of the Crown.

JOHN (ST.), county of York.—See LETWELL.

JOHN (ST.) CASTLERIGG, a joint chapelry with Wythburn, in that part of the parish of Crosthwaite which is in Allerdale ward below Darwent, county of Cumberland, 4½ miles (E. S. E.) from Keswick, containing 566 inhabitants. The living is a perpetual curacy, in the archdeaconry and diocese of Carlisle, endowed with £1200 royal bounty, and £200 parliamentary grant, and in the patronage of the Vicar of Crosthwaite. Here is a small rent-charge for the instruction of poor children.

JOHNBY, a township in the parish of Greystock, Leath ward, county of Cumberland, 7½ miles (W.N.W.) from Penrith, containing 99 inhabitants.

JULIOT (ST.), a parish in the hundred of Lesnewth, county of Cornwall, 6 miles (N. by E.) from Camelford, containing 263 inhabitants. The living is a perpetual curacy, in the archdeaconry of Cornwall, and diocese of Exeter, endowed with £800 royal bounty. —Rawl, Esq. was patron in 1810. Here was a small cell of Benedictine or Cluniac monks from the time of Richard I., subordinate to the priory of Montacute in Somersetshire.

JUST (ST.), a parish in the hundred of Penwith, county of Cornwall, 7 miles (W. by N.) from Penzance, containing 3666 inhabitants. The living is a vicarage, in the archdeaconry of Cornwall, and diocese of Exeter, rated in the king's books at £11.11.0½., and in the patronage of the Crown. There is a school with a small endowment. Mines were worked here at a very early period ; and near the spot about one hundred copper coins were found, in the early part of the last century. On the Botallock estate is a famous tin and copper mine, which extends a considerable distance under the sea. Here are the ruins of Chapel Carne Bré, built on a very large cairn, or tumulus; and on the plain above Cape Cornwall, which is the extreme western point, are those of an ancient chapel, called Parken chapel, with a cemetery. The parish is bounded on the west by the Western ocean. Dr. William Borlase, the Cornish antiquary and naturalist, was a native of Pendeen, in this parish, where his family resided.

JUST (ST.) in ROSELAND, a parish in the western division of the hundred of Powder, county of Cornwall, 1½ mile (N.) from St. Mawes, comprising the borough town of St. Mawes, and containing 1648 inhabitants. The living is a rectory, in the archdeaconry of Cornwall, and diocese of Exeter, rated in the king's books at £37, and in the patronage of Sir Christopher Hawkins, Bart. This parish lies on the eastern margin of

Carrick road, and has a small harbour, on the south of which the village is situated. The castle of St. Mawes, which is kept in repair by the government, was erected by Henry VIII. A modern battery of eight guns has been constructed on the cliff below the castle. Here are the remains of an amphitheatre for the ancient Cornish interludes, one hundred and twenty-six feet in diameter, with stone benches; and on the summit of Bartini hill are the remains of a circular fortification.

K.

KABER, a township partly in the parish of BROUGH, but chiefly in that of KIRKBY-STEPHEN, EAST ward, county of WESTMORLAND, 2 miles (S.) from Brough, containing 164 inhabitants. A school was founded and endowed by Thomas Waller and others, in 1689; the annual income is £12. 16. 6., and twenty children are instructed. In 1663 an insurrection of the republican party being contemplated, preparatory meetings were held at Kaber Rigg by the disaffected, several of whom were eventually executed at Appleby.

KEA, a parish in the western division of the hundred of POWDER, county of CORNWALL, 3½ miles (S. S. E.) from Truro, containing, with the manor of Tregavethan, 3208 inhabitants. The living is a vicarage, with that of Kenwyn, in the archdeaconry of Cornwall, and diocese of Exeter, and in the patronage of the Bishop of Exeter. The church, dedicated to St. Kea, was built about 1803. The Wesleyan Methodists have a place of worship here. There is a small endowment for the instruction of children; and an almshouse for eight poor persons was founded by a bequest from Mr. John Lanyon in 1724, and endowed with an estate now producing about £50 per annum. This parish lies on the west of the Mopas roadstead.

KEADBY, a township in the parish of ALTHORP, western division of the wapentake of MANLEY, parts of LINDSEY, county of LINCOLN, 12 miles (W. N. W.) from Glandford-Bridge, containing 279 inhabitants.

KEAL (EAST), a parish in the eastern division of the soke of BOLINGBROKE, parts of LINDSEY, county of LINCOLN, 1¾ mile (S. W.) from Spilsby, containing 313 inhabitants. The living is a discharged rectory, in the archdeaconry and diocese of Lincoln, rated in the king's books at £17. 11. 3., and in the patronage of Mrs. Mary Pine Gates. The church is dedicated to St. Helen. There is a place of worship for Wesleyan Methodists. Some springs in this parish are slightly chalybeate.

KEAL (WEST), a parish in the western division of the soke of BOLINGBROKE, parts of LINDSEY, county of LINCOLN, 3 miles (S. W. by W.) from Spilsby, containing 502 inhabitants. The living is a rectory, in the archdeaconry and diocese of Lincoln, rated in the king's books at £20. 1. 8., and in the patronage of Robert Cracroft, Esq. The church is dedicated to St. Helen. There is a place of worship for Wesleyan Methodists. The springs here are impregnated with iron.

KEARSLEY, a township in the parish of DEAN, hundred of SALFORD, county palatine of LANCASTER, 5 miles (S. E.) from Great Bolton, containing 1833 inhabitants. High Style school was erected by Henry Mather about 1752, and endowed with land for the education of orphans and other poor children of the towns or hamlets of Kearsley, Bolton le Moors, and Tonge with Haulgh : the annual income is £249. 15. 11., and fifteen boys are boarded, clothed, and educated. The poor inhabitants of this township, and of the precinct of the chapelry of Ringley, have the privilege of sending their children for free instruction to Ringley school, founded by Nathaniel Walworth. Here are establishments for making vitriol and for spinning and bleaching yarn, besides numerous coal pits.

KEARSLEY, a township in the parish of STAMFORDHAM, north-eastern division of TINDALE ward, county of NORTHUMBERLAND, 10¾ miles (N. E.) from Hexham, containing 11 inhabitants.

KECKWICK, a township in the parish of RUNCORN, hundred of BUCKLOW, county palatine of CHESTER, containing 56 inhabitants. The Duke of Bridgewater's canal passes through this township.

KEDDINGTON, a parish in the Wold division of the hundred of LOUTH-ESKE, parts of LINDSEY, county of LINCOLN, 1½ mile (N. E.) from Louth, containing 179 inhabitants. The living is a discharged vicarage, in the archdeaconry and diocese of Lincoln, rated in the king's books at £3. 6. 8., endowed with £400 royal bounty. Sir W. E. Welby, Bart. was patron in 1816. The church is dedicated to St. Margaret.

KEDINGTON, or KETTON, a parish partly in the hundred of HINCKFORD, county of ESSEX, but chiefly in that of RISBRIDGE, county of SUFFOLK, 4½ miles (W. N. W.) from Clare, containing 607 inhabitants. The living is a rectory, in the archdeaconry of Sudbury, and diocese of Norwich, rated in the king's books at £16. 8. 6½., and in the patronage of the Rev. Barrington Syer. The church is dedicated to St. Peter and St. Paul. The river Stour passes through the parish.

KEDLESTON, a parish in the hundred of APPLETREE, county of DERBY, 4½ miles (N. W.) from Derby, containing 109 inhabitants. The living is a discharged rectory, in the archdeaconry of Derby, and diocese of Lichfield and Coventry, rated in the king's books at £3. 19. 7., and in the patronage of Lord Scarsdale. The church, dedicated to All Saints, has a Norman south door, and contains several ancient monuments of the Curzon family. The poor of this parish are entitled to the benefit of the school at Quarndon. Here is an endowment of £4 per annum, for apprenticing poor children, the gift of Mr. Baskerville. The noble mansion of Lord Scarsdale, called Kedleston hall, was erected about 1765, from a design by Adam : in the park is a sulphureous spring, with a convenient bath, the waters of which are considered serviceable in cutaneous and scorbutic disorders.

KEELBY, a parish in the eastern division of the wapentake of YARBOROUGH, parts of LINDSEY, county of LINCOLN, 7 miles (N. E. by N.) from Caistor, containing 462 inhabitants. The living is a discharged vicarage, in the archdeaconry and diocese of Lincoln, endowed with £200 royal bounty. Lord Yarborough was patron in 1792. The church is dedicated to St. Bartholomew. There is a place of worship for Wesleyan Methodists.

KEELE, a parish in the northern division of the hundred of PIREHILL, county of STAFFORD, 2½ miles (W. by S.) from Newcastle under Line, containing 1061 inhabitants. The living is a perpetual curacy, in the archdeaconry of Stafford, and diocese of Lichfield and Coventry, endowed with £200 private benefaction, £200 royal bounty, and £600 parliamentary grant, and in the patronage of William Sneyd, Esq. The church, dedicated to St. Michael, is a neat embattled stone edifice, not built due east and west. There are two places of worship for Wesleyan Methodists. A small shcool is supported by voluntary contributions, aided by £5 per annum bequeathed by Madam Frances Sneyd. In the neighbourhood are iron-stone mines, collieries, and smelting-furnaces, which afford employment to upwards of four hundred persons; and about one hundred and seventy are engaged in a silk-throwing mill.

KEEVIL, a parish comprising the tything of Bulkington, in the hundred of MELKSHAM, but chiefly in the hundred of WHORWELSDOWN, county of WILTS, 4 miles (E.) from Trowbridge, containing 802 inhabitants. The living is a vicarage, in the archdeaconry of Wilts, and diocese of Salisbury, rated in the king's books at £12. 7. 1., and in the patronage of the Dean and Chapter of Winchester. The church is dedicated to St. Leonard.

KEGWORTH, a parish in the western division of the hundred of GOSCOTE, county of LEICESTER, 6 miles (N. W. by N.) from Loughborough, containing, with the chapelry of Isley-Walton, 1672 inhabitants. The living is a rectory, in the archdeaconry of Leicester, and diocese of Lincoln, rated in the king's books at £25. 15. 7½., and in the patronage of the Master and Fellows of Christ College, Cambridge. The church is dedicated to St. Andrew. There are places of worship for Baptists and Wesleyan Methodists. A free school was founded here, in 1575, by license of Queen Elizabeth. Many of the females are employed in frame-work knitting, and in figuring lace. Fairs are held on February 18th, on Easter-Monday, April 30th, and October 10th.

KEIGHLEY, a market town and parish in the eastern division of the wapentake of STAINCLIFFE and EW-CROSS, West riding of the county of YORK, 4 miles (W.) from Bingley, 39 (W. by S.) from York, and 210 (N. N. W.) from London, containing 9223 inhabitants. According to Dr. Whitaker, *Kihel*, or *Kikel*, is a Saxon proper name, and Keighley, anciently *Kigheley*, is "the field of Kihel." This place, according to Camden, gave name to the family of Kigheley, Henry Kigheley having obtained from Edward I. the privilege of a market and a fair, and free warren for his manor here. During the reign of Charles I., this town being occupied by the parliamentary troops, was entered by a detachment of the royalist army, consisting of one hundred and fifty horse, when about one hundred prisoners, with a number of horses and other booty, were captured, on which General Lambert, who was in the neighbourhood, advancing unexpectedly, attacked the royalists, recovered the prisoners and the principal part of the plunder, killed fifteen of the enemy, took about thirty prisoners, and pursued the rest to the gates of Skipton castle, where they eventually found refuge. The town is situated in a deep valley, near the south-western bank of the river Aire, over which is a stone bridge; the streets are tolerably well paved, and lighted with gas; the houses, which are chiefly of stone, present a mean appearance; the inhabitants are supplied with water from two springs, at the east and west ends of the town, according to the regulations of an act of parliament

passed in 1816. A mechanics' institute was established in 1823, to which is attached an excellent library. The cotton, linen, and worsted manufactures are carried on with great activity, particularly the last, which affords employment to a great number of persons: the goods are chiefly sold at Bradford and Halifax in an unfinished state, the purchasers being principally foreigners, and merchants from Leeds and Manchester. The modern improvements in the adjacent roads, and the vicinity of the Leeds and Liverpool canal, which passes within a mile of the town, thus opening a communication with the counties of York and Lancaster, have greatly advanced the commercial interests of the town. The market is on Wednesday; and fairs are held on the 7th of November and the 8th of May, for cattle and pedlary. A meeting of the neighbouring magistrates is held here on the first Wednesday in every month; and a court baron, the jurisdiction of which was extended, by act of parliament passed in the 20th of George III., to debts not exceeding £5, is held before the steward of the manor, on the Thursday in every third week.

The living is a rectory, in the archdeaconry and diocese of York, rated in the king's books at £21. 0. 7½., and in the patronage of the Duke of Devonshire. The church, dedicated to St. Andrew, is a neat and spacious edifice, and was repaired in the year 1805: the tower, which is octagonal and in the Grecian style of architecture, contains a peal of eight bells, and a clock of very curious workmanship. There are places of worship for Baptists, Independents, Wesleyan Methodists (both of the Old and the New connexion), and Swedenborgians. A free grammar school was founded and endowed with messuages and lands by John Drake, in the year 1713, for the instruction of children: all boys born and residing in the town are admitted on the foundation, and instructed in English, Latin, and Greek, if required: the yearly income is £162. 9. 6., and there are about fifty scholars: the master has £100 per annum, and a residence rent-free. In 1716, Jonas Tonson conveyed to trustees a dwelling-house and land, the proceeds of which now amount to £40. 15. per annum, which is paid to an usher for teaching children preparatory to their admission into the grammar school. At Harehill, in this parish, a school was erected and endowed by means of a bequest by Mrs. Sarah Heaton, in 1738, for the support of a master who should teach English and Latin gratuitously: the income is £33 per annum: the children of inhabitants are taught to read, but must pay for additional instruction. A National school for one hundred and twenty girls is supported by voluntary contributions. Five poor boys are apprenticed annually from the proceeds of property devised to trustees by Isaac Bowcock, by will dated February 11th, 1669, for this and other charitable purposes. In the year 1775 a large quantity of Roman coins was found at Elam Grange, near this town.

KEINTON-MANSFIELD, a parish in the hundred of CATSASH, county of SOMERSET, 4¼ miles (E. N. E.) from Somerton, containing 349 inhabitants. The living is a discharged rectory, in the archdeaconry of Wells, and diocese of Bath and Wells, rated in the king's books at £6. 13. 9., and endowed with £200 private benefaction, and £200 royal bounty. The Rev. George Stone was patron in 1810. The church is dedicated to St. Mary Magdalene, and consists of a nave and a chancel, with an arched passage on the north side of the former, which leads to an octagonal tower at the west end. In this parish is dug a kind of hard blue stone, much used for paving. The old Roman Fosse-way passes on the south-east of the parish.

KEISBY, a hamlet in the parish of LAVINGTON, wapentake of BELTISLOE, parts of KESTEVEN, county of LINCOLN, 5 miles (N.E.) from Corby, containing 80 inhabitants.

KELBY, a chapelry in that part of the parish of HAYDOR which is in the wapentake of ASWARDHURN, parts of KESTEVEN, county of LINCOLN, 5½ miles (S.W. by W.) from Sleaford, containing 124 inhabitants. The church, dedicated to St. Andrew, comprises portions in the Norman style, with decorated and later insertions ; the font is very ancient.

KELDHOLME, a hamlet in the parish of KIRKBY-MOORSIDE, wapentake of RYEDALE, North riding of the county of YORK, 6½ miles (W. by N.) from Pickering. The population is returned with the parish. A Cistercian nunnery was founded here in the time of Henry I., by Robert Stuteville, the revenue of which, at the dissolution, was valued at £29. 6. 1.

KELFIELD, a hamlet in the parish of OWSTON, western division of the wapentake of MANLEY, parts of LINDSEY, county of LINCOLN. The population is returned with the chapelry of West Butterwick.

KELFIELD, a township in that part of the parish of STILLINGFLEET which is in the wapentake of OUZE and DERWENT, East riding of the county of YORK, 6¼ miles (N. by W.) from Selby, containing 286 inhabitants. There is a place of worship for Wesleyan Methodists. A free school was founded by Mrs. Mary Stillingfield, who devised £400 by will, dated in May 1802, to trustees, for the instruction of poor children of this township : the annual income is about £21. 6., and twenty children are taught gratuitously.

KELHAM, a parish in the northern division of the wapentake of THURGARTON, county of NOTTINGHAM, 2 miles (N.W. by W.) from Newark, containing 199 inhabitants. The living is a rectory, annexed to that of Averham, in the archdeaconry of Nottingham, and diocese of York, rated in the king's books at £19. 8. 4., and in the patronage of John Henry Manners Sutton, a minor. The church, dedicated to St. Wilfrid, is in the later style of English architecture, with a little screenwork, and some ancient stained glass. Here is a bridge across the Trent, on the left bank of which river the village is situated.

KELK (GREAT), a township in the parish of Foston upon WOLDS, wapentake of DICKERING, East riding of the county of YORK, 6½ miles (E.) from Great Driffield, containing 158 inhabitants.

KELK (LITTLE), an extra-parochial liberty, in the wapentake of DICKERING, East riding of the county of YORK, 5¾ miles (E. by N.) from Great Driffield, containing 51 inhabitants.

KELLASNERGH, a joint township with Bryning, in the parish of KIRKHAM, hundred of AMOUNDERNESS, county palatine of LANCASTER, 2¾ miles (S.W.) from Kirkham. The population is returned with Bryning.

KELLAWAYS, a parish in the hundred of CHIPPENHAM, county of WILTS, 3 miles (N.E.) from Chippenham, containing 15 inhabitants. The living is a discharged rectory, in the archdeaconry of Wilts, and diocese of Salisbury, rated in the king's books at £2. 13. 4., endowed with £200 private benefaction, and £800 royal bounty. R. G. Long, Esq. was patron in 1819. The church is dedicated to St. Giles. A causeway, constructed on brick arches, well paved and in good order, runs through this parish from Chippenham to Wickhill ; the expense having been defrayed by a bequest from one Maud Heath, in the fifteenth century, charged upon land, and vested in feoffees. This parish is bounded on the west by the river Avon.

KELLET (NETHER), a township in the parish of BOLTON le SANDS, hundred of LONSDALE, south of the sands, county palatine of LANCASTER, 4¼ miles (N.N.E.) from Lancaster, containing 358 inhabitants. Here is a curious natural cave half a mile in length.

KELLET (OVER), a chapelry in the parish of BOLTON le SANDS, hundred of LONSDALE, south of the sands, county palatine of LANCASTER, 6¼ miles (N. N. E.) from Lancaster, containing 531 inhabitants. The living is a perpetual curacy, in the archdeaconry of Richmond, and diocese of Chester, endowed with £400 private benefaction, and £400 royal bounty, and in the patronage of the Bishop of Chester. The church is dedicated to St. Cuthbert. The school was endowed, in 1802, with an annuity of £11, by Thomas Wilson, which, being subsequently augmented by the inhabitants, now produces an income of £60 per annum : from sixty to seventy children are taught to read gratuitously, but they pay for further instruction. The best limestone in the kingdom is produced here in abundance.

KELLEYTHORPE, a joint township with Emswell, in the Bainton-Beacon division of the wapentake of HARTHILL, East riding of the county of YORK, 2 miles (S.W.) from Great Driffield, containing 93 inhabitants.

KELLING, a parish in the hundred of HOLT, county of NORFOLK, 2 miles (N. by E.) from Holt, containing 163 inhabitants. The living is a discharged rectory, in the archdeaconry and diocese of Norwich, rated in the king's books at £12, and in the patronage of Mrs. Girdlestone. The church is dedicated to St. Mary. There is a mineral spring in the parish.

KELLINGTON, a parish in the lower division of the wapentake of OSGOLDCROSS, West riding of the county of YORK, comprising the townships of Beaghall, Egbrough, Kellington, and Whitley, and containing 1328 inhabitants, of which number, 283 are in the township of Kellington, 7 miles (E. by N.) from Pontefract. The living is a discharged vicarage, in the archdeaconry and diocese of York, rated in the king's books at £9. 8. 11½., and in the patronage of the Master and Fellows of Trinity College, Cambridge. The church is dedicated to St. Edmund.

KELLOE, a parish in the southern division of EASINGTON ward, county palatine of DURHAM, comprising the townships of Cassop, Coxhoe, Church-Kelloe, Quarrington, Thornley, and Wingate, and containing 679 inhabitants, of which number, 101 are in the township of Church-Kelloe, 6½ miles (S.E. by E.) from Durham. The living is a vicarage, in the archdeaconry and diocese of Durham. rated in the king's books at £20, and in the patronage of the Bishop of Durham. The church, dedicated to St. Helen, has some portions in the decorated style, and others of earlier date.

3 P 2

KELLY, a parish in the hundred of LIFTON, county of DEVON, 4¾ miles (E. S. E.) from Launceston, containing 218 inhabitants. The living is a rectory, in the archdeaconry of Totness, and diocese of Exeter, rated in the king's books at £9. 8. 9. The Trustees of — Kelly, a minor, were patrons in 1823. The church is dedicated to St. Mary. In the vicinity is Romsden Castle, an ancient encampment with a single vallum.

KELMARSH, a parish in the hundred of ROTH-WELL, county of NORTHAMPTON, 5½ miles (W. S. W.) from Rothwell, containing 172 inhabitants. The living is a rectory, in the archdeaconry of Northampton, and diocese of Peterborough, rated in the king's books at £23. 1. 5¼. W. Hanbury, Esq. was patron in 1812. The church is dedicated to St. Denis.

KELMSCOTT, a chapelry in the parish of BROAD-WELL, hundred of BAMPTON, county of OXFORD, 2 miles (E.) from Lechlade, containing 118 inhabitants. The chapel is dedicated to St. George.

KELSALE, a parish in the hundred of HOXNE, county of SUFFOLK, 1 mile (N.) from Saxmundham, containing 1060 inhabitants. The living is a rectory, consolidated in 1679 with that of Carlton, in the archdeaconry of Suffolk, and diocese of Norwich, rated in the king's books at £20. 0. 5. The church is dedicated to St. Mary. A free school for the instruction of the children of all the inhabitants is supported by various ancient grants : the salary of the master is £50 per annum, for which he likewise teaches the scholars of a Sunday school : from the same funds poor children are also apprenticed.

KELSALL, a township in that part of the parish of TARVIN which is in the second division of the hundred of EDDISBURY, county palatine of CHESTER, 4¼ miles (N. W. by N.) from Tarporley, containing 598 inhabitants. Here is a place of worship for Wesleyan Methodists. Kelsall was formerly a military post of great importance, commanding the principal approach to Chester. Here is a quarry of excellent freestone ; also a chalybeate spring.

KELSEY (NORTH), a parish in the southern division of the wapentake of YARBOROUGH, parts of LIND-SEY, county of LINCOLN, 5 miles (W.) from Caistor, containing 573 inhabitants. The living is a discharged vicarage, in the peculiar jurisdiction of the Dean and Chapter of Lincoln, rated in the king's books at £8, endowed with £200 private benefaction, and £400 royal bounty, and in the patronage of the Prebendary of North Kelsey in the Cathedral Church of Lincoln. There is a place of worship for Wesleyan Methodists.

KELSEY (SOUTH), a parish in the northern division of the wapentake of WALSHCROFT, parts of LIND-SEY, county of LINCOLN, 5¾ miles (W. by S.) from Caistor, comprising the united parishes of St. Mary and St. Nicholas, and containing 623 inhabitants. The living is a discharged rectory, in the archdeaconry and diocese of Lincoln, rated jointly in the king's books at £19. 15., and in the alternate patronage of the Crown and the Lord of the Manor. The church of St. Nicholas is a modern edifice attached to the ancient tower : that of St. Mary has gone to ruins. Here was formerly an Alien priory, a cell to the abbey of Seize in Normandy, but there are no remains. The river An-cholme passes through the parish.

KELSHALL, a parish in the hundred of ODSEY,

county of HERTFORD, 3½ miles (S. W. by S.) from Royston, containing 208 inhabitants. The living is a rectory, in the archdeaconry of Huntingdon, and diocese of Lincoln, rated in the king's books at £21, and in the patronage of the Bishop of Ely. The church is dedicated to St. Faith.

KELSTERN, a parish in the Wold division of the wapentake of LOUTH-ESKE, parts of LINDSEY, county of LINCOLN, 5½ miles (W. N. W.) from Louth, containing, with the hamlet of Lambcroft, 179 inhabitants. The living is a discharged vicarage, in the archdeaconry and diocese of Lincoln, rated in the king's books at £6. 11. 10. John Denison, Esq. was patron in 1806. The church is dedicated to St. Faith : in the chancel is a monument erected by Sir Francis South, Knt., to the memory of his wife Elizabeth, who died in 1604, which is curiously ornamented with emblematical figures and inscriptions. There is a place of worship for Wesleyan Methodists.

KELSTON, a parish in the hundred of BATH-FO-RUM, county of SOMERSET, 3¼ miles (W. N. W.) from Bath, containing 248 inhabitants. The living is a rectory, in the archdeaconry of Bath, and diocese of Bath and Wells, rated in the king's books at £15. 9. 4½., and in the patronage of Sir J. C. Hawkins. The church is dedicated to St. Nicholas. A small sum was given by John Harrington, in 1725, for the instruction of children. The river Avon passes on the west and south of the parish. Sir John Harrington, a distinguished writer in the reign of Elizabeth, whose family seat was in this parish, died in 1612, and was interred in the church.

KELVEDON, a parish in the hundred of WITHAM, county of ESSEX, 12¾ miles (N. E.) from Chelmsford, containing 1328 inhabitants. The living is a vicarage, in the archdeaconry of Colchester, and diocese of London, rated in the king's books at £9. 4. 2., and in the patronage of the Bishop of London. The church is dedicated to St. Mary. The Independents have a place of worship here. The village, situated on the line of the main road through Essex, is neat and well built, and contains several highly respectable dwelling-houses : the Blackwater river runs on the eastern and southern sides of it. There is a small endowment for the instruction of children, with a school-house for the master.

KELVEDON-HATCH, a parish in the hundred of ONGAR, county of ESSEX, 2¾ miles (S. by E.) from Chipping-Ongar, containing 336 inhabitants. The living is a rectory, in the archdeaconry of Essex, and diocese of London, rated in the king's books at £12. A. Serle, Esq. was patron in 1798. The church is dedicated to St. Nicholas.

KEMBERTON, a parish in the Shiffnall division of the hundred of BRIMSTREE, county of SALOP, 3 miles (S. S. W.) from Shiffnall, containing 260 inhabitants. The living is a rectory, with the vicarage of Sutton-Maddock, in the archdeaconry of Salop, and diocese of Lichfield and Coventry, rated in the king's books at £5. 6. 5½., and in the patronage of H. Oakes, Esq. The church is dedicated to St. Andrew. Veins of coal are occasionally discovered in this parish.

KEMBLE, a parish in the hundred of MALMESBURY, county of WILTS, 7½ miles (N. E. by N.) from Malmesbury, containing, with the tythings of Ewen and Wick, 435 inhabitants. The living is a vicarage, in the archdeaconry of Wilts, and diocese of Salisbury, rated in the king's books at £11. 4. 7., and in the patronage of C. W. Cox, Esq. The church is dedicated to All Saints.

KEMERTON, a parish in the lower division of the hundred of TEWKESBURY, county of GLOUCESTER, 4½ miles (N.E.) from Tewkesbury, containing 520 inhabitants. The living is a rectory, in the archdeaconry and diocese of Gloucester, rated in the king's books at £17. 13. 1½., and in the patronage of the Mayor and Corporation of Gloucester. The church has portions in the early, and some in the later, style of English architecture. There are places of worship for Wesleyan Methodists. The parish contains an excellent quarry of freestone, and several petrifying springs.

KEMEYS COMMANDER, a parish in the upper division of the hundred of USK, county of MONMOUTH, 4 miles (N.W. by N.) from Usk, containing 72 inhabitants. The living is a perpetual curacy, in the archdeaconry and diocese of Llandaff, endowed with £800 royal bounty, and in the patronage of — Gore, Esq. The church is dedicated to All Saints.

KEMEYS-INFERIOR, a parish in the upper division of the hundred of USK, county of MONMOUTH, 2 miles (E. N. E.) from Caerleon, containing 109 inhabitants. The living is a discharged rectory, in the archdeaconry and diocese of Llandaff, rated in the king's books at £6. 10. 5., endowed with £400 royal bounty, and in the patronage of Mrs. Rebecca Cotton. The church is dedicated to All Saints. The parish, which is bounded on the north by the river Usk, contains quarries of paving-stone and tile-stone.

KEMPLEY, a parish in the hundred of BOTLOE, county of GLOUCESTER, 5½ miles (N. W. by N.) from Newent, containing 301 inhabitants. The living is a vicarage, in the archdeaconry of Hereford, and diocese of Gloucester, rated in the king's books at £5. 6. 5½., and in the patronage of the Dean and Chapter of Hereford, as masters of Ledbury Hospital. The church is in the Norman style. There is a small endowment for the instruction of children, the bequest of Elizabeth Pyndar in 1755.

KEMPSEY, a parish in the lower division of the hundred of OSWALDSLOW, county of WORCESTER, 4¼ miles (S.) from Worcester, containing 1129 inhabitants. The living is a discharged vicarage, in the archdeaconry and diocese of Worcester, rated in the king's books at £6. 18. 9., and in the patronage of the Bishop of Worcester. The church is dedicated to St. Mary. The village is agreeably situated near the eastern bank of the river Severn, and contains several genteel dwelling-houses. There is an unendowed free school, in which ten boys are taught to read and write. A monastery which existed here so early as 799, was subsequently united to the church of Worcester. At this place Henry II. held his court; and in 1265, shortly before the battle of Evesham, Simon de Montfort was quartered at the Bishop's palace here, with his prisoner, Henry III. Near to the church are the remains of an ancient encampment.

KEMPSFORD, a parish in the hundred of BRIGHT-WELLS-BARROW, county of GLOUCESTER, 3 miles (S.) from Fairford, containing 838 inhabitants. The living is a vicarage, in the archdeaconry and diocese of Gloucester, rated in the king's books at £19, and in the patronage of the Bishop of Gloucester. The church is

dedicated to St. Mary. A school was built by subscription, in 1750, upon a site given by Thomas, Lord Viscount Weymouth, who likewise endowed it with £10 per annum for the instruction of children. The rivers Coln, Thames, and Severn, run through the parish.

KEMPSHOT, a tything in the parish of WINSLADE, hundred of BASINGSTOKE, Basingstoke division of county of SOUTHAMPTON, 3¾ miles (S. W. by W.) from Basingstoke. The population is returned with the parish.

KEMPSTON, a parish in the hundred of REDBORNE-STOKE, county of BEDFORD, 2¼ miles (S. W. by W.) from Bedford, containing 1419 inhabitants. The living is a vicarage, in the archdeaconry of Bedford, and diocese of Lincoln, rated in the king's books at £12, and in the patronage of the Rev. G. Ousley Fenwicke. The church is dedicated to All Saints. There is a place of worship for Wesleyan Methodists. Within the parish are the sites of several moated buildings.

KEMPSTON, a parish in the hundred of LAUN-DITCH, county of NORFOLK, 6¾ miles (N. E.) from Swaffham, containing 56 inhabitants. The living is a discharged vicarage, in the archdeaconry and diocese of Norwich, rated in the king's books at £4. 18. 4., and endowed with £600 royal bounty. T. W. Coke, Esq. was patron in 1809. The church is dedicated to St. Paul.

KEMSING, a parish in the hundred of CODSHEATH, lathe of SUTTON at HONE, county of KENT, 4 miles (N. E. by N.) from Seven Oaks, containing 359 inhabitants. The living is a vicarage, in the archdeaconry and diocese of Rochester, rated in the king's books at £19. 13. 4., and in the patronage of the Heirs of the Dorset family. The church is dedicated to St. Mary. There is a chapel of ease at Seal, in this parish. The village is situated at the junction of four roads which diverge from St. Edith's well, formerly esteemed for its miraculous efficacy : an image of the saint was long placed on a pedestal in the church, and much resorted to, being supposed to possess the power of dissipating mildew and blights of corn. A market was anciently held here, and an annual fair is now held on Easter-Monday. A rent-charge of £20 was bequeathed by Lady Sarah Smythe, for educating and clothing eight poor girls.

KENARDINGTON, a parish in the hundred of BLACKBOURNE, lathe of SCRAY, county of KENT, 7 miles (E. by S.) from Tenterden, containing 196 inhabitants. The living is a rectory, in the archdeaconry and diocese of Canterbury, rated in the king's books at £12. 1. 0½., and in the patronage of the Rev. J. Billington. The church is dedicated to St. Mary. Here are extensive remains of ancient military earth-works, including a high breast-work, and a small circular mount, supposed to have been thrown up by Alfred against the Danes, in 893, when a division of them sailed up the Rother, and intrenched themselves in the adjoining parish of Apple-dore. The Shorncliff and Rye canal passes through the parish.

KENCHESTER, a parish in the hundred of GRIMS-WORTH, county of HEREFORD, 5 miles (W. N. W.) from Hereford, containing 94 inhabitants. The living is a discharged vicarage, in the archdeaconry and diocese of Hereford, rated in the king's books at £6. 5. 7., endowed with £200 private benefaction, and £200 royal bounty, and in the patronage of the Crown. The church is dedicated to St. Michael. According to Camden this place was the *Ariconium*, but Dr. Horsley considers it as the *Magna*, of the Romans. The form of the station is that of an irregular hexagon, the site comprising fifty or sixty acres; there are two openings on the west side, and two on the north; some traces of the walls, which entirely surrounded the city, are discernible, but no vestiges of any foss or ditch. The remains principally consist of fragments of a temple at the eastern end, with a niche of Ròman brick and mortar, called the Chair; around this are foundations and holes, similar to vaults: at different periods large vaults, tesselated pavements, a fine Mosaic floor, relics of pottery, urns, and large bones, have been discovered. An hypocaust, about seven feet square, with the leaden pipes entire, and those of brick a foot in length and three inches square, was found in 1670. At the close of the last century, a stone altar was dug up from the foundation of the northern wall, bearing an inscription implying its dedication to the Emperor Cæsar Marcus Aurelius, and now in the possession of the Rev. J. C. Bird, rector of Dindon and Mordiford.

KENCOTT, a parish in the hundred of BAMPTON, county of OXFORD, 5 miles (S.) from Burford, containing 174 inhabitants. The living is a rectory, in the archdeaconry and diocese of Oxford, rated in the king's books at £6. 19. 4½. H. Hammersley, Esq. was patron in 1801. The church is dedicated to St. George. Here is a small sum for the instruction of poor children, the gift of Goddard Carter, in 1723.

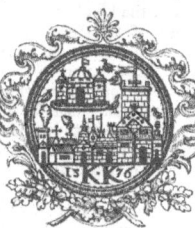
Corporate Seal.

KENDAL, a parish comprising the incorporated market town of Kirkby-Kendal, the chapelries of Crook, Grayrigg, Helsington, Hugil, Kentmere, Long Sleddale, Natland, New Hutton, Over-Staveley, Old Hutton with Holmescales, which last is a township of the parish of Burton in Kendal, Selside with Whitwell, Underbarrow with Bradley-field, and Winster, and the townships of Docker, Kirkland, Lambrigg, Nether Graveship, Nether Staveley, Patton, Scathwaiterigg-Hay with Hutton in the Hay, Skelsmergh, Kettle-Strickland, Strickland-Roger, Whinfell, and a portion of Fawcet-Forest, in KENDAL ward, and the township of Dilliker in LONSDALE ward, county of WESTMORLAND, and containing, exclusively of the chapelry of Winster, which is returned with Undermilbeck, 17,417 inhabitants, of which number, 8984 are in the town of Kendal, 23 miles (S.W. by S.) from Appleby, and 262 (N.W. by N.) from London, on the great north road. This place, which, from the various relics of antiquity discovered, was evidently a Roman station, is supposed by Dr. Gale to have been the *Brovonacis* of Antoninus; but the correctness of this opinion has been doubted by other antiquaries. The town, which is the largest in the county, is very pleasantly situated in a valley on the western bank of the river Kent, which passes through it, and over which there are three stone bridges, of three arches each, one of them erected by the corporation in 1744, and the others by the county: from one of these bridges a spacious street leads up a gentle acclivity to the centre of the town, where it meets another principal street, a mile in length, called Stramongate, extending from north to south; from this a third main street leads down to the water side: these streets, which contain good houses of hewn freestone, roofed with blue slate, are intersected at right angles by several narrower streets, in which the houses are chiefly of rough stone, plastered, and in the ancient style. The town is well lighted with gas, but the streets are badly paved with pebbles; the inhabitants are well supplied with water. On the west side the view is enriched by a long tier of gardens and terraces, and ornamented with tall Lombardy poplars; on the opposite bank of the river are the ruins of an old castle, the baronial seat of the Lords of Kendal, and the birthplace of Catherine Parr, last queen of Henry VIII.: the remains of this ancient structure, which was probably raised on the site of the Roman station, consist of the outer walls, with two square and two round towers: opposite the castle, and overlooking the town, is Castle-how hill, an artificial circular mount, thirty feet in height, surrounded at its base by a deep fosse and a high rampart, strengthened by two bastions on the east; the summit, which is flat, is crossed by a ditch, and defended by a breast-work of earth: it is of greater antiquity than the castle, and, as its name imports, was one of the spots on which, in ancient times, justice was dispensed to the people. On this eminence an obelisk, commemorative of the revolution of 1688, was erected by the inhabitants of Kendal, in 1788. Races are held in August, and generally well attended. A mechanics' institute and library was established in April 1824. There are also a news-room, a free library, a book club, and a natural history society, with a splendid museum containing a collection of antiquities and natural curiosities. The assembly-rooms, erected by Mr. Webster of this town, and opened December 31st, 1827, consist of two fronts, one in Lowther-street, the other in Highgate; the latter is ornamented with a receding balcony, fronted with columns and pilasters of the Ionic order, supporting a pediment, and surmounted by a handsome lantern: the interior contains a library and apartments for the librarian, on the ground-floor; and on the principal floor is an elegant ball-room. The news-room communicates with a balcony in the front, facing Highgate-street, above which is a billiard-room: the building was erected by shares of £100 each, and the total expenditure amounted to £6000.

The manufacture of woollen cloth was introduced in the reign of Edward III., by emigrants from the Low Countries skilled in making cloth; and it appears to have flourished as, in the reigns of Richard II. and Henry IV., several provisions were made by parliament for the regulation of the " Kendal cloths." Previously to the establishment of these manufactories, all the wool of the country was exported to the Netherlands, and manufactured there, affording such a source of gain as to induce the Duke of Burgundy to institute the order of the " Golden fleece." The green druggets made here and at other places were the common clothing of the poor in London and elsewhere, for several centuries, so that " Kendal Green " became proverbial. The chief articles of manufacture at present are, coarse woollen cloth, linsey, and knit worsted stockings: there are an extensive tannery and a manufactory for fish-hooks and wool-cards, which last have been greatly improved by a machine invented for the purpose ; likewise mills for scouring, fulling, and friezing cloth, and for rasping dye-wood, together with corn and paper-mills. Combs of all descriptions are made here, and the manufacture of this article has been greatly facilitated by the introduction of a machine for sawing ivory, and cutting the teeth of ivory combs. In addition to these, several persons are employed in working and polishing marble, which is remarkable for the beauty and variety of its colours, and is obtained from the adjacent mountainous district, and imported from Italy, to be wrought and re-shipped. The neighbourhood abounds with limestone, of which the houses in general are built, and which was first polished here in 1788 : the stone presents a hard surface variegated with petrified shells, and has a very beautiful appearance. At some mills below the town a large quantity of gunpowder is manufactured. The neighbourhood abounds with orchards, which are still increasing, and afford a considerable supply of fruit. A canal extends from the river Kent to Lancaster, thus affording a communication with the extensive inland navigation in that part of the kingdom ; it was opened in 1819 : fly-boats are despatched daily, and a packet-boat leaves every morning at six o'clock, during the summer months, for the conveyance of passengers to Lancaster, Garstang, and Preston. The market, established by charter of Richard I., and confirmed by subsequent sovereigns, is held on Saturday, and is principally for corn, which is pitched in large quantities. Fairs are held annually, at a place called Beast-banks, on the 22nd of March, the 29th of April, and on the 8th of November and the following day, for horses, cattle, and sheep : a statute fair for hiring servants is held on the Saturday in Whitsun-week. The market-place, now used almost exclusively for corn, is near the centre of the town ; very convenient shambles were opened · in 1804, on its southern side : the fish market is at the head of Finkle-street, and vegetables are sold in Stramongate.

This town received its charter of incorporation from Queen Elizabeth, which was afterwards extended by Charles I. The corporate body consists of a mayor, twelve aldermen, and twenty capital burgesses, assisted by a recorder, deputy recorder, town clerk, and other officers : the mayor is chosen annually on the Monday after Michaelmas-day, by the mayor for the preceding year and the senior aldermen ; the aldermen, capital burgesses, and all the officers of the corporation, are chosen in a similar manner : the mayor, the two senior aldermen, and the recorder, or, in his absence, the deputy recorder, are justices of the peace by virtue of their office ; they have power, by charter of 1684, to hold sessions quarterly, to hear and determine on all offences except felony and cases involving the loss of life or limb ; and to hold, every three weeks, a court of record for the recovery of debts from 40s. to £40. The members of the corporation are exempt from being empannelled on juries : the mayor, who is clerk of the market, and the senior aldermen, act as coroners. The adjourned sessions from Appleby, for the Kendal and Lonsdale wards, are held here ; as is also, occasionally, a court baron under the Earl of Lonsdale, and one annually by the Hon. F. Greville Howard : there is a court of requests for the

recovery of debts under 40s., the jurisdiction of which extends over the whole parish. The town-hall is a handsome and spacious building, originally erected in 1591, and rebuilt on the same site in 1758. Near the house of industry, a commodious edifice at the east end of the town, erected in 1771, is the house of correction, built in 1786, and which has recently undergone considerable alterations. Kendal is the head of a barony, which, prior to the Conquest, was included in the principality of Cumberland, and was in the possession of the Scottish crown : it comprises the whole of the Kendal and Lonsdale wards, and several other places within the county, and was given by William the Conqueror to Ivo de Talbois, who thus became its first baron.

The living is a vicarage, in the archdeaconry of Richmond, and diocese of Chester, rated in the king's books at £92. 5., and in the patronage of the Master and Fellows of Trinity College, Cambridge. The church, dedicated to the Holy Trinity, stands in Kirkland, a hamlet without the liberties : it is principally in the later style of English architecture with a low square tower ; the roof is supported by four rows of pillars, which divide the interior into five aisles, and there is a little screen-work ; it contains many ancient monuments. A church, dedicated to St. George, and standing in the centre of the town, was erected, in 1754, as a chapel of ease to the parish church. The living is a perpetual curacy, endowed with £400 private benefaction, and £400 royal bounty, and in the patronage of the Vicar of Kendal. There are places of worship for Baptists, the Society of Friends, Glassites, Independents, Inghamites, Primitive and Wesleyan Methodists, Scotch Seceders, Unitarians, and Roman Catholics : the meeting-houses for the Society of Friends and the Independents are spacious and handsome buildings. The free grammar school was founded and endowed with houses and land in Kendal, by Adam Pennington, of Boston in Lincolnshire, in 1525 : the site was given, in 1588, by Miles Phillipson, and the school-room was rebuilt in 1592 : it has been successively endowed by Edward VI., Queens Mary and Elizabeth, the last of whom transferred to it the revenues of two dissolved chantries ; the whole endowment producing about £37 per annum : the nomination of the master and the usher is vested in the mayor and aldermen. The school has three exhibitions of £5 each to Queen's College, Oxford, payable out of the tithes of the parish of Farlton, by a bequest from Henry Wilson, in 1638 ; another exhibition of £8 to the same college, paid by the Chamber of Kendal, the exhibitioner being appointed by the corporation, and receiving the stipend for four years ; one of £5 per annum for four years, to any college in Oxford, the bequest of Mr. Alderman Park, in 1631, the candidate to be of the parishes of Kendal, Millom, or Heversham ; also twenty shillings per annum, the gift of Mr. Joseph Smith, and forty shillings per annum, the gift of Mr. Jobson, for two exhibitioners to Queen's College, Oxford. The system of education in this school, which is open to boys of the parish indefinitely, is strictly classical. Ephraim Chambers, the writer of the Cyclopædia ; Dr. Edmund Law, Bishop of Carlisle ; and Dr. Shaw, the celebrated traveller, were educated here. The Blue-coat school and hospital were founded and endowed with estates by Thomas Sandes, an inhabitant of this town, in 1670 ; the former for the education of forty boys, who are taught the art of carding and weaving, and thirty girls, being children of the inhabitants of Kendal; the latter as the residence of eight poor widows, six to be chosen from Kendal, one from Skelsmergh, and the other from Strickland, and all to be nominated by the mayor and aldermen, as trustees of the charity: the inmates receive the weekly sum of five shillings each, and a provision is made for a schoolmaster to read prayers to the widows twice a day, and to teach poor children preparatory to their entering the free-school : the founder bequeathed a library to the Blue-coat school, which has been increased by subsequent additions. The permanent income belonging to the school and almshouse has been augmented by various benefactions, and amounts to £283. 12. per annum, besides which a collection is made at an annual sermon for the benefit of the charity. A school of industry was established in 1799, and is supported partly from the interest of two bequests, and partly by voluntary contributions; one hundred and thirty children of both sexes are instructed and employed. A National school for boys was built by subscription in 1818, at an expense of £700, and munificently endowed with £2000 in the five per cent. annuities, by Matthew Piper, Esq., of Whitehaven, a member of the Society of Friends, who, dying in 1821, at the advanced age of ninety-three, was interred by his own request in the interior of the building; one hundred and eighty-six boys are educated. The National school for girls, adjoining the preceding edifice, was built in 1824; and the expense, amounting to £500, was defrayed by subscription : it is supported by voluntary contributions, and contains about one hundred children. The Green-coat Sunday school was founded, in 1813, by Mr. W. Sleddal, and endowed with the interest of £525, for providing green hats and coats for the boys, gowns and bonnets for the girls, and a weekly stipend of two shillings to a master, for their instruction on the Sunday: two junior aldermen and two senior burgesses are appointed trustees. A dispensary was established in 1783, to which a fever-house has been recently annexed : the medical establishment consists of a physician, five surgeons, and an apothecary. A savings bank, established in 1816, is held at the committee-room of the school of industry. Kendal has conferred the title of earl on John, Duke of Bedford, brother of Henry V., Prince George of Denmark, Prince Charles, third son of James II., and other illustrious persons : the present Earl of Pembroke has the title of Baron Ross and Parr of Kendal. The following eminent persons were natives of the town : Dr. Thomas Shaw, a celebrated oriental traveller, the son of an alderman of Kendal, born in 1692; Dr. Anthony Askew, a learned physician and classical scholar, born in 1722; John Wilson, a journeyman shoemaker, who distinguished himself as a botanist, and published a "Synopsis of British plants;" William Hudson, the author of "Flora Anglica," who was an apothecary in London, where he died in 1797; and John Gough, a member of the Society of Friends, who, though blind, attained considerable eminence by his researches in natural philosophy.

KENDER-CHURCH, a parish in the hundred of Webtree, county of Hereford, 11¼ miles (S. W.) from Hereford, containing 77 inhabitants. The living is a perpetual curacy, in the archdeaconry and diocese of Hereford, rated in the king's books at £2. 5. 2½.,

endowed with £1000 royal bounty, and in the patronage of the Earl of Oxford. The church is dedicated to St. Mary.

KENELM (ST.), a chapelry in the parish of Hales-Owen, Hales-Owen division of the hundred of Brimstree, county of Salop, though locally in the lower division of the hundred of Halfshire, county of Worcester, 2½ miles (S. W. by S.) from Hales-Owen, with which the population is returned. The living is a curacy with the rectory of Hagley, in the archdeaconry and diocese of Worcester.

KENILWORTH, a market town and parish, in the Kenilworth division of the hundred of Knightlow county of Warwick, 5 miles (N.) from Warwick, and 101 (N. W by N.) from London, containing 2577 inhabitants. This place, anciently called *Kenelworda*, is supposed to have derived its name from Kenelm, or Kenulph, one of its Saxon possessors, who had on the bank of the Avon a strong hold or fortress, which was demolished in the war between Edmund Ironside and Canute. After the Conquest, Henry I. bestowed the manor upon Geoffrey de Clinton, his treasurer and chamberlain, who built the church and founded a priory for canons regular of the order of St. Augustine, which he dedicated to the Blessed Virgin, the revenue of which, at the dissolution, was £643. 14. 9¼. The same Geoffrey, soon after the establishment of his monastery, erected the earlier portion of that stately castle, for the magnificent and picturesque remains of which the town is principally distinguished. This castle, which was sold by his grandson to Henry III., was greatly enlarged and strongly fortified by Simon de Montfort, to whom that monarch gave it as a marriage portion with his sister Eleanor. Simon de Montfort afterwards rebelling against his sovereign, and joining the discontented barons who had taken up arms against the king, took that monarch prisoner at the battle of Lewes, but was afterwards defeated and slain by Prince Edward at the battle of Evesham. After the defeat of this baron, his younger son Simon shut himself up with a party of his adherents in the castle, which sustained a siege for six months against the royal forces commanded by the king in person; but the garrison being reduced by famine, the castle was surrendered to the king, by whom it was bestowed upon his younger son Edmund, afterwards created Earl of Leicester. Upon this occasion was issued the "*Dictum de Kenilworth*," enacting that all who took up arms against the king should pay them the value of their lands for five years. In the 7th of Edward I. the Earl of Leicester held a splendid tournament here, at which one hundred knights and as many ladies assisted. Edward II., having been made prisoner by the Earl of Lancaster, was confined in the castle of Kenilworth, and, on his deposition being voted by parliament, a deputation was sent to extort from him an abdication of the throne, soon after the signing of which he was removed to Berkeley castle, where he was inhumanly put to death. In the reign of Edward III. the castle was considerably enlarged, and in that of Richard II. many additional buildings were erected by John of Gaunt, Duke of Lancaster, whose son becoming king, the castle reverted to the crown. Queen Elizabeth gave it to her favourite, Dudley, Earl of Leicester, by whom the magnificent gate-house was built, and who also erected the Gallery tower and Mortimer's tower, at each extremity of the tilt-yard, and after having completed and embellished the castle at a prodigious expense, entertained Queen Elizabeth and her whole court for seventeen days, with the most splendid pageants and costly magnificence : the expense of these sumptuous entertainments, which included every variety of luxurious gratification, was not less than £1000 each day. During the civil war in the reign of Charles I., Cromwell took possession of the castle, which he gave up to his soldiers, who plundered it of every thing valuable, destroyed the walls and the park, drained the lake, and divided the lands among themselves into small farms, and after wantonly defacing the building, left it in a state of ruin and desolation. The present remains bear evident testimony of its ancient grandeur and formidable strength : the entrance into the outer ward is through a lofty arch under the Gateway-tower, a square building of great beauty, with angular turrets, now occupied as a farmhouse ; in one of the parlours is preserved an ancient mantel-piece of alabaster richly sculptured, and surmounted with finely-carved oak, which, having escaped the destructive ravages of the soldiery, was removed from one of the state apartments. The ruins occupy three sides of a spacious quadrangle forming the inner ward, and consist of Cæsar's tower, built by Geoffrey de Clinton, a lofty and massive square structure, the walls of which are sixteen feet in thickness, beyond which are the keep, or strong tower, and part of the kitchens ; the banquet-hall, eighty-six feet long, and forty-four feet wide, with a range of windows of excellent symmetry, ornamented with rich tracery, and a triangular recess of three very beautiful windows almost entire ; and the Water tower and Lion's tower, which are in good preservation. Opposite to Cæsar's tower, with which it was connected by a range of buildings forming the fourth side of the quadrangle, but of which only the vestiges of the arched entrance are discernible, is Mortimer's tower, extending from which was the tilt-yard, two hundred and forty feet in length, and terminated by the Gallery tower. The prevailing character of the architecture is the Norman, intermixed with the decorated and later English styles : the walls included an area of more than seven acres, and the venerable ruins, in many parts overspread with ivy, form one of the most extensive, superb, and interesting memorials of baronial splendour and feudal magnificence. Of the monastery, situated to the east of the castle, only some fragments of the walls and part of the gateway entrance are remaining. The town consists principally of one street, extending for more than a mile along the turnpike-road, and divided into two parts by a small valley, in which are situated the church and the remains of the ancient monastery ; on the higher grounds are some handsome well-built houses, and crowning the summit are the magnificent remains of the castle. A stream, tributary to the Avon, and abounding with excellent trout, after passing under an ancient stone bridge, divides into two branches, enclosing the castle and the town. There is a subscription book society ; and assemblies are held occasionally at the principal inn. The chief articles of manufacture are, horn combs, Prussian blue, Glauber salts, and sal ammoniac. The market is on Wednesday, and a fair for cattle is held on the last day in April. The town is within the jurisdiction of the county magistrates ; and two constables and two headboroughs are appointed at the court leet of the lord of the manor.

The living is a discharged vicarage, in the archdeaconry of Coventry, and diocese of Lichfield and Coventry, rated in the king's books at £6. 13. 4., and in the patronage of the Crown. The church, dedicated to St. Nicholas, is a venerable structure, exhibiting portions in the Norman and in the early and decorated styles of English architecture, with a square embattled tower, strengthened with angular buttresses, and surmounted by a lofty spire : the western entrance is through a very fine and richly-moulded Norman archway, and the north porch has two finely-pointed and richly-moulded arched doorways, above which is a small window with elegant tracery ; the interior contains an ancient circular font supported on a single Norman column, and some ancient and interesting monuments. There are places of worship for Baptists, Independents, and Presbyterians. The free school was founded, in 1724, by Dr. Edwards of Kenilworth, who endowed it with twenty acres of land in the parish, producing about £70 per annum : it is under the direction of five trustees, who appoint the master, with a salary of £68 per annum, a house, and garden : the scholars are instructed in reading, writing, and arithmetic ; the number at present on the foundation is about fifty. A school for teaching eight poor boys to read, prior to their admission into Dr. Edwards's school, is endowed with £5 per annum, from a bequest by William Turner, in 1790 ; and there is a school of industry for thirty girls, supported by the interest of £200 left by the Earl of Clarendon, in 1775, with the aid of voluntary contributions. Under Dr. Edwards's endowment eight almshouses also have been erected for aged widows, to which Alicia, Duchess Dudley, was a considerable benefactress ; and eight additional almshouses are now being built. Several benefactions have been made for apprenticing poor children, and for other charitable purposes.

KENLEY, a parish in the hundred of CONDOVER, county of SALOP, 4½ miles (W. by N.) from Much Wenlock, containing 321 inhabitants. The living is a perpetual curacy, with the rectory of Harley, in the archdeaconry of Salop, and diocese of Lichfield and Coventry.

KENN, a parish in the hundred of EXMINSTER, county of DEVON, 4¼ miles (S.) from Exeter, containing 906 inhabitants. The living is a rectory, in the archdeaconry and diocese of Exeter, rated in the king's books at £46. 13. 4. Henry Ley, Esq. was patron in 1805. The church, dedicated to St. Andrew, has a stone font in the early style, and a good wooden screen. The lord of this manor holds his court at Kenneford, where a portreeve, two constables, and a tythingman, are sworn in at Michaelmas.

KENN, a parish in the hundred of WINTERSTOKE, county of SOMERSET, 10 miles (N.) from Axbridge, containing 276 inhabitants. The living is a perpetual curacy, in the peculiar jurisdiction and patronage of the Prebendary of Yatton. Thomas Kenn, created Bishop of Bath and Wells by Charles II., was a member of the family that possessed this manor for many generations : this prelate was one of the seven committed to the tower by James II., and, on the accession of William and Mary, refusing to transfer his allegiance, he relinquished his preferment, and retired from public life : his remains are interred in the parish church of Frome.

KENNERLEY, a parish in the hundred of CRE-

DITON, county of DEVON, 5 miles (N. by W.) from Crediton, containing 93 inhabitants. The living is a perpetual curacy, in the jurisdiction of the Consistorial Court of the Bishop of Exeter, endowed with £200 private benefaction, and £200 royal bounty, and in the patronage of the Governors of the Crediton charity. The church is dedicated to St. John the Baptist.

KENNET (EAST), a parish in the hundred of SELKLEY, county of WILTS, 5¼ miles (W. S. W.) from Marlborough, containing 94 inhabitants. The living is a perpetual curacy, in the archdeaconry of Wilts, and diocese of Salisbury, endowed with £200 royal bounty, and in the patronage of Richard Mathews, Esq. The river Kennet rises near the village, and is noted for the excellence of its water, which is used in brewing the famous ale known by that name. Within the parish is a barrow terminating in a point, and called Selbury hill.

KENNETT, a parish in the hundred of STAPLOE, county of CAMBRIDGE, 5 miles (N. E.) from Newmarket, containing 164 inhabitants. The living is a rectory, in the archdeaconry of Sudbury, and diocese of Norwich, rated in the king's books at £11. 10. 10. O. Godfrey, Esq. was patron in 1813. The church is dedicated to St. Nicholas. In June 1647, this place was the headquarters of the parliamentarian army.

KENNINGHALL, a parish in the hundred of GUILT-CROSS, county of NORFOLK, 3 miles (E. by S.) from East Harling, containing 1273 inhabitants. The living is a discharged vicarage, in the archdeaconry of Norfolk, and diocese of Norwich, rated in the king's books at £5. 17 1., and in the patronage of the Bishop of Ely. The church, dedicated to St. Mary, has a door in the Norman style, and a large square tower at the west end. There is a place of worship for Baptists. The name of this place is derived from the Saxon words Cyning, king, and Halla, palace; it having been the residence of the kings of East Anglia, the site of whose castle is clearly visible. The demesne was granted by the Conqueror to De Albini and his heirs, to be held by service of chief butler at the coronation of the kings of England. Here was formerly a weekly market, now disused. On the site of the ancient palace was erected the manorial residence, which was afterwards destroyed by Thomas, Duke of Norfolk, who built a most magnificent edifice to the north-east, with two noble fronts: it was forfeited to the crown by the attainder of Thomas Howard, Duke of Norfolk, in the reign of Henry VIII., and given to the Princess Mary, who, as well as her successor, Queen Elizabeth, often resided here: in the seventeenth century it was taken down and the materials were sold. The only remaining traces are a few bricks in the walls of the houses in the village, bearing the arms of Arundel and Howard.

KENNINGTON, a chapelry partly in the parish of RADLEY, and partly in that of SUNNINGWELL, hundred of HORMER, county of BERKS, 4 miles (N. E.) from Abingdon, containing 171 inhabitants. The chapel, dedicated to St. Swithin, fell down some years since, and has been recently rebuilt.

KENNINGTON, a parish in the hundred of CHART and LONGBRIDGE, lathe of SCRAY, county of KENT, 2 miles (N. E. by N.) from Ashford, containing 447 inhabitants. The living is a discharged vicarage, in the archdeaconry and diocese of Canterbury, rated in the king's books at £12, endowed with £200 private benefaction, and £200 royal bounty, and in the patronage of the Archbishop of Canterbury. The church, dedicated to St. Mary, is principally in the early style of English architecture.

KENNINGTON, a district in the parish of LAMBETH, eastern division of the hundred of BRIXTON, county of SURREY, 2½ miles (S. S. W.) from London. The population is returned with Lambeth. This place consists principally of several ranges of handsome houses in the line of road leading from the metropolis towards Clapham and Brixton. The name is said to be of Saxon origin, there having been a royal palace here prior to the Conquest, whence the appellation Cynington, from the Saxon Cyning, a king. Kennington is distinguished in history as the scene of the banquet, or marriage festival, of a Danish nobleman, at which Hardicanute, the son of Canute the Great, became the victim of his own intemperance, or, according to some writers, was poisoned; and, in commemoration of his death, the festival called Hocktide is supposed to have been instituted. The palace was subsequently the favourite residence of the Black Prince, and the occasional resort of Henry VIII. and some of his predecessors; but it was at length superseded by the manor-house, which was inhabited by Charles I., when Prince of Wales; and the site, called Park Place, is now covered by modern buildings. Kennington common, an unenclosed tract of ground belonging to the duchy of Cornwall, was formerly the place of execution for criminals convicted at the Surrey assizes; and here several of the adherents of the Pretender underwent the sentence of the law as traitors, in 1746. This place is lighted with gas, and is supplied with water from the South London Water-works. Here are manufactories for oil of vitriol and wadding. Kennington is within the jurisdiction of a court of requests held in the borough of Southwark, for the recovery of debts under 40s.; also within the limits of the New Police. The church, dedicated to St. Mark, is a spacious edifice, with a Grecian Doric portico, tower, and cupola, at the west end, erected in 1824, at an expense, including the purchase of the site and furniture, of £22,719. 19. 11., of which sum the parliamentary commissioners gave £7651. 1. 10., lent without interest £8442. 2 6., and the remainder with interest. The living is a perpetual curacy, in the archdeaconry of Surrey, and diocese of Winchester, and in the patronage of the Rector of Lambeth. This is one of the four districts into which the parish of Lambeth has lately been divided, each of which, on the decease of the present incumbent of Lambeth, will be constituted a distinct rectory. There is an episcopal chapel in Kennington-lane; and those at Stockwell and South Lambeth are within this district. The Independents have two places of worship, and the Baptists and Wesleyan Methodists have one each. There is a school in Kennington-lane under the patronage of the Company of Licensed Victuallers, in which eighty-nine boys and eighty-nine girls are clothed and educated. A National school, in which two hundred boys and one hundred and sixty girls are instructed, was erected in Kennington-oval, in 1824, at an expense of £2500; and an infant school for this district was instituted in 1828.

KENNYTHORPE, a township in the parish of LANGTON, wapentake of BUCKROSE, East riding of the county of YORK, 4 miles (S. by E.) from New Malton, containing 83 inhabitants.

KENSINGTON, a parish in the Kensington division of the hundred of OSSULSTONE, county of MIDDLESEX, 2 miles (W. by S.) from London, containing, with that part of the chapelry of Knightsbridge which is within this parish, 14,428 inhabitants. This place, which since the reign of William III. has been a royal residence, consists of a long street of respectable houses, forming, with the numerous ranges of buildings in its vicinity, one of the most interesting, populous, and extensive appendages to the metropolis. The salubrity of the air, the pleasantness of its situation, the beauty of the gardens belonging to the palace, and its proximity to the parks, render it highly desirable as a place of residence. The village, which extends for a considerable distance on the great western road, consists of several ranges of handsome and well-built houses, is well paved, and lighted with gas, and amply supplied with water by the West Middlesex Company, who have a capacious reservoir at Kensington Gravel Pits, elevated more than one hundred and twenty feet above the level of the Thames. The palace, which stands within the parish of St. Margaret, Westminster, was originally built by Heneage Finch, Lord High Chancellor, and afterwards Earl of Nottingham, and was purchased from his son, the second earl, by King William III., who made it his principal residence: it was subsequently inhabited by Queen Anne, George I., and George II., whose queen, Caroline, made many additions to it, and very much extended and improved the gardens and pleasure grounds, which, under certain regulations, are open to the public, and are frequented as the most fashionable and favourite promenade in the environs of the metropolis. The late Duke of Kent had apartments in this palace, which are now occupied by his Duchess ; and the Duke of Sussex resides in the south wing of the more ancient building, in which His Royal Highness has collected an extensive library of the most valuable authors in every department of literature, particularly in Theology. The palace comprises three quadrangles, neatly and substantially built of red brick, and ornamented with columns, quoins, and cornices of stone, and though externally wanting uniformity of design, and destitute of architectural interest, they contain a noble and extensive suite of apartments, and a splendid collection of pictures by the most eminent Flemish and English artists. The walls and ceilings of the halls and staircases are finely painted in chiaro-oscuro, with allegorical devices and subjects from mythology and history. The gardens are beautifully laid out, in some of its minuter details : the living is a perpetual walks are spacious, and the grounds, which are more than three miles in circuit, comprehend the stately scenery of Hyde park, from which more than three hundred acres, included within a sunk wall and separated by a fosse, were added to the gardens by Queen Caroline, and a view of the serpentine river, over which a handsome stone bridge of five arches was erected in 1824. Detachments of the foot guards and of the lancers are stationed here in barracks. Holland house, originally built by Sir Walter Cope, and now the seat of Lord Holland, though much enlarged with additional buildings, under the superintendence of Inigo Jones, retains much of its Elizabethan character ; and Campden house, erected by Baptist Hicks, Viscount Campden, is a good specimen in the same style of domestic architec-

ture. Hale house, now in a dilapidated state, is said to have been the residence of Oliver Cromwell; and there are some other remains of ancient buildings in various parts of the parish. On Campden-hill and Notting-hill are several stately mansions and elegant villas. Kensington is famous for its manufacture of candles; and at Little Chelsea, in this parish, is a mill for the preparation of cotton flocks for the use of paper-hanging manufacturers. A creek from the Thames has been widened within the last two years, and made navigable to Counter's bridge ; and the Paddington canal passes through the northern extremity of the parish, near Kensal Green. Kensington is within the jurisdiction of the court of requests held in Kingsgate-street, Holborn, for the recovery of debts under 40s., and within the limits of the new police establishment.

The living is a vicarage, in the archdeaconry of Middlesex, and diocese of London, rated in the king's books at £18. 8. 4., and in the patronage of the Bishop of London. The church, dedicated to St. Mary, is a large modern brick building ; in the window of the chancel are whole-length figures of St. Peter, St. Paul, St. John, and St. Andrew, in stained glass, and on the south side of the altar is the sepulchral monument of Edward Henry Rich, Earl of Warwick and Holland, who died in 1721, and whose statue in white marble is finely sculptured. William Courten, a celebrated virtuoso, who died in 1702; Dr. Jortin, vicar of this parish, and an eminent theological writer ; the Rev. Martin Madan, author of Thelypthora; George Colman, sen., a dramatic writer; Dr. Richard Warren, an eminent physician; Samuel Pegge, F. S. A.; and James Elphinstone, a writer on grammar and elocution, were interred here. The church in Addison-road, dedicated to St. Barnabas, and containing one thousand three hundred and thirty sittings, of which five hundred and twelve are free, was erected, in 1829, by subscription among the inhabitants, aided by a grant of £5000 from the parliamentary commissioners ; it is a handsome edifice of Suffolk brick, in the later style of English architecture, with four campanile turrets : the living is a perpetual curacy, in the patronage of the Vicar. The church, or chapel, at Brompton, dedicated to the Holy Trinity, intended as a district church for Old and New Brompton and Little Chelsea, and containing one thousand five hundred and five sittings, of which six hundred and six are free, was erected at the same time and by the same means as that of St. Barnabas, from which it differs principally in having a square embattled tower at the western extremity, and curacy, in the patronage of the Vicar. A chapel of ease to the vicarage was erected at Brompton in 1769. There are places of worship for Baptists and Independents, and a Roman Catholic chapel. The National school was originally founded as a parochial free school, in 1645, by Roger Pimble, who endowed it with tenements in the parish, the rents of which, augmented by subsequent benefactions, produce an income of more than £250 per annum : the premises, situated in High-street, are handsomely built of brick in the ancient style of English architecture, and comprise two ample school-rooms, capable of receiving five hundred children, with apartments for the master and the mistress ; there are now in the school one hundred and thirty boys, and one hundred girls, of whom, fourteen boys and sixty girls are completely clothed. From the same funds, and by subscription, a Sunday school is supported in connexion with the above, which affords instruction to one hundred other children ; and, when the funds will afford it, three girls are boarded, clothed, and instructed by the schoolmaster and mistress, by means of an income of £50 per annum, arising from a benefaction of £1500 five per cent. Bank Annuities, bequeathed in trust for that purpose, by Mrs. Margaret Leach, in 1799. Lord and Lady Campden, in 1635, bequeathed £200, with which, including a benefaction of £45 supposed to have been given by Oliver Cromwell, and called Cromwell's gift, an estate was purchased producing nearly £200 per ann., of which one moiety was to be given to the poor, and the other appropriated to the apprenticing of children. There are Sunday schools in connexion with the established church and the several dissenting congregations. Six almshouses were built, in 1652, by William Methwold, Esq., who endowed them with sixteen acres of land, for the support of six aged women, of whom three are nominated by the vestry, and three by the owner, or inhabitant, of Hale house. The lying-in charity was established in 1817, and there are numerous charitable bequests for the relief of the poor. There are several chalybeate springs in different parts of the parish, of which some were formerly in repute, though now little noticed. Charles Boyle, Earl of Orrery, born in 1674; and Charles Pratt, Earl Camden, Lord High Chancellor in 1766, were natives of Kensington.

KENSWICK, a chapelry in the parish of KNIGHT-WICK, lower division of the hundred of OSWALDSLOW, county of WORCESTER, 4½ miles (N. W. by W.) from Worcester, containing 15 inhabitants.

KENSWORTH, a parish in the hundred of DACO-RUM, county of HERTFORD, 2½ miles (N.W.) from Market-Street, containing 615 inhabitants. The living is a vicarage, in the archdeaconry of Huntingdon, and diocese of Lincoln, rated in the king's books at £9. 13. 4., and in the patronage of the Dean and Chapter of St. Paul's, London. The church, dedicated to St. Mary, has some portions in the early style of English architecture, with some of later date : the capital of the western pillars exhibits the fable of the Wolf and the Crane on one side, and that of the Eagle and the Hare on the other : the doorway within the tower has capitals representing birds and human heads; both doorways are built of Caen stone. A school for teaching sixteen poor children to read was endowed, in 1754, by Mr. and Mrs. Burgis, with a rent-charge : the present income is £12. 10. per annum.

KENT, a maritime county, situated at the south-eastern extremity of the kingdom, and bounded on the north by the river Thames, which separates it from Essex (except for about two miles opposite to Woolwich, a part of which parish lies on the Essex side of the river), and by the German ocean; on the east and southeast by the German ocean, the straits of Dovor, and the British channel ; on the south-west by Sussex ; and on the west by Surrey : it extends from 50° 53′ to 51° 28′ (N. Lat.), and from 3′ (W. Lon.) to 1° 22′ (E. Lon.); and contains nine hundred and eighty-three thousand six hundred and eighty acres, or one thousand five hundred and thirty-seven square miles. The population, in 1821, amounted to 426,016. The name Cantium, by which that part of England now forming the county

of Kent is first distinctly noticed, was, doubtless, a Latinization of the ancient British appellation of the same territory. By the Saxons it was called at first Kant-wara-rike, meaning the Kentish men's country. The present name is an evident variation of the first word of the Saxon compound. The situation of the county at that point of the island which lies nearest to the European continent (the cliffs in the vicinity of Dovor being constantly visible from the opposite coast of France), has given it an importance in the general history of England nearly corresponding with the prominence of its geographical aspect, as forming a sort of advanced post or van-guard of the English territory, considered in its relations with the continental states, and more particularly with those of France and the Netherlands, the ancient Gaul and Belgium. From this proximity it was exposed to, and sustained, the first attack made by Julius Cæsar upon the aboriginal inhabitants of the isle. In his first expedition, the Kentish Britons immediately opposed him, and compelled him to fight upon his landing in the vicinity of Dovor, combating, even amidst the waves, with singular courage ; and although Cæsar, observing his troops to be dispirited by the attacks of the enemy, ordered up the vessels with his artillery, and poured from their sides, stones, arrows, and other missiles, yet the natives sustained these unusal discharges with unshaken intrepidity, and the invaders made no impression, until the standard-bearer of the tenth legion rushed forward, exclaiming, "Follow me, unless you mean to betray your standard to your enemies ;" upon which the Roman legions were incited to that desperate and closer battle which at length forced back the Britons and secured a landing. The inhabitants of the neighbourhood then sent a message of peace; but four days afterwards, a tempest dispersing the enemy's fleet, they attacked the Romans afresh. Cæsar's invasion in the ensuing summer was more formidable : it was made with five well-appointed legions, and two thousand cavalry, amounting to a force of thirty thousand of the best-disciplined troops then known, under the ablest commander. Terrified at the menacing approach of such a force, the inhabitants of the coast retired among the hills, and Cæsar, having effected a landing without opposition, and chosen a proper place to encamp his army, when he had learned from the prisoners where the British forces were posted, marched about midnight in quest of them, leaving ten cohorts and three hundred cavalry, under the command of Q. Atrius, to guard the ships. Having proceeded about twelve miles, he discovered the Britons, who had advanced with their horse and chariots to the banks of a river, where they began from a rising ground to oppose the passage of the Romans, and to give them battle; but being repulsed by the Roman cavalry, they retired to a place in the woods, which was fortified both by art and nature in an extraordinary manner, and which seemed to have been so prepared some time before, on account of their own civil wars. All the passages to it were blocked up by heaps of trees cut down for that purpose, and the Britons seldom venturing to skirmish out of the woods, prevented the Romans from entering their works ; but the soldiers of the seventh legion having cast themselves into a testudo, and raised a mound opposite their works, took the place, and drove them out of the woods; "Various," says Hasted, "have been the conjectures of

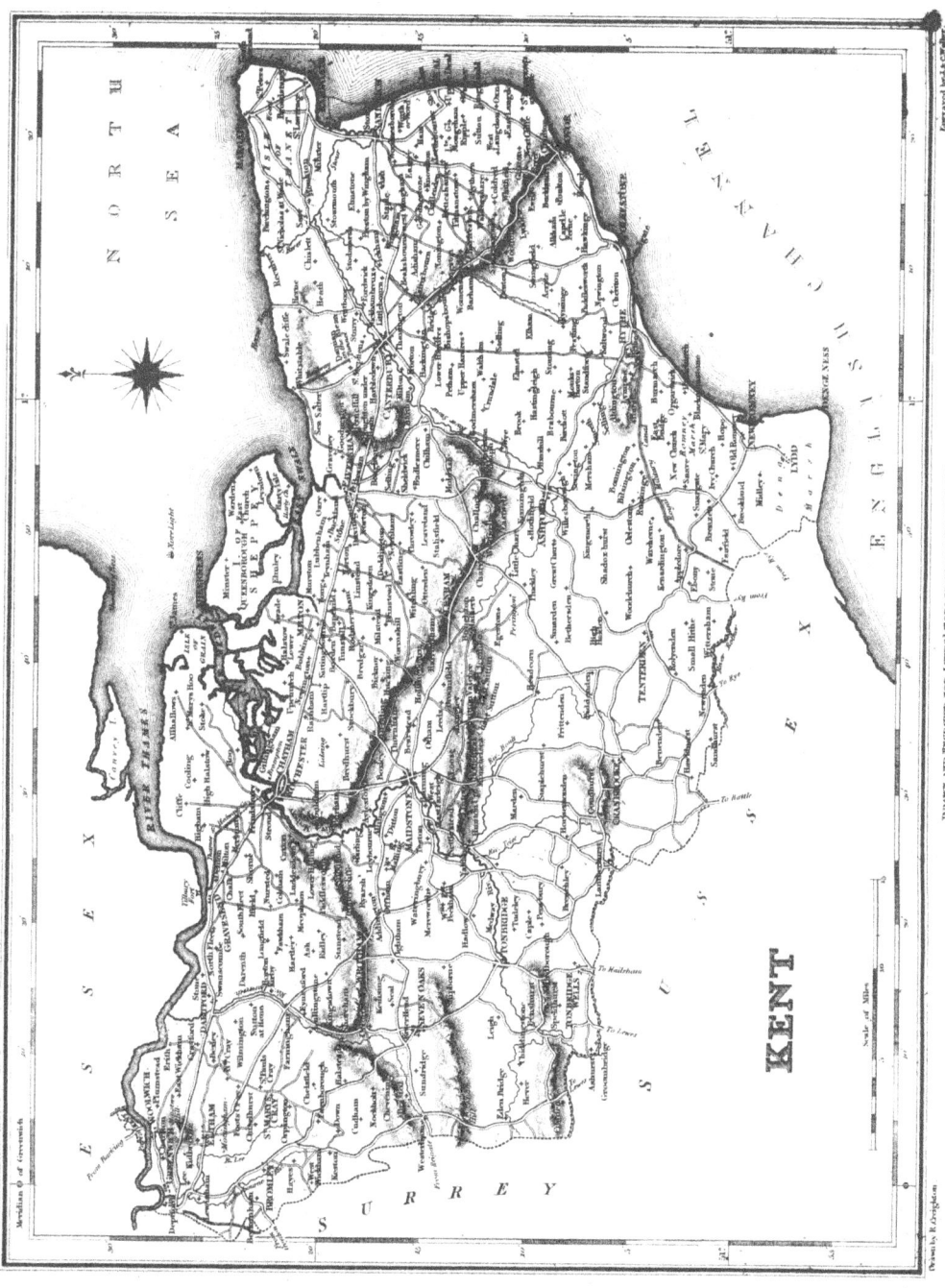

KENT

our antiquaries concerning this place of the Britons, fortified both by art and nature. Horsley thinks it likely that this engagement was on the banks of the river Stour, a little to the north of *Durovernum*, or Canterbury, in the way towards Sturry, which is about fourteen English miles from the Downs; others, well acquainted with this part of Kent, have conjectured it to have been on the banks of the rivulet below Barham-downs, and that the fortification of the Britons was in the woods behind Kingston, towards Bearstead; and the distance as well as the situation of this place, and the remains of Roman works about it, almost in a continued line to Deal, add some strength to this conjecture. Some have placed this encounter below Swerdling-downs, three miles north-west from Bearstead, and the intrenchment in the woods above the downs behind Heppington, where many remains of intrenchments,&c., are still visible." The next morning, having divided his army into three bodies, Cæsar sent both his horse and foot in pursuit of the Britons; soon after which, before the rear of them had got out of sight, some horse-men arrived from Q. Atrius, to inform him that the night before there had happened a dreadful storm, which had shattered almost all his ships, and cast them on shore. Upon this intelligence, the Roman general, countermanding his orders, returned himself in person to the fleet, and there found that about forty of his ships were entirely lost, and that the rest of them were so much damaged as not to be refitted without great labour. Wherefore, having chosen some workmen from among his soldiers, and sent for others from the continent, he wrote to Labienus, in Gaul, to build him as many ships as he could with those legions that were left him; and he himself determined to have his fleet hauled on shore, and to enclose it, with his camp, within the same fortification. In the execution of this, the soldiers laboured ten days and nights without intermission; and at this day, upon the shore about Deal, Sandown, and Walmer, there is a long range of heaps of earth, where Camden supposes this ship camp to have been, and which, in his time, he says, was called by the people, as he was told, Rome's work; though some have conjectured that the place of Cæsar's naval camp was where the town of Deal now stands. This work having been completed, Cæsar returned to the scene of conflict, and found on his arrival that the Britons had assembled in greater numbers from all parts. Whilst the Romans were on their march they were briskly attacked by the British horse and chariots, whom they repulsed with great slaughter, and drove them into the woods. Not long after this, the Britons made a sudden sally out of the woods, and sharply attacked the advanced guard of the Romans, who, not expecting it, were employed in fortifying their camp; upon which, Cæsar immediately despatched the two first cohorts of his legions to their assistance: but the Britons, whilst the soldiers stood amazed at their new mode of fighting, boldly broke through the midst of them, and returned again without the loss of a single man. Quintus Laberius Durus was slain in this action, but some fresh cohorts coming up, the Britons were at last repulsed. The next day the Britons shewed themselves on the hills at some distance from the Roman camp, appearing but seldom, and with less eagerness to harrass the enemy's horse than the day before. But about noon, when

Cæsar had sent out three legions and all the cavalry, under the command of C. Trebonius, to forage, they suddenly rushed on the foragers from all parts, insomuch as to fall in with the legions and their standards. The Romans, however, returning the attack briskly, drove them back, and their cavalry did not desist from the pursuit until they had utterly routed them and slain a great number. Upon this rout, the British auxiliaries, which had come from all parts, left them, nor did the Britons ever after this engage the Romans with their united forces. Cæsar then led his army to the river Thames, towards the territories of Cassivelaunus, the principal leader of the defeated Britons. In the mean time, Cassivelaunus, to make a diversion, sent his messengers into Kent, which was then governed by four petty princes, whom Cæsar styles Kings, and commanded them to raise what forces they could, and suddenly attack the camp where the Roman ships were laid up; which they did, but were repulsed with great slaughter in a sally made by the Romans, who made prisoner one of the kings named Cingetorix, and returned without loss to their trenches. On the submission of Cassivelaunus, which followed this defeat, Cæsar, having imposed an annual tribute on the vanquished, and received the hostages which he demanded, marched back through Kent to the sea-shore, from which he shortly after took his last leave of Britain. In the course of the second invasion and first effectual conquest of Britain by the Romans, in the reign of Claudius, their first descent appears to have been on the south-western coast, but it is plain, from Dion Cassius's account, that Plautius, who commanded this expedition, waited for the promised assistance of the emperor on the southern, or Kentish, side of the Thames; and it has been thought by many, that the place of his encampment was where those large remains of a Roman camp, or intrenchment, are still to be seen at Keston down, near Bromley. In the division of Britain by Constantine, Kent was included in Britannia Prima; and, after the Saxon pirates had begun to infest the south-eastern coast, this was one of the maritime districts placed under the command of the officer called *Comes Littoris Saxonici*, or Count of the Saxon shore, under whom there were, within the limits of this county, according to the Notitia, the commander of the Tungrian soldiers stationed at Dovor; the commander of the detachment of soldiers of Tournay, at Limne; the commander of the first cohort of Vetascians, at Reculver; the commander of the second legion, called Augusta, at Richborough; and the commander of the detachment of the Albuci, at Anderida. The Romans also built several watch-towers, forts, and castles, on the coast, as well to overawe the Britons, and preserve a safe intercourse with the continent, as to guard against the assaults of the Saxon pirates. They made three public, or consular, ways in Kent, the principal of which led from Dovor to London, forming part of the great military way, afterwards denominated by the Saxons, Watling-street.

Ebbs-fleet, in the Isle of Thanet, near Richborough, in this county, is remarkable as having been the place of landing, in 449, of the Saxon chiefs Hengist and Horsa, who, with their followers, were retained by the British sovereign, Guorteyrn, or Vortigern, to serve against the northern invaders, the Picts and Scots. It was about the year 455 that Hengist, aiming at an independent sovereignty in Britain, began the conquest of the territory in the immediate vicinity of the Isle of Thanet, his original station. A series of battles ensued between Hengist and Horsa on the one side, and Guortemir and Catigern, two sons of Vortigern, on the other : the first of these was fought on the banks of the Darent; the next at a place called Eagle's-ford, now Aylesford, which is memorable for the death of Horsa, on the side of the Saxons, and of Catigern on that of the Britons; and a third was fought at Stonar, from which last defeat the Saxons fled to their ships ; and it is asserted that Hengist and his followers remained absent from Britain until the death of Guortemir, which happened not long after. The great battle which, according to the Saxon chroniclers, completed the establishment of Hengist in Kent, was fought at Crayford in 457 : the Britons, being defeated in this with great slaughter, abandoned Kent, and fled in terror to London. Eight years afterwards, the Britons attacked Hengist again, but were utterly routed; and in 473 they attempted another battle with him, but with such a calamitous issue, that they are declared to have fled from the Saxons as from fire. All the battles of Hengist, particularised by the Saxon chroniclers, were fought in Kent ; one of the last of them having occurred at Wippeds-Fleot, or Wipped-fleet, in the Isle of Thanet. Hengist was succeeded in the sovereignty of Kent by his son Esca, who reigned twenty-four years. No subsequent event of importance is recorded of this small kingdom until the reign of Ethelbert, the fourth successor of Hengist, who acceded in 560, and held the sceptre for upwards of half a century : this latter monarch was defeated at Wimbledon in Surrey, by Ceawlin, King of Wessex, whose territories he had invaded, in the first battle which occurred among the sovereigns of the Anglo-Saxon octarchy. Ethelbert also became afterwards remarkable as the first of the Anglo-Saxon kings converted to Christianity by the Roman missionaries, who, in 596, landed in the Isle of Thanet, already memorable for the first disembarkation of the Saxon conquerors of Britain. Kent now became a Christian kingdom, and its metropolis, Canterbury, acquired that ecclesiastical pre-eminence over the other English cities which it has retained to the present day. This kingdom, however, owing in a great measure to its narrow limits, and its situation in an angle of the island, was one of the weaker powers of the octarchy ; and after first becoming tributary to the kingdom of Mercia, about the year 800, was finally annexed to that of Wessex, by Egbert, in 823, who had sent his son Ethelwulf and Bishop Ealstan thither with a competent army, by which the last of the Kentish sovereigns was expelled beyond the Thames.

Although the Danes had, for some years before the accession of Egbert to the sovereignty of all England, harassed the coast of Britain, yet this shire, or earldom, as it was then denominated, remained free from their piratical incursions until the year 832, when they invaded it with a numerous fleet, landing in the Isle of Sheppy, and plundering that island and the neighbouring country. In 838 they landed, and extended their ravages as far as Canterbury, Rochester, and even to London. In 851, having been driven from Essex, they retired to the Isle of Thanet, where they wintered ; but King Athelstan attacking them at Sandwich, both by sea and land, defeated them, and

took nine of their ships. The next spring, having advanced up the æstuary of the Thames with three hundred and fifty ships, they landed in Kent, and pillaged Canterbury ; and in 853 they invaded the Isle of Thanet with a considerable force, where, being attacked by Earl Alcher with the men of Kent, and Earl Huda with those of Surrey, an obstinate battle ensued, in which the two English commanders lost their lives. In 865, in the reign of King Ethelbert, they again landed in the Isle of Thanet, where they wintered, in order to commence their incursions in the spring : the Kentish men offered them a large sum of money to depart peaceably, which, however, they had no sooner received, than they laid waste all the eastern part of the county with fire and sword. In the reign of Alfred, one division of the Danish fleet, under the piratical chief Hesting, on Hastings, sailed up the Medway to Rochester, in order to take that city by surprise ; but failing in this design, they closely besieged it, until it was relieved by the arrival of Alfred with his army, on whose approach they fled hastily to their ships, leaving their plunder behind them. In 893, entering the mouth of the river Limene, or Rother, and sailing up as high as Appledore, they strongly intrenched themselves there, while another division entering the Thames, landed at Milton near Sittingbourne, and built the castle, the site of which is now called the Castle-ruff, after which they mercilessly ravaged the adjoining country. In 902, in the reign of Edward the Elder, a battle was fought between the Kentish men and the Danes, at a place called Holme, or Holme-wood, in Sussex, in which the latter were defeated. During the three years' peace which shortly after ensued, King Edward provided a hundred sail of ships on the Kentish coast, as a security against the Danish descents. In 980, in the calamitous reign of Ethelred II., they again laid waste the Isle of Thanet ; and, in 992, they landed and plundered several parts of the county. In 994, Sweyn, King of Denmark, and Olave, King of Norway, came to Sandwich, with a fleet of ninety-three ships, and having plundered it and the coast of Kent, returned with their booty : the next year they entered the Thames, and having been repulsed in an attack on London, they ravaged the coasts of Kent and Essex. In 998, the Danish forces under Sweyn sailed up the Medway, and attacked Rochester : the Kentish men assembled to defend the city, but were overpowered after a furious battle, upon which the Danes utterly devastated the western parts of the county. In 1006, after the general massacre of the English Danes, King Sweyn again arrived at Sandwich, and laid waste the neighbouring country. At length King Ethelred assembled at Sandwich, in order to oppose to the Danes the most powerful fleet that England had yet possessed, which, however, by the treachery and dissensions of its principal commanders, was rendered of no avail ; and in the next spring, the Danes again landed in the Isle of Thanet, under Heming and Anlaf, from the former of whom several places in this county still retain the name of Heming's Dane : these leaders, joining their forces in Kent, plundered the country, and then laid siege to Canterbury ; but the inhabitants purchased their departure with the sum of £3000. After wintering in the Isle of Thanet, they refitted their ships in Kent, and after various expeditions into different parts of England, they crossed the Thames, in 1010, and marching into the marshes of Kent, burned and destroyed whatever they met with. One of the most memorable events of this disastrous period was the siege, capture, and destruction of the city of Canterbury and its inhabitants, which speedily followed, and from which they returned to their fleet lying in the Thames at Greenwich, carrying with them the Archbishop Elfeg, or Alphage, whom they had made prisoner, and whom they afterwards barbarously murdered there. In the contest between Canute and Edmund Ironside, Canute, having been obliged to raise the siege of London to sail down the Thames with his fleet, and thence up the Medway, in order to secure his navy, Edmund, passing the Thames, marched after him through Surrey into Kent, and encountering him at Otford, in this county, put the Danes to flight, and pursued them as far as Aylesford, in their retreat to the Isle of Sheppy. The last incursion of the Danish pirates in this county was in 1046, in the reign of Edward the Confessor, when twenty-five of their ships arrived unexpectedly at Sandwich, plundered the neighbouring country, and immediately retired.

At the battle of Hastings the Kentish men formed the van of the English army, according to ancient privilege conferred upon them by former sovereigns, for the prowess by which they had distinguished themselves in battle. During the time that the English and the Norman armies were encamped in sight of each other, prior to that memorable engagement, some fresh vessels from Normandy having crossed the strait, in order to join the great fleet stationed off Hastings, their commanders landed, by mistake, several miles further to the north-east, in the neighbourhood of Romney, when the inhabitants of the neighbourhood assembled to oppose them, and a conflict ensued, in which the Normans were overpowered. William was apprised of their defeat when in the midst of his triumph, and, to prevent a similar disaster befalling the rest of the recruits which he expected from the continent, he resolved, without loss of time, to secure the possession of the south-eastern shores. Accordingly, he marched along the Kentish coast from south-west to north-east, ravaging the country in his way, and revenging the rout of his soldiers at Romney, by burning the houses there, and slaughtering the inhabitants. From Romney he proceeded to Dovor, which was at that time the strongest place on the whole coast : the garrison, however, speedily surrendered; and at this place William passed eight days in repairing and strengthening the fortifications ; then changing the direction of his route, he turned aside from the coast, and marched towards London, along the great Roman way, called Watling-street, which led to the capital through the middle of the Kentish territory. On his departure from Dovor, according to the historians of the age, William was met by the inhabitants of Kent with offers of submission, and received from them hostages in token of their allegiance. In 1088, this county was thrown into disturbance, and the crown lands within it ravaged, in consequence of the intrigues of Eudes, or Odo, Bishop of Bayeux, and Earl of Kent, which ended with the capture of Rochester by William Rufus, after a siege of six weeks, that city having been held against him by Eustace, Earl of Boulogne, and the other partisans of his uncle. The year 1170 is memorable for the return of the primate,

Thomas à Becket, from his long exile, and still more so for his murder at Canterbury ; nor is the year 1172 less remarkable for the voluntary penance which Henry II. underwent at his tomb. The additional celebrity which the ecclesiastical metropolis of England now derived from the elevation of Becket to the dignity of a saint and martyr extended itself to the whole county, so that "St. Thomas of Kent" became a popular designation for the most renowned of the English saints, and the principal roads to Canterbury, more especially that from London, were thronged with pilgrims from all parts of England, and even from the continent, to pay their devotions and make their offerings at his shrine. In 1215, Rochester castle was held by the barons against King John, who took it after a two-months' siege, and had all the common soldiers of the garrison hanged. In the following year, Louis the Dauphin landed his army at Stonar, from a fleet of six hundred and eighty vessels, and advanced to Rochester, which he took, and then proceeded to London ; Dovor castle being at the same time successfully defended against him by Hubert de Burgh, Earl of Kent. In 1381, the insurrection under Wat Tyler commenced at Dartford, and the insurgents encamped on Blackheath, whence they proceeded to London. In 1450, also, the rebels under Jack Cade encamped upon Blackheath, from which place, on the approach of Henry VI. with fifteen thousand men, they retired to Sevenoaks, where they defeated and slew Sir Humphrey Stafford and his brother William, who commanded a detachment of the royal army, after which Cade re-encamped on Blackheath, and from that place entered London : on the same heath, in the February following, a great number of his partisans craved pardon of the king upon their knees. In 1459, four thousand French troops, under Marshal de Breze, landed on the coast, and burned the town of Sandwich. In 1471, Thomas Neville, the bastard Fauconbridge, encamped his army of seventeen thousand men upon Blackheath, whence he proceeded to his unsuccessful attack upon London. In 1497, the Cornish insurgents, under Lord Audley and others encamped on Blackheath, where they were surprised by the Earl of Oxford, two thousand being killed, and their leaders made prisoners. In January 1554 the insurrection under Sir Thomas Wyat, to oppose the intended marriage of Queen Mary with Philip II., King of Spain, commenced at Maidstone. On the breaking out of the civil war, in 1642, ten or twelve parliamentarians contrived to possess themselves of Dovor castle by surprise, on the 1st of August; and in 1648, on the formation of the celebrated Kentish Association, the royalists, under Sir John Mayney and Sir William Brockman, were defeated by General Fairfax, at Maidstone. The year 1677 is memorable in the Kentish annals for the daring attack made by a part of the Dutch fleet, under Admiral de Ruyter, on the shipping in the Medway. In December 1688, the fugitive king, James II., was seized at Sheerness, on board a small vessel bound for France, and conveyed, by Captain William Amis, to Faversham. In the course of the last continental war, when apprehensions were entertained of an invasion by the French emperor, every precaution was taken for the protection of this exposed point of the kingdom, by strengthening the different forts, forming a line of Martello towers along the coast, cutting the Grand Military canal, &c. The main route between the English metropolis and the continent of Europe having lain for so many centuries through the heart of this county, the various landings and embarkations of sovereigns and other remarkable personages, whether native or foreign, upon its shores are too numerous for recital: among the most memorable occurrences of this kind are, the landing of the Emperor Charles V. at Dovor, from Corunna, May 16th, 1520, on a visit to Henry VIII.; that of Charles II. at the same place, May 26th, 1660, on his being recalled to the British throne; the embarkation of Louis XVIII. at the same port, in April 1814, at the time of the restoration of his family to the sovereignty of France; and the landing, on June 6th of the same year, also at Dovor, of Alexander I., Emperor of Russia, and Frederic William III., King of Prussia, on a visit to his late Majesty George IV., while Prince Regent, on the occasion of the general peace.

This county comprises the two dioceses of Canterbury and Rochester, in the province of Canterbury, the former consisting of the southern, the latter of the northern, part of the county. The diocese of Canterbury forms an archdeaconry, containing the eleven deaneries of Bridge, Canterbury, Charing, Dovor, Elham, Limne, Ospringe, Sandwich, Sittingbourne, Sutton, and Westbere, in which are two hundred and eighty-two parishes. The diocese of Rochester contains the three deaneries of Dartford, Malling, and Rochester, which form the archdeaconry of Rochester, and the deanery of Shoreham, which is a peculiar belonging to the Archbishop of Canterbury: the whole diocese contains one hundred and thirty-two parishes, making the total number of parishes in the county four hundred and fourteen, of which, one hundred and sixty-nine are rectories, one hundred and sixty-two vicarages, and the remainder perpetual curacies, or united to other parishes. For the purposes of civil government the whole county is divided into five great districts, called lathes, namely, those of St. Augustine, Aylesford, Scray, Shepway, and Sutton at Hone. The lathe of St. Augustine comprises the hundreds of Bewsborough, Bleangate, Bridge and Petham, Cornilo, Downhamford, Eastry, Kinghamford, Preston, Ringslow, or the Isle of Thanet, Westgate, Whitstable, and Wingham. The lathe of Aylesford comprises the hundreds of Brenchley and Horsemonden, Chatham and Gillingham, Eyhorne, Hoo, Larkfield, Littlefield, Maidstone, Shamwell, Toltingtrough, Twyford, Washlingstone, and Wrotham, and the lowey of Tonbridge. The lathe of Scray comprises the hundreds of East Barnfield, Barclay, Blackbourne, Boughton under Blean, Calehill, Chart and Longbridge, Cranbrooke, Faversham, Felborough, Marden, Milton, Rolvenden, Selbrittenden, Tenterden, Teynham, and Wye, and the liberty of the Isle of Sheppy. The lathe of Shepway comprises the hundreds of Aloesbridge, Folkestone, Ham, Hayne, Hythe, Langport, Loningborough, Martin-Pountney, Newchurch, Oxney, Stouting, Street, and Worth, the franchise and barony of Bircholt, the cinque-port of Romney, and the liberty of Romney-Marsh. The lathe of Sutton at Hone comprises the hundreds of Axton, Dartford, and Wilmington; Blackheath; Bromley and Beckingham; Codsheath; Lessness; Ruxley; and Westerham. This county includes the cities of Canterbury and Rochester; the cinque-ports of Dovor, Hythe, New Romney, and Sand-

wich; the borough of Queenborough, and the market towns of Ashford, Bromley, Chatham, Cranbrooke, Dartford, Deal, Elham (the market of which is held only once in five or six years, to prevent the forfeiture of the charter), Faversham, Folkestone, Gravesend, Greenwich, Lydd, Maidstone, Margate, Milton, Ramsgate, Sevenoaks, Sittingbourne (the market of which is held monthly), Smarden, Tenterden, Tunbridge (this market being also held monthly), Westerham, Woolwich, and Wrotham. Of the above, Deal, Dovor, Faversham, Folkestone, Margate, Ramsgate, and Sandwich, are sea-ports; and, besides those at Chatham and Woolwich, there are extensive dock-yards for the Royal navy at Deptford and Sheerness. Two knights are returned to parliament for the county, two citizens for each of the cities, two barons for each of the cinque-ports, and two burgesses for each of the boroughs. Kent is included in the Home circuit: the assizes are held at Maidstone, at which place are the county gaol and house of correction: there are one hundred and sixty-eight acting magistrates. By long usage this county is divided into two great districts of nearly equal extent, commonly called East Kent and West Kent; the former, comprising the lathes of St. Augustine and Shepway, and the upper division of the lathe of Scray; the latter, the lathes of Sutton at Hone and Aylesford, and the lower division of the lathe of Scray; and it is usual for the justices of the peace for the county to confine the exercise of their authority, except upon extraordinary occasions, to the division in which they respectively reside. The quarter sessions for the county are also held four times in the year in each of these divisions, that is, twice originally, and twice by adjournment, as follows: they are held originally, for East Kent, at Canterbury, on the Tuesday after Epiphany and on the Tuesday after the feast of St. Thomas à Becket; and by adjournment, for West Kent, at Maidstone, on the Thursday next after each of those days: they are also held originally, for West Kent, at Maidstone, on the Tuesday after Easter and the Tuesday after Michaelmas; and by adjournment, for East Kent, at Canterbury, on the Friday next after each of those days. The following places, together with others of minor importance, are exempt from the jurisdiction of the county magistrates, as lying within the liberty of the cinque-ports, viz.; Sandwich, Deal, Dovor, New Romney, Hythe, Folkestone, Faversham, and Tenterden: the other places which have a separate jurisdiction are, the cities of Canterbury and Rochester, the corporate town of Maidstone, and the liberty of Romney-Marsh, which last is under the jurisdiction of a bailiff and jurats. The rates raised in the county for the year ending March 25th, 1827, amounted to £384,120. 11., and the expenditure to £392,253. 16., of which £337,832. 18. was applied to the relief of the poor.

The contiguity of Kent to the German ocean and the British channel subjects it to cold sea-winds, which in the spring season, and more especially when they blow from the north-east, frequently injure vegetation in the vicinity of the coast. The winds which mostly prevail are the north-easterly and south-westerly, the chilling effects of the former being often severely felt. The south-western part of the county is more enclosed, and, being sheltered by hills on the north-east, the climate is something milder; but in consequence of the soil being principally a cold wet clay, the harvest is later there than in other parts of the county, which are more exposed. The air of the Isle of Sheppy is very thick, and the district is much subject to noxious vapours, which rise from the vast tracts of marshes adjoining, rendering it very unhealthy: from this cause the country there is not very populous, and, in the marshes more especially, the few inhabitants are chiefly men employed in taking care of the cattle, who are provincially called *lookers:* nearly the same may be said of Romney-Marsh. The effect of the climate on the agriculture of Kent will be seen from a statement of the respective periods of the commencement of the wheat harvest in different parts of the county: in the Isles of Sheppy and Thanet, which are the most forward parts of the county, it usually commences in the last week of July; between Canterbury and Dovor, six or seven days later; and later still by ten or twelve days on the cold hills which run through the centre of the county, as well as in the Weald.

The surface of the county is divided by two nearly parallel chains of hills, called the Upper and the Lower, or the Chalk and the Gravel hills, which run through the middle of it from west to east; extending from the neighbourhoods of Folkestone and Hythe on the eastern, to the vicinity of Westerham on the western, border. The northern range, and the substratum of the whole northern side of the county, are composed chiefly of chalk and flints; the southern range of iron and rag-stone; and below these last-mentioned hills lies the Weald of Kent, an extensive and nearly level tract, occupying the whole southern side of the county, from the border of Surrey to that of the marshy tract at the south-eastern extremity of the county, of which Romney-Marsh forms the principal portion, and being in some places rich and fertile, is productive of excellent pasturage and fine timber. It has already been observed that the county is commonly divided into the two grand districts of East Kent and West Kent. East Kent includes two tracts of land, one very dry and open, the other much sheltered by woods and coppices; the open part lies between the city of Canterbury and the towns of Dovor and Deal; the enclosed part extends in length from Dovor, by Elham and Ashford, to Rochester, and in breadth from the Isle of Sheppy to Lenham, &c. All that portion of East Kent which lies in the vicinity of Faversham, Sandwich, and Deal, is very fertile, and for the most part under tillage. The Isle of Thanet, at the north-eastern extremity of the county, is now only insulated by a small sewer, which communicates both with the river Stour and the sea: the bed of the once famous harbour of the *Portus Rutupensis* now forms a valuable marshy tract of above twenty-five thousand acres in extent. Including Stonar, Thanet isle contains nearly forty-one square miles, or about twenty-seven thousand acres, of which three thousand five hundred are excellent marsh land, and twenty-three thousand arable. It is in a high state of cultivation, and has always been celebrated for its fertility, which has been greatly increased by the inexhaustible supply of sea-weed, a most valuable species of manure, constantly thrown on its shore by the tides. The Isle of Sheppy lies eastward from the mouth of the Medway, and is separated from the rest of the county by an arm of the sea, called the Swale, which is navigable for ships of two hundred tons' burden. It is about

eleven miles long, and eight miles across, in the broadest part, and contains seven parishes, including the borough of Queenborough and the naval station of Sheerness. The southern side of the island, where there are two streams running into the Swale, and forming the islets of Elmley and Harty, is for the most part low and marshy: the land rises gradually towards the centre of the isle, on its south-eastern and western sides; but on the north is a range of cliffs about six miles in length, which gradually decline in height at each extremity, the more elevated parts continuing for about two-thirds of their whole extent. The highest of them, which are in the neighbourhood of Minster, are not less than ninety feet perpendicularly above the level of the shore: they consist of clay, and being washed at their base by the tides, which beat against them with uncommon violence when driven by strong north-east winds, they are continually wasting and falling down upon the beach at the highest parts, occasioning a great loss of land, as sometimes nearly an acre has sunk down in one mass. These cliffs belong to the three manors of Minster, Shurland, and Warden, the owners of which let them out to the proprietors of copperas works, who employ the neighbouring poor to collect the pyrites, or copperas stones, from the shore.

About four-fifths of this island consist of pasture land of two sorts; *viz.,* marsh land, which includes a large tract of rich fattening land; and upland pasture, a great part of which is very poor, and is used for breeding sheep. Most of the arable land is very productive of wheat and beans, especially towards the northern side, in the parishes of Minster and East Church. The enclosures on the hills are small, and are surrounded by thick hedge-rows; and as the country is finely varied with hill and dale, and the prospects are very pleasing and extensive, in fine weather the Isle of Sheppy is remarkably pleasant. Good fresh water is very scarce in most parts of it: the roads throughout are very good, owing to the abundance of materials, and the limited travelling on them. The Isle of Grain, situated between the mouth of the Medway and the mouth of the Thames, is no longer an island; the channel which separated it from the main-land, and communicated with the two rivers, being now filled up: the tract still called the Isle of Grain is about three miles and a half long, and two and a half wide, being low and marshy. West Kent, comprehending the Weald, a great part of the rag-stone shelf, between the Weald and the chalk range, together with all the district lying between the towns of Westerham, Deptford, Rochester, and Maidstone, and their vicinities, forms a great variety of country, having soils and features of almost every description, with many varied and beautiful prospects. The rag-stone shelf of land is chiefly enclosed, having much of its surface undulating, the hills shelving in different directions, but mostly across the rag-stone shelf, so that the little rills of the vales are collected into larger rivulets, which run nearly along the middle of the range; those rising eastward of Lenham discharging themselves into the Stour, and those rising westward of that town into the Medway: the sides of these rag-stone hills descending to the Weald, are thickly covered with villages. The Weald of Kent was, in ancient times, one immense forest; but it has by degrees been cleared of a great part of its wood and cultivated, though it is yet more thinly peopled than any other portion of the county. When viewed from the adjoining hills, in consequence of the few and slight elevations in its surface, this tract has the appearance of an immense plain of great richness and beauty, in which the meadows, seats, and villages, seem dispersed among the stately oaks which still abound in every part of it. At its southeastern extremity is the Isle of Oxney, which is formed by the different channels of the Rother, of which, however, the northernmost is now forsaken by the waters of that river, and is about ten miles in circumference, having an upland ridge running through the middle of it, and low fertile marshes next the river. Great quantities of hops and fruit are grown in this western district; and the surplus of corn not consumed in it is exported, chiefly to London. Romney-Marsh is an extensive tract of rich land, enclosed from the sea by a strong earthen wall thrown up between the towns of Romney and Hythe. In form it is an irregular oblong quadrangle, of about twelve miles long, and eight broad, containing about forty-four thousand acres, and including sixteen parishes, with the corporate towns of Romney and Lydd. The embankment of Romney-Marsh is of very ancient date: it is divided into three districts, viz., Romney-Marsh, properly so called, containing about twenty-four thousand acres; Walland-Marsh, about twelve thousand; and Denge-Marsh, about eight thousand. The bank which protects the first of these portions from the sea, called Dimchurch Wall, is upwards of three miles in length: the side next the sea is covered with common fagots and rag-stone, fastened down by oak piles and overlaths, which prevents the sea from washing away the earth. The expense of repairing this wall and the drainage amounts to the annual sum of four thousand pounds, which is raised by scot on the acreage of the whole of Romney-Marsh. The other two districts, Walland-Marsh and Denge-Marsh, are rated separately, to defray their own expenses of drainage, &c. Few oxen are fed in this tract compared with those kept on other rich marsh lands; but the number of sheep bred and fattened is thought to exceed that of any other district of the same extent in the kingdom. The fences are either ditches, or oak posts and rails, there being hardly any hedges or trees, excepting a few in the neighbourhood of some of the villages: immense quantities of oak posts and rails are annually brought into these marshes from the woodlands of the Weald. The chalk district occupies the whole northern side of the county, from the range of chalk hills which intersects it from east to west, to the Thames and the sea, excepting only the marshy tracts, which form a narrow stripe along the whole course of the Thames, lie in greater breadth about the mouths of the Thames and Medway, and the borders of the Swale, run thence in a narrow line along the coast as far as the high grounds of the Isle of Thanet, and stretch in a wider expanse across that corner of the county to the eastern coast; and to this may be added the lower part of the vallies, through which flow the Medway and the Greater and the Lesser Stour. The most westerly portion of this large district possesses some of the most pleasing scenery in the county, being, from its vicinity to the metropolis, one of the most ornamented as well as most populous parts, and commanding, from Shooter's Hill and other eminences, fine prospects over the Thames on one side, and

over a richly-cultivated country on the other, beautifully diversified with numerous handsome seats and pleasant villages.

The soils of East Kent are various; the principal being chalk, loam, strong cledge, hazel mould, and stiff clay. The chalk soil consists of loose chalky mould on a substratum of rock chalk, and is mostly found on the tops and sides of the ridges of this district: its depth is from three to six or seven inches; in some places there is a slight mixture of small flints, and in others of black light mould, provincially called *black hover*. The whole of these chalky soils are naturally of little value, but where they have been improved, they have become excellent turnip-land: the chalk soil in the Isle of Thanet is found on the tops of the poor chalky ridges, about sixty feet above the level of the sea, its depth being from six to eight inches; but the vales between the ridges and the flat lands on the hills have a depth of dry loamy soil of from one to three feet, with less chalk, and of a much better quality. The west end of the Isle of Thanet, even on the hills, has a good mould from one to two feet deep, a little inclining to stiffness; but the deepest and best soil is that which lies on the south side of the southernmost ridge, running westward from Ramsgate to Monkton, where it is a deep, rich, sandy loam: the lowlands are mostly dry enough to be ploughed flat, without any water-furrows: the soil of the marshes is a stiff clay, mixed with sea-sand and small marine shells: the substratum of the whole of the isle is the dry chalk rock. The loamy soil is a very dry, soft, light mould, from six to ten inches deep, on a stratum of red soft clay, from three to seven feet deep, under which is generally a layer of chalky marl, and then the chalk rock; this soil may be made to produce good crops of every kind of grain and grass. The strong cledge is a stiff tenacious earth, with a small proportion of flints, and, in some places, small particles of chalk; it is from six to ten inches deep, lies on the chalk rock, which is the substratum of almost all this district, and in favourable seasons produces good crops of wheat, clover, beans, and oats. The hazel mould is a light dry soil on a clay bottom, more or less mixed with flints or sand. The stiff clay lies on the tops of the highest hills, and is generally a wet soil: in some places it has a layer of a yellow clay between the surface mould and the chalk rock. In the vallies about Dovor, and Stockbury near Maidstone, are small tracts of land consisting of beds of flint with hardly any mould to be seen. There is very little gravel and not much sand in this district; a little of the latter is found in the vicinity of Hythe and Folkestone. The rich flat lands in the vicinity of Faversham, Sandwich, and Deal, have two kinds of soil; a rich, sandy loam, seven or eight inches deep, having a sub-soil of strong loam, clay, or chalk, of various depths; and a stiff clay, some of which, in the lower parts, is rather wet. Almost the whole of the Isle of Sheppy is a deep, strong, stiff clay; but some of the upper parts of the island have a few gravelly fields: the soil of the marshes is a stiff clay, having on its surface a rich vegetable mould, an inch or two deep.

The various soils of West Kent are chalk, loam, clay, gravel, sand, and hazel mould. The chalky soils are like those of East Kent, and are found on the sides of the hills, and at different places along the borders of the Thames, between Dartford and Rochester. The loamy soils are of various depths, and are found chiefly in the vallies, being all fertile : what in Kent is called hassock, or stone-shatter, is a mixture of sandy loam with a large proportion of light-coloured Kentish rag-stone; it is from six inches to several feet deep, the substratum being the solid stone rock: great quantities of fruit and hops are produced on this soil. The principal part of Romney-Marsh is a fine soft loam with a mixture of sea-sand, and the herbage it produces is of the first quality for fattening. The inferior parts of this marsh, being those which are used in breeding, are such as have a less portion of sea-sand, and are a stiff clay; and such as have too much of sand and gravel, which latter lie near the sea-shore : the sub-soil is frequently seen in alternate layers of clay and sand, and sometimes beach and sand. The clay of the western part of Kent is of different sorts ; one is cold, much mixed with flints, from eight to fourteen inches deep, and extremely tenacious ; it is found on the top of the chalk-hills, having in some places a yellow clay between it and the chalk ; another is cold, wet, and stiff, with a small mixture of rag-stone, and is found chiefly in the low grounds of the western part of the county. An extremely stiff moist clay, mixed with stones and flints of different sorts, and found about Seal and Wrotham, is provincially called coomb. Pinnock, too, is a provincial name for a red sticky clay, mixed with small stones, the substratum of which is the rag-stone rock. The clay, which is by far the most predominant kind of soil in the Weald, is there either stiff and exceedingly heavy, or a wet sort which ploughs somewhat lighter : the first, chiefly found on eminences, or their declivities, is seven or eight inches deep, and rests on a stratum of stiff yellow clay, which has in some places a substratum of excellent marl ; the other lies in lower situations, and is seven or eight inches deep, the sub-soil being in some places a yellow clay, and in others a soft sand-stone rock. Gravelly soils are chiefly found about Dartford and Blackheath ; they are from five to eight inches deep, with a sub-soil of rocky gravel or sand : there are other soils, called gravel, in the lower part of this district, which are a mixture of the small pieces of Kentish rag-stone, with sand and loam. The sandy soils of West Kent are mostly black, and are found chiefly on commons and heaths : in the Weald there is some white sandy land, which is much improved by marl and lime. A fine hazel mould is found on the sides of the hills at different places throughout the whole district.

The crops most commonly cultivated are wheat, barley, beans, oats, peas, canary-seed, radish-seed, turnips, and cole-wort. In a county where soils are so various, it is very difficult to make an accurate estimate of produce : of wheat, in some places, two quarters per acre is a very good crop, while in others, double that quantity is a very indifferent one : about twenty two bushels per acre is estimated as the general average crop. The produce of barley is from one and a half to seven quarters per acre. Of beans the common tick is the sort most cultivated in Kent ; and it produces from two to six quarters per acre, according to the quality and condition of the land. The produce of oats is from three to six or seven quarters per acre; that of peas, from one and a half to five quarters

per acre. Potatoes, cabbages, tares, clover, trefoil, sainfoin, lucerne, and burnet, are also cultivated, but less generally than the crops above-mentioned. The produce of canary-seed is from three to five quarters per acre, and it is sold to seedsmen in London, who export it to all parts of Europe. Radish-seed is much cultivated on the best loamy soils of the Isle of Thanet and East Kent, for the supply of the London seedsmen, who retail it to all parts of the kingdom ; the produce is from eight to twenty-four bushels per acre. For the London seedsmen are also grown spinach-seed, in the Isle of Thanet and East Kent, the produce of which is from two to five quarters per acre; kidney beans, in the Isle of Thanet and the vicinity of Sandwich, the produce being from ten to twenty bushels per acre ; and cresses and white mustard-seed, which produce from eight to twenty bushels per acre. Some flax is cultivated, and produces per acre from eight to twelve bushels of seed, and from one to two packs of flax of two hundred and forty pounds each, the quality of which is somewhat similar to that imported from Holland, but inferior. Woad for dyeing is much cultivated in the western part of the county, on poor and stiff, and in some instances on chalky, soils. The quantity of land in natural meadow in the uplands of East Kent is comparatively small, and the greater part of the hay used in that district is produced in the marshes. The Weald abounds in natural grass land, which produces a vast quantity of hay of excellent quality. Other parts of the county have scattered parcels of meadow land, some of which are of good quality ; but in general the meadows of Kent are much inferior to those of many other counties : the downland sheep-walks on the chalky hills of East Kent can hardly be called pasture. The grass land of the marshes, which are situated along the borders of the rivers, or of the sea, is of very considerable extent : Romney-Marsh contains forty-four thousand acres ; the marshes on the borders of the Stour comprise twenty-seven thousand ; and those on the Medway, the Thames, and the Swale, about eleven thousand five hundred collectively. The whole of these tracts is appropriated to the fattening of cattle and sheep, or to the breeding of sheep : the system of grazing in the marsh lands of the Isle of Thanet and East Kent is generally to buy in lean cattle and sheep, and keep them till they are fit for the butcher : the inferior parts of the marshes, and the whole of the upland pasture, which is generally very poor, are assigned to the breeding of lambs, or the feeding of young lean sheep, which latter are sold out to the fattening graziers at about two years and a half old. The grass lands at the western part of the county are fed off in various ways. There is no breed of cattle peculiar to this county; those bought in by the graziers to be fattened in the marshes of East Kent are chiefly from Wales, and are brought by the Welch drovers to Canterbury and other markets. The majority of the dairy cows are selected from these droves, while others are a mixture of these and home-bred cattle : in West Kent the dairies are small. In the Weald, the cattle, whether for the dairy or for the plough, are chiefly of the Sussex breed. The principal part of the cattle fed in Romney-Marsh are the property of farmers in the upland districts, who, in return, take lambs for the graziers to keep during winter. Oxen are not so generally used in the labours of agriculture in East Kent as in the western part. Kent has long been famous for a fine breed of sheep, called in that county Romney-Marsh sheep, the greater number of them being bred in that district; but in Smithfield market, where numbers of them are constantly sold, they are called Kent sheep: their carcasses and legs are rather long, their bones large, compared with other breeds, and their faces and legs white. These sheep are remarkable for arriving at an extraordinary degree of fatness at an early age, and for possessing large fleeces of very long fine wool: the fat wethers, at two years old, weigh from twenty-two to twenty-eight pounds per quarter. Many fold flocks of lean sheep are kept in the uplands of East Kent, and are mostly of this breed, as also are all the sheep of the Isle of Sheppy; but the latter, in consequence of the inferiority of the soil, are somewhat smaller than those of Romney-Marsh, and their wool is lighter and finer. Many South-Down sheep are bred and kept in the eastern part of the county, and in the uplands of that district are also flocks of the Wiltshire and Dorsetshire breeds: the Romney-Marsh sheep, in some few flocks, have been crossed with the new Leicester. Several flocks of the sheep kept in West Kent are of the South-Down breed: Wiltshire and Dorsetshire sheep are also found there. There are considerable fairs for the sale of fat and lean cattle, at Maidstone and Ashford, as well as at other places in the Weald: fortnight markets for the sale of fat cattle and sheep have also been established at different places, and from these unsold stock is frequently taken away by drovers, being then consigned to salesmen at Smithfield market. The hogs of East Kent are of various sorts, the smaller of which are those that have been intermingled with the Chinese breed: many pigs are reared in this district, and having been fed on the corn stubbles for the butchers, are killed in the autumn for roasting pork. In the western part of the county are some of the large Berkshire breed. Many hogs are fed on acorns in the woods of the Weald, and fattened on corn in the winter. In the Isle of Sheppy the horses are chiefly bred from a sort that has been in the island from time immemorial; in the other parts they have been crossed with other breeds. West Kent is principally supplied with cart horses by dealers who bring them at three, four, or five years old, from the midland counties: in the Weald, horses and oxen are not unusually yoked together. The chief hop plantations are situated around Canterbury and Maidstone. Those near Canterbury, called the City Grounds, surround it to the distance of two or three miles, and comprise between two and three thousand acres. The best portion of the plantations of East Kent, the hops growing in which are esteemed of a very rich quality, are upon a deep, rich, loamy soil, with a thick sub-soil of loamy brick-earth. The plantations in the vicinity of Maidstone extend through the several parishes on the rag-stone shelf of land which lie below the hills that border on the Weald: the quality of the hops grown here is somewhat inferior to that of the hops of Canterbury and East Kent. The hop plantations of the central parts of the county are so extensive, that thrice the labouring population of the district is required to gather the crops; so that numbers of people are employed from London and other places. No certain report can be made of the produce of the hop-plantations, it being

so variable: the average is considered not to exceed seven hundred weight per acre. In the neighbourhood of Gravesend and Deptford a great quantity of vegetables is raised for the supply of the metropolis. Great quantities of fruit, chiefly apples, cherries, and filberts, are grown in the vicinity of Maidstone, the young trees being frequently planted among the hops; and it is doubted, whether a soil more adapted to the growth of corn, fruit, and hops, conjointly, exists in the kingdom. This fruit is chiefly sent to the London market by water, and some of it is taken to the north of England by the coal vessels. Besides the manures in common use in other counties, chalk is employed in Kent, for the improvement of wet stiff soils which possess no calcareous particles: lime burned from chalk is much applied to the lands of the Weald. Immense quantities of seaweed are thrown on the shores of the Isle of Thanet, and the farmers are very diligent in removing it to the top of the cliffs, lest the next succeeding tide should wash it away: this manure is mixed with that of the farm-yard. Woollen rags, sprats and other fish, and rape cake, are used as manure in the hop plantations. A society for the encouragement of agriculture and industry was established at Canterbury, in January 1793, under the patronage of the late Sir Edward Knatchbull, Bart. and the late Filmer Honywood, Esq., at that time members of parliament for the county.

The waste lands of Kent consist of about twenty thousand acres, dispersed in various parts of the county, in commons, heaths, &c. The soil of a few of these is a cold sterile loam, that of others a wet stiff clay, but of most of them it is gravel and sand. They are generally covered with furze and fern, interspersed with patches of grass, and are grazed by lean cattle and sheep. The chief woodlands of East Kent are scattered between the great road from Rochester to Dovor, and the range of chalk hills that runs from Folkestone, by Charing, to Debtling: besides the immense quantity of hop-poles cut for the neighbouring plantations, which are their chief produce, they also furnish piles for securing the sea-walls of the marshes, and props to be used in the Newcastle coal mines. West Kent abounds in woods and coppices, of which there are about thirteen thousand acres; some of those of the Weald are still in their original forest state. The kinds of wood which grow in this county are chiefly oak, beech, ash, hornbeam, chesnut, birch, and hazel. Faggots for fuel are plentiful in West Kent; coal from Newcastle and Sunderland is brought to the sea-ports of the county, and thence distributed through the interior. The manufacture of silk has been carried on to a great extent at Canterbury, but is now giving way to that of cotton. At Dovor and at Maidstone are extensive mills for the manufacture of paper of all kinds, the white paper made at the latter place having long been in high repute: at Maidstone also the woollen manufacture is carried on. There are salt-works at Stonar, near Sandwich, and in the Isle of Grain. At Whitstable and Deptford are large copperas works: gunpowder is made at Dartford and Faversham. At Crayford are extensive works for the printing of calico and the bleaching of linen. And in the Weald of Kent, bordering on Sussex, were formerly furnaces for the casting of iron. A quantity of sacking and hop-bagging is manufactured within the limits of the county. Under this head may be noticed the ship-building for the Royal navy, carried on at Deptford, Woolwich, Chatham, and Sheerness.

The two great rivers of Kent are the Thames and the Medway. The Thames forms the northern boundary of the county for a distance of upwards of forty miles, and first touches it at Deptford, about three miles below London bridge, where it is joined by the Ravensbourne, whence, flowing by Greenwich, Woolwich, and Erith, it receives the united waters of the Cray and the Darent, and continues its course, by Greenhythe and Northfleet, to Gravesend, immediately below which town it passes through the road called the Hope, and joins the waters of the Medway and the German ocean at the Nore : in the whole of this course it is navigable for merchant vessels of the largest burden. The Medway is formed by the confluence of four streams, two of which rise in Sussex, one in Surrey, and the other in Kent : that which rises in Surrey enters this county a little above Eaton bridge, and flowing to Penshurst joins another of the principal branches, and then continues its course past Tunbridge to Yalding, where it forms a junction with a very considerable stream from the other two of its sources, and, having received the waters of various other minor streams, it passes by Maidstone and Aylesford to the towns of Stroud, Rochester, and Chatham ; below which, having formed numerous creeks and islands, it falls into the German ocean at the mouth of the Thames, between the Isle of Grain and the naval station of Sheerness. This river was made navigable for small barges as high as Tunbridge, about the middle of the last century, under the provisions of an act passed in the year 1740 : up to Chatham it is navigable for vessels of the largest burden. The Medway is well stocked in the higher part of its course with the usual river fish, and lower down with smelts, soals, flounders, dabs, thornbacks, &c. But its principal fishery is that of oysters, which is also carried on in the various creeks which are formed towards its mouth, and is under the jurisdiction of the corporation of Rochester, the mayor and citizens holding a yearly court, called the Admiralty court, for its regulation. There are six smaller rivers ; the Greater Stour, the Lesser Stour, the Rother, the Darent, the Cray, and the Ravensbourne. The Greater Stour rises from two principal heads in the eastern part of the county, and flowing to Ashford, there takes a north-easterly course to Canterbury, whence it runs to the Isle of Thanet, and takes a south-easterly course between the island and the main land to Sandwich, where it becomes navigable for coasting vessels, and having made a circuit to the north, falls into the British channel at Pepperness. The Lesser Stour, rising from various heads, flows along the western side of Barham Downs, and passing through a line of beautiful country, nearly parallel with the higher course of the Greater Stour, falls into the last-mentioned river in its course round the southern part of the Isle of Thanet, about a mile from Stourmouth. The trout in both these rivers is remarkably fine : there is a peculiar kind of trout which frequents the Greater Stour in the latter part of the year, and appears to be of the salmon species, the ordinary weight being about nine pounds, though it is sometimes much more. Towards the mouth of this river there is yet another sort, commonly called " Fordwich trout," the weight of which varies from four to twelve pounds ; but it is now much less abundant than formerly. The Rother rises

at Gravel-hill, in the parish of Rotherfield, in the county of Sussex, and flowing eastward, becomes the boundary between this county and Sussex, near Sandhurst, and having skirted the south side of the Isle of Oxney, quits Kent, and empties its waters into Rye harbour. The Darent, which pursues its entire course through this county, rises on the borders of Surrey, near Westerham, and flows in a north-easterly direction to Riverhead ; then taking a northerly course, it passes through a considerable extent of country to Dartford, where it becomes navigable, and assumes the name of Dartford creek, falling into the Thames between two and three miles further down, at Long Reach. The Cray rises at Newell, in the parish of Orpington, and flowing through the district called the Crays and through Crayford marshes, it falls into Dartford creek, half way between Dartford and the Thames. The Ravensbourne rises on Keston common, and running through the parishes of Hayes, Bromley, Lee, and Lewisham, on the north-western border of Kent, it falls into the Thames at Deptford, where it receives the name of Deptford creek, and is navigable for small craft for the distance of about a mile from its mouth. In different parts of the county are numerous springs, the water of which is chalybeate, but those of Tunbridge Wells are the most celebrated. At Sydenham, in the parish of Lewisham, are some springs of medicinal purgative water, resembling those of Epsom, which, from their proximity to Dulwich, have received the name of Dulwich Wells.

Owing to the peninsular situation of this county, between the English channel and the long æstuary of the Thames, it has little connexion, except through the medium of that great river, with the grand system of canal navigation which branches through the midland districts of England. The only work of this nature that can be regarded as belonging exclusively to Kent, is the cut from the Thames at Gravesend to the Medway at Rochester, which saves, for barges, a circuitous navigation by the mouths of those two great rivers. The canal extending from the Thames at Deptford, to Croydon in Surrey, runs through a small portion of the western border of the county ; and the Grand Surrey canal touches its north-western extremity. The Grand Military canal, constructed as a defensive work during the last continental war, at the time of the threatened invasion from France, commences eastward near Hythe, and quits this county for Sussex, near Fairfield. The great road from London to Dover enters Kent near New-cross turnpike, and pursues its course for the most part along the line of the ancient Watling-street, over Blackheath, and through Dartford, Gravesend, Stroud, Rochester, Chatham, and Canterbury. A long line of road branches from the former near New-cross, and passes through Lewisham, Eltham, Foot's Cray, Wrotham, Maidstone, and Ashford, to Hythe and Folkestone ; and another diverges from the same spot through Lewisham, Bromley, Sevenoaks, and Tunbridge, to Rye and Winchelsea in Sussex.

Among the more remarkable features of the coast of Kent may be specified the North and South Forelands, the promontory of Dungeness, and the cliffs of Dover. In connexion with this coast should also be noticed the well-known road, or anchorage-place, called the Downs, which lies opposite to the town of Deal, the southern boundary being formed by the Goodwin Sands: its width is about six miles, its length about eight, and its depth varies from eight to twelve fathoms. This is the common rendezvous of the East India and other fleets, both on their outward and homeward bound voyages; and in certain states of the wind nearly four hundred sail have anchored there at one time. The situation of the Goodwin Sands (supposed to have derived their name from Goodwin, the celebrated Anglo-Saxon earl of Kent,) forms the principal security of this much-frequented road, serving as a break-water during the prevalence of southerly winds. These sands extend in length about ten miles, the north sand head being nearly opposite to Ramsgate, and the south sand head to Kingsdown: at low water they are dry in many places, and parties frequently land on them. Several years ago, in consequence of the numerous accidents to shipping, the corporation of the Trinity-house formed the design of erecting a light-house on them; but after the sand had been penetrated by boring to a great depth, the scheme was given up as impracticable, as no solid foundation could be obtained. A floating light, however, has been placed on the eastern side of the north sand head, and has proved of important service. The county abounds with rich, extensive, and interesting prospects; the most striking of which are those from the heights of Greenwich and Woolwich, Dovor castle and cliffs, Gad's hill near Rochester, Maram's Court, Wrotham and River hills, the high grounds in the parish of Minster, Wye down, and the hills of Boughton, Boxley, Gravesend, Hampton, Holwood, Oldbury, and Shottington.

Kent having been the portion of Britain from which, both in the Roman and in the Saxon conquest, the Britons were first expelled, contains few remains of antiquity purely British. Brass celts and other weapons have been dug up in places supposed to have been the scenes of conflicts between the Britons and their invaders; and a very few cromlechs are still to be found within the limits of the county; the most remarkable of which, for its magnitude and good preservation, is that commonly called Kit's Coty House, which, from its name and situation, some antiquaries have conjectured to have been a monument over the grave of the British prince, Certigern, slain in one of the battles with Hengist. The Roman stations here were *Anderida*, supposed to have been at Newenden; *Dubris*, Dovor; *Durobrivæ*, Rochester; *Durolevum*, Judde Hill, Newington, or Sittingbourne; *Durovernum*, Canterbury; *Lemania*, Lymne; *Noviomagus*, Keston, or Crayford; *Regulbium*, Reculver; *Rutupium*, Richborough; and *Vagniacæ*, Northfleet, or Southfleet. The principal remains of Roman buildings are at Canterbury, Dovor, and Richborough; and numerous other remains, such as weapons, utensils, &c., have been dug up in various parts of the county, on or near the sites of the several stations.

Owing to the great number of parishes into which the county is divided, the churches are numerous; but, excepting the ancient cathedrals of Canterbury and Rochester, its ecclesiastical buildings are in general more remarkable for the number of interesting monuments which they contain, than for architectural grandeur or beauty. Besides the church of Barfreston, which is one of the most perfect specimens of pure Saxon in the kingdom, the following are worthy of no-

tice for their antiquity or curiosity, *viz.*, St. Mary's Dovor, and those of Maidstone, Minster, Patrixbourne, Reculver, Romney, and Sandwich. In this county was made the first settlement in England of the four following monastic orders, *viz.*, of Augustine canons at Canterbury, in 605; of Grey friars, or Franciscans, at the same place, in 1224; of Trinitarian friars at Mottenden, in the same year; and of White friars, or Carmelites, at Aylesford, in 1240. The religious houses in Kent before the Reformation were, of the Benedictine order, two abbeys, three priories, and five nunneries; of the Cluniac, one priory; of the Cistercian, one abbey; of Secular canons, five colleges; of canons Regular, four abbeys and five priories; of Dominicans, one priory and one nunnery; of Franciscans, two priories; of Trinitarians, one priory; of Carmelites, three priories: the number of Alien priories was four: there were two commanderies of the Knights of St. John of Jerusalem, and fifteen hospitals, besides several hermitages, chantries, and free chapels. The principal remains of monastic buildings are those of St. Augustine's abbey, Canterbury, and the abbeys of Boxley, Bradsole, or St. Radegund's, and West Malling. Of ancient castles, the most interesting specimens are at Canterbury, Chilham, Rochester, and Dovor; besides which, there are similar remains at Allington, Cooling, Hever, Leeds, Leybourne, Limne, Saltwood, Stutfall, Sutton-Valence, and Tunbridge. The great hall of the ancient royal palace at Eltham is, perhaps, the noblest specimen remaining in the county of the domestic architecture of the middle ages. Besides the magnificent buildings of the naval hospital at Greenwich, with its fine park, anciently and so long a favourite residence of the English sovereigns, this pleasant and fertile county abounds with elegant mansions, fine parks, and thriving plantations. Among the most distinguished of the former may be noticed Knowle park, anciently a stately residence of the Archbishops of Canterbury, and now that of the Earl of Plymouth; Penshurst, the ancient seat of the Sidney family; Waldershare park, that of the Earl of Guildford; and Lee priory, that of Sir S. E. Brydges, Baronet. Charlton house, the seat of Sir T. M. Wilson, Bart.; and Summer Hill, that of —— Alexander, Esq., are very perfect specimens of the domestic architecture of the reigns of Elizabeth and James I.

A peculiar custom respecting the descent of real property having always prevailed in this county, has produced a marked distinction between Kent and almost every other county in England, with regard to the occupation of land and the number of freeholders, the latter being very numerous in it, so that the Kentish yeomanry have long formed one of the strongest and most independent divisions of that important class of British subjects. The name Gavelkind, by which this custom is generally known, is merely a modern pronunciation of the Saxon compound *Gafel-kind, Gafel* signifying a rent, or acknowledgment in money or in kind, and Gafel-kind lands, those for which a rent was paid, or, in other words, lands held by socage tenure, in contradistinction from those which were held by military service. And so predominant has the former of these tenures anciently been in this county, that all lands within it are in the courts presumed to be "of the nature of gavelkind," that is, to have been anciently and originally holden in socage tenure, unless the contrary can be proved; such being regarded and designated "the common law of Kent." The descent of gavelkind land, in the right line, is to all the sons equally, "but the harth for fire shall remain to the youngest sonne;" if there be one son only, then wholly to such only son, as at common law. In default of a son the descent is, as at common law, to all the daughters; if there be but one daughter, to such daughter alone. The partible quality in the descent amongst males is not limited to the right or lineal line, but extends likewise throughout the collateral line. So also the right of '-representation' prevails both lineally and collaterally, as in common law inheritances. This customary descent is not confined to an estate in fee-simple; it extends also to an estate tail in gavelkind land. The most important of the customary privileges annexed to all lands of this nature within the county of Kent are the following :—I. That the husband is tenant by the courtesy of only a moiety of the wife's land of inheritance, whether he has issue by her or not, and this estate continues during the period of his widowhood only; whereas, by the common law, to make a tenancy by the courtesy there must have been issue born alive of the wife during the existence of the marriage, and the husband is tenant of the whole of such lands during his life absolutely.—II. That the wife has dower of a moiety of such lands of inheritance, whereof the husband was seized during espousals, but if she commit fornication, or afterwards marry, her dower is forfeited ; whereas, by the common law she is endowed of one-third only, to continue for her life absolutely. III. That the heir should continue in wardship until fifteen years old, and at that age he has power to alienate his lands ; whereas, by the common law, the wardship in socage continues only until the infant attains fourteen years, and he is incapable of alienating until twenty-one. IV. In a writ of right touching gavelkind land, the Grand Assize is not chosen by four knights, but by four tenants in gavelkind, who do not associate to themselves twelve knights, but twelve tenants in gavelkind. Statutes have at times been made for disgavelling particular lands in Kent ; but these statutes, although strongly drawn, declaring that the lands should thenceforth be to all intents as lands at common law, and that they should descend as such lands do, yet it has been adjudged that they took away the partibility in descent only, and not the other qualities and customs appertaining to the tenure ; inasmuch as these last are merely collateral, and not essential to the nature of gavelkind. Another legal custom is peculiar to the Weald, within the limits of which the proof of woodlands having ever paid tithe lies on the parson to entitle him to take tithe of it, contrary to the general custom in other places, where proof of the exemption lies upon the owner ; nor has the lord waste within the Weald, the timber growing thereon belonging to the tenant : the custom which excludes the lord from the waste is called Land-peerage. The title of Duke of Kent was borne by the deceased Prince Edward, fourth son of George III., brother of his present Majesty, and father of the Princess Victoria of Kent, now heir presumptive to the British crown.

KENT-CHURCH, a parish in the hundred of WEBTREE, county of HEREFORD, 13 miles (S. W. by S.) from Hereford, containing 311 inhabitants. The living is a rectory, in the archdeaconry and diocese of Here-

ford, rated in the king's books at £10. 12. 3½., and in the patronage of the Crown. The church is dedicated to St. Mary. A school here has an endowment of £8 per annum. A rail-road runs through the parish.

KENTFORD, a parish partly in the hundred of LACKFORD, but chiefly in that of RISBRIDGE, county of SUFFOLK, 4½ miles (N. E. by E.) from Newmarket, containing 109 inhabitants. The living is a perpetual curacy, with the vicarage of Gazeley, in the archdeaconry of Sudbury, and diocese of Norwich, rated in the king's books at £7. 3. 4., and in the patronage of the Master and Fellows of Trinity Hall, Cambridge. The church is dedicated to St. Mary.

KENTISBERE, a parish in the hundred of HAYRIDGE, county of DEVON, 3¾ miles (E. by N.) from Cullompton, containing, with the parish of Blackborough, 1143 inhabitants. The living is a rectory, in the archdeaconry and diocese of Exeter, rated in the king's books at £27. 18. 11½., and in the patronage of the Wyndham family. The church, dedicated to St. Mary, has a fine wooden screen and rood-loft.

KENTISBURY, a parish in the hundred of BRAUNTON, county of DEVON, 8 miles (E. by S.) from Ilfracombe, containing 307 inhabitants. The living is a rectory, in the archdeaconry of Barnstaple, and diocese of Exeter, rated in the king's books at £12. 10. 7½. Mr. and Mrs. Sweet were patrons in 1776. There is a place of worship for Baptists. Mary Jones, in 1783, gave a small rent-charge for the instruction of children.

KENTISH-TOWN, a chapelry in the parish of ST. PANCRAS, Holborn division of the hundred of OSSULSTONE, county of MIDDLESEX, 3 miles (N.) from London. The population is returned with the parish. This is a pleasant and populous village between London and Highgate : it consists of several handsome detached houses, with gardens and lawns, and a line of buildings along the road, which is not regularly paved, but lighted with gas. To the south of the village passes the Paddington canal, on the banks of which are coal wharfs. there is a public brewery, and the adjoining fields are chiefly occupied by cow-keepers. The chapel is a neat modern building. There are places of worship for Independents and Wesleyan Methodists. A National school for three hundred children of both sexes, belonging to this place and Camden Town, is supported by subscription.

KENTMERE, a chapelry in that part of the parish of KENDAL which is in KENDAL ward, county of WESTMORLAND, 9 miles (N. N. W.) from Kendal, containing 212 inhabitants. The living is a perpetual curacy, in the archdeaconry of Richmond, and diocese of Chester, endowed with £200 private benefaction, and £600 royal bounty, and in the patronage of the Land-owners. There are quarries of blue slate and limestone in this township. The river Kent, which rises a little to the northward, forms a lake here one mile in length. Bernard Gilpin, an eminent divine, was born at this place in 1517.

KENTON, a parish in the hundred of EXMINSTER, county of DEVON, 8¾ miles (S. S. E.) from Exeter, containing 1891 inhabitants. The living is a vicarage, in the archdeaconry and diocese of Exeter, rated in the king's books at £34. 13. 4., and in the patronage of the Dean and Chapter of Salisbury. The church, dedicated to All Saints, is a handsome structure in the later style of

English architecture, and has a rich wooden screen, on which is inscribed the Creed, in Latin. There is a chapel of ease at Star-cross, in this parish. The river Ex is navigable for large ships along the eastern boundary of the parish. Kenton was once an ancient borough, and had a weekly market and an annual fair. Courts leet and baron are held annually by the lord of the manor. A curious custom prevails here regarding tenancy, by which the heirs of a tenant, retaining their occupancy for three descents in succession, establish their claim to the inheritance.

KENTON, a township comprising East and West Kenton, in that part of the parish of Gosforth which is in the western division of Castle ward, county of Northumberland, 3¾ miles (N. W. by N.) from Newcastle upon Tyne, containing 1204 inhabitants.

KENTON, a parish in the hundred of Loes, county of Suffolk, 2¾ miles (N. N. E.) from Debenham, containing 252 inhabitants. The living is a vicarage, in the archdeaconry of Suffolk, and diocese of Norwich, rated in the king's books at £8, and in the patronage of Lord Henniker. The church is dedicated to All Saints.

KENWYN, a parish in the western division of the hundred of Powder, county of Cornwall, ½ a mile (N. W.) from Truro, containing, with a portion of the town of Truro, which is in this parish, 6221 inhabitants. The living is a vicarage, united to that of St. Kea, in the archdeaconry of Cornwall, and diocese of Exeter, rated in the king's books at £16. The church, dedicated to St. Cuby, has lately received an addition of one hundred sittings, of which sixty are free, the Incorporated Society for the enlargement of churches and chapels having granted £50 towards defraying the expense. This parish comprises a considerable part of the environs of the town of Truro.

KENYON, a township in the parish of Winwick, hundred of West Derby, county palatine of Lancaster, 1 mile (E. N. E.) from Newton in Mackerfield, containing 396 inhabitants.

KEPWICK, a township in the parish of Over Silton, wapentake of Birdforth, North riding of the county of York, 7½ miles (N. N. E.) from Thirsk, containing 170 inhabitants.

KERDISTON, a parish in the hundred of Eynsford, county of Norfolk, 1½ mile (N. W. by N.) from Reepham, containing 160 inhabitants. The living is a discharged rectory, with that of Reepham, not rated in the king's books, in the archdeaconry of Norfolk, and diocese of Norwich. The church is dedicated to St. Mary.

KERESLEY, a hamlet in that part of the parish of St. Michael which is in the county of the city of Coventry, 3 miles (N. N. W.) from Coventry, containing 386 inhabitants.

KERMINCHAM, a township in the parish of Swettenham, hundred of Northwich, county palatine of Chester, 5½ miles (N. W.) from Congleton, containing 176 inhabitants.

KERSALL, a hamlet in that part of the parish of Kneesall which is in the northern division of the wapentake of Thurgarton, county of Nottingham, 6 miles (S. E.) from Ollerton, containing 82 inhabitants. This place is in the honour of Tutbury, duchy of Lancaster, and within the jurisdiction of a court of pleas held at Tutbury every third Tuesday, for the recovery of debts under 40s.

KERSEY, a parish in the hundred of Cosford, county of Suffolk, 1¾ mile (N. W. by W.) from Hadleigh, containing 621 inhabitants. The living is a perpetual curacy, in the archdeaconry of Sudbury, and diocese of Norwich, and in the patronage of the Provost and Fellows of King's College, Cambridge. The church is dedicated to St. Mary. In 1580, Robert Nightingale bequeathed 40s. per annum for the instruction of poor children, also a tenement, since rebuilt by the parish, for the residence of three poor families. Here was a priory of canons of the order of St. Augustine, dedicated to St. Mary and St. Anthony, but the periods of its foundation and dissolution are unknown.

KERSWELL (ABBOT'S), a parish in the hundred of Haytor, county of Devon, 1¾ mile (S.) from Newton-Bushel, containing 437 inhabitants. The living is a vicarage, in the archdeaconry of Totness, and diocese of Exeter, rated in the king's books at £11. 1. 3., and in the patronage of the Crown. The church is dedicated to St. Mary. A Cluniac priory was founded here subordinate to the priory of Montacute in Somersetshire.

KERSWELL (KING'S), a parish in the hundred of Haytor, county of Devon, 2¾ miles (S. E. by S.) from Newton-Bushel, containing 679 inhabitants. The living is a perpetual curacy, with the vicarage of St. Mary Church, in the archdeaconry of Totness, and diocese of Exeter, and in the patronage of the Dean and Chapter of Exeter. The church is dedicated to St. Mary. There is a place of worship for Independents, and another for Wesleyan Methodists. A school-house, built by the Rev. A. Hick, is supported by voluntary contributions.

KESGRAVE, a parish in the hundred of Carlford, county of Suffolk, 3¾ miles (E. by N.) from Ipswich, containing 102 inhabitants. The living is a perpetual curacy, in the archdeaconry of Suffolk, and diocese of Norwich, endowed with £800 royal bounty, and £400 parliamentary grant, and in the patronage of Sir J. G. Shaw, Bart.

KESSINGLAND, a parish in the hundred of Mutford and Lothingland, county of Suffolk, 5¼ miles (S. S. W.) from Lowestoft, containing 579 inhabitants. The living is a discharged vicarage, in the archdeaconry of Suffolk, and diocese of Norwich, rated in the king's books at £10, and in the patronage of the Bishop of Norwich. The church is dedicated to St. Edmund. There is a place of worship for Wesleyan Methodists. This parish is bounded by the North sea on the east, where there is a signal station.

KESTON, a parish in the hundred of Ruxley, lathe of Sutton at Hone, county of Kent, 5 miles (S. by E.) from Bromley, containing 252 inhabitants. The living is a discharged rectory, in the exempt deanery of Shoreham, which is under the peculiar jurisdiction and patronage of the Archbishop of Canterbury, rated in the king's books at £6. 10. Holwood hill, the residence of the late Rt. Hon. William Pitt, occupies an eminence in this parish, and commands a delightful prospect of the surrounding country: here are traces of a camp nearly two miles in circumference, supposed to have been a *Castra æstiva* of the Romans, and Roman coins, tiles, and bricks, with two stone coffins, have been found at different periods. Here is a fine cold spring, called Ravensbourne, the water of which is considered to possess excellent tonic properties.

KESWICK, a market town in that part of the parish of CROSTHWAITE which is in ALLERDALE ward below Darwent, county of CUMBERLAND, 27 miles (S.S.W.) from Carlisle, and 291 (N.W. by N.) from London, containing 1901 inhabitants. This place is more celebrated for the picturesque beauty of its lake, and the magnificent scenery by which it is surrounded, than for historical interest. Prior to the time of Edward I. it was the property of an ancient family, one of whose descendants in the female line, in the reign of James II., was created Earl of Derwentwater. James, the third earl, having taken part in the rebellion of 1715, was, in the early part of the following year, beheaded on Tower hill, and his large estates being forfeited to the crown, were settled upon the commissioners of Greenwich hospital, to whom the manor now belongs. The town is romantically situated in a deep valley, on the banks of the lake Derwentwater, embosomed in hills of various elevations, and sheltered by the towering Skiddaw, which crowns the lofty range of mountains that bounds the northern extremity of the vale. The houses, though chiefly of stone and generally well built, are rather neat than handsome in their appearance. A neat market-house, crowned with a turret, was erected, in 1814, by the commissioners of Greenwich hospital, for the transaction of the public business; and there are some good inns and respectable lodging-houses for the accommodation of the numerous parties that make this town the principal station in their tour of the Lakes. There are two museums, both well supplied with specimens of the most curious and valuable minerals and fossils with which this part of the country abounds. An annual regatta takes place on the last Thursday and Friday in August, the sports chiefly consisting of rowing, horse-racing, and wrestling.

The lake Derwentwater, which is within less than a mile of the town, and separated from it by rising ground, is nearly three miles and a half in length, and one mile and a half in breadth, of an irregularly elliptical form, and equally remarkable for the perfect tranquillity and brilliant transparency of its waters, which reflect with additional lustre the beautiful and sublime scenery that adorns its banks. On the bosom of the lake are some picturesque islands, of the richest verdure and most luxuriant foliage. Lord's island, of five acres in extent, was formerly the site of a noble mansion belonging to the Earls of Derwentwater, the foundations of which, now the only remains, may, with difficulty, be distinguished in the woods by which they are overspread. Vicar's island, containing six acres, anciently belonged to the abbey of Fountains, at the dissolution of which it was given, by Henry VIII., to John Williamson, Esq., and was for some time inhabited by a company of Dutch miners: it is now elegantly laid out in plantations and pleasure grounds, in the centre of which is a handsome villa, the residence of General Peachy. Herbert's island, comprising four acres, was so called from its having been for many years the site of a hermitage occupied by that saint, of whose cell there are still some faint remains, though almost concealed in the recesses of a thick grove: in honour of the saint, Appleby, Bishop of Carlisle, granted forty days remission of penance to all who should visit the hermitage on the anniversary of his decease. About twenty years since, the late Sir Wilfred Lawson, Bart. built a small grotto, or fishing-

cottage, on this beautiful island, which is almost in the centre of the lake. There is also an island, called the Floating island, which occasionally rises from the bottom, but constantly adhering by its sides to the earth beneath, it never changes its position: it is covered with reeds and rushes interspersed with a variety of aquatic plants, and forms by its sterility a striking contrast to the others. The smooth surface of the lake is occasionally disturbed by a visible agitation of the water, when there is not a breath of wind in any part, and when the atmosphere is perfectly calm: this phenomenon is called the "Bottom Wind," but the cause of it has not been satisfactorily ascertained. The lake, through which the river Derwent has its course, also receives the waters which in heavy rains issue in torrents from the fells of Borrowdale, by which it is bounded on the south: these falls present a spectacle of awful grandeur, the torrent tumbling over huge abrupt masses of rugged cliffs, separated by a tremendous chasm; and near the south-east extremity of the lake are the falls of Lowdore, an immense amphitheatre of precipices, from which the waters, rushing with impetuosity, and frequently interrupted in their descent by projecting rocks, form a stupendous cataract, the roar of which, when the violence is aggravated in rainy seasons, may be heard for many miles. At the extremities of the fall are Gowder crag, five hundred feet in height, of rude and terrific aspect, and Shepherd's crag, in the fissures of which are almost every variety of forest trees, plants, and flowers, growing with wild luxuriance. Within this concave range of rugged cliffs is a powerful echo, of which the numerous reverberations are repeated with great force and distinctness of articulation; a cannon discharged in this situation produces, on its explosion, an effect equal to that of a park of artillery, the successive reverberations continuing with diminished force until they gradually die away. The northern extremity of the lake is characterised by features of majestic grandeur and romantic beauty, the more prominent of which are the Skiddaw and Saddleback mountains; the former, three thousand and twenty-two feet above the level of the sea, of a dark-coloured slate interspersed with verdure, in several parts affording pasturage for sheep, and terminating with a double apex almost constantly enveloped in mist; the latter, undulating with graceful curve to the height of two thousand seven hundred and eighty-nine feet, of similar hue with Skiddaw, and having its northern declivity covered with herbage, and overspread with various mountain plants. In the distance, the Carrock Fell, two thousand two hundred and ninety feet in height, is seen among the interesting group of objects which add so much beauty and magnificence to the scenery for which Keswick and its vicinity are so deservedly celebrated.

The manufacture of woollen goods is carried on to some extent, consisting chiefly of kerseys, swansdowns, toilinets, blankets, &c.: there are also a carpet manufactory, and a manufactory for black-lead pencils, the material for which is obtained in the celebrated mine at Borrowdale, in this neighbourhood. The mountains abound in mineral wealth: a mine of lead is now in successful operation a little below the lake; and upon Greta river, which passes by the town, are corn-mills, and a forge for the manufacture of spades, scythes, and edge tools. The market, held on Saturday, is very considerable for corn, which is pitched; and, in addition to the varieties of fish which the lake produces in abundance, it is supplied with mutton of superior flavour, and with provisions of every description. The old shambles, which stood at the northern end of the town-hall, were pulled down in 1815, when new ones were erected. The fairs are on the Saturdays before Whitsuntide and Martinmas, for hiring servants; and on the Saturday next after October 29th, for cheese and sheep: on the first Thursday in May, and every other Thursday for six weeks following, there are small fairs for horses and cattle, and a large cattle market is held on the 11th of October. The commissioners of the hospital hold a copyhold court, and a court baron in May and October, for the recovery of debts under 40s. The parish church stands about three quarters of a mile north-westward from the town. There are places of worship for Independents and Wesleyan Methodists in the town, and adjoining it is a building formerly used as a place of worship by the Society of Friends, but now a school of industry for girls. About a mile to the south, on an eminence, the summit of which forms a level plain of considerable extent, is a supposed Druidical temple. Sir John Banks, Lord Chief Justice in the reign of Charles I., was born here, in 1589; during his absence from home, Corfe Castle, where he then resided, was defended against the parliamentarians by the intrepidity of Lady Banks and her daughters, who, assisted only by their domestics, kept possession of it until relieved by the royal forces. The workhouse for the parish was founded by Sir John Banks, who in 1644 bequeathed £200 for building a manufactory, and lands now producing £200 per annum, for employing the poor. Robert Southey, L.L.D., the poet-laureat, resides at Greta hall, near Keswick. William Green, an eminent landscape painter, who published, in two volumes, a description of the Lakes in Cumberland, Lancashire, and Westmorland, was for sixteen years a resident at this place.

KESWICK, a parish in the hundred of HUMBLE-YARD, county of NORFOLK, 3 miles (S. S. W.) from Norwich, containing 104 inhabitants. The living is a rectory, with that of Intwood, in the archdeaconry of Norfolk, and diocese of Norwich, rated in the king's books at £5. J. Musket, Esq. was patron in 1789. The church is dedicated to St. Mary.

KESWICK (EAST), a township in that part of the parish of HAREWOOD which is in the lower division of the wapentake of SKYRACK, West riding of the county of YORK, 4 miles (S. W.) from Wetherby, containing 296 inhabitants. Here is a place of worship for Wesleyan Methodists.

KETSBY, a parish in the hundred of HILL, parts of LINDSEY, county of LINCOLN, 8½ miles (N. N. W.) from Spilsby, containing, with the parish of South Ormsby, 261 inhabitants. The living is a rectory, with that of South Ormsby, united in 1774 to the vicarage of Calceby and the rectory of Driby, in the archdeaconry and diocese of Lincoln. The church, which was dedicated to St. Margaret, is in ruins.

KETTERING, a market town and parish in the hundred of HUXLOE, county of NORTHAMPTON, 15 miles (N. E. by N.) from Northampton, and 75 (N. W.) from London, on the high road from London to Leeds, containing 3668 inhabitants. The Saxon name of this town was *Cytringham*, the etymology of which is uncertain. At the Norman survey the manor and church belonged to the abbey of Burgh, or Peterborough, and continued in the possession of that house until the dissolution. The town, which is but indifferently built, is situated on the declivity of a hill, at the foot of which flows a small stream, that joins the Ice brook, a branch of the river Nen. The market-place is a spacious area, surrounded by good private houses and respectable shops. A reading-society, or book-club, has been established for half a century; and another has recently been formed, for the middling and lower classes of the inhabitants. The manufacture of shoes has been carried on for many years, affording employment to a considerable number of persons: wool stapling and combing, and the spinning of worsted yarn, are extensively pursued; the weaving of silk shag for hats has been recently introduced, and a few persons are employed in the weaving of ribands and Persians: there are also two brush manufactories. The market is on Friday; and fairs are held on the Thursday before Easter, Friday before Whit-Sunday, Thursday before Old Michaelmas-day, and the Thursday before the festival of St. Thomas. Courts leet and baron are held annually for the appointment of constables and other officers; and the petty sessions for Kettering division are holden usually once a fortnight. The living is a discharged rectory, in the archdeaconry of Northampton, and diocese of Peterborough, rated in the king's books at £34. 13. 4., endowed with £200 private benefaction, and £200 royal bounty, and in the patronage of Lord Sondes. The church, which is dedicated to St. Peter, is a handsome edifice in the later style of English architecture, with a fine tower at the west end, having double buttresses, and octagonal turrets at the angles, and surmounted by an octagonal crocketed spire: round the base of the spire, and connected with the angular turrets, is an embattled parapet, enclosing a walk which commands an extensive and beautiful prospect. There are places of worship for Baptists, the Society of Friends, Independents, and Wesleyan Methodists. A free grammar school for poor children of this parish is endowed with land producing about £120 per annum, the benefaction of a person unknown. There is likewise a small charity school for girls; and a National school is supported by voluntary contributions. An hospital for six poor widows was founded by Mr. Sawyer, in 1688, and subsequently endowed by Martha Baker and others. Mrs. Rachael Sawyer bequeathed £100, directing the interest to be applied in apprenticing poor children; and there are several other bequests for charitable purposes. In 1726, several coins were discovered here of Trajan, Marcus Aurelius, Constantine, and other Roman emperors; also of Carausius, who assumed the purple in Britain; together with a brass seal having the figure of St. Michael engraved on it, and other antique remains. Dr. John Gill, an eminent oriental and biblical scholar, was born here in 1697.

KETTERINGHAM, a parish in the hundred of HUMBLEYARD, county of NORFOLK, 3¾ miles (E. by N.) from Wymondham, containing 175 inhabitants. The living is a discharged vicarage, in the archdeaconry of Norfolk, and diocese of Norwich, rated in the king's books at £6. E. Atkins, Esq. was patron in 1786. The church is dedicated to St. Peter.

KETTLEBASTON, a parish in the hundred of Cosford, county of SUFFOLK, $2\frac{1}{4}$ miles (N. W. by W.) from Bildeston, containing 190 inhabitants. The living is a discharged rectory, in the archdeaconry of Sudbury, and diocese of Norwich, rated in the king's books at £13. 6. 8. The Rev. Thomas Fiske was patron in 1801. The church is dedicated to St. Mary. The children of a Sunday school in this parish are partially clothed by means of a small rent-charge.

KETTLEBURGH, a parish in the hundred of LOES, county of SUFFOLK, $2\frac{1}{4}$ miles (S. W. by S.) from Framlingham, containing 360 inhabitants. The living is a rectory, in the archdeaconry of Suffolk, and diocese of Norwich, rated in the king's books at £16, and in the patronage of the Earl of Gosford. The church is dedicated to St. Andrew. The river Deben runs through this parish.

KETTLEBY, a hamlet in the parish of WRAWBY, southern division of the wapentake of YARBOROUGH, parts of LINDSEY, county of LINCOLN, $2\frac{3}{4}$ miles (E. by N.) from Glandford-Bridge. The population is returned with the parish.

KETTLESHULME, a township in the parish of PRESTBURY, hundred of MACCLESFIELD, county palatine of CHESTER, $6\frac{3}{4}$ miles (N. E.) from Macclesfield, containing 354 inhabitants. The Wesleyan Methodists have a place of worship here. There is a small endowment for the instruction of children.

KETTLESTON, a parish in the hundred of GALLOW, county of NORFOLK, $3\frac{1}{4}$ miles (E. N. E.) from Fakenham, containing 230 inhabitants. The living is a discharged rectory, in the archdeaconry of Norfolk, and diocese of Norwich, rated in the king's books at £10, and in the patronage of the Crown. The church is dedicated to All Saints.

KETTLETHORPE, a parish in the wapentake of WELL, parts of LINDSEY, county of LINCOLN, $9\frac{1}{2}$ miles (W. N. W.) from Lincoln, containing, with the hamlets of Fenton and Laughton, 399 inhabitants. The living is a rectory, in the archdeaconry of Stow, and diocese of Lincoln, rated in the king's books at £28. Sir W. A. Ingilby, Bart. was patron in 1806. The church is dedicated to St. Peter and St. Paul.

KETTLEWELL, a parish in the eastern division of the wapentake of STAINCLIFFE and EWCROSS, West riding of the county of YORK, 16 miles (N. E.) from Settle, containing, with the township of Starbotton, 663 inhabitants. The living is a discharged vicarage, in the archdeaconry and diocese of York, rated in the king's books at £5, endowed with £200 private benefaction, and £200 royal bounty. R. Tennant, Esq. was patron in 1786. The church, dedicated to St. Mary, has lately received an addition of one hundred and fourteen sittings, of which seventy-one are free, the Incorporated Society for the enlargement of churches and chapels having granted £100 towards defraying the expense. A school was built by Solomon Swale, and endowed with property for its repair; three children are instructed by means of a rent-charge of 30s. per annum, the donor of which is unknown.

KETTON, a township in the parish of LAMPLUGH, ALLERDALE ward above Darwent, county of CUMBERLAND, 8 miles (E.) from Whitehaven. The population is returned with the parish.

KETTON, a parish in EAST hundred, county of RUTLAND, 4 miles (S. W. by W.) from Stamford, containing 797 inhabitants. The living is a discharged vicarage, with the curacy of Tixover, rated in the king's books at £8, endowed with £200 private benefaction, and £200 royal bounty, and in the peculiar jurisdiction and patronage of the Prebendary of Ketton in the Cathedral Church of Lincoln. The church, dedicated to St. Mary, is principally in the early style of English architecture, but at the west end is an intermixture of Norman; the date of the south porch is 1232. Here is a place of worship for Independents. In 1791, Sophia Eliz. Edwards gave £1000 three per cents. for the support of a school of industry.

KEVERNE (ST.), a parish in the hundred of KERRIER, county of CORNWALL, $9\frac{1}{2}$ miles (S. by W.) from Falmouth, containing 2505 inhabitants. The living is a vicarage, in the archdeaconry of Cornwall, and diocese of Exeter, rated in the king's books at £18. 11. $5\frac{1}{2}$. The Rev. James Pascoe was patron in 1817. There is a place of worship for Wesleyan Methodists. A school was founded and endowed, in 1698, by Sampson Sandys, for teaching and apprenticing poor children, which has received subsequent augmentations: the master receives a stipend of £15 per annum; and there are six reading-schools in the parish, with small salaries for the teachers. In this parish also are three fishing coves, named Coverack, Porthalla, and Porthonstock, at the first of which there is a good pier for small vessels. A fair for cattle is held on the first Tuesday after Twelfth-day. The English channel bounds the parish on the east and south: there is a signal station at the extreme southern point, called Blackhead. Here was formerly a college of Secular canons, dedicated to St. Achelran, and subsequently a cell of Cistercian monks, subordinate to Beaulieu abbey in Hampshire.

KEVERSTONE, a joint township with Raby, in the parish of STAINDROP, south-western division of DARLINGTON ward, county palatine of DURHAM, 7 miles (N. E. by E.) from Barnard-Castle, containing 203 inhabitants.

KEW, a parish in the second division of the hundred of KINGSTON, county of SURREY, $6\frac{1}{2}$ miles (W. by S.) from London, containing 683 inhabitants. The village is pleasantly situated on the southern bank of the Thames, over which a handsome stone bridge of seven arches, replacing a former structure of wood, was erected in 1789, connecting it with Brentford. George III., who resided for a considerable length of time in a mansion since called the Nursery, in which most of the royal family were brought up, and in which his consort Queen Charlotte died, greatly improved and extended the gardens, which he united to those of Richmond, and began to erect a royal palace in the ancient style of English architecture, which, after remaining for several years in an unfinished state, was taken down in 1828. The royal gardens, which are supposed to contain one of the most extensive and complete collections of exotic plants in Europe, are tastefully laid out, and embellished with temples of the various orders of Grecian architecture, a Turkish mosque, and a Chinese pagoda of considerable elevation, from the summit of which a most extensive prospect is obtained of the scenery on the banks of the Thames, and of the surrounding country. The Dukes of Cumberland and Cambridge have residences on the south side of the green, and in the environs are several handsome villas. Kew, formerly a chapelry to Kingston, was constituted a separate parish by act of parliament in 1770. The living is a vicarage, with the perpetual curacy of Petersham, in the archdeaconry of Surrey, and diocese of Winchester, endowed with £600 private benefaction, and £600 royal bounty, and in the patronage of the Provost and Fellows of King's College, Cambridge. The church, dedicated to St.Anne, was built by subscription among the inhabitants, in 1714, on a site given by Queen Anne, as a chapel of ease to the vicarage of Kingston, and made parochial in 1770 : it was enlarged by George III., who built the side aisles and the portico; and his late Majesty, George IV., erected the organ gallery, and presented to the parish the organ on which his royal father had been accustomed to play. The free school was founded, in 1721, by Dorothy, Lady Capel, who endowed it with one-twelfth part of an estate at Faversham, at present producing about £450 per annum, which sum is divided by her trustees in the church at Kew among twelve parishes, of which Kew is one: the sum arising to each is £37.10., which, augmented by annual subscriptions, is appropriated to the instruction of nineteen boys, of whom two are apprenticed yearly : the school-house was erected in 1824, to which his late Majesty munificently contributed, and granted it the appellation of "The King's Free School."

KEW (ST.), a parish in the hundred of TRIGG, county of CORNWALL, 4¼ miles (N. E. by N.) from Wade Bridge, containing 1218 inhabitants. The living is a vicarage, in the archdeaconry of Cornwall, and diocese of Exeter, rated in the king's books at £19. 11. 0½., T. Pitt, Esq. was patron in 1777. The church, dedicated to St. Kew, has considerable remains of painted glass. There is a small sum for the instruction of children. The river Camel, on the south of this parish, is navigable to Padstow and the Bristol channel.

KEWSTOKE, a parish in the hundred of WINTERSTOKE, county of SOMERSET, 9½ miles (N.W.) from Axbridge, containing 429 inhabitants. The living is a discharged vicarage, in the archdeaconry of Wells, and diocese of Bath and Wells, rated in the king's books at £9. 12. 6., and in the patronage of the Crown. The church, dedicated to St. Paul, is in the later style of English architecture, with Norman portions. A priory of Augustine canons was founded here about 1210, by William de Courtenay, and dissolved in 1534, when its revenue was valued at £110. 18. 4¾.: the remains of the monastic buildings, now principally converted into a farm-house, are the chapel, refectory, and barn.

KEXBOROUGH, a township in the parish of DARTON, wapentake of STAINCROSS, West riding of the county of YORK, 3½ miles (N. W. by W.) from Barnesley, containing 440 inhabitants. John Sylvester, Esq. erected a school, and endowed it with a rent-charge of £5 per annum, for which eight children are instructed.

KEXBY, a township in the parish of UPTON, wapentake of WELL, parts of LINDSEY, county of LINCOLN, 5½ miles (S.E.) from Gainsborough, containing 171 inhabitants.

KEXBY, a township in that part of the parish of CATTON which is in the wapentake of OUZE and DERWENT, East riding of the county of YORK, 6 miles (E.) from York, containing 149 inhabitants.

KEYHAM, a chapelry in that part of the parish of

ROTHLEY which is in the eastern division of the hundred of GOSCOTE, county of LEICESTER, 5¾ miles (E. by N.) from Leicester, containing 210 inhabitants. This chapelry is within the peculiar jurisdiction of the Lord of the Manor of Rothley.

KEYHAVEN, a tything in that part of the parish of MILFORD which is in the hundred of CHRISTCHURCH, New Forest (West) division of the county of SOUTHAMPTON, 2¼ miles (S. S. W.) from Lymington. The population is returned with the parish.

KEYINGHAM, a parish in the southern division of the wapentake of HOLDERNESS, East riding of the county of YORK, 5 miles (S. E. by E.) from Hedon, containing 639 inhabitants. The living is a discharged vicarage, in the archdeaconry of the East riding, and diocese of York, rated in the king's books at £12, endowed with £600 royal bounty, and £1200 parliamentary grant, and in the patronage of the Archbishop of York. The church is dedicated to St. Nicholas. There is a place of worship for Wesleyan Methodists. In 1802, Edward Ombler, Esq. bequeathed £200, directing the interest to be appropriated to the education of children ; and in 1807, Edward Marriott bequeathed the residue of his estate, amounting to £255 four per cents. for a similar purpose.

KEYMER, a parish comprising North and South Keymer, in the hundred of BUTTINGHILL, rape of LEWES, county of SUSSEX, 2¼ miles (E. S. E.) from Hurstpierrepoint, containing 679 inhabitants. The living is a perpetual curacy, annexed to the rectory of Clayton, in the archdeaconry of Lewes, and diocese of Chichester. The church is in the early style of English architecture.

KEYNE (ST.), a parish in the hundred of WEST, county of CORNWALL, 2½ miles (S.) from Leskeard, containing 153 inhabitants. The living is a discharged rectory, in the archdeaconry of Cornwall, and diocese of Exeter, rated in the king's books at £5. 18. 6½., and in the patronage of Lieut. Cory, R. N. The church is dedicated to St. Kayne, who lived in the fifth century, and is said to have been the daughter of Braganus, Prince of Brecknockshire. Near the church is St. Kayne's well, long celebrated in legendary tales for its peculiar virtues : the roof of the enclosure supports, in a singular manner, five trees, two of oak, two of ash, and one of elm, planted more than half a century ago. The Looe navigation passes on the eastern side of this parish.

KEYNSHAM, a parish (formerly a market town) in the hundred of KEYNSHAM, county of SOMERSET, 7¼ miles (W. N. W.) from Bath, containing 1761 inhabitants. The living is a discharged vicarage, in the archdeaconry of Bath, and diocese of Bath and Wells, rated in the king's books at £11. 19.'7., endowed with £200 royal bounty, and in the patronage of the Duke of Buckingham. The church is a spacious edifice in the later style of English architecture. The town is situated upon the river Avon, which is navigable hence to Bath, and across it is a bridge leading into Gloucestershire : on this river are some mills belonging to a brass and copper company at Bristol. A court leet is held for the hundred ; also a hundred court for the recovery of debts under 40s. There are places of worship for Baptists and Wesleyan Methodists. A schoolroom was built, in 1705, by Sir Thomas Bridges, and endowed with £500, for the education of twenty poor boys : he likewise founded an almshouse for six poor widows, who receive £4 each per annum. An abbey of Black canons was founded, by William, Earl of Gloucester, about 1170, and dedicated to the Virgin Mary, St. Peter, and St. Paul : its revenue, at the dissolution, was valued at £450. 3. 6. In this parish is a mineral spring of reputed efficacy in ophthalmia.

KEYSOE, a parish in the hundred of STODDEN, county of BEDFORD, 4½ miles (S.S.W.) from Kimbolton, containing 649 inhabitants. The living is a discharged vicarage, in the archdeaconry of Bedford, and diocese of Lincoln, rated in the king's books at £8, endowed with £200 private benefaction, and £200 royal bounty, and in the patronage of the Master and Fellows of Trinity College, Cambridge. The church is dedicated to St. Mary. There is a place of worship for Baptists.

KEYSTON, a parish in the hundred of LEIGHTON-STONE, county of HUNTINGDON, 3¼ miles (S.E. by E.) from Thrapston, containing 196 inhabitants. The living is a rectory, in the archdeaconry of Huntingdon, and diocese of Lincoln, rated in the king's books at £29. 5. Earl Fitzwilliam was patron in 1807. The church is dedicated to St. John the Baptist.

KEYTHORPE, a liberty in that part of the parish of TUGBY which is in the hundred of GARTREE, county of LEICESTER, 9 miles (N. by E.) from Market-Harborough, containing 26 inhabitants.

KEYWORTH, a parish in the northern division of the wapentake of RUSHCLIFFE, county of NOTTINGHAM, 6¾ miles (S.S.E.) from Nottingham, containing 454 inhabitants. The living is a rectory, in the archdeaconry of Nottingham, and diocese of York, rated in the king's books at £7. 5., and in the patronage of H. Keyworth, Esq. The church, dedicated to St. Mary Magdalene, has a curious tower, with one smaller erected upon it. There are places of worship for Independents. This parish is in the honour of Tutbury, duchy of Lancaster, and within the jurisdiction of a court of pleas held at Tutbury every third Tuesday, for the recovery of debts under 40s.

KIBBLESTONE, a liberty in the parish of STONE, southern division of the hundred of PIREHILL, county of STAFFORD, containing 1089 inhabitants. This was anciently a large park, and there are still the vestiges of some large fish-ponds, one of which supplies a stream that falls into the Trent at Walton bridge, turning in its course several mills for grinding flints used at the potteries. At Meaford, within this liberty, is an old mansion, long possessed by the Jervis family, in which the gallant admiral, Earl St. Vincent, was born, and which is now occupied by his nephew, Viscount St. Vincent, Baron Meaford. There is a petrifying spring issuing out of the rocks near Catwalton.

KIBBLESWORTH, a township in that part of the parish of CHESTER le STREET which is in the middle division of CHESTER ward, county palatine of DURHAM, 5 miles (S.) from Gateshead, containing 237 inhabitants.

KIBWORTH-BEAUCHAMP, a parish in the hundred of GARTREE, county of LEICESTER, 5¼ miles (N. W.) from Market-Harborough, comprising the chapelry of Kibworth-Harcourt, and the township of Smeeton-Westerby, and containing 1372 inhabitants. The living is a rectory, in the archdeaconry of Leicester, and diocese of Lincoln, rated in the king's books at £39. 15., and in the patronage of the Warden and Fellows of Merton College, Oxford. The church, dedicated

to St. Wilfrid, is a spacious edifice, with a tower supporting a spire nearly one hundred and sixty feet high. There are places of worship for Independents and Wesleyan Methodists. A free grammar school was founded, in 1709, by Sir Nathaniel Edwards; the school-house was rebuilt in 1775. The Union canal passes through the parish ; and at Smeeton-Westerby there is a small chalybeate spring. Dr. John Aikin, an ingenious physician and public writer, (brother of Mrs. Barbauld and of Lucy Aikin, likewise celebrated authoress of several valuable works,) was born here in 1747, and died at Stoke-Newington in 1822.

KIBWORTH-HARCOURT, a chapelry in the parish of KIBWORTH-BEAUCHAMP, hundred of GARTREE, county of LEICESTER, 5½ miles (N.W. by N.) from Market-Harborough, containing 396 inhabitants. The chapel has been demolished. In this chapelry are the remains of an ancient encampment, consisting of a large mount encompassed by a moat.

KIDBROOKE, a liberty (anciently a parish) in the hundred of BLACKHEATH, lathe of SUTTON at HONE, county of KENT, 2 miles (S.S.W.) from Woolwich, containing 73 inhabitants. Cecilia, Countess of Hereford, in the 5th of Henry VI., gave this place to the prior and convent of St. Mary Overy, in Southwark, who obtained from the Bishop of Rochester a grant of impropriation. In old records, the church, which has long been demolished, is described as a rectory, but a few years since the civil authorities of Charlton endeavoured to shew that Kidbrooke was only a hamlet belonging to that parish : it now chooses its own officers, and maintains its own poor. A free chapel has lately been erected by Dr. Greenlaw, who is the officiating minister. Kidbrooke gives the title of baron to the family of Hervey, Marquises of Bristol.

KIDDAL, a joint township with Potterton, in the parish of BARWICK in ELMETT, lower division of the wapentake of SKYRACK, West riding of the county of YORK, 7½ miles (N.E. by E.) from Leeds, containing 124 inhabitants.

KIDDERMINSTER, a parish in the lower division of the hundred of HALF-SHIRE, county of WORCESTER, comprising the incorporated market town of Kidderminster, having separate jurisdiction, the chapelry of Lower Mitton, and the hamlet of Wribbenhall, and containing 15,296 inhabitants, of which number, 10,709 are in the town of Kidderminster, 14 miles (N.) from Worcester, and 126 (N. W. by N.) from London. Its ancient name was *Chiderminster, Kid, or Chid,* signifying, in ancient British, the brow of a hill, *Dwr,* water, and *Minster,* a church ; an etymology highly characteristic of its situation. At the time of the Conquest it was a royal manor, and continued so until the reign of Henry II., when it passed into private hands, and among its possessors was Waller the poet. The town is situated on the eastern bank of the river Stour, about three miles from its confluence with the Severn : it is of an irregular form, contains several good and well-built houses, but the greater part consists of

Seal and Arms.

small dwellings inhabited by the workmen employed in the different factories. The entrances to the town are spacious; in those from Worcester, Bridgenorth, and Bewdley, where improvements have been made by cutting away the rock to lower the road, houses have been excavated in the sides of the rock. The town is well paved, and lighted with gas, and the inhabitants are amply supplied with water. In the reign of Henry VIII. Kidderminster was noted for the manufacture of broad cloths, to which, at different periods, succeeded linsey-woolseys, friezes, and tammies and flowered stuffs. About the year 1735 the manufacture of carpets was introduced, which has continued to flourish with progressive improvement, and now constitutes the staple trade of the town. On its introduction the Scotch carpets were the principal articles made, but the Wilton and Brussels carpets (the former begun by the grandfather of the present Mr. Broom, in 1745,) have been within the last few years brought to a high degree of perfection : the elegance and variety of the patterns, the brilliancy and permanency of the colours, arising, as it is supposed, from the peculiar property of the water of the Stour in fixing the dyes, and the great improvement in their texture, have given to the carpets of Kidderminster a decided superiority over those of every other place. In 1772, the number of carpet-looms was about two hundred and fifty; at present there are nearly one thousand six hundred. A considerable quantity of carpets is constantly being exported to almost every part of the kingdom. From a return to parliament it appears that, of the whole quantity of wool produced in the kingdom, one twenty-eighth part is consumed here in the weaving of carpets. The trade in bombazines is also carried on, but not to the same extent as formerly : in 1772, here were one thousand seven hundred silk and worsted looms ; at present there are not more than one-fifth of that number. In the town and neighbourhood are five spinning-mills ; but a great quantity of the yarn is obtained from Halifax, and other towns in Yorkshire. On the banks of the Stour are several dye-houses, in connexion with the various manufactories. The Staffordshire and Worcestershire canal passes through the town to Stourport, where it joins the river Severn, by which a medium of conveyance by water is afforded to all parts of the kingdom, and a supply of coal and other useful commodities is obtained. The market days are Thursday, chiefly for corn, and Saturday for provisions : the fairs are, the last Monday in January, the Monday before Easter, Ascension-day, June 20th, September 4th, and the last Monday in November. The market-place [has been greatly enlarged by the corporation, at an expense of £10,000, and is arranged in separate divisions for the various kinds of goods exposed for sale.

Kidderminster was a borough by prescription, and sent members to parliament in the 23rd of Edward I., since which time it has made no return. It received a charter of incorporation in the twelfth year of the reign of Charles I., but the charter at present in force was granted August 31st, 1827, by which the government of the town is vested in a high steward, a recorder, a high bailiff, a low bailiff, twelve aldermen (exclusively of the high bailiff) twenty-five assistants, with a town clerk, constables, &c. The high bailiff is elected annually by the aldermen, from among their own body. A sin-

gular custom has prevailed at the election of this chief magistrate, when the people assemble in the principal streets to throw cabbage stalks at each other : the bell at the town-hall gives the signal for the commencement of the municipal affray, which, from its duration and the mode of procedure, is called the "lawless hour." When it is over, the bailiff elect and the other members of the corporation, in their robes, parade the streets, preceded by flags, drums, and trumpets, inviting the principal families in the neighbourhood to meet and throw apples at them : but this custom has of late been falling into disuse. The high bailiff, the late bailiff, the recorder, and the three senior aldermen, are justices of the peace, and hold quarterly courts of session for the borough, on the Friday in the week in which the general quarter sessions for the county are held, for the trial of all offenders not charged capitally. A court of requests is also held every fortnight, by commissioners appointed under an act passed in the 12th of George III., for the recovery of debts under 40s., the jurisdiction of which extends over the whole parish. The town-hall is a neat building of brick ; the lower part is appropriated as shops, and the upper part to the holding of the courts and the transaction of the public business of the corporation : it also contains a spacious assembly-room, and under the building is a small prison for the confinement of malefactors prior to their committal to the county gaol.

The living is a vicarage with the curacy of Mitton, in the archdeaconry and diocese of Worcester, rated in the king's books at £30. 15. 7½., and in the patronage of Lord Foley. The church, dedicated to St. Mary, is a spacious and venerable structure, partly in the decorated, and partly in the later, style of English architecture, with a handsome square embattled tower, strengthened with buttresses, and crowned with pinnacles : the walls of the nave and aisles are finished with panelled battlements, and the whole exterior of the building, which occupies the summit of a hill overlooking the river, has an imposing grandeur of appearance ; the chancel, which is in the decorated style, contains several ancient monuments and recumbent figures ; the nave is separated from the aisles by a beautiful series of pointed arches and clustered columns, and lighted by a fine range of clerestory windows enriched with elegant tracery. A new church, dedicated to St. George, and containing two thousand and three sittings, of which one thousand two hundred and eighty-nine are free, was built by grant from the parliamentary commissioners, in 1824, at an expense of £16,131. 4. 2., to which was added £2000 raised by the inhabitants : it is a handsome structure in the later style of English architecture, with a lofty and richly-ornamented tower, and, standing on an eminence, forms a prominent feature in the view of the town : the altar-piece is embellished with a representation of the Descent from the Cross, woven in carpet-work, with exquisite brilliancy of colour and elegance of design, by Mr. Bowyer, a manufacturer in the town, and by him presented to the parish ; but this characteristic piece of workmanship has been wantonly cut in different places by a sacrilegious outrage, of which the perpetrator and his motive have not yet been discovered. The living is a perpetual curacy, in the patronage of the Vicar. Besides the chapel at Mitton, there is a proprietary chapel at Wribbenhall, the living of which is a donative, in the gift of Lord Foley. There are places of worship for Baptists, Independents, Wesleyan Methodists, and Unitarians.

The free grammar school is of uncertain origin: it was made a royal foundation by charter of Charles I., and has an endowment in lands and tenements, from the produce of which the head master receives a salary of £260, and the second master one of £130 per annum: they are chosen by trustees appointed under the charter, and have each a house rent-free, and the privilege of taking private pupils: this school is entitled to the fifth of six scholarships founded in Worcester College, Oxford, by Sir Thomas Cookes, from which the candidates for his fellowships in that college are chosen. An ancient chapel adjoining St. Mary's church has been for many years appropriated to the use of the school. A free school was also founded, in 1795, by Mr. Nicholas Pearsall, who endowed it with a sum of money for providing a salary for the master, by whom twenty-five boys, chiefly dissenters, receive the rudiments of a classical and commercial education. A National school for boys was erected in 1817; and there is one for girls, originally founded as a small charity school in 1730: in the former two hundred and thirty boys, and in the latter one hundred and ninety girls, are taught reading, writing, and arithmetic, and about twenty in each are clothed. St. George's National school was built, in 1827, by subscription, aided by a grant from the National Society, for the instruction of two hundred and fifty children of each sex; and there are various other institutions of a similar kind, supported by subscription, some of which have small endowments. An infant school has been recently established, in which are one hundred and fifty children, but no building has yet been erected for the purpose. The dispensary was established in 1824, and the building erected on a site near the old church, given for that purpose by William Lea, Esq., of Stone: the institution is under the direction of a president, vice-president, and a committee of governors, by whom a resident surgeon is appointed, with a salary of £100 per annum: it receives also the gratuitous attendance of the members of the medical profession in the vicinity. There are six almshouses, founded in 1629, by Sir Edward Blount, for six aged men and their wives, who receive £8 per annum each. H. Higgins, Esq., in 1684, bequeathed four messuages for the same purpose, to which a fifth has been added, for aged persons nominated by the corporation: the inmates live rent-free, but have no pecuniary allowance. Two houses were also given in trust to the corporation for the same use, by Sir Ralph Clare, K.B. There are various charitable donations and bequests for distribution among the poor. On Wassall hill, about half a mile from the bank of the Severn, are the remains of a small camp, supposed by Dr. Nash to have been occupied by Henry IV., in his pursuit of Owen Glyndwr, after the burning of the city of Worcester; and at Blackstone rock, between Stourport and Bewdley, are the remains of a hermitage and chapel, now converted into an out-house for agricultural implements. There are several chalybeate springs in the parish, of which the most strongly impregnated is at Round hill, near the town; and the dropping well, on Burlish common, is celebrated for its efficacy in curing diseases of the eye. Richard Baxter, the celebrated nonconformist, was for some time vicar of this parish;

on being ejected from his ministry, he established an Independent congregation, consisting of a number of his parishioners who, having adhered to his ministry when ejected from his living, are supposed to have formed the first separate church of that denomination.

KIDDINGTON, a parish comprising the hamlet of Over Kiddington in the hundred of CHADLINGTON, and that of Nether Kiddington in the hundred of WOOTTON, county of OXFORD, and containing 252 inhabitants. Nether Kiddington is 3¼ miles (E. S. E.), and Over Kiddington 3¼ (S.E. by E.), from Neat Enstone. The living is a rectory, in the archdeaconry and diocese of Oxford, rated in the king's books at £7. 9. 4½., and in the patronage of Lord Viscount Dillon. The church, dedicated to St. Nicholas, and situated in Nether Kiddington, is supposed to have been built about the year 1400; but the chancel is evidently of earlier date, having probably belonged to the original edifice. In 1466, the emoluments of the ancient rectory of Asterley being considered inadequate for the support of an incumbent, they were formally incorporated with those of this rectory, and thenceforth both parishes became united under the name of Kiddington. There is a farm-house still called Asterley, which claims the privilege of being extra-parochial; and in a large field, termed Chapelbreke, are the supposed sites of the ancient church, mansion-house, and village of Asterley; foundations, mouldings of lancet windows, and other fragments of old masonry, having from time to time been discovered on the spot. A branch of the river Isis runs through the parish. In the gardens of a private mansion in this village is an ancient stone font, found in the chapel of Edward the Confessor at Islip, where was a royal palace, stated, by tradition, to have been that in which the monarch was baptized, in 1010. The ancient road Akeman-street runs through the parish. In Hill wood are visible traces of a Roman encampment; and at other places in the neighbourhood are vestiges of earth-works.

KIDLAND, an extra-parochial liberty, in the western division of COQUETDALE ward, county of NORTHUMBERLAND, 12 miles (N.W. by W.(from Rothbury, containing 62 inhabitants.

KIDLINGTON, a parish in the hundred of WOOTTON, county of OXFORD, 4 miles (E.S.E.) from Woodstock, comprising the townships of Gosford, and Water-Eaton, and the hamlet of Thrup, and containing 1153 inhabitants. The living is a vicarage not in charge, in the archdeaconry and diocese of Oxford, and annexed to the Headship of Exeter College, Oxford. The church is dedicated to St. Mary. There is a small endowment, the bequest of Roger Almont, for teaching two children.

KIGBEAR, a hamlet in that part of the parish of OAKHAMPTON which is in the hundred of BLACK TORRINGTON, county of DEVON, 3½ miles (W. by N.) from Oakhampton, containing 116 inhabitants.

KILBOURNE, a township in the parish of HORSLEY, hundred of MORLESTON and LITCHURCH, county of DERBY, 6¾ miles (N.N.E.) from Derby, containing 498 inhabitants.

KILBURN, a hamlet in the parish of ST. JOHN, HAMPSTEAD, Holborn division of the hundred of OSSULSTONE, county of MIDDLESEX, 3 miles (W.N.W.) from London. The population is returned with the parish. The village, which is situated on the ancient Watling-street, on the road to Edgware, contains some good houses occupied by genteel families, the short distance from the metropolis rendering it a desirable place of residence. There is a medicinal spring, called Kilburn wells, the water of which possesses aperient properties. Near the close of the reign of Henry I., a Benedictine nunnery, dedicated to the Blessed Virgin Mary and St. John the Baptist, was founded here on the site of an ancient hermitage, the revenue of which, at the dissolution, was estimated at £121. 16.

KILBURN, a parish partly in the wapentake of BIRDFORTH, North riding, and partly within the liberty of RIPON, West riding, of the county of YORK, comprising the township of Hood with Osgoodby-Grange, and Kilburn, and containing 530 inhabitants, of which number, 500 are in the township of Kilburn, 7 miles (N. by W.) from Easingwould. The living is a perpetual curacy, in the archdeaconry of Cleveland, and diocese of York, endowed with £200 private benefaction, £200 royal bounty, and £1000 parliamentary grant, and in the patronage of the Archbishop of York. The church is dedicated to St. Mary. There is a trifling sum, the gift of Ann Berry, in 1768, for the education of one girl.

KILBY, a parish in the hundred of GUTHLAXTON, county of LEICESTER, 6½ miles (S.S.E.) from Leicester, containing 409 inhabitants. The living is a perpetual curacy, in the archdeaconry of Leicester, and diocese of Lincoln, endowed with £500 private benefaction, £1000 royal bounty, and £600 parliamentary grant, and in the patronage of Sir H. Halford, Bart. The church is dedicated to St. Mary Magdalene.

KILDALE, a parish in the western division of the liberty of LANGBAURGH, North riding of the county of YORK, 5¾ miles (E. by N.) from Stokesley, containing 209 inhabitants. The living is a discharged rectory, in the archdeaconry of Cleveland, and diocese of York, rated in the king's books at £10. 3. 4. R. Bell Livesay, Esq. was patron in 1811. The church, dedicated to St. Cuthbert, is a very ancient structure, said to have been founded at an early period of the Saxon octarchy : near it is the site of an old castle. About 1312, the friars of the order of the Holy Cross began to erect an oratory here, but the work having been interdicted by Archbishop Grenfield, it was abandoned.

KILDWICK, a parish in the eastern division of the wapentake of STAINCLIFFE and EWCROSS, West riding of the county of YORK, comprising the chapelry of Silsden, and the townships of Bradley's Both, Cowling, Farnhill with Conoley, Glusburn, Kildwick, Steeton with Easburn, Stirton with Thorlby, and Sutton, and containing 8605 inhabitants, of which number, 175 are in the township of Kildwick, 4 miles (S.S.E.) from Skipton. The living is a discharged vicarage, in the peculiar jurisdiction of the Dean of York, rated in the king's books at £10. 8. 1½., endowed with £200 private benefaction, and £200 royal bounty, and in the patronage of the Dean and Canons of Christ Church, Oxford. The church, dedicated to St. Andrew, is principally in the later style of English architecture.

KILGWRRWG, a parish in the upper division of the hundred of RAGLAND, county of MONMOUTH, 5¾ miles (E.S.E.) from Usk, containing 113 inhabitants. The living is a perpetual curacy, in the archdeaconry and diocese of Llandaff, endowed with £800 royal bounty,

and £200 parliamentary grant, and in the patronage of the Rev. Mr. Birkin.

KILHAM, a township in the parish of KIRK-NEWTON, western division of GLENDALE ward, county of NORTHUMBERLAND, 7½ miles (W.N.W.) from Wooler, containing 246 inhabitants.

KILHAM, a parish partly within the liberty of ST. PETER of YORK, and partly in the wapentake of DICKERING, East riding of the county of YORK, 5¼ miles (N. N. E.) from Great Driffield, containing 971 inhabitants. The living is a discharged vicarage, in the peculiar jurisdiction and patronage of the Dean of York, rated in the king's books at £6. 13. 4. The church, dedicated to All Saints, is a stately edifice. There are places of worship for Baptists and Wesleyan Methodists. The town, pleasantly situated on a declivity of the Wolds, now consists of one irregular street, extending from east to west nearly one mile and a quarter, but was once a much larger place, vestiges of foundations having been often discovered. It had anciently a market, which, from the vicinity and greater convenience of that at Great Driffield, had long been declining, and is now entirely discontinued. Fairs for cattle are held on August 21st and November 12th; the latter is also a statute fair. A free school was founded, in the 9th of Charles I., by John, Lord D'Arcy, who endowed it with a rent-charge of £30, for which sum, and trifling quarterages paid by the pupils, from eighty to one hundred children are instructed. A branch of the river Hull has its source in the parish; and at Hempit Hole a remarkable intermittent spring, called the Gipsey, issues with such violence from the earth as to form an arch sufficiently elevated for a man on horseback to pass beneath it. Near the Rudston road is a fine mineral spring, possessing medicinal properties.

KILKHAMPTON, a parish in the hundred of STRATTON, county of CORNWALL, 3½ miles (N. by E.) from Stratton, containing 1024 inhabitants. The living is a rectory, in the archdeaconry of Cornwall, and diocese of Exeter, rated in the king's books at £26. 3. 11½. Lord Carteret was patron in 1810. The church, dedicated to St. James, is remarkable for the singular richness of its architecture, particularly the south doorway, which is a beautiful specimen of the Norman style, exhibiting shafts and bands of zig-zag mouldings, with the beak-headed ornaments; some other portions of the fabric are of much later date : it contains an enriched pulpit, a very ancient font, and several handsome monuments, the most striking of which is one to the memory of the renowned warrior Sir Beville Grenville, Earl of Corbill, and Lord of Thorigny and Grenville, in France and Normandy, descended in a direct line from Robert, second son of Rollo, first Duke of Normandy, and slain in the parliamentary war, at the battle of Lansdown, July 5th, 1643. One of his ancestors, who came over with the Conqueror, is said to have founded the church. This place had anciently a market. There are fairs on Holy Thursday, the third Thursday following, and on August 28th; the first and last are considerable cattle fairs. It is stated that the pious Hervey conceived his "Meditations among the Tombs" at Kilkhampton.

KILLAMARSH, a parish in the hundred of SCARSDALE, county of DERBY, 9 miles (N. E.) from Chesterfield, containing 779 inhabitants. The living is a perpetual curacy, with the rectory of Eckington, in the archdeaconry of Derby, and diocese of Lichfield and Coventry. The church, dedicated to St. Giles, is partly in the Norman style. At the Norman survey this place was called *Chinewoldemaresc*, and the manor was formerly held by the tenure of providing a horse of the value of five shillings, with a sack and a spur, for the king's army in Wales. Robert Turie, in 1720, bequeathed a rent-charge of £7. 10.; which sum, with the produce of sundry other gifts, amounting together of about £22, is paid for the instruction of twenty-five children. The Chesterfield canal, and a railway communicating with the coal mines in the vicinity, pass through the parish.

KILLCOT, a joint tything with Boulsdon, in the parish of NEWENT, hundred of BOTLOE, county of GLOUCESTER, containing 408 inhabitants.

KILLERBY, a township in the parish of HEIGHINGTON, though entirely surrounded by that of Gainford, south-eastern division of DARLINGTON ward, county palatine of DURHAM, 7 miles (N. W. by W.) from Darlington, containing 107 inhabitants.

KILLERBY, a township in that part of the parish of CATTERICK which is in the eastern division of the wapentake of HANG, North riding of the county of YORK, 2 miles (S. E. by E.) from Catterick, containing 48 inhabitants.

KILLINGHALL, a township in that part of the parish of RIPLEY which is in the lower division of the wapentake of CLARO, West riding of the county of YORK, 1 mile (S. by E.) from Ripley, containing 519 inhabitants. There is a place of worship for Wesleyan Methodists.

KILLINGHOLME, a parish comprising North and South Killingholme, in the eastern division of the wapentake of YARBOROUGH, parts of LINDSEY, county of LINCOLN, 12 miles (N. W. by W.) from Great Grimsby, containing 438 inhabitants. The living is a discharged vicarage, with that of Harbrough, in the archdeaconry and diocese of Lincoln, rated in the king's books at £7. 18. 4. Lord Yarborough was patron in 1792. The church is dedicated to St. Denis. There are places of worship for Baptists and Wesleyan Methodists.

KILLINGTON, a chapelry in the parish of KIRKBY-LONSDALE, LONSDALE ward, county of WESTMORLAND, 7¼ miles (N.) from Kirkby-Lonsdale, containing 335 inhabitants. The living is a perpetual curacy, in the archdeaconry of Richmond, and diocese of Chester, endowed with £400 private benefaction, and £600 royal bounty, and in the patronage of the Vicar of Kirkby-Lonsdale. The chapel was re-pewed in 1824. A school is endowed with £7 per annum, for which, and trifling quarterages, sixteen children receive instruction: the school-room was built by subscription. Killington hall, now a farm-house, is an ancient tower-building, long the residence of the Pickerings.

KILLINGWORTH, a township in the parish of LONG BENTON, eastern division of CASTLE ward, county of NORTHUMBERLAND, 5½ miles (N. E. by N.) from Newcastle upon Tyne. The population is returned with the parish. There is a place of worship for Wesleyan Methodists. Coal is obtained here. On Killingworth moor the Newcastle races were held till 1790, when it was enclosed for cultivation.

KILLPECK, a parish in the upper division of the hundred of WORMELOW, county of HEREFORD, 8¾

miles (S. W.) from Hereford, containing 265 inhabitants. The living is a perpetual curacy, in the archdeaconry and diocese of Hereford, rated in the king's books at £4. 11. 8., and in the patronage of the Bishop of Gloucester. The church, dedicated to St. David, has some fine portions in the Norman style of architecture. It was given by Hugh Fitzwilliam (whose family assumed the name of Kilpec), son of the Conqueror, to the abbey of St. Peter, Gloucester, in 1134, and became a cell of Black monks subordinate thereto till its suppression. The ancient castle of the Kilpecs fell early to ruin, since, in the time of Edward I. a part only of the walls was remaining.

KILMERSDON, a parish in the hundred of KILMERSDON, county of SOMERSET, 6 miles (N. W. by W.) from Frome, comprising the hamlets of Charlton, Coleford, Kilmersdon, Kilmersdon-Common, Luckington, and Lypeat, and containing 1991 inhabitants. The living is a discharged vicarage, with the perpetual curacies of Ashwick and Coleford annexed, in the archdeaconry of Wells, and diocese of Bath and Wells, rated in the king's books at £6. 18. 6½., and in the patronage of the Crown. The church, dedicated to St. Peter and St. Paul, is extremely light and elegant, and has a lofty tower. A new church is in progress of erection at Coleford. There are two places of worship for Methodists and one for Presbyterians. The Rev. Thomas Shute, in 1719, gave a rent-charge of £20 towards the support of a school for forty children, to which Mrs. Mary Freeman, in 1760, bequeathed £100, to be placed at interest for repairs and for the purchase of books.

KILMESTON, a parish in the hundred of FAWLEY, Fawley division of the county of SOUTHAMPTON, 4½ miles (S.) from New Alresford, containing 212 inhabitants. The living is a perpetual curacy, with the rectory of Cheriton, in the peculiar jurisdiction of the incumbent. Eight poor children are instructed for a trifling sum left by Dame Mary Sadler. Kilmeston is within the jurisdiction of the Cheyney Court held at Winchester every Thursday, for the recovery of debts to any amount.

KILMINGTON, a parish in the hundred of AX-MINSTER, county of DEVON, 1¾ mile (W. by S.) from Axminster, containing 484 inhabitants. The living is a perpetual curacy, annexed to the vicarage of Axminster, in the archdeaconry and diocese of Exeter. The church is dedicated to St. Giles. The river Axe runs through the parish. There is a fair for cattle on the first Wednesday in September. Kilmington has the privilege of sending two boys to Axminster free school.

KILMINGTON, a parish in, and forming a detached portion of, the hundred of NORTON-FERRIS, county of SOMERSET, 6½ miles (E. by N.) from Bruton, containing 556 inhabitants. The living is a rectory, in the archdeaconry of Wells, and diocese of Bath and Wells, rated in the king's books at £21. 9. 4½. The Earl of Ilchester was patron in 1811. The church is dedicated to St. Mary: in it lie the remains of Mr. Hartgill and his son, both murdered, in the reign of Queen Mary, by Lord Stourton and four others, who were convicted and executed; his lordship at Salisbury, in a silken halter, and his accomplices near the spot where the foul deed was perpetrated. About two miles south-west from the church is a small oval intrenchment, called Jack's Castle, supposed to have been the site of a Danish camp or fortress ; and at the south-western extremity of the parish, near Stourhead, is a triangular brick tower, one hundred and fifty-five feet high, erected, in 1772, by Henry Hoare, Esq., with an inscription commemorative of Alfred the Great and his victories over the Danes.

KILNSAY, a hamlet in the parish of BURNSALL, eastern division of the wapentake of STAINCLIFFE and EWCROSS, West riding of the county of YORK, 11 miles (E. N. E.) from Settle. The population is returned with the chapelry of Coniston.

KILNSEA, a parish in the southern division of the wapentake of HOLDERNESS, East riding of the county of YORK, 8½ miles (S. E. by E.) from Patrington, containing, with Spurn, 196 inhabitants. The living is a discharged vicarage, in the archdeaconry of the East riding, and diocese of York, rated in the king's books at £6. 8. 6½., endowed with £600 royal bounty. L. Thompson, Esq. was patron in 1813. The church, dedicated to St. Helen, has been suffered to fall to ruin, being situated so near the brink of the cliff, upon which the sea is continually encroaching, that it must ultimately have been swept away ; a part of the cemetery having already disappeared.

KILNWICK, a parish in the Bainton-Beacon division of the wapentake of HARTHILL, East riding of the county of YORK, comprising the chapelry of Beswick, and the townships of Bracken, Kilnwick, and a portion of Lockington, and containing 576 inhabitants, of which number, 230 are in the township of Kilnwick, 7 miles (S.S.W.) from Great Driffield. The living is a perpetual curacy, in the archdeaconry of the East riding, and diocese of York. Charles Grimston, Esq. was patron in 1817. The church is dedicated to All Saints.

KILNWICK-PERCY, a parish in the Wilton-Beacon division of the wapentake of HARTHILL, East riding of the county of YORK, 2 miles (E. N. E.) from Pocklington, containing 43 inhabitants. The living is a discharged vicarage, in the peculiar jurisdiction and patronage of the Dean of York, rated in the king's books at £4. 16. 3., and endowed with £600 royal bounty. The church is dedicated to St. Helen.

KILPIN, a township in the parish of HOWDEN, wapentake of HOWDENSHIRE, East riding of the county of YORK, 2 miles (S. E. by E.) from Howden, containing 318 inhabitants.

KILSBY, a parish in the hundred of FAWSLEY, county of NORTHAMPTON, 5½ miles (N. by W.) from Daventry, containing 690 inhabitants. The living is a rectory, annexed to the Precentorship in the Cathedral Church of Lincoln, in the archdeaconry of Northampton, and diocese of Peterborough, rated in the king's books at £14, and endowed with £200 royal bounty : there is also a discharged vicarage, rated in the king's books at £7, and in the patronage of the Precentor. The church is dedicated to St. Faith. There is a place of worship for Independents. The Oxford canal passes through the parish, and the ancient Watling-street marks its western boundary. A bequest from Abraham Cowley, Esq., in land producing £18 a year, is given to the poor in money and bread, a small portion of it being applied also to the instruction of children.

KILTON, a parish in the hundred of WILLITON and FREEMANNERS, county of SOMERSET, 10½ miles (N. W. by W.) from Bridg-water, containing 149 inha-

bitants. The living is a discharged vicarage, in the archdeaconry of Taunton, and diocese of Bath and Wells, rated in the king's books at £7. 6. 10., and in the patronage of the Crown. The church is dedicated to St. Nicholas.

KILTON, a township in the parish of BROTTON, eastern division of the liberty of LANGBAURGH, North riding of the county of YORK, 6¾ miles (N. E. by E.) from Guilsbrough, containing 100 inhabitants. There was formerly a castle, which, with the lordship, belonged to the ancient family of Thwengs.

KILVE, a parish in the hundred of WILLITON and FREEMANNERS, county of SOMERSET, 11½ miles (N. W. by W.) from Bridg-water, containing 263 inhabitants. The living is a rectory, united with the vicarage of Stringston, in the archdeaconry of Taunton, and diocese of Bath and Wells, rated in the king's books at £9. 16. 8. The church is dedicated to St. Mary.

KILVERSTONE, a parish in the hundred of SHROP-HAM, county of NORFOLK, 1¾ mile (E. N. E.) from Thetford, containing 31 inhabitants. The living is a discharged rectory, in the archdeaconry of Norfolk, and diocese of Norwich, rated in the king's books at £7. 14. 9., and in the patronage of the Crown.

KILVINGTON, a parish in the southern division of the wapentake of NEWARK, county of NOTTINGHAM, 7 miles (S.) from Newark, containing, with a portion of the hamlet of Alverton, 24 inhabitants. The living is a discharged rectory, in the archdeaconry of Nottingham, and diocese of York, rated in the king's books at £6. 12. 1., and in the patronage of the Rector of Staunton in Vale. The church is dedicated to St. Mary.

KILVINGTON (NORTH), a township in the parish of THORNTON le STREET, wapentake of ALLERTON-SHIRE, North riding of the county of YORK, 2½ miles (N.) from Thirsk, containing 68 inhabitants. There is a chapel for Roman Catholics.

KILVINGTON (SOUTH), a parish in the wapentake of BIRDFORTH, North riding of the county of YORK, comprising the townships of South Kilvington, Thornbrough, and Upsal, and containing 405 inhabitants, of which number, 260 are in the township of South Kilvington, 1½ mile (N.) from Thirsk. The living is a rectory, in the archdeaconry of Cleveland, and diocese of York, rated in the king's books at £17. 10. 10., and in the patronage of the Master and Fellows of Sidney Sussex College, Cambridge. The church is dedicated to St. Wilfrid.

KILWORTH (NORTH), a parish in the hundred of GUTHLAXTON, county of LEICESTER, 5 miles (E. by S.) from Lutterworth, containing 391 inhabitants. The living is a rectory, in the archdeaconry of Leicester, and diocese of Lincoln, rated in the king's books at £15. 0. 5. The Rev. T. Belgrave was patron in 1811. The church is dedicated to St. Andrew. The Grand Union canal passes through the north-eastern part of the parish.

KILWORTH (SOUTH), a parish in the hundred of GUTHLAXTON, county of LEICESTER, 5 miles (E.S.E.) from Lutterworth, containing 450 inhabitants. The living is a rectory, in the archdeaconry of Leicester and diocese of Lincoln, rated in the king's books at £10. 8. 11½., and in the patronage of the Crown. The church is dedicated to St. Nicholas. There is a place of worship for Wesleyan Methodists.

KIMBERLEY, a parish in the hundred of FOREHOE, county of NORFOLK, 3½ miles (N.W.) from Wymondham, containing 145 inhabitants. The living is a discharged vicarage, with the rectory of Barnham-Broom, in the archdeaconry of Norfolk, and diocese of Norwich, rated in the king's books at £6. 12. 3., endowed with £200 private benefaction, and £200 royal bounty. Lord Wodehouse was patron in 1820. The church is dedicated to St. Peter. There is a place of worship for Wesleyan Methodists. In the time of Henry III. there was a chapel in the church-yard, the ruins of which are still visible. Kimberley hall formerly belonged to the family of Fastolf, but in the reign of Henry IV. it came into the possession of Sir John Wodehouse, who took it down and erected a noble mansion upon its site. Subsequently he was appointed gentleman of the privy chamber to Henry V., attended that monarch into France, and conducted himself in the field with so much bravery, that the king granted an augmentation to his arms, with leave to bear the motto "AGINCOURT." Here the family resided till 1659, when they removed to the present seat, in which are preserved the fragments of a large old sword and a poniard, used by their ancestor at the battle of Agincourt; also a costly pair of necklaces of coral and gold, the gift of Catherine, Queen of Henry V.

KIMBERLEY, a hamlet (formerly a chapelry) in the parish of GREASLY, southern division of the wapentake of BROXTOW, county of NOTTINGHAM. The population is returned with the parish. The chapel has been demolished.

KIMBERWORTH, a township in that part of the parish of ROTHERHAM which is in the northern division of the wapentake of STRAFFORTH and TICKHILL, West riding of the county of YORK, 1¼ mile (W.) from Rotherham, containing 3797 inhabitants. There are places of worship for Independents and Wesleyan Methodists. A school has been erected partly by subscription and partly by the produce of the old school-room; the annual income, arising from sundry donations, is about £8, for which sum eight poor children are instructed.

KIMBLE (GREAT), a parish in the hundred of AYLESBURY, county of BUCKINGHAM, 3½ miles (W. S. W.) from Wendover, containing 360 inhabitants. The living is a discharged vicarage, consolidated, in 1799, with the rectory of Great Hampden, in the archdeaconry of Buckingham, and diocese of Lincoln, rated in the king's books at £6. 10. 5., endowed with £400 private benefaction, and £400 royal bounty, and in the patronage of the Earl of Buckinghamshire. The church is dedicated to St. Nicholas. A school for boys is supported by voluntary contributions. Kimble, according to old records, was anciently called Kunebel, from Cunobelin, or Cymbeline, the British king, whose sons here gallantly opposed the Romans, but were defeated and one of them slain. There are still the remains of several intrenchments on the supposed field of battle; and on a circular mound in the neighbourhood are vestiges of a fortification, termed Belinus' Castle, where it is said Cunobelin resided.

KIMBLE (LITTLE), a parish in the hundred of AYLESBURY, county of BUCKINGHAM, 3 miles (W. by S.) from Wendover, containing 165 inhabitants. The living is a rectory, in the archdeaconry of Buckingham, and diocese of Lincoln, rated in the king's books at

£6. 2. 11. The Rev. S. T. Chapman was patron in 1810. The church is dedicated to All Saints.

KIMBLEWORTH, formerly a parish, in the western division of CHESTER ward, county palatine of DURHAM, 3 miles (N. by W.) from Durham, containing 32 inhabitants. The living, a rectory rated in the king's books at £3. 6. 8., and endowed with £200 royal bounty, was united, in 1593, to the perpetual curacy of Witton-Gilbert, in the peculiar jurisdiction of the Dean and Chapter of Durham. The church has long since fallen to decay, and the place is now considered an extra-parochial liberty.

KIMBOLTON, a parish in the hundred of WOLPHY, county of HEREFORD, 3 miles (N.E. by E.) from Leominster, containing 634 inhabitants. The living is a perpetual curacy, in the archdeaconry and diocese of Hereford, endowed with £200 private benefaction, £400 royal bounty, and £600 parliamentary grant, and in the patronage of the Bishop of Hereford. The church is dedicated to St. James.

KIMBOLTON, a market town and parish in the hundred of LEIGHTONSTONE, county of HUNTINGDON, 10½ miles (W. by S.) from Huntingdon, and 63 (N.N.W.) from London, containing 1562 inhabitants. The town is pleasantly situated on the verge of the county, amidst sloping hills and woodlands diversified with fertile valleys. There are a few lace-makers, but general employment of the inhabitants is in agriculture. The market is on Friday; and fairs are held on the Friday in Easter week, for sheep and pedlary, and on the 11th of December, for cattle and hogs. A constable is appointed at the courts leet and baron held under the Duke of Manchester, who is lord of the manor. The living is a vicarage, in the archdeaconry of Huntingdon, and diocese of Lincoln, rated in the king's books at £5, and in the patronage of the Duke of Manchester. The church, dedicated to St. Andrew, is surmounted by a lofty spire. There are places of worship for Baptists, Independents, Moravians, and Wesleyan Methodists. A grammar school is endowed for a master and an usher; and there is an almshouse for four poor widows. Kimbolton castle, the magnificent residence of the Duke of Manchester, an ancient stone edifice, situated in a spacious park, was the residence of Catherine of Arragon, first wife of Henry VIII., subsequently to her divorce, where she also died. In this parish are the remains of Stonely priory, a convent of canons of the order of St. Augustine, founded by William Mandeville, Earl of Essex, about 1180, and dedicated to the Blessed Virgin Mary, the revenue of which, at the dissolution, was valued at £62. 12. 3. Kimbolton gives the inferior title of baron to the Duke of Manchester: it was the birth-place of Lord Kimbolton, afterwards Earl of Manchester, a parliamentary general in the civil war.

KIMCOTE, a parish in the hundred of GUTHLAXTON, county of LEICESTER, 3½ miles (E.N.E.) from Lutterworth, containing, with the hamlet of Cotes de Val, 505 inhabitants. The living is a rectory, in the archdeaconry of Leicester, and diocese of Lincoln, rated in the king's books at £20. 16. 3. Lord Willoughby de Broke was patron in 1811. The church is dedicated to All Saints.

KIMMERIDGE, a parish in the hundred of HASILOR, Blandford (South) division of the county of DORSET, 4¼ miles (S.W. by W.) from Corfe-Castle, containing 90 inhabitants. The living is a donative, in the patronage of the Clavell family. The parish is bounded on the south by Botteridge pool, or Kimmeridge bay, the entrance to which, between two high cliffs, is defended by a battery of two pieces of cannon. Here was formerly a pier, one hundred feet long, sixty broad, and fifty high, constructed, by Sir William Clavell, for the convenience of vessels which resorted to his alum, salt, and glass works, in the vicinity. It was, however, demolished by a great storm in 1745, and in 1748 the ruins of buildings and heaps of ashes were all that remained. On the shore are copperas stones in abundance; and in the cliffs of this and the neighbouring parishes is found a sort of coal, of a bituminous nature, which burns with a strong light, and emits a sulphureous smell; it is naturally a hard substance, but, on exposure to the air, splits into pieces like slate, and is sold to the poor at a moderate price.

KIMPTON, a parish in the hundred of HITCHIN and PIRTON, county of HERTFORD, 4½ miles (N. W. by W.) from Welwyn, containing 866 inhabitants. The living is a vicarage, in the archdeaconry of Huntingdon, and diocese of Lincoln, rated in the king's books at £12, and in the patronage of Lord Dacre. The church, dedicated to St. Peter and St. Paul, is situated on an acclivity rising from the north of the village: it has a square western tower, embattled, and surmounted by a short spire, and contains a fine screen of oak, with almost perfect remains of the ancient rood-loft.

KIMPTON, a parish in the hundred of ANDOVER, Andover division of the county of SOUTHAMPTON, 3 miles (S. S. E.) from Ludgershall, containing 366 inhabitants. The living is a rectory, in the archdeaconry and diocese of Winchester, rated in the king's books at £25. 12. 1. George Foyle, Esq. was patron in 1785.

KINDER, a hamlet in the parish of GLOSSOP, hundred of HIGH PEAK, county of DERBY, 4½ miles (N.) from Chapel en le Frith, containing 129 inhabitants.

KINDERTON, a joint township with Hulme, in that part of the parish of MIDDLEWICH which is in the hundred of NORTHWICH, county palatine of CHESTER, 1½ mile (E. S. E.) from Middlewich, containing 469 inhabitants. The early and powerful Barons of Kinderton had possessions here at the time of the Conquest; and until about the end of the sixteenth century, they exercised the right of inflicting capital punishment for crimes committed within the barony.

KINFARE, or KINVER, a parish in the southern division of the hundred of SEISDON, county of STAFFORD, 4 miles (W. S. W.) from Stourbridge, containing 1735 inhabitants. The living is a perpetual curacy, in the archdeaconry of Stafford, and diocese of Lichfield and Coventry, endowed with £600 parliamentary grant, and in the patronage of certain Trustees. The church is dedicated to St. Peter. The Staffordshire and Worcestershire and the Stourbridge canals form a junction here. There is a free grammar school, of ancient and obscure foundation, in support of which, William Vynsent, in the 34th of Elizabeth, bequeathed certain land, which, with subsequent gifts, produces £112. 12. 11. a year to the master, for the instruction of an unlimited number of children. Within the parish is an ancient fortification, forming a parallelogram three hundred yards long by two hundred broad, deeply intrenched on two sides, and on the other two defended by a hill.

In the neighbourhood is a tumulus, also a large block of stone, called Battlestone, six feet high, and about twelve in girth.

KINGCOMBE, a tything, consisting of Nether and Over Kingcombe, in that part of the parish of TOLLERPORCORUM which is in the hundred of BEAMINSTERFORUM and REDHONE, Bridport division of the county of DORSET, 6 miles (E. by S.) from Beaminster, containing 159 inhabitants.

KINGERBY, a parish in the northern division of the wapentake of WALSHCROFT, parts of LINDSEY, county of LINCOLN, 5 miles (N. W.) from Market-Raisen, containing 84 inhabitants. The living is a vicarage, in the archdeaconry and diocese of Lincoln, rated in the king's books at £5. The University of Cambridge presented in 1811. The church is dedicated to St. Peter.

KINGHAM, a parish in the hundred of CHADLINGTON, county of OXFORD, 4¼ miles (W. S. W.) from Chipping-Norton, containing 464 inhabitants. The living is a rectory, in the archdeaconry and diocese of Oxford, rated in the king's books at £17. 11. 8., and in the patronage of the Rev. J. C. Lockwood. The church is dedicated to St. Andrew. The river Evenlode bounds the parish on the west, and separates it from Gloucestershire.

KINGMOOR, an extra-parochial liberty, in ESKDALE ward, county of CUMBERLAND, 2 miles (N. W. by N.) from Carlisle, containing 162 inhabitants. It belongs to the corporation of Carlisle, the freemen of which city hold their guild races here annually on Ascensionday. There is a small donation in support of a school.

KINGSBRIDGE, a market town and parish, in the hundred of STANBOROUGH, county of DEVON, 34 miles (S. S. W.) from Exeter, and 207 (W. S.W.) from London, containing 1430 inhabitants. This place is pleasantly situated at the head of the bay, or haven, of Salcombe, on the summit and declivity of a hill, surrounded by others

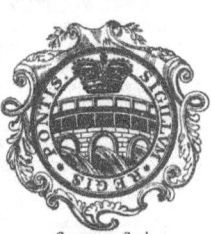

Corporate Seal.

of greater elevation; and consists chiefly of a long street, in which are some good houses. The town, which is partially paved but not lighted, is bounded on the east by a brook, which separates it from the town of Dodbrook. A mechanics' institute has been established. Races are held in the neighbourhood, generally once a year, but at no fixed period. The woollen manufacture was formerly carried on here very extensively, but it is now inconsiderable: the principal branches of trade at present are in malt and leather, especially the former, a considerable quantity of malt and grain being annually sent from this place. Various articles of commerce are brought coastwise, chiefly in vessels of from fifty to sixty tons' burden, though the haven is navigable for ships of a larger size: about thirty of these vessels belong to Kingsbridge and Salcombe. The market is on Saturday; and there is a fair on the 20th of July, unless that day falls later in the week than Thursday, when the fair is postponed to the following Tuesday, and continued for three successive days, for the sale of woollen cloth, toys, &c. The town is under the jurisdiction of the county magistrates, but a port-reeve, or chief officer, is appointed annually at Michael-mas, at which period a court leet is held by the lord of the manor.

The living is a discharged vicarage, with that of Churchstow, in the archdeaconry of Totness, and diocese of Exeter, endowed with £200 private benefaction, and £200 royal bounty, and in the patronage of the Crown. The church, originally founded about 1330, was con-siderably enlarged and improved in 1827, when it re-ceived an addition of two hundred and eighty-six sittings, of which, one hundred and sixty-five are free, the Incor-porated Society for the enlargement of churches and chapels having granted £160 towards defraying the expense. There are places of worship for Baptists, the Society of Friends, Independents, and Wesleyan Me-thodists. A free grammar school was founded pur-suant to the will of Thomas Crispin, who, in 1689, be-queathed to trustees an estate for its endowment, and also made provision for teaching gratuitously, in addition to the classics, reading, writing, and arith-metic : the number of boys in the grammar school is restricted to fifteen, and if so many are not to be found in the town, the trustees may complete the num-ber from any other place. William Duncombe, in 1691, gave by will property now producing about £350 per annum, for the support of four exhibitioners from this school to Oxford or Cambridge ; for apprenticing boys educated in the school ; and for the salary of a lecturer at the parish church : by order of the court of Chancery, in 1819, the stipends of the exhibitioners were extended from £10 to £50 per annum. Almshouses for four poor persons were founded by Robert Myd-wynter, in the reign of Elizabeth ; and a considerable income for the repair of the church, &c., arising from the rents of the town-lands, is vested in trustees.

KINGSBURY, a parish in the hundred of Gore, county of Middlesex, 7½ miles (W.N.W.) from London, containing 360 inhabitants. The living is a perpetual curacy, in the peculiar jurisdiction and patronage of the Dean and Chapter of St. Paul's, London. The church, dedicated to St. Andrew, is principally in the later style of English architecture.

KINGSBURY, a parish in the Tamworth division of the hundred of Hemlingford, county of Warwick, 5¼ miles (N. by E.) from Coleshill, containing 1345 in-habitants. The living is a vicarage, in the archdeacon-ry of Coventry, and diocese of Lichfield and Coventry, rated in the king's books at £8. 10., endowed with £200 parliamentary grant, and in the patronage of the Crown. The church, dedicated to St. Peter and St. Paul, has lately received an addition of one hundred and fifty sittings, of which one hundred are free, the Incorporated Society for the enlargement of churches and chapels having granted £100 towards defraying the expense.

KINGSBURY-EPISCOPI, a parish forming one of the four unconnected portions which constitute the eastern division of the hundred of Kingsbury, county of Somerset, 4¾ miles (S. byE.) from Langport, comprising the tythings of Barrow, Kingsbury-Episcopi, East Lam-brook, West Lambrook with Lake, and Stembridge, and containing 1470 inhabitants. The living is a vicarage, in the archdeaconry of Taunton, and diocese of Bath and Wells, rated in the king's books at £17. 18. 1½., and in

the peculiar jurisdiction and patronage of the Chancellor of the Cathedral Church of Wells. The church, dedicated to St. Martin, is a stately structure, with an elegant west-ern tower one hundred and twenty feet high, ornamented with eleven statues of kings, and crowned with twenty open-worked pinnacles. The parish anciently belonged to the Bishop of Wells, whence the adjunct to its name. There is a place of worship for Wesleyan Methodists.

KING'S-CAPLE, a parish in the upper division of the hundred of Wormelow, county of Hereford, 5¼ miles (N. W. by N.) from Ross, containing 271 inhabit-ants. The living is a perpetual curacy with the vicarage of Sellack, in the archdeaconry and diocese of Hereford. The church is dedicated to St. John the Baptist.

KINGSCLERE, a parish comprising the market town of Kingsclere and the chapelry of Sidmonton, in the hundred of Kingsclere, and the chapelry of Ec-chinswell in the hundred of Evingar, Kingsclere divi-sion of the county of Southampton, and containing 2851 inhabitants, of which number, 2296 are in the town of Kingsclere, 9 miles (N. E. by N.) from Whitchurch, 21 (N.) from Winchester, and 55 (W. by S.) from London. This place, as the name implies, was anciently a seat of the West Saxon kings ; and at Freemantle park, a short distance to the south of the town, was a man-sion said to have been a royal residence in the reigns of John and Elizabeth. The town is situated on the edge of the downs, near the northern extremity of the county; the streets are neither lighted nor paved ; the inha-bitants are well supplied with water. The trade is principally in malt, for making which the fine barley produced in the vicinity is peculiarly adapted. A small spring near the town turns four flour-mills within a mile and a half from its source. The market is on Tuesday ; and fairs are held on the first Tuesday after Easter, and the first Tuesday after October 10th, principally for sheep. Kingsclere is within the juris-diction of the Cheyney Court held at Winchester every Thursday, for the recovery of debts to any amount ; and petty sessions for the division of Kingsclere are held here and at Overton alternately. The living is a vi-carage, in the archdeaconry and diocese of Winchester, rated in the king's books at £17. 19. 7., and in the patronage of Lord Bolton. The church, dedicated to St. Mary, is a large stuccoed building, with a low tower. There is a place of worship for Wesleyan Methodists, and at Ecchinswell one for Independents. A free grammar school, supposed to have been of ancient foundation, was endowed by Sir James Lancaster, in 1618, with £20 per annum : the school-room was rebuilt in 1820, when the institution was converted into a National school open to all applicants. A bequest from Robert Higham, in 1722, is appropriated towards the clothing, maintenance, edu-cation, and apprenticing, of four boys. A quantity of clothes is annually distributed among the poor, by means of various benefactions. Here is a slightly chalybeate spring ; and on the adjacent hills are the remains of two Roman encampments, near which the fragments of two or three human skeletons, and several Roman copper coins, were recently discovered.

KINGSCOTE, a parish in the upper division of the hundred of Berkeley, county of Gloucester, 4¾ miles (N. W. by W.) from Tetbury, containing 266 inhabitants. The living is a perpetual curacy, annexed to the rectory of Beverstone, in the archdeaconry and diocese of Gloucester, and in the patronage of the Crown. The church, dedicated to St. John the Baptist, is a small edifice with a low embattled tower. A branch of the river Frome rises here. There are quarries of stone full of petrifactions called Clay-rags, which take a polish, and resemble the Derbyshire marble. At a supposed Roman station, called Chestles, in this parish, have been found coins, tesselated pavements, and a curiously-enamelled fibula.

KINGSDON, a parish in the hundred of SOMERTON, county of SOMERSET, 2¼ miles (S. E. by E.) from Somerton, containing 536 inhabitants. The living is a rectory, in the archdeaconry of Wells, and diocese of Bath and Wells, rated in the king's books at £27.3.1½. John Tucker, Esq. was patron in 1827. The church is dedicated to All Saints. There is a place of worship for Independents. The old Roman Fosse-way forms the south-eastern boundary of the parish.

KINGSDOWN, a parish partly in the hundred of CODSHEATH, but chiefly in that of AXTON, DARTFORD, and WILMINGTON, lathe of SUTTON at HONE, county of KENT, 2¾ miles (N. W. by N.) from Wrotham, containing 438 inhabitants. The living is a rectory, with that of Maplescombe, in the archdeaconry and diocese of Rochester, rated in the king's books at £9.1.8., and in the patronage of the Dean and Chapter of Rochester. The church, dedicated to St. Edmund, is a small building romantically situated in the bosom of a wood of about one hundred acres in extent. Kingsdown was anciently a chapelry in the parish of Sutton at Hone, and appropriated to the priory of St. Andrew in Rochester. Woodland, or Week, now only a hamlet to Kingsdown, was formerly a distinct parish.

KINGSDOWN, a parish in the hundred of MILTON, lathe of SCRAY, county of KENT, 3½ miles (S.) from Sittingbourne, containing 75 inhabitants. The living is a discharged rectory, in the archdeaconry and diocese of Canterbury, rated in the king's books at £5.9.2., and in the patronage of — Lushington, Esq. The church is dedicated to St. Catherine.

KINGSEY, a parish in the hundred of ASHENDON, county of BUCKINGHAM, 3 miles (E. by N.) from Thame, containing 204 inhabitants. The living is a vicarage, in the archdeaconry of Buckingham, and diocese of Lincoln, rated in the king's books at £8.10.5., and in the patronage of the Dean and Chapter of Rochester. The church is dedicated to St. Nicholas.

KINGSFORD, a hamlet in that part of the parish of WOLVERLEY which is in the lower division of the hundred of HALFSHIRE, county of WORCESTER, 4½ miles (N. by W.) from Kidderminster. The population is returned with the parish.

KINGSHOLME, a hamlet adjacent to the city of Gloucester, partly in those portions of the parishes of ST. CATHERINE and ST. MARY de LODE, GLOUCESTER, which are in the middle division of the hundred of DUDSTONE and KING's-BARTON, county of GLOUCESTER. The population is returned with the respective parishes.

KINGSLAND, a parish in the hundred of STRETFORD, county of HEREFORD, 4½ miles (N. W. by W.) from Leominster, containing 989 inhabitants. The living is a rectory, in the archdeaconry and diocese of Hereford, rated in the king's books at £31.3.6½., and in the patronage of the Rev. W. Evans. The church, dedicated to St. Michael, is a massive edifice, built in the

reign of Edward I., by Edward Lord Mortimer, whose relict obtained a grant for a market and a fair, the former of which has been long discontinued, but the latter is still held on October 10th, for horses, cattle, hops, cheese, &c. A free school has been endowed with £15 per annum, by Thomas Woodhouse. Kingsland formerly comprised part of the dower of Catherine, Queen of Charles II.: and tradition relates that near the glebe-house is the site of an ancient castle, the burial-place of King Merwald. In West Field there is a pedestal, erected by the neighbouring gentry, commemorative of the celebrated battle of Mortimer's Cross, fought in 1461, in which the Earl of Pembroke was defeated by the Duke of York, afterwards Edward IV., with the loss of about four thousand men: the earl escaped, but his father, Sir Owen Tudor, was taken prisoner and immediately beheaded.

KINGSLAND, a chapelry partly in the parish of ISLINGTON, Finsbury division, and partly in that of HACKNEY, Tower division, of the hundred of OSSULSTONE, county of MIDDLESEX, 1 mile (N. E.) from London. The population is returned with the parishes. This place consists principally of several ranges of buildings, extending a considerable distance along the road from London to Tottenham and Edmonton. Here are brick-fields, and some part of the ground is occupied by nurserymen and market-gardeners. Previously to the middle of the fifteenth century there was at Kingsland an hospital, or house for lepers, which, after the Reformation, became annexed to St. Bartholomew's hospital, and was used as a kind of out-ward to that institution; but, in 1761, the patients were removed from Kingsland, and the site of the establishment there was let on a building lease, though the chapel, on the petition of the inhabitants, was suffered to stand, as a proprietary chapel in the patronage of the Governors of the hospital: it is a small edifice in the early style of English architecture. Here are places of worship for Independents.

KINGSLEY, a township in the parish of FRODSHAM, second division of the hundred of EDDISBURY, county palatine of CHESTER, 3¾ miles (S.E.) from Frodsham, containing 924 inhabitants. There is a place of worship for Wesleyan Methodists. A school is endowed with four acres and a half of land.

KINGSLEY, a parish in the hundred of ALTON, Alton (North) division of the county of SOUTHAMPTON, 4½ miles (E. S.E.) from Alton, containing 373 inhabitants. The living is a perpetual curacy, in the archdeaconry and diocese of Winchester, and in the patronage of the Vicar of Alton. The church is dedicated to St. Nicholas.

KINGSLEY, a parish comprising the township of Whiston in the northern, but chiefly in the southern, division of the hundred of TOTMONSLOW, county of STAFFORD, 2¾ miles (N. by E.) from Cheadle, and containing 1320 inhabitants. The living is a rectory, in the archdeaconry of Stafford, and diocese of Lichfield and Coventry, rated in the king's books at £16.15., and in the patronage of the Duke of Devonshire. The church, dedicated to St. Werburgh, has lately received an addition of two hundred and six sittings, of which, one hundred and ninety-two are free, the Incorporated Society for the enlargement of churches and chapels having granted £100 towards defraying the expense. There is a place of worship for Wesleyan Methodists. The river Churnet and the Uttoxeter canal run parallel to each other through the parish. Here are several coal mines, and a furnace for smelting copper-ore. A free school was founded, in 1703, by John Stubbs, who endowed it with houses and land now producing about £60 per annum, for which one hundred and twenty children are instructed on the National system. Kingsley is in the honour of Tutbury, duchy of Lancaster, and within the jurisdiction of a court of pleas held at Tutbury every third Tuesday, for the recovery of debts under 40s.

KINGSMARSH, an extra-parochial liberty, in the higher division of the hundred of BROXTON, county palatine of CHESTER, 5½ miles (N. W.) from Malpas, containing 46 inhabitants.

KINGSNORTH, a parish in the hundred of CHART and LONGBRIDGE, lathe of SCRAY, county of KENT, 2¾ miles (S.) from Ashford, containing 372 inhabitants. The living is a rectory, in the archdeaconry and diocese of Canterbury, rated in the king's books at £11. 9. 9½. W. S. Coast, Esq. was patron in 1798. The church is dedicated to St. Michael.

KINGS-NORTON, county of WORCESTER. — See NORTON (KINGS).

KINGSTHORPE, a parish in the hundred of SPELHOE, county of NORTHAMPTON, 2 miles (N. by W.) from Northampton, containing 1226 inhabitants. The living is a perpetual curacy, annexed to the rectory of St. Peter's, Northampton, in the archdeaconry of Northampton, and diocese of Peterborough. The church, dedicated to St. John the Baptist, is partly Norman, and partly in the later style of English architecture. There is a place of worship for Baptists. This was anciently a royal demesne, having been governed by a bailiff, and had a common seal, the impress of which was a crowned head between two fleur de lis, with the motto *Sigillum Commune Kingsthorpe*. Among other privileges formerly possessed by the inhabitants was exemption from toll. At present a certain number of freeholders, under the payment of a fixed annual rent to the grantee, hold the manor in trust for the town : the trustees transact all manorial business in a small building called the townhouse, erected by Lady Pritchard. Within this lordship are extensive quarries of fine white freestone. Elizabeth Cooke and Margaret Fremeaux, in 1753, assigned to trustees an estate for the support of a free school, the annual rental of which, amounting to £20, is applied towards the instruction of fifteen boys and fifteen girls.

KINGSTON, a parish in the hundred of LONGSTOW, county of CAMBRIDGE, 3¾ miles (E. S. E.) from Caxton, containing 278 inhabitants. The living is a rectory, in the archdeaconry and diocese of Ely, rated in the king's books at £11. 15. 5., and in the patronage of the Provost and Fellows of King's College, Cambridge. The church is dedicated to All Saints and St. Andrew. Here were anciently a market and two fairs. A charity school was founded, in 1702, by Mr. Francis Todd, who endowed it with a rent-charge of about £13.

KINGSTON, a parish in the hundred of ERMINGTON, county of DEVON, 3½ miles (S. W. by S.) from Modbury, containing 525 inhabitants. The living is a perpetual curacy, annexed to the vicarage of Ermington, in the archdeaconry of Totness, and diocese of Exeter. There is a place of worship for Wesleyan Methodists. The parish is bounded on the west by the river Erme, and on the south by the English channel.

KINGSTON, or KINSON, a chapelry in the parish of CANFORD-MAGNA, hundred of COGDEAN, Shaston (East) division of the county of DORSET, 1¾ mile (S.) from Corfe-Castle, containing 619 inhabitants. It is within the peculiar jurisdiction of the Dean of Sarum. The chapel is dedicated to St. Andrew. The navigable river Stour runs on the northern side of this chapelry.

KINGSTON, a parish in the hundred of TAUNTON and TAUNTON-DEAN, county of SOMERSET, comprising the tythings of the Eastern division and the Western division, and the hamlet of Hestercombe, 3¾ miles (N.) from Taunton, and containing 954 inhabitants. The living is a vicarage, with the curacy of Cothelston annexed, in the archdeaconry of Taunton, and diocese of Bath and Wells, rated in the king's books at £18. 17. 11., endowed with £400 private benefaction, £600 royal bounty, and £700 parliamentary grant, and in the patronage of the Dean and Chapter of Bristol. The church, dedicated to St. Mary, is a fine structure in the later English style, with a western tower ornamented with sculpture, and crowned with pinnacles. There is a place of worship for Independents. Copper mines were formerly worked in the parish, but they have been discontinued. There are sundry bequests for the instruction of the poor, amounting to £16 per annum, which, with voluntary contributions, is applied in supporting a Sunday school.

KINGSTON, a parish in the hundred of TINTINHULL, though locally in the southern division of the hundred of Petherton, county of SOMERSET, 1½ mile (S.E.) from Ilminster, containing, with the hamlet of Allowenshay, 264 inhabitants. The living is a rectory, in the archdeaconry of Wells, and diocese of Bath and Wells, rated in the king's books at £5. 19. 2. W. Harbin, Esq. was patron in 1817. The church is dedicated to All Saints. At Allowenshay, a place of great antiquity, now a hamlet in this parish, there was formerly a church or chapel. Here was born Henry Jeanes, a learned divine and theological writer in the seventeenth century.

KINGSTON, a parish in the liberty of WEST MEDINA, Isle of Wight division of the county of SOUTHAMPTON, 6½ miles (S.S.W.) from Newport, containing 68 inhabitants. The living is a rectory, in the archdeaconry and diocese of Winchester, rated in the king's books at £5. 6. 8., and in the patronage of G. Ward, Esq.

KINGSTON, a parish in the southern division of the hundred of TOTMONSLOW, county of STAFFORD, 3½ miles (S.W. by S.) from Uttoxeter, containing 355 inhabitants. The living is a perpetual curacy, in the archdeaconry of Stafford, and diocese of Lichfield and Coventry, endowed with £400 private benefaction, and £400 royal bounty, and in the patronage of —— Sneyd, Esq.

KINGSTON, a parish in the hundred of POLING, rape of ARUNDEL, county of SUSSEX, 4¼ miles (E. by S.) from Little Hampton, containing 43 inhabitants. The living is a vicarage, in the archdeaconry of Lewes, and diocese of Chichester. The church is demolished.

Arms.

KINGSTON upon HULL, a sea-port, borough, and county of itself, locally in the East riding of the county of York, comprising, within the borough, the parishes of St. Mary and the Holy Trinity, and in the county of the town, the parishes of Kirk-Ella, North Ferriby, Hessle, and the extra-parochial district of Garrison-Side, and containing 31,425 inhabitants, of which number, 28,591 are in the borough of Hull, 39 miles (S.E.) from York, and 170 (N.) from London. This town has arisen since the Norman Conquest; for, at the time of the general survey, the principal place in the neighbourhood was Myton, of which there are now no remains. Edward I., on his return from the battle of Dunbar, where he had defeated the Scottish king, John Balliol, and deprived him of his crown, visited Baynard castle, the seat of the lords of Wake, in this vicinity: while staying there, being engaged one day in the amusements of the chase, he was led to the hamlet of Myton and Wyke, the present site of the town of Hull, and contemplating the advantages of its situation, determined on the foundation of a fortified town and commercial port. He consequently negociated an exchange with the abbot of Meaux in Holderness, to whom the property belonged, for lands productive of a higher revenue. He then issued a proclamation inviting settlers, to whom he offered advantages sufficient to induce several to accept his proposals. He next built a manor-house, and in a little time had the satisfaction of seeing the town erected, which he dignified with the appellation of *King's Town*, now Kingston, distinguished, by its situation on the river Hull, from Kingston upon Thames, and other places of the same name. In the twenty-seventh year of his reign the harbour was completed, and in the same year he granted a royal charter constituting the place a free borough. From this period its increase and prosperity have been remarkable. A ferry was soon after established over the Humber, and, in 1316, vessels began to sail at fixed periods between Hull and Barton, for the conveyance of passengers, cattle, and articles of traffic, which intercourse has continued to the present day. Ten years afterwards the town was fortified; and so rapid was its improvement, that in the reign of Edward III. it supplied sixteen sail of ships and four hundred and sixty-six men towards an armament for the invasion of France; when the city of London furnished only twenty-five ships and six hundred and sixty-two men. From the earliest period of its history, this town had suffered through the want of a proper supply of fresh water, which the inhabitants were compelled to bring from a considerable distance; and, in 1376, the people of Hessle, Anlaby, Cottingham, and other neighbouring places, conspired to withhold from them this necessary of life. After a long and violent contest, an appeal was made to the pope, who issued his mandate, July 20th, 1413, to prevent all further interruption of the supply of water. In the reign of Richard II., when the Scots were making incursions into England, and threatening the country between the Tweed and the Humber, the fortifications of Hull under-

went considerable repairs, and a strong castle, for the security of the town and harbour, was erected on the eastern side of the river. During the contests between the houses of York and Lancaster, this town continued faithful to the latter, whose cause they resolutely maintained in the battles of Wakefield and Towton. Such indeed was their loyalty, that when the public treasury of the borough was exhausted by the expenses of the war, the corporation took down a stately market-cross, erected at a great expense about thirty years before, to raise money by the sale of the materials for the support of the royal cause. At different periods in the fifteenth and sixteenth centuries this place suffered greatly, in common with many others, from pestilential diseases, which swept away vast numbers of the inhabitants, and materially checked the increase of population; yet it continued to prosper and extend its commerce. On the suppression of the monasteries, a strong spirit of discontent manifested itself at Hull; and at the time of the insurrection called the Pilgrimage of Grace, in 1537, while one division took Pontefract, and another entered York, a third took Hull by surprise, and reinstated the monks and friars who had been ejected from their convents. The triumph of the insurgents, however, was but transient, for the main body of them, under Aske, having been dispersed in the neighbourhood of Doncaster, the magistrates of Hull seized Hallam, the ringleader of the insurrection there, and many of his associates, who, being soon after tried by a special commission, were convicted of rebellion and executed. Not long after this a fresh insurrection broke out in Hull, in consequence of the alterations made by Henry VIII. in the established religion. On this occasion the town was besieged by the insurgents, and taken by stratagem, but the successful party, with Sir Robert Constable at their head, after keeping possession of the castle during thirty days, were compelled to surrender it into the hands of the mayor; when numbers of the rebels were tried for high treason under a special commission, and, being convicted, were hanged and quartered; among whom was their leader, Sir Robert Constable, whose body was exposed on Beverley gate. In the year 1541, Henry VIII. visited Hull, where he was most hospitably received by the body corporate, who presented him with a purse of £100: after taking an accurate survey of the town, the king gave directions for building a castle and two strong block-houses, with other fortifications, for the security of the place. He also gave orders for cutting a new ditch, from Newland to Hull, and that the manor-house, formerly called Suffolk's palace, should be repaired and improved. In 1527, and again in 1549, the town suffered greatly from inundation: the Humber overflowed its banks, and overspread all the low lands, doing immense damage both to town and country. But the commerce of the place continued to flourish, and the merchants increased in wealth and importance.

On the accession of Charles I., in 1625, Hull cheerfully contributed its quota for the prosecution of the war with France; and though the plague, by which it was again visited in this monarch's reign, swept away, in the space of three years, nearly three thousand persons, or one-half of its population, it rose superior to this check, and in a few years regained its former prosperity. Charles I., on his way towards the Scottish border, in 1639, visited Hull, which had been made a depôt for arms and military stores; on the 29th of March he inspected the fortifications, and having received the homage of the inhabitants, proceeded to Beverley, and thence to York. At the commencement of the parliamentary war during this reign, each party became anxious to obtain possession of the town, it being at that time not only a place of considerable strength by nature, but surrounded with walls and strongly fortified by art, and its importance still further augmented by the immense magazine of arms, ammunition, and military stores which had been collected there. The king, who was then at York, relying upon the assurances of loyalty and attachment which he had received from the mayor, aldermen, and burgesses, on his visit to the town, sent the Earl of Northumberland with a party of the royalists to take possession of it, but the mayor refused to receive the king's general, and, after a short consultation, admitted Sir John Hotham, who had been sent down to take upon himself the office of governor for the parliament. The ammunition and stores, which at that time exceeded the quantity in the Tower of London, became an object of great solicitude, and the two houses of parliament addressed a petition to the king at York, requesting that they might be removed to London, to which request his Majesty peremptorily refused to accede. On the 23rd of April, 1642, the king, with his son, Prince Charles, attended by many gentlemen of the county, advanced from York to Hull, and when within a few miles of the town despatched an officer to inform the governor, Sir John Hotham, that he would dine with him that day; to which the governor replied, that he could not, without betraying the trust reposed in him by the parliament, open the gates to the king's retinue, and requested to be excused from receiving the honour of his Majesty's visit. The king having arrived at Beverley gate, demanded admission for himself and twenty of his retinue, which the governor, with renewed protestations of loyalty, persisted in refusing. He then retired with his party to Beverley, where he passed the night, and on the following morning sent a herald to the governor to demand entrance into the town, threatening to proclaim him as a traitor in case of his refusal, and promising indemnity for the past in the event of his compliance; but the herald returned without success, and the king retired to York, whence he despatched a message to the two houses of parliament, complaining of the insult offered to his authority, and demanding punishment of the governor for his disobedience to the royal commands. The parliament, however, so far from attending to the message of the king, passed a vote of thanks to Sir John Hotham, for the resolution with which he had maintained the post committed to his charge. The king having assembled a force of three thousand infantry and eight hundred cavalry, and procured a supply of arms and ammunition from Holland by the sale of the crown jewels, and through the assiduity of the queen, resolved upon the reduction of the town by force, and advanced with this force to besiege it in form; but the governor, in order to prevent the near approach of the assailants, cut the banks of the Humber and Hull rivers, and raising the sluices, laid the country adjoining the town for a considerable distance under water. In order the more effectually to provide for the internal defence, he pulled down the Charter-house hos-

pital, and several buildings in Myton-lane, and erected batteries with the materials, and planted cannon on the walls. But notwithstanding these precautions, the king's troops erected several batteries in the vicinity, and brought their cannon to bear upon the town, which for some time sustained a vigorous attack, and was as resolutely defended. The garrison, inflamed with desperation at a report industriously circulated by the parliamentarians, that the king would give no quarter, if he took the town, sallied out to the number of five hundred, with a determination to compel the royalists to raise the siege, and made a furious attack on the besiegers, headed by Sir John Meldrum, a Scotch officer, whom the parliament had sent down to the assistance of the governor, obliging them to retreat with considerable loss to Beverley, where, after holding a council of war, the siege was abandoned, and the royal forces retired to York. It appears that in this siege, the king relied for success less upon the efficiency of his own troops than upon the treachery of Sir John Hotham, with whom he had previously entered into a private treaty for surrendering the town; but the plot being prematurely discovered by the mayor, was frustrated before it could take effect, and the governor and his son, Captain Hotham, being arrested, were sent prisoners to London, where, after trial in the guildhall, they were convicted of treason, and executed upon Tower Hill. After the seizure of the governor, the custody of the town was entrusted to the mayor and eleven commissioners, appointed by the parliament, who retained it till the arrival of Lord Fairfax, who was afterwards appointed governor. The Marquis of Newcastle having subsequently made himself master of Gainsborough and Lincoln for the king, and driven Sir Thomas Fairfax from Beverley, with considerable loss, appeared before Hull with all his forces, and having cut off all supplies of provisions from the adjoining parts of Yorkshire, and diverted the supply of fresh water, succeeded, under a heavy fire from the walls, in erecting a battery called the King's fort, within half a mile of the town, mounted with heavy ordnance, and provided with a furnace for heating balls, which being fired red hot into the town, threw the inhabitants into the greatest consternation. The prudent precautions of the governor, however, counteracted their efficacy, and having again inundated the country surrounding the town, he compelled the assailants to abandon the greater part of their works, and the Marquis of Newcastle soon after raised the siege, and having destroyed the bridges and broken up the roads in the line of his retreat, to prevent pursuit, retired with his forces to York, and Lord Fairfax ordered the day on which he retreated to be observed as a day of public thanksgiving. From this time Hull remained in a state of tranquillity till 1645, when the Liturgy of the church of England being abolished, the soldiers quartered in the town entered the churches, collected the prayer-books, and committed them to a fire kindled for the purpose, amidst the acclamations of the spectators. After the decapitation of Charles I., the Protector visited Hull, and was received by the corporation with a congratulatory address.

The town is situated at the confluence of the rivers Hull and Humber: the streets in the older part are narrow and incommodious; but in other parts of the town they are spacious and more regularly formed.

The houses in general are built of brick: the streets are well paved with excellent durable stone, brought from Iceland as ballast in the ships employed in the whale fishery, and lighted with gas by two companies; one for oil-gas, established in 1821; the other for coal-gas, in 1826: the inhabitants are well supplied with water from copious springs which rise near Kirk-Ella, about four miles from the town, conveyed by a sluice called Spring Dyke, to the confines of the town, and supplied to the houses by means of pipes. The whole town consists of three unequal divisions: that which was first built is completely insulated by the docks, which have been constructed on the site of the ancient military works: on the north side of the old dock is the parish of Sculcoates, in which are several handsome streets that have risen up within the last forty years: and of still more recent date is that part which lies westward from the Humber dock, occupying the supposed site of the ancient hamlet of Myton, which name it still retains: the Garrison side is extra-parochial, and is connected with the principal part of the town by a bridge of four arches, with a draw-bridge in the centre over the river Hull. In 1443, the town was divided into six wards, which number was increased to eight, in 1824. The exchange is a neat building, with a portico in front; the area is divided by two Doric pillars, which help to support the ceiling; above is a news-room. A subscription library was established in 1775, and the present building in Parliament-street, having a spacious reading-room, was erected in 1800: it contains about twenty thousand volumes; and there are about five hundred subscribers, who pay £1. 5. each annually. The Lyceum library was instituted in 1807; and the members, in 1830, completed the erection of a handsome hall in Charlotte-street: the number of subscribers, at 12s. 6d. each, is about two hundred. The Theological library contains many scarce volumes of great value; a building on the south side of Trinity church, formerly used as a chapel, was appropriated to its use in 1669. The Literary and Philosophical Society, established in 1822, has a museum attached, comprising a good collection of specimens in natural history and the arts. The public rooms, of which the first stone was laid on the day on which his present Majesty King William IV. was proclaimed, form a handsome edifice of brick, ornamented with quoins and cornices of stone; the west, which is the principal front, has an elegant portico of the Grecian Ionic order, and the south front, in all other respects, is of corresponding character. The basement story will contain a regular arrangement of baths, fitted up with every accommodation, and the various offices connected with the institution: the principal floor contains a spacious and splendid public room, ninety-one feet and a half in length, forty-one feet wide, and forty feet in height, to be elegantly fitted up for assemblies, concerts, and public meetings; the vestibule leading to this room is forty-one feet long and sixteen feet and a half wide, attached to which is a cloak-room, twenty-three feet long and eighteen feet wide. On the same floor are a handsome dining-room, forty-eight feet long and twenty-four feet wide; an elegant drawing-room, forty feet long and twenty-four feet wide; and a committee-room, sixteen feet long and ten feet wide, all of which have communication with the large room. The attic floor contains a lecture-room, forty-five feet long and forty-one feet in width, adjoining which are an apartment for the lecturer and a room for apparatus, and a museum, one hundred and twenty-one feet long and twenty-four feet wide, which is lighted from the roof, and will contain valuable specimens of antiquity and natural history, of which the society, since its formation, have accumulated a numerous and highly interesting collection. The geological department comprises an extensive assortment of the various specimens of rock and fossil remains of the Yorkshire coast, the bones of various animals formerly common to this part of the country, but now peculiar to the tropical climates, lately discovered at Cliff, near Cave, by the honorary curator, Mr. Dikes, and a large collection of bones from the celebrated cavern at Kirkdale: the zoological department contains numerous fine specimens of birds and fish, and various other curiosities which the confined state of the room in which they are for the present deposited excludes from public inspection. There is also a mechanics' institute, formed June 1st, 1825, which possesses a good library. The botanical garden was opened in June 1812; it is in the environs of the town, and comprises about five acres of land, suitably laid out in compartments for alpine, aquatic, and other plants: the proprietors, in number two hundred and seventy, are holders of four hundred and seventy-nine transferable shares, of the value of five guineas each, subject to an annual subscription of a guinea and a half. There are also a few subscribers who are not shareholders. The entrance lodges, of which one is appropriated to the use of a botanical library, and the other as a residence for the curator, were erected in 1813, when the centre and the east wing of the green-house were also built, and in 1825 completed by the addition of the west wing; the property of the institution is vested in sixteen trustees, and the garden, established principally through the exertions of J. C. Parker, Esq. has become a valuable and interesting object of attention. The Hull Medical and Chirurgical Society, to which a museum is attached in the infirmary, was instituted in 1821. Wallis's museum, in Myton-gate, contains many natural and artificial curiosities, collected by the proprietor during the last sixty years. There is also a Florists' and Horticultural Society of recent establishment. The theatre royal, situated in Humber-street, is a neat and well-arranged building, erected in 1809. There is also an olympic circus, in Humber-street; and assembly-rooms have been fitted up and recently opened in North-street. The public baths are situated on the bank of the Humber, the water of which, by an improved method of filtration, is raised without sediment, and visitors enjoy the benefit arising from the use of it in every possible way.

Hull has long been famed for its trade and shipping, for which its situation is peculiarly favourable; the port is situated on the northern shore of the æstuary of the Humber, and on the left bank of the river Hull: its jurisdiction extends from the mouth of the river to Bridlington harbour on the north, including all the intermediate coast. It carries on a considerable foreign trade with Norway, Sweden, Holland, Hamburgh, France, Spain, and America, to which it exports the manufactured goods and produce of the counties of York, Nottingham, Derby, Stafford, and

Chester, with which it has great facility of intercourse, by means of the Aire, Calder, Ouse, Trent, and other large rivers which fall into the Humber, and the numerous canals communicating with them ; in consequence of which it possesses greater advantages for inland traffic than any other port in the kingdom : the manufactured goods and produce brought into this port from the West riding of the county of York alone are estimated at five millions sterling per annum. It carries on also a very extensive coasting trade in corn, wool, manufactured goods, and other articles of merchandise. The whale fishery originated at this place in 1589, when the merchants fitted out two vessels for Greenland ; this branch of commerce was attended with progressive increase, and soon formed a considerable part of the staple trade : at present no ships are sent from this port to Greenland, the whole being fitted out for Davies' straits : one thousand three hundred and eighteen ships have been fitted out from Hull since the year 1800, averaging nearly forty-four annually ; of this number forty-seven have been lost, nine of them during the past year (1830) ; the quantity of oil produced from the blubber exceeds that of all other ports in the kingdom, one hundred and thirty-three thousand one hundred and fifty-seven tons having been brought in during the above period, exclusively of the year 1830.

The harbour was constructed in the reign of Richard II., but the principal source of the commercial prosperity of the town arises from the capacious docks with which the port is now provided. In 1774, a subscription was opened for making a wet dock on the north side of the town, now called the Old dock, and an act of parliament was obtained for carrying the project into execution, by which act the shareholders were incorporated under the name of "The Dock Company of Kingston upon Hull," and received from the crown a grant of the military works of the town, and a vote from parliament of £15,000, towards defraying the expense of the undertaking. The first stone was laid October 19th, 1775, and the whole undertaking completed in four years. The length of this dock is six hundred yards, its width eighty-five yards, and depth twenty-three feet, and it occupies forty-eight thousand one hundred and fifteen square yards of excavated land. Originally the number of shares was one hundred and twenty, but the trade of the port requiring further accommodation, two other acts of parliament were obtained, one in 1802, and the other in 1805, by which the company were empowered to increase the number to one hundred and eighty : the money arising from the sixty additional shares amounted to £82,300, which sum was appropriated towards making a new dock. The first stone of this dock was laid on the 13th of April, 1807, and having been completed at an expense of £220,000, it was opened on the 30th of June, 1809 : it is called the Humber dock, and communicates with the river from which it takes its name, by a lock of excellent construction, large enough to admit a fifty-gun ship : it is three hundred yards in

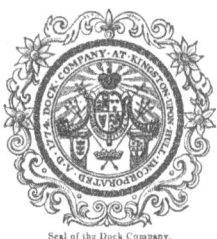

Seal of the Dock Company.

length, one hundred and fourteen yards wide, and thirty feet deep, and occupies thirty-five thousand four hundred and ninety-eight square yards. A dredging machine, worked by a steam-engine of six-horse power, is used to cleanse this dock from the mud which accumulates : this machine raises fifty tons of mud in an hour, which is transferred to barges, and conveyed to a situation in the Humber where it can be washed away by the current. The Old dock is cleansed by a similar machine worked by two horses. These two docks are capable of holding six hundred sail of vessels. A Junction dock, uniting the two former, has lately been completed, by which means vessels are enabled to pass round the town : it occupies thirty thousand three hundred and sixty-two square yards of land, and is capable of containing sixty sail of ships, leaving sufficient room for others to pass. Besides these wet docks, there are two basins, the Old dock basin, and the Humber dock basin, the former occupying an area of one thousand eight hundred and seventy-six square yards, and the latter thirteen thousand three hundred and ninety-three, the total area of water of the several docks and basins is twenty-six acres and three roods, for the convenience of repairing vessels. In the year ending October 30th, 1830, one thousand one hundred and eighty-six vessels entered inwards from foreign parts, and one thousand and thirty-seven cleared outwards. The tonnage upon which dock duties were paid for the same period was three hundred and thirteen thousand eight hundred and fifteen, including coasters. The number of ships employed in the coasting trade in 1829 was one thousand four hundred and seventy-seven, entered inwards, and one thousand six hundred and seventy-nine, cleared outwards. The number of vessels belonging to the port in 1829 was five hundred and seventy-nine, averaging a burden of one hundred and twenty-seven tons ; and eleven ships were built in the dock-yards at this port in the same year. The docks, to which are two entrances, one from the river Humber on the south, and the other from the river Hull, or the harbour, on the east, are amply provided with extensive quays, and spacious and commodious warehouses, and, under the judicious regulations of the Dock Company, are carefully guarded from accident by fire ; an engine, with lighters for floating it to any part of the docks, is constantly in readiness in case of need, and firemen, constables, and watchmen, are constantly on duty day and night. The greatest caution is also used to prevent any depredation from being committed on the very valuable cargoes which are transhipped at this port by the company, who keep a sufficient number of known and responsible labourers for loading and unloading the vessels. To facilitate the passing and repassing of vessels from the several docks, signals are used by the dock-master, under the authority of the Trinity House, by which body also, to obviate any irregularity, or partiality, in discharging the ships, the master and all his assistants are appointed. No fees or gratuities are allowed to the officers or servants employed in the docks, and heavy penalties are inflicted for partiality or neglect in the discharge of their duties. Of the ancient fortifications there remain only two of the forts erected by Henry VIII, by which, and by several batteries on the east side of the river, the town and harbour are defended. The citadel commands the entrance of the Hull roads and the Humber. The ma-

3 U 2

gazine is capable of containing twenty-thousand stand of arms, and ordnance stores for twelve or fifteen sail of the line, defended by a regular garrison under the command of a governor, who is generally a nobleman of high military rank. The custom-house is a large and handsome edifice, in Whitefriar-gate, originally built by the Corporation of the Trinity House, for the purpose of an inn, with a room for public entertainments, fifty-two feet long by twenty-four feet wide, and twenty-two high, which is now the long room for the transaction of the general official business. The pilot office, situated opposite the ferry-boat dock, consists of a modern lofty brick building : the pilots attended the observatory by turns, from six in the morning till nine in the evening, from the vernal to the autumnal equinox, and the remainder of the year from nine in the morning till six in the evening : it is under the direction of commissioners appointed by the Humber Pilot act. A life-boat was established at Spurn in 1810, and the crew resident there are maintained and regulated by the Wardens of the Trinity House. The excise office is situated in a street called The Land of Green Ginger. The principal articles of manufacture are turpentine and tar, white lead, soap, tobacco and snuff, sails, sail-cloth, ropes, and chain-cables; and there are several mills worked by steam and by wind, for the extraction of oil from linseed and rape seed, and the preparation of the residuum of the former for feeding cattle. There is an extensive sugar-refinery, which has been conducted by the Thornton family for one hundred and thirty years, and affords employment to about eighty persons. A large portion of the produce is exported to Germany, Prussia, and the Mediterranean. There are also some large breweries. The market days are Tuesday and Friday; the former for corn, which is sold in the corn exchange : there is also a customary market for provisions, on Saturday : in the marketplace, which has been recently improved, is a fine equestrian statue of William III.

The town was incorporated by charter of Edward I. in which the inhabitants are styled " free burgesses," and the chief magistrate the warden. Richard II. confirmed and extended the charter of Edward I., and vested the government in a mayor and four bailiffs; and Henry VI., who erected the town and liberties into a county of itself, under the designation of "The Town

Corporate Seal.

and County of the Town of Kingston upon Hull," empowered the inhabitants to elect thirteen aldermen, one of whom was to be mayor. Under this charter, which has been confirmed and enlarged with additional privileges in succeeding reigns, the government is vested in a mayor, recorder, twelve aldermen, sheriff, chamberlain, &c. assisted by a town clerk, sword-bearer, two mace-bearers, and subordinate officers. The mayor is chosen annually on the 30th of September, by the burgesses generally, from two aldermen nominated to that office : the recorder is appointed by the king, on the nomination of the mayor and aldermen, and holds his office for life : the sheriff is chosen annually, by the

burgesses at large, from two burgesses nominated by the mayor and aldermen ; and the chamberlain and water-bailiff in the same manner, from burgesses nominated by the mayor : the town clerk is appointed by the king, on the nomination of the mayor and aldermen, and holds his office for life : there are other officers appointed by the mayor and aldermen, of which the principal is the " town's husband," who keeps the accounts of the corporation, and receives their rents. There is also an annual officer of the corporation, called the water-bailiff, who collects the port dues belonging to that body. The mayor, recorder, and aldermen are justices of the peace, and have exclusive jurisdiction within the town and county of the town. The corporation possess admiralty jurisdiction within the limits of the port, and hold general quarter sessions of the peace. They hold a court of record for civil actions to any amount, under the charter of the 18th of Henry VI., at which the mayor and sheriff preside, and of which the town clerk is prothonotary; and a court of requests is held every fortnight, by commissioners appointed under an act passed in the 48th of George III., for the recovery of debts not exceeding £5. The jurisdiction of both these courts extends over the whole of the town and county of the town. The freedom of the borough is inherited by birth, acquired by servitude, and obtained by purchase or gift of the corporation : every son of a burgess, born after the father has taken up his freedom, is entitled to be admitted at the age of twenty-one, whether he was born within the borough or not ; and an apprentice, having served his time to a burgess, is entitled, though the master resides without the limits of the borough. On the gift of the freedom it is necessary there should be present, in order to constitute a court, the mayor and seven aldermen. The assizes for the town and county of the town were formerly held here by the judges when on their circuits, but an arrangement has long since been entered into, by which the business is transferred to the assizes at York. A new gaol and house of correction, situated on the Humber bank, has lately been erected, at an expense of £22,000, upon the plan recommended by Mr. Howard, which thus supersedes the old prison and former house of correction, both of which were exceedingly defective. In the parish of Sculcoates is a neat hall for the administration of justice, and for other public purposes, where the petty sessions for the Hunsley-Beacon division and other parts of the East riding are held every Tuesday. This borough returned burgesses to parliament in the 33rd of Edward I., but from that time it omitted sending till the 12th of Edward II., since which it has regularly returned two members : the right of election is vested in the burgesses at large : the sheriff is the returning officer. Andrew Marvel, a man of stern uncompromising integrity, represented this borough in parliament from 1658 to 1678, in which year he died, and was interred in the church of St. Giles' in the Fields, London, at the expense of the corporation, having been the last member of parliament who received pay from his constituents.

Hull, about the year 1534, was made the see of a suffragan bishop, who had a stately palace in the High-street, but it did not long retain that distinction, as the office was abolished on the death of Edward VI. The borough comprises the parishes of St. Mary and the Holy Trinity, both in the archdeaconry of the East riding, and diocese of York. The living of St. Mary's is a perpetual curacy, endowed with £200 royal bounty, and in the patronage of S. Thornton, Esq. : the church, of which the greater part was demolished in the reign of Henry VIII., consists principally of the chancel of the original structure, which was enlarged in 1570, and to which a steeple was added in 1696 : it contains some good windows in the later style of English architecture. The living of the parish of the Holy Trinity is a vicarage not in charge, in the patronage of the Mayor and Corporation : the church is an ancient and spacious cruciform structure, with a lofty and every beautiful tower rising from the intersection, and supported on piers and arches of elegant proportion : the east end is in the decorated style of English architecture, the transepts being fine specimens of the earliest period of that style; and the window in the south transept is filled with tracery, and enriched with mouldings of curious character : the nave is separated from the aisles by slender piers and graceful arches, and, being only partly pewed, affords a fine open view of the chancel, in which are some beautiful niches and stalls, and a superb monument in the decorated style, with a rich canopy and buttresses. The church, dedicated to St. John, in this parish, was completed, in 1792, at the sole expense of the Rev. Thomas Dikes, L.L.B.: it is a neat edifice of brick, to which a tower has been subsequently added. The living is a perpetual curacy, the right of presentation to which, on the demise of the founder, will belong to the Vicar. The parliamentary commissioners for the erection of churches have also granted a sum for building a church, or chapel, in Myton, within this parish, which is now in progress. There are places of worship for General and Particular Baptists, the Society of Friends, those in the late Countess of Huntingdon's Connexion, Independents, Primitive, Wesleyan, and New Connexion of Methodists, Swedenborgians, Unitarians, a Roman Catholic chapel, and a synagogue : there is a mariners' chapel, also a floating chapel in the junction dock, supported by the contributions of churchmen and dissenters.

The grammar school was founded, in 1486, by Dr. Alcock, a native of Beverley, and successively Bishop of Rochester, Worcester, and Ely ; and the present schoolhouse was rebuilt in 1583 : the school is open to all the sons of burgesses, on the payment of 40s. annually, for classical instruction only : writing and arithmetic have been recently introduced, and are now taught at a charge of four guineas per annum for the sons of freemen, and eight guineas for the sons of non-freemen. An exhibition to Oxford or Cambridge was founded in its behalf, by Thomas Ferres, alderman, in 1630 ; and a scholarship in one of the colleges at Cambridge, by Thomas Bury, in 1627, which have been for a long time consolidated : the total yearly income of the property in trust for this purpose is £82. 2. 2½. Among the distinguished masters of this school may be enumerated John Clarke, M.A., author of the Essay on Study, and translator of some of the classics ; and Joseph Milner, M.A., author of the History of the Christian Church. Of the eminent men educated here may be noticed, Andrew Marvel ; Mason, the poet ; Isaac Milner, D.D., late Dean of Carlisle ; W. Wilberforce, Esq., the senator and philanthropist ; and

Archdeacon Wrangham. The Vicar's chool, in which upwards of fifty boys are educated, was founded about 1737, by the Rev. William Mason, vicar of this parish, and father of the poet : the sum of £400 was originally raised for its endowment, and several legacies have since been added. The Marine school, near the Trinity House, was established in 1786, and is supported by the funds of that fraternity ; thirty-six boys are completely clothed, and instructed in writing, arithmetic, and navigation. Cogan's charity school for girls was founded, in 1753, by an aldermen of that name, who endowed it with about £2000 three per cent. consols., for clothing and instructing twenty poor girls. A further sum of £500 in the same stock was added by the founder, in 1760 : the property produces annually upwards of £400. In 1822 the number was increased to forty, and a marriage portion is given to those girls who remain in respectable service seven years. National schools, open to children of all denominations, were erected, in 1806, at an expense of £3000, and afford instruction to three hundred boys, and one hundred and seventy girls, each of whom pays one shilling per quarter. The Church of England Sunday School Association, and the Sunday School Union, both founded in 1819, instruct not fewer than seven thousand children, who are superintended by one thousand six hundred and thirty teachers. The Dissenters also support a considerable number of schools, and their Sunday schools are upon an extensive scale.

The " Guild of the Holy Trinity," established by the masters, pilots, and seamen of the Trinity House in Hull, in 1369, for the relief of decayed seamen and their widows, was incorporated by charter of the 20th of Henry VI., which has been renewed and confirmed by seven others. This corporate body consists of twelve elder brethren, six assistants, and an indefinite number of younger brethren, who are pilots of a superior class : from the former two wardens, and from the latter two stewards, are annually chosen. The annual expenditure exceeds £11,500 ; the revenue arises from property in land and the funds, from tolls, imposts, and duties on goods brought into or conveyed out of the port of Hull, and various other sources ; of this amount, the primage of threepence per ton on goods yields about £3400 annually, on an average ; the property given by Alderman Ferres, of which the brethren of the Trinity House are trustees, produces about £1660 annually ; a levy of sixpence per month on the wages of all seamen employed in vessels belonging to the port, produces an additional £700 per annum, which last sum is appropriated to the relief of distressed members of the Merchant Seamen's hospital, and the remainder arises from the funded property and other sources. The Trinity House was originally founded in 1457, and was rebuilt in 1753 : the building forms a handsome quadrangle surrounding a spacious area : the north, south, and east sides consist of single apartments for thirty-four pensioners : the front is ornamented with a freestone pediment of the Tuscan order, in the tympanum of which are the king's arms, with the figure of Neptune on one side, and that of Britannia on the other. On the side towards the west are the hall and housekeeper's rooms, with kitchens and other offices, over which are two elegant council-chambers, for transacting public business. The various apartments of this building contain several curiosities brought from foreign countries, and are decorated with a number of paintings. Adjoining the front of the Trinity House is a handsome chapel, built in 1772, and fitted up in an elegant manner for the purpose of divine worship. Robinson's hospital contains six rooms for younger brethren and their wives: it was granted to the corporation in 1682, by the founder, William Robinson, Esq., then sheriff of Hull, and in 1769 rebuilt and enlarged with six additional rooms, for the reception of as many widows. The Marine hospital contains nine rooms, of which eight are occupied by seamen and their wives, the other by an unmarried seaman. Watson's hospital affords accommodation for six widows. Ferres's hospital, recently erected at an expense of £2000, has accommodation for twenty or thirty inmates. The Merchant Seamen's hospital supplies accommodation for twenty seamen and their wives: there are also several out-pensioners of various classes; and temporary relief is afforded to poor shipwrecked mariners and their families. A marine school is also supported by this society, in which thirty-six boys are clothed and educated for the sea service. The charter-house was founded in the year 1384, by Michael de la Pole, first Earl of Suffolk of that name: having been destroyed in the time of Charles I., it was rebuilt at the end of the civil war; this building was taken down in 1780, and the present spacious and handsome structure was erected in its stead: it was enlarged in 1803, and now furnishes accommodation for twenty-eight men and twenty-nine women: the establishment is under the direction of a master, who has a stipend of £200 per annum, with a house and garden. The revenue of this hospital, which in 1660 amounted to no more than £54, now amounts to more than £5000, arising from the rental of land, and a share in the Hull Dock Company's concerns. Gregg's hospital was founded in 1416, for twelve poor women. Harrison's hospital, founded in 1550, for ten poor women, was enlarged in 1795, by Mrs. Mary Fox, who increased the number to fourteen. Gee's hospital, built about the year 1600, affords an asylum to ten poor aged women. Sir John Lister, alderman, and M.P. for Hull, founded an hospital, in 1641, for the reception of twelve aged persons, with suitable apartments for a lecturer: in 1775, Mr. John Buttery assigned to the mayor and burgesses three mortgages, amounting in value to £410, in trust for the benefit of Weaver's hospital, which is occupied by six poor women. Crowle's hospital was established in 1661, for twelve poor women of the age of fifty and upwards. Dr. Thomas Watson, Bishop of St. David's, erected almshouses for fourteen aged persons, about 1687, which were endowed with £300 by his brother, William Watson, in 1721. The hospital in Salthouse-lane contains rooms for four poor persons; and the indigent receive extensive benefit from sums bequeathed for the purpose of employing them, for putting out apprentices, and for occasional distributions in money and bread. The charity hall, or workhouse, established by an act passed in the 9th and 10th of William III., is under the direction of the mayor and aldermen, with twenty-four other persons chosen from the six wards of the town, who are incorporated by the name of "The Governor, Deputy Governor, Guardians, and Assistants of the Poor:" the provisions of the original act were confirmed and extended by the 8th of Queen Anne, and again by the 15th and 28th of George II.

The general infirmary, a short distance from the town, on the Beverley road, was erected in 1782, at an expense of £4126: it has accommodations for seventy in-patients; the average expenditure is £1400, annually raised by subscription: three physicians and three surgeons attend gratuitously. The dispensary for Hull and Sculcoates was instituted, Sept. 1st, 1814, at an annual expense of £350: and there are, an asylum for the insane, established in the same year, and capable of containing from eighty to ninety patients; a lying-in charity, instituted in 1802; a dispensary for curing diseases of the eye and ear, in 1822; the Poor and Strangers' Friend Society, established in 1795; an Educational Clothing Society, in 1820; a Humane Society, in 1800; and other associations of a similar kind, which confer important benefits. There is an Annuitant Society; and a savings bank was established in 1818.

A few religious houses existed here previously to the general suppression; but their remains have all been swept away by the tide of modern improvement. In 1331, Gilfred de Hotham, a devout knight, founded a priory for Black monks, in the street called Blackfriargate. Of this religious house, a square tower, and a pile of buildings used as an inn, remained about half a century ago, behind the old guildhall, at the top of the market-place: these were removed when the house of correction was built; and when, subsequently, the hall itself was pulled down, and the present range of buildings erected for shambles, in 1806, some groined arches of brick were discovered under the hall. Hull is the birthplace of several persons of distinction, among whom are Dr. Thomas Johnson, an eminent physician and botanist; Sir John Lawson, a distinguished naval officer in the reign of Charles II.; the Rev. W. Mason, the poet, and the friend and biographer of Gray; William Wilberforce, Esq.; Mr. Porden, the architect; Charles Frost, Esq., F.S.A., author of some tracts on legal subjects; John Crosse, Esq., F.S.A., and John Broadley, Esq., F.S.A., the patrons of literature and science; A.H. Haworth, Esq., F.R.S., author of "Lepidoptera Britannica, &c.;" William Spence, Esq., F.L.S., author of tracts on Political Economy, and an Introduction to Entomology; Thomas Thompson, Esq., author of tracts on the Poor Laws, &c.; and P.W. Watson, Esq., the author of "Dendrologia Britannica:" all these were natives of the town or neighbourhood, and residents in Hull. Andrew Marvel, M.P. for this borough in the reign of Charles II., is also commonly supposed to have been born here, but the place of his nativity was Winestead, near Partington, in the East riding, of which place his father was rector. The titles of Duke of Kingston, and Earl of Kingston upon Hull, formerly belonged to the Pierrepoint family, but in 1773 they became extinct.

KINGSTON near LEWES, a parish in the hundred of SWANBOROUGH, rape of LEWES, county of SUSSEX, 2 mile (S.W.) from Lewes, containing 172 inhabitants. The living is a vicarage, with which that of Iford is united, in the archdeaconry of Lewes, and diocese of Chichester, rated in the king's books at £8. 13. 9. Mrs. Jackson was patroness in 1822.

KINGSTON by SEA, otherwise KINGSTON-BOWSEY, a parish in the hundred of FISHERGATE, rape of BRAMBER, county of SUSSEX, 1½ mile (E.) from New Shoreham, containing 56 inhabitants. The living is a rectory, in the archdeaconry of Lewes, and diocese of Chichester, rated in the king's books at £12. 19. 2. W. Goring, Esq. was patron in 1809. This place is situated opposite to the entrance to Shoreham new harbour, which bounds it on the south.

KINGSTON upon SOAR, a parish in the southern division of the wapentake of RUSHCLIFFE, county of NOTTINGHAM, 1¼ mile (W. S. W.) from Kegworth, containing 166 inhabitants. The living is a perpetual curacy, annexed to the vicarage of Ratcliffe upon Soar, in the archdeaconry and diocese of York, endowed with £1000 royal bounty. William Strutt, and William Harrison, Esqrs. were patron in 1827. The church is dedicated to St. Wilfrid : the doorway of the western porch is Norman, and the east end is in the latter style of English architecture, built for the reception of a monument of uncommon splendour to one of the Babyngton family, the remains of whose ancient mansion are still visible in the neighbourhood.

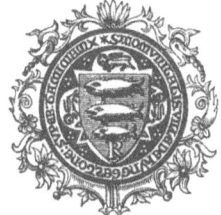

Seal and Arms.

KINGSTON upon THAMES, a parish in the first division of the hundred of KINGSTON, county of SURREY, comprising the market town of Kingston, which has a separate jurisdiction, and the hamlets of Ham with Hatch, and Hook, and containing 6091 inhabitants, of which number, 4908 are in the town of Kingston, 17½ miles (N. E.) from Guildford, and 12½ (S. W.) from London, on the road to Portsmouth. This town, which, according to Leland, was built in the time of the Saxons, appears to have derived its name *Kyningestun* from its having been held in royal demesne, and the place in which many of the Saxon kings were crowned, among whom were Athelstan, Edwin, Ethelred, Edward the Elder, Edmund, Edward the Martyr, and Edred. Near the town-hall is a large stone, on which, according to tradition, the ceremony of coronation was performed, and statues of several of those monarchs were preserved in the chapel of St. Mary near the spot, which, having been undermined by the digging of a grave, fell down in 1730. The present town appears to have risen from the ruins of a more ancient one, called Moreford, from a ford across the Thames, and which Dr. Gale supposes to have been the *Tamesa* of the geographer of Ravenna, a conjecture resting chiefly on the frequent discovery of numerous relics of Roman antiquity in the immediate vicinity. Vestiges of the old town, a little to the east of the present, were till very lately discernible in the foundations of houses and other buildings ; and the site of a Roman cemetery seems to have been ascertained by the numerous sepulchral urns, containing ashes and other relics, that have been found on the spot. Recently, on digging the foundation for a new bridge across the river, several Roman military weapons, consisting of spear-heads and swords, of beautiful workmanship and in a good state of preservation, were discovered, and are now in the possession of a gentleman resident in the neighbourhood : about the same time also were found several human skeletons, with Roman ornaments lying near them, in a field near the spot, on the Surrey side of the

river ; these discoveries have given rise to an opinion that Cæsar, on quitting his encampment on Wimbledon common, crossed the Thames at Kingston, and not at Weybridge, as has hitherto been imagined ; the skeletons being those of some of his troops that fell in endeavouring to force the passage of the river against the opposing Britons, whose slain are supposed to be interred in a tumulus (not yet opened) in a field called the Barrow field, on the Middlesex side of the river, and about half a mile from the spot where the weapons were found. In the latter part of the reign of Egbert, an ecclesiastical council was held at Kingston, at which that prince was present, together with most of the dignitaries of the Anglo-Saxon church, and the nobility. During the parliamentary war, the inhabitants embraced the cause of their sovereign, and suffered severely for their loyalty and attachment to the interests of the king.

The town is pleasantly situated on the southern bank of the Thames, over which was a very ancient wooden bridge, noticed in a record of the 8th of Henry III., and, with the exception of Old London bridge, the oldest of that river ; it has been replaced by an elegant structure of Portland-stone, consisting of five spacious elliptical arches, completed in 1828, at an expense of £40,000, and surmounted by a handsome cornice and balustrade, with galleries projecting over the piers. The houses are in general indifferently built, and the appearance of the town, which is paved and lighted under the provisions of a local act of parliament, passed in the 13th of George III., is by no means prepossessing : the inhabitants are supplied with water by pumps attached to their houses, and from a conduit on Combe hill, the water of which is conveyed also by pipes under the river Thames, laid down by Cardinal Wolsey for the supply of Hampton Court palace. The air is very salubrious, and the environs abound with beautiful scenery. The trade is principally in malt, a great quantity of which is made : there are also an extensive distillery and brewery, and several flour and oil mills. The market days are Wednesday and Saturday, but the former has nearly fallen into disuse : the fairs are on the Thursday, Friday, and Saturday in Whitsun-week; for horses, cattle, and toys; August 2nd and the following day, for horses ; and November 13th and seven following days, which is a large fair for sheep, of which generally about twenty thousand are exposed for sale ; also for horses, of which there are seldom less than a thousand ; and for cattle, of which frequently ten thousand head are sold.

Kingston returned members to parliament from the 4th of Edward II. until the 47th of Edward III., since which time it has made no return. The first charter of privileges was granted by King John, in the 10th year of his reign, which was confirmed and extended by succeeding sovereigns; under that of the 14th of Charles I. the government is vested in a corporation, consisting of two bailiffs, high steward, recorder, and an indefinite number of gownsmen and peers, and a council of fifteen, assisted by a town clerk, two coroners, four serjeants at mace, and other officers : James II., in 1685, granted a new charter for a mayor and twelve aldermen; but, in October 1688, this charter was annulled, the preceding one of Charles I. remaining in force. The bailiffs, who are also clerks of the market, are chosen from four of the peers and gownsmen nominated by the council of fifteen, the bailiffs and recorder selecting one, and the peers the other : the fifteen also elect two free tenants of the manor to the office of ale-conner, which forms their introduction into the corporation, and two of their own body become peers, and are eligible to the office of bailiff. The bailiffs, the late bailiffs, and the recorder, are justices of the peace within the town and liberties, and have power to hold sessions for the trial of all offenders not accused of capital crimes. The freedom of the town is inherited by the eldest son on the death of his father, or acquired by servitude of seven years apprenticeship to a member of either of the three companies of Mercers, Vintners, and Cordwainers. Among the privileges which the freedom confers is exemption from tolls throughout the realm, from serving on juries for the county, and, anciently, from contributing to the expenses of the knights of the shire. A singular custom connected with the election of the members of the corporation is observed, and is said to be sanctioned by the charter. A match at foot-ball takes place, in which the lower orders engage with so much zeal and activity, that the inhabitants of the principal streets find it expedient to barricade all the windows in front of their houses.

The corporation hold general courts of session in April and October, and a petty session every Saturday ; at which time they also hold a court of record for the recovery of debts to any amount, at which the bailiffs and recorder preside: the steward of this court is the attorney general, for the time being, and its jurisdiction extends over the hundreds of Kingston, Elmbridge, Copthorne, and Effingham. A court for the hundred of ancient demesne is held every third Saturday, before the bailiffs ; and as lords of the manor, they hold courts leet and baron on the Tuesday in Whitsun-week. The town-hall is an ancient building erected in the reign of Elizabeth, and partly rebuilt in that of James I., or more probably of Queen Anne, whose statue is set up on the outside of the building, and whose portrait is placed in the hall : the lower part is appropriated to the use of the market, and the upper part comprises rooms for the several courts, and for the general business of the corporation ; the windows are ornamented with stained glass, in which are the arms of James I. surrounded by small shields, containing the armorial bearings, or devices of the Saxon and other kings. The town gaol is a small neat building, erected in 1829, at an expense of £1100, for the confinement of debtors. The Winter and the Lent assizes for the county are held in this town, which is included in the home circuit : the court-house in which they are held was built by the corporation, in 1811, at an expense of £10,000, and contains two spacious courts for the crown and nisi prius causes: a grand jury room and requisite offices, attached to which is a house for the accommodation of the judges. The house of correction for the county comprises seven wards, one work-room, two day-rooms, and two airing-yards, for the classification of prisoners.

The living is a discharged vicarage, in the archdeaconry of Surrey, and diocese of Winchester, rated in the king's books at £20. 6. 3., endowed with £1000 royal bounty, and in the patronage of the Provost and Fellows of King's College, Cambridge. The church, dedicated to All Saints, is an ancient cruciform struc-

ture, in the decorated style of English architecture, with a tower rising from the intersection, formerly surmounted by a spire, which having been greatly injured by a storm in November 1703, was taken down. There are places of worship for Baptists, the Society of Friends, and Independents. The free grammar school was founded by Queen Elizabeth, who endowed it with lands and tenements producing about £100 per annum, for a head master and an usher appointed by the bailiffs, with the approval of the bishop of the diocese : there are about fourteen scholars, who are instructed in the classics and mathematics : the remains of an ancient chapel, dedicated to St. Mary Magdalene, are appropriated to the use of the school, and are at present undergoing a course of repair, in which due regard is paid to the preservation of the original architecture. The Bluecoat school for boys, of whom thirty-two are clothed, and that for girls, of whom thirty-six are clothed, are supported by a share of the funds bequeathed for charitable uses by Messrs. Smith, Tiffin, Belitha, Mrs. Elizabeth Brown, and others. A National school, in which two hundred and sixty boys, and one hundred and fifty girls, are instructed, and for which school-rooms were built, in 1819, by N. Pallmer, Esq., at an expense of £1200 ; and an infant school for one hundred and fifty children, for which a building was erected, in 1828, at an expense of £600, are supported by subscription. Almshouses for six aged men and six aged women were founded, in 1665, by William Cleave, Esq., alderman of London, who endowed them with houses and lands producing upwards of £400 per annum, to which was added £1000 in the three per cent. reduced annuities, by John Tilsley, Esq., the dividends on which are appropriated weekly in sums of four shillings each, to the almspeople, in addition to £1. 16. per month from the original endowment : the buildings comprise twelve neat tenements under one roof, with a large common hall in the centre. A dispensary is supported by subscription : and there are numerous charitable bequests for the relief of the indigent poor. An hospital, with a chapel dedicated to St. Mary Magdalene, was founded here, in 1309, by Edward Lovekin, of which the original endowment was considerably augmented by his son, John Lovekin, four times lord mayor of London between the years 1348 and 1356. Dr. George Bate, physician to Charles II. ; Dr. William Battie, a physician of considerable repute in cases of insanity ; and Judge Hardinge, were interred here.

KINGSTON-BAGPUZE, a parish in the hundred of OCK, county of BERKS, 6¼ miles (W.) from Abingdon, containing 327 inhabitants. The living is a rectory, in the archdeaconry of Berks, and diocese of Salisbury, rated in the king's books at £10. 6. 5½., and in the patronage of the President and Fellows of St. John's College, Oxford. The church is dedicated to St. James. At New-Bridge, in this parish, are held two annual fairs, on March 31st and September 28th. A sharp skirmish took place here between the army of the parliament and the royalists, when the former were defeated and driven back, on May 27th, 1644. A charity school has been founded here, but it has no permanent endowment, being supported by annual donations, amounting to about £20.

KINGSTON-BLOUNT, a liberty in the parish of

ASTON-ROWANT, hundred of LEWKNOR, county of Oxford, 4 miles (E.S.E.) from Tetsworth. The population is returned with the parish.

KINGSTON-DEVERILL, a parish in the hundred of MERE, county of WILTS, 3½ miles (N.E. by N.) from Mere, containing 328 inhabitants. The living is a rectory, in the archdeaconry and diocese of Salisbury, rated in the king's books at £19. 15., and in the patronage of the Marquis of Bath. The church is dedicated to St. Mary.

KINGSTON-LISLE, a joint chapelry with Farlow, in that part of the parish of SPARSHOLT which is in the hundred of SHRIVENHAM, county of BERKS, 5 miles (W.) from Wantage, containing 357 inhabitants. The chapel, which was dedicated to St. James, has been demolished. There is a place of worship for Baptists.

KINGSTON-RUSSELL, an extra-parochial liberty, in the hundred of UGGSCOMBE, Dorchester division of the county of DORSET, 1¾ mile (E. by N.) from Dorchester, containing 79 inhabitants. Here was formerly a free chapel, dedicated to St. James, of which a part of the walls only is now remaining. Since its demolition the inhabitants have been permitted, on payment of £4 per annum to the rector of Long Bredy, to bury in the church-yard there. In ancient records this place is stated to have been in the parish of Whitchurch-Canonicorum: it had formerly a weekly market, and a fair annually on the eve, day, and morrow of St. Matthew.

KINGSTON-SEYMOUR, a parish in the hundred of CHEWTON, though locally in that of Winterstoke, county of SOMERSET, 8½ miles (N. by W.) from Axbridge, containing 320 inhabitants. The living is a rectory, in the archdeaconry of Bath, and diocese of Bath and Wells, rated in the king's books at £29. 3. 11½., and in the patronage of John Hugh Smyth Pigott, Esq. The church is dedicated to All Saints: the altar-piece is adorned with a painting of the Transfiguration, by Smirke. The parish is bounded on the south by the river Yeo, and on the west by the Bristol channel, the waters of which make frequent irruptions into the adjoining lands, two of which, in 1606 and 1703, are commemorated by inscriptions in the church. The manor-house, erected in the reign of Edward IV., though it has undergone many alterations, is still interesting on account of its antiquity.

KINGSTON-WINTERBOURNE, county of DORSET.—See WINTERBOURNE (KINGSTON).

KINGSTONE, a parish in the hundred of WEBTREE, county of HEREFORD, 7 miles (W. S. W.) from Hereford, containing 406 inhabitants. The living is a discharged vicarage, consolidated with the rectory of Thruxton, rated in the king's books at £6. 6. 8., endowed with £200 royal bounty, and in the peculiar jurisdiction and patronage of the Dean of Hereford. The church is dedicated to St. Michael.

KINGSTONE, a parish in the hundred of KINGHAMFORD, lathe of ST. AUGUSTINE, county of KENT, 5¼ miles (S. E. by S.) from Canterbury, containing 301 inhabitants. The living is a rectory, in the archdeaconry and diocese of Canterbury, rated in the king's books at £16. Sir E. Bridges, Bart. was patron in 1816. The church, dedicated to St. Giles, is principally in the decorated style of architecture.

KINGSWEAR, a parish in the hundred of HAYTOR,

county of DEVON, 3¼ miles (S. W. by S.) from Brixham, containing 328 inhabitants. The living is a perpetual curacy, annexed to the vicarage of Brixham, in the archdeaconry of Totness, and diocese of Exeter, endowed with £200 private benefaction, £200 royal bounty, and £300 parliamentary grant. The church is dedicated to St. Thomas à Becket. Kingswear is situated on the eastern side of Dartmouth harbour, near the mouth of which are vestiges of a castle, and on the brow of a hill near the village are some remains of military earth-works. From Dartmouth castle opposite to the ruins of a fort here, a chain was formerly stretched to prevent ships entering the harbour: this fort was taken from Sir Henry Carew by General Fairfax, in January 1646.

KINGSWINFORD, county of STAFFORD. —— See SWINFORD (KING'S).

KINGSWOOD, a hamlet in the parish of LUDGERSHALL, hundred of ASHENDON, county of BUCKINGHAM, 9 miles (W. N. W.) from Aylesbury, containing 56 inhabitants.

KINGSWOOD, a township in the parish of SHOTWICK, higher division of the hundred of WIRRALL, county palatine of CHESTER, containing 44 inhabitants.

KINGSWOOD, a parish in the upper division of the hundred of LANGLEY and SWINESHEAD, county of GLOUCESTER, 4 miles (E. by N.) from Bristol. The population is returned with the parish of Bitton, in which the village of Kingswood Hill is partly situate. The living is a perpetual curacy, in the archdeaconry of Dorset, and diocese of Bristol, endowed with £2400 parliamentary grant, and in the patronage of Trustees. The chapel is dedicated to the Holy Trinity. Here is a free school, founded in 1748, by the Rev. John Wesley, for clothing and educating in the classics one hundred boys, the sons of Wesleyan ministers, under the direction of a governor and six assistants, and supported chiefly by the voluntary contributions of the Methodist societies. Here are some extensive collieries, from which the city of Bristol and its vicinity are principally supplied with coal.

KINGSWOOD, a liberty in that part of the parish of EWELL which is in the first division of the hundred of REIGATE, county of SURREY, 2½ miles (N. N. W.) from Gatton, containing 187 inhabitants. Here was formerly a chapel, which has been demolished.

KINGSWOOD, a hamlet partly in the parish of LAPWORTH, Warwick division of the hundred of KINGTON, and partly in the parish of ROWINGTON, Henley division of the hundred of BARLICHWAY, county of WARWICK, 5 miles (N. E. by N.) from Henley in Arden. The population is returned with the respective parishes. Here is a place of worship for Unitarians.

KINGSWOOD, a parish in the hundred of CHIPPENHAM, county of WILTS, though locally in the hundred of Grumbald's Ash, county of Gloucester, 5¼ miles (S. by W.) from Dursley, containing 1391 inhabitants. The living is a perpetual curacy, in the archdeaconry and diocese of Gloucester, endowed with £200 private benefaction, £200 royal bounty, and £1000 parliamentary grant, and in the patronage of the Inhabitants. The church is dedicated to St. Mary. There are places of worship for Independents and Wesleyan Methodists. The parish is watered by the Middle Avon, on the banks of which river are several extensive cloth manufactories. A free school for teaching children to read and write was endowed with £50 per annum, in 1674, by John Mayo, Esq. An abbey of Cistercian monks from Tintern was founded here, in 1139, by William de Berkeley, in honour of the Blessed Virgin, but the society afterwards removed to Tetbury. In 1170 they once more removed, and settled at Mireford in Kingswood, near the old site, and at the dissolution possessed a revenue of £254. 11. 2. The only remains of the monastic buildings are the foundations of the two churches and a gate-house of the gable form, with a range of ruins on each side.

KINGTHORP, a township in the parish and lythe of PICKERING, North riding of the county of YORK, 2 miles (N. E. by E.) from Pickering, containing 52 inhabitants.

KINGTON, a tything in the parish and lower division of the hundred of THORNBURY, county of GLOUCESTER, ¾ of a mile (W.N.W.) from Thornbury, containing 831 inhabitants.

KINGTON, a parish in the hundred of HUNTINGTON, county of HEREFORD, comprising the market town of Kington, and the townships of Barton and Bradnor with Rustrock, Chickward and Pembers-Oak with Lilwall, and Both-Hergists, and containing 2813 inhabitants, of which number, 1980 are in the town of Kington, 19 miles (W.N.W.) from Hereford, and 154 (W. by N.) from London. The town, which is of considerable antiquity, is situated on the banks of the river Arrow, and consists of two spacious streets. Charles II. is said to have visited it prior to the fatal battle of Worcester, and to have slept at an inn then called the Lion, but now the Talbot. In a barn still standing here, the celebrated tragic actress, Mrs. Siddons, made her first public appearance on the stage. The manufacture of woollen cloth, which was formerly carried on very extensively, has entirely ceased; and glove-making, which, until a very recent period, furnished employment to a considerable number of the inhabitants, has much declined: there is an iron-foundry and nail manufactory, established in 1815, in which about one hundred persons are employed. A rail-road has been constructed from the foundry to Brecon, joining the canal at Newport. An act of parliament was obtained, in 1791, for making a canal from Kington, by Leominster, to join the Severn at Stourport; but it has been left unfinished for want of capital. There is a good market for provisions on Wednesday: fairs are held on Whit-Monday, August 2nd, and September 19th, and annual cattle markets take place on the Wednesdays previously to February 2nd, Easter Sunday, Old Michaelmas-day, October 11th, and Christmas-day. Courts leet and baron for the manor, at the former of which a bailiff is appointed, are held annually. The county magistrates hold here petty sessions for the hundreds of Huntington and Wigmore every Friday. A court for the recovery of debts under 40s. is held once in three weeks.

The living is a vicarage, with the curacies of Brilley, Huntington, and Michaelchurch, in the archdeaconry and diocese of Hereford, rated in the king's books at £25. 2. 11., and in the patronage of the Bishop of Hereford. The church, dedicated to St. Michael, is an ancient structure. Here are places of worship for Baptists and Wesleyan Methodists. A free grammar school was founded pursuant to the will of Lady Hawkins, who, in 1619, bequeathed money for the purchase of an estate

producing £224. 10. per annum, of which the master receives three-fourths as his salary, and the usher onefourth: the school is open to the children of Kington, Brilley, Huntington, and Michaelchurch, and the present number of free scholars is forty-two. On Bradnor hill, about a mile north of the town, are traces of an ancient camp; and there is a rocky eminence in the vicinity, called Castle hill, though it does not appear that any castle ever stood there, or that it was the site of an encampment.

KINGTON, or KINETON, a parish in the Kington division of the hundred of KINGTON, county of WARWICK, comprising the market town of Kington, and the chapelry of Combrook, and containing 1071 inhabitants, of which number, 782 are in the town of Kington, 10½ miles (S. S. E.) from Warwick, and 82 (N. W. by W.) from London. This place, which gives name to the hundred, is so called from its having been a royal residence. About a quarter of a mile to the south-west, on a spot still called Castle hill, was a castle, in which King John is said to have held his court, but there are no vestiges of the building, traces of the moat by which it was surrounded being the only discernible remains; the site is planted with trees, and at a short distance from the spot is a well called King John's well, the water of which, though very pure, possesses no remarkable qualities. The name Kineton, which is the more ancient, is thought by some to have been obtained from its having been at a very early period a considerable mart for cattle, or kine: by this name it was given by Henry I., to the monks of Kenilworth, and coming afterwards into the possession of Milo de Kineton, it was taken from him by Stephen, and restored to the monks. The memorable battle of Edgehill took place near this town, and within half a mile of it, a great quantity of bullets was dug up in 1800: about a mile further, on the road to Edgehill, is a place called Battle Farm, where several of the slain were interred; and in a field about a mile to the west of the town is a tumulus covering several hundred of them: a gold ring was found in the neighbourhood, and the skeletons of human bodies are frequently discovered.

The town is irregularly built: the houses, in general ancient, are of stone, with thatched roofs, and bear some resemblance to the rudest features of the Elizabethan style; but in detached situations there are some handsome modern houses, built of stone and of brick: the inhabitants are amply supplied with water from wells; the air is salubrious, and the environs abound with pleasant walks. There is no branch of trade or manufacture carried on, the inhabitants being principally employed in agriculture. The market, which has almost fallen into disuse, is on Tuesday, and was formerly very considerable for grain; the fairs are, February 5th, which formerly regulated the price of beans for seed, but is now very thinly attended; and October 2nd, which is principally a statute fair for the hiring of servants. The market-place is a small area in which is an old building, or rather a shed, supported on arches of brick, in one angle of which there is a small prison for the temporary confinement of offenders. A constable and head-borough are annually appointed at the court leet of the lord of the manor, held in October. The living is a discharged vicarage, in the archdeaconry and diocese of Worcester, rated in the king's books at £8. 6. 8., endowed with £200 private benefaction, £400 royal bounty, and £1400 parliamentary grant, and in the patronage of Lord Willoughby de Broke. The church, dedicated to St. Peter, is an ancient cruciform structure, in the early and decorated styles of English architecture, with some remains of the later Norman style, and having a square embattled tower crowned with pinnacles, some of which are wanting; in the tower are windows of elegant tracery, and under the battlements is a band of antique heads and bosses. The western entrance is through a richly-moulded and deeply-receding arch, in the most finished style of later Norman architecture : the chancel was rebuilt in 1315, and the nave, aisles, and transepts in 1755 : under an arch at the western extremity of the north aisle is the recumbent figure of a monk, removed from the chancel on the rebuilding of the church. A National school, in which forty boys and thirty girls are instructed in reading, writing, and arithmetic, is supported by subscription ; and there is a small endowment in land for apprenticing poor boys. At Combrook, a chapelry in this parish, is a free school, with a house for the master.

KINGTON, a parish in the upper division of the hundred of HALFSHIRE, though locally in the middle division of the hundred of Oswaldslow, county of WORCESTER, 9¾ miles (E.) from Worcester, containing 148 inhabitants. The living is a discharged rectory, in the archdeaconry and diocese of Worcester, rated in the king's books at £8. Mr. and Mrs. Phillips were patrons in 1804. The church is dedicated to St. James.

KINGTON (MAGNA), a parish in the hundred of REDLANE, Sturminster division of the county of DORSET, 6½ miles (W.) from Shaftesbury, containing 486 inhabitants. The living is a rectory, in the archdeaconry of Dorset, and diocese of Bristol, rated in the king's books at £13. 4. 7., and in the patronage of the Duke of Portland. The church is dedicated to the Holy Trinity.

KINGTON (ST. MICHAEL), a parish in the northern division of the hundred of DAMERHAM, county of WILTS, comprising the tythings of Easton-Percey, Kingston, St. Michael, and Langley, and containing 969 inhabitants, of which number, 436 are in the tything of Kington, St. Michael, 3 miles (N.N.W.) from Chippenham. The living is a vicarage, in the archdeaconry of Wilts, and diocese of Salisbury, rated in the king's books at £8. 9. 4½., and in the patronage of the Hon. W. T. L. P. Wellesley. The church is dedicated to St. Michael. An annual fair for horses and cattle is held on October 6th. In this parish are considerable remains of three religious houses, the principal of which, a Benedictine nunnery, in honour of the Blessed Virgin Mary, was founded before the time of Henry II., as a cell to the abbey of Glastonbury, the revenue of which, at the dissolution, was £38. 3. 10. ; the remains have been converted into a farm-house. A free school is endowed with an annuity of £5, given by Mrs. S. Bowerman in 1730. Isaac Lyte, Esq., an alderman of London, who died in 1659, erected six almshouses, which he endowed with £20 per annum.

KINGTON (WEST), a parish in the hundred of CHIPPENHAM, county of WILTS, 8½ miles (W.N.W.) from Chippenham, containing 285 inhabitants. The living is a rectory, in the archdeaconry of Wilts, and diocese of Salisbury, rated in the king's books at

£11. 9. 9½., and in the patronage of the Bishop of Salisbury. The church is dedicated to St. Mary. Near Ebbedown are vestiges of a small Roman camp. In the walk to the glebe-house is a small hollow oak, a favourite resort of Latimer, when that celebrated prelate held the incumbency.

KINGWATER, a township in the parish of LANERCOST-ABBEY, ESKDALE ward, county of CUMBERLAND, 9 miles (N.E.) from Brampton, containing 331 inhabitants. It derives its name from a stream formed by several rills issuing from the mountains, which unite to the northward of Gilsland.

KINGWESTON, a parish in the hundred of CATS-ASH, county of SOMERSET, 3½ miles (N.E.) from Somerton, containing 111 inhabitants. The living is a discharged rectory, in the archdeaconry of Wells, and diocese of Bath and Wells, rated in the king's books at £10. 6. 3. W. Dickenson, Esq. was patron in 1827. The church is dedicated to All Saints.

KINLET, a parish in the hundred of STOTTESDEN, county of SALOP, 5¼ miles (N.E. by N.) from Cleobury-Mortimer, containing 552 inhabitants. The living is a discharged vicarage, in the archdeaconry of Salop, and diocese of Hereford, rated in the king's books at £8. 2. 4. William Child, Esq. was patron in 1814. The church, dedicated to St. Peter, is an ancient cruciform structure in the Norman style, and contains several splendid monuments of the family of Blount, whose ancestors came over with the Conqueror.

KINNERLEY, a parish in the hundred of OSWESTRY, county of SALOP, 6½ miles (S.E. by S.) from Oswestry, containing 1167 inhabitants. The living is a discharged vicarage, in the archdeaconry and diocese of St. Asaph, rated in the king's books at £7. 6. 8., and in the patronage of the Crown. The church is dedicated to St. Mary. The ancient castle was demolished during the minority of Henry III., by Llewellyn, Prince of Wales, who agreed to make reparation for the act, though it was never habitable afterwards.

KINNERSLEY, a parish comprising the township of Newchurch in the hundred of WOLPHY, but chiefly in the hundred of STRETFORD, county of HEREFORD, 4½ miles (W. by S.) from Weobly, containing 340 inhabitants. The living is a rectory, in the archdeaconry and diocese of Hereford, rated in the king's books at £13. 8. 4., and in the patronage of J. A. G. Clarke, Esq. The church is dedicated to St. James.

KINNERSLEY, a parish in the Newport division of the hundred of BRADFORD (South), county of SALOP, 4¾ miles (N. N. E.) from Wellington, containing 253 inhabitants. The living is a rectory, in the archdeaconry of Salop, and diocese of Lichfield and Coventry, rated in the king's books at £6. 1. 8. Earl Gower was patron in 1816. The church is dedicated to St. Chad.

KINNERTON (LOWER), a township in the parish of DODDLESTON, lower division of the hundred of BROXTON, county palatine of CHESTER, 5¾ miles (S. W. by W.) from Chester, containing 85 inhabitants.

KINNEYSIDE, a township in the parish of ST. BEES, ALLERDALE ward above Darwent, county of CUMBERLAND, 3¾ miles (N.E. by N.) from Egremont, containing 225 inhabitants, of whom many are employed in the extensive lead mines worked here, and others at the smelting-mill belonging to the London Lead Company.

KINOULTON, a parish in the southern division of the wapentake of BINGHAM, county of NOTTINGHAM, 9 miles (S. E.) from Nottingham, containing, with the extra-parochial liberty of Lodge on the Woulds, 370 inhabitants. The living is a discharged vicarage, in the peculiar jurisdiction of the Vicar, rated in the king's books at £7. 18. 11., and in the patronage of the Archbishop of York. The church is dedicated to St. Wilfrid. There was anciently a chapel at Newbold, in this parish, but no vestiges of it are now visible. The Grantham canal passes through the parish, and the old Fosse road forms its western boundary. Kinoulton is in the honour of Tutbury, duchy of Lancaster, and within the jurisdiction of a court of pleas held at Tutbury every third Tuesday, for the recovery of debts under 40s. In the neighbourhood is an excellent chalybeate spring, called the Spa. Here was formerly a palace belonging to the Archbishops of York, but there are now no vestiges of it.

KINSHAM, a parish comprising Lower and Upper Kinsham, in the hundred of WIGMORE, county of HEREFORD, 3½ miles (E.) from Presteigne, containing 107 inhabitants. The living is a perpetual curacy, in the archdeaconry and diocese of Hereford, and in the patronage of the Earl of Oxford.

KINSHAM, a hamlet in that part of the parish of BREDON which is in the middle division of the hundred of OSWALDSLOW, county of WORCESTER. The population is returned with the parish.

KINTBURY, a parish (formerly a market town) in the hundred of KINTBURY-EAGLE, county of BERKS, 3¼ miles (E. S. E.) from Hungerford, containing 1763 inhabitants. The living is a vicarage, in the archdeaconry of Berks, and diocese of Salisbury, rated in the king's books at £20. Charles Dundas, Esq. was patron in 1798. The church, dedicated to St. Mary, is partly in the Norman style of architecture. There is a place of worship for Wesleyan Methodists. The Kennet and Avon canal passes through the parish; and on the banks of the river Kennet there is a silk-throwing mill, affording employment to about one hundred persons. Kintbury had formerly a market on Friday, and two annual fairs, one on the festival of the Nativity of the Virgin Mary, the other on that of St. Simon and St. Jude, granted, in 1268, to the nuns of Shaftesbury. In digging a grave here, in 1762, a considerable number of Saxon coins of Edred, Edwy, and Edmund, was discovered under a scull.

KINTON, a township in the parish of LEINTWARDINE, hundred of WIGMORE, county of HEREFORD, containing 197 inhabitants.

KINVASTON, a township in that part of the parish of WOLVERHAMPTON which is in the eastern division of the hundred of CUTTLESTONE, county of STAFFORD, containing 19 inhabitants. Dr. James, a distinguished physician, was born here in 1703; he died in 1776.

KINVER, county of STAFFORD.—See KINFARE.

KINWALSEY, a hamlet in the parish of HAMPTON in ARDEN, Solihull division of the hundred of HEMLINGFORD, county of WARWICK, containing 20 inhabitants.

KINWARTON, a parish in the Alcester division of the hundred of BARLICHWAY, county of WARWICK, 1¼ mile (N. E.) from Alcester, containing 41 inhabitants. The living is a rectory, with the curacies of Great Alne and

Weethley, in the archdeaconry and diocese of Worcester, rated in the king's books at £17. 11. 0½., and in the patronage of the Bishop of Worcester. The church is dedicated to St. Mary.

KIPLIN, a township in that part of the parish of CATTERICK which is in the eastern division of the wapentake of GILLING, North riding of the county of YORK, 2¾ miles (E. S. E.) from Catterick, containing 100 inhabitants.

KIPPAX, a parish in the lower division of the wapentake of SKYRACK, West riding of the county of YORK, comprising the townships of Allerton-Bywater, Kippax, and Great and Little Preston, and containing 1765 inhabitants, of which number, 958 are in the township of Kippax, 6½ miles (N. W. by N.) from Pontefract. The living is a discharged vicarage, in the archdeaconry and diocese of York, rated in the king's books at £5. 7. 1., endowed with £200 private benefaction, and £200 royal bounty, and in the patronage of the Crown. The church is dedicated to St. Mary. There is a place of worship for Wesleyan Methodists. This place is said to have derived its name from a mount raised by the Saxons, called the Keep, whereon the village now stands, and from a remarkable ash which grew near it, hence Keep-Ash, since corrupted to Kippax. There are extensive coal mines in the parish, through which runs the river Air. George Goldsmith, in the 36th of Henry VIII., founded a free school here, and endowed it with cottages and land now producing £22 a year, for which eight children are instructed.

KIRBY, a parish in the hundred of TENDRING, county of ESSEX, 11¼ miles (S. E.) from Manningtree, containing 853 inhabitants. The living is a discharged vicarage, consolidated with those of Thorpe le Soken, and Walton le Soken, in the peculiar jurisdiction of the Sokens, the wills and records being deposited at the residence of the Lord of the Manor, at Harwich; it is rated in the king's books at £10, and in the patronage of W. P. Honeywood, Esq. The church is dedicated to St. Michael. There is a place of worship for Wesleyan Methodists. The parish is bounded on the north by a creek of the North sea, which runs up to Landermere. Here is a wharf for loading and unloading small craft, which occasionally sail to London with corn. A fair is held on the festival of St. Ann, when the lord of the manor holds his annual court.

KIRBY (COLD), a parish in the wapentake of BIRDFORTH, North riding of the county of YORK, 7¼ miles (E. N. E.) from Thirsk, containing 185 inhabitants. The living is a perpetual curacy, in the archdeaconry of Cleveland, and diocese of York, endowed with £800 royal bounty, and in the patronage of Lord Feversham.

KIRBY (MONKS), a parish in the Kirby division of the hundred of KNIGHTLOW, county of WARWICK, 7 miles (N. N. W.) from Rugby, containing, with the chapelry of Copston-Magna, and the hamlets of Easenhall, Paitton, and Stretton under Foss with Newbold-Revel, 1659 inhabitants. The living is a discharged vicarage, in the archdeaconry of Coventry, and diocese of Lichfield and Coventry, rated in the king's books at £22. 9. 7., and in the patronage of the Master and Fellows of Trinity College, Cambridge. The church is dedicated to St. Edith. There is a place of worship for Baptists. Dugdale fixes here the town of *Cyrcbirig*, built by Ethelfreda, Countess of Mercia; but Gibson places it at Chirbury in Shropshire, on the frontier of the ancient kingdom of Mercia. A priory of Benedictine monks, a cell to the abbey of Angiers in Normandy, was founded here about 1077, by Gosfred de Wirchia, the possessions of which, after its suppression, were annexed to the Carthusian priory of Axholme, and valued at £220. 3. 4. per annum.

KIRBY on the MOOR, a parish in the wapentake of HALLIKELD, North riding of the county of YORK, comprising the townships of Kirby on the Moor, Langthorp, and a portion of Humberton with Milby, and containing 458 inhabitants, of which number, 190 are in the township of Kirby on the Moor, 1¼ mile (N. by W.) from Boroughbridge. The living is a discharged vicarage, in the archdeaconry of Richmond, and diocese of Chester, rated in the king's books at £7. 13. 6½., endowed with £200 private benefaction, and £200 royal bounty and in the patronage of the Crown. The church is dedicated to All Saints.

KIRBY (WEST), a parish in the lower division of the hundred of WIRRALL, county palatine of CHESTER, comprising the townships of Great and Little Caldey, Frankby, Grange, Greasby, Hoose, Great Meolse, Little Meolse, Newton with Larton, and West Kirby, and containing 1140 inhabitants, of which number, 172 are in the township of West Kirby, 7½ miles (N. W. by N.) from Great Neston. The living is a rectory, in the archdeaconry and diocese of Chester, rated in the king's books at £28. 13. 4., and in the patronage of the Dean and Chapter of Chester. The church, dedicated to St. Bridget, was rebuilt in 1786. A free grammar school was founded at Caldey-Grange, in 1636, by William Clegg, Esq., who endowed it with premises now producing from £30 to £40 a year, to which an annuity of £30 was added in 1677, by a Mr. Bennett, who also left £24 per annum to buy gowns for twenty-four poor persons, and an estate at Neston *cum* Larton, the annual proceeds of which, amounting to £200, are distributed among the poor on Good Friday. The parish lies at the entrance to the river Dee, which bounds it on the west, and on the north is the Irish sea. At Little Meolse are two hotels well frequented, and affording good accommodation for visitors during the bathing season.

KIRBY-BEDON, a parish in the hundred of HENSTEAD, county of NORFOLK, 3¾ miles (S. E.) from Norwich, comprising the consolidated parishes of St. Andrew and St. Mary, and containing 201 inhabitants. The living is a discharged rectory, in the archdeaconry of Norfolk, and diocese of Norwich, rated in the king's books at £6. 4. 9½. Mrs. Muskett was patroness in 1822. The church of St. Mary has been demolished.

KIRBY-BELLARS, a parish in the hundred of FRAMLAND, county of LEICESTER, 3½ miles (W. by S.) from Melton-Mowbray, containing 203 inhabitants. The living is a perpetual curacy, in the archdeaconry of Leicester, and diocese of Lincoln, endowed with £600 royal bounty, and £200 parliamentary grant. Sir F. Burdett, Bart. was patron in 1813. The church is dedicated to St. Peter. A college for a warden and twelve priests was founded here, in the reign of Edward II., by Roger Beller, which, in 1359, was made conventual, for a prior and canons regular of the order of St. Augustine, and so continued to the dissolution, when its revenue was estimated at £178. 7. 10.

KIRBY-CANE, a parish in the hundred of CLAVERING, county of NORFOLK, 4 miles (N. W.) from Beccles, containing 340 inhabitants. The living is a discharged rectory, in the archdeaconry of Norfolk, and diocese of Norwich, rated in the king's books at £10. R. Wilson, Esq. was patron in 1820. The church is dedicated to All Saints.

KIRBY-GRINDALYTH, a parish in the wapentake of BUCKROSE, East riding of the county of YORK, comprising the townships of Duggleby, Kirby-Grindalyth, and Thirkleby, and containing 376 inhabitants, of which number, 178 are in the township of Kirby-Grindalyth, 9 miles (E. S. E.) from New Malton. The living is a discharged vicarage, in the archdeaconry of the East riding, and diocese of York, rated in the king's books at £8. 9. 7. Sir Tatton Sykes, Bart. was patron in 1789. The church is dedicated to St. Andrew.

KIRBY-KNOWLE, a parish in the wapentake of BIRDFORTH, North riding of the county of YORK, comprising the chapelry of Bagby, and the townships of Balk and Kirby-Knowle, and containing 505 inhabitants, of which number, 138 are in the township of Kirby-Knowle, 4¾ miles (N. E. by N.) from Thirsk. The living is a rectory, in the archdeaconry of Cleveland, and diocese of York, rated in the king's books at £8. 2. 1. Sir T. Frankland, Bart. was patron in 1797.

KIRBY-UNDERDALE, a parish in the wapentake of BUCKROSE, East riding of the county of YORK, 6½ miles (N.) from Pocklington, containing 335 inhabitants. The living is a rectory, in the archdeaconry of the East riding, and diocese of York, rated in the king's books at £6. 3. 4., and in the patronage of the Crown. The church is dedicated to All Saints.

KIRBY-WISK, a parish comprising the joint township of Newsham with Breckenbrough in the wapentake of BIRDFORTH, and the townships of Kirby-Wisk, Maunby, and Newby-Wisk, in the eastern division of the wapentake of GILLING, North riding of the county of YORK, and containing 841 inhabitants, of which number, 197 are in the township of Kirby-Wisk, 4¾ miles (W. by N.) from Thirsk. The living is a rectory, in the archdeaconry of Richmond, and diocese of Chester, rated in the king's books at £27. 16. 5½. The Duke of Northumberland was patron in 1808. The church is dedicated to St. John the Baptist. In this parish were born Roger Ascham, the learned and accomplished tutor of Queen Elizabeth; Dr. George Hickes, author of the *Thesaurus Linguarum Septemptrionalium*; and Dr. John Palliser, Archbishop of Tuam.

KIRDFORD, a parish in the hundred of ROTHERBRIDGE, rape of ARUNDEL, county of SUSSEX, 4½ miles (N. E. by N.) from Petworth, containing 1602 inhabitants. The living is a vicarage, in the archdeaconry and diocese of Chichester, rated in the king's books at £11, and in the patronage of the Earl of Egremont. The church, dedicated to St. John the Baptist, is principally in the early style of English architecture.

KIRK-ANDREWS upon EDEN, a parish in the ward and county of CUMBERLAND, 3¼ miles (W. N. W.) from Carlisle, containing 141 inhabitants. The living is a discharged rectory, with that of Beaumont, in the archdeaconry and diocese of Carlisle. The church has long been demolished, and the ruins, removed upwards of sixty years since, were used in the erection of the glebe house. The inhabitants attend divine service at

Beaumont, but bury their dead in the church-yard here. There was a still more ancient church at Kirksteads, about one mile from the site of this, which was attended by the inhabitants of Kirk-Andrews, Beaumont, Grinsdale, and Orton, but at what period it was destroyed is unknown; the cemetery, in which stones curiously carved, and human bones have been found, may yet be traced. The river Eden and the Carlisle canal run through this parish, which is parcel of the barony of Burgh. There is a trifling endowment for the instruction of children. On the common is a triple intrenchment, near which several urns were discovered about forty years ago. The Roman wall passed through this parish.

KIRK-ANDREWS upon ESK, a parish in ESKDALE ward, county of CUMBERLAND, comprising the chapelry of Nichol-Forest, and the townships of Middle Kirk-Andrews, Nether Kirk-Andrews, and Moat, and containing 2235 inhabitants, of which number, 624 are in the township of Middle Kirk-Andrews, 3 miles (N. by E.) from Longtown. The living is a discharged rectory, in the archdeaconry and diocese of Carlisle, rated in the king's books at £3. 11. 5.. endowed with £200 royal bounty, and in the patronage of Sir James Graham, Bart. The church, dedicated to St. Andrew, is a very picturesque object, standing alone on the western bank of the Esk: it was erected by Sir Richard Graham upon the site of a more ancient structure, in 1637, at which period Kirk-Andrews was made a distinct parish, having previously been only a chapelry in that of Arthuret, or Easton. Here are four charity schools, with endowments of £5 each bequeathed by Lady Widdrington, in 1754. This parish, which is separated from Scotland by the rivers Liddel, Kershope, and Sark, and by the Scots' dyke, forms a large portion of the English border, and was the scene of almost constant warfare before the union of the two crowns. Near the church is one of the ancient tower fortresses erected for the defence of the border; and on the steep banks of the Liddel is a moated place, called Liddel's Strength, believed to have been the site of the castle of the ancient barons of Liddel. William, King of Scotland, took this castle in 1174; and David Bruce captured it by assault in 1346. About a mile from the church is a quarry of good freestone: over the Esk is a bridge, where many of the rebels, in 1745, were slaughtered by the army of the Duke of Cumberland. There is a cast-iron bridge across the same river at Garristown, also two of stone over the Sark. In this parish is Solway Moss, celebrated for the victory obtained there over the Scots in the reign of Henry VIII., and for its extraordinary irruption in November 1771, when a large tract of land was inundated, though it was afterwards recovered and brought again into cultivation.

KIRK-ANDREWS (NETHER), a township in the parish of KIRK-ANDREWS upon ESK, ESKDALE ward, county of CUMBERLAND, containing 516 inhabitants. This township, lying between the rivers Sark and Esk, comprises Solway Moss and a portion of the once debateable lands.

KIRK-BRIDE, a parish in the ward and county of CUMBERLAND, 5¾ miles (N.N.W.) from Wigton, containing 308 inhabitants. The living is a discharged rectory, in the archdeaconry and diocese of Carlisle, rated in the king's books at £5, and in the patronage of the

Rev. Francis Metcalfe. The church, dedicated to St. Bride, or Brydoch, an Irish woman of great sanctity, was built before the Conquest. The Society of Friends have a meeting-house here. The parish is watered by the Wampool, which bounds it on the east and north; the village being situated on the south side of the æstuary of that river, in which the sand banks are so often shifted by the violent meeting of the tides and freshes, that no bridge hitherto erected has been found to withstand their united force.

KIRK-BURN, a parish in the Bainton - Beacon division of the wapentake of HARTHILL, East riding of the county of YORK, comprising the townships of East Burn, Kirk-Burn, South Burn, and Tibthorp, and containing 455 inhabitants, of which number, 119 are in the township of Kirk-Burn, 4 miles (S.W. by W.) from Great Driffield. The living is a discharged vicarage, in the archdeaconry of the East riding, and diocese of York, rated in the king's books at £4. 10. 2½., endowed with £600 royal bounty, and in the patronage of the Crown. The church is dedicated to St. Mary.

KIRK-BURTON, county of YORK. — See BURTON (KIRK).

KIRKBY, a chapelry in the parish of WALTON on the HILL, hundred of WEST DERBY, county palatine of LANCASTER, 5¾ miles (N.W.) from Prescot, containing 1035 inhabitants. The living is a perpetual curacy, in the archdeaconry and diocese of Chester, endowed with £200 private benefaction, and £600 royal bounty, and in the patronage of the Rector of Walton. The church is dedicated to St. Chad. A school has been erected here by Lord Sefton, the master receiving £8 a year, the produce of an ancient bequest. There is also a bequest from Thomas Aspe, in 1698, for apprenticing poor children.

KIRKBY, a joint parish with Osgodby, in the northern division of the wapentake of WALSHCROFT, parts of LINDSEY, county of LINCOLN, 4¼ miles (N.W.) from Market-Raisen, containing, with Osgodby, 214 inhabitants. The living is a discharged vicarage with that of Owersby, in the archdeaconry and diocese of Lincoln, rated in the king's books at £8. 18. 4., and endowed with £200 royal bounty. The church, dedicated to St. Andrew, though much modernised, appears to have been originally of Norman architecture; in the chancel are some ancient tombs. Thomas Goodrich, Bishop of Ely, and Lord Chancellor in the reign of Edward VI., was born here.

KIRKBY, a joint township with Netherby, in the parish of KIRKBY-OVERBLOWS, upper division of the wapentake of CLARO, West riding of the county of YORK, 4½ miles (w. by S.) from Wetherby, containing, with Netherby, 226 inhabitants. There is a place of worship for Wesleyan Methodists.

KIRKBY in ASHFIELD, a parish in the northern division of the wapentake of BROXTOW, county of NOTTINGHAM, 5¼ miles (S.W.) from Mansfield, containing 1420 inhabitants. The living is a rectory, in the archdeaconry of Nottingham, and diocese of York, rated in the king's books at £18. 1. 8., and in the patronage of the Duke of Portland. The church, dedicated to St. Wilfrid, is a large stone structure, with a lofty steeple. The rivers Erewash and Maun rise in this parish; and the Mansfield and Pinxton railway, in passing through it, affords a medium of conveyance for the coal and lime which are obtained here in considerable quantities. Several of the inhabitants are employed in frame-work knitting. A free school, erected by subscription in 1826, is chiefly supported by the Duke of Portland and the rector.

KIRKBY upon BAIN, a parish in the southern division of the wapentake of GARTREE, parts of LINDSEY, county of LINCOLN, 6 miles (S. S. W.) from Horncastle, containing, with the township of Tumby, 591 inhabitants. The living is a rectory, in the peculiar jurisdiction of the manor court of Kirkstead, rated in the king's books at £13. 13. 6½., and in the patronage of the Crown. The church is dedicated to St. Mary. There is a place of worship for Wesleyan Methodists. A school for the instruction of poor children is endowed with land bequeathed by Richard Brocklesby, in 1713.

KIRKBY in CLEVELAND, a parish in the western division of the liberty of LANGBAURGH, North riding of the county of YORK, comprising the townships of Great and Little Broughton, and Kirkby in Cleveland, and containing 685 inhabitants, of which number, 168 are in the township of Kirkby in Cleveland, 2 miles (S. E. by S.) from Stokesley. The living comprises a discharged vicarage and a sinecure rectory, in the archdeaconry of Cleveland, and diocese of York, the former rated in the king's books at £5. 6. 3., and the latter at £21. 8. 6½. The Archbishop of York appoints to the rectory, and the Rector to the vicarage. The church, dedicated to St. Augustine, was erected, in 1815, upon the site of a smaller cruciform structure. A free grammar school was founded, in 1683, by Henry Edmunds, Esq., who endowed it with a school-house, garden, and an estate at Broughton, producing £50 per annum, for the benefit of all the poor children of the parish. A Sunday school, established and supported by subscription, is attended by about sixty of both sexes. There is also a library for the use of the parishioners, selected from books recommended by the Society for propagating Christian Knowledge.

KIRKBY (EAST), a parish in the western division of the soke of BOLINGBROKE, parts of LINDSEY, county of LINCOLN, 5 miles (W. S. W.) from Spilsby, containing 347 inhabitants. The living is a discharged vicarage, in the archdeaconry and diocese of Lincoln, rated in the king's books at £5. 12. 1., endowed with £200 royal bounty, and in the patronage of William Thimbleby, Esq. The church is dedicated to St. Nicholas. A charity school is endowed with land bequeathed by Gregory and Margaret Croft, in 1712.

KIRKBY on the HILL, a township in the parish of KIRKBY-RAVENSWORTH, western division of the wapentake of GILLING, North riding of the county of YORK, 4 miles (N. N. W.) from Richmond, containing 161 inhabitants.

KIRKBY in MALHAM-DALE, a parish comprising the township of Calton in the eastern division, and the townships of Airton, Hanlith, Kirkby in Malham-Dale, Malham, Malham-Moor, Otterburn, and Scosthorpe, in the western division, of the wapentake of STAINCLIFFE and EWCROSS, West riding of the county of YORK, and containing 1005 inhabitants, of which number, 204 are in the township of Kirkby in Malham-Dale, 5½ miles (E. S. E.) from Settle. The living is a vicarage, in the archdeaconry and diocese of York, rated in the king's books at £6. 13. 4., endowed with

£200 private benefaction, £400 royal bounty, and £1200 parliamentary grant, and in the patronage of the Duke of Devonshire. A free grammar school was founded here, in 1606, by John Topham, who endowed it with certain lands which, with subsequent bequests, produce an income of £21 a year, for which, and moderate quarterages, from twenty to thirty children receive an English education; but the classics are taught free to those who apply.

KIRKBY (SOUTH), a parish in the upper division of the wapentake of OSGOLDCROSS, West riding of the county of YORK, comprising the townships of North Elmsall, South Elmsall, South Kirkby, and Shelbrooke, and containing 1314 inhabitants, of which number, 633 are in the township of South Kirkby, 8½ miles (S.) from Pontefract. The living is a discharged vicarage, in the archdeaconry and diocese of York, rated in the king's books at £15. 10. 2½. The Rev. James Allott was patron in 1813. The church is dedicated to All Saints.

KIRKBY le THORPE, a parish in the wapentake of ASWARDHURN, parts of KESTEVEN, county of LINCOLN, 2 miles (E. by N.) from Sleaford, containing 166 inhabitants. The living is a rectory in medieties, united, in 1737, to that of Asgarby, in the archdeaconry and diocese of Lincoln, rated jointly in the king's books at £9. 12. 6. The church, dedicated to St. Denis, has a Norman door, with some portions in the early, and a font and wooden porch in the later, style of English architecture.

KIRKBY-FLEETHAM, a parish in the eastern division of the wapentake of HANG, North riding of the county of YORK, 4 miles (S. E. by E.) from Catterick, containing 566 inhabitants. The living is a discharged vicarage, in the archdeaconry of Cleveland, and diocese of Chester, rated in the king's books at £9. 18. 2., and in the patronage of the Crown. The church is dedicated to St. Mary.

KIRKBY-FRITH, a liberty in the parish of GLENFIELD, hundred of SPARKENHOE, county of LEICESTER, 3½ miles (W. by N.) from Leicester, containing 18 inhabitants.

KIRKBY-GREEN, a parish in the first division of the wapentake of LANGOE, parts of KESTEVEN, county of LINCOLN, 7¾ miles (N. by E.) from Sleaford, containing 68 inhabitants. The living is a discharged vicarage, in the archdeaconry and diocese of Lincoln, rated in the king's books at £11. 7. 6., and in the patronage of the Crown. The church is dedicated to the Holy Cross.

KIRKBY-HALL, a township in that part of the parish of LITTLE OUSEBURN which is in the lower division of the wapentake of CLARO, West riding of the county of YORK, 4½ miles (S.E.) from Aldborough, containing 55 inhabitants.

KIRKBY-IRELETH, a parish in the hundred of LONSDALE, north of the sands, county palatine of LANCASTER, 4½ miles (N. W. by W.) from Ulverstone, comprising the market town and chapelry of Broughton in Furness, the chapelries of Dunnerdale, Seathwaite, and Woodland with Heathwaite, and the townships of Low Quarter, and Middle Quarter, and containing 2947 inhabitants. The living is a discharged vicarage, in the archdeaconry of Richmond, and diocese of Chester, rated in the king's books at £5. 6. 8., endowed with £200 private benefaction, £400 royal bounty, and

£1200 parliamentary grant, and in the peculiar jurisdiction and patronage of the Dean and Chapter of York. The church, dedicated to St. Cuthbert, contains several ancient monuments, and the windows exhibit some beautiful specimens of stained glass. Here are extensive quarries of a dark blue slate of excellent quality, with which vessels are laden at the mouth of the river Duddon, which, after separating this parish from that of Millom in Cumberland, empties itself into the Irish sea. There is a small bequest by Samuel Wilson, in 1769, towards the support of a schoolmaster.

KIRKBY-LONSDALE, a parish in LONSDALE ward, county of WESTMORLAND, comprising the market town of Kirkby-Lonsdale, with the chapelries of Barbon, Firbank, Hutton-Roof, Killington, Mansergh, and Middleton, and the townships of Casterton and Lupton, and containing 3769 inhabitants, of which number, 1643 are in the town of Kirkby-Lonsdale, 30 miles (S. by W.) from Appleby, and 252 (N.W. by W.) from London, on the great road from Kendal to Leeds. The name of this place is derived from its having been the chief town of the district which had a church, and the adjunct from its situation in a dale, or valley, on the western bank of the river Lon, or Lune. The town is one of the largest in the county, and consists of several handsome streets, which are lighted, but not paved; the three principal ones meeting nearly in the centre, where is the market-place: the houses are well built of white hewn stone, and roofed with blue slate; many of them have fine gardens attached: the inhabitants are supplied with water from a spring at Totley wood, one mile distant, by means of pipes, under the direction of a joint stock company. The surrounding scenery is highly picturesque, to which the distant mountains, particularly Ingleborough, the loftiest of them, give a grandeur of effect rarely excelled: the peculiar beauty of the valley of Lonsdale, and the eligible society of the neighbourhood, have rendered the town a favourite residence. A book society, supported by subscription, was founded in 1794, to which a small permanent library belongs. The manufacture of knit stockings, for which this place was formerly famous, has greatly declined; and the weaving of carpets, blankets, coarse linen, calicoe, and gingham, is now carried on to a small extent. Several mills, built on the steep banks of the hills, are worked by the Lune, which here turns machinery consisting of seven wheels placed almost perpendicularly under each other, by which two threshing and grinding-mills, a wool-carding mill, and two tanneries, are kept in action. This river, which winds round the town, is crossed by a lofty stone bridge of exquisite workmanship and great antiquity: it is founded on a rock, and consists of three semicircular ribbed arches, the centre arch being much higher than the others: the road-way is inconveniently narrow. The market is on Thursday; and fairs are held on Holy Thursday, and October 5th and 6th, for horned cattle and horses, and on St. Thomas's day for woollen cloth. The new market-place, formed in 1822, is a spacious quadrangle: in the fish market is an ancient market cross. A court leet and view of frankpledge for the manor are held annually in October; and petty sessions for the Lonsdale ward are held every Thursday. The living is a discharged vicarage, in the archdeaconry of Richmond, and diocese of Chester, rated in the king's

books at £20. 15. 2., endowed with £200 private benefaction, and £200 royal bounty, and in the patronage of the Master and Fellows of Trinity College, Cambridge. The church, which is dedicated to St. Mary, is a noble structure of great antiquity, with a square tower nearly seventy feet in height, which was rebuilt in 1705: the interior is divided into four great aisles, by three rows of pillars which support the roof: the arched doorway under the tower is evidently of Norman architecture, the bases of some of the pillars, and the shafts of others, are also Norman, and the east window, with light detached pillars, is in the early style of English architecture: the pulpit, which is curiously carved, was erected, in 1619, at the expense of Mr. Henry Wilson, who also founded a library attached to the church, and bequeathed various sums for charitable uses. There are places of worship for Independents, Wesleyan Methodists, and Glassites, or Sandemanians The free grammar school was founded, in 1591, by letters patent of Queen Elizabeth, and endowed by Mr. Godshalfe and others: it is under the direction of twenty-four governors, and, by means of several subsequent benefactions, the endowment has been augmented, and produces about £50 per annum, which is received by the master, who has a house for his residence, and instructs in Greek and Latin about forty boys, who pay for being taught writing and arithmetic, besides which he is allowed to take stipendiary pupils: the school has the benefit of four exhibitions, of £5 per annum each, to Queen's College, Oxford, founded by Henry Wilson, in 1638; three, of about £20 each, to Christ's College, Cambridge, on the foundation of the Rev. Thomas Wilson, in 1626; and three at the same college, founded by Dr. Thomas Otway, Bishop of Ossory, who died in 1692. At Sellet Bank, about a mile and a half from the town, is a chalybeate spring; and, according to tradition, an artificial mount in the neighbourhood, called " Cock Pit Hill," is the tumulus of one of the British kings. Lonsdale gives the title of earl to the family of Lowther.

KIRKBY-MALLORY, a parish in the hundred of SPARKENHOE, county of LEICESTER, 4½ miles (N.N.E.) from Hinckley, containing, with the chapelry of Earl-Shilton, 2067 inhabitants. The living is a rectory, in the archdeaconry of Leicester, and diocese of Lincoln, rated in the king's books at £15, and in the patronage of Lady Byron. The church is dedicated to All Saints.

KIRKBY-MALZEARD, a parish in the lower division of the wapentake of CLARO, West riding of the county of YORK, comprising the market town of Kirkby-Malzeard, the chapelries of Hartwith with Winsley, and Middlesmoor, and the townships of Cozenley, Fountains Earth, Gravelthorpe, Laverton, Down Stonebeck, and Upper Stonebeck, and containing 4263 inhabitants, of which number, 682 are in the town of Kirkby-Malzeard, 6 miles (W.N.W.) from Ripon. The market is on Wednesday; and fairs are held on Whit-Monday and October 2nd; all which, after long disuse, have been recently revived. The living is a vicarage, with that of Masham, either in the peculiar jurisdiction of the Dean and Chapter of York, or in that of the manor court of Masham, being claimed by both, and the matter not determined; it is in the patronage of the Master and Fellows of Trinity College, Cambridge. The church is dedicated to St. Andrew. A school, in which fifteen children are instructed and five clothed annually, is supported by the proceeds of a rent-charge of £5, the benefaction of Gilbert Horseman, in 1640, subsequently augmented with the interest of £100 given by Gregory Elsley, in 1716.

KIRKBY-MISPERTON, a parish in Pickering lythe, North riding of the county of York, comprising the townships of Barugh-Ambe, Great Habton, Little Habton, Kirkby-Misperton, and Ryton, and containing 809 inhabitants, of which number, 170 are in the township of Kirkby-Misperton, 3¾ miles (S. W. by S.) from Pickering. The living is a rectory, in the archdeaconry of Cleveland, and diocese of York, rated in the king's books at £25. 1. 10½., and in the patronage of Lord Feversham. The church is dedicated to St. Lawrence. William Smithson, in 1637, bequeathed a rent-charge of £10 per annum towards the support of a school for all the poor children of the parish.

KIRKBY-MOORSIDE, a parish in the wapentake of Ryedale, North riding of the county of York, comprising the market town of Kirkby-Moorside, and the townships of Bransdale (East Side), Fadmore, Farndale (Low Quarter), and Gillimoor, and containing 2903 inhabitants, of which number, 1878 are in the town of Kirkby-Moorside, 29 miles (N. by E.) from York, and 224 (N. by W.) from London. This is a small and irregularly built town, situated on the banks of the river Dove, and almost surrounded by steep hills. In the vicinity are several corn-mills; a considerable quantity of malt is made here, and there is a small linen manufactory. Near the town are limestone and freestone quarries, and coal mines. The market is on Wednesday; and fairs are held on the Wednesday in Whitsun-week, and September 18th for cattle, sheep, &c. The living is a discharged vicarage, in the archdeaconry of Cleveland, and diocese of York, rated in the king's books at £14. 0. 10., and in the patronage of the Crown. The church, which contains some ancient portions, with later insertions, is dedicated to All Saints. There are places of worship for the Society of Friends, Independents, and Wesleyan Methodists. Here is a Sunday school, with an endowment of £4 per annum, the gift of the Rev. W. Comber, in 1800, but principally supported by subscription. The manor of Kirkby-Moorside was given by James I. to his favourite, the Duke of Buckingham, whose son, the second Duke, having retired hither, died at the manor-house, in 1687.

KIRKBY-MUXLOE, a chapelry in the parish of Glenfield, hundred of Sparkenhoe, county of Leicester, 4½ miles (W.) from Leicester, containing 256 inhabitants. Here are the ruins of an ancient moated and castellated mansion, formerly belonging to the family of Hastings.

KIRKBY-OVERBLOWS, a parish in the upper division of the wapentake of Claro, West riding of the county of York, comprising the chapelry of Stainburn, and the townships of Kirkby with Netherby, Kirkby-Overblows, Rigton, Sicklinghall, and a portion of Swindon, and containing 1646 inhabitants, of which number, 318 are in the township of Kirkby-Overblows, 6 miles (W.) from Wetherby. The living is a rectory, in the archdeaconry and diocese of York, rated in the king's books at £20. 1. 0½., and in the patronage of the Earl of Egremont. The church, dedicated to All Saints, was

made collegiate previously to 1364, for a provost and four chaplains. A school was erected by subscription in 1782, and £10 a year is paid for teaching six boys.

KIRKBY-RAVENSWORTH, a parish in the western division of the wapentake of Gilling, North riding of the county of York, 4¾ miles (N. N. W.) from Richmond, comprising the townships of Gayles, Kirkby on the Hill, New Forest, Newsham, Ravensworth, Whashton, and a portion of Dalton, and containing 1685 inhabitants. The living is a perpetual curacy, in the archdeaconry of Richmond, and diocese of Chester, endowed with £400 private benefaction, £400 royal bounty, and £200 parliamentary grant, and in the patronage of the Bishop of Chester, as impropriator of the rectory, which is rated in the king's books at £25. 5. 2½. The church, dedicated to St. Peter and St. Felix, is a handsome edifice, built, in 1397, on the supposed site of a more ancient one erected by the Saxons. Near it are the grammar school, and hospital of St. John the Baptist, founded, in 1556, by Dr. Dakyn, then rector, who endowed them with lands, &c., at East Coulton, now producing about £1300 per annum. The school is free for all who apply for instruction in the classics; the master receives a salary of £200, and the usher about £70 per annum. The hospital is for the reception and maintenance of twenty-four aged persons of both sexes, who must either be natives of the parish, or resident for ten years within it. The government of the whole is vested in two wardens, elected biennially by ballot, who, with the master of the school, and the inmates of the hospital, form a body corporate, and have a common seal. Here are extensive remains of a castle built by Bodin, ancestor of the Fitz-Hughs.

KIRKBY-STEPHEN, a parish in East ward, county of Westmorland, comprising the market town of Kirkby-Stephen, the chapelries of Mallerstang and Soulby, and the townships of Hartley, Kaber, Nateby, Smardale, Waitby, Wharton, and Winton, and containing 2712 inhabitants, of which number, 1312 are in the town of Kirkby-Stephen, 11 miles (S. E. by S.) from Appleby, and 268 (N.N.W.) from London. This town, which derives the adjunct to its name from the saint to whom its church is dedicated, is pleasantly situated in a fertile plain, on the western bank of the river Eden, opposite the hills which separate this county from Yorkshire on the north and south; it consists of one good street, the houses in which are well built, and the inhabitants abundantly supplied with water; but the town is neither paved nor lighted. Races are held annually, on Hartley Ings, about the middle of April. The inhabitants are partly employed in the woollen manufacture; and in knitting stockings, of which a great quantity was formerly exposed for sale at the market, but the trade in this article is on the decline: a silk manufactory has lately been established on a limited scale, and there is a manufactory for spinning and carding wool. In the parish are mines of lead, copper, and coal, which are all worked, though the coal mines are not very productive; a kind of spotted stone is also found here, which is polished to make watch-seals and other ornaments. The market is on Monday, for corn, flour, oatmeal, and provisions. Fairs are held on the first Monday in Lent, the Monday before March 20th, April 25th, and October 2nd, for horned cattle, horses, woollen cloth, blankets, cotton goods, &c.; on the 29th of September chiefly

†

for horses, and on the 29th of October for cattle and sheep: there are statute fairs for hiring servants on the last Monday in June and the first Monday in July. On the north side of the market-place, which is spacious and convenient, is a market-house, with a piazza, called the cloister: the upper part of the edifice is supported on eight stone pillars, the whole having been erected in 1810, in pursuance of the will of Mr. John Waller, who left a sum of money for the express purpose. The county magistrates formerly held petty sessions here, which, although of late discontinued, it is in contemplation to revive.

The living is a vicarage, in the archdeaconry and diocese of Carlisle, rated in the king's books at £48. 19. 2., and in the patronage of the Rev. T. P. Williamson. The church, which is dedicated to St. Stephen, is an ancient and spacious building, surmounted by a lofty square tower ; the interior is divided into three principal aisles, by two rows of plain round-shafted columns which support the roof: there are sepulchral chapels belonging to Smardale hall, Wharton hall, and Hartley castle ; in the second of these is a fine alabaster monument, with the effigies of Thomas, Lord Wharton, and his first and second wives; and in the last a monumental figure of a man in armour, supposed to have been erected to the memory of Sir Andrew Harcla, Earl of Carlisle, and governor of Hartley castle, who was beheaded for treason in the reign of Edward II. Here are places of worship for Independents and Wesleyan Methodists. The free grammar school, which stands eastward from the church, was founded, in the 8th of Elizabeth, by Thomas, Lord Wharton, and endowed with property producing £52. 3. per annum: there are two exhibitions, of £3. 6. 8. each, to either of the Universities, and one especially to St. John's College, Cambridge, for a scholar from this school, or that at Appleby, but these have not been claimed for several years. The school is held in an ancient edifice, formerly the rectory house, and is under the direction of eight governors, who appoint the master: it is open to the boys of Kirkby-Stephen and the vicinity, at a small quarterage. Several poor children are instructed in the Sunday school, which is held at the poor-house, and is supported by voluntary contributions. There are divers small bequests for the poor of this parish.

KIRKBY-THORE, a parish in East ward, county of Westmorland, comprising the chapelries of Milburn with Milburn-Grange, and Temple-Sowerby, and the township of Kirkby-Thore, and containing 1051 inhabitants, of which number, 377 are in the township of Kirkby-Thore, 5¼ miles (N. W. by N.) from Appleby. The living is a rectory, in the archdeaconry and diocese of Carlisle, rated in the king's books at £37. 17. 11., and in the patronage of the Earl of Thanet. The church is dedicated to St. Michael. There is a place of worship for Wesleyan Methodists; also a school with a trifling endowment bequeathed by Mr. John Horn, in 1823. This place received its adjunct designation from Thor, the chief of the Saxon idols, to whose honour a temple was raised here. The rivers Eden and Troutbeck run through the parish, and unite their streams at the village, a great part of which, with the hall, was built out of the ruins of Whelp castle, an ancient fortress formerly occupying an adjacent eminence, where, in

1687, were discovered, on turning up its site for cultivation, a four-fold wall, arched vaults, leaden pipes, an altar inscribed "Fortvnae Servatrici," with many other antiquities, the supposed relics of a Roman station called Brovonacæ, as fixed by Horsley An ancient well, several urns, curious earthen vessels, and other relics, are recorded as having been discovered in 1684, near the bridge ; and, about 1770, the horn of a moose deer was dug up near the confluence of the two rivers. Not far from the village is a spring slightly sulphureous, termed Pots Well, which rises from an alabaster rock lying at a considerable depth below the surface.

KIRKBY-UNDERWOOD, a parish in the wapentake of Aveland, parts of Kesteven, county of Lincoln, 5 miles (N. N. W.) from Bourne, containing 167 inhabitants. The living is a rectory, in the archdeaconry and diocese of Lincoln, rated in the king's books at £6. 3. 4., and in the patronage of the Bishop of Lincoln. The church is dedicated to St. Mary and All Saints.

KIRKBY-WHARFE, a parish comprising the township of Ulleskelf within the liberty of St. Peter of York, East riding, and the townships of Grimston and Kirkby-Wharfe with Milford (a portion of which latter is also within the liberty of St. Peter of York), upper division of the wapentake of Barkstone-Ash, West riding, of the county of York, and containing 574 inhabitants, of which number, 86 are in the township of Kirkby-Wharfe with Milford, 2¼ miles (S. E. by S.) from Tadcaster. The living is a discharged vicarage, rated in the king's books at £3. 16. 8., endowed with £500 private benefaction, and £200 royal bounty, and in the peculiar jurisdiction and patronage of the Prebendary of Wetwang in the Cathedral Church of York. The church, dedicated to St. John the Baptist, has lately received an addition of eighty-six sittings, of which forty-three are free, the Incorporated Society for the enlargement of churches and chapels having granted £20 towards defraying the expense. The river Wharfe runs through the parish.

KIRKDALE, a township in the parish of Walton on the Hill, hundred of West Derby, county palatine of Lancaster, 1½ mile (N. by E.) from Liverpool, containing 1273 inhabitants. The petty sessions for the Kirkdale division of the hundred of West Derby are held here.

KIRKDALE, a parish comprising the township of Norton, with a portion of Wombleton, within the liberty of St. Peter of York, East riding, and the townships of Beadlam, Bransdale (West Side), Muscoates, Nawton, North Holme, Skiplam, Welburn, and a portion of Wombleton, in the wapentake of Ryedale, North riding, of the county of York, 4¼ miles (E. by N.) from Helmsley, and containing 1616 inhabitants. The living is a perpetual curacy, in the archdeaconry of Cleveland, and diocese of York, endowed with £400 royal bounty, and £1400 parliamentary grant, and in the patronage of the Chancellor, Masters, and Scholars of the University of Oxford. The church contains some Norman portions, and the chancel is in the early style of English architecture : there is also some ancient stained glass. In the wall over the south door is a stone bearing a Saxon inscription commemorative of the purchase and repairs of St. Gregory's church here in the reign of the Confessor. From this circumstance the church has been called a Saxon edifice, but it is allowed that the stone has been removed from its original situation, and inserted in the wall for its preservation: the church has lately received an addition of eighty free sittings, the Incorporated Society for the enlargement of churches and chapels having granted £30 towards defraying the expense. In a cave near this place, three hundred feet in extent, and from two to five feet in height and breadth, various fossil remains of an hyena, elephant, rhinoceros, hippopotamus, and other animals, were found in 1820.

KIRK-ELLA, county of York. —— See ELLA (KIRK).

KIRKHAM, a parish in the hundred of AMOUNDER-NESS, county palatine of LANCASTER, comprising the market town of Kirkham, the chapelries of Goosnargh, Hambleton, Ribby with Wrea, Singleton, and Warton, and the townships of Bryning with Kellasnergh, Clifton with Salwick, Little Eccleston with Larbrick, Freckleton, Greenhalgh with Thistleton, Medlar with Wesham, Newsham, Newton with Scales Treales, with Roseacre and Wharles, Weeton, Westby with Plumptons, and Whittingham, and containing 11,925 inhabitants, of which number, 2735 are in the town of Kirkham, 22 miles (S. by W.) from Lancaster, and 226 (N. W. by N.) from London. This place, which is of Saxon origin, derived its name from its church, which, soon after the Conquest, was given by Roger de Poictou to the abbey of St. Peter and St. Paul in Shrewsbury, from which it was, by Edward I., transferred to the monks of Vale Royal in Cheshire, in whose patronage it remained till the dissolution. The town, which may be considered as the capital of a surrounding district called the Fylde country, though small, is neatly built, and the houses in general respectable. The manufacture of sail-cloth, sacking, and cordage, originally formed the principal source of employment, and is still carried on to a limited extent; the manufacture of cotton has been recently introduced, and a considerable number of handlooms is employed in the town and neighbourhood. At Wardless, within eight miles of the town, a small port on the north-east bank of the river Wyre, which is accessible to vessels of three hundred tons, several of the principal manufacturers have warehouses for supplying the town with the produce of the countries bordering on the Baltic. The Lancaster canal passes at the distance of about three miles from the town, which suffers from the want of a more varied and extensive course of inland navigation. Within three miles is the æstuary of the Ribble, near the mouth of which, a guide is stationed to conduct travellers across the sands at low water to Hesketh bank, the passage of which is dangerous to persons attempting it without such assistance. The market is on Thursday: the fairs are, February 4th and the following day, April 29th, and October 18th. The town is within the jurisdiction of the county magistrates, who hold a petty session for the hundred of Amounderness every alternate Thursday; and a constable and other officers are appointed annually at the court leet of the lord of the manor: a court of requests is held monthly, under an act passed in the 10th year of the reign of George III., for the recovery of debts under 40s., the jurisdiction of which extends over the parishes of Kirkham, Bispham, Lytham, and Poulton, and the townships of Preesall and Stalmine, in the parish of Lancaster.

VOL. II.

The living is a vicarage, in the archdeaconry of Richmond, and diocese of Chester, rated in the king's books at £21. 1. 0½., and in the patronage of the Dean and Canons of Christ Church, Oxford. The church, dedicated to St. Michael, was, with the exception of the tower, which is in the Norman style of architecture, rebuilt in 1822, at an expense of £5000, defrayed by a rate on the parishioners: it contains several ancient portions of its original character, and some interesting monuments. There are places of worship for Independents and Swedenborgians, and a Roman Catholic chapel. The free grammar school, originally founded by Isabel Wildinge, was, in 1655, endowed with a portion of the proceeds of the rectory of Kirkham, purchased by the Drapers' Company, with funds bequeathed in trust to them by Henry Colborne, Esq.; the endowment was further augmented by the Rev. James Barker in 1670, by Dr. Grimbaldson, and other benefactors, the aggregate income now being about £550 per annum: it is conducted by a head master and two under masters, appointed by the Drapers' Company, and is under the management of trustees appointed pursuant to the will of the Rev. James Barker; it is open to all boys of the parish, and has an exhibition of about £100 per annum to either of the Universities, founded by Mr. Barker, who also left £80 per annum for apprenticing boys, to which purpose the endowment of the exhibition is also applied when there is no exhibitioner from the school. There are similar schools at Newton with Scales, and at Treales, townships in this parish; and in the chapelry of Goosnargh is an hospital for decayed gentlemen and gentlewomen, with a considerable endowment. A parochial school for girls, established in 1760, has an endowment in houses and land producing about £80 per annum, which is appropriated to the clothing and instruction of forty girls. A National school is supported by subscription; and there are Sunday schools connected with the established church and the dissenting congregations.

KIRKHAM, an extra-parochial liberty, in the wapentake of BUCKROSE, East riding of the county of York, 5½ miles (S. W. by S.) from New Malton, containing 7 inhabitants. A priory of Augustine canons was founded, in 1121, by Sir Walter L'Espec, Knt., and Adelina his wife, and dedicated to the Holy Trinity, the revenue of which, at the dissolution, was estimated at £300. 15. 6.: the ruins of this splendid establishment stand in a delightful vale watered by the Derwent; the fine Gothic tower, covered with ivy, was blown down in 1784; the remaining vestiges are the northern part of the gate, with fragments of the walls.

KIRKHAMMERTON, county of York. — See HAMMERTON (KIRK).

KIRKHARLE, county of NORTHUMBERLAND.—See HARLE (KIRK).

KIRKHAUGH, a parish in the western division of TINDALE ward, county of NORTHUMBERLAND, 2¾ miles (N. W. by N.) from Alston-Moor, containing 286 inhabitants. The living is a discharged rectory, in the archdeaconry of Northumberland, and diocese of Durham, rated in the king's books at £4. 7. 8½., endowed with £200 private benefaction, and £300 parliamentary grant, and in the patronage of Miss Wilkinson. Here is a small sum for the instruction of children. Castle Nook, in this parish, is the site of a Roman station

3 Y

which occupies an area of nearly nine acres, being defended on the west by ten breastworks and trenches. At the north-east corner a sudatory was discovered, in 1813, from which flows a copious spring of clear water: near to the eastern wall is the Maiden-way, and in the vicinity, a Roman altar, with fragments of a colossal statue, was found some few years since; here, according to Camden, an inscription was erected, and a palace built, in honour of the Emperor Antoninus, about 213, by the third cohort of the Nervii. Over the stable door of a public house in the vicinity is an altar, on which are carved a *patera* and *urceolus*. An altar, dedicated to Minerva and Hercules, was also found in the church-yard, but has been lost.

KIRKHEATON, a chapelry in the parish of KIRKHARLE, north-eastern division of TINDALE ward, county of NORTHUMBERLAND, 11½ miles (N. E. by N.) from Hexham, containing 140 inhabitants. The chapel was rebuilt in 1755. The school was endowed by William Lyley, in 1685, with a rent-charge of £5 per annum, which was augmented by a bequest of £100 from Mrs. Frances Beaumont, in 1713: ten children are instructed gratuitously, and the rest pay a quarterage. In 1703, Richard Beaumont, Esq. devised £10 per annum to trustees, for apprenticing poor children of this chapelry. Here are some lime-kilns and a colliery.

KIRKLAND, a joint township with Blennerhasset, in the parish of TORPENHOW, ALLERDALE ward below Darwent, county of CUMBERLAND, 7¾ miles (N.E. by E.) from Cockermouth. The population is returned with Blennerhasset.

KIRKLAND, a parish in LEATH ward, county of CUMBERLAND, comprising the chapelry of Culgaith, and the townships of Kirkland with Blencarn, and Skirwith, and containing 712 inhabitants, of which number, 217 are in the township of Kirkland with Blencarn, 10½ miles (E. by N.) from Penrith. The living is a vicarage, in the archdeaconry and diocese of Carlisle, rated in the king's books at £8. 10., and in the patronage of the Dean and Chapter of Carlisle. The church is dedicated to St. Lawrence. A school was established in 1775, and endowed with land by the commissioners under the enclosure act; the income is about £60 per annum: from forty to fifty children are educated. Coal was wrought at Ardale Head by the late Sir Michael le Fleming; and on Cross fell a lead mine, called Bullman Hills Vein, is in operation, which also yields copper and silver: there is also a smelting-mill. The circumference of the mountain is twenty miles at the base, and its height two thousand nine hundred and one feet above the level of the sea: on its summit and declivities are various kinds of moss, herbs, and minerals. During a great part of the year this mountain is covered with snow, and enveloped in clouds: a little below the apex is Gentleman's well; and from the summit is a fine view over a great part of six counties.

KIRKLAND, a township in the parish of GARSTANG, hundred of AMOUNDERNESS, county palatine of LANCASTER, 2 miles (S.W.) from Garstang, containing 511 inhabitants. In 1778, Margaret Butler gave £200 for the erection of a school-house, and endowed it with £100; augmentations were made, in 1788, by Jane Butler's bequest of £240, and in 1813, by Mrs. Elizabeth Cromholme's gift of £200: the annual income is £36, and eleven children are instructed gratuitously.

KIRKLAND, a township adjoining the town, and in the parish and ward, of KENDAL, county of WESTMORLAND, containing 1378 inhabitants.

KIRK-LEATHAM, a parish in the eastern division of the liberty of LANGBAURGH, North riding of the county of YORK, comprising the townships of Kirk-Leatham and Wilton, and containing 1091 inhabitants, of which number, 686 are in the township of Kirk-Leatham, 4½ miles (N. N. W.) from Guilsborough. The living is a discharged vicarage, in the archdeaconry of Cleveland, and diocese of York, rated in the king's books at £13. 6. 8., endowed with £200 royal bounty, and £1200 parliamentary grant, and in the patronage of Henry Vansittart, Esq. The church is dedicated to St. Cuthbert. A free grammar school was founded by means of a bequest of £5000 from Sir W. Turner, lord mayor of London in 1669, and erected, in 1709, by his nephew, Cholmeley Turner, Esq.; the income is about £350 per annum, of which a master receives a stipend of £100, and an usher one of £50 per annum, but for a very considerable length of time no scholars have been admitted, the building being occupied in separate tenements, rent-free, by poor families. Sir W. Turner likewise erected and endowed a splendid hospital, for the maintenance of forty poor people, viz., ten men and ten women, and an equal number of boys and girls. John Turner, Esq., serjeant at law, bequeathed a sum of money for clothing each child on leaving the institution, which is under the sole direction of Henry Vansittart, Esq., in right of his wife: there are a chaplain, a master and a mistress, a surgeon, and a nurse, who have handsome salaries, and apartments in the hospital, the annual income of which is about £1600. An elegant chapel adorns the centre of the building, the roof being supported by four light Ionic pillars; and from the centre is suspended a chandelier of burnished gold: over the altar is one of the finest paintings on glass in the world, representing the offerings of the Magi. A commodious library is furnished with valuable works, and in a handsome case is a likeness of Sir W. Turner in wax, with the wig and band he used to wear: he was buried in the chancel of the church among the poor of the hospital, and a monument has been erected to his memory at Lazenby in this parish. A chapel in honour of the Virgin Mary, with a chantry or hospital, was founded, in the reign of Edward I., by John de Lythegraynes, and Alice his wife, for a master and six chaplains; the revenue, at the dissolution, was valued at £9. 6. 8.

KIRK-LEAVINGTON, county of YORK. — See LEAVINGTON (KIRK).

KIRK-LEES, a hamlet in that part of the parish of DEWSBURY which is in the wapentake of MORLEY, West riding of the county of YORK, 5 miles (N. N. E.) from Huddersfield. The population is returned with the parish. Here was a Cistercian nunnery, erected in the reign of Henry II., by Reynerus Flandrensis, and dedicated to the Virgin and St. James, the revenue of which, at the suppression, was valued at £20. 7. 8.: the celebrated Robin Hood was buried here, where his tomb is yet to be seen.

KIRKLEY, a township in the parish of PONTELAND, western division of CASTLE ward, county of NORTHUMBERLAND, 10¼ miles (N. W. by N.) from Newcastle upon Tyne, containing, with Benridge and Cartermoor, 146 inhabitants. Here is a place of worship for Presbyterians.

KIRKLEY, a parish in the hundred of MUTFORD and LOTHINGLAND, county of SUFFOLK, 1½ mile (S. W.) from Lowestoft, containing 337 inhabitants. The living is a discharged rectory, in the archdeaconry of Suffolk, and diocese of Norwich, rated in the king's books at £5. 6. 10½., and endowed with £400 royal bounty. Robert Reeve, Esq. was patron in 1812. The church is dedicated to All Saints. This parish is bounded on the east by the North sea, and on the north by Lake Lothing. Kirkley is a small fishing village, in which are three schools supported by the rector.

KIRKLINGTON, a parish in that part of the liberty of SOUTHWELL and SCROOBY which separates the northern from the southern division of the wapentake of THURGARTON, county of NOTTINGHAM, 3½ miles (N. W. by N.) from Southwell, containing 240 inhabitants. The living is a discharged vicarage, in the peculiar jurisdiction and patronage of the Chapter of the Collegiate Church of Southwell, rated in the king's books at £3. 13. 4., endowed with £600 royal bounty, and £200 parliamentary grant. The church is dedicated to St. Swithin.

KIRKLINGTON, a parish in the wapentake of HALLIKELD, North riding of the county of YORK, comprising the townships of Kirklington with Upsland, Sutton with Howgrave, and East Tanfield, and containing 491 inhabitants, of which number, 337 are in the township of Kirklington with Upsland, 6¼ miles (S. E. by S.) from Bedale. The living is a rectory, in the archdeaconry of Richmond, and diocese of Chester, rated in the king's books at £25. 7. 3½., and in the patronage of the Countess of Ormond. The church is dedicated to St. Mary. Here is a small endowment for a school, the bequest of Lady Ormond. In the neighbourhood are vestiges of a Roman or Danish encampment.

KIRK-LINTON, or KIRK-LEVINGTON, a parish in ESKDALE ward, county of CUMBERLAND, 4¾ miles (E. by S.) from Longtown, comprising the townships of Hethersgill, Middle Quarter, and West Linton, or Levington, and containing 1931 inhabitants. The living is a rectory, in the archdeaconry and diocese of Carlisle, rated in the king's books at £1. 1. 0½., endowed with £1000 parliamentary grant, and in the patronage of Mrs. Dacre. The church, dedicated to St. Cuthbert, is a good and uniform specimen of the Norman style. Here is a place of worship for the Society of Friends. This parish is bounded on the north by the river Line. Near Kirk-Linton hall are the remains of an ancient fortress. The celebrated watchmaker, George Graham, esteemed the best mechanic of his time, was a native of this place.

KIRK-OSWALD, a parish in LEATH ward, county of CUMBERLAND, comprising the market town of Kirk-Oswald, and the township of Staffield, or Staffol, and containing 1069 inhabitants, of which number, 760 are in the town of Kirk-Oswald, 15½ miles (S. E.) from Carlisle, and 292 (N.N.W.) from London. This place, which derived its name from St. Oswald, the canonized King of Northumberland, belonged, in the reign of John, to Hugh de Morville, one of the murderers of Thomas à Becket : it was burnt by the Scots in 1314, since which period it has not been distinguished by any events of historical importance. The town is pleasantly situated on the eastern bank of the river Eden, in a beautiful and fertile vale, which gradually widens towards the south, and expands into a large tract of open country. The houses, which are in general well built, are irregularly scattered along the declivities of the hills which enclose the vale. The castle, of which only one square tower and some dark vaults are remaining, occupies a bold eminence to the east of the town, and is said to have been a very noble structure, of which the great hall was more than three hundred feet in length, and embellished with a series of portraits of ancient British kings : it was built by Ranulph d'Engaine, enclosed with a quadrangular rampart by Hugh de Morville, enlarged and fortified by Thomas de Multon, and beautified by Thomas Dacre ; the acclivities are richly wooded, and defended by a deep ditch on all sides, except that which overlooks the river : the castle was demolished by the Howards, and the furniture and antiquities removed to Naworth castle. The Raven beck, over which is a bridge of one arch, intersects the town ; and the inhabitants are supplied with water from a reservoir at the market-cross, into which it is conveyed by pipes from an eminence at a short distance. Within half a mile westward of the town is a bridge of six arches over the river Eden, built in 1762. There are flour-mills, a paper-mill, and a mill for carding wool. The parish contains several quarries of freestone, and one of marble, of a blue colour spotted with white. The market, granted in the 2nd year of the reign of King John, is on Thursday, and a market for corn was established a few years since on Monday ; the corn is pitched in the market-place : the fairs are on the Thursday before Whitsuntide, and August 5th for cattle.

The living is a discharged vicarage, in the archdeaconry and diocese of Carlisle, rated in the king's books at £8, endowed with £400 private benefaction, and £400 royal bounty, and in the patronage of the Crown. The church, dedicated to St. Oswald, was, about the year 1523, made collegiate for twelve secular priests ; but this society did not subsist for more than ten or twelve years ; at the dissolution, the revenue was £78. 17. : the building, situated at a little distance from the town, is very irregular and ill proportioned, and was probably enlarged by the Dacres and the Cliffords, whose arms appear in the windows ; it has no teeple, but on the summit of an adjoining eminence a tower has been erected, which is used as a belfry. There is a place of worship for Wesleyan Methodists in the town, and one for Independents at Park-head, near the eastern extremity of the parish. The free school is endowed with a house and some land producing £10 per annum, to which John Lowthian bequeathed £100 : fifteen boys are instructed at a trifling expense. A benefit society, said to have been the first established in the country, has existed here for a considerable time. On the side of a hill, in a field about one mile from the town, are two cairns of moderate size.

KIRKSTEAD, a parish in the southern division of the wapentake of GARTREE, parts of LINDSEY, county of LINCOLN, 8 miles (S. W. by S.) from Horncastle, containing 132 inhabitants. The living is a donative, in the peculiar jurisdiction of the manor court of Kirkstead, and in the patronage of the Trustees of R. Ellison, Esq. There is a place of worship for Unitarians.

Daniel Disney, about the year 1736, bequeathed a rent-charge of £6 for the instruction of children. A Cistercian abbey was founded here, in 1139, by Hugo Brito, and dedicated to the Virgin Mary : at the dissolution it was valued at £338. 13. 11. per annum.

KIRKTON, a parish in the South-clay division of the wapentake of BASSETLAW, county of NOTTINGHAM, 2¾ miles (N. E. by E.) from Ollerton, containing 200 inhabitants. The living is a rectory, in the peculiar jurisdiction of the Sub-Dean of Lincoln, rated in the king's books at £7. 14. 9½., and in the patronage of the Duke of Newcastle. The church is dedicated to the Holy Trinity.

KIRMINGTON, a parish in the eastern division of the wapentake of YARBOROUGH, parts of LINDSEY, county of LINCOLN, 8 miles (N.) from Caistor, containing 243 inhabitants. The living is a discharged vicarage, in the archdeaconry and diocese of Lincoln, rated in the king's books at £4. 18. 4., and endowed with £600 royal bounty. Lord Yarborough was patron in 1812. The church is dedicated to St. Helen.

KIRMOND le MIRE, a parish in the eastern division of the wapentake of WRAGGOE, parts of LINDSEY, county of LINCOLN, 6¼ miles (E. N. E.) from Market-Raisen, containing 71 inhabitants. The living is a discharged vicarage, in the archdeaconry and diocese of Lincoln, rated in the king's books at £5, endowed with £400 royal bounty, and £200 parliamentary grant. Edmund Turnor, Esq. was patron in 1825. The church is dedicated to St. Martin.

KIRSTEAD, a parish in the hundred of LODDON, county of NORFOLK, 7¼ miles (N. N. W.) from Bungay, containing 230 inhabitants. The living is a rectory, with that of Langhale, in the archdeaconry of Norfolk, and diocese of Norwich, rated in the king's books at £10, and in the patronage of the Master and Fellows of Caius College, Cambridge. The church is dedicated to St. Margaret.

KIRTLING, a parish in the hundred of CHEVELEY, county of CAMBRIDGE, 4¼ miles (S. E.) from Newmarket, containing 627 inhabitants. The living is a vicarage, in the archdeaconry of Sudbury, and diocese of Norwich, rated in the king's books at £10, and in the patronage of Lord Guildford. The church, which is dedicated to All Saints, is principally in the Norman style, and contains various monuments of the noble family of North : the only relic of antiquity is the gateway of an ancient mansion which belonged to that family.

KIRTLINGTON, a parish in the hundred of PLOUGHLEY, county of OXFORD, 5 miles (E. N. E.) from Woodstock, containing 697 inhabitants. The living is a discharged vicarage, in the archdeaconry and diocese of Oxford, rated in the king's books at £11. 9. 4., and endowed with £200 private benefaction, and £200 royal bounty, and in the patronage of the President and Fellows of St. John's College, Oxford. The church is dedicated to St. Mary. About twenty children are clothed and educated at the expense of Sir Henry Dashwood, aided by a rent-charge of £4. 4. per annum from an unknown benefactor.

KIRTON, a parish in the wapentake of KIRTON, parts of HOLLAND, county of LINCOLN, 4¼ miles (S. S. W.) from Boston, containing, with the chapelry of Brothertoft, 1803 inhabitants. The living is a discharged vicarage, in the archdeaconry and diocese of Lincoln, rated in the king's books at £21. 10. 10., endowed with £200 private. benefaction, and £200 royal bounty, and in the patronage of the Master and Wardens of the Mercers' Company, London. The church, dedicated to St. Peter and St. Paul, is a noble cruciform structure in the decorated style, with a square tower at the intersection, and ornamented with battlements and pinnacles : the western entrance seems to have formed part of an earlier edifice, which was probably erected in the thirteenth century. Here were a market and an annual fair, but both disused.

KIRTON, a parish in the hundred of COLNEIS, county of SUFFOLK, 7½ miles (E. S. E.) from Ipswich, containing 578 inhabitants. The living is a discharged rectory, in the archdeaconry of Suffolk, and diocese of Norwich, rated in the king's books at £10. 13. 4., and in the patronage of the Crown. The church is dedicated to St. Mary. The navigable river Deben runs on the north-east of this parish.

KIRTON in LINDSEY, a market town and parish, in the wapentake of CORRINGHAM, parts of LINDSEY, county of LINCOLN, 18 miles (N. by W.) from Lin·coln, and 147 (N. by W.) from London, containing 1480 inhabitants. The manor was granted by the Conqueror to his half-brother, Robert of Mortaigne, the first Earl of Cornwall, subsequently bestowed by Edward II. on the widow of his favourite, Piers Gavestone, and, having again reverted to the crown, was given by Edward III. to William, Earl of Huntingdon, at whose death it became the property of Edward the Black Prince, who gave a third part to Elizabeth, the widow of the late earl, and the remainder to the Earl of Chandos. It again became attached to the duchy of Cornwall, to which it now belongs. The town is situated on the western declivity of an eminence commanding an extensive view of the surrounding country. On Kirton Green stands the duchy court-house, where the manorial courts are held, and where the records are kept. The quarter sessions for the parts of Lindsey are held in the second whole week after Epiphany and Easter, on the first Friday after July 7th, and on the Friday in the first week after the 11th of October. The house of correction is a large stone building, consisting of a centre and two wings ; in the centre is the court-room, also used as a chapel, and over it the grand jury-room ; the gaoler's apartments are in the western division ; the male prisoners occupy the south, and the females the north, wing. This place is within the jurisdiction of a court of requests for the recovery of debts not exceeding £5, the jurisdiction of which extends over the borough and parish of Boston, and the wapentake of Skirbeck and Kirton, excepting the parishes of Gosburton and Surfleet. The market is on Saturday ; and fairs are held on the 18th of July and the 11th of December, for cattle and pedlary.

The living is a discharged vicarage, in the peculiar jurisdiction and patronage of the Sub-Dean of Lincoln, rated in the king's books at £6. 13. 4. The church, dedicated to St. Peter and St. Paul, has a considerable portion in the early style of English architecture, with later insertions ; it contains some circular-headed windows, and in the interior are some curious oak seats, screen-work, and piscinæ. There is a chapel of ease at Brothertoft, in this parish. There are places of worship for Baptists and Wesleyan Methodists, both of the New and Old Connexion. The free grammar school, endowed with about £70 per annum, is now conducted on the National system, and contains about eighty scholars. About one hundred children are instructed in a Sunday school.

KISLINGBURY, a parish in the hundred of No-BOTTLE-GROVE, county of NORTHAMPTON, 3½ miles (W. by S.) from Northampton, containing 643 inhabitants. The living is a rectory, in the archdeaconry of Northampton, and diocese of Peterborough, rated in the king's books at £18. 9. 7., and in the patronage of Mrs. Hughes. The church, dedicated to St. Luke, has some portions in the decorated style, an embattled tower surmounted by a spire, and a fine octagonal font. There is a place of worship for Baptists. A considerable annual income, the produce of divers benefactions, is applied in instructing and apprenticing children.

KITTISFORD, a parish in the hundred of MILVERTON, county of SOMERSET, 4¾ miles (W. by N.) from Wellington, containing 175 inhabitants. The living is a rectory, in the archdeaconry of Taunton, and diocese of Bath and Wells, rated in the king's books at £11. 10. 5. The Rev. T. Sweet Escott was patron in 1824. The church is dedicated to St. Nicholas.

KNAITH, a parish in the wapentake of WELL, parts of LINDSEY, county of LINCOLN, 3½ miles (S. by E.) from Gainsborough, containing 59 inhabitants. The living is a perpetual curacy, in the archdeaconry of Stow, and diocese of Lincoln, endowed with £400 royal bounty. The church, formerly belonging to the Cistercian monastery of Heyninges, has two windows, richly ornamented with tracery, in the decorated style of English architecture. The monastery was founded about 1180, and valued at the dissolution at £58. 13. 4. per annum. The river Trent bounds this parish on the west. Thomas Sutton, founder of the Charter-house in London, was a native of this place.

KNAPP, a tything in the parish of NORTH CURRY, northern division of the hundred of CURRY, county of SOMERSET, 5¼ miles (E. by N.) from Taunton. The population is returned with the parish. Here was formerly a chapel.

KNAPTOFT, a parish comprising the chapelry of Mowsley in the hundred of GARTREE, the chapelry of Shearsby, and the hamlet of Walton, in the hundred of GUTHLAXTON, county of LEICESTER, 7 miles (N.E. by E.) from Lutterworth, and containing 864 inhabitants. The living is a rectory, in the archdeaconry of Leicester, and diocese of Lincoln, rated in the king's books at £32. 12. 6. The Duke of Rutland was patron in 1817. The church is dilapidated. There are traces of an ancient encampment in the parish. Dr. Richard Watson, late Bishop of Llandaff, was one of the incumbents.

KNAPTON, a parish in the northern division of the hundred of ERPINGHAM, county of NORFOLK, 3¼ miles (N. E. by N.) from North Walsham, containing 312 inhabitants. The living is a rectory, in the archdeaconry of Norfolk, and diocese of Norwich, rated in the king's books at £13. 7. 1., and in the patronage of Lord Suffield and the Master of Peter House, Cambridge, alternately. The church is dedicated to St. Peter and St. Paul.

KNAPTON, a township in the parish of ACOMB, ainsty of the city, and East riding of the county, of YORK, 3¼ miles (W. by N.) from York, containing 137 inhabitants.

KNAPTON, a chapelry in the parish of WINTRING-HAM, wapentake of BUCKROSE, East riding of the county of YORK, 6¼ miles (N.E. by E.) from New Malton, containing 206 inhabitants. The living is a perpetual curacy, in the archdeaconry of the East riding, and diocese of York, endowed with £600 royal bounty, and £200 parliamentary grant. John Tindale, Esq. was patron in 1804. The navigable river Derwent runs within a short distance of the village.

KNAPWELL, a parish in the hundred of PAPWORTH, county of CAMBRIDGE, 4½ miles (N.E. by N.) from Caxton, containing 136 inhabitants. The living is a rectory, in the archdeaconry and diocese of Ely, rated in the king's books at £6. 17. 11. The Rev. F. Gunniss was patron in 1786. The church is dedicated to All Saints.

KNARESBOROUGH, a parish comprising the manor of Beach Hill within the liberty of ST. PETER of York, East riding, and the borough and market town of Knaresborough, a portion of which is also within the above liberty, the chapelry of Arkendale, and the townships of Bilton with Harrogate, Brearton, and Scriven with Tentergate, in the lower division of the wapentake of CLARO, West riding, of the county of YORK, and containing 9101 inhabitants, of which number, 5283 are in the borough of Knaresborough, 18 miles (W. by N.) from York, and 197 (N.N.W.) from London. This place is supposed to derive its name from the German word *Knares*, a rocky mountain, thus indicating the situation of its ancient castle, erected by Serlo de Burgh, who accompanied William the Conqueror to England, and became lord of this manor. During the civil war in the reign of Charles I., the castle was garrisoned for the king, but was eventually taken by Lord Fairfax, after the battle of Marston Moor. A priory was founded in the thirteenth century, by Robert Flower, whose father was mayor of York, who was afterwards canonized: it was endowed by Richard, Earl of Cornwall, the brother of Henry III., for friars of the order of the Holy Trinity, the revenue of which, at the dissolution, was £35. 10. 11. The town is situated on the north-eastern bank of the river Midd, and is surrounded by picturesque and beautiful scenery; the streets are well paved, and lighted with gas; the houses, many of which are handsome buildings, are in general constructed of stone found in the immediate vicinity. There are a subscription library and a news-room. Knaresborough was formerly a favourite watering-place, but has been of late years superseded by Harrogate. The linen and cotton manufactures, which were formerly very extensive, yet employ a considerable number of the inhabitants, though they have somewhat declined, in consequence of the inland situation of the town and the want of facilities for the carriage of goods, and for obtaining coal. The market, held on Wednesday, is one of the principal corn markets in the county: fairs, chiefly for horses, cattle, and sheep, are on the first Wednesdays after January 13th, March 12th, May 5th, August 12th, October 11th, and December 10th, for cattle, horses, and sheep. A statute fair for hiring

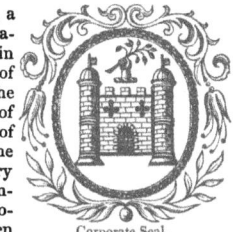

Corporate Seal.

servants is held on the Wednesday before November 23rd. The county magistrates hold petty sessions weekly for the wapentake of Claro. Courts of record, for the recovery of debts to any amount within the honour of Knaresborough, comprising the borough, the Forest, and the Forest liberty, are held once a fortnight, before the steward (a barrister), and the under steward, who are appointed by the Duke of Devonshire, lessee of the honour under the duchy of Lancaster. Attached to this court is a gaol for debtors, consisting of a single room, part of the remains of Knaresborough castle, which will afford accommodation for two prisoners only. Sessions for the West riding are held here annually at Michaelmas. Borough courts are held after Michaelmas and Easter, by the Duke of Devonshire. The elective franchise was granted in the first year of the reign of Mary; two representatives are sent to parliament: the right of election is in the proprietors of burgage tenements, eighty-eight in number, who are chiefly non-resident: the bailiff, in whom the government of the borough is vested, is the returning officer; and the influence of the Duke of Devonshire is predominant.

The living is a vicarage, in the peculiar jurisdiction of the court of the honour of Knaresborough, rated in the king's books at £9. 9. 4½., and in the patronage of the Dean and Chapter of York. The church, which is dedicated to St. John the Baptist, has been erected at various periods: it is an extensive edifice, with a tower between the nave and the chancel, and a decorated east window. There are places of worship for the Society of Friends, Independents, and Wesleyan Methodists, and a Roman Catholic chapel. A free grammar school was founded and endowed by Dr. Robert Chaloner, in 1616, with a rent-charge of £20 per annum, for the education of boys, but there are none on the foundation. A school for boys and girls was endowed by Thomas Richardson, in 1765, with £400 and a dwelling-house, which donation, with subsequent legacies and benefactions, produces an annual income of £101. 16.: thirty boys and girls are educated. A National school for children of both sexes was erected in 1814; and, in 1823, Charles Marshall left £500 to trustees, to apply the interest in providing four suits of clothes every Easter for four scholars who have made the greatest proficiency; the surplus to be used at their discretion in support of the school. Various Sunday schools are well supported and numerously attended. There is a charitable fund of £200 per annum for apprenticing poor children; and another of £150 per annum, distributed in gratuities of £5 each to indigent persons, arising from the joint benefactions of Mrs. Alice Shepherd, in 1806, and Dr. William Craven, in 1812.

The ruins of the castle extend over a circular area about three hundred feet in diameter, and consist of part of the keep and some round towers of excellent masonry, with arches and windows displaying the decorated English style of building. Southward of the castle is an excavation in the rock, called St. Robert's Chapel, founded, in the reign of Richard I., by a native of York; and above it is a hermitage, which contains a figure of the hermit in monastic attire, surrounded by his books. A little higher up is Fort Montagu, an ornamental structure consisting of excavations in the rock, and so called in honour of the Duchess of Buccleuch, with appropriate arbours, green-house, and tea-rooms:

in the vicinity is St. Robert's cave, remarkable in modern times as the scene of a horrible murder committed on the body of Daniel Clarke, by Eugene Aram, a schoolmaster in this town. About a mile from the town are the remains of an ancient encampment, on the point of a hill two hundred feet above the surface of the river, whence there is a fine view of the town and castle. In this parish there are four mineral springs: the sweet, or vitriolic spa, in Knaresborough Forest, discovered in 1620; the sulphureous spa, which is very foetid, and changes silver to the colour of copper; St. Mungo's cold bath; and a dropping well, the water of which is the most noted petrifying spring in England.

KNARESDALE, a parish in the western division of TINDALE ward, county of NORTHUMBERLAND, 6 miles (N. W. by N.) from Alston Moor, containing 564 inhabitants. The living is a discharged rectory, in the archdeaconry of Northumberland, and diocese of Durham, rated in the king's books at £4. 18. 9., and endowed with £600 parliamentary grant, and in the patronage of the Crown. The church is an ancient structure, surrounded by vestiges of other buildings. It is believed that the Romans had a lead mine in this parish: on the side of a fell is a medicinal spring called Snope's well. The South Tyne runs through the parish. Knaresdale gives the title of baron to the family of Wallace.

KNAYTON, a joint township with Brawith, in that part of the parish of LEAK which is in the wapentake of ALLERTONSHIRE, North riding of the county of YORK, 4 miles (N.) from Thirsk, containing, with Brawith, 377 inhabitants. The Wesleyan Methodists have here a place of worship. There is a small endowment for the instruction of children.

KNEBWORTH, a parish in the hundred of BROADWATER, county of HERTFORD, 4 miles (N.) from Welwyn, containing 266 inhabitants. The living is a rectory, in the archdeaconry of Huntingdon, and diocese of Lincoln, rated in the king's books at £13. 1. 10½. R. W. Lytton, Esq. was patron in 1788. The church is dedicated to St. Mary.

KNEDLINGTON, a township in the parish of HOWDEN, wapentake of HOWDENSHIRE, East riding of the county of YORK, 1 mile (W. by S.) from Howden, containing 118 inhabitants.

KNEESALL, a parish comprising the township of Ompton in the South-clay division of the wapentake of BASSETLAW, and the hamlet of Kersall in the northern division of the wapentake of THURGARTON, county of NOTTINGHAM, 4 miles (S. E. by E.) from Ollerton, and containing 602 inhabitants. The living is a discharged vicarage, in the archdeaconry of Nottingham, and diocese of York, rated in the king's books at £10, and in the patronage of the Chapter of the Collegiate Church of Southwell. The church is dedicated to St. Bartholomew. There is also a chapel of ease in the parish. Here is a place of worship for Wesleyan Methodists.

KNEESWORTH, a hamlet in the parish of BASSINGBOURNE, hundred of ARMINGFORD, county of CAMBRIDGE, 2¾ miles (N. W.) from Royston, containing 171 inhabitants.

KNEETON, a parish in the northern division of the wapentake of BINGHAM, county of NOTTINGHAM, 7¾ miles (S. W. by W.) from Newark, containing 104 inhabitants. The living is a discharged vicarage, in the archdeaconry of Nottingham, and diocese of York, rated in the king's books at £4. 9. 4½., endowed with £800 royal bounty, and £200 parliamentary grant. Sir. F. Molyneux, Bart. was patron in 1804. The church is dedicated to St. Peter. The river Trent is here crossed by a ferry to Hoveringham, and the Fosse road passes along the south-eastern boundary of the parish.

KNEIGHTON, a township in that part of the parish of MUCKLESTON which is in the northern division of the hundred of PIREHILL, county of STAFFORD, 5½ miles (N. E. by N.) from Drayton in Hales, containing 148 inhabitants.

KNETTISHALL, a parish in the hundred of BLACKBOURN, county of SUFFOLK, 5 miles (S. by W.) from East Harling, containing 70 inhabitants. The living is a discharged rectory, in the archdeaconry of Suffolk, and diocese of Norwich, rated in the king's books at £6. 7. 11. Thomas Thornhill, Esq. was patron in 1826. The church is dedicated to All Saints.

KNIGHTLEY, a township in the parish of GNOSALL, western division of the hundred of CUTTLESTONE, county of STAFFORD, 3½ miles (S. S. W.) from Eccleshall, containing 322 inhabitants.

KNIGHTON, a chapelry in that part of the parish of ST. MARGARET, LEICESTER, which is in the hundred of GUTHLAXTON, county of LEICESTER, 2½ miles (S. S. E.) from Leicester, containing 383 inhabitants. There is a place of worship for Wesleyan Methodists.

KNIGHTON upon TEAME, a chapelry in the parish of LINDRIDGE, lower division of the hundred of OSWALDSLOW, but locally in the upper division of the hundred of Doddingtree, county of WORCESTER, 3¾ miles (E. N. E.) from Tenbury, containing, with Newnham, 526 inhabitants.

KNIGHTON (WEST), a parish in the hundred of CULLIFORD-TREE, Dorchester division of the county of DORSET, 3½ miles (S. E.) from Dorchester, containing 229 inhabitants. The living is a rectory, annexed to that of Broadmayne, in the archdeaconry of Dorset, and diocese of Bristol, rated in the king's books at £8. 15. 5. The church is dedicated to St. Peter. Here is a small sum for the instruction of children.

KNIGHTSBRIDGE, a chapelry partly in the parish of ST. MARGARET, WESTMINSTER, but chiefly in the parishes of KENSINGTON and CHELSEA, Kensington division of the hundred of OSSULSTONE, county of MIDDLESEX, 1 mile (W.) from London. The population is returned with the respective parishes. This place consists principally of a long street on the line of the great western road from the metropolis : it is partially paved, lighted with gas, and supplied with water from the Chelsea Water Works. There are many good houses, and a few large and handsome mansions, with gardens and pleasure grounds attached. Great improvement has been recently effected by the removal of a large portion of the wall which separates Hyde Park from the road, and the erection of iron palisades, thus affording a fine prospect over the park from the houses on the opposite side. On the north side, adjoining Hyde Park, are extensive and commodious barracks for cavalry. At the entrance to Knightsbridge from London, on the south side of the road, is St. George's Hospital. Here are a very considerable ale brewery, and two large floor-cloth manufactories, one of which was established in 1754, and is said to have been the first in the kingdom. Knightsbridge is within the jurisdiction of the court of requests for the recovery of debts under 40s., held in Kingsgate-street, Holborn. The chapel, dedicated to the Holy Trinity, belonged originally to an ancient hospital, or lazar-house, under the patronage of the abbot and convent of Westminster; it was rebuilt, in 1629, at the cost of the inhabitants, by a license from Dr. Laud, then Bishop of London, as a chapel of ease to St. Martin's in the Fields, within the precincts of which parish it was situated, but the site was subsequently assigned to the parish of St. George, Hanover-square, and at present forms a part of that of Kensington : the present building was erected in 1789. Adjoining the chapel is a charity school, which was founded in 1783, and is supported by voluntary contributions. Here is a place of worship for Baptists.

KNIGHT-THORPE, a township in the parish of LOUGHBOROUGH, western division of the hundred of GOSCOTE, county of LEICESTER, containing 52 inhabitants.

KNIGHTWICK, a parish in the lower division of the hundred of OSWALDSLOW, though locally in the upper division of the hundred of Doddingtree, county of WORCESTER, 5½ miles (E.) from Bromyard, containing, with the chapelry of Kenswick, 170 inhabitants. The living is a rectory, in the archdeaconry and diocese of Worcester, rated in the king's books at £13. 13. 4., and in the patronage of the Dean and Chapter of Worcester. The church is dedicated to St. Mary : the two daughters of Colonel Lane, who were supposed to have been instrumental in secreting Charles II., on his flight from Worcester, are interred in it. There is a curious knife, for cutting the sacramental bread, with an agate handle, given about one hundred and fifty years since for the use of the church, by Mr. Clent. There is a chapel of ease at Doddenham, in this parish.

KNILL, a parish in the hundred of WIGMORE, county of HEREFORD, 2¾ miles (N. N. W.) from Kington, containing 79 inhabitants. The living is a discharged rectory, in the archdeaconry and diocese of Hereford, rated in the king's books at £4. 10., and in the patronage of Mrs. A. M. Garbett Walsham. The church is dedicated to St. Michael.

KNIPTON, a parish in the hundred of FRAMLAND county of LEICESTER, 7 miles (S. W. by W.) from Grantham, containing 310 inhabitants. The living is a rectory, in the archdeaconry of Leicester, and diocese of Lincoln, rated in the king's books at £16. 12. 3½., and in the patronage of the Duke of Rutland. The church is dedicated to All Saints. In this parish is a very extensive reservoir for the Grantham canal.

KNITSLEY, a joint township with Conside, in that part of the parish of LANCHESTER which is in the western division of CHESTER ward, county palatine of DURHAM, 11 miles (W. N. W.) from Durham. The population is returned with Conside.

KNIVETON, a parish in the hundred of WIRKSWORTH, county of DERBY, 3½ miles (N. E.) from Ashbourn, containing 394 inhabitants. The living is a perpetual curacy, endowed with £600 royal bounty, and £200 parliamentary grant, and in the peculiar jurisdiction and patronage of the Dean and Chapter of Lichfield and Coventry. The church is dedicated to St. John the Baptist. A school was endowed by John Hurd, in 1715, with a small rent-charge for the instruction of poor children, twelve of whom are educated gratuitously.

Kniveton is in the honour of Tutbury, duchy of Lancaster, and within the jurisdiction of a court of pleas held at Tutbury every third Tuesday, for the recovery of debts under 40s.

KNOCKIN, a parish in the hundred of OSWESTRY, county of SALOP, 5¾ miles (S.S.E.) from Oswestry, containing 225 inhabitants. The living is a discharged rectory, in the archdeaconry and diocese of St. Asaph, and in the patronage of the Earl of Bradford. The church is dedicated to St. Mary. This parish derives its name from a castle founded here by the family of L'Estrange, who possessed the manor in the reigns of Henry II. and Henry III., the latter of whom directed a precept to the sheriff of this county, commanding the aid thereof, to enable John L'Estrange to erect part of the "Castle of Cnukyn," and to repair the rest for the defence of the borders : his son received from the same monarch the grant of a weekly market, and a fair on the eve and morrow of the festival of St. John the Baptist, both of which are disused. In the reign of Edward III., Madoc, a Welch nobleman, headed an insurrection, and defeated Lord Strange at Cnukyn. Thomas Staveley, first earl of Derby of that name, was, in his father's lifetime, summoned to parliament by the name of Lord Strange of Knokyn. Few vestiges of the old castle remain, except the keep, which may still be seen.

KNODISHALL, a parish in the hundred of BLYTHING, county of SUFFOLK, 3 miles (E. by S.) from Saxmundham, containing 316 inhabitants. The living is a discharged rectory with Buxlow, in the archdeaconry of Suffolk, and diocese of Norwich, rated in the king's books at £11, endowed with £200 private benefaction, and £200 royal bounty. John Vernon, Esq. was patron in 1801. The church is dedicated to St. Lawrence.

KNOOK, a parish in the hundred of HEYTESBURY, county of WILTS, 1 mile (E. S. E.) from Heytesbury, containing 268 inhabitants. The living is a perpetual curacy, with that of Heytesbury, in the peculiar jurisdiction of the Dean of Salisbury, endowed with £400 private benefaction, and £1000 royal bounty. The church is dedicated to St. Margaret.

KNOSSINGTON, a parish in the hundred of GARTREE, though locally in that of Guthlaxton, county of LEICESTER, 4½ miles (W. by S.) from Oakham, containing 193 inhabitants. The living is a rectory, in the archdeaconry of Leicester, and diocese of Lincoln, rated in the king's books at £6. 11. 8., and in the patronage of the Rev. Thomas Wartnaby. The church is dedicated to St. Peter. An hospital for four widows of beneficed clergymen, who have each a stipend of £30 per annum, was founded by William Scott of Croxton, in this county, but the date of its foundation is unknown.

KNOTTING, a parish in the hundred of STODDEN, county of BEDFORD, 4½ miles (S. E.) from Higham-Ferrers, containing 135 inhabitants. The living is a rectory, united, in 1735, to that of Souldrop, in the archdeaconry of Bedford, and diocese of Lincoln, rated in the king's books at £10. 6. 8. The Rev. J. W. Hawksley uo.s patron in 1792. The church is dedicated to St. Margaret.

KNOTTINGLY, a chapelry in the parish of PONTEFRACT, upper division of the wapentake of OSGOLDCROSS, West riding of the county of YORK, 1¼ mile (E. S. E.) from Ferry-Bridge, containing 3753 inhabitants. The living is a perpetual curacy, in the archdeaconry and diocese of York, endowed with £600 private benefaction, £600 royal bounty, and £200 parliamentary grant, and in the patronage of the Vicar of Pontefract. The chapel is dedicated to St. Botolph. There are places of worship for Independents and Wesleyan Methodists. A school, in which thirty poor girls are instructed, is supported by bequests of £200 each, from Mrs. Banks in 1792, and Mrs. Eliz. Brown in 1811. The village is situated on the banks of the river Aire, and has long been noted for its great production of limestone. A canal hence to Goole is in progress of formation.

KNOTT-LANES, a district in the parish of ASHTON under LINE, hundred of SALFORD, county palatine of LANCASTER, 5¼ miles (N. E. by E.) from Manchester, containing 3827 inhabitants.

KNOWLE, a tything in that part of the parish of CREDITON which is in the hundred of CREDITON, county of DEVON, 3 miles (W. N. W.) from Crediton, with which the population is returned.

KNOWLE, a joint tything with Brockhampton, in the parish of BUCKLAND-NEWTON, Cerne subdivision of the county of DORSET. The population is returned with Brockhampton.

KNOWLE, a chapelry in the parish of HAMPTON in ARDEN, Solihull division of the hundred of HEMLINGFORD, county of WARWICK, 2½ miles (S. E. by E.) from Solihull, containing 1082 inhabitants. The living is a perpetual curacy, in the peculiar jurisdiction of the manor court of Knowle, endowed with £400 private benefaction, £400 royal bounty, and £800 parliamentary grant, and in the patronage of H. Greswold Lewis, Esq. The chapel, dedicated to St. Ann, is in the later style of English architecture, and contains some ancient stalls and fragments of stained glass : it was built and a chantry established here by Walter Cook, canon of Lincoln, in the reign of Richard II., and was valued, at the dissolution, at £18. 5. 6. per annum. The name is a corruption of Cnolle, or Knoll, the summit of a hill : this is supposed to have been the site of a Roman station ; an urn, containing coins of the Lower Empire, and weighing 15lb., was discovered in an adjoining field. The petty sessions for the division are held here during the winter months, in conjunction with Solihull. From twenty to twenty-five children of this chapelry are clothed and educated, conjointly with others in the parishes of St. Mary and St. Nicholas, in Warwick, on the foundation of the Hon. Sarah Greville, by a bequest in 1718 ; at the same time the Hon. Algernon Greville bequeathed £500 for the education of boys and girls, the income arising from which is £25 per annum. There are various benefactions for the relief of the poor, the principal of which is by Fulk Greville, Esq., in 1742, a small portion of the income being also applied towards the instruction of children. A fair for cattle and sheep is held on the first Monday after St. Ann's day. The Warwick and Birmingham canal passes through this parish.

KNOWLE (CHURCH), a parish in the hundred of HASILOR, Blandford (South) division of the county of DORSET, 1 mile (W.) from Corfe-Castle, containing, with the tythings of Bradle and Creech, 400 inhabitants. The living is a discharged rectory, in the archdeaconry of Dorset, and diocese of Bristol, rated in the king's books at £17. 17. 6. W. Richards, Esq. was patron in 1782. The church is dedicated to St. Peter.

KNOWLE (ST. GILES), a parish in the southern division of the hundred of PETHERTON, county of SOMERSET, 2¾ miles (S. by W.) from Ilminster, containing 91 inhabitants. The living is a perpetual curacy, in the archdeaconry of Taunton, and diocese of Bath and Wells, endowed with £200 private benefaction, and £200 royal bounty, and in the peculiar jurisdiction and patronage of the Prebendary of Cudworth in the Cathedral Church of Wells.

KNOWL-END, a township in the parish of AUD-LEY, northern division of the hundred of PIREHILL, county of STAFFORD, containing 208 inhabitants.

KNOWLTON, a parish in the hundred of EASTRY, lathe of ST. AUGUSTINE, county of KENT, 4¼ miles (S. E.) from Wingham, containing 34 inhabitants. The living is a rectory, in the archdeaconry and diocese of Canterbury, rated in the king's books at £6. 5. 2½., and in the patronage of G. W. H. D'Aeth, Esq. The church is dedicated to St. Clement.

KNOWSLEY, a township in the parish of HUYTON, hundred of WEST DERBY, county palatine of LANCASTER, 3¼ miles (N. W.) from Prescot, containing 1174 inhabitants. There is a place of worship for Unitarians.

KNOWSTONE, a parish in the southern division of the hundred of MOLTON, county of DEVON, 8¼ miles (W.) from Bampton, comprising East and West Knowstone, and containing 444 inhabitants. The living is a vicarage with Molland, in the archdeaconry of Barnstaple, and diocese of Exeter, rated in the king's books at £26. 10. 10., and in the patronage of Mr. Courtenay. The church, dedicated to St. Peter, has a plain Norman door.

KNOYLE (EAST), a parish in the hundred of DOWN-TON, though locally in that of Mere, county of WILTS, 2¼ miles (S. W.) from Hindon, containing 954 inhabitants. The living is a rectory, in the archdeaconry and diocese of Salisbury, rated in the king's books at £30, and in the patronage of the Bishop of Winchester. The church is dedicated to St. Mary. There is a place of worship for Baptists. The sum of about £10 per annum, arising from bequests by Charles Trippet, in 1707, and Mary Shaw, is applied towards the instruction of children. The celebrated architect, Sir Christopher Wren, was a native of this parish, of which his father, Christopher Wren, D.D., was rector.

KNOYLE (WEST), a parish in the hundred of MERE, county of WILTS, 3 miles (E.) from Mere, containing 208 inhabitants. The living is a perpetual curacy, annexed to the vicarage of Newenton, in the archdeaconry and diocese of Salisbury: the prebend of West Knoyle, which is an appendage to that of Newenton, is rated in the king's books at £8. 12. 11.

KNUTSFORD, a parish in the hundred of BUCK-LOW, county palatine of CHESTER, comprising the market town of Knutsford, and the townships of Bexton, Over Knutsford, Ollerton, and Toft, and containing 3535 inhabitants, of which number, 2753 are in the town of Nether Knutsford, 24¼ miles (N. E. by E.) from Chester, and 172½ (N. W. by N.) from London. This place, which is of great antiquity, is situated on the banks of a small stream, and near a ford, over which Canute the Dane is said to have passed with his army

for the conquest of the northern parts of the kingdom, in the reign of Ethelred II., or that of Edmund Ironside, and thence called Canute's Ford, from which the town derives its name. At the Conquest, Knutsford formed part of the barony of Halton, but in the reign of Edward I. it came into the possession of William de Tableigh, who obtained for it a charter of incorporation and various privileges, all which are become obsolete.

The town consists principally of two long streets, and is well paved and supplied with water. The houses are in general indifferently built, and of mean appearance; but in the immediate neighbourhood are several handsome villas: the environs are pleasant; and near the town is a good race-course, the races being held on the last Tuesday in July. Assemblies take place in the town, in November and December. The manufacture of thread, which formerly flourished here to a considerable extent, has, since the introduction of machinery, given place to the weaving of cotton, in which the principal part of the population is employed, working with hand-looms, for the manufacturers at Manchester and the adjacent towns. The Trent and Mersey canal passes within five miles of the town, affording a communication with Liverpool, and thence with various other parts of the kingdom. The market is on Saturday: the fairs, to which a small number of cattle are brought from the neighbouring villages, are, April 23rd, July 10th, and November 8th; a cattle fair is also held at Over Knutsford, on the Tuesday in Whitsun-week. Constables and other officers are appointed at the court leet of the lord of the manor, who also holds a court baron: the hundred court, and the Midsummer and Michaelmas quarter sessions for the county, are held in the town. The sessions-house and house of correction for the county were erected in 1817: the former is an elegant edifice, comprising spacious court-rooms, with the requisite accommodation for the business of the sessions; the latter, a spacious and commodious building, contains a governor's house, infirmary, and schools, eight day-rooms, seven airing-yards, in some of which are tread-mills, and one hundred and fifty separate cells, for the classification, employment, and instruction of the prisoners.

Knutsford, with its several townships, was formerly included in the parish of Rostherne, from which it was severed by act of parliament, in 1714, and formed into a separate parish. The living is a vicarage, in the archdeaconry and diocese of Chester, endowed with £16 per annum private benefaction, and £400 royal bounty, and in the alternate patronage, according to the following order, of the Lords of the Manors of Over Knutsford, Nether Knutsford, Ollerton, Toft, and Bexton. The church, erected in 1744, and dedicated to St. John the Baptist, is a neat edifice of brick, with a stone tower. There are places of worship for Independents, Wesleyan Methodists, and Unitarians. The free grammar school was founded and endowed with sixteen marks per annum, in the reign of Edward VI., by an ancestor of the family of Peter Leigh, Esq., of Over Knutsford, who appoints the master and nominates the scholars, with the exception of three, who, under a special endowment, are appointed by the vicar. A parochial school has lately been established, in which seventy boys are taught reading, writing, and arithmetic; and a school, in which one hundred girls are instructed in reading and needlework, is supported by Mrs. Egerton of Tatton. There are also various charitable bequests for distribution among the poor, the proceeds of which, about £100 per annum, are divided by the vicar, churchwardens and overseers of the parish.

KNUTSFORD (OVER), a township in the parish of KNUTSFORD, hundred of BUCKLOW, county palatine of CHESTER, ¼ of a mile (S. E. by S.) from Nether Knutsford, containing 231 inhabitants.

KNUTTON, a township in the parish of WOLSTANTON, northern division of the hundred of PIREHILL, county of STAFFORD, containing 809 inhabitants. Knutton is in the honour of Tutbury, duchy of Lancaster, and within the jurisdiction of a court of pleas held at Tutbury every third Tuesday, for the recovery of debts under 40s.

KYLOE, a parish in ISLANDSHIRE, county palatine of DURHAM, though locally northward of the county of Northumberland, adjoining Berwick upon Tweed, and containing 990 inhabitants. The living is a perpetual curacy, in the archdeaconry of Northumberland, and diocese of Durham, endowed with £200 private benefaction, £400 royal bounty, and £200 parliamentary grant, and in the patronage of the Dean and Chapter of Durham. The church was rebuilt in 1792. Coal and lime are found in this parish.

KYME (NORTH), a township in that part of the parish of SOUTH KYME which is in the first division of the wapentake of LANGOE, parts of KESTEVEN, county of LINCOLN, 7¾ miles (N. E. by E.) from Sleaford, containing 283 inhabitants.

KYME (SOUTH), a parish comprising the township of North Kyme in the first division of the wapentake of LANGOE, but chiefly in the wapentake of ASWARDHURN, parts of KESTEVEN county of LINCOLN, 8½ miles (S. W. by S.) from Tattershall, and containing 799 inhabitants. The living is a perpetual curacy, in the archdeaconry and diocese of Lincoln, endowed with £600 royal bounty, and £200 parliamentary grant. Sir A. Hume, Bart. was patron in 1806. The church is dedicated to All Saints. A priory of Black canons was founded, in honour of the Virgin Mary, in the reign of Henry II., which was valued at the dissolution at £138. 4. 9. Sir Gilbert Talbois, created Baron of Kyme in the reign of Henry VIII., is interred in the church.

KYNNERSLEY, county of SALOP. — See KINNERSLEY.

KYO, a township in that part of the parish of LANCHESTER which is in the western division of CHESTER ward, county palatine of DURHAM, 10½ miles (N.W.) from Durham, containing 448 inhabitants.

KYRE (GREAT), a parish in the upper division of the hundred of DODDINGTREE, county of WORCESTER, 4 miles (S. E. by S.) from Tenbury, containing 162 inhabitants. The living is a discharged rectory, in the archdeaconry of Salop, and diocese of Hereford, rated in the king's books at £6. 17. 8½., and in the patronage of Mrs. Pitts. The church is dedicated to St. Mary. An almshouse for eight poor widows, who are partly clothed and receive 2s. 6d. per week, was founded by Mr. Fettiplace.

KYRE (LITTLE), a chapelry in that part of the parish of STOKE-BLISS which is in the upper division of the hundred of DODDINGTREE, county of WORCESTER, 4½ miles (S. E. by S.) from Tenbury, containing 121 inhabitants.

THE END OF VOLUME II.

www.ingramcontent.com/pod-product-compliance
Lightning Source LLC
Chambersburg PA
CBHW072038020426
42334CB00017B/1309